Advances in Studies of Aging and Health

Volume 5

This book series is a theme-driven compilation, publishing the latest international research findings by key topics upon roles of social, behavioral, psychological, and contextual factors in associating or determining health and wellbeing of older people, with biomedical components taken into consideration. It applies an internationally comparative perspective and a biopsychosocial framework to understand healthy, active, productive, and successful aging, in order to build up a comprehensive and practical source of knowledge for researchers and practitioners in the field of aging and health.

This book series publishes original studies and tracks new research progresses by the major topics in the field of aging and health; systematically reviews recent research advancements of new concepts, frameworks, and methodology; and frameworks; explores the aging issues through an interdisciplinary perspective, and provides fresh empirical findings and theoretical insights in an internationally comparative manner. The goal is to effectively disseminate new policies and intervention practices on aging, in order for the improvement of quality of life of older persons.

The major themes of this book series include but are not limited to disability, cognitive function, chronic diseases and conditions, happiness and psychological wellbeing, self-rated health, frailty, mortality, living arrangements and intergenerational transfers, retirement and pension reforms, financial health and poverty, elderly abuse and human rights, ageism, long-term care, end-of-life care, aging in place, environmental health, age-friendly cities/communities, social participation, centenarian studies, big data in aging research, resilience and vulnerability, health life expectancies, active aging, successful aging, and healthy longevity.

Kun Wang • Hee Yun Lee • Qiushi Feng
Danan Gu
Editors

ICT Use and Healthy Longevity

Empirical Data and Perspectives

Springer

Editors
Kun Wang
Department of Social Work, College of Arts and Sciences
University of Alabama at Birmingham
Birmingham, AL, USA

Qiushi Feng
Centre for Family and Population Research/
Department of Sociology and Anthropology
National University of Singapore
Singapore, Singapore

Hee Yun Lee
School of Social Work
University of Georgia
Athens, GA, USA

Danan Gu
Population Division
UN Department of Economic and Social Affairs
New York, NY, USA

ISSN 2522-5146 ISSN 2522-5154 (electronic)
Advances in Studies of Aging and Health
ISBN 978-3-031-98963-6 ISBN 978-3-031-98964-3 (eBook)
https://doi.org/10.1007/978-3-031-98964-3

This Springer imprint is published by the registered company Springer Nature Switzerland AG
The registered company address is: Gewerbestrasse 11, 6330 Cham, Switzerland

Preface

The rapid aging of populations worldwide has brought into sharp focus the critical role of information and communication technologies (ICT) in shaping the health and well-being of older adults. This volume, *ICT Use and Healthy Longevity: Empirical Data and Perspectives*, emerges at a pivotal moment when digital technologies are transforming aging experiences of the world's older persons while creating new forms of inequality and new opportunities for healthy aging. Drawing on empirical research from diverse global contexts, this book offers a comprehensive examination of how ICT use is affected by various factors in later life and thus lead to significant disparities and inequalities under different contexts, and how it influences various dimensions of healthy aging, from cognitive function and social connectedness to health behaviors and quality of life.

The impetus for this work stems from three significant gaps in current knowledge. First, while numerous studies have explored ICT use among older populations, most have focused on Western, educated, industrialized, rich, and democratic (WEIRD) societies, leaving crucial questions about technology adoption and impacts in low- and middle-income countries largely unanswered. Second, existing research has often documented correlations between ICT use and health outcomes without sufficiently illuminating the underlying mechanisms and contextual factors that shape these associations. Third, there have been limited translation efforts of research findings into practical, actionable strategies for policymakers, practitioners, and technology designers working to promote digital inclusion and healthy aging.

This volume is organized into five thematic sections that collectively address these gaps. The first section establishes the conceptual foundation by reviewing major theoretical frameworks and global patterns of ICT adoption among older adults. Building on this foundation, the second section provides rigorous analyses of inequalities in ICT access and use across different populations, with particular attention to how factors such as race, gender, education, and rural/urban residence create digital divides. The third section shifts focus to examine how ICT influences health-related behaviors and perceptions of aging, including detailed case studies from rural communities in the United States and Southeast Asia. The fourth section presents compelling evidence of ICT's cognitive and psychosocial benefits while examining how these effects vary across demographic subgroups. Finally, the fifth section synthesizes these insights into concrete recommendations for policy and practice while identifying promising directions for future research.

The contributions to this volume reflect the work of an international, interdisciplinary team of scholars who bring diverse methodological approaches and theoretical perspectives to bear on these critical issues. Their collective efforts have produced findings that are both academically rigorous and practically relevant. For researchers in gerontology, public health, social work, and related fields, this book offers novel theoretical insights and empirical models that advance understanding of the technology-aging nexus. For practitioners developing interventions to support older adults' digital engagement or harness technology for health promotion, it provides evidence-based guidance tailored to different populations and settings. For policymakers addressing the societal challenges of population aging such as the digital divide, it highlights both the potential of ICT to support healthy longevity and the structural barriers that must be overcome to realize this potential equitably.

We are profoundly grateful to the many individuals and organizations who made this work possible. Our deepest appreciation goes to the older adults who participated in the studies featured in this volume, sharing their experiences and perspectives. We also thank our contributing authors for their scholarly rigor and commitment to advancing knowledge in this field. The editorial team at Springer Nature provided invaluable support throughout the publication process, and we particularly acknowledge Evelien Bakker, Prasad Tangudu, and other colleagues at Springer Nature for their guidance and patience. Finally, we thank our families and colleagues for their encouragement and understanding during the intensive work of compiling and editing this volume.

As the digital transformation of societies continues to accelerate, understanding how technology shapes and is shaped by the aging process becomes increasingly urgent. It is our hope that this book will stimulate further research, inform more effective policies and practices, and ultimately contribute to creating a digital landscape that supports healthy, meaningful aging for all.

Birmingham, AL, USA Kun Wang
Athens, GA, USA Hee Yun Lee
Singapore, Singapore Qiushi Feng
New York, NY, USA Danan Gu

Contents

Section I
Introduction & Theoretical Framework

Chapter 1
Healthy Aging: Concept, Global Actions, and the Role of ICT

Danan Gu, Qiushi Feng, Kun Wang, and Hee Yun Lee

Healthy aging is a vital concept in contemporary public health and gerontology, which emphasizes the importance of promoting the health and well-being of older individuals to ensure active and fulfilling later lives. This concept considers various aspects of health and health-related issues, including physical health, mental health, social connectedness, and access to healthcare services and support systems, etc. The importance of healthy aging has been increasingly recognized by international communities, most notably the United Nations, which has recently launched the "*Decade of Healthy Ageing*" initiative (2021–2030) (United Nations, 2020).

This chapter explores the concept of healthy aging, examines its related initiatives and actions undertaken by the international community, particularly the United Nations, and highlights the critical role of Information and Communication Technologies (ICTs) in achieving healthy aging. With the global population aging rapidly, implementing strategies to enhance ICT use among older people and thus promoting healthy aging is becoming crucial for societies worldwide.

D. Gu (✉)
Population Division, UN Department of Economic and Social Affairs, New York, NY, USA
e-mail: gudanan@yahoo.com

Q. Feng
Centre for Family and Population Research/Department of Sociology and Anthropology, National University of Singapore, Singapore, Singapore
e-mail: socfq@nus.edu.sg

K. Wang
Department of Social Work, College of Arts and Sciences, University of Alabama at Birmingham, Birmingham, AL, USA
e-mail: kw2@uab.edu

H. Y. Lee
School of Social Work, University of Georgia, Athens, GA, USA
e-mail: heeyunlee@uga.edu

K. Wang et al. (eds.), *ICT Use and Healthy Longevity*, Advances in Studies of Aging and Health 5, https://doi.org/10.1007/978-3-031-98964-3_1

1.1 Concept of Healthy Aging

1.1.1 Evolution of the Concept of Healthy Aging

Over time, the concept of healthy aging has originated and evolved in response to shifts in demographic trends, scientific advancements, and public health priorities. The initial idea of this concept can be traced back to the early 1960s when researchers began examining the health status of the aging population in the United States (Bortz, 1963; Davidson et al., 1962). The early discussions were mainly grounded in the World Health Organization's (WHO) 1948 definition of health, which emphasized physical, mental, and social well-being. By then, no formal definition was proposed, and healthy aging was largely understood as the absence of pathological disease conditions in later life.

The formal recognition of healthy aging as a public health priority emerged in the 1990s, when WHO launched the *Global Programme on Health of the Elderly*. To address challenges posed by declining fertility rates and increased life expectancy, this international initiative laid the groundwork for a more structured approach to population aging (United Nations, 1993). The concept of healthy aging gained further momentum with the 2002 *Madrid International Plan of Action on Ageing*, which further expanded this concept by emphasizing the importance of promoting active participation, independence, and dignity of older adults (United Nations, 2002).

Moving away from the old focus on disease, healthy aging has increasingly shifted the focus toward enhancing the quality of life in older adults. In 2015, WHO provided a formal definition of healthy aging in its *World Report on Ageing and Health*, describing it as "the process of developing and maintaining the functional ability that enables well-being in older ages." This definition encapsulates a broader perspective, emphasizing not just the absence of disease but also the preservation of physical, mental, and social well-being (WHO, 2015, p. 28).

The concept of healthy aging overlaps significantly with other related concepts such as successful aging, active aging, aging well, and productive aging, though nuanced differences exist across these terms (Foster & Walker, 2015; Michel & Sadana, 2017; Rowe & Kahn, 1997). In many cases, these terms are used interchangeably (Bowling & Dieppe, 2005; Bülow & Söderqvist, 2014), reflecting the multifaceted and multidimensional nature of human aging.

1.1.2 Scope of Healthy Aging

Healthy aging, as defined by WHO, emphasizes the importance of enabling older individuals to age with physical, mental, and social well-being. This highlights the importance of ensuring a person's capability in older ages to meet their basic needs, to maintain mobility, to learn and develop, to make decisions, to build and sustain relationships, and to contribute to family, community, and society.

Maintaining physical health is crucial for healthy aging. This domain of healthy aging entails preventing and managing chronic diseases and conditions, maintaining physical functioning, and promoting healthy lifestyles. Regular exercise, a balanced diet, and preventive healthcare are essential components (Rowe & Kahn, 1997; WHO, 2015). Physical health is not merely the absence of disease but also the maintenance of mobility, strength, and endurance. As people age, they are more likely to experience chronic conditions such as arthritis, diabetes, and cardiovascular diseases. Effective management of these conditions through medication, lifestyle changes, and regular medical check-ups is vital for maintaining quality of life at older ages (Centers for Disease Control and Prevention [CDC], 2022; Hines & Pandol, 2024).

Mental well-being is equally important. Cognitive health and emotional resilience are key aspects of healthy aging (Sterina et al., 2022). Cognitive health involves maintaining memory, attention, and problem-solving skills. Emotional resilience refers to the ability to cope with stress, loss, and change, which are common in later life. Mental health interventions, such as cognitive-behavioral therapy, psychotherapy, mindfulness practices, and social support groups (Niclasen et al., 2019), can effectively enhance healthy aging (Charles & Carstensen, 2010). Additionally, recent studies have highlighted the effectiveness of digital mental health interventions, such as online cognitive training programs and telehealth psychotherapy, in improving mental health outcomes for older adults (Lau et al., 2024; Piera-Jiménez et al., 2021).

Social relationships and community engagement also play a vital role in healthy aging. Social isolation and loneliness are significant risk factors for poor health outcomes in older adults. Maintaining social connections and participating in community activities can enhance well-being in later life (Holt-Lunstad et al., 2015). Social connectedness can be fostered through strengthening family relationships, expanding social networks, and participating in community activities, all of which can provide emotional support, reduce stress, and promote a sense of belonging and purpose (Li et al., 2021).

Access to healthcare services, including preventive care, treatment, and rehabilitation, is essential for healthy aging. Preventive care includes regular health screening, vaccination, and health education. Treatment involves managing chronic conditions and acute illnesses, while rehabilitation focuses on recovering from falls, injuries, stroke, or surgeries, etc. Recent advancements in telemedicine and digital health platforms have improved access to healthcare services for older adults, particularly in rural and underserved areas (Hailey, 2021). Support systems, such as family, caregivers, and community resources, also contribute to the overall well-being of older adults (Berkman et al., 2000), which can provide instrumental assistance and emotional support, and can also advocate for the benefits of older adults.

1.2 Global Actions and Initiatives of Healthy Aging

1.2.1 *The United Nations Decade of Healthy Ageing (2021–2030)*

The recognition of healthy aging as a global priority over the past several decades has led to the development of various initiatives and actions, both globally and locally, aimed at ensuring that older adults can maintain their well-being and independence as they age. One of the most significant initiatives is the United Nations' *Decade of Healthy Ageing* (2021–2030), which seeks to promote health and well-being among older persons by addressing age-related disparities and fostering an age-friendly environment, emphasizing the need for a global commitment to improving the lives of older persons (United Nations, 2020). The call highlights the importance of accessible housing, transportation, and public spaces (WHO, 2007). The initiative also aims to combat ageism by seeking to change the stereotypes of aging and older individuals that hinder their full participation in society, thus promoting a more inclusive and respectful society (United Nations, 2020; Jönson & Larsson, 2021). Another objective is to deliver person-centered integrated care and primary health services to ensure that older adults receive comprehensive and coordinated healthcare services at the right time, in the right place, and from the right sources (Hoh et al., 2021). The initiative mentioned long-term care that involves services and support for individuals who need assistance with daily activities over an extended period, emphasizing the importance of high-quality, affordable long-term care services to support older adults in maintaining independence and dignity (United Nations, 2020).

WHO has been playing a central role behind this key initiative. Its Global Strategy and Action Plan on Ageing and Health, adopted in 2016, laid the foundation for the *Decade of Healthy Ageing* by emphasizing the need for long-term care systems, integrated health services, and community-based support to enhance the quality of life for older adults (WHO, 2017). Additionally, the WHO Age-Friendly Cities and Communities Initiative has encouraged local governments to develop environments that promote active aging through improved infrastructure, accessible healthcare, and more social participation opportunities (Buffel et al., 2018).

Beyond WHO, regional organizations and national governments have also implemented strategies to support healthy aging. For example, the European Union (EU) has developed the *European Innovation Partnership on Active and Healthy Ageing* (EIP on AHA) to foster collaboration among policymakers, researchers, and healthcare professionals in developing innovative solutions for aging populations (European Commission, 2018). Similarly, in Asia, China has implemented comprehensive policies under its *"Home and Community-Based Integrated Care System"* to ensure that older adults receive coordinated health and social services within their homes and communities, promoting aging in place (Zou et al., 2024). In North America, initiatives such as the *Age-Friendly Communities Movement* in Canada and the U.S. aim to create environments that enhance older adults' mobility, safety, and social inclusion (Golant, 2014). Meanwhile, in low- and middle-income countries, efforts have focused on addressing challenges such as inadequate healthcare infrastructure and social protection. In this regard, the WHO's *Integrated Care for Older People* (ICOPE) framework has been instrumental in guiding countries to implement cost-effective, community-based interventions that support older adults' health and functional ability (WHO, 2019).

These country and continental level programs often involve multi-sectoral partnerships, including government agencies, non-profit organizations, and private organizations. Domestic partnerships between the public and private sectors have led to innovations in assistive technologies, telehealth, and digital literacy programs that empower older adults to actively engage with healthcare services and social networks (Chen et al., 2022). Moreover, international collaboration has become a major force in advancing healthy aging. Organizations such as the International Federation on Ageing (IFA) and HelpAge International have advocated for policy reforms and capacity-building initiatives that address age-related inequalities on a global scale (Beard et al., 2016).

Despite these efforts, challenges remain in ensuring equitable access to healthcare, reducing ageism, and addressing disparities in aging experiences across different socio-economic groups. Continued investment in research, policy development, and cross-sector collaboration are necessary to build resilient health and social systems that support healthy aging for all.

1.2.2 Global Initiatives and Frameworks

There are several prominent global initiatives and frameworks supporting the goals of the *Decade of Healthy Ageing. The Madrid International Plan of Action on Ageing* (MIPAA), adopted in 2002, provides a comprehensive framework for addressing the challenges of population aging. It emphasizes the importance of health promotion, social inclusion, and empowerment of older adults, and proposes "mainstreaming aging" to integrate aging issues into the national development agenda and implementation (United Nations, 2002). Calling for action at the national and international levels to promote the rights and well-being of older adults, MIPAA outlines three priority areas for policymaking: older adults and development, advancing health and well-being into old age, and ensuring enabling and supportive environments.

The Sustainable Development Goals (SDGs), adopted in 2015, include specific targets related to healthy aging, in which Goal 3 (*Good Health and Well-being*) and Goal 10 (*Reduced Inequalities*) are particularly relevant (United Nations, 2015). Goal 3 aims to ensure healthy lives and promote well-being for all at all ages, while Goal 10 focuses on reducing inequalities within and among countries. These goals emphasize the importance of addressing the health and social needs of older adults in achieving sustainable development.

Another key framework supporting healthy aging is the WHO's Global Strategy and Action Plan on Ageing and Health as noted earlier (WHO, 2017). This strategy advocates a life-course approach to aging, emphasizing the need for health systems that support older people's health and well-being throughout their lives. It encourages governments to adopt policies that promote aging in place, combat ageism, and improve the quality of life for older adults. The framework also stresses the importance of integrating aging into public health and social policies and enhancing global collaboration to ensure that older people can fully participate in society.

These initiatives and frameworks represent the joint efforts of the international community to promote healthy aging and address the challenges faced by older adults worldwide. By aligning with the goals set forth in these initiatives and frameworks, governments and organizations can work together to create a world where older individuals are empowered, supported, and able to enjoy healthy and fulfilling lives.

1.3 The Role of ICT in Healthy Aging

1.3.1 ICT as a Tool for Healthy Aging

ICTs have the potential to significantly enhance the healthy aging of older adults. First, ICTs provide older adults with access to a wealth of health information and educational resources. Health information online, such as news, articles, videos, and digital tools, and health educational resources, such as online courses, webinars, and virtual support groups, help to increase health and medical literacy, recommend healthy lifestyles, and support health management. Health-related online platforms and mobile applications can enable older adults to learn about medical knowledge, preventive measures, and treatment options, thus facilitating informed decisions on health (Czaja et al., 2018; van Dijk, 2005).

Next, telemedicine and remote monitoring technologies allow older adults to receive medical services from the comfort of their homes. This is particularly beneficial for individuals with mobility issues or those living in areas without good medical resources. Remote monitoring devices, such as wearable sensors, can track vital signs such as blood pressure, heart rate, and glucose level, provide real-time data to healthcare providers, and alert them to emergency situation or potential health issues (Bashshur et al., 2016). Telemedicine involves video conferencing, phone calls, and online messaging to provide medical consultations, follow-ups, and support.

ICTs can also help older adults maintain social connections. Social media platforms and online communities enable older adults to stay connected with family, friends, peers, and society. This social connectivity can combat loneliness, maintain mental health and overall well-being (Nordin et al., 2021; Seifert et al., 2021), and promote positive attitudes toward aging (Wang & Gu, 2023). Social media platforms such as Facebook and Twitter allow older adults to share updates, photos, and messages with their social networks. The other tools, such as *WeChat*, *TikTok*, and *WhatsApp*, enable face-to-face communication with loved ones, even when they are far away. Online communities and forums also provide opportunities for older adults to connect with people with similar interests and thus enhance broader social connectedness (Xie et al., 2020).

Moreover, digital cognitive training programs and brain health applications are developing fast to enhance cognitive functioning at older ages and delay cognitive decline. Targeting memory, attention, and problem-solving skills, these interventions and programs often rely on games and exercises through computers, tablets, and smartphones, which are convenient and accessible. They can be tailored and customized to meet the individual's specific situation, providing a personalized approach to cognitive health. Research has shown promising evidence that these training sessions can effectively improve cognitive performance in older adults (Lampit et al., 2014).

Assistive digital technologies, such as hearing aids, mobility aids, and smart home devices, can enhance independence for older adults and thus promote their quality of life. Smart home technologies, including voice-activated assistants and automated lighting systems, can help older persons manage daily tasks and maintain their autonomy (Mitzner et al., 2010). Hearing aids and mobility aids can improve communication and mobility of older people, and the development of these technologies directly benefits the older people suffering from sensory and physical limitations, reducing their burden of daily tasks and enhancing safety and comfort.

1.3.2 Challenges and Barriers to ICT Adoption

While ICTs offer numerous benefits to later life, there are significant challenges and barriers for older adults in adoption. This makes up the so-called digital gap, which has been broadly used to highlight the disparity in access to, skills, and usage of ICTs across subpopulations, notably between young and older people (Sims et al., 2017).

Some older people in the world are still struggling with access to ICTs. Underdeveloped digital infrastructure is still haunting many developing societies. Besides the macro-level factors, socioeconomic disadvantages at the individual level prove to play a crucial role in limiting access to ICTs among older adults (Wang et al., 2024, 2025). Affordability can be an issue for older adults with limited incomes, while usability challenges may arise for those with limited experience with digital technology (Jøranson et al., 2023; Yusif et al., 2016). Providing subsidies, discounts, and low-cost options can increase accessibility, while designing intuitive and simple user interfaces can improve usability. Therefore, ensuring access to affordable and user-friendly technology and reliable internet connections is essential in this regard (Heart & Kalderon, 2013).

Even with access to ICTs, some people yet lack the digital literacy and skills needed to use ICTs effectively. It is necessary to provide training and support of

ICTs, such as hands-on workshops, online tutorials, and one-on-one consultation, to help older adults in using ICTs (Czaja et al., 2018). On the other hand, informal learning should also be encouraged, especially through family members and social networks, since older adults may not effectively master the knowledge and skills taught only through formal channels. Notably, with ICTs advancement, digital literacy involves not only the ability to use digital devices but also to navigate online platforms and understand digital content. This raised new requirements for the training and support programs of ICTs.

Privacy and security concerns are becoming another major barrier to ICTs adoption among older adults, who may hesitate to use ICTs due to the fear and anxiety over the risk of leaking their personal confidential information (Zaman et al., 2022). These concerns are often about the risk of data breaches, identity theft, and unauthorized access to personal information. Security measures, such as encryption, secure login procedures, and regular software updates, can enhance protection. However, older adults need to learn how to safeguard their personal information, recognize phishing attempts, and use privacy settings. These issues have become more prominent in recent years with the development and prevalence of ICTs and should be addressed through educating older people on robust security measures (Mitzner et al., 2010).

In sum, healthy aging is a holistic concept that encompasses physical, mental, and social well-being, representing the ideal model of human aging. The *Decade of Healthy Ageing* (2021–2030) highlights the global commitment to promoting the well-being of older adults. In advancing the goals of healthy aging, promoting the adoption of ICTs among older adults is crucial. ICTs can provide access to health information, enable telemedicine and remote monitoring, foster social connectedness, support cognitive health, and enhance independence through assistive technologies. In this sense, addressing challenges related to digital access, literacy, and privacy is key to fully realizing the potential of ICTs in promoting healthy aging. As the global population continues to age, the integration of ICTs into aging policies and interventions will be vital in ensuring that older adults can lead healthy, active, and fulfilling lives.

Disclaimer Views expressed in the chapter are solely those of the authors and do not necessarily reflect those of the United Nations, the National University of Singapore, the University of Alabama at Birmingham, and the University of Georgia.

References

Bashshur, R. L., Shannon, G. W., Smith, B. R., & Alverson, D. C. (2016). The empirical foundations of telemedicine interventions for chronic disease management. *Telemedicine Journal and E-Health, 22*(9), 769–800.

Beard, J. R., Officer, A., de Carvalho, I. A., Sadana, R., Pot, A. M., Michel, J. P., Chatterji, S., et al. (2016). The world report on ageing and health: A policy framework for healthy ageing. *The Lancet, 387*(10033), 2145–2154.

Berkman, L. F., Glass, T., Brissette, I., & Seeman, T. E. (2000). From social integration to health: Durkheim in the new millennium. *Social Science & Medicine, 51*(6), 843–857.
Bortz, E. L. (1963). Healthy aging. *Journal of Michigan State Medical Society, 62*, 664–666.
Bowling, A., & Dieppe, P. (2005). What is successful ageing and who should define it? *BMJ, 331*(7531), 1548–1551.
Buffel, T., Handler, S., & Phillipson, C. (2018). *Age-friendly cities and communities: A global perspective*. Policy Press.
Bülow, M. H., & Söderqvist, T. (2014). Successful aging: A historical overview and critical analysis of a successful concept. *Journal of Aging Studies, 31*, 139–149.
Centers for Disease Control and Prevention (CDC). (2022). *Living with a chronic disease*. Retrieved from https://www.cdc.gov/chronic-disease/living-with/index.html
Charles, S. T., & Carstensen, L. L. (2010). Social and emotional aging. *Annual Review of Psychology, 61*, 383–409.
Chen, J., Spencer, M. R. T., & Buchongo, P. (2022). Strengthening the public health partnership and telehealth infrastructure to reduce health care disparities. *Population Health Management, 25*(6), 814–821.
Czaja, S. J., Boot, W. R., Charness, N., & Rogers, W. A. (2018). *Designing for older adults: Principles and creative human factors approaches*. CRC Press.
Davidson, C. S., Livermore, J., Andersen, P., & Kaufman, S. (1962). The nutrition of a group of apparently healthy aging persons. *American Journal of Clinical Nutrition, 10*(3), 181–199.
European Commission. (2018). *The European innovation partnership on active and healthy ageing: Strategic implementation plan*. https://ec.europa.eu/eip/ageing
Foster, L., & Walker, A. (2015). Active and successful aging: A European policy perspective. *The Gerontologist, 55*(1), 83–90.
Golant, S. M. (2014). Age-friendly communities: Are we expecting too much? *IRPP Insight, 5*, 1–16.
Hailey, D. (2021). Telemedicine. In D. Gu & M. E. Dupre (Eds.), *Encyclopedia of gerontology and population aging* (pp. 4946–4951). Springer Nature.
Heart, T., & Kalderon, E. (2013). Older adults: Are they ready to adopt health-related ICT? *International Journal of Medical Informatics, 82*(11), e209–e231.
Hines, O. J., & Pandol, S. J. (2024). Management of chronic pancreatitis. *BMJ, 384*, e070920.
Hoh, J. W. T., Feng, Q., & Gu, D. (2021). Aging in the right place. In D. Gu & M. E. Dupre (Eds.), *Encyclopedia of gerontology and population aging* (pp. 299–303). Springer Nature.
Holt-Lunstad, J., Smith, T. B., Baker, M., Harris, T., & Stephenson, D. (2015). Loneliness and social isolation as risk factors for mortality: A meta-analytic review. *Perspectives on Psychological Science, 10*(2), 227–237.
Jönson, H., & Larsson, A. T. (2021). Ableism and ageism. In D. Gu & M. E. Dupre (Eds.), *Encyclopedia of gerontology and population aging* (pp. 4–9). Springer Nature.
Jøranson, N., Zechner, M., Korkmaz, Y. N., Efthymiou, A., & Silva, R. (2023). Experienced barriers in the use of ICT for social interaction in older adults ageing in place: A qualitative systematic review protocol (SYSR-D-22-00848). *Systematic Review, 12*(1), 192.
Lampit, A., Hallock, H., & Valenzuela, M. (2014). Computerized cognitive training in cognitively healthy older adults: A systematic review and meta-analysis of effect modifiers. *PLoS Medicine, 11*(11), e1001756.
Lau, C. K. Y., Saad, A., Camara, B., Rahman, D., & Bolea-Alamanac, B. (2024). Acceptability of digital mental health interventions for depression and anxiety: Systematic review. *Journal of Medical Internet Research, 26*, e52609.
Li, Y., Feng, Q., Zhu, H., Dupre, M., & Gu, D. (2021). Social participation. In D. Gu & M. E. Dupre (Eds.), *Encyclopedia of gerontology and population aging* (pp. 4592–4601). Springer Nature.
Michel, J. P., & Sadana, R. (2017). "Healthy aging" concepts and measures. *Journal of the American Medical Directors Association, 18*(6), 460–464.

Mitzner, T. L., Boron, J. B., Fausset, C. B., Adams, A. E., Charness, N., Czaja, S. J., Sharit, J., et al. (2010). Older adults talk technology: Technology usage and attitudes. *Computers in Human Behavior, 26*(6), 1710–1721.

Niclasen, J., Lund, L., Obel, C., & Larsen, L. (2019). Mental health interventions among older adults: A systematic review. *Scandinavian Journal of Public Health, 47*(2), 240–250.

Nordin, S., Sturge, J., Ayoub, M., Jones, A., McKee, K., Dahlberg, L., et al. (2021). The role of information and communication technology (ICT) for older adults' decision-making related to health, and health and social care services in daily life: A scoping review. *International Journal of Environmental Research and Public Health, 19*(1), 151.

Piera-Jiménez, J., Etzelmueller, A., Kolovos, S., Folkvord, F., & Lupiáñez-Villanueva, F. (2021). Guided internet-based cognitive behavioral therapy for depression: Implementation cost-effectiveness study. *Journal of Medical Internet Research, 23*(5), e27410.

Rowe, J. W., & Kahn, R. L. (1997). Successful aging. *The Gerontologist, 37*(4), 433–440.

Seifert, A., Cotten, S. R., & Xie, B. (2021). A double burden of exclusion? Digital and social exclusion of older adults in times of COVID-19. *The Journals of Gerontology: Series B, 76*(3), e99–e103.

Sims, T., Reed, A. E., & Carr, D. C. (2017). Information and communication technology use is related to higher well-being among the oldest-old. *Journals of Gerontology: Social Scienes, 72*(5), 761–770.

Sterina, E., Hermida, A. P., Gerberi, D. J., & Lapid, M. I. (2022). Emotional resilience of older adults during COVID-19: A systematic review of studies of stress and well-being. *Clinical Gerontology, 45*(1), 4–19.

United Nations. (1993). World Health Organization. In *The yearbook of the United Nations 1991* (pp. 953–959). United Nations.

United Nations. (2002). *Madrid international plan of action on aging*. Retrieved from https://www.un.org/esa/socdev/documents/ageing/MIPAA/political-declaration-en.pdf

United Nations. (2015). *Sustainable development goals*. Retrieved from https://www.un.org/sustainabledevelopment/sustainable-development-goals/

United Nations. (2020). *Decade of Healthy Aging (2021–2030)*. Retrieved from https://www.who.int/initiatives/decade-of-healthy-ageing

van Dijk, J. A. G. M. (2005). *The deepening divide: Inequality in the information society*. Sage.

Wang, K., & Gu, D. (2023). Reciprocal associations between social media use and self-perception of aging among older adults: Do men and women differ? *Social Science & Medicine, 321*, 115786.

Wang, K., Chen, X., Gu, D., Smith, B. D., Dong, Y., & Peet, J. Z. (2024). Examining first and second-level digital divide at the intersection of race/ethnicity, gender, and socioeconomic status: An analysis of the National Health and aging trends study. *The Gerontologist, 64*(gnae079), 1–11.

Wang, K., Chen, X. S., Dong, Y., Sanabria Véaz, K., & Gu, D. (2025). Bridging the access gap: A decade of narrowing the digital divide for Hispanic older adults in the United States. *Journal of Aging and Health, 37*(3/4), 182–191.

World Health Organization. (2007). *Global age-friendly cities: A guide*. Retrieved from https://www.who.int/publications/i/item/9789241547307

World Health Organization. (2015). *World report on aging and health*. Retrieved from https://www.who.int/publications/i/item/9789241565042

World Health Organization. (2016). *Global strategy and action plan on aging and health (2016–2020)*. Retrieved from https://www.who.int/ageing/global-strategy/en/

World Health Organization. (2017). *Global strategy and action plan on ageing and health*. Retrieved from https://www.who.int/ageing/global-strategy

World Health Organization. (2019). *Integrated care for older people: Guidelines on community-level interventions to manage declines in intrinsic capacity*. Retrieved from https://www.who.int/ageing/health-systems/icope/en/

Xie, B., Charness, N., Fingerman, K., Kaye, J., Kim, M. T., & Khurshid, A. (2020). When going digital becomes a necessity: Ensuring older adults' needs for information, services, and social inclusion during COVID-19. *Journal of Aging & Social Policy, 32*(4–5), 460–470.

Yusif, S., Soar, J., & Hafeez-Baig, A. (2016). Older people, assistive technologies, and the barriers to adoption: A systematic review. *International Journal of Medical Informatics, 94*, 112–116.

Zaman, S. B., Khan, R. K., Evans, R. G., Thrift, A. G., Maddison, R., & Islam, S. M. S. (2022). Exploring barriers to and enablers of the adoption of information and communication technology for the care of older adults with chronic diseases: Scoping review. *JMIR Aging, 5*(1), e25251.

Zou, Y., Chen, W., Shen, K., Huang, K., Gui, J., Zhang, G., Feng, Q., & Liu, H. (2024). Embrace the past and forge ahead: The China report on the 30th anniversary of the international conference on population and development (ICPD). *China Population and Development Studies, 8*(3), 239–286.

Chapter 2
ICT Use Among Older Adults Around the World

Danan Gu, Qiushi Feng, Kun Wang, and Hee Yun Lee

The global landscape of information and communication technology (ICT) use among older adults has undergone a significant transformation in recent years, with adoption rates steadily increasing across diverse demographic groups and various nations. This shift reflects broader societal trends toward digitalization, driven by rapid technological advancements; and it is further accelerated by the COVID-19 pandemic, which underscored the vital importance of digital connectivity for accessing health care, maintaining social connections, and obtaining essential services. Although older adults have historically lagged behind younger populations in ICT adoption, recent data indicate a narrowing digital divide, as growing numbers of older individuals embrace smartphones, internet, video conferencing, and telehealth solutions. This chapter examines recent global trends in ICT use among older adults, with attention to specific regions and countries both in developed and developing worlds, to identify general usage patterns, key drivers, persistent barriers, and implications for future digital inclusion. Understanding these issues provides not

D. Gu (✉)
Population Division, UN Department of Economic and Social Affairs, New York, NY, USA
e-mail: gudanan@yahoo.com

Q. Feng
Centre for Family and Population Research/Department of Sociology and Anthropology, National University of Singapore, Singapore, Singapore
e-mail: socfq@nus.edu.sg

K. Wang
Department of Social Work, College of Arts and Sciences, University of Alabama at Birmingham, Birmingham, AL, USA
e-mail: kw2@uab.edu

H. Y. Lee
School of Social Work, University of Georgia, Athens, GA, USA
e-mail: heeyunlee@uga.edu

K. Wang et al. (eds.), *ICT Use and Healthy Longevity*, Advances in Studies of Aging and Health 5, https://doi.org/10.1007/978-3-031-98964-3_2

only a foundational backdrop for the discussions in subsequent chapters, but also critical insights for developing inclusive policies and technologies that address the evolving needs of the global aging population.

2.1 Trends in ICT Use

2.1.1 Global Trend and Digital Divide

Over the past two or three decades, the global adoption of ICT has grown significantly. This upward trend has been fueled by the increasing availability of affordable internet services, the widespread use of user-friendly digital devices, and a growing awareness of the benefits of digital inclusion. As of February 2025, approximately 5.56 billion people, equivalent to 67.9% of the global population, had internet access. In comparison, the number of mobile phone users reached 5.78 billion (70.5%), while social media users numbered 5.24 billion (63.9%) (Kemp, 2025). Figure 2.1 illustrates the trajectory of internet adoption from 1990 to 2025, in terms of both the absolute number of internet users (blue bars, left Y-axis) and their proportion of the global population (orange line, right Y-axis). As can be seen, in 2000, there were 396 million internet users worldwide, comprising merely 6.5% of the global population. Yet this figure rose to 1.91 billion by 2010, 27.4% of the global population, and further surged to 4.5 billion by 2020, 57.3% of the global population.

The number of internet users aged 65 years or older worldwide has not been directly reported; however, based on the global age distribution of internet users (Petrosyan, 2024), it is estimated that approximately 235 million individuals aged 65 years or older were online in 2024. In conjunction with age-specific population data from the World Population Prospects 2024 (United Nations, 2024), we estimate that globally, about 28% of older adults aged 65 years or older were internet users

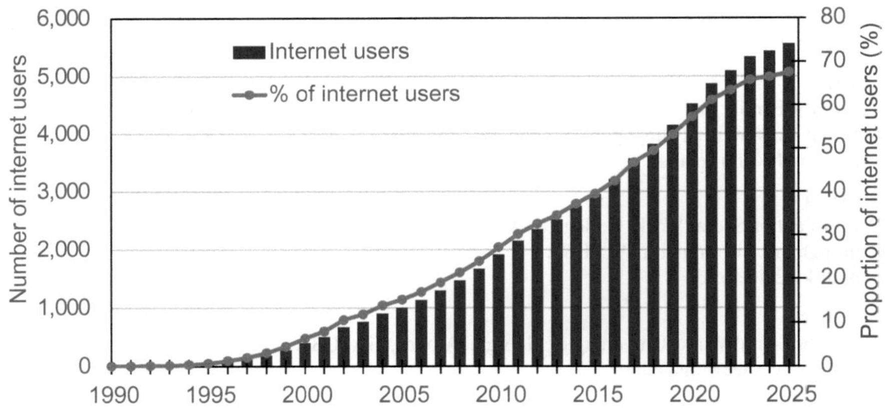

Fig. 2.1 Numbers of internet users worldwide and their proportions in the total population, 1990 to 2025. Source: Kemp (2025) and United Nations (2024)

in 2024. This proportion is significantly lower than the internet penetration rate for the total population, which stood at 66.5% (Kemp, 2025). Such a large digital gap can be further shown in Figure 2.2, which compares the proportions of internet use between the total population and people aged 55–74 years in the European Union (EU).

The digital divide between older adults and younger populations is particularly evident. A study by the International Telecommunication Union (ITU, 2022) found that in over half of 31 countries surveyed, including France and Italy, the gap in internet use prevalence exceeded 50 percentage points between individuals aged 75 years or older and those aged 15–74. Figure 2.3 presents the age-specific prevalence of internet use in the United States from 2000 to 2024, showing that in the early 2000s, older adults lagged considerably behind other younger age groups. Encouragingly, this gap has steadily diminished over time, especially in the recent 3 years when the overall internet penetration rate surpassed 80% and reached over 90%.

However, in many developing countries, the age-related digital divide remains substantial and persistent. In China, for example, only about half of individuals aged 60 years or older were internet users in 2024, compared to the rate of over 90% among those aged 20–29 (CNNIC, 2025). In India, merely 11% of older adults reported having ICT skills, in stark contrast to the rate of nearly 80% in younger adults aged 20–29 (Waghmare, 2025). The disparity is likely more pronounced in many African countries, where the overall ICT access remains significantly lower than in China and India.

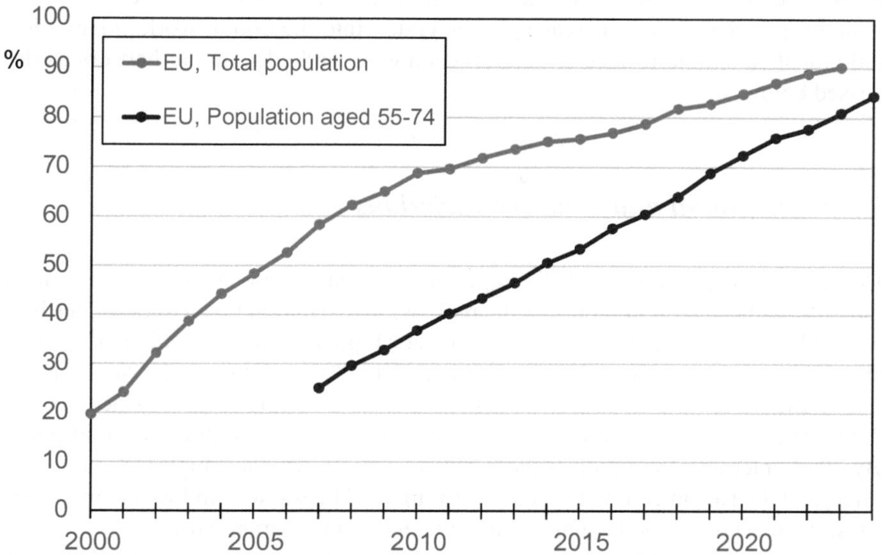

Fig. 2.2 Proportions of internet use among the total population and people aged 55–74 years in European Union (EU) countries, 2000–2024. Source: UNECE Statistical Database (2025)

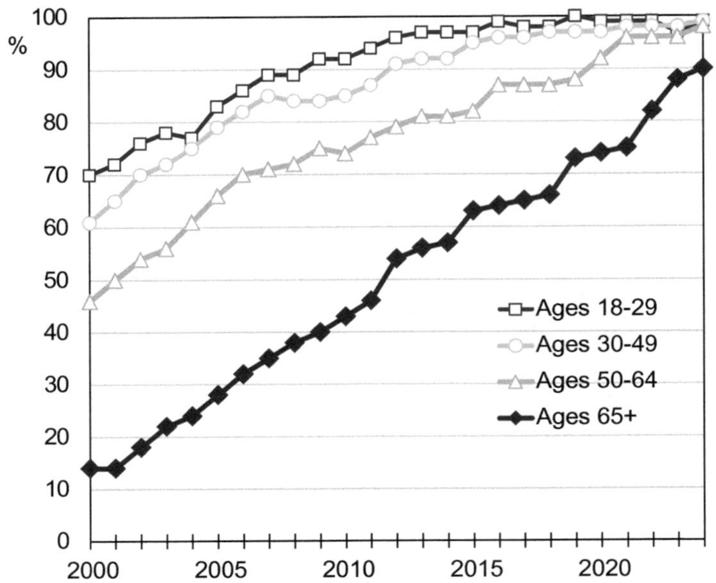

Fig. 2.3 Prevalence of internet use by age groups for American adults, 2000–2024. Source: Pew Research Center (2024). Note: The missing values for the years 2017, 2020, and 2022 were linearly interpolated

All these suggest that, despite a global upward trend in ICT adoption, older adults remain consistently disadvantaged in digital access and literacy. While younger populations are increasingly integrated into the digital world, many older individuals continue to face structural, economic, and educational barriers as discussed below.

2.1.2 Regional and Country Variations

Despite global progress in ICT adoption, significant regional disparities remain. Growth has been seen in high-income regions, where internet penetration rates have reached near-universal levels, while many developing countries continue to suffer a slow and uneven progress in ICT adoption (ITU, 2024; Kemp, 2025; World Bank, 2025). Figure 2.4 shows trends in internet use across selected regions since the year 2000. The world has seen upward changes everywhere, though at different paces. By 2023, internet penetration exceeded 90% in North America, high-income economies, and the EU; in contrast, usage rates remained below 40% in low-income countries, the least developed countries, and much of sub-Saharan Africa.

For older adults, comprehensive data on ICT or internet use are primarily limited to North America and Europe, or more broadly, to OECD and other developed

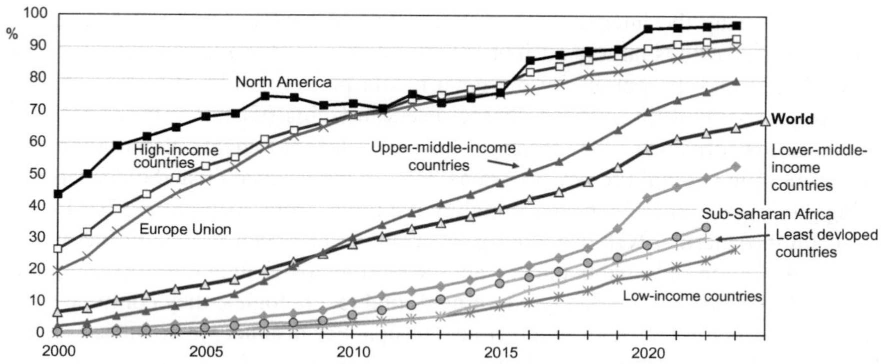

Fig. 2.4 Prevalence of internet access among the total population for selected regions, 2000–2023. Source: World Bank (2025)

countries. In most other regions, such data are scarce, particularly time series statistics. According to the available data, ICT use among older adults in North America and Europe is prevalent and has continued to grow in recent years, attributable to high internet penetration, advanced technological infrastructure, and supportive government policies promoting digital inclusion (European Union Agency for Fundamental Rights, 2023; ITU, 2025a, 2025b; Seifert & Cotton, 2022). For instance, in the United States, 75% of adults aged 65 years or older used the internet in 2021, with 61% owning a smartphone and 45% using social media, up from 63%, 30%, and 35% in 2015, respectively (Pew Research Center, 2022). Similarly, in Canada, 71% of adults aged 65 years or older reported internet use in 2018 (Wavrock et al., 2021), rising to nearly 83% by 2022 (Statistics Canada, 2023).

In Europe, the trends are similar but vary by country. For instance, in the EU, as noted in Figure 2.2, the prevalence rate of internet use among persons aged 55–74 years reached nearly 85% by 2024 (UNECE, 2025). However, there is notable variation across countries. Northern European countries like Sweden and Denmark have some of the highest rates of internet use among older adults, with over 90% of those aged 55–74 years since 2020. By contrast, Southern and Eastern European countries like Greece and Bulgaria have relatively lower rates, with only less than 65% of older adults using the internet (UNECE, 2025). These differences are attributed to regional variations in economic development, digital literacy programs, and cultural attitudes toward technology (Elena-Bucea et al., 2021; Mohan et al., 2024; Oh et al., 2021; Zhang, 2023).

In developing countries, ICT use among older adults is growing but remains limited when compared to developed regions. Barriers such as low internet penetration, high costs of devices and data, and lack of digital literacy programs hinder widespread adoption in these countries (Donner, 2008; Chinn & Fairlie, 2007; ITU, 2022; Li, 2024). In Asia, countries like China and South Korea have recently seen significant increases in ICT use among older adults. According to the China Internet Network Information Center (CNNIC) (2025), 53% of Chinese aged 60 years or older were using the internet in 2024, up from just 15% in 2015 (CNNIC, 2016, 2022). This growth is largely attributed to the widespread availability of affordable smartphones and the popularity of social media platforms like *WeChat*, which is currently used by 80% of older internet users in China (CNNIC, 2022, 2025). In South Korea, driven by the country's advanced technological infrastructure and government-led digital literacy programs, 80% of adults aged 60 and older reported using the internet in 2023, nearly doubling the figure from 2015 (Jobst, 2024).

In Latin America, ICT use among older adults has been gradually increasing, though the progress remains uneven and generally slower than developed regions. While older adults are gradually adopting digital technologies, they continue to lag significantly behind those of younger age groups. For instance, in countries such as Uruguay, Chile, Brazil, Peru, Bolivia (Plurinational State of), and Mexico, internet use among individuals aged 60 or older remained below 10% in 2014, despite some growth since 2010 (ECLAC, 2016). By contrast, rates of internet use among those aged 16–31 ranged from 30% to 50% across these countries (Barrantes & Vargas, 2019; ECLAC, 2016). For comparison, during the same period, internet usage in the United States reached 57% for adults aged 65 and older and 97% for those aged 18–29 (Pew Research Center, 2024). Since 2015, internet penetration in Latin America has improved markedly in some countries. In Brazil, for example, the proportion of older adults aged 60 and above using the internet reached approximately 60% in 2024, while usage among individuals under 45 exceeded 90% (Bianchi, 2025).

In Africa, the limited data available indicate that internet penetration among older adults remains low, largely due to underdeveloped infrastructure, high connectivity costs, and limited digital literacy resources. According to the Pew Research Center's Global Attitudes Survey conducted in 2017 across six sub-Saharan African countries (Kenya, Nigeria, Ghana, Senegal, South Africa, and Tanzania), fewer than 30% of individuals aged 50 and above reported going online at least occasionally or owning a smartphone. In contrast, internet use among those aged 18–29 ranged from 34% in Tanzania to 75% in South Africa (Pew Research Center, 2018).

In sum, while ICT use among older adults has grown globally, stark regional disparities persist. High-income regions lead in both ICT access and adoption, supported by established infrastructure and inclusive policies. In contrast, older populations in many developing countries face persistent barriers to digital engagement. To ensure that older adults worldwide can benefit equitably from digital transformation, bridging these gaps call for targeted investments in infrastructure, affordable access, and tailored digital literacy initiatives.

2.1.3 Role of the COVID-19 Pandemic

The COVID-19 pandemic significantly accelerated the adoption of ICT among older adults worldwide, as lockdowns and social distancing measures necessitated digital solutions for communication, healthcare and service access, and daily life management (Pew Research Center, 2021, 2025; Seifert, 2020). For many older individuals who were previously hesitant to use digital tools, the pandemic created both a practical need and a social impetus for them to adopt. Sixsmith et al. (2022) found that older adults in Canada began engaging with technologies such as smartphones and internet-based services out of necessity during the pandemic, resulting in notable increases in usage. In the United Kingdom, the proportion of older adults using video calling platforms like Zoom and Skype more than doubled during the pandemic (Ofcom, 2021), illustrating a widespread behavioral shift.

In the United States, one study (Kakulla, 2021) reported that during the pandemic, older Americans actively used various digital communication tools, such as text messaging, social media, emails, and video chat, to maintain social connections, with many using them daily. Notably, about 70% of older adults reported using video chat across multiple devices during the pandemic, a 20 percentage-point increase from 2019, although usage rates for other digital tools remained stable. And the age-based differences in ICT use were generally modest, with only a slight decline among those aged 70 and older (Kakulla, 2021). More importantly, the study reveals that while approximately half of the participants reported no change in their ICT habits, 44% viewed the role of technology in their lives more positively than before (Kakulla, 2021). These attitudinal shifts appear to persist beyond the acute phase of the pandemic (Kakulla, 2025), leading to longer-term changes in digital engagement among older populations. Telehealth adoption also increased dramatically. Among older Medicare beneficiaries in the United States, telehealth use rose from 4.6% before the pandemic to 21.1% during its peak (Choi et al., 2022).

Overall, the COVID-19 pandemic has been a powerful catalyst for digital adoption among older adults. However, the extent and sustainability of this shift remain closely tied to broader efforts of infrastructure development and policy initiatives aimed at closing the digital divide.

2.2 Profiles of the Internet and Social Media Users

2.2.1 Primary Purposes of Using the Internet and Social Media

People are using the internet and social media for various reasons. Based on the data from the 2025 Revision of the Global Digital Overview Report (Kemp, 2025), Table 2.1 reveals that nearly 82% of adults aged 65 years or older worldwide reported information-seeking as their primary reason for using the internet. This motivation also ranks highest among the 35–44, 45–54, and 55–64 age groups. Among older adults (65+), the second most common reason for internet use is keeping up with news and current events, followed by connecting with friends and family, reported by approximately two-thirds and 63% of users, respectively. Learning how to do things ranks fourth. Notably, the top four reasons for going online are

Table 2.1 Rankings of primary reasons for using the internet by age group, worldwide

Rankings of the age group 65+	**Purposes of internet use**	**Age groups**					
		65+	**55-64**	**45-54**	**35-44**	**25-34**	**16-24**
1	Find information	81.7	68.1	65.2	62.1	58.5	61.1
2	Follow news & events	66.9	61.2	58.9	56.3	51.5	49.5
3	Contact friends & family	62.7	61.1	59.3	59.7	58.7	62.1
4	Learn how to do things	60.9	53.2	51.8	50.0	48.6	51.7
5	Research brands	57.0	47.5	47.4	46.1	43.4	49.3
6	Research places & travel	50.7	41.7	40.5	39.5	44.1	
7	Research health	46.9	40.5				
8	Manage finances	42.3					
9	Fill spare time & browsing	40.9	44.8	44.4	43.6		
10	Watch videos & shows	35.6	49.3	53.6	55.1	56.2	59.3
	Find new ideas		41.5	45.7	48.0	48.4	50.5
	Listen to music			43.1	45.4	47.8	55.3
	Education & study					39.5	52.4
	Gaming						42.8

Source: Kemp (2025). The pink shadowed values are the top rank for each age group, while the numbers in grey shadows refer to the 10th rank (or the lowest rank) of each age group

consistent between the 65+ and 55–64 age groups, although a higher proportion of the 65+ group reported each of these motivations. By contrast, entertainment-related use, such as watching videos and shows, ranks tenth among those aged 65+, indicating a decline in using the internet for entertainment with age. This differs from younger age groups, for whom it usually ranks within the top five. Similarly, purposes such as finding new ideas, listening to music, learning/training or studying, and playing games that are common in the top ten for adults under 45 do not appear in the top ten for older adults. One interesting pattern is that the most reported motivation (or the leading reason of internet use) has a much larger percentage among the age 65+ group than in other age groups, so does the percentage gap between the most and least reported top ten reasons, indicating that the motivation of older adults in using the internet is more focused and less diversified.

Based on the same data, Table 2.2 further presents the primary reasons for using social media, revealing a pattern that differs markedly from that of internet use. Contacting friends and family was identified as the most common reason for using social media, reported by 58% of respondents. Notably, this motivation is consistently reported as the top among all age groups. Reading news and filling spare time ranked second and third, respectively, reported by just over one-quarter of respondents. Among older adults aged 65 years or older, posting about one's life is ranked tenth, a purpose not included in the top ten for other age groups. By contrast, purposes such as watching or following sports, watching live streams, viewing branded content, avoiding missing out, and following influencers or celebrities that are common in the top ten among younger users do not appear on the list for those aged 65 years or older. Similar to patterns observed in internet use, as compared with younger people, older adults aged 65 years or older engage with social media with a narrower scope of purposes but higher concentration, as shown by the dominance

Table 2.2 Primary reasons of using social media by age group, worldwide

Rankings of age group 65+	Purposes of social media use	Age groups					
		65+	**55-64**	**45-54**	**35-44**	**25-34**	**16-24**
1	Contact friends & family	58.1	56.2	53.1	50.8	48.1	48.3
2	Read news stories	27.1	40.6	38.2	36.4	33.2	29.1
3	Fill up spare time	25.8	35.8	37.0	37.9	39.5	44.3
4	Find content (e.g. videos)	14.0	26.1	29.4	30.8	31.7	33.9
5	See trending topics	14.0	24.3	27.2	30.3	30.9	32.2
6	Find like-minded people	13.5					
7	Ideas: things to do & buy	12.9	24.4	26.8	28.2	28.2	28.6
8	Find products to buy	12.9	26.7	28.7	29.4	27.7	26.1
9	Share & discuss opinions	12.1	21.9	22.5	25.6	25.3	24.9
10	Post about your life	10.6					
	Watch or follow sports		20.1	22.7	24.7	25.2	
	Watch live streams		19.8	22.9	25.6		
	See branded content					24.2	
	Avoid missing out						24.7
	Influencers & celebrities						24.3

Source: Kemp (2025). The pink shadowed values are the top rank for each age group, while the numbers in grey shadows refer to the 10th rank (or the lowest rank) of each age group

of a single purpose and the large proportion gap between the most and least cited top-ten reasons.

Although older adults tend to have a less diversified scope in online activities compared to younger age groups, they are found to be more likely to use the internet for financial services, such as online banking and digital payments. According to the 2025 Global Digital Overview Report, 43% of women and 47% of men, aged 65 or older, regularly use online banking, compared to 32–38% of women and 39–40% of men in younger age groups (Kemp, 2025). This phenomenon deserves further investigations but may indicate a growing digital proficiency and comfort with financial technology among older adults, a shift that banks and financial service providers can strategically leverage by offering tailored products and services for this demographic. It also underscores the importance of designing accessible, user-friendly, and secure online banking platforms that address the specific needs of older users.

2.2.2 *Devices of Internet Use*

According to the 2025 Revision of the Global Digital Overview Report (Kemp, 2025), by February 2025, 98.0% and 97.8% of the global internet users were using mobile phones and smartphones, respectively; nearly 60% of internet users also adopted desktop or laptop computers; nearly half used a Smart TV or a tablet; and nearly one-third wore smart wrist devices.

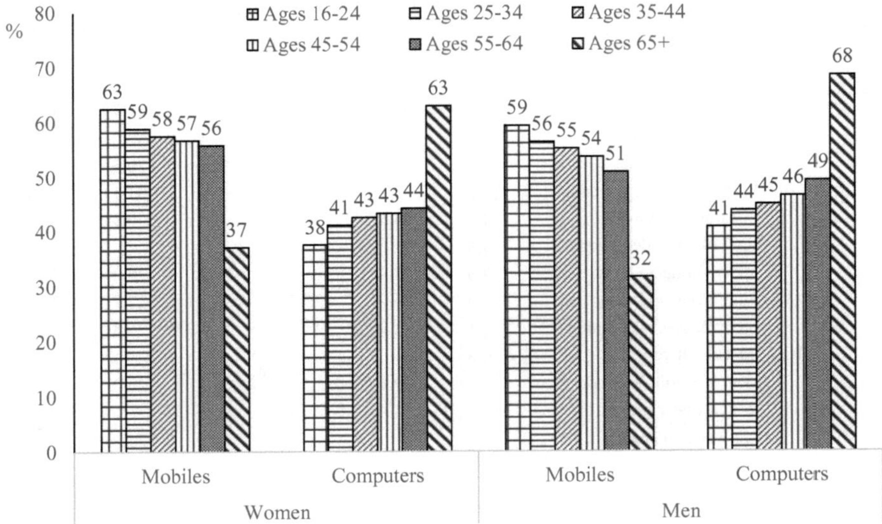

Fig. 2.5 Proportions of daily time spent on mobile phones and computers in the total daily internet time, worldwide. Source: Kemp (2025)

Figure 2.5 presents the proportion of daily time spent either on a mobile phone or on a computer in the total daily internet time, based on data from the 2025 Revision of the Global Digital Overview Report (Kemp, 2025). The results reveal that online activities of older adults aged 65 years or older used almost twice as much time using computers as using mobile phones. Men and older ages were associated with more computer use, which may relate to generational differences in technology adoption, ergonomic preference, or types of online activities. Older adults, for example, may favor computers due to larger screens and keyboards, while younger users may prefer the mobility and convenience of smartphones.

This disparity of age groups is well evidenced in the United States. While smartphone ownership among adults aged 65 and older rose significantly, from 13% in 2012 to 61% in 2021 (Pew Research Center, 2022) and further to 76% in 2023 (Laricchia, 2024), the corresponding figures for younger adults aged 18 to 29 has consistently exceeded 90% since 2015 (Laricchia, 2024).

2.2.3 *Favorite Apps or Platforms in Using Social Media*

While using social media, older individuals often exhibit diverse preferences in selecting their favorite platforms or apps, and understanding these choices can reveal valuable insights into their digital behavior. Table 2.3 presents the percentage distribution of reported favorite social media platforms/apps by sex among active users of social media across different age groups. Here, "active users" are defined as

Table 2.3 Percentages of active social media users who say that each option is their favorite social media platforms, worldwide, 2024

Favorite media platform	Age groups 16-24	25-34	35-44	45-54	55-64
Women					
WhatsApp	12.7	14.3	15.4	17.3	21.1
Facebook	5.9	10.6	13.2	14.9	17.1
WeChat	8.2	11.7	15.5	13.6	12.0
Instagram	24.8	20.8	16.0	13.9	10.2
Douyin	6.6	8.1	9.8	6.4	5.4
TikTok	15.5	11.3	7.8	6.9	5.0
Line	0.5	0.8	1.2	2.6	3.5
Messenger	1.7	2.5	2.5	2.7	3.0
Telegram	2.6	2.1	2.0	2.1	2.2
X (formerly Twitter)	3.1	2.1	1.8	1.6	1.7
Men					
WhatsApp	14.1	14.7	17.3	19.5	21.9
Facebook	7.8	13.5	14.7	16.4	17.5
WeChat	6.2	11.8	16.0	14.4	14.4
Douyin	6.5	8.5	8.2	6.8	6.6
Instagram	26.6	18.4	11.7	9.4	6.1
TikTok	9.6	7.1	5.7	5.3	4.3
X (formerly Twitter)	4.2	4.6	4.0	3.8	3.3
Line	0.7	1.0	1.2	2.4	2.9
Telegram	4.0	3.2	3.2	2.6	2.5
Messenger	1.8	2.4	2.2	2.4	2.3

Note: Pink shadowed numbers refer to the top rank in a given age group, while the gray shadowed numbers refer to the 10th rank (or the lowest rank) of a given age group. The data for the age group 65+ are not available
Source: Kemp (2025)

individuals who regularly interact with social media through activities such as posting, liking, commenting, sharing, or engaging with others (Godard & Holtzman, 2024).

The results show that globally, among women, WhatsApp is the most favored platform in the two older age groups (45–54 and 55–64), whereas Instagram remains the most popular among those younger than age 45. Among men, WhatsApp is the preferred platform across the three older age groups (35–44, 45–54 and 55–64), while Instagram dominates among users under the age 35. Line is consistently the least favored platform among individuals under age 45, regardless of sex, while X (formerly Twitter) is the least favored among older women and Messenger is the least favored among older men.

These results suggest that social media preferences among older adults are not only shaped by age but also by gender, and that platforms facilitating direct, private communication, such as WhatsApp, are especially valued among users of older ages. This underscores the need for platform design and digital inclusion strategies that consider the evolving communication preferences of aging populations.

2.2.4 *Time/frequencies of Internet Use*

The frequency of internet use varies considerably among older adults depending on individual needs, preferences, and circumstances. While some older adults engage with digital technology as a daily routine for communication, accessing information, or managing health, others may use it less frequently or selectively. Key factors influencing the usage frequency include levels of digital literacy, perceived usefulness of technology, accessibility of devices and internet services, and physical or cognitive limitations.

Based on the latest Global Digital Overview Report (Kemp, 2025), Fig. 2.6 compares the average daily time spent online, regardless of device type, across different age groups for both men and women. Globally, internet users aged 65 or older spend an average of 4 h online per day, with women spending approximately 8 min more than their male counterparts. By contrast, younger adults under the age of 45 years typically spend over 7 h online each day. This contrast reveals a digital gap in online engagement, in which younger individuals are more deeply embedded in online environments due to demands and needs from work, social participation; by contrast, the internet use of older adults may be less driven by the constant economic and social motivations, being more task- or functional- specific.

2.3 Barriers of ICT Use

As previously noted, internet penetration has increased at an unprecedented pace over the past two decades. However, this rapid growth has not resulted in equitable digital engagement across age groups. Older adults, in particular, continue to

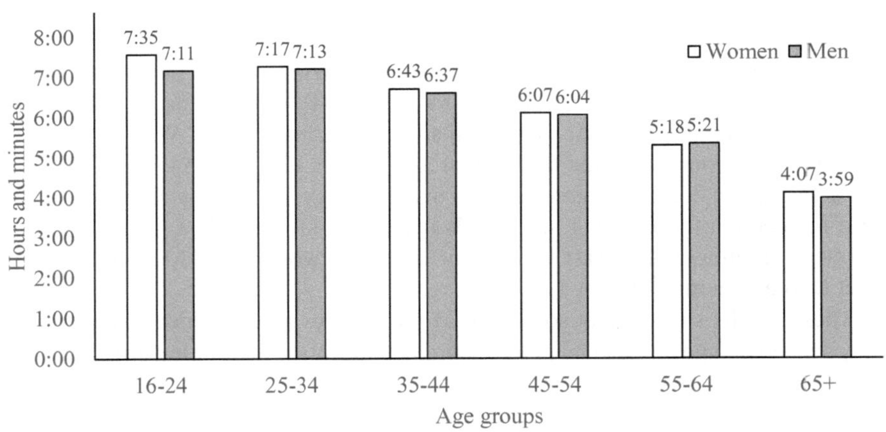

Fig. 2.6 Daily Averages of internet use time on any device in hours and minutes by age groups. Source: Kemp (2025)

encounter distinct and multifaceted barriers that hinder their adoption and effective use of ICTs, limiting the sustained integration of digital tools into their daily lives. A widely recognized framework categorizes these barriers into four key dimensions: accessibility (or coverage), affordability, capability (particularly digital literacy), and concerns related to privacy and security. Research consistently shows that these barriers are interrelated and often mutually reinforcing. For instance, limited digital literacy can heighten concerns about privacy, while financial constraints may restrict access to devices that could otherwise support digital competence in later life (Choi et al., 2025). This section examines the complex landscape of ICT-related barriers experienced by older adults globally, contrasts these challenges with those faced by younger generations, and identifies potential strategies to help close the digital divide.

2.3.1 Accessibility or Coverage

Although nearly 70% of the global population now has internet access, significant disparities persist across regions, countries, and even within nations. As explored in this book, these digital divides are driven by structural and demographic factors, including race, ethnicity, socioeconomic status, and urban–rural residence. Older adults, in particular, face pronounced gaps in access and adoption compared to younger populations. Even in the United States, where internet usage surpassed 95% in 2024, only 90% of adults aged 65 or older reported being online, falling far short of the near-universal 99% adoption rate among adults aged 18–54 (Pew Research Center, 2025). The disparity is even starker in smartphone ownership: in 2023, just 76% of older Americans owned a smartphone, compared to 97% of younger adults, a 21-point gap (Laricchia, 2024).

The Mobile Connectivity Index (MCI), developed by the Global System for Mobile Communications Association (GSMA), offers a more granular understanding of cross-national disparities in this regard. It evaluates the enabling a country's environment for mobile internet adoption. The index scores ranges from 0 to 100 across four key dimensions of infrastructure, affordability, consumer readiness, and the availability of relevant content and services. According to GSMA (2024), Singapore topped the index with a score above 93, followed closely by several Northern and Western European countries, the United States, Australia, and the United Arab Emirates, all scoring above 90. At the other end of the spectrum, South Sudan recorded the lowest score (<10), joined by many other developing countries. The significant disparities reflect daunting challenges in digital infrastructure and readiness (GSMA, 2024), underscoring the urgent need for targeted policies and initiatives to bridge the digital divide and ensure inclusive access to digital technologies for older adults worldwide.

2.3.2 Affordability

Affordability, encompassing the cost of digital devices and internet access, remains a significant barrier to ICT adoption among older adults worldwide. The high purchase cost is often a primary obstacle to mobile ownership. A GSMA survey covering 12 countries found that the device cost is the most frequently cited barrier among mobile users who are aware of mobile internet (GSMA, 2023). For many older adults, who rely on fixed incomes such as retirement pensions or social security benefits, these technology-related expenses are difficult to accommodate. By contrast, younger individuals often prioritize technology-related spending, or have access to devices through workplaces, educational institutions, or family support (Choi & DiNitto, 2013).

Internet subscription costs further exacerbate the affordability challenge. According to the ITU, internet usage declines sharply when mobile broadband access costs exceed 10% of the average monthly income of potential users (ITU, 2024). Older adults are disproportionately affected by this threshold due to their limited and often fixed financial resources. Affordability challenges are particularly severe in low- and middle-income countries (LMICs). Mobile internet prices in Africa were 12 times higher than in Europe in 2023 and rose to 14 times higher in 2024 (ITU, 2024). In these regions, an entry-level smartphone costs 16% of the average monthly income, and this proportion even rises dramatically among poorer groups, 40% for the poorest 40% and 55% for the poorest 20%. In Sub-Saharan Africa, home to a quarter of the global unconnected population, the price of an entry-level device can reach up to 95% of the average monthly income for the poorest 20% (GSMA, 2022, 2023). Moreover, rural older adults usually face higher handset prices than their urban counterparts, due to increased transportation and logistics costs, intermediary commissions, and limited local distributor presence, further deepening the affordability gap (GSMA, 2022).

2.3.3 Digital Literacy

Digital literacy, which refers to the ability to use digital technologies, communication tools, and networks to locate, evaluate, and create information, remains one of the most persistent barriers for older adults in our digital era. Unlike younger "digital natives" who grow up with digital technology, older adults often encounter it later life, requiring intentional adaptation. This generational gap leads to several challenges, such as understanding digital terminology, navigating through changing interfaces, troubleshooting issues, and transferring skills across platforms (Kakulla, 2021, 2025).

According to data from the EU-27, as of 2021, 54% of adults aged 16–74 possessed at least basic digital skills, compared to just 37% among older adults aged 55–74 (Eurostat, 2023). A similar pattern is observed in the United States, where only 66% of adults aged 50 and older report feeling comfortable with their digital skills, a sense of confidence that declines with increasing age (Kakulla, 2025). This digital skills gap is even more pronounced in low- and middle-income countries (LMICs). A 2022 GSMA survey conducted across 12 LMICs found that a lack of literacy and digital skills was the second most commonly cited barrier to mobile internet adoption among individuals who were aware of mobile internet but not using it. In one-third of the countries surveyed, it was identified as the primary barrier (GSMA, 2023).

2.3.4 Privacy and Security Concerns

Privacy and security concerns pose significant psychological barriers to ICT adoption among older adults. These concerns are identified as some of the most critical factors preventing older adults from embracing new technologies (Knight et al., 2024). An AARP report, for example, shows that data privacy worries constitute the biggest barrier to technology adoption for about one-third of older Americans (Kakulla, 2025).

Fear of data breaches, scams, and unauthorized information sharing often discourages seniors from using ICT. Globally, concerns about personal information leakage are notably high among older adults. The latest Global Digital Overview Report indicates that 47% of women and 44% of men aged 65 years or older worldwide express worries about such privacy issues. In comparison, younger age groups report lower levels of concern, ranging between 28 to 36% for women and 26 to 35% for men (Kemp, 2025).

These findings underscore the urgent need for more effective and transparent data protection policies and user-centered privacy safeguards, tailored to older users. Building trust through better primary protections is essential to promote digital inclusion for older adult populations.

Overall, these barriers of affordability, digital literacy, and privacy concerns are consistently cited across countries. For example, a 2020 nationwide survey in the United States found that older adults identified cost, knowledge gaps, and privacy concerns as the main reasons for hesitation in adopting new technologies (Kakulla, 2021). Addressing these challenges is essential for ensuring that older adults are not excluded from an increasingly digital world.

2.4 Conclusions

By examining the complex landscape of ICT use among older adults, this chapter reveals that despite the dramatic global surge in internet penetration, older populations continue to face persistent and disproportionate exclusion from the digital world. This exclusion is driven by a constellation of interlinked barriers, including limited accessibility, high costs of devices and connectivity, insufficient digital literacy, and psychological concerns such as fears over privacy breaches and cybersecurity threats. These obstacles are further compounded by broader geographic, structural and socioeconomic inequalities, all of which restrict older adults' opportunities to benefit meaningfully from digital technologies. The resulting digital divide not only limits their access to critical services such as healthcare, financing, and social support but also undermines their independence, dignity, civic engagement, and overall quality of life.

To bridge this widening gap, policymakers must adopt inclusive, equity-driven strategies. These should include expanding access to affordable and reliable broadband, subsidizing user-friendly digital devices tailored to the needs of older adults, and promoting lifelong digital learning opportunities. Equally important is the systematic collection and availability of age-disaggregated data on ICT use, which are essential for conducting evidence-based analyses, designing targeted interventions, and monitoring progress over time. Improving data infrastructure in this area is not only critical for deepening our understanding of the digital divide experienced by older adults, but also for advancing their meaningful digital inclusion in line with broader sustainable development goals. This is particularly true for those goals related to reducing inequalities, ensuring healthy lives, and fostering inclusive communities. All these efforts should contribute directly to the achievement of healthy and active aging in an increasingly digital world.

Disclaimer Views expressed in the chapter are solely those of the authors and do not necessarily reflect those of the United Nations, the National University of Singapore, the University of Alabama at Birmingham, and the University of Georgia.

References

Barrantes, R., & Vargas, E. (2019). Different paths and same destinations? An analysis of the convergence in internet usage patterns between different age groups. *Electronic Journal of Information Systems in Developing Countries, 85*(1), e12105.

Bianchi, T. (2025). *Brazil: Share of internet users 2024, by age group*. Retrieved from https://www.statista.com/statistics/254724/age-distribution-of-internet-users-in-brazil/

China Internet Network Information Center (CNNIC). (2016). *The 37th China Statistical Report on Internet Development* [in Chinese].

China Internet Network Information Center (CNNIC). (2022). *The 49th China Statistical Report on Internet Development*. [in Chinese].

Chinn, M. D., & Fairlie, R. W. (2007). The determinants of the global digital divide: A cross-country analysis of computer and internet penetration. *Oxford Economic Papers, 59*(1), 16–44.

Choi, N. G., & DiNitto, D. M. (2013). The digital divide among low-income homebound older adults: Internet use patterns, eHealth literacy, and attitudes toward computer/internet use. *Journal of Medical Internet Research, 15*(5), e93.

Choi, N. G., DiNitto, D. M., Marti, C. N., & Choi, B. Y. (2022). Telehealth use among older adults during COVID-19: Associations with sociodemographic and health characteristics, technology device ownership, and technology learning. *Journal of Applied Gerontology, 41*(3), 600–609.

Choi, N. G., Choi, B. Y., & Marti, C. N. (2025). Digital divide among homebound and semi-homebound older adults. *Journal of Applied Gerontology, 44*(6), 970–980.

Donner, J. (2008). Research approaches to mobile use in the developing world: A review of the literature. *The Information Society, 24*(3), 140–159.

Economic Commission for Latin America and the Caribbean (ECLAC). (2016). *State of Broadband in Latin America and the Caribbean 2016* [in Spanish]. Retrieved from https://repositorio.cepal.org/entities/publication/c5199e7b-97ca-441d-b5f9-2a3ccba5a388

Elena-Bucea, A., Cruz-Jesus, F., Oliveira, T., & Coelho, P. S. (2021). Assessing the role of age, education, gender and income on the digital divide: Evidence for the European Union. *Information Systems Frontiers, 23*(4), 1007–1021.

European Union Agency for Fundamental Rights. (2023). *Fundamental rights of older people: Ensuring access to public services in digital societies*. Retrieved from https://fra.europa.eu/en/publication/2023/older-people-digital-rights

EuroStat. (2023). *EuroStat Database*. Retrieved from https://ec.europa.eu/eurostat

Global System for Mobile Communications Association (GSMA). (2022). *The State of Mobile Internet Connectivity 2022*. Retrieved from https://www.gsma.com/r/somic-2022/

Global System for Mobile Communications Association (GSMA). (2023). *The State of Mobile Internet Connectivity 2023*. Retrieved from https://www.gsma.com/r/wp-content/uploads/2023/10/The-State-of-Mobile-Internet-Connectivity-Report-2023.pdf

Global System for Mobile Communications Association (GSMA). (2024). *Mobile Connectivity Index version 1.0*. Retrieved from www.gsma.com/connected-society

Godard, R., & Holtzman, S. (2024). Are active and passive social media use related to mental health, wellbeing, and social support outcomes? *Journal of Computer-Mediated Communication, 29*(1), zmad055.

International Telecommunication Union (ITU). (2022). *Global connectivity report 2022*. Retrieved from https://www.itu.int/itu-d/reports/statistics/global-connectivity-report-2022/

International Telecommunication Union (ITU). (2024). *Measuring digital development: Facts and figures 2024*. Retrieved from https://www.itu.int/en/ITU-D/Statistics/pages/facts/default.aspx

International Telecommunication Union (ITU). (2025a). *Measuring digital development: State of digital development and trends in the Americas region: Challenges and opportunities*. Retrieved from https://www.itu.int/hub/publication/d-ind-sddt_ams-2025/

International Telecommunication Union (ITU). (2025b). *Measuring digital development: State of digital development and trends in the Europe region: Challenges and opportunities*. Retrieved from https://www.itu.int/hub/publication/D-IND-SDDT_EUR-2025/

Jobst, N. (2024). *South Korea: Internet penetration 2015–2023, by age group*. Retrieved from https://www.statista.com/statistics/226740/age-composition-of-internet-users-in-south-korea/

Kakulla, B. (2021). *Tech Trends and the 50-Plus: Top 10 biggest trends*. AARP Research, April 2021. https://doi.org/10.26419/res.00420.001

Kakulla, B. (2025). *Technology adoption continues as older adults integrate tech into daily life*. AARP Research. Retrieved from https://www.aarp.org/pri/topics/technology/internet-media-devices/2025-technology-trends-older-adults/

Kemp, S. (2025). *Digital 2025: Global overview report*. Retrieved from https://datareportal.com/reports/digital-2025-global-overview-report

Knight, T., Yuan, X., & Bennett Gayle, D. (2024). Illuminating privacy and security concerns in older adults' technology adoption. *Work, Aging and Retirement, 10*(1), 57–60.

Laricchia, F. (2024). *Smartphone ownership in the U.S. 2015–2023, by age group*. Retrieved from https://www.statista.com/statistics/489255/percentage-of-us-smartphone-owners-by-age-group/

Li, L. (2024). Internet use and frailty in middle-aged and older adults: Findings from developed and developing countries. *Globalization and Health, 20*, 53.

Mohan, R., Saleem, F., Voderhobli, K., & Sheikh-Akbari, A. (2024). Ensuring sustainable digital inclusion among the elderly: A comprehensive analysis. *Sustainability, 16*(17), 7485.

Ofcom. (2021). *Online Nations Report 2021*. Retrieved from https://www.connectivityuk.org/2021/06/09/ofcom-online-nation-report-2021/

Oh, S. S., Kim, K. A., Kim, M., Oh, J., Chu, S. H., & Choi, J. (2021). Measurement of digital literacy among older adults: Systematic review. *Journal of Medical Internet Research, 23*(2), e26145.
Petrosyan, A. (2024). *Age distribution of internet users worldwide 2024*. Retrieved from https://www.statista.com/statistics/272365/age-distribution-of-internet-users-worldwide/
Pew Research Center. (2018). *Internet connectivity seen as having positive impact on life in Sub-Saharan Africa*. Retrieved from https://www.pewresearch.org/global/2018/10/09/internet-use-is-growing-across-much-of-sub-saharan-africa-but-most-are-still-offline/
Pew Research Center. (2021). *The internet and the pandemic*. Retrieved from https://www.pewresearch.org/internet/2021/09/01/the-internet-and-the-pandemic/
Pew Research Center. (2022). *Share of those 65 and older who are tech users has grown in the past decade*. Retrieved from https://www.pewresearch.org/short-reads/2022/01/13/share-of-those-65-and-older-who-are-tech-users-has-grown-in-the-past-decade/
Pew Research Center. (2024). *Internet, broadband fact sheet*. Retrieved from https://www.pewresearch.org/internet/fact-sheet/internet-broadband/
Pew Research Center. (2025). *5 years later: America looks back at the impact of COVID-19*. Retrieved from https://www.pewresearch.org/wp-content/uploads/sites/20/2025/02/PRC_2025.02.12_Covid-5-Year_REPORT.pdf
Seifert, A. (2020). The digital exclusion of older adults during the COVID-19 pandemic. *Journal of Gerontological Social Work, 63*(6–7), 674–676.
Seifert, A., & Cotten, S. R. (2022). Use of information and communication technologies among older adults: Usage differences, health-related impacts, and future needs. In D. A. Rohlinger & S. Sobieraj (Eds.), *The Oxford handbook of digital media sociology* (pp. 291–315). Oxford University Press.
Sixsmith, A., Horst, B. R., Simeonov, D., & Mihailidis, A. (2022). Older people's use of digital technology during the COVID-19 pandemic. *Bulletin of Science, Technology & Society, 42*(1–2), 19–24.
Statistics Canada. (2023). *Internet use by province and age group*. Retrieved from https://www150.statcan.gc.ca/t1/tbl1/en/tv.action?pid=2210013501
United Nations. (2024). *World population prospects 2024*. Retrieved from https://population.un.org/wpp/
United Nations Economic Commission for Europe (UNECE). (2025). *UNECE Statistical Database: Science and ICT*. Retrieved from https://w3.unece.org/PXWeb2015/pxweb/en/STAT/STAT__30-GE__09-Science_ICT/
Waghmare, A. (2025). *ICT skills*. Retrieved from https://www.dataforindia.com/ict-skills/
Wavrock, D., Schellenberg, G., & Schimmele, C. (2021). *Internet-use typology of Canadians: Online activities and digital skills*. Statistics Canada. 11F0019M- No.465. Retrieved from https://www150.statcan.gc.ca/n1/pub/11f0019m/11f0019m2021008-eng.htm
World Bank. (2025). *World development indicators*. Retrieved from https://databank.worldbank.org/source/world-development-indicatorsexes
Zhang, M. (2023). Older people's attitudes towards emerging technologies: A systematic literature review. *Public Understanding of Science, 32*(8), 948–968.

Chapter 3
Key Theories and Frameworks Related to ICT and Healthy Aging

Danan Gu, Kun Wang, Qiushi Feng, and Hee Yun Lee

With societies aging and digital technologies advancing, understanding the role of Information and Communication Technology (ICT) in supporting healthy aging has become increasingly important. As Chap. 4 reviewed and later chapters illustrated, ICT has the potential to enhance older adults' social participation, cognitive engagement, and access to health information, ultimately contributing to their overall well-being. Understanding the theoretical foundations of ICT use among older adults is essential for promoting healthy aging in an increasingly digital world as it is influenced by various individual, social, and technological factors, and thus it requires a theoretical lens to analyze these dynamics systematically. This chapter provides a comprehensive review of key theories related to ICT use and healthy aging. The first section explores theories that explain patterns of ICT adoption and purposes of ICT use among older adults. The second section delves into theories that illuminate the relationship between ICT use and healthy aging. Finally, the concluding section reflects research gaps of current theories and points out future directions, offering

---

D. Gu (✉)
Population Division, UN Department of Economic and Social Affairs, New York, NY, USA
e-mail: gudanan@yahoo.com

K. Wang
Department of Social Work, College of Arts and Sciences, University of Alabama at Birmingham, Birmingham, AL, USA
e-mail: kw2@uab.edu

Q. Feng
Centre for Family and Population Research/Department of Sociology and Anthropology, National University of Singapore, Singapore, Singapore
e-mail: socfq@nus.edu.sg

H. Y. Lee
School of Social Work, University of Georgia, Athens, GA, USA
e-mail: heeyunlee@uga.edu

K. Wang et al. (eds.), *ICT Use and Healthy Longevity*, Advances in Studies of Aging and Health 5, https://doi.org/10.1007/978-3-031-98964-3_3

insights for policymakers, practitioners, and researchers. The present chapter underscores the significance of theoretical perspectives in designing effective ICT interventions that promote digital inclusion among older adults, ultimately contributing to a more age-friendly digital society.

3.1 Theories and Frameworks Related to ICT Use

3.1.1 Theories and Frameworks of ICT Adoption

Over the past few decades, scholars have developed various theories to explain how individuals accept and use ICT, which are foundational in understanding behaviors of ICT use, especially in the rapidly evolving digital environment. This section highlights three influential theories/frameworks: the Technology Acceptance Model (TAM), the Unified Theory of Acceptance and Use of Technology (UTAUT), and the Senior Technology Acceptance Model (STAM). These models emphasize different psychological, contextual, and demographic factors influencing ICT adoption, offering valuable insights for designing inclusive technologies and promoting effective digital engagement, particularly among older populations and other underserved groups.

Technology Acceptance Model

TAM is a widely used framework for understanding how individuals adopt and use technology. Developed by Fred Davis in 1989, TAM posits that two key factors influence technology acceptance: Perceived Usefulness (PU) and Perceived Ease of Use (PEOU) (Davis, 1989). PU refers to the extent to which a person believes that using a particular technology will enhance his/her activity performance (e.g., job performance), whereas PEOU reflects how effortless they perceive the use of technology. According to TAM, these factors shape an individual's attitude toward using technology, which in turn influences their intention to use it and ultimately determines actual usage. By identifying barriers and facilitators to technology adoption, TAM helps developers and policymakers design user-friendly technologies that meet the needs of older adults, healthcare professionals, and students in digital learning environments.

While TAM has been widely adopted for its simplicity and validity, it has also drawn criticisms for its limited scope. The model primarily focuses on cognitive perceptions on usefulness and ease of use and often overlooks emotional, social, and contextual factors that may influence technology adoption as well (Venkatesh & Bala, 2008). Moreover, TAM assumes a rational decision-making process in the adoption of technology, which may not fully reflect the diverse motivations, needs, and experiences of those with varying levels of digital exposure and limited digital literacy. Despite these limitations, TAM remains a foundational model and has been successfully extended and adapted in numerous studies across healthcare, education, and aging research (Chen & Chan, 2014; Holden & Karsh, 2010).

In response to the criticisms of TAM, Venkatesh and Davis (2000) extended the original TAM, called TAM2, by incorporating additional determinants of perceived usefulness and technology adoption, including social influence processes (subjective norm, voluntariness, and image) and cognitive instrumental processes (e.g., job relevance, output quality, and result demonstrability). These factors shape perceived usefulness and ultimately influence users' intention to adopt technology. TAM2 provides a more comprehensive framework for understanding technology adoption in various contexts, including workplace settings and emerging digital tools (King & He, 2006).

However, while TAM2 enhances the original model by incorporating social and cognitive factors, it has also been criticized for maintaining a strong emphasis on rational decision-making and for its limited consideration of affective and environmental influences (Lee et al., 2003; Venkatesh & Bala, 2008). Moreover, the model assumes that social influence is primarily relevant in mandatory settings, potentially overlooking its significance in voluntary contexts. In response to these criticisms, particularly the model's limited practical guidance for implementation (Lee et al., 2003), Venkatesh and Bala (2008) proposed TAM3. This iteration integrates a broader range of antecedents influencing perceived usefulness and perceived ease of use within a unified framework. By systematically analyzing the distinct effects of these antecedents while minimizing crossover influences, TAM3 aims to construct a coherent nomological network for understanding technology adoption. This approach not only seeks to bring greater conceptual clarity to the literature (Marikyan & Papagiannidis, 2024) but also addresses inconsistencies in previous research regarding the predictors of the two central perception variables (Agarwal & Karahanna, 2000; Venkatesh & Davis, 2000). Ultimately, TAM3 aspires to provide a more comprehensive and actionable model for both researchers and practitioners.

Unified Theory of Acceptance and Use of Technology

UTAUT, introduced by Venkatesh et al. (2003), provides a comprehensive framework for understanding the factors influencing user acceptance of information technology. It synthesizes key constructs from eight models of technology acceptance, including TAM, the Theory of Reasoned Action (TRA), the Theory of Planned Behavior (TPB), and others (see the next section). UTAUT identifies four primary determinants of technology acceptance: performance expectancy, effort expectancy, social influence, and facilitating conditions.

Performance expectancy refers to the degree to which a person believes that using technology will improve their ability to accomplish valued tasks, which has been shown to be a strong predictor of technology adoption. Effort expectancy reflects the perceived ease of using the technology, closely aligned with the ease-of-use component in TAM. Social influence captures the extent to which individuals believe that important others (e.g., family, peers, colleagues) think they should use technology. Finally, facilitating conditions refer to the resources and support available to use the technology, such as technical assistance and training.

Venkatesh et al. (2003) argue that individual characteristics (e.g., age, gender, prior experience, and voluntariness of use) moderate the effects of key determinants on technology adoption. For instance, performance expectancy tends to exert a stronger influence on older users, while effort expectancy is more pronounced among those with limited experience. These moderating factors help explain the varied adoption patterns observed across different user groups. Building on this framework, subsequent research has explored its applicability across diverse cultural contexts. For example, Venkatesh and Zhang (2010) examined the model in both the U.S. and China, uncovering national differences in the relative weight of specific determinants. In the U.S., social influence was found to be less significant, whereas in China, societal norms and familial expectations played a more prominent role in shaping technology use.

Building on the original UTAUT, Venkatesh et al. (2012) introduced UTAUT2 to better understand technology acceptance in consumer contexts. This extended model incorporates three additional components: hedonic motivation, price value, and habit, which correspondingly reflect the experiential, economic, and behavioral dimensions of consumer decision-making. By integrating these factors, UTAUT2 provides a more comprehensive framework that captures the complexities of individual technology use beyond organizational settings, enhancing its applicability to real-world consumer environments.

Overall, UTAUT and UTAUT2 offer a unified and comprehensive approach to understanding technology adoption, accounting for both individual factors and external influences. An important contribution of UTAUT and UTAUT2 is to incorporating *mediating* factors such as attitudes and behavioral intention to use ICT. Its flexibility and evolvability have made it a widely adopted framework in research across different technologies, industries, and cultures. Despite its strengths, UTAUT and UTAUT2 have limitations as well. Critics argue that it overly emphasizes extrinsic motivation while neglecting psychological and affective factors like emotions and trust (Bagozzi, 2007). Additionally, its reliance on self-reported intentions may not always translate into actual behavior, limiting its predictive power (Straub & Burton-Jones, 2007).

Senior Technology Acceptance Model

STAM is the application of TAM and/or UTAUT to older adults. There are mainly two versions of STAMs. One is proposed by Renaud and Biljon (2008), which focuses on smart phone use. The other is proposed by Chen and Chan (2014), focusing on the use of gerontechnology. These two models may be more appropriate to study ICT use among aging populations.

Renaud and van Biljon's STAM focuses on a multi-stage adoption process that recognizes the unique pathway older adults take when engaging with technology. Unlike younger users, older adults are often introduced to new technologies by family members or caregivers rather than actively seeking them out on their own. This dynamic influences their initial perception of usefulness and ease of learning that shape older adult's behavioral intention to use technology. Another critical component of STAM is the ease of learning, which is a stronger determinant for older users than it is for younger populations. The model identifies key stages in the adoption process, including an experimentation phase, where older users test a new technology, and a confirmation phase, where they assess whether it meets their needs. The ultimate outcome may be either acceptance or rejection, with usability and learning difficulties often being the primary barriers to full adoption.

By contrast, Chen and Chan's STAM (2014) refines the TAM framework by introducing aging-specific determinants that influence technology acceptance. Their model incorporates three major additional factors: perceived health conditions, computer self-efficacy, and facilitating conditions. Recognizing that older adults may face physical or cognitive declines that impact their ability to use technology, this STAM includes perceived health conditions as a direct factor influencing perceived ease of use and perceived usefulness. This means that older adults with deteriorating vision, reduced dexterity, or cognitive decline may find technology more difficult to use, affecting their overall willingness to adopt it. Another critical factor in their model is computer self-efficacy, which refers to an individual's confidence in their ability to use technology effectively. Older adults with greater self-efficacy are more likely to perceive technology as useful and easy to use, leading to higher adoption rates. Lastly, facilitating conditions, such as technical support, training opportunities, and user-friendly interfaces, play a crucial role in shaping acceptance. Unlike Renaud and van Biljon's model, which emphasizes a staged adoption process, Chen and Chan's framework presents a more predictive approach, identifying how specific age-related characteristics interact with traditional technology acceptance factors to determine an individual's likelihood of adoption.

In short, the key distinction of the two models lies in their focus and application. Renaud and van Biljon's STAM is more process-driven, underscoring how older adults engage with technology in phases and how ease of learning and social influence play pivotal roles in determining whether they continue to use a device. By contrast, Chen and Chan's STAM is more factor-oriented, aiming to quantify and predict acceptance by incorporating aging-specific variables. Their model provides a clearer explanation of why certain older individuals may struggle with or resist technology, particularly due to health conditions and self-efficacy issues, which are less explicitly addressed in Renaud and van Biljon's framework.

In application, the two models serve different purposes. Renaud and van Biljon's model is more useful for understanding the adoption process and how external influences shape older adults' technology engagement over time. On the other hand, Chen and Chan's model offers a framework with more predictors, which policymakers and designers can target to improve adoption rates. Together, these models complement each other, offering a comprehensive understanding of the complex factors influencing technology acceptance among older adults.

While both STAM models offer valuable insights into older adults' technology acceptance, they have limitations. Renaud and van Biljon's model may oversimplify the adoption process by focusing heavily on social influence while underemphasizing individual psychological factors. Conversely, Chen and Chan's model, while incorporating aging-specific determinants, may not fully capture cultural and socioeconomic influences on adoption (Barnard et al., 2013). Additionally, both models could benefit from integrating emerging factors such as digital literacy interventions and AI-driven accessibility tools, which are developing rapidly to enhance older adults' engagement with technology (Charness & Boot, 2009; Mo et al., 2025).

3.1.2 Theories and Frameworks of Purposes of ICT Use

In this section, we review three theories that focus on the purposes of ICT use, providing insights into why individuals engage with different forms of technology. These theories explore the motivations behind media consumption and technology adoption, illustrating the diverse needs and goals that drive people to use ICT. By understanding these theoretical frameworks, we can better grasp how people use technology as a tool to achieve personal, social, and professional objectives, obtaining a comprehensive view of factors that influence ICT use.

Uses and Gratifications Theory
The Uses and Gratifications Theory (UGT), proposed by Katz et al. in 1973, explains how individuals actively seek media to fulfill specific needs. Unlike traditional models in media studies that view audiences as passive, UGT asserts that people make deliberate media choices based on their personal desires (Katz et al., 1973). UGT identifies several key needs: cognition (seeking information), affection (emotional satisfaction or entertainment), personal integration (self-esteem and recognition), and social integration (fostering relationships). This implies that individuals select media to pursue their goals, such as education, relaxation, or socialization.

The theory has played a significant role in media research by guiding studies on the diverse needs that drive media use. For instance, television is typically associated with entertainment, while the internet serves as a tool for information gathering and social interaction. Social media platforms like Facebook are often used to fulfill social needs, as demonstrated by Raacke and Bonds-Raacke (2008). Nonetheless, critics argue that UGT may oversimplify media use by emphasizing individual motivations while overlooking broader societal and cultural influences. Its focus on active users also tends to neglect the growing role of media producers and algorithmic curation in shaping user behavior. Despite these limitations, UGT remains a foundational framework in media studies, offering valuable insight into how media consumption satisfies human needs, particularly in an age of increasingly personalized content. It helps explain a wide range of media behaviors, from news consumption and entertainment to social engagement.

Theory of Planned Behavior
The Theory of Planned Behavior (TPB), proposed by Icek Ajzen in 1991, focuses on intentions in explaining human behavior, which are influenced by attitude (evaluation of the behavior), subjective norms (social pressure to engage or not engage), and perceived behavioral control (belief in one's ability to perform the behavior,

considering resources and obstacles) (PBC). TPB extends TRA by adding PBC, and acknowledges external factors that may affect behavior.

TPB is widely applicable in fields such as health behaviors (e.g., smoking cessation), environmental behaviors (e.g., recycling), and consumer behaviors. Research has shown that PBC is particularly important for behaviors, which are influenced by external constraints like time or financial limitations. However, TPB has been criticized for focusing on cognitive factors and the assumption of rationality, which overlooks emotional and unconscious influences on behavior. Despite these critiques, TPB remains a widely used and effective model for understanding human behaviors in contexts like social media, where users' behavior is shaped by attitudes, social influences, and perceived ease of engaging in activities like commenting or sharing posts (Conner & Armitage, 1998).

Media Richness Theory

The Media Richness Theory (MRT), proposed by Daft and Lengel in 1986, suggests that communication effectiveness depends on the richness of the medium, defined by its ability to convey information. Richer media, like face-to-face communication, are more effective for complex, ambiguous messages, as they allow immediate feedback, personal interaction, and non-verbal cues. In contrast, leaner media, such as emails, are better for clear, straightforward communication due to their lack of interpersonal elements. The theory thus posits that the choice of communication medium should match the task's complexity. For more ambiguous tasks requiring nuanced understanding, richer media are essential. This theory has significantly influenced organizational communication and decision-making (Daft & Lengel, 1986).

Although MRT is criticized by overemphasizing media richness and neglects contextual factors like technological advancements and individual preferences (Dennis et al., 2008), it remains a key framework in understanding how media characteristics affect communication and decision-making dynamics. For example, video calls provide more social interaction cues than text-based communication, making them more suitable for tasks requiring rich interaction (Daft & Lengel, 1986).

Overall, the theories of UGT, TPB, and MRT have significantly contributed to the development of models like TAM, UTAUT, and STAM as we reviewed above, which has helped enrich our understanding of users' behaviors, especially reminding that ICT solutions should align with the users' needs and motivations.

3.1.3 Theories and Frameworks for Barriers to ICT Use

Barriers to ICT adoption are often closely tied to perceived ease of use, a central component in models such as TAM, UTAUT, and STAM, which, along with perceived usefulness, can significantly influence technology acceptance. In the case of older adults, their adoption of new technologies is frequently impeded by factors such as unfamiliarity with digital interfaces, complex designs, and perceived difficulty in mastering technological tools. Additionally, according to these theories, external factors, such as the availability of user-friendly designs, training, and support from caregivers or family members, can also greatly influence older adults' willingness to engage with ICT.

In contrast to these psychologically and environmentally focused frameworks, the digital divide theory offers a broader lens by incorporating structural factors, particularly socioeconomic and geographical disparities, that affect both access to and effective use of digital technologies.

Digital Divide Theory

The digital divide is commonly defined as the gap between those who access and use ICT devices and those who do not (van Dijk, 2005, 2017, 2020). The digital divide theory examines the disparities in access to and use of ICT that are influenced by various socioeconomic factors such as income, education, and geographical location (van Dijk, 2005, 2006). As van Dijk (2006) argues, the digital divide is not only about physical access but also the ability to make use of technology in a meaningful way. In reality, the digital divide often leaves older adults at a disadvantage, limiting their opportunities for digital engagement, including access to healthcare, social networks, and educational resources, which are increasingly dependent on digital platforms. According to the digital divide theory, socioeconomic factors play a critical role in determining the access and ability of older adults to engage with technology.

There are three levels of the digital divide according to the existing literature. The first level of the digital divide theory emphasizes disparities in access to ICT, which are frequently shaped by factors such as income, infrastructure, and location (Norris, 2001). Older adults in rural areas or low-income households, for example, are often faced with significant challenges in accessing the necessary technology, whether due to limited availability of internet infrastructure, high costs of devices, or geographic isolation. Norris (2001) suggests that these barriers are especially pronounced among marginalized groups who may lack the financial resources to purchase and maintain digital devices and services. For people suffering from this digital gap, technology adoption is less of a matter of choice.

The second level addresses the gaps in digital skills and literacy that persist even when access to technology is not an issue (Hargittai, 2002). From this perspective, having access to ICT does not automatically translate into the ability to use it effectively. Many older individuals struggle with digital literacy due to a lack of prior exposure to technology or insufficient training. Hargittai (2002) points out that digital skills are unevenly distributed, and those with limited experience are less likely to engage with online platforms. This disparity results in older adults being unable to take full advantage of digital tools, which further lead to social isolation and exclusion from the digital economy. Bridging this second-level divide requires targeted efforts in education, training, and skills development to ensure that older users can navigate and benefit from technology.

The third level of the digital divide focuses on the impact of digital engagement on important outcomes like social participation, health, and well-being (van Deursen

& Helsper, 2015). While bridging the access and skills gaps is important, it is also essential to consider how technology use influences the quality of life for older adults. According to van Deursen and Helsper (2015), older adults who overcome the first- and second-level divides also need to become digitally engaged, which can enhance social participation and improve cognitive functioning. For example, engaging online platforms can help combat isolation by facilitating communication with family and peers, while also providing access to health resources and services that are increasingly delivered digitally. However, those who remain excluded from digital engagement may face a widening gap in health and social outcomes, leading to further marginalization.

In sum, the digital divide theory offers a comprehensive framework for understanding the multifaceted barriers to digital engagement. Its multi-level approach, which encompasses access, skills, and meaningful use, provides valuable insights into the complex interplay between technological availability and broader societal impacts in affecting older people in using ICT, advanced our understanding of digital barriers, and informed interventions that improve digital inclusion for aging populations. This theory also faces several criticisms. Scholars argue that it can be overly reductive, often concentrating on access alone while overlooking critical nuances such as digital skills, user motivations, and the sociocultural contexts in which technology is used (Helsper, 2021). Moreover, the theory is sometimes criticized for failing to address the evolving nature of digital technologies, such as smartphones and social media, and their varied impacts on digital inclusion (Robinson et al., 2020; Helsper, 2021). Importantly, it has been noted that digital inclusion is not solely about having access but about using technology effectively and meaningfully, a challenge particularly relevant to older adults (Friemel, 2016; Neves & Vetere, 2019). Despite these critiques, the digital divide framework remains an essential starting point for identifying barriers or inequities in digital use and designing more inclusive digital policies and practices.

3.1.4 Other Theories Related to ICT Use

In addition to the major theories and frameworks reviewed above, numerous other theories have been proposed to elucidate various aspects of ICT adoption, including acceptance, usage, motivation, behaviors, barriers, and objectives. These theories further enrich our understanding of ICT-related behaviors, particularly among older adults, by offering diverse perspectives grounded in psychology, sociology, gerontology, and communication studies. Below is a short review of selected theories and frameworks.

1. The Diffusion of Innovation Theory (DIT): This theory categorizes individuals based on their willingness to adopt new innovations, identifying groups such as innovators, early adopters, early majority, late majority, and laggards. According to DIT, factors influencing innovation adoption include age, social networks, and

perceived benefits. DIT has been widely applied to understand how technological innovations spread within societies (Rogers, 2003; Czaja et al., 2006).

2. The Gerontechnology Theory (GTT): Emphasizing the intersection of aging, technology, and the environment, GTT advocates for the design of technologies that are age-friendly, accessible, and tailored to the unique needs of older adults. This has been applied to facilitate the successful adoption and utilization of ICT among older adults, particularly for health-related purposes (Bouma et al., 2007; van Bronswijk et al., 2002).
3. The Ecological Model of Aging and Technology (EMAT): This model presents multiple levels of factors, including individual, interpersonal, organizational, community, and societal elements, which affect ICT usage among older adults. Aligned with EMAT, effective interventions and policies promoting healthy aging through ICT should address barriers and facilitators at each of these levels (Mylonopoulou et al., 2022; Wahl et al., 2012).
4. The Intersectionality Theory: This theory, developed by Crenshaw (1989), highlights how multiple social identities, such as age, gender, race, socio-economic status, and disability, intersect to shape individuals' experiences and opportunities. When applied in ICT adoption, this framework helps explain how these identities interactively impact the use of technology (Wang et al., 2024). This theory recognizes that individuals experience overlapping layers of privilege and disadvantages, which influence their access to resources, technological literacy, and social networks.
5. The Age-Related Positivity Bias Theory (ARPBT): This theory proposes that older adults tend to focus more on positive information and experiences, thus they may be more inclined to use ICT to engage with uplifting content, such as positive videos, music, and photos, as well as to maintain emotionally meaningful connections. They may also prefer platforms that enable the curation and sharing of positive experiences. These activities can enhance their emotional well-being and contribute to overall psychological health (Mather & Carstensen, 2005; Reed & Carstensen, 2012).
6. The Stereotype Embodiment Theory (SET): SET posits that individuals internalize age-related stereotypes over time, which can influence their self-perception and behaviors. Therefore, negative stereotypes about aging may lead to self-limiting behaviors, such as reduced engagement with ICT, whereas positive stereotypes can encourage greater participation (Levy, 2009; Levy et al., 2002).
7. The Aging Identity Theory (AIT): Similar to SET, AIT suggests that older adults who maintain a positive identification with their age group and view aging as a meaningful life stage are more open to engaging with ICT. In contrast, those who internalize negative stereotypes about aging may be less likely to adopt new technologies (Levy, 2003; Barrett, 2005).
8. The Self-Efficacy Theory: This theory emphasizes the role of an individual's belief in their ability to perform specific tasks. For older adults, confidence in using ICT and the perceived ability to learn and adapt to new technologies significantly impact their engagement levels (Bandura, 1997; Eastin & LaRose, 2000).

9. The Expectation-Confirmation Theory (ECT): ECT explains post-adoption satisfaction as a function of initial expectations, perceived performance, and confirmation or disconfirmation of beliefs. For older adults, positive initial expectations about ICT, such as beliefs about its relevance and ease of use, combined with satisfying experiences, can lead to continued and increased use of ICTs (Bhattacherjee, 2001; Hong & Tam, 2006; Kim & Crowston, 2011).

These theories summarized here further offer valuable insights into the multifaceted factors associated with ICT use in later life. By integrating these theoretical perspectives, together with those reviewed in earlier sections, researchers and policymakers can better design and implement policies and interventions that support digital engagement among older adults. A holistic understanding of ICT use at older ages helps promote inclusive digital participation, reduce technology-related inequalities, and ultimately improve the quality of life for aging populations.

3.2 Theories and Frameworks Related to the Relationships Between ICT Use and Healthy Aging

Understanding the interplay between ICT use and healthy aging requires insights from a range of interdisciplinary theories, which have shed light on how digital engagement can promote social inclusion, cognitive vitality, autonomy, and overall well-being among older adults. Drawing from psychology, gerontology, and communication studies, this section categorizes relevant theories into thematic areas, highlighting how they help explain the mechanisms through which ICT use supports healthy aging in different dimensions, including social connectivity, cognitive and health benefits, and the ability to age in place.

3.2.1 ICT and Social Connectivity in Aging

Activity Theory of Aging

The Activity Theory of Aging (ATA), one of the three major psychosocial theories of aging, posits that sustained engagement in meaningful activities, particularly social interactions, enhances life satisfaction in later life (Havighurst, 1961). Based on the idea that older adults share similar psychological and social needs with middle-aged adults, the theory emphasizes the importance of maintaining active roles for emotional well-being. However, age-related health declines and the loss of social roles due to retirement or bereavement can reduce opportunities for engagement, leading to loneliness, depression, and self-evaluation crises (Hawkley & Kocherginsky, 2017; Li et al., 2021). In this context, ICT offers a promising solution by facilitating online social networking, learning, entertainment, and access to services such as shopping and banking. These digital interactions help older adults overcome physical and social limitations, reduce loneliness and depression, and may even support cognitive health (Chopik, 2016; Yu & Fiebig, 2020). Activity Theory thus provides a useful framework for understanding the psychological and social benefits of ICT use in promoting active and satisfying aging.

Socioemotional Selectivity Theory

The Socioemotional Selectivity Theory (SEST), proposed by Carstensen (1995), posits that as individuals age and perceive time as more limited, they become increasingly motivated to focus on emotionally meaningful goals and relationships, which drive them to prioritize quality over quantity in their social interactions. In the context of ICT use, SEST provides a valuable framework for understanding why older adults may be drawn to technologies, such as video calls, messaging apps, or social networking platforms, in order to help maintain close ties with family and friends. These digital tools can thus enhance emotional well-being by enabling sustained social connection and reducing feelings of loneliness and isolation. Recent studies have supported SEST's applicability in the field, demonstrating that ICT use aligned with emotionally meaningful interactions contributes positively to life satisfaction and mental health among older adults (Chen & Schulz, 2016; Chopik, 2016; Quan-Haase et al., 2017).

Social Network Theory

The Social Network Theory (SNT) emphasizes the structural and functional aspects of social connections, illustrating how individuals are embedded within social networks that influence their behaviors and access to resources (Granovetter, 1973). For older adults, ICT use has been shown to enhance their social networks by facilitating both the maintenance of strong ties (e.g., close family) and the formation of weak ties (e.g., acquaintances or community members), both of which are important for accessing diverse forms of social support. Through platforms like social media, email, and video conferencing, older adults can sustain existing relationships and forge new ones, even if they face physical decline or geographic separation. These digital interactions can reduce feelings of loneliness, promote engagement, and help older adults remain socially integrated in later life (Wright, 2000; Hogan, 2009). The application of SNT in the field thus provides a useful lens to understand how ICT functions not just as a communication tool, but as a mechanism for building and maintaining relational capital that supports healthy aging.

3.2.2 ICT and Cognitive/Health Benefits

Cognitive Reserve Theory

The Cognitive Reserve Theory (CRT) posits that individual differences in cognitive processing, often shaped by life experiences such as education, occupational complexity, and leisure activities, contribute to resilience against age-related cognitive decline and neuropathology (Stern, 2002). ICT use, particularly those involving cognitively stimulating activities like online learning, digital games, or web navigation, can play a role in building or maintaining this reserve in older adults. Engaging with ICT may thus promote executive functioning, memory, and problem-solving, thus enhancing the brain's capacity to compensate for age-related changes. Empirical studies have supported the view that sustained digital engagement is associated with slower cognitive decline and higher cognitive functioning in aging populations (Small et al., 2009; Tun & Lachman, 2010). These findings support that digital technologies are not merely tools for communication or convenience but can serve as meaningful interventions in cognitive health promotion. Thus, CRT offers a valuable framework for understanding the mechanism of how digital engagement can contribute to healthy cognitive aging in an increasingly digital society.

Self-Determination Theory

The Self-Determination Theory (SDT) posits that fulfilling the psychological needs of autonomy, competence, and relatedness enhances motivation and well-being. In the context of ICT use among older adults, engaging with ICT can support these needs. For instance, a study by Cotter et al. (2024) examined how eHealth systems can promote autonomy by allowing older adults to access health information independently, competence through user-friendly interfaces that enhance their technological skills, and relatedness by facilitating social connections through online communities. Similarly, the study by Schreurs et al. (2017) highlighted that older adults' participation in ICT-based activities can lead to a sense of empowerment, aligning with the principles of SDT. These findings also suggest that thoughtfully designed ICT interventions can support meeting the psychological needs of older adults, outlined in SDT, thereby promoting greater engagement and well-being among older adults.

Life-Span Theory of Control

The Life-Span Theory of Control, proposed by Heckhausen and Schulz (1995), highlights the central role of perceived control in promoting personal development and well-being throughout the life course, including in later adulthood. The theory distinguishes between primary control (i.e., efforts to actively shape the external environment to achieve personal goals) and secondary control (i.e., internal strategies that support and sustain primary control). In the context of aging, perceived control has been consistently associated with better cognitive outcomes and slower memory decline (Infurna & Gerstorf, 2013; Lachman & Andreoletti, 2006). As older adults encounter age-related physical declines and shifts in social roles, internet use can serve as a valuable tool for exercising or regaining control over daily life. Acquiring digital skills reflects adaptability and agency, while access to online services can help preserve autonomy, particularly amid physical limitations (Bernardo et al., 2022). By supporting both primary and secondary control processes, ICT use may mitigate the adverse effects of diminished control, thereby enhancing psychological and cognitive well-being in later life.

Model of Selection, Optimization, and Compensation

The Model of Selection, Optimization, and Compensation (SOC), introduced by Baltes and Baltes (1993), offers a dynamic framework for understanding successful aging by focusing on adaptive processes rather than fixed outcomes. According to this model, older adults can respond to age-related challenges by selecting meaningful and achievable goals, optimizing their internal and external resources to pursue those goals, and compensating for losses by adopting alternative strategies. In later life, goals such as maintaining social relationships and personal autonomy often become central, yet physiological declines may limit the ability to pursue them through traditional means. ICT offers a promising avenue for compensation, enabling older adults, especially those with mobility or sensory impairments, to maintain social engagement, manage daily tasks, and access health services virtually. From online shopping and bill payments to telehealth and video calls, digital tools help older adults adapt to age-related changes while continuing to pursue valued goals. SOC thus provides a useful lens to understand how ICT use supports autonomy, emotional well-being, and active engagement in the face of aging-related challenges.

3.2.3 ICT and Aging-in-Place

Person-Environment Fit Theory

The Person-Environment Fit Theory (PEFT) argues that optimal well-being occurs when there is a good match between an individual's needs and the characteristics of their environment (Kahana, 1974). Older adults may face physical, cognitive, and emotional changes that affect their ability to live independently, and ICT solutions can mitigate these challenges by offering tools for monitoring health, managing daily tasks, and providing access to social networks and medical care. In this sense, PEFT suggests that aging-in-place can be supported through ICT-based solutions, such as smart home technologies and telehealth platforms, which adapt the environment to the needs of older adults, enabling them to maintain independence and quality of life (Hu et al., 2024). Research has shown that these technologies can enhance older adults' autonomy, reduce reliance on caregivers, and promote their engagement in the community (Aggar et al., 2023). Moreover, the integration of smart technologies within the home environment has been linked to improved mental health, reduced feelings of isolation, and greater overall well-being (Hu et al., 2024). Overall, PEFT provides a useful framework for understanding how technology can enable older adults to thrive while aging in place.

Technology-Enabled Aging (Aging 2.0)

The Technology-Enabled Aging (Aging 2.0), proposed by Katy Fike and Stephen Johnston, who co-founded the organization Aging 2.0 in 2012 (https://www.aging2.com/about-us), is a framework that underscores how technological innovations, particularly in ICT, can enable older adults to live independently and age in place. This framework emphasizes that personalized healthcare services, such as remote monitoring, telemedicine, and smart home technologies, can significantly enhance the quality of life for older individuals (Peek et al., 2014). The adoption of ICT solutions not only supports the independence of older adults but also provides continuous access to health services and promotes social inclusion by reducing isolation. However, the successful implementation of these technologies depends on factors such as ease of use, accessibility, and the perceived benefits of the technology for older adults (Ollevier et al., 2020). These technologies, when tailored to the specific needs of older adults, can increase autonomy, improve health outcomes, and facilitate aging in place (Chang et al., 2024; Mu et al., 2022). Overall, the Aging 2.0 framework offers a valuable perspective on how ICT can empower older adults to maintain their independence and improve their overall well-being.

3.2.4 Other Theories on ICT Use and Healthy Aging

There are numerous other theories related to the relationship between ICT use and healthy aging, helping explain how technology can contribute to older adults' physical, cognitive, and social well-being. Below is summary of selected ones that highlight the diverse ways in which ICT can influence healthy aging in older populations.

1. The Positive Aging Theory (PAT): Developed by Fernández-Ballesteros (2011), PAT emphasizes optimizing physical, cognitive, and social functioning to enhance well-being in later life. It advocates proactive engagement in meaningful activities to foster resilience and life satisfaction. In the context of ICT use, studies show that older adults who use technology for social connection, learning, or health management report higher subjective well-being. For example, Chen and Schulz (2016) found that ICT interventions reduced loneliness and improved mental health by enabling social participation online.
2. The Active Aging Theory (AAT): Proposed by the WHO (2002), AAT prioritizes health, participation, and security to enhance quality of life. Under this framework, ICT can support active aging by enabling lifelong learning (e.g., online courses), remote work, and civic engagement. Likewise, Heart and Kalderon (2013) also linked technology use to greater autonomy in managing health and social activities among older adults.
3. The Successful Aging Theory (SAT): The concept of successful aging was first articulated by Havighurst (1961), who emphasized the importance of continued social roles and active engagement in later life. Building on this, Rowe and Kahn (1987, 1997) offered a more structured model, defining successful aging as a combination of low probability of disease and disability, high cognitive and physical functioning, and active engagement with life. Within this framework, ICT tools, such as brain-training apps, telehealth services, and social networking platforms, can serve as valuable resources for promoting cognitive vitality,

access to care, and social connectedness. Research shows that ICT adoption is associated with improved cognitive outcomes and enhanced social engagement among older adults (Charness & Boot, 2009).

4. The Social Capital Theory: Rooted in Putnam's (2000) work, this theory highlights the value of social networks and trust in fostering community well-being. Applied to ICT, online platforms can strengthen bonding (close ties) and bridging (diverse networks) social capital among older adults. Winstead et al. (2013) demonstrated that older adults using social media maintained stronger intergenerational connections, which enhanced emotional support and reduced feelings of isolation.
5. The Social Support Theory (SST): House (1981) defined social support as emotional, informational, or instrumental aid from social networks, which are essential for the health and well-being of older adults. In this sense, ICT facilitates social support exchange for older adults through telehealth, online forums, and messaging apps. Chen and Schulz (2016) showed that ICT-mediated support improved coping strategies for chronic illnesses, particularly for geographically isolated seniors.
6. The Social Compensation Theory (SCT): This theory explains how individuals with limited offline social resources or skills use the internet to compensate for social deficits. Unlike the "rich-get-richer" hypothesis, which suggests that socially active individuals benefit most from online interactions, SCT proposes that those who are socially isolated or less confident offline may gain more from digital communication because the internet provides a low-pressure environment for building relationships and enhancing well-being (Kraut et al., 1998, 2002; Peter et al., 2005). While SCT was initially applied to non-older adults, it has since been extended to older adults seeking to overcome challenges such as reduced mobility and shrinking social networks (Nimrod, 2010).
7. The Social Cognitive Theory: Bandura (1986) emphasized the roles of self-efficacy and observational learning in behavior change. Applied to ICT use, older adults with higher technology self-efficacy are more likely to adopt and benefit from digital tools. Supporting this, Czaja et al. (2006) showed that tailored training programs improved older adults' confidence and promoted sustained engagement with technology.
8. The Use-It-or-Lose-It Hypothesis: This hypothesis asserts that cognitive abilities decline without regular stimulation (Salthouse, 2006). ICT use, such as video games or apps, provides mental exercise. Boot et al. (2013) found that older adults using brain-training apps showed improved processing speed and working memory.

In summary, the diverse theoretical frameworks presented in Sects. 3.2.1–3.2.4 provide a rich and multi-dimensional understanding of how ICT use can support healthy aging. The Social Support Theory and Cognitive Reserve Theory emphasize the ability of digital tools to enhance social inclusion and cognitive health by fostering social connectivity and providing cognitive stimulation, both critical for maintaining autonomy and resilience in later life. The Self-Determination Theory and

Person-Environment Fit Theory highlight how ICT can meet older adults' psychological needs for autonomy, competence, and relatedness while adapting their environments to enhance independence and well-being.

The Activity Theory of Aging further contributes by suggesting that continued engagement in social, physical, and mental activities is essential for well-being as people age. In this context, ICT facilitates ongoing participation in meaningful activities, such as online learning, social interactions, and health management, that are integral to maintaining an active lifestyle. The Socioemotional Selectivity Theory, on the other hand, posits that as people age, they prioritize emotionally fulfilling relationships. ICT offers a means to maintain and deepen these relationships, particularly when face-to-face interaction becomes more challenging due to mobility issues or geographical distance.

From a more functional perspective, the Life-Span Theory of Control and the Model of Selection, Optimization, and Compensation underscore the importance of maintaining control over one's life through adaptive strategies. In this light, ICT tools empower older adults to select the activities that are most meaningful to them, optimize their use of resources (such as health information or social networks), and compensate for age-related declines in physical or cognitive function. These theories align with the Active Aging Theory, which stresses health, participation, and security as key to quality of life, further supported by ICT's ability to promote lifelong learning, civic participation, and health management.

Furthermore, the Positive Aging Theory, the Successful Aging Theory, and the Social Capital Theory emphasize the importance of maintaining social roles, life satisfaction, and social networks in later life, suggesting that ICT can be a catalyst for these aspects. The Social Network Theory further enriches this perspective by emphasizing the importance of social ties and connections in influencing the health and well-being of older adults. According to this theory, maintaining and expanding one's social network through digital means can offer emotional support, improve mental health, and reduce isolation, which are crucial for aging well. ICT platforms, including social media and messaging apps, can help older adults stay connected with family, friends, and communities, strengthening both bonding and bridging social capital.

In addition, Social Compensation Theory and Social Cognitive Theory provide insights into how technology can be especially beneficial for older adults who face social isolation or have lower self-efficacy, helping them build confidence and establish meaningful connections in a low-pressure digital environment. The Use-It-or-Lose-It Hypothesis and Selection-Optimization-Compensation model further reinforce the cognitive benefits of ICT use by promoting mental exercise through digital tools, such as brain-training apps or virtual health consultations, which can preserve and enhance cognitive function.

Finally, the Technology-Enabled Aging (Aging 2.0) concept integrates all these theories by framing ICT not only as a tool for health management but as a transformative force in aging. This modern approach to aging sees technology as a central enabler of aging with dignity and independence, offering solutions that support older adults' needs in all aspects of life socially, cognitively, and physically.

Together, these integrated theories demonstrate the transformative potential of ICT in promoting healthy aging. They reveal how ICT not only fosters social connections and cognitive stimulation but also supports autonomy, resilience, and a sense of purpose in later life. By leveraging these theoretical frameworks, interventions and policies can be designed to enhance the well-being and quality of life of older adults, ensuring they remain engaged, healthy, and autonomous. Ultimately, these frameworks provide essential guidance for developing age-inclusive technologies and strategies that address the complex, evolving needs of aging populations.

3.3 Conclusions and Prospects

This chapter, based on the established theoretical framework, illustrated a complicated scenario consisting of various conditions, drivers, barriers, and procedures, in which ICT is adopted among older people, and also a broad scope of benefits of using ICT in later life in social connectivity, cognitive and health benefits, and the ability to age in place. These insights have laid down a firm foundation for future studies.

As aging societies face challenges related to increased dependency and social isolation among the older population, these frameworks, as discussed in this chapter, offer valuable perspectives on the ICT use and its essential role in later life. Future research should pay attention to the integration of artificial intelligence in supporting older adults, such as AI-driven health monitoring systems, and investigate how interdisciplinary studies can further our understanding of digital inclusion for aging populations. Additionally, examining how AI can enhance cognitive health, social engagement, and overall well-being through personalized interventions could be a promising area for exploration.

From a policy standpoint, addressing the digital divide remains crucial. Policies that focus on improving access to ICT for older adults, particularly those in underserved communities, can significantly reduce inequalities and enhance the impact of digital technologies. Ensuring that older individuals have skills, resources, and support to engage with ICT is essential for maximizing their potential to age healthily and autonomously. Policies aimed at bridging this divide are vital for ensuring the inclusion of older adults in the digital age, fostering greater independence, and improving quality of life.

Disclaimer Views expressed in the chapter are solely those of the authors and do not necessarily reflect those of the United Nations, the University of Alabama at Birmingham, the National University of Singapore, and the University of Georgia.

References

Agarwal, R., & Karahanna, E. (2000). Time flies when you're having fun: Cognitive absorption and beliefs about information technology usage. *MIS Quarterly, 24*(4), 665–694.

Aggar, C., Sorwar, G., Seton, C., Penman, O., & Ward, A. (2023). Smart home technology to support older people's quality of life: A longitudinal pilot study. *International Journal of Older People Nursing, 18*(1), e12489.

Ajzen, I. (1991). The theory of planned behavior. *Organizational Behavior and Human Decision Processes, 50*(2), 179–211.

Bagozzi, R. P. (2007). The legacy of the technology acceptance model and a proposal for a paradigm shift. *Journal of the Association for Information Systems, 8*(4), 12.

Baltes, P. B., & Baltes, M. M. (1993). *Successful aging: Perspectives from the behavioral sciences* (Vol. 4). Cambridge University Press.

Bandura, A. (1986). *Social foundations of thought and action: A social cognitive theory.* Prentice-Hall.

Bandura, A. (1997). *Self-efficacy: The exercise of control.* W. H. Freeman.

Barnard, Y., Bradley, M. D., Hodgson, F., & Lloyd, A. D. (2013). Learning to use new technologies by older adults: Perceived difficulties, experimentation behavior, and usability. *Computers in Human Behavior, 29*(4), 1715–1724.

Barrett, A. E. (2005). Gendered experiences in midlife: Implications for age identity. *Journal of Aging Studies, 19*(2), 163–183.

Bernardo, J., Apóstolo, J., Loureiro, R., Santana, E., Yaylagul, N. K., Dantas, C., et al. (2022). eHealth platforms to promote autonomous life and active aging: A scoping review. *International Journal of Environmental Research and Public Health, 19*(23), 15854.

Bhattacherjee, A. (2001). Understanding information systems continuance: An expectation-confirmation model. *MIS Quarterly, 25*(3), 351–370.

Boot, W. R., Champion, M., Blakely, D. P., Wright, T., Souders, D. J., & Charness, N. (2013). Video games as a means to reduce age-related cognitive decline: Attitudes, compliance, and effectiveness. *Frontiers in Psychology, 4*, 31.

Bouma, H., Fozard, J. L., Bouwhuis, D. G., & Taipale, V. (2007). Gerontechnology in perspective. *Gerontechnology, 6*(4), 190–216.

Carstensen, L. L. (1995). Evidence for a life-span theory of socioemotional selectivity. *Current Directions in Psychological Science, 4*(5), 151–156.

Chang, F., Wang, G., & Gu, Z. (2024). Navigating challenges and opportunities in community-based interventions for promoting active aging: A systematic review of the roles of technology. *Innovation in Aging, 8*(10), igae077.

Charness, N., & Boot, W. (2009). Aging and information technology use: Potential and barriers. *Current Directions in Psychological Science, 18*(5), 253–258.

Chen, K., & Chan, A. H. (2014). Gerontechnology acceptance by elderly Hong Kong Chinese: A senior technology acceptance model (STAM). *Ergonomics, 57*(5), 635–652.

Chen, Y.-R. R., & Schulz, P. J. (2016). The effect of information communication technology interventions on reducing social isolation in the elderly: A systematic review. *Journal of Medical Internet Research, 18*(1), e18.

Chopik, W. J. (2016). The benefits of social technology use among older adults are mediated by reduced loneliness. *Cyberpsychology, Behavior, and Social Networking, 19*(9), 551–556.

Conner, M., & Armitage, C. J. (1998). Extending the theory of planned behavior: A review and avenues for further research. *Journal of Applied Social Psychology, 28*(15), 1429–1464.

Cotter, L. M., Shah, D., Brown, K., Mares, M.-L., Landucci, G., Saunders, S., Johnston, D. C., Pe-Romashko, K., Gustafson, D., Maus, A., Thompson, K., & Gustafson, D. H. (2024). Decoding the influence of eHealth on autonomy, competence, and relatedness in older adults: Qualitative analysis of self-determination through the motivational technology model. *JMIR Aging, 7*(1), e56923.

Crenshaw, K. (1989). Demarginalizing the Intersection of Race and Sex: A Black Feminist Critique of Antidiscrimination Doctrine, Feminist Theory and Antiracist Politics. *University of Chicago Legal Forum, 1989*(1), 139–167.

Czaja, S. J., Charness, N., Fisk, A. D., Hertzog, C., Nair, S. N., Rogers, W. A., & Sharit, J. (2006). Factors predicting the use of technology: Findings from the Center for Research and Education on aging and technology enhancement (CREATE). *Psychology and Aging, 21*(2), 333–352.

Daft, R. L., & Lengel, R. H. (1986). Organizational information requirements, media richness, and structural design. *Management Science, 32*(5), 554–571.

Davis, F. D. (1989). Perceived usefulness, perceived ease of use, and user acceptance of information technology. *MIS Quarterly, 13*(3), 319–340.

Dennis, A. R., Fuller, R. M., & Valacich, J. S. (2008). Media, tasks, and communication processes: A theory of media synchronicity. *MIS Quarterly, 32*(3), 575–600.

Eastin, M. S., & LaRose, R. (2000). Internet self-efficacy and the psychology of the digital divide. *Journal of Computer-Mediated Communication, 6*(1).

Fernández-Ballesteros, R. (2011). Positive ageing: Objective, subjective, and combined outcomes. *Electronic Journal of Applied Psychology, 7*(1), 22–30.

Friemel, T. N. (2016). The digital divide has grown old: Determinants of a digital divide among seniors. *New Media & Society, 18*(2), 313–331.

Granovetter, M. S. (1973). The strength of weak ties. *American Journal of Sociology, 78*(6), 1360–1380.

Hargittai, E. (2002). Second-level digital divide: Mapping differences in people's online skills. *First Monday, 7*(4). https://doi.org/10.5210/fm.v7i4.942

Havighurst, R. J. (1961). Successful aging. *The Gerontologist, 1*, 8–13.

Hawkley, L. C., & Kocherginsky, M. (2017). Transitions in loneliness among oder adults: A 5-year follow-up in the National Social Life, health, and aging project. *Research on Aging, 40*(4), 365–387.

Heart, T., & Kalderon, E. (2013). Older adults: Are they ready to adopt health-related ICT? *International Journal of Medical Informatics, 82*(11), e209–e231.

Heckhausen, J., & Schulz, R. (1995). A life-span theory of control. *Psychological Review, 102*(2), 284–304.

Helsper, E. J. (2021). *The digital disconnect: The social causes and consequences of digital inequalities*. Sage.

Hogan, B. (2009). Networking in everyday life. In A. H. Quan-Haase & L. Lievrouw (Eds.), *The handbook of new media* (pp. 143–155). Sage.

Holden, R. J., & Karsh, B.-T. (2010). The technology acceptance model: Its past and its future in health care. *Journal of Biomedical Informatics, 43*(1), 159–172.

Hong, S.-J., & Tam, K. Y. (2006). Understanding the adoption of multipurpose information appliances: The xase of mobile data services. *Information Systems Research, 17*(2), 162–179.

House, J. S. (1981). *Work stress and social support*. Addison-Wesley.

Hu, M., Han, S., Ghorbany, S., & Zhang, K. (2024). Healthy aging in place with the aid of smart technologies: A systematic review. *Encyclopedia, 4*(4), 1918–1932.

Infurna, F. J., & Gerstorf, D. (2013). Linking perceived control, physical activity, and biological health to memory change. *Psychology and Aging, 28*(4), 1147–1163.

Kahana, E. (1974). A congruence model of person-environment interaction. *The Gerontologist, 14*(3), 267–272.

Katz, E., Blumler, J. G., & Gurevitch, M. (1973). Uses and gratifications research. *Public Opinion Quarterly, 37*(4), 509–523.

Kim, Y., & Crowston, K. (2011). Technology adoption and use theory review for studying scientists' continued use of cyber-infrastructure. *Proceedings of the American Society for Information Science and Technology, 48*(1), 1–14.

King, W. R., & He, J. (2006). A meta-analysis of the technology acceptance model. *Information & Management, 43*(6), 740–755.

Kraut, R., Patterson, M., Lundmark, V., Kiesler, S., Mukopadhyay, T., & Scherlis, W. (1998). Internet paradox: A social technology that reduces social involvement and psychological well-being? *American Psychologist, 53*(9), 1017–1031.

Kraut, R., Kiesler, S., Boneva, B., Cummings, J., Helgeson, V., & Crawford, A. (2002). Internet paradox revisited. *Journal of Social Issues, 58*(1), 49–74.

Lachman, M. E., & Andreoletti, C. (2006). Strategy use mediates the relationship between control beliefs and memory performance for middle-aged and older adults. *Journal of Gerontology Psychological Sciences, 61*(2), P88–P94.

Lee, Y., Kozar, K. A., & Larsen, K. R. (2003). The technology acceptance model: Past, present, and future. *Communications of the Association for Information Systems, 12*, 752–780.

Levy, B. R. (2003). Mind matters: Cognitive and physical effects of aging self-stereotypes. *Journals of Gerontology Psychological Sciences, 58*(4), 203–211.

Levy, B. R. (2009). Stereotype embodiment: A psychosocial approach to aging. *Current Directions in Psychological Science, 18*(6), 332–336.

Levy, B. R., Slade, M. D., & Kasl, S. V. (2002). Longitudinal benefit of positive self-perceptions of aging on functional health. *Journals of Gerontology Psychological Sciences, 57*(5), P409–P417.

Li, W., Ye, X., Zhu, D., & He, P. (2021). The longitudinal association between retirement and depression: A systematic review and meta-analysis. *American Journal of Epidemiology, 190*(10), 2220–2230.

Marikyan, D., & Papagiannidis, S. (2024). Technology acceptance model: A review. In S. Papagiannidis (Ed), *TheoryHub Book*. Retrieved from https://open.ncl.ac.uk/theories/1/technology-acceptance-model/

Mather, M., & Carstensen, L. L. (2005). Aging and motivated cognition: The positivity effect in attention and memory. *Trends in Cognitive Sciences, 9*(10), 496–502.

Mo, Y., Liu, Y., Yeung, J. Koh, W-P., Gu, D., & Feng, Q. (2025). From digital divide to digital equality: The role of leaning in older Singaporeans. *Journal of Gerontology: Social Sciences*, Resubmitted.

Mu, J., Zhang, S., & Wu, Y. (2022). The influence of physical environmental factors on older adults in residential care facilities in Northeast China. *Health Environments Research & Design Journal, 15*(1), 131–149.

Mylonopoulou, V., Weilenmann, A., Buratti, S., Torgersson, O., & Rost, M. (2022). A socioecological approach to ICT use by adults over 65 and its implication on design. In *Proceedings of the 25th International Academic Mindtrek Conference. Academic Mindtrek 2022* (pp. 203–218).

Neves, B. B., & Vetere, F. (Eds.). (2019). *Ageing and digital technology: Designing and evaluating emerging technologies for older adults*. Springer.

Nimrod, G. (2010). Seniors' online communities: A quantitative content analysis. *The Gerontologist, 50*(3), 382–392.

Norris, P. (2001). *Digital divide: Civic engagement, information poverty, and the Internet worldwide*. Cambridge University Press.

Ollevier, A., Aguiar, G., Palomino, M., et al. (2020). How can technology support ageing in place in healthy older adults? A systematic review. *Public Health Reviews, 41*, 26.

Peek, S. T., Wouters, E. J., van Hoof, J., et al. (2014). Factors influencing acceptance of technology for aging in place: A systematic review. *International Journal of Medical Informatics, 83*(4), 235–248.

Peter, J., Valkenburg, P. M., & Schouten, A. P. (2005). Developing a model of adolescent friendship formation on the internet. *Cyberpsychology & Behavior, 8*(5), 423–430.

Putnam, R. D. (2000). *Bowling alone: The collapse and revival of American community*. Simon & Schuster.

Quan-Haase, A., Mo, G. Y., & Wellman, B. (2017). Connected seniors: How older adults in East York exchange social support online and offline. *Information, Communication & Society, 20*(7), 967–983.

Raacke, J., & Bonds-Raacke, J. M. (2008). MySpace and Facebook: Applying the uses and gratifications theory to exploring friend-networking sites. *Cyberpsychology & Behavior, 11*(2), 169–174.

Reed, A. E., & Carstensen, L. L. (2012). The theory behind the age-related positivity effect. *Frontiers in Psychology, 3*, 339.

Renaud, K., & van Biljon, J. (2008). Predicting technology acceptance and adoption by the elderly: A qualitative study. In *Proceedings of the 2008 annual research conference of the south African Institute of Computer Scientists and Information Technologists* (pp. 210–219).

Robinson, L., Schulz, J., Dunn, H. S., Casilli, A. A., Tubaro, P., Carvath, R., Khilnani, A., et al. (2020). Digital inequalities 3.0: Emergent inequalities in the information age. *First Monday, 25*(7). https://doi.org/10.5210/fm.v25i7.10844

Rogers, E. M. (2003). *Diffusion of innovations* (5th ed.). Free Press.

Rowe, J. W., & Kahn, R. L. (1987). Human aging: Usual and successful. *Science, 237*(4811), 143–149.

Rowe, J. W., & Kahn, R. L. (1997). Successful aging. *The Gerontologist, 37*(4), 433–440.

Salthouse, T. A. (2006). Mental exercise and mental aging: Evaluating the validity of the "use it or lose it" hypothesis. *Perspectives on Psychological Science, 1*(1), 68–87.

Schreurs, K., Quan-Haase, A., & Martin, K. (2017). Problematizing the digital literacy paradox in the context of older adults' ICT use: Aging, media discourse, and self-determination. *Canadian Journal of Communication, 42*(2), 359–377.

Small, G. W., Moody, T. D., Siddarth, P., & Bookheimer, S. Y. (2009). Your brain on Google: Patterns of cerebral activation during internet searching. *The American Journal of Geriatric Psychiatry, 17*(2), 116–126.

Stern, Y. (2002). What is cognitive reserve? Theory and research application of the reserve concept. *Journal of the International Neuropsychological Society, 8*(3), 448–460.

Straub, D., & Burton-Jones, A. (2007). Veni, vidi, vici: Breaking the TAM logjam. *Journal of the Association for Information Systems, 8*(4), 14.

Tun, P. A., & Lachman, M. E. (2010). The association between computer use and cognition across adulthood: Use it so you won't lose it? *Psychology and Aging, 25*(3), 560–568.

van Bronswijk, J. E. M. H., Bouma, H., & Fozard, J. L. (2002). Technology for quality of life: An enriched framework for gerontechnology. *Gerontechnology, 2*(2), 169–172.

van Deursen, A. J., & Helsper, E. J. (2015). The third-level digital divide: Who benefits most from being online? *Communication and Information Technologies Annual: Digital Distinctions and Inequalities Studies in Media and Communications, 10*, 29–52.

van Dijk, J. A. (2005). *The deepening divide: Inequality in the information society*. Sage.

van Dijk, J. (2006). Digital divide research, achievements and shortcomings. *Poetics, 34*(4–5), 221–235.

van Dijk, J. (2017). Afterword: The state of digital divide theory. In M. Ragnedda & G. W. Muschert (Eds.), *Theorizing digital divides* (pp. 199–206). Routledge.

Van Dijk, J. (2020). *The digital divide*. Polity Press.

Venkatesh, V., & Bala, H. (2008). Technology acceptance model 3 and a research agenda on interventions. *Decision Sciences, 39*(2), 273–315.

Venkatesh, V., & Davis, F. D. (2000). A theoretical extension of the technology acceptance model: Four longitudinal field studies. *Management Science, 46*(2), 186–204.

Venkatesh, V., & Zhang, X. (2010). Unified theory of acceptance and use of technology: U.S. vs. China. *Journal of Global Information Technology Management, 13*(1), 5–27.

Venkatesh, V., Morris, M. G., Davis, G. B., & Davis, F. D. (2003). User acceptance of information technology: Toward a unified view. *MIS Quarterly, 27*(3), 425–478.

Venkatesh, V., Thong, J. Y. L., & Xu, X. (2012). Consumer acceptance and use of information technology: Extending the unified theory of acceptance and use of technology. *MIS Quarterly, 36*(1), 157–178.

Wahl, H.-W., Iwarsson, S., & Oswald, F. (2012). Aging well and the environment: Toward an integrative model and research agenda for the future. *The Gerontologist, 52*(3), 306–316.

Wang, K., Chen, X., Gu, D., Smith, B. D., Dong, Y., & Peet, J. Z. (2024). Examining first and second-level digital divide at the intersection of race/ethnicity, gender, and socioeconomic status: An analysis of the National Health and Aging Trends Study. *The Gerontologist, 64*(gnae079), 1–11.

Winstead, V., Anderson, W. A., Yost, E. A., Cotten, S. R., Warr, A., & Berkowsky, R. W. (2013). You can teach an old dog new tricks: A qualitative analysis of how residents of senior living communities may use the web to overcome spatial and social barriers. *Journal of Applied Gerontology, 32*(5), 540–560.

World Health Organization. (2002). *Active ageing: A policy framework*. WHO.

Wright, K. B. (2000). Computer-mediated social support, older adults, and coping. *Journal of Communication, 50*(3), 100–118.

Yu, D., & Fiebig, D. G. (2020). Internet use and cognition among middle-aged and older adults in China: A cross-lagged panel analysis. *The Journal of the Economics of Ageing, 17*, 100262.

Chapter 4
A Literature Review on Linkages Between ICT Use and Healthy Aging

Danan Gu, Qiushi Feng, Kun Wang, and Hee Yun Lee

4.1 Introduction

The relationship between Information and Communication Technology (ICT) use and health outcomes in older adults has emerged as an important area of research, particularly in the context of global population aging and the increasing integration of digital technologies into healthcare, social services, and daily living (see Chaps. 1–3). As the digital landscape evolves, understanding how older individuals engage with technology, and how such engagement influences their physical, mental, and social well-being, holds critical implications for clinical practice, public health strategies, and the design of inclusive digital tools (Charness & Boot, 2016; Czaja et al., 2018; van Dijk, 2020; Yao & Dong, 2025). Researchers have increasingly recognized that ICT use in older age is not simply a matter of access, but also involves more issues of efficacy, relevance, and impact, especially as governments

D. Gu (✉)
Population Division, UN Department of Economic and Social Affairs, New York, NY, USA
e-mail: gudanan@yahoo.com

Q. Feng
Centre for Family and Population Research/Department of Sociology and Anthropology, National University of Singapore, Singapore, Singapore
e-mail: socfq@nus.edu.sg

K. Wang
Department of Social Work, College of Arts and Sciences, University of Alabama at Birmingham, Birmingham, AL, USA
e-mail: kw2@uab.edu

H. Y. Lee
School of Social Work, University of Georgia, Athens, GA, USA
e-mail: heeyunlee@uga.edu

K. Wang et al. (eds.), *ICT Use and Healthy Longevity*, Advances in Studies of Aging and Health 5, https://doi.org/10.1007/978-3-031-98964-3_4

and health systems start to promote digital inclusion as a pillar of healthy aging policy (Marston & van Hoof, 2019; van Deursen & van Dijk, 2014).

As stated in Chap. 1, the concept of healthy aging refers to a dynamic process of developing and maintaining the functional ability that enables well-being in older ages (World Health Organization [WHO], 2015, p. 28). This multidimensional framework encompasses cognitive health, physical functioning, psychological well-being, and social connectedness, each of which may be positively or negatively affected by ICT use, depending on individual capacities, digital environments, and broader societal factors (Berkowsky et al., 2013).

These relationships fall within what van Dijk (2005, 2020) identifies as the "third level of the digital divide", that is, the differential outcomes that arise from ICT use after access and digital skills are accounted for. While the first level of the digital divide concerns disparities in physical access to digital tools and the second level relates to inequalities in digital literacy and usage skills, the third level centers on the extent to which individuals benefit from their engagement with ICT. For older adults, this may mean experiencing improved health monitoring through wearable devices, enhanced social connections via communication platforms, or increased autonomy through online services; yet these benefits are not equally realized. Such Inequities in benefit can reinforce or even exacerbate pre-existing health and social disparities (Hargittai et al., 2019; van Dijk, 2020). This chapter thus focuses on reviewing the current state of evidence regarding how ICT use affects health outcomes in older adults, critically examining not just if ICT is used, but how it is used and what it affects.

The evidence regarding ICT use and health outcomes has evolved substantially over the past two decades, with increasing methodological rigor, larger sample sizes, and more diverse research approaches (Balki et al., 2022; Charness & Boot, 2016; Czaja et al., 2018; Hargittai et al., 2019; van Dijk, 2020). Early research in this field often focused on basic questions about access and adoption, while more recent work has examined health impacts, mechanisms of these effects, and factors that may mediate or moderate these relationships. This evolution reflects both the rapid development of digital technologies and growing recognition of their potential importance for health in later life.

This chapter synthesizes findings from systematic reviews, meta-analyses, and key primary studies to provide a comprehensive overview of current knowledge regarding ICT use and health outcomes in older adults. The review is organized around major domains of healthy aging, such as cognitive health, physical health, social engagement, and psychological well-being. For each domain, the review considers both observational evidence regarding associations between everyday technology use and health outcomes, and intervention research examining the effectiveness of specific technology-based approaches for improving health.

4.2 ICT Use and Cognitive Health

4.2.1 Associations Between ICT Use and Cognitive Function

Multiple cross-sectional and longitudinal studies have examined relationships between everyday ICT use and various aspects of cognitive function in older adults. A systematic review by Klimova et al. (2018) found consistent evidence of positive associations between computer and internet use and cognitive function across multiple domains, including executive function, attention, and memory. These associations persisted after controlling for potential confounding factors such as age, education, and socioeconomic status. Longitudinal research provides stronger evidence regarding potential cognitive benefits of ICT use. Almeida et al. (2012), for instance, conducted a 6-year follow-up study of 5506 Australian older adults aged 70 years or older and found that regular computer use was associated with a 30% reduction in the risk of mild cognitive impairment, even after adjusting for demographic factors, physical activity, and social engagement. Similarly, Ihle et al. (2017) found that diverse internet use was associated with slower cognitive decline over a 7-day period in a sample of 868 Brazilian older adults aged 57–92 years old.

Based on 57 studies involving over 411,000 individuals aged 50 years or older, a recent meta-analysis and systematic review examined whether lifelong digital technology use helps or harms cognitive health in older adults (Benge & Scullin, 2025). Researchers found that digital technology use was associated with a significantly reduced risk of cognitive impairment and slower cognitive decline. These findings support the "technological reserve" hypothesis, suggesting technology use may help preserve cognition. Results held even after controlling for demographic and health factors (Benge & Scullin, 2025).

The mechanisms underlying these associations may include cognitive stimulation, as suggested by Firth et al. (2019), who proposed that the novel and complex cognitive demands of technology use may exercise neural networks and promote cognitive reserve. Social stimulation may also play a role, as technology-enabled social interaction may provide cognitive benefits through meaningful engagement with others. Additionally, Xavier et al. (2014) noted that technology use may facilitate access to health information and services that support cognitive health indirectly through better management of conditions that affect brain health, such as hypertension and diabetes.

However, the relationship between ICT use and cognitive function is likely bidirectional, with better cognitive function predisposing individuals to adopt and continue using digital technologies (Kamin & Lang, 2020; Wang et al., 2024). This bidirectionality complicates the interpretations of observational findings and highlights the importance of intervention studies for establishing causal relationships.

4.2.2 ICT-Based Interventions for Cognitive Health

Research on ICT-based cognitive interventions has expanded substantially in recent years, with numerous randomized controlled trials examining the effectiveness of various approaches. A meta-analysis by Chiu et al. (2017) of 31 randomized controlled trials found that computerized cognitive training produced moderate improvements in the overall cognitive function, executive function, memory, and attention among healthy older adults.

More recent research has focused on specific types of cognitive interventions. Hill et al. (2017) conducted a systematic review of 17 studies examining various digital cognitive interventions and found that multi-domain training programs targeting multiple cognitive functions simultaneously showed stronger and more sustained effects than single-domain approaches. They also noted that adaptive training that can adjust levels of difficulty based on individual performance appeared more effective than non-adaptive approaches.

Recent studies have shown promising results for virtual reality (VR) applications in cognitive health. Liu et al. (2019) reviewed nine studies of VR-based cognitive interventions for older adults and found significant improvements in spatial cognition, executive function, and episodic memory. The immersive nature of VR may enhance engagement and ecological validity compared to traditional computerized approaches, potentially improving the transfer to real-world functioning (García-Betances et al., 2015). Social computing platforms that combine cognitive activities with social interaction have also demonstrated cognitive benefits. Dodge et al. (2020), for example, conducted a randomized controlled trial of an online social platform with integrated cognitive games and found significant improvements in both cognitive function and social connectedness compared to a wait-list control group. This suggests potential synergistic effects of combining social and cognitive stimulation through technology.

Despite these promising findings, several limitations in the current studies should be noted. Zhang et al. (2019) highlighted significant heterogeneity in intervention approaches, outcome measures, and study populations across the literature, making direct comparisons challenging. Additionally, many studies have relatively short follow-up periods, limiting the understanding of long-term effects. Questions also remain about the optimal "dose" (frequency, duration, intensity) of cognitive interventions and how to match these approaches to specific individual needs and characteristics.

4.3 ICT Use and Physical Health

4.3.1 Associations Between ICT Use and Physical Activity

The relationship between everyday technology use and physical activity levels in older adults appears complex. A systematic review by Stockwell et al. (2019) found mixed associations, with some studies reporting positive relationships between mobile technology use and physical activity, while others found negative or null associations. The authors noted that the nature of technology use (e.g., active versus passive, purpose-specific versus general) appeared to moderate these relationships.

Wearable activity monitors and fitness trackers have been specifically examined for their associations with physical activity. In a longitudinal study of 32 older adults aged 52–84 years old, Mercer et al. (2016) found that consistent use of activity trackers was associated with increased daily step counts and moderate-to-vigorous physical activity over a 5-month period. The mechanisms linking technology use to physical activity may include enhanced awareness and motivation. As noted by Lyons et al. (2017), activity trackers provide immediate feedback that can increase awareness of activity levels and sedentary behaviors. Goal-setting features and social comparison elements in these devices may also motivate increased activity through gamification and social reinforcement. However, Kononova et al. (2019) found that these motivational effects often diminished over time without additional supporting strategies.

4.3.2 ICT-Based Interventions for Physical Health

Digital exercise games (exergames) and virtual reality applications designed to promote physical activity have been extensively studied in older adults. A meta-analysis by Taylor et al. (2018) of 18 randomized controlled trials found that exergame interventions produced significant improvements in balance, functional mobility, and lower limb strength compared to non-intervention controls. Exergames that specifically targeted balance and incorporated whole-body movements showed the strongest effects. More recent research has examined specific types of exergames and their differential effects. Pacheco et al. (2020) examined the effects of two types of exergaming on mobility and balance in 1520 older adults with impairments but without neurological conditions from 12 randomized controlled trials. They found that in comparison to non-intervention controls, exergames improved participants' balance and mobility, whereas two types of exergames (commercial or serious games) yielded very similar effects.

Telerehabilitation, that is, the delivery of rehabilitation services via digital communication technologies, has shown effectiveness for various conditions common in older adults. A systematic review and meta-analysis by Xiang et al. (2023) of 6 randomized controlled trials found that telerehabilitation for musculoskeletal conditions produced outcomes comparable to in-person rehabilitation for pain reduction and functional improvement. The authors noted that telerehabilitation may be particularly valuable for older adults with mobility limitations or those living in rural areas with limited access to rehabilitation services. In addition, remote monitoring systems for chronic disease management have demonstrated positive effects on clinical outcomes. A systematic review by Nieuwenhuys et al. (2024) of 41 studies involving 16,512 heart failure patients found that remote patient monitoring significantly reduced both mortality and heart failure-related rehospitalizations compared to patients under usual care.

The mechanisms through which these interventions improve physical health outcomes may include increased engagement in health behaviors, as gamified elements and social features enhanced adherence to physical activity interventions (Patel et al., 2019). Improved self-management may also play a role, as digital tools can support medication adherence, symptom monitoring, and appropriate help-seeking. Additionally, Batsis et al. (2021) noted that technology-enabled care may facilitate more consistent monitoring and earlier intervention for emerging health problems, potentially preventing serious complications.

Despite these promising findings, several challenges and limitations should be acknowledged. Accessibility barriers of ICT-based interventions may limit benefits for those with physical or sensory impairments. As noted by Gordon and Hornbrook (2018), many health technologies were not designed to meet the needs of older adults with disabilities. Challenges in integration with existing healthcare systems may also limit the effectiveness of ICT-based interventions, as the impact of remote monitoring depends significantly on appropriate clinical response protocols. Additionally, questions remain about cost-effectiveness and sustainability of technology-based physical health interventions in real-world settings.

4.4 ICT Use and Social Engagement

4.4.1 Associations Between ICT Use and Social Connectivity

Research examining associations between ICT use and social outcomes suggests several important patterns. A systematic review by Chen and Schulz (2016) found consistent evidence that internet use was associated with reduced loneliness and social isolation among older adults across 25 studies. The authors also identified several mechanisms through which technology supported social connection, including interacting with family and friends, forming new social connections, and engaging with community activities. A scoping review by Petersen et al. (2023) examined 54 studies on how ICT use affects loneliness and social connectedness among older adults, reporting that ICT use is linked to reduced loneliness and improved well-being, facilitated communication, and enhanced social connectedness.

Social media use shows positive relationships with social connection outcomes in older adults. Kusumota et al. (2022) synthesized 11 studies on the use of social media and its impact on loneliness and social isolation in older adults. Their review showed that 63.6% of these 11 studies reported that social media use helped reduce loneliness and isolation in older adults, and internet use facilitated greater family contact, social support, and a stronger sense of community. However, Yu et al. (2016b) emphasized that passive consumption of social media content without active engagement was associated with increased loneliness, suggesting that how older adults use social media may matter. The frequency of social media use also matters. Wang and Gu (2023) found that more frequent social media use marginally predicted more positive self-perceived aging (SPA), but the impact was only significant for older men but not for older women.

The COVID-19 pandemic highlighted the value of technology use for maintaining social connections during periods of physical distancing. Kotwal et al. (2021) found that older adults who increased their use of video communication during the pandemic reported better maintenance of social relationships and lower increases in loneliness compared to those who did not adopt these technologies. However, they also noted persistent disparities in technology access and use, with socioeconomically disadvantaged older adults less able to benefit from digital social connections.

4.4.2 ICT-Based Interventions for Social Isolation and Loneliness

Interventions providing video communication technology and related training to older adults have shown promising results for reducing social isolation and loneliness. A randomized controlled trial by Czaja et al. (2017) of the PRISM (Personal Reminder Information and Social Management) system, which included video chat, email, and other features, found significant reductions in loneliness and increases in perceived social support compared to a paper-based information control condition over a 12-month period. Virtual group activities facilitated through digital platforms have also demonstrated positive psychosocial outcomes. A randomized pilot trial of 37 older adults by Baez et al. (2017) found that older adults engaging in online group exercises after 8 weeks experienced improvements in physical, psychological, and social well-being, highlighting the effectiveness of virtual group interactions in enhancing social connectedness among seniors. According to the study, participants particularly valued the sense of shared experience and routine social contact provided by the virtual groups.

Social networking platforms designed specifically for older adults have shown mixed results. A systematic review by Chipps et al. (2017) of 22 studies found modest positive effects on social connectedness and loneliness, but noted significant heterogeneity in intervention approaches and outcomes. The authors concluded that social networking interventions were most effective when they included structured activities, facilitated interaction, and adequate technical support rather than simply providing access to platforms.

Multicomponent interventions that simultaneously address multiple barriers to social engagement appear particularly promising. A randomized controlled trial by Balki et al. (2022) of a comprehensive digital social engagement program that combined technology provision, training, technical support, and facilitated group activities revealed significant improvements in social network size, frequency of social contact, and reduced loneliness compared to a technology-only condition. This suggests that technology alone may be insufficient to address social isolation without appropriate support and structured opportunities for meaningful interaction. The mechanisms through which these interventions improve social outcomes may include reduced barriers to social interaction, as technology can overcome physical limitations, geographic distance, and transportation challenges. Enhanced communication options may also play a role, as digital tools provide multiple channels for maintaining relationships through different modalities (text, voice, video) to meet varying preferences and circumstances. Additionally, technology-enabled social activities can provide a sense of purpose and structure that contributes to well-being beyond the direct social benefits (Barbosa Neves et al., 2019).

Despite these promising findings, several challenges and considerations should be acknowledged. The quality of technology-mediated social interaction may differ from in-person engagement in important ways. While digital communication was valued by older adults, many still preferred face-to-face interaction for emotionally meaningful exchanges (Hülür & Macdonald, 2020). Digital literacy barriers may also limit benefits, as those with limited technology experience may find digital social platforms challenging to navigate without appropriate support. Additionally, concerns about privacy, security, and online safety may affect willingness to engage with ICT.

4.5 ICT Use, Subjective Well-being, and Quality of Life

4.5.1 Associations Between ICT Use and Subjective Well-being

Studies examining associations between everyday technology use and subjective well-being have yielded several important insights. For example, Forsman et al. (2018) reviewed 18 interventional studies and found generally positive associations between internet use as an interventional tool and various indicators of psychological well-being in older adults, including life satisfaction, positive affect, and purpose in life. However, the authors noted significant heterogeneity in their findings, suggesting that the relationship between technology use and well-being is complex and likely moderated by multiple factors.

The nature and purpose of technology use, for instance, appear to influence its relationship with well-being. In this regard, Sims et al. (2017) found that internet use for communication, information seeking, and instrumental activities was associated with higher life satisfaction, yet internet use primarily for entertainment showed weaker associations. Similarly, research specific to older adults suggests that active, purposeful technology use (e.g., video calls, online learning, or digital hobbies) is more strongly linked to well-being than passive consumption. A longitudinal study by Hunsaker and Hargittai (2018) found that older adults who used the internet for communication (e.g., email, Skype) reported significantly lower loneliness and higher social connectivity over time, while passive browsing had no such benefits. Supporting this, Boucher et al. (2022) demonstrated that older adults who actively engaged in digital activities reported greater improvements in subjective well-being than those who are less actively. Conversely, Cotten et al. (2022) found that passive social media use in older adults correlated with increased depressive symptoms, particularly when replacing in-person social interactions.

The relationship between social media use and well-being in older adults appears particularly nuanced. A longitudinal study by Yu et al. (2016a) found that Facebook use was associated with reduced depression among older adults, but this relationship was mediated by perceived social support and reduced loneliness. In contrast, Steers et al. (2014) found that social comparison processes on social media platforms could negatively affect well-being through unfavorable comparisons with others' presented lives.

Digital technology use may influence the well-being of older people by enhancing autonomy and independence. Peek et al. (2016) found that technology use supported aging in place and reduced dependence on others for daily activities with physical limitations. This suggests that the well-being benefits of technology may be particularly important for those experiencing age-related functional declines.

4.5.2 ICT-Based Interventions for Subjective Well-being and Quality of Life

Digital applications based on positive psychology principles have shown promising results for enhancing well-being in older adults. A randomized controlled trial by Proyer et al. (2014) of an online positive psychology intervention that included gratitude exercises, strength identification, and positive reminiscence found significant improvements in life satisfaction and positive affect compared to a placebo control condition. These effects were maintained at 6-month follow-up, suggesting the potential durability of benefits.

Reminiscence and life review applications have demonstrated effectiveness for enhancing well-being and reducing depression. A meta-analysis by Pinquart and Forstmeier (2012) found that digital reminiscence interventions produced significant improvements in life satisfaction, emotional well-being, and purpose in life among older adults. The structured nature of digital reminiscence platforms may enhance the therapeutic benefits of life review by providing guided prompts, multimedia capabilities, and opportunities to share memories with others.

Entertainment and leisure applications designed for enjoyment rather than specific health outcomes have also shown well-being benefits at older ages. A study by Allaire et al. (2013) found that digital game play was associated with higher positive affect, lower depression, and better social functioning among older adults who regularly engaged with these activities. The authors suggested that cognitive stimulation, sense of achievement, and immersive nature of digital games may contribute to these well-being effects.

Multicomponent well-being platforms that integrate multiple evidence-based approaches have shown particular promise. A randomized controlled trial by Fanning et al. (2020) of a comprehensive digital well-being program that combined mindfulness exercises, positive psychology activities, social connection features, and health behavior support found significant improvements in psychological well-being, perceived stress, and health-related quality of life compared to a health education control condition. The integrated nature of this approach may address multiple determinants of well-being simultaneously.

The mechanisms through which these interventions improve well-being may include enhanced positive emotions, as digital activities that generate enjoyment, interest, and engagement may increase the frequency of positive emotional experiences. A sense of meaning and purpose may also be enhanced, as technology can facilitate continued engagement with valued activities and roles despite physical or geographic limitations. Additionally, Lazar et al. (2014) noted that technology use may support a sense of competence and mastery that contributes to well-being through successful navigation of digital environments and acquisition of new skills.

Despite these promising findings, several challenges and considerations should be acknowledged. Individual differences in technology attitudes and experiences may moderate effects on well-being, as suggested by Vroman et al. (2015), who found that pre-existing views about technology influenced the psychological impact of technology adoption. The potential for technology-induced stress ("technostress") should also be considered, as difficulties with technology use may create frustration and anxiety that undermine potential well-being benefits (Di Giacomo et al., 2020). Additionally, questions remain about how to optimize technology-based well-being interventions for diverse older adult populations with varying preferences, capabilities, and cultural backgrounds.

4.6 Research Trends and Future Directions

As shown by the previous sessions, research on ICT use and health outcomes in older adults has evolved significantly over the past two decades, with notable trends in research focus, methodology, and theoretical approaches. Understanding these trends provides a precondition for interpreting current evidence and identifying promising directions for future investigation.

4.6.1 Evolution of Research Focus

Early Research (2000–2010)

Early research in this field focused on foundational questions about technology access and adoption among older adults, with limited exploration of direct health impacts. Studies during this period often examined correlations between basic technology use (e.g., computer, email) and broad health indicators like social engagement or self-reported well-being, though underlying mechanisms were rarely investigated. For example, Czaja et al. (2006) identified key barriers to technology adoption, such as perceived complexity and lack of perceived relevance, emphasizing the need for user-centered design to improve usability. Building on this, Charness and Boot (2009) highlighted age-related cognitive and physical challenges in technology interaction, advocating for adaptive interface designs to accommodate sensory and motor declines. These works laid the groundwork for understanding how design influences adoption, but offered limited insights into health outcomes.

Middle Period (2010–2015)
This period saw a shift toward investigating the health impacts of specific health applications, particularly cognitive training and social connectivity tools. Rebok et al. (2014) conducted a landmark 10-year longitudinal study (the ACTIVE trial) showing that computerized cognitive training could improve memory and reasoning skills in older adults, though the context of transfer to real-world functioning remained debated. Concurrently, research on technology-mediated social connections expanded. Cotten et al. (2013) demonstrated that internet use for communication reduced depression and loneliness among older adults in assisted living facilities. Mobile health tools also began gaining traction, though early studies like Free et al. (2013) tended to focus on younger populations. This period marked growing methodological rigor but limited diversity in participant demographics.

Recent Period (2016–Present)
Recent research emphasizes holistic, tailored, technology-enabled care models and real-world implementation challenges. The COVID-19 pandemic accelerated studies on telehealth and remote monitoring. Mariano et al. (2021) documented that rapid adoption of video consultations among older adults, though disparities persisted for those with low digital literacy. In the post-pandemic era, attention has shifted to the long-term sustainability and equity of benefits. Chopik (2016) found sustained benefits of technology use for social connectedness, but warned of widening gaps for marginalized groups. Surveys like AARP's 2025 Tech Trends report note that over 90% of older adults own smartphones, with growing interest in aging-in-place technologies (AARP, 2025). Multimodal interfaces are now a priority: Mitzner et al. (2019) demonstrated that voice-activated assistants (e.g., Amazon Alexa) improved medication adherence and daily task management for older adults with mobility limitations. Meanwhile, Seifert et al. (2018) identified generational differences in social media acceptance, showing that perceived usefulness, not ease of use, was the strongest predictor of ICT adoption among adults aged 65–100. Current research also critiques "one-size-fits-all" approaches, calling for culturally tailored interventions that consider diverse aging experiences.

4.6.2 Methodological Evolution

The methodological approaches employed in research on ICT use and health outcomes have evolved significantly. Early studies were predominantly descriptive and cross-sectional, with limited ability to establish causal relationships or examine changes over time. Sample sizes were often small, and convenience sampling was commonly used, limiting generalizability. For example, Wagner et al. (2010) analyzed 151 studies on older adults' technology use and found that most studies relied on cross-sectional designs and used convenience samples of under 100 participants.

Recent years have seen movement toward more rigorous designs, including longitudinal studies with extended follow-up periods, randomized controlled trials (RCTs) with active comparison conditions, and mixed method approaches that integrate quantitative outcomes with qualitative insights (Tappen et al., 2022). Sample sizes have generally increased, though many intervention studies still have limited statistical power. There has been greater inclusion of diverse participant populations, though underrepresentation of racial/ethnic minority groups, those with lower socioeconomic status, and the oldest-old remains a significant limitation. For example, when analyzing U.S. national data, Choi and Dinitto (2013) found that adults over 85 and those with less than a high school education were consistently excluded from technology-health studies.

Measurement approaches have also improved, with greater use of validated, standardized measures to facilitate comparison across studies (Wild et al., 2008). Increased incorporation of objective measures of technology use (e.g., device logs, sensor metrics) rather than relying solely on self-reported usage has enhanced measurement precision (Fausset et al., 2013). After all, Fausset et al. (2013) demonstrated that older adults' self-reported internet use overestimated actual usage by 40% compared to browser history data. Beyond the narrow focus on single health outcome, comprehensive assessments across multiple domains of health (e.g., physical, cognitive, psychosocial) have become standard in many studies.

Analytical approaches have become more sophisticated, with increased use of advanced statistical techniques, such as structural equation modeling, multilevel modeling, and growth curve analysis to examine complex relationships and trajectories (Klasnja et al., 2015). Greater attention paid on factors that may mediate or moderate the relationship between technology use and health outcomes (e.g., digital literacy, baseline health status) has provided a more nuanced understanding of these relationships (Choi & Dinitto, 2013).

4.6.3 Current Research Gaps

Despite substantial progress, critical gaps remain. Research on the long-term effects of technology use on health outcomes is limited, as most existing studies have relatively short follow-up periods (Koo & Vizer, 2019). Additionally, a limited understanding of the factors influencing successful implementation and the scalability of effective interventions in diverse real-world settings continues to hinder translation into practice (Kvedar et al., 2016). Moreover, the lack of direct comparisons between different technological approaches for similar objectives makes it challenging to identify the most effective strategies for specific populations or outcomes.

Significant underrepresentation of oldest-old adults aged 80 or older in research persists, despite this being the fastest-growing segment of the older adult population in many countries (United Nations, 2024). Similarly, research involving older adults with cognitive impairments remains limited, despite the potential for technology to enhance support and quality of life in this population (Lazar et al., 2014). Insufficient research in non-Western contexts and among ethnically diverse populations within Western countries restricts the generalizability of established findings (Peek et al., 2014).

There is also limited research on factors affecting the discontinuation of technology use and strategies to support sustained engagement (Berkowsky & Czaja, 2018). Insufficient attention to potential negative consequences of technology use, including privacy concerns, dependency, and displacement of beneficial offline activities, presents an unbalanced view of ICT use (Choi & DiNitto, 2013; Hargittai et al., 2019). An underdeveloped understanding of the role of caregivers in supporting beneficial technology use among older adults with varying levels of independence leaves out important stakeholders (Mitzner et al., 2019).

4.6.4 Future Research Directions

Based on current trends and identified gaps, several promising directions for future research emerge. Greater use of pragmatic clinical trials that balance internal validity with real-world applicability could accelerate the translation of findings into practice. A more systematic application of implementation science frameworks to understand and address barriers to widespread adoption of effective technology approaches would improve the practical impact of digital tools. Development and evaluation of adaptive intervention approaches that can be personalized based on individual characteristics, preferences, and response patterns would enhance relevance and effectiveness. Focused research on strategies to ensure equitable access to beneficial technologies across diverse older population groups, with particular attention to those at risk of digital exclusion, is urgently needed. Development and evaluation of models for integrating technology-based approaches with existing healthcare and social service systems would enhance practical implementation.

Theoretical development is also needed to advance this field. Application of life course theoretical frameworks to understand how technology experiences across the lifespan influence ICT adoption and health outcomes in later life would provide a developmental lens. Development of ecological models that account for the multiple levels of influence on technology use and its health impacts, from individual factors to policy environments, would enhance comprehensive understanding. Integration of technological factors into biopsychosocial models of health and aging to guide comprehensive research and intervention approaches would enhance further theoretical integration.

4.7 Conclusions

This chapter briefly reviewed the current evidence regarding relationships between ICT use and health outcomes in older adults across multiple domains, including cognitive health, physical health, social engagement, and subjective well-being. The evidence, as reviewed, suggests that technology use has significant potential to support various aspects of health in later life, though the strength of evidence varies across domains and specific applications.

As digital technologies continue to evolve and become more deeply integrated into healthcare systems and daily life, ensuring their appropriate design, evaluation, and implementation will be essential for realizing their potential to support health and well-being in the context of population aging. By addressing current limitations and pursuing promising new directions, a stronger evidence base of research is taking form to guide the development of technology-based approaches that effectively support diverse aspects of health in later life.

Disclaimer Views expressed in the chapter are solely those of the authors and do not necessarily reflect those of the United Nations, the National University of Singapore, the University of Alabama at Birmingham, and the University of Georgia.

References

AARP. (2025). *2025 Tech trends and adults 50-plus.* AARP Research. Retrieved from https://www.aarp.org/content/dam/aarp/research/topics/technology/internet-media-devices/2025-technology-trends-older-adults.doi.10.26419-2fres.00891.001.pdf

Allaire, J. C., McLaughlin, A. C., Trujillo, A., Whitlock, L. A., LaPorte, L., & Gandy, M. (2013). Successful aging through digital games: Socioemotional differences between older adult gamers and non-gamers. *Computers in Human Behavior, 29*(4), 1302–1306.

Almeida, O. P., Yeap, B. B., Alfonso, H., Hankey, G. J., Flicker, L., & Norman, P. E. (2012). Older men who use computers have lower risk of dementia. *PLoS One, 7*(8), e44239.

Baez, M., Khaghani Far, I., Ibarra, F., Ferron, M., Didino, D., & Casati, F. (2017). Effects of online group exercises for older adults on physical, psychological and social wellbeing: A randomized pilot trial. *PeerJ, 5*, e3150.

Balki, E., Hayes, N., & Holland, C. (2022). Effectiveness of technology interventions in addressing social isolation, connectedness, and loneliness in older adults: Systematic umbrella review. *JMIR Aging, 5*(4), e40125.

Barbosa Neves, B., Franz, R., Judges, R., Beermann, C., & Baecker, R. (2019). Can digital technology enhance social connectedness among older adults? A feasibility study. *Journal of Applied Gerontology, 38*(1), 49–72.

Batsis, J. A., Daniel, K., Eckstrom, E., Goldlist, K., Kusz, H., Lane, D., Loewenthal, J., Coll, P. P., & Friedman, S. M. (2021). Promoting healthy aging during COVID-19. *Journal of the American Geriatrics Society, 69*(3), 572–580.

Benge, J. F., & Scullin, M. K. (2025). A meta-analysis of technology use and cognitive aging. *Nature Human Behaviour.* Online first. https://doi.org/10.1038/s41562-025-01835-4

Berkowsky, R. W., & Czaja, S. J. (2018). Factors predicting decisions about technology adoption among older adults. *Innovation in Aging, 2*(3), igy002.

Berkowsky, R. W., Cotten, S. R., Yost, E. A., & Winstead, V. P. (2013). Attitudes towards and limitations to ICT use in assisted and independent living communities: Findings from a specially-designed technological intervention. *Educational Gerontology, 39*(11), 797–811.

Boucher, E., Honomichl, R., Ward, H., Powell, T., Stoeckl, S. E., & Parks, A. (2022). The effects of a digital well-being intervention on older adults: Retrospective analysis of real-world user data. *JMIR Aging, 5*(3), e39851.

Charness, N., & Boot, W. R. (2009). Aging and information technology use: Potential and barriers. *Current Directions in Psychological Science, 18*(5), 253–258.

Charness, N., & Boot, W. R. (2016). Technology, gaming, and social networking. In K. W. Schaie & S. L. Willis (Eds.), *Handbook of the psychology of aging* (8th ed., pp. 389–407). Academic.

Chen, Y. R., & Schulz, P. J. (2016). The effect of information communication technology interventions on reducing social isolation in the elderly: A systematic review. *Journal of Medical Internet Research, 18*(1), e18.

Chipps, J., Jarvis, M. A., & Ramlall, S. (2017). The effectiveness of e-Interventions on reducing social isolation in older persons: A systematic review of systematic reviews. *Journal of Telemedicine and Telecare, 23*(10), 817–827.

Chiu, H. L., Chu, H., Tsai, J. C., Liu, D., Chen, Y. R., Yang, H. L., & Chou, K. R. (2017). The effect of cognitive-based training for the healthy older people: A meta-analysis of randomized controlled trials. *PLoS One, 12*(5), e0176742.

Choi, N. G., & Dinitto, D. M. (2013). The digital divide among low-income homebound older adults: Internet use patterns, eHealth literacy, and attitudes toward computer/Internet use. *Journal of Medical Internet Research, 15*(5), e93.

Chopik, W. J. (2016). The benefits of social technology use among older adults are mediated by reduced loneliness. *Cyberpsychology, Behavior, and Social Networking, 19*(9), 551–556.

Cotten, S. R., Anderson, W. A., & McCullough, B. M. (2013). Impact of internet use on loneliness and contact with others among older adults: Cross-sectional analysis. *Journal of Medical Internet Research, 15*(2), e39.

Cotten, S. R., Schuster, A. M., & Seifert, A. (2022). Social media use and well-being among older adults. *Current Opinion in Psychology, 45*, 101293.

Czaja, S. J., Charness, N., Fisk, A. D., Hertzog, C., Nair, S. N., Rogers, W. A., & Sharit, J. (2006). Factors predicting the use of technology: Findings from the Center for Research and Education on Aging and Technology Enhancement (CREATE). *Psychology and Aging, 21*(2), 333–352.

Czaja, S. J., Boot, W. R., Charness, N., Rogers, W. A., & Sharit, J. (2017). Improving social support for older adults through technology: Findings from the PRISM randomized controlled trial. *The Gerontologist, 58*(3), 467–477.

Czaja, S. J., Boot, W. R., Charness, N., & Rogers, W. A. (2018). *Designing for older adults: Principles and creative human factors approaches* (3rd ed.). CRC Press.

Di Giacomo, D., Guerra, F., Perilli, E., & Ranieri, J. (2020). Technophobia as an emerging risk factor in aging: Investigation on computer anxiety dimension. *Health Psychology Research, 8*(1), 8207.

Dodge, H. H., Zhu, J., Mattek, N. C., Bowman, M., Ybarra, O., Wild, K. V., Loewenstein, D. A., & Kaye, J. A. (2020). Web-enabled conversational interactions as a method to improve cognitive functions: Results of a 6-week randomized controlled trial. *Alzheimer's & Dementia: Translational Research & Clinical Interventions, 1*(1), 1–12.

Fanning, J., Brooks, A. K., Ip, E., Nicklas, B. J., & Rejeski, W. J. (2020). A mobile health intervention to reduce pain and improve health (MORPH) in older adults with obesity: Protocol for the MORPH trial. *JMIR Research Protocols, 7*(5), e128.

Fausset, C. B., Harley, L., Farmer, S., & Fain, B. (2013). Older adults' perceptions and use of technology: A novel approach. In: C Stephanidis & M. Antona (eds) *Universal access in human-computer interaction. User and context diversity. UAHCI 2013. Lecture notes in computer science* (Vol. 8010, pp. 51–58). Springer.

Firth, J., Torous, J., Stubbs, B., Firth, J. A., Steiner, G. Z., Smith, L., Alvarez-Jimenez, M., Gleeson, J., Vancampfort, D., Armitage, C. J., & Sarris, J. (2019). The "online brain": How the Internet may be changing our cognition. *World Psychiatry, 18*(2), 119–129.

Forsman, A. K., Nordmyr, J., Matosevic, T., Park, A.-L., Wahlbeck, K., & McDaid, D. (2018). Promoting mental wellbeing among older people: Technology-based interventions. *Health Promotion International, 33*, 1042–1054.

Free, C., Phillips, G., Watson, L., Galli, L., Felix, L., Edwards, P., Patel, V., & Haines, A. (2013). The effectiveness of mobile-health technologies to improve health care service delivery processes: A systematic review and meta-analysis. *PLoS Medicine, 10*(1), e1001363.

García-Betances, R. I., Jiménez-Mixco, V., Arredondo, M. T., & Cabrera-Umpiérrez, M. F. (2015). Using virtual reality for cognitive training of the elderly. *American Journal of Alzheimer's Disease & Other Dementias, 30*(1), 49–54.

Gordon, N. P., & Hornbrook, M. C. (2018). Older adults' readiness to engage with eHealth patient education and self-care resources: A cross-sectional survey. *BMC Health Services Research, 18*, 220.

Hargittai, E., Piper, A. M., & Morris, M. R. (2019). From internet access to internet skills: Digital inequality among older adults. *Universal Access in the Information Society, 18*, 881–890.

Hill, N. T. M., Mowszowski, L., Naismith, S. L., Chadwick, V. L., Valenzuela, M., & Lampit, A. (2017). Computerized cognitive training in older adults with mild cognitive impairment or dementia: A systematic review and meta-analysis. *The American Journal of Psychiatry, 174*(4), 329–340.

Hülür, G., & Macdonald, B. (2020). Rethinking social relationships in old age: Digitalization and the social lives of older adults. *American Psychologist, 75*(4), 554–566.

Hunsaker, A., & Hargittai, E. (2018). A review of internet use among older adults. *New Media & Society, 20*(10), 3937–3954.

Ihle, A., Gouveia, É. R., Gouveia, B. R., & Kliegel, M. (2017). The cognitive telephone screening instrument (COGTEL): A brief, reliable, and valid tool for capturing interindividual differences in cognitive functioning in epidemiological and aging studies. *Dementia and Geriatric Cognitive Disorders Extra, 7*(3), 339–345.

Kamin, S. T., & Lang, F. R. (2020). Internet use and cognitive functioning in late adulthood: Longitudinal findings from the Survey of Health, Ageing and Retirement in Europe (SHARE). *Journals of Gerontology: Social Sciences, 75*(3), 534–539.

Klasnja, P., Hekler, E. B., Shiffman, S., Boruvka, A., Almirall, D., Tewari, A., & Murphy, S. A. (2015). Microrandomized trials: An experimental design for developing just-in-time adaptive interventions. *Health Psychology, 34*(S), 1220–1228.

Klimova, B., Valis, M., & Kuca, K. (2018). Exploring assistive technology as a potential beneficial intervention tool for people with Alzheimer's disease – a systematic review. *Neuropsychiatric Disease and Treatment, 14*, 3151–3158.

Kononova, A., Li, L., Kamp, K., Bowen, M., Rikard, R. V., Cotten, S., & Peng, W. (2019). The use of wearable activity trackers among older adults: Focus group study of tracker perceptions, motivators, and barriers in the maintenance stage of behavior change. *JMIR mHealth and uHealth, 7*(4), e9832.

Koo, B. M., & Vizer, L. M. (2019). Examining mobile technologies to support older adults with dementia through the lens of personhood and human needs: Scoping review. *JMIR mHealth and uHealth, 7*(11), e15122.

Kotwal, A. A., Holt-Lunstad, J., Newmark, R. L., Cenzer, I., Smith, A. K., Covinsky, K. E., Escueta, D. P., Lee, J. M., & Perissinotto, C. M. (2021). Social isolation and loneliness among San Francisco Bay Area older adults during the COVID-19 shelter-in-place orders. *Journal of the American Geriatrics Society, 69*(1), 20–29.

Kusumota, L., Diniz, M. A. A., Ribeiro, R. M., Silva, I. L. C. D., Figueira, A. L. G., Rodrigues, F. R., & Rodrigues, R. A. P. (2022). Impact of digital social media on the perception of loneliness and social isolation in older adults. *Revista Latino-Americana de Enfermagem, 30*, e3573.

Kvedar, J. C., Fogel, A. L., Elenko, E., & Zohar, D. (2016). Digital medicine's march on chronic disease. *Nature Biotechnology, 34*(3), 239–246.

Lazar, A., Thompson, H., & Demiris, G. (2014). A systematic review of the use of technology for reminiscence therapy. *Health Education & Behavior, 41*(1 Suppl), 51S–61S.

Liu, Y., Tan, W., Chen, C., Liu, C., Yang, J., & Zhang, Y. (2019). A review of the application of virtual reality technology in the diagnosis and treatment of cognitive impairment. *Frontiers in Aging Neuroscience, 11*, 280.

Lyons, E. J., Swartz, M. C., Lewis, Z. H., Martinez, E., & Jennings, K. (2017). Feasibility and acceptability of a wearable technology physical activity intervention with telephone counseling for mid-aged and older adults: A randomized controlled pilot trial. *JMIR mHealth and uHealth, 5*(3), e28.

Mariano, J., Marques, S., Ramos, M. R., Gerardo, F., da Cunha, C. L., Girenko, A., de Vries, H., et al. (2021). Too old for technology? Stereotype threat and technology use by older adults. *Behaviour & Information Technology, 41*(7), 1503–1514.

Marston, H. R., & van Hoof, J. (2019). Who doesn't think about technology when designing urban environments for older people? A case study approach to a proposed extension of the WHO's age-friendly cities model. *International Journal of Environmental Research and Public Health, 16*(19), 3525.

Mercer, K., Giangregorio, L., Schneider, E., Chilana, P., Li, M., & Grindrod, K. (2016). Acceptance of commercially available wearable activity trackers among adults aged over 50 and with chronic illness: A mixed-methods evaluation. *JMIR mHealth and uHealth, 4*(1), e7.

Mitzner, T. L., Savla, J., Boot, W. R., Sharit, J., Charness, N., Czaja, S. J., & Rogers, W. A. (2019). Technology adoption by older adults: Findings from the PRISM trial. *The Gerontologist, 59*(1), 34–44.

Nieuwenhuys, W. W., De Lathauwer, I. L. J., Regis, M., Hafkamp, F. J., Brouwers, R. W. M., Funk, M., & Kemps, H. M. C. (2024). Remote patient monitoring in heart failure: A comprehensive meta-analysis and systematic review analyzing efficacious program components for hospitalization reduction. *European Journal of Preventive Cardiology, 31*(Suppl_1), zwae175.115.

Pacheco, T. B. F., de Medeiros, C. S. P., de Oliveira, V. H. B., Vieira, E. R., & de Cavalcanti, F. A. C. (2020). Effectiveness of exergames for improving mobility and balance in older adults: A systematic review and meta-analysis. *Systematic Reviews, 9*(1), 163.

Patel, M. S., Small, D. S., Harrison, J. D., Fortunato, M. P., Oon, A. L., Rareshide, C. A. L., et al. (2019). Effectiveness of behaviorally designed gamification interventions with social incentives for increasing physical activity among overweight and obese adults across the United States: The STEP UP randomized clinical trial. *JAMA Internal Medicine, 179*(12), 1624–1632.

Peek, S. T., Wouters, E. J., van Hoof, J., et al. (2014). Factors influencing acceptance of technology for aging in place: A systematic review. *International Journal of Medical Informatics, 83*(4), 235–248.

Peek, S. T. M., Luijkx, K. G., Rijnaard, M. D., Nieboer, M. E., van der Voort, C. S., Aarts, S., et al. (2016). Older adults' reasons for using technology while aging in place. *Gerontology, 62*(2), 226–237.

Petersen, B., Khalili-Mahani, N., Murphy, C., Sawchuk, K., Phillips, N., Li, K. Z. H., & Hebblethwaite, S. (2023). The association between information and communication technol-

ogies, loneliness and social connectedness: A scoping review. *Frontiers in Psychology, 14*, 1063146.
Pinquart, M., & Forstmeier, S. (2012). Effects of reminiscence interventions on psychosocial outcomes: A meta-analysis. *Aging & Mental Health, 16*(5), 541–558.
Proyer, R. T., Gander, F., Wellenzohn, S., & Ruch, W. (2014). Positive psychology interventions in people aged 50-79 years: Long-term effects of placebo-controlled online interventions on well-being and depression. *Aging & Mental Health, 18*(8), 997–1005. https://doi.org/10.1080/13607863.2014.899978
Rebok, G. W., Ball, K., Guey, L. T., Jones, R. N., Kim, H.-Y., King, J. W., ACTIVE Study Group, et al. (2014). Ten-year effects of the advanced cognitive training for independent and vital elderly cognitive training trial on cognition and everyday functioning in older adults. *Journal of the American Geriatrics Society, 62*(1), 16–24.
Seifert, A., Hofer, M., & Rössel, J. (2018). Older adults' perceived sense of social exclusion from the digital world. *Educational Gerontology, 44*(12), 775–785.
Sims, T., Reed, A. E., & Carr, D. C. (2017). Information and communication technology use is related to higher well-being among the oldest-old. *Journals of Gerontology: Social Sciences, 72*(5), 761–770.
Steers, M. L. N., Wickham, R. E., & Acitelli, L. K. (2014). Seeing everyone else's highlight reels: How Facebook usage is linked to depressive symptoms. *Journal of Social and Clinical Psychology, 33*(8), 701–731.
Stockwell, S., Schofield, P., Fisher, A., Firth, J., Jackson, S. E., Stubbs, B., & Smith, L. (2019). Digital behavior change interventions to promote physical activity and/or reduce sedentary behavior in older adults: A systematic review and meta-analysis. *Experimental Gerontology, 120*, 68–87.
Tappen, R. M., Cooley, M. E., Luckmann, R., & Panday, S. (2022). Digital health information disparities in older adults: A mixed methods study. *Journal of Racial and Ethnic Health Disparities, 9*(1), 82–92.
Taylor, L. M., Kerse, N., Frakking, T., & Maddison, R. (2018). Active video games for improving physical performance measures in older people: A meta-analysis. *Journal of Geriatric Physical Therapy, 41*(2), 108–123.
United Nations. (2024). *World Population Prospects 2024*. https://population.un.org/wpp/
van Deursen, A. J., & van Dijk, J. (2014). The digital divide shifts to differences in usage. *New Media & Society, 16*(3), 507–526.
van Dijk, J. (2005). *The deepening divide: Inequality in the information society*. Sage.
van Dijk, J. (2020). *The digital divide*. Polity Press.
Vroman, K. G., Arthanat, S., & Lysack, C. (2015). "Who over 65 is online?" Older adults' dispositions toward information communication technology. *Computers in Human Behavior, 43*, 156–166.
Wagner, N., Hassanein, K., & Head, M. (2010). Computer use by older adults: A multi-disciplinary review. *Computers in Human Behavior, 26*(5), 870–882.
Wang, K., & Gu, D. (2023). Reciprocal associations between social media use and self-perception of aging among older adults: Do men and women differ? *Social Science & Medicine, 321*, 115786.
Wang, K., Chen, X., Kang, S.-Y., Smith, B. D., & Gu, D. (2024). Older adults' online activities and cognition: Investigating the psychological mechanisms and age and gender differences. *Social Science & Medicine, 352*(116988), 1–12.
Wild, K., Boise, L., Lundell, J., & Foucek, A. (2008). Unobtrusive in-home monitoring of cognitive and physical health: Reactions and perceptions of older adults. *Journal of Applied Gerontology, 27*(2), 181–200.
World Health Organization. (2015). *World report on aging and health*. Retrieved from https://www.who.int/publications/i/item/9789241565042

Xavier, A. J., d'Orsi, E., de Oliveira, C. M., Orrell, M., Demakakos, P., Biddulph, J. P., & Marmot, M. G. (2014). English longitudinal study of aging: Can internet/e-mail use reduce cognitive decline? *Journals of Gerontology: Medical Sciences, 69*(9), 1117–1121.

Xiang, W., Wang, J. Y., Ji, B. J., Li, L. J., & Xiang, H. (2023). Effectiveness of different telerehabilitation strategies on pain and physical function in patients with knee osteoarthritis: Systematic review and meta-analysis. *Journal of Medical Internet Research, 25*, e40735.

Yao, Y., & Dong, E. (2025). Internet use and mental wellbeing in older adults. *Nature Human Behaviour, 9*, 24–25.

Yu, R. P., Ellison, N. B., McCammon, R. J., & Langa, K. M. (2016a). Mapping the two levels of digital divide: Internet access and social network site adoption among older adults in the USA. *Information, Communication & Society, 19*(10), 1445–1464.

Yu, R. P., McCammon, R. J., Ellison, N. B., & Langa, K. M. (2016b). The relationships that matter: Social network site use and social wellbeing among older adults in The United States of America. *Ageing and Society, 36*(9), 1826–1852.

Zhang, H., Huntley, J., Bhome, R., Holmes, B., Cahill, J., Gould, R. L., et al. (2019). Effect of computerised cognitive training on cognitive outcomes in mild cognitive impairment: A systematic review and meta-analysis. *BMJ Open, 9*(8), e027062.

Section II
Associated Factors with ICT Use

Chapter 5
Internet Engagement Patterns in African American Older Adults: Unraveling Gender and Age Disparities

Kun Wang, Kefentse P. Malele, and Saumya Tripathi

5.1 Introduction

The widespread adoption of Information, Communication, and Technology (ICT) among older adults has become essential for accessing various services. The swift evolution of technology, coupled with smart electronics, has the potential to significantly enhance the quality of life for older individuals by fostering connectivity, activity, and independence. This rapid evolution opens avenues for successful aging, overcoming constraints like distance and space. ICT can expand social networks, provide healthcare treatments at home, offer accessible resources, and improve living standards (Berde, 2019; Harper et al., 2020). Recent studies emphasize the

---

Note on Reuse of Published Materials
This chapter incorporates a revised and expanded version of material originally published in the article "Correlates of internet Use Among African American Older Adults: Gender and Age Differences" by Wang, K., & Kubanga, K. (2020), published in *International Journal of Population Studies*, 6(2), 26–38. The original work has been adapted and updated in accordance with the publisher's policies

---

K. Wang (✉)
Department of Social Work, College of Arts and Sciences, University of Alabama at Birmingham, Birmingham, AL, USA
e-mail: kw2@uab.edu

K. P. Malele
University of Botswana, Gaborone, Botswana
e-mail: malelek@ub.ac.bw

S. Tripathi
Binghamton University, Binghamton, NY, USA
e-mail: stripathi@binghamton.edu

K. Wang et al. (eds.), *ICT Use and Healthy Longevity*, Advances in Studies of Aging and Health 5, https://doi.org/10.1007/978-3-031-98964-3_5

positive impact of the internet on older populations, increasing social interactions, reducing isolation, aiding in managing chronic diseases, and enhancing the overall quality of life (Cotten et al., 2013; Yu et al., 2020). The internet also facilitates the delivery of traditional interventions online, with evaluation studies confirming effectiveness in reducing loneliness, depression, and promoting healthy lifestyles (Choi et al., 2012; Sriramatr et al., 2014).

Despite these benefits, navigating these technologies poses a challenge for the older generation. These challenges are further compounded by gender and racial ethnicity disparities. Findings from the China Longitudinal Ageing Social Survey suggest that digital exclusion exhibits gender variation, with rural females experiencing higher levels of exclusion, possibly due to lower capital endowment (Yang & Du, 2021). Socio-economic background also moderates this relationship to some extent, with socio-economic status remaining a primary factor influencing quality of life (Ihm & Hsieh, 2015). Cotten et al. (2016) argue that potential sub-divides exist within traditionally digitally divided populations. The digital divide is particularly pronounced within marginalized communities, where factors such as race and ethnicity, socioeconomic status, gender, and rural-urban disparities contribute to uneven access and utilization of the internet. Investigating correlates of internet use among older adults and promoting their adoption is crucial for addressing this disparity (Anderson & Perrin, 2017). This chapter provides a particular focus on the utilization of the internet in the lives of older African Americans to reduce digital inequality.

5.1.1 *Internet Use Among Older African Americans*

In the last two decades, internet use among U.S. older adults increased by 55% (Anderson & Perrin, 2017). However, African American older adults trail their White counterparts in internet adoption (Choi & DiNitto, 2013; Elliot et al., 2014; Yoon et al., 2018). Choi and DiNitto's (2013) national study on Medicare beneficiaries aged over 65 found African Americans 0.41 times less likely to use the internet than non-Hispanic Whites. The California Health Interview Survey reported a 0.54 times lower likelihood for African American older adults to use the internet for health information (Yoon et al., 2018).

Despite overall internet use growth among older adults, they lag behind the general adult population. In 2016, 67% of older adults (aged 65+) were online, compared to 90% of all U.S. adults (Anderson & Perrin, 2017). Breakdown by age shows a decline: 82% for 65–69-year-olds, 75% for 70–74-year-olds, 60% for 75–79-year-olds, and 44% for those 80 and above (Anderson & Perrin, 2017). This age-related decline is consistent across studies (Hargittai & Dobransky, 2017; König et al., 2018). Friemel (2014) noted an exponential drop after age 70, indicating a "grey digital divide" (Millward, 2003; Morris & Brading, 2007). Generational differences impact internet use, with those born during/after World War II more likely to engage online (Gilleard & Higgs, 2008). Hargittai and Dobransky (2017) found the oldest-old (80–97) least likely to be online due to completing careers before internet mass diffusion. Pre-retirement computer use predicts later-age internet access, highlighting cohort effects on digital connectivity (Friemel, 2014).

Digital disparities, including variations in internet access and use, have been observed among different racial and ethnic groups in the United States. African Americans, along with other minority groups, have faced challenges related to digital access and technology utilization. Prior research suggests that the limited adoption of the internet among African American older adults may be attributed to factors such as lower educational attainment, higher poverty rates, and increased prevalence of health and mental health-related conditions (Carpenter & Buday, 2007; Berde, 2019; Kim et al., 2017; Mitchell et al., 2019). While numerous studies have investigated ICT use among older adults, particularly examining racial and ethnic disparities, most have treated race or ethnicity as categorical variables. Few studies have delved into the specific correlates of internet use among African American older adults, such as factors influencing their digital engagement (Choi & DiNitto, 2013; Mitchell et al., 2019; Yoon et al., 2018). Understanding these correlates can help policymakers pinpoint target factors and explore causal associations. It is also valuable for practitioners seeking to identify issues, design tailored interventions, and promote internet use. Given the unique life experiences of African American older adults, including distinct social support networks, experiences of depressive symptoms, and encounters with systemic discrimination (Ayalon & Young, 2003; Peek & O'Neill, 2001; Sarkisian & Gerstel, 2004), the correlates of internet use in this population may differ from those of other racial or ethnic groups. For instance, resilience to discrimination may vary between White and African American older adults, impacting their internet use differently. Additionally, due to the relatively smaller population of African Americans compared to Whites among racial or ethnic minorities, aggregating results may lead to misleading conclusions.

Given the recognized advantages of internet use in enhancing health, mental health, and overall quality of life for older adults, the underutilization of internet resources among this demographic could exacerbate existing health and mental health disparities. Therefore, it is crucial to prioritize efforts aimed at increasing internet adoption and utilization within the African American older adult population.

5.1.2 Gender Differences Among Older Adults

Internet usage patterns may fluctuate based on gender, contingent upon their cultural and national contexts. However, existing findings on the moderating role of gender remain inconclusive. While some researchers identify gender-related disparities in internet use (Morahan-Martin, 1998; Lee, 2006), others, like Shaw and Gant (2002) and Ono and Zavodny (2003), do not discern any significant differences between genders. Notably, in the United States and Australia, internet usage is nearly equal between men and women, while in Japan, India, and China, men dominate internet use (Singh, 2001). Women in Bangladesh are more likely to experience digital exclusion compared to other countries (Rashid, 2016). These conflicting outcomes underscore the need for a comprehensive exploration of factors contributing to the gender gap in internet use that remains insufficiently illuminated.

Empirical evidence suggests that older men are more inclined to access and utilize the internet than older women (Kim et al., 2017; Marston et al., 2016). Attempts to explain these differences have proposed factors such as higher self-confidence, positive attitudes towards the internet, or greater proficiency in computer use among older men (Chu, 2010; Hunsaker & Hargittai, 2018). However, recent studies have produced inconsistent results, with some finding no differences in internet use between genders (Friemel, 2014; König et al., 2018) and others indicating higher internet use among older women than men (Yu et al., 2016). These conflicting findings underscore the need for further exploration into correlates of internet use among older adults to gain a more nuanced understanding of gender differences, particularly among older African American adults. Inclusion needs to be seen in terms of the unique information needs of various socioeconomic groups and in specific social contexts.

Moreover, aging experiences differ between older women and men (Xie, 2003). Notably, menopause and widowhood serve as distinctive social markers of aging for older women (Osorio-Parraguez, 2013). Women experiencing menopause may intensify their internet use to seek consultations and other relevant information online; however, this may not be true for women living in poverty or different cultural contexts. Considering the widely acknowledged longer life expectancy of older women and their caregiving roles, the adverse effects of widowhood may impact widowers more significantly than widows. A widower living alone may allocate more time to household chores and self-care after bereavement, potentially reducing their online activity. Conversely, a widow may increase online engagement for additional social interaction and support. Consequently, the influences of correlates may vary between older men and women. Chiu and Liu (2017), in their analysis of internet withdrawal reasons among older adults in Taiwan, discovered that health factors more strongly affected older women than men. Therefore, examining internet use correlates by gender among older adults is valuable in the US context, where overlapping identities in the form of different socioeconomic, racial, ethnic, and immigration statuses exist. Additionally, given women's longer life expectancy and their higher representation in study samples, analyzing results without gender separation may lead to misconceptions about older men. Hence, our analysis will separately investigate correlates among older African American men and women.

5.1.3 Age Differences Among Older Adults

Scholars have extensively documented age-related disparities in internet use among older adults (Anderson & Perrin, 2017; Chang et al., 2015). Old-old adults, in comparison to their young-old counterparts, exhibit a lower likelihood of utilizing the internet. Simultaneously, they face elevated risks of loneliness, cognitive decline, and increased functional limitations (Cohen-Mansfield et al., 2013; Koo et al., 2017). Several studies highlight the potential of internet use in mitigating loneliness and depression, enhancing cognitive functioning, and fostering psychological well-being, particularly among old-old adults (Sims et al., 2017; Fang et al., 2018). Therefore, fostering the adoption and use of the internet among old-old adults holds significant value.

However, recognizing distinctions between young-old and old-old adults, especially concerning health and mental health conditions, suggests potential differences in correlates of internet use. Internet use is intricate and demands high cognitive functioning. Consequently, compared to young-old adults with superior cognitive abilities, acquiring the necessary skills for internet use may pose greater challenges for old-old adults. Hence, investigating correlates of internet use based on age groups becomes crucial for informing the design and implementation of age-tailored interventions aimed at enhancing internet use among African American older adults.

5.1.4 Current Study

The review of current literatures reveals significant research gaps concerning the internet adoption and utilization of African American older adults. Existing studies often treated race or ethnicity as categorical variables, lacking specific exploration of correlates within the African American older adult subgroup. Furthermore, gender and age differences in internet use emphasize the need for tailored interventions and further investigation of subgroups. Consequently, this study focuses on older African American adults to (1) compare internet use prevalence based on gender and age group and (2) examine correlates of internet use among this population, considering gender and age groups. This research aims to address the unique challenges faced by African American older adults, fostering targeted interventions for a more equitable digital landscape.

5.2 Method

5.2.1 Study Sample

Data were drawn from the 2016 Wave of the Health and Retirement Study (HRS). The HRS is a nationally representative longitudinal panel survey of U.S. individuals aged over 50 and their spouses. Questions about participants' health, family structure, retirement, subjective well-being, and lifestyles have been collected. HRS is funded by the National Institute on Aging (grant number NIA U01AG009740) and is conducted by the University of Michigan. The Institutional Review Board at the

University of Michigan and the National Institution on Aging provided ethical approval for the HRS.

Internet use and perceived daily discrimination were obtained from the Left-Behind Questionnaire module of the 2016 Wave of HRS. In the 2016 Wave, 20,912 adults participated in the survey. First, since the Left-Behind Questionnaire was assigned to a rotating (random) 50% of participants who completed the enhanced face-to-face interview, 10,674 participants who were ineligible for the Left-Behind Questionnaire were removed from this study. Second, among the total eligible sample, 3882 participants who did not return or complete the questionnaire and 32 questionnaires completed by those who were not the assigned respondents were excluded from this study. Third, after removing participants who were not older than 50 or did not report their age, a subsample of 1117 African American older adults was included as the final analytic sample.

5.2.2 Measures

Internet Use The dependent variable, internet use, was measured by a single-item question, "How often do you use a computer for e-mail, internet or other tasks?" Responses to this question were reversely coded as 1 = never/not relevant, 2 = not in the last month, 3 = once a month, 4 = several times a month, 5 = once a week, 6 = several times a week, and 7 = daily.

Health-Related Factors Previous studies have indicated that health-related factors, such as self-rated health, number of diseases, activities of daily living (ADL), and instrumental activities of daily living (IADL) are correlates of internet use among older adults (Ang et al., 2020; Choi & DiNitto, 2013). Self-rated health was measured by a 5-point Likert Scale (1 = poor, 2 = fair, 3 = good, 4 = very good, 5 = excellent). Number of chronic illnesses was the sum of doctor diagnosed illnesses, including high blood pressure, diabetes, cancer, lung disease, heart condition, stroke, and arthritis, ranging from 0 to 7. Difficulties in ADL and IADL were measured by the total number of limited activities, including ADL, such as bathing, dressing, eating, getting in/out of bed, and walking across a room, and IADL, such as using a phone, using money, taking medications, shopping for groceries and preparing for hot meals. Both difficulties in ADL and IADL ranged from 0 to 5.

Mental Health-Related Factors Based on previous studies, depression, discrimination, and cognitive functioning were included as mental health-related factors in this study (Ang et al., 2020; Choi & DiNitto, 2013; Choi et al., 2020; Elliot et al., 2014). Depression was measured by the Center for Epidemiological Studies Depression (CESD) scale (Radloff, 1977). Participants were asked to indicate whether they "felt depressed", "felt activities were efforts", "slept restless", "was happy", "felt lonely", "enjoyed life", "felt sad", and "could not get going" in much of the time during the past week (0 = no, 1 = yes). The items, "was happy" and "enjoyed life", were reversely recoded in this study (0 = yes, 1 = no). Depression was assessed by the unweighted sum of the 8 binary items, ranging from 0 to 8, with higher score indicating higher levels of depression. Perceived everyday discrimination was measured by a six-item scale. Participants were asked to indicate how often they experienced the following things, “You are treated with less courtesy or respect than other people”, “You receive poorer service than other people at restaurants or stores”, “People act as if they think you are not smart”, “People as if they are afraid of you”, “You are threatened or harassed”, and “You receive poorer service or treatment than other people from doctors or hospitals”. Responses to these items were reversely recoded (1 = never, 2 = less than once a year, 3 = a few times a year, 4 = a few times a month, 5 = at least once a week, and 6 = almost every day). Perceived everyday discrimination was assessed by the average of six items, ranging from 1 to 6, with higher scores indicating higher levels of discrimination. Cognitive functioning was measured by a reduced version of the Telephone Interview for Cognitive Status (TIC) scale (Brandt et al., 1988). Cognitive functioning is a composite score of immediate (0–10) and delayed word recall (0–10), Serial 7s (0–5), backwards counting (0–2), date naming (month, day, year, day of week; 0–4), object naming (scissors & cactus; 0–2), naming the President (0–1) and Vice President of the United States (0–1). Cognitive functioning ranged from 0 to 35 with higher scores indicating higher cognitive functioning.

Socioeconomic Factors Education, marital status, retirement status, and poverty were included as socioeconomic factors for internet use in this study (Ang et al., 2020; Chang et al., 2015; Choi & DiNitto, 2013). Education was a continuous variable and measured as years of education. Marital status (0 = divorced, widowed, never married, or others, 1 = married or partnered), retirement status (0 = not retired or partially retired, 1 = completely retired), and living in poverty (0 = no, 1 = yes) were measured dichotomously.

Demographic Factors Previous studies have found that age, gender, and living arrangements were important correlates of internet use among older adults (Ang et al., 2020; Chang et al., 2015; Choi & DiNitto, 2013; Choi et al., 2020; Elliot et al., 2014). The Pew Research Center Survey indicated that internet use among older adults dropped dramatically around 75 years of age (Anderson & Perrin, 2017). Consequently, in this study, age was categorized into a binary variable (0 = less than 75 years, young-old; 1 = 75 years or older, old-old). Gender (0 = men, 1 = women) and living arrangements (0 = living alone, 1 = living with others) were dichotomous variables.

5.2.3 Analytic Strategies

The study utilized Stata 14.2 for the analyses, employing a systematic sequential approach. Initially, descriptive statistics were employed to characterize African American older adults and comprehend their internet usage. Following this, bivariate analysis investigated gender and age discrepancies in internet use. Recognizing the ordinal nature of the dependent variable (internet use), ordinal logistic regressions were employed. Two distinct sets of sequential ordinal logistic regressions were carried out, categorized by gender and age. Each set comprised four models: Model 1 integrated only demographic factors, Model 2 included both demographic and socioeconomic factors, Model 3 incorporated demographic, socioeconomic, and health-related factors, and Model 4 considered demographic, socioeconomic, health-related, and mental health-related factors.

5.3 Results

5.3.1 Sample Characteristics

Table 5.1 shows descriptive characteristics of the African American older adults in the study sample. About 18% of the sample was aged 75 years or older, 63% were women and about 29% were living alone. The participants had about 13 years of education on average (SD = 2.73), or just above high school completion. Less than half of the participants were married/partnered (45%) or retired (46%), and about 22% were living in poverty. As for their health, the mean self-rated health was 3 (SD = 0.99), and on average participants had 2 chronic illness (SD = 1.39). Participants had very low difficulties in ADL (M = 0.41, SD = 0.98) and IADL (M = 0.27, SD = 0.77). Regarding mental health-related factors, African American

Table 5.1 Sample characteristics of African American Older Adults (N = 1117)

	Mean	SD	N	%
Demographic				
Old-old			200	17.9
Women			707	63.3
Living alone			327	29.3
Socioeconomic				
Years of education (0–17)	12.84	2.728		
Married or partnered			506	45.3
Retired			509	45.6
Living in poverty			242	21.7
Health-related				
Self-rated health (1–5)	2.94	0.994		
Number of chronic illness (0–7)	2.19	1.390		
Difficulties in activities of daily living (0–5)	0.41	0.981		
Difficulties in instrumental activities of daily living (0–5)	0.27	0.767		
Mental health-related				
Depression (0–8)	1.68	2.003		
Discrimination (1–6)	1.75	0.838		
Cognitive functioning (0–35)	20.28	4.613		

older adults had relatively low levels of depression (M = 1.68, SD = 2.00) and perceived daily discrimination (M = 1.75, SD = 0.83). Cognitive functioning scores among participants was about 20 (SD = 4.61), indicating no cognitive impairment.

5.3.2 *Internet Use Differences by Gender and Age Group*

Descriptive and bivariate analyses of internet use are presented in Table 5.2. About 56% of older African American adults in the study sample used the internet at least once a week, whereas about 31% never used the internet or reported "not relevant". Chi-square tests showed significant gender differences in internet use ($\chi^2 = 13.05$, $p < 0.05$). About 42% of sampled older women used the internet daily, and 28% never used the internet or reported "not relevant". By contrast, about 38% of older men used the internet daily, and 37% never used the internet or reported "not relevant". Significant age differences were also found ($\chi^2 = 94.82$, $p < 0.001$). Among sampled old-old adults, about 16% used the internet daily, and 59% never used the internet or reported "not relevant". However, among young-old adults, about 45% used the internet daily, and 25% never used the internet or reported "not relevant".

5.3.3 *Sequential Ordinal Logistic Regression on Internet Use*

Findings from the sequential ordinal logistic regressions by gender are summarized in Table 5.3. In Model 1, being old-old was associated with lower odds of frequent internet use for both men and women, while living alone was only associated with lower odds of frequent internet use for older men. In Model 2, more years of education was associated with higher odds of more frequent internet use for both older men and women, whereas being retired and living in poverty were associated with lower odds for both older men and women. Age and living alone were not significant covariates among older men, while age was still significant among older

Table 5.2 Descriptive and bivariate analysis of the internet use by gender and age group

	Total		Men	Women	Young-old	Old-old
	N	%	%	%	%	%
Internet use			$\chi^2 = 13.05^{*}$		$\chi^2 = 94.82^{***}$	
Never/not relevant	341	30.94	35.89	28.08	25.00	58.76
Not in the last month	55	4.99	2.97	6.16	4.85	5.67
Once a month	38	3.45	2.97	3.72	3.63	2.58
Several times a month	56	5.08	4.21	5.59	5.51	3.09
Once a week	38	3.45	3.47	3.44	3.52	3.09
Several times a week	132	11.98	12.87	11.46	12.33	10.31
Daily	442	40.11	37.62	41.55	45.15	16.49

* $p < 0.05$; *** $p < 0.001$

Table 5.3 Ordinal logistic regression on internet use by gender

	Model 1		Model 2		Model 3		Model 4	
	Men	Women	Men	Women	Men	Women	Men	Women
Demographic								
Old-old (ref = young-old)	0.33***	0.20***	0.58	0.28***	0.54	0.28***	0.69	0.35***
Living alone (ref = yes)	0.57*	0.87	1.21	0.99	1.18	0.97	0.38	1.15
Socioeconomic								
Years of education			1.32***	1.42***	1.32***	1.41***	1.18**	1.28***
Married/partnered (ref = yes)			1.52	0.99	1.61	0.99	0.76	1.32
Retired (ref = yes)			0.42***	0.39***	0.44**	0.50***	0.39**	0.39***
Living in poverty (ref = yes)			0.26***	0.39***	0.27***	0.42***	0.12***	0.57+($p = 0.53$)
Health-related								
Self-rated health					1.14	1.19	1.12	1.15
Number of diseases					1.07	0.98	1.05	1.07
Difficulties in activities of daily living					1.19	0.75*	0.86	0.72*
Difficulties in instrumental activities of daily living					0.62	0.93	0.97	1.18
Mental health-related								
Depression							0.77*	0.91
Discrimination							1.13	1.18
Cognitive functioning							1.17***	1.12***
R Square	0.022	0.034	0.115	0.141	0.125	0.151	0.212	0.168
-Log likelihood	575.95***	1038.79***	500.78***	892.61***	472.57***	841.84***	238.65***	476.83***

Note: Effect sizes stand for odds ratio
* $p < 0.05$; ** $p < 0.01$; *** $p < 0.001$

women. In Model 3, more difficulties in ADL was associated with lower odds of frequent internet use among older women. None of the health-related factors were significant among older men. Other significant demographic and socioeconomic variables retained the same directions as in the prior model. In Model 4, better cognitive functioning was associated with higher odds of frequent internet use both among older men and women. Depression was a significant predictor only among older men. To be more specific, for one-unit increase in the level of depression, the odds of having more frequent internet use would decrease by 23%. All other significant variables in Model 3 remained significant or marginally significant.

Ordinal logistic regression results by age groups were presented in Table 5.4. In Model 1, only among young-old adults, being women was associated with higher odds of more frequent internet use, and living alone was associated with lower odds. In Model 2, more years of education was associated with increased odds of more frequent internet use among both young-old and old-old adults. Being retired and living in poverty were associated with lower odds and being women was associated with higher odds among young-old adults. In Model 3, no health-related factors were significant both among young-old and old-old adults. Significant variables in Model 2 remained the same direction in Model 3. In Model 4, better cognitive functioning was associated with higher odds of more frequent use of the internet for both young-old and old-old adults. Among young-old adults, depression was also a significant predictor. For a one-unit increase in the level of depression, the odds of more frequent use of the internet would decrease by 13%. All other significant variables remained the same directions as in Model 3.

5.3.4 Sensitivity Analysis

Sensitivity analyses were conducted and presented in Tables 5.5, 5.6 and 5.7. First, the outcome variable, internet use, was analyzed as a continuous variable, and multilinear regressions were conducted (Table 5.5). Second, the ordinal internet use variable (1–7) was recoded into two categories: internet nonuser (1) and user (2–7), and binary logistic regressions were performed and reported in Table 5.6. Third, the ordinal internet use variable (1–7) was categorized into a binary variable: active internet user (5–7) versus non-active user (1–4), and its binary logistic regressions were conducted and summarized in Table 5.7. Results from all the three analyses remained largely the same.

Table 5.4 Ordinal logistic regression on internet use by age group

	Model 1		Model 2		Model 3		Model 4	
	Young-old	Old-old	Young-old	Old-old	Young-old	Old-old	Young-old	Old-old
Demographic								
Women	1.38*	0.94	1.47**	0.92	1.50**	1.14	2.19**	1.05
Living alone	0.73*	0.90	0.98	1.11	0.99	0.98	0.91	0.91
Socioeconomic								
Years of education			1.38***	1.35***	1.37***	1.38***	1.22***	1.26**
Married or partnered			1.03	1.76	1.02	2.18	1.15	1.71
Retired			0.38***	0.48	0.46***	0.61	0.37***	0.45
Living in poverty			0.32***	0.51	0.32***	0.66	0.27***	0.75
Health-related								
Self-rated health					1.15	1.18	1.11	1.21
Number of diseases					1.00	1.21	1.03	1.32
Difficulties in activities of daily living					0.89	0.78	0.77	0.76
Difficulties in instrumental activities of daily living					0.81	0.86	1.15	1.05
Mental health-related								
Depression							0.87*	0.90
Discrimination							1.19	1.02
Cognitive functioning							1.15***	1.14**
R Square	0.004	0.000	0.111	0.081	0.118	0.097	0.156	0.124
-Log likelihood	1364.58***	255.20***	1165.23***	233.20***	1102.75***	217.71***	526.80***	194.56***

Note: Effect sizes stand for odds ratio

* $p < 0.05$; ** $p < 0.01$; *** $p < 0.001$

Table 5.5 Multilinear regression on internet use by gender and age groups

	Gender		Age	
	Men	Women	Old-old	Young-old
Demographic				
Female			1.01**	0.29
Old-old	−0.25	−1.15***		
Living alone	−0.80	0.11	−0.48	−0.06
Socioeconomic				
Years of education	0.15**	0.23***	0.26***	0.26**
Married or partnered	−0.05	0.20	0.10	0.51
Retired	−1.18**	−0.78**	−1.00**	−0.43
Living in poverty	−1.95***	−0.68*	−1.10**	−0.52
Health-related				
Self-rated health	0.12	0.14	0.17	0.11
Number of diseases	0.11	0.05	0.12	0.31
Difficulties in activities of daily living	−0.31	−0.29*	−0.19	−0.34
Difficulties in instrumental activities of daily living	0.14	0.19	0.03	0.16
Mental health-related				
Depression	−0.21*	−0.09	−0.13	−0.09
Discrimination	0.18	0.11	0.19	0.35
Cognitive functioning	0.16***	0.12***	0.17***	0.14**

* $p < 0.05$; ** $p < 0.01$; *** $p < 0.001$

Table 5.6 Binary logistic regression on internet user by gender and age groups

	Gender		Age	
	Men	Women	Old-old	Young-old
Demographic				
Female			2.75**	1.34
Old-old	0.53	0.31***		
Living alone	0.37	1.03	0.62	0.94
Socioeconomic				
Years of education	1.25**	1.39***	1.30***	1.30**
Married or partnered	1.27	1.17	1.11	1.67
Retired	0.32*	0.43*	0.37**	0.65
Living in poverty	0.15**	0.66	0.33**	0.60
Health-related				
Self-rated health	1.22	1.12	1.19	1.12
Number of diseases	1.17	1.12	1.13	1.36+
Difficulties in activities of daily living	0.94	0.71+	0.82	0.71
Difficulties in instrumental activities of daily living	1.28	1.03	1.03	1.17
Mental health-related				
Depression	0.70**	0.96	0.88	0.91
Discrimination	1.29	1.27	1.20	1.42
Cognitive functioning	1.22***	1.13**	1.19***	1.15***

* $p < 0.05$; ** $p < 0.01$; *** $p < 0.001$

Table 5.7 Binary logistic regression on active internet user by gender and age groups

	Gender		Age	
	Men	Women	Old-old	Young-old
Demographic				
Female			1.93*	0.93
Old-old	0.94	0.41**		
Living alone	0.48	1.12	1.09	0.70
Socioeconomic				
Years of education	1.17*	1.24***	1.18**	1.20*
Married or partnered	0.92	1.54	1.51	1.32
Retired	0.16***	0.59+	0.34***	0.76
Living in poverty	0.04***	0.47*	0.19***	0.61
Health-related				
Self-rated health	1.20	1.11	1.09	1.22
Number of diseases	1.26	0.92	1.03	1.23
Difficulties in activities of daily living	0.75	0.67*	0.68*	0.69
Difficulties in instrumental activities of daily living	0.99	1.28	1.32	0.99
Mental health-related				
Depression	0.77+	0.91	0.86*	0.82
Discrimination	1.51+	1.06	1.31	0.83
Cognitive functioning	1.17**	1.12**	1.16***	1.12*

* $p < 0.05$; ** $p < 0.01$; *** $p < 0.001$

5.4 Discussion

The purpose of this study was to examine internet use among African American older adults and investigate gender and age differences on correlates of internet use. Internet users among older African American adults in this study were less than 70%, and the active users, those who used the internet at least once a week, was only about 55%. Gender and age differences in the internet use were identified in this study: older women and young-old adults had higher percentages of active internet users and lower percentages of non-users than older men and old-old adults, respectively. Gender and age differences on the correlates of internet use among older African Americans were revealed: being old-old and having difficulties in ADL were significant factors only for older women, whereas depression was predictive only for older men. Education and cognition were the only two significant predictors for old-old adults. By contrast, for young-old adults, besides education and cognition, being retired, living in poverty, and depression all affected their internet use.

Consistent with Wilson et al. (2021), digital exclusion presents itself through three levels: access, skills, and usage, as well as tangible offline benefits derived from technology use. This study emphasizes that individuals, even with access to technology, may face digital exclusion due to physical, psychological, and social barriers, coupled with perceptions of social technology and online communication.

These barriers to skills and usage impede technology utilization, amplifying inequalities, even among those with access to this technology.

Findings in this study indicated that membership within the old-old category was associated with decreased odds of more frequent use of the internet only among older African American women but not men. This difference may be explained by gender differences on internalized ageist stereotypes. Choices are also influenced by domestic as well as workplace components and other social contexts such as sex regimes in the society, family structures and employment cultures. Compared to older men, older women are more susceptible to internalized ageist stereotypes and are more likely to feel helpless, dependent, and weak, and have reduced self-esteem and self-efficacy because of their older age (Chrisler et al., 2016; Choi et al., 2020). Due to the negative effects of internalized ageist stereotypes, older women may have lower self-confidence and believe that they are not capable of using the internet when they become older, especially when they have functional difficulties. This discovery aligns with research proposing that engagement with digital technologies in later life should not be viewed as a binary choice between use and non-use but, instead, as a continuum (Gallistl et al., 2021). Older women may be more likely to interpret their limitations in ADL as results of older age, internalize ageist stereotypes and believe that they are too old, and act out those stereotypes in the form of a self-fulfilling prophecy (Chrisler et al., 2016). Consequently, they might reduce the use of the internet, which is consistent with a recent study (Choi et al., 2020). Choi et al. (2020) also used the 2016 Wave of the HRS data and found that negative self-perception of aging was associated with reduced internet use only among older women but not older men, despite using a different analytical method.

Prior research suggests that older adults experiencing depressive symptoms tend to possess fewer social resources, including living alone, lacking or losing close relationships, and having low social support, potentially driving them towards using the internet for social interactions (Bessiere et al., 2008; Choi & DiNitto, 2013). However, in this study, depression was linked to a reduced likelihood of more frequent internet use among older African American men and was not significant among women. This disparity may be attributed to distinct influences of depression on older men and women, along with their different coping strategies. Depression's adverse effects on daily functioning appear more pronounced for men, impacting primary activities, mobility, and household chores (Forlani et al., 2014). Consequently, older men affected by depression may lack the time or competence for internet use. On the other hand, older women's internet use, while affected by depression, might involve seeking social support, such as engaging in online chats with family and friends, sharing experiences on social media, or exploring coping strategies online (Girgus et al., 2017).

Age difference on correlates of internet use were also revealed in this study. Among old-old adults, those who aged 75 or older, more years of education and better cognitive functioning were the only two significant correlates of more frequent use of the internet. However, among young-old adults, being retired, living in poverty, and depression were also predictive of internet use frequency besides education and cognition. Different from retirement, poverty, and depression, education and cognition are relevant to one's capacity to use the internet. It seemed that compared to young-old adults, the capacity to use the internet may be more essential for internet use among old-old adults. This could be explained by the complexity of the internet and the required technology knowledge and skills to use it. Older adults with higher education may have previous training, use experience, or have more self-confidence and capacity to use the internet (Carpenter & Buday, 2007; Choi & DiNitto, 2013; Elliot et al., 2014; Hung et al., 2020). Cognitive function decreases with age, so compared to young-old adults, old-old adults may have lower cognitive functioning or even cognitive impairment, which may be the biggest challenge for them to use the internet (Choi & DiNitto, 2013; Elliot et al., 2014; Hunsaker & Hargittai, 2018).

To address the gaps in internet use among older adults, the government should proceed with its plan by implementing programs and interventions aimed at promoting internet adoption and enhancing digital skills. Additionally, improving digital accessibility and implementing incentive systems can contribute to narrowing this gap. Policymakers should prioritize creating an environment that fosters the digital inclusion of older adults, aligning with sociocultural structures of this demographic.

Subsequent investigations should subject these findings to experimental scrutiny to discern key distinctions among smartphone, tablet, and computer devices. Directly comparing the impacts of smartphone internet access with multimodal internet access on social and informational activities would provide valuable insights. Additionally, exploring whether diverse demographic groups perceive distinct affordances for smartphones could offer an additional rationale for the observed usage gap. This result highlights the challenges in equating digitalization solely with efficiency, convenience, and inclusion. Such a perspective may unfairly label resistance or inability to participate in digitalization processes as unproductive, inconvenient, and contributory to exclusion (Hakkarainen, 2012; Kania-Lundholm, 2019).

5.4.1 Limitations

This study has several limitations. Firstly, the cross-sectional design hinders the estimation of causal associations. Future longitudinal studies are essential for a comprehensive examination of the causal predictors of technology use among older African Americans. Secondly, due to the constraints of the archival questionnaires, internet use in this study was gauged solely by use frequency through a single question. Subsequent studies should consider incorporating more detailed information on computer/internet use, encompassing types of activities, time spent online, and internet use efficiency (Berde, 2019). Thirdly, while this study uncovered gender and age differences in internet use correlates among older African Americans, the underlying mechanisms of these differences remain unclear. Subsequent research should delve deeper into understanding why certain correlates exhibited variations between gender and age groups. Lastly, the non-response rate for the 2016 Wave of HRS was notably high, nearly 40%, and 47% for African Americans. Given that the non-response pattern among African Americans was linked to factors like gender, living alone, and better ADL and IADL functioning, potential biases in the present findings could exist. Further research is warranted to accurately quantify and address such biases.

5.4.2 Implications

Despite its limitations, this study significantly contributes to the intersection of gerontology and technology use in several ways. Notably, it stands out as one of the few studies specifically delving into the correlates of technology use among older African Americans, a marginalized demographic in the country. This focus provides valuable insights and expands the limited existing literature on this population. Furthermore, the study offers crucial information for shaping future interventions aimed at promoting computer literacy and internet use among older African Americans, particularly those with low socioeconomic status. Recommendations include implementing more computer classes in senior centers and establishing free training programs to boost computer and smartphone internet use in this demographic. The identification of gender differences in correlates of internet use emphasizes the need for gender-tailored interventions. For instance, initiatives targeting older African American women should focus on those at advanced ages facing difficulties in activities of daily living (ADL). These interventions should work towards dispelling internalized negative ageist stereotypes and empowering them technologically. In contrast, interventions for older men should address those experiencing depressive symptoms. Given the observed age differences in correlates and recognition of internet use as a cognitive stimulation activity, there's a call for more innovative computer training programs. These programs should be designed to support the cognitive stimulation of older African Americans, both with and without mild cognitive impairment.

5.4.3 Conclusions

The literature on technology use by older adults is extensive, but studies specifically focusing on African American older adults are notably scarce and exhibit disparate results. This study revealed a low prevalence of internet use among older African Americans compared to other ethnicities and races. Implementing interventions that incorporate technology could significantly benefit African American older adults in accessing day-to-day care and non-care services. The study identified similarities and gender and age differences among older African American adults. Consequently, practitioners should take these variations into account when promoting computer/internet use in this demographic. Moreover, designing and implementing gender-specific interventions is crucial, recognizing that the needs and pathways of male versus female older adults differ significantly. Women, in particular, face greater marginalization due to time constraints in caregiving roles, which impacts their ability to use or access the internet. This discrepancy is more pronounced for women in low-income situations, impoverished neighborhoods, those who are single or widowed, and those facing depression barriers.

Authors' Contributions KW conceived the research question, conducted the analysis, drafted the introduction, methods, results, and discussions of the manuscript, and reviewed the manuscript. KK advised on the research question, drafter the introduction, and reviewed the manuscript. ST revised the manuscript and updated with new references for the book chapter.

Ethics Statement The Health and Retirement Study data used in this study is publicly available and is waived from the oversee of the authors' Institutional Review Board.

Conflict of Interest No conflict of interest was reported by all others.

Funding This study was not supported by any grant. Thank Alexandra Marbut for providing gramma checking.

Disclaimer The views expressed in this chapter are solely those of the authors and do not necessarily reflect the views of the University of Alabama at Birmingham, the University of Botswana, or Binghamton University.

References

Anderson, M., & Perrin, A. (2017). *Technology use among seniors*. Pew Research Center for Internet & Technology. Retrieved December 2, 2020, from https://www.pewresearch.org/internet/2017/05/17/technology-use-among-seniors/

Ang, S., Lim, E., & Malhotra, R. (2020). Health-related difficulty in internet use among older adults: Correlates and mediation of its association with quality of life through social support networks. *The Gerontologist, 61*, 693–702. https://doi.org/10.1093/geront/gnaa096

Ayalon, L., & Young, M. A. (2003). A comparison of depressive symptoms in African Americans and Caucasian Americans. *Journal of Cross-Cultural Psychology, 34*(1), 111–124. https://doi.org/10.1177/0022022102239158

Berde, E. (2019). Digital divide and robotics divide. In D. Gu & M. E. Dupre (Eds.), *Encyclopedia of gerontology and population aging*. Springer. https://doi.org/10.1007/978-3-319-69892-2_184-1

Bessiere, K., Kiesler, S., Kraut, R., et al. (2008). Effects of internet use and social resources on changes in depression. *Information, Community & Society, 11*(1), 47–70. https://doi.org/10.1080/13691180701858851

Brandt, J., Spencer, M., & Folstein, M. (1988). The telephone interview for cognitive status. *Neuropsychiatry, Neuropsychology, and Behavioral Neurology, 1*(2), 111–117.

Carpenter, B. D., & Buday, S. (2007). Computer use among older adults in a naturally occurring retirement community. *Computers in Human Behavior, 23*(6), 3012–3024. https://doi.org/10.1016/j.chb.2006.08.015

Chang, J., McAllister, C., & McCaslin, R. (2015). Correlates of, and barriers to, internet use among older adults. *Journal of Gerontological Social Work, 58*(1), 66–85. https://doi.org/10.1080/01634372.2014.913754

Chiu, C. J., & Liu, C. W. (2017). Understanding older adult's technology adoption and withdrawal for elderly care and education: Mixed method analysis from national survey. *Journal of Medical Internet Research, 19*(11), e374. https://doi.org/10.2196/jmir.7401

Choi, N. G., & DiNitto, D. M. (2013). Internet use among older adults: Association with health needs, psychological capital, and social capital. *Journal of Medical Internet Research, 15*(5), e97. https://doi.org/10.2196/jmir.2333

Choi, M., Kong, S., & Jung, D. (2012). Computer and internet interventions for loneliness and depression in older adults: A meta-analysis. *Healthcare Informatics Research, 18*(3), 191–198. https://doi.org/10.4258/hir.2012.18.3.191

Choi, E. Y., Kim, Y., Chipalo, E., et al. (2020). Does perceived ageism widen the digital divide? And does it vary by gender? *The Gerontologist, 60*(7), 1213–1223. https://doi.org/10.1093/geront/gnaa066

Chrisler, J. C., Barney, A., & Palatino, B. (2016). Ageism can be hazardous to women's health: Ageism, sexism, and stereotypes of older women in the healthcare system. *Journal of Social Issues, 72*(1), 86–104. https://doi.org/10.1111/josi.12157

Chu, R. J. (2010). How family support and internet self-efficacy influence the effects of e-learning among higher aged adults–analyses of gender and age differences. *Computers & Education, 55*(1), 255–264. https://doi.org/10.1016/j.compedu.2010.01.011

Cohen-Mansfield, J., Shmotkin, D., Blumstein, Z., et al. (2013). The old, old-old, and the oldest old: Continuation or distinct categories? An examination of the relationship between age and changes in health, function, and wellbeing. *The International Journal of Aging and Human Development, 77*(1), 37–57. https://doi.org/10.2190/AG.77.1.c

Cotten, S. R., Anderson, W. A., & McCullough, B. M. (2013). Impact of internet use on loneliness and contact with others among older adults: Cross-sectional analysis. *Journal of Medical Internet Research, 15*(2), e39. https://doi.org/10.2196/jmir.2306

Cotten, S. R., Francis, J., Kadylak, T., Rikard, R. V., Huang, T., Ball, C., & DeCook, J. (2016). A tale of two divides: Technology experiences among racially and socioeconomically diverse older adults. *Human Aspects of IT for the Aged Population. Design for Aging, 9754*, 167–177.

Elliot, A. J., Mooney, C. J., Douthit, K. Z., et al. (2014). Predictors of older adults' technology use and its relationship to depressive symptoms and well-being. *Journals of Gerontology Series B: Psychological Sciences and Social Sciences, 69*(5), 667–677. https://doi.org/10.1093/geronb/gbt109

Fang, Y., Chau, A. K., Wong, A., et al. (2018). Information and communicative technology use enhances psychological well-being of older adults: The roles of age, social connectedness, and frailty status. *Aging and Mental Health, 22*(11), 1516–1524. https://doi.org/10.1080/13607863.2017.1358354

Forlani, C., Morri, M., Ferrari, B., et al. (2014). Prevalence and gender differences in late-life depression: A population-based study. *The American Journal of Geriatric Psychiatry, 22*(4), 370–380. https://doi.org/10.1016/j.jagp.2012.08.01

Friemel, T. N. (2014). The digital divide has grown old: Determinants of a digital divide among seniors. *New Media & Society, 18*(2), 313–331. https://doi.org/10.1177/1461444814538648

Gallistl, V., Rohner, R., Hengl, L., & Kolland, F. (2021). Doing digital exclusion – Technology practices of older internet non-users. *Journal of Aging Studies, 59*, 100973.

Gilleard, C., & Higgs, P. (2008). Internet use and the digital divide in the English longitudinal study of ageing. *European Journal of Ageing, 5*(3), 233–239.

Girgus, J. S., Yang, K., & Ferri, C. V. (2017). The gender difference in depression: Are elderly women at greater risk for depression than elderly men? *Geriatrics, 2*(4), 35. https://doi.org/10.3390/geriatrics2040035

Hakkarainen, P. (2012). No good for shovelling snow and carrying firewood: Social representations of computers and the internet by elderly Finnish non-user. *New Media & Society, 14*(7), 1198–1215. https://doi.org/10.1177/1461444812442663

Hargittai, E., & Dobransky, K. (2017). Old dogs, new clicks: Digital inequality in skills and uses among older adults. *Canadian Journal of Communication, 42*(2), 195–212.

Harper, M. G., Wellman, B., & Quan-Haase, A. (2020). Older adults and information and communication technologies in the Global North. In D. Gu & M. E. Dupre (Eds.), *Encyclopedia of gerontology and population aging*. Springer. https://doi.org/10.1007/978-3-319-69892-2_902-1

Hung, L. Y., Lyons, J. G., & Wu, C. H. (2020). Health information technology use among older adults in the United States, 2009–2018. *Current Medical Research and Opinion, 36*(5), 789–797. https://doi.org/10.1080/03007995.2020.1734782

Hunsaker, A., & Hargittai, E. (2018). A review of internet use among older adults. *New Media & Society, 20*(10), 3937–3954. https://doi.org/10.1177/1461444818787348

Ihm, J., & Hsieh, Y. P. (2015). The implications of information and communication technology use for the social well-being of older adults. *Information, Communication & Society, 18*(10), 1123–1138.

Kania-Lundholm, M. (2019). Slow side of the divide? Older ICT non- and seldom-users discussing social acceleration and social change Digital. *Culture and Society, 5*(1), 85–103. https://doi.org/10.14361/dcs-2019-0106

Kim, J., Lee, H. Y., Christensen, M. C., et al. (2017). Technology access and use, and their associations with social engagement among older adults: Do women and men differ? *Journals of Gerontology Series B: Psychological Sciences and Social Sciences, 72*(5), 836–845. https://doi.org/10.1093/geronb/gbw123

König, R., Seifert, A., & Doh, M. (2018). Internet use among older Europeans: An analysis based on SHARE data. *Universal Access in the Information Society, 17*(3), 621–633. https://doi.org/10.1007/s10209-018-0609-5

Koo, Y. W., Kõlves, K., & De Leo, D. (2017). Suicide in older adults: Differences between the young-old, middle-old, and oldest old. *International Psychogeriatrics, 29*(8), 1297–1306. https://doi.org/10.1017/S1041610217000618

Lee, Y. C. (2006). An empirical investigation into factors influencing the adoption of an e-learning system. *Online Inform Rev, 30*(5), 517–541.

Marston HR, Kroll M, Fink D, et al. (2016). Technology use, adoption and behavior in older adults: Results from the iStoppFalls project. *Educational Gerontology, 42*(6), 371–387. https://doi.org/10.1080/03601277.2015.1125178

Millward, P. (2003). The "grey digital divide": Perception, exclusion and barriers of access to the internet for older people. *First Monday, 8*(7). Accessed September 4, 2017, from http://journals.uic.edu/ojs/index.php/fm/article/view/1066

Mitchell, U. A., Chebli, P. G., Ruggiero, L., et al. (2019). The digital divide in health-related technology use: The significance of race/ethnicity. *The Gerontologist, 59*(1), 6–14. https://doi.org/10.1093/geront/gny138

Morahan-Martin, J. (1998). The gender gap in internet use: Why men use the internet more than women—A literature review. *Cyber Psychol Behav, 1*(1), 3–10.

Morris, A., & Brading, H. (2007). E-literacy and the grey digital divide: A review with recommendations. *Journal of Information Literacy, 1*(3), 13–28.

Ono, H., & Zavodny, M. (2003). Gender and the internet. *Social Science Quarterly, 84*(1), 111–121.

Osorio-Parraguez, P. J. H. (2013). Health and widowhood: Meanings and experience of elderly women in Chile. *Health, 05*, 1272–1276. https://doi.org/10.4236/health.2013.58173

Peek, M. K., & O'Neill, G. S. (2001). Networks in later life: An examination of race differences in social support networks. *The International Journal of Aging and Human Development, 52*(3), 207–229. https://doi.org/10.2190/F1Q1-JV7D-VN77-L6WX

Radloff, L. S. (1977). The CES-D scale: A self-report depression scale for research in the general population. *Applied Psychological Measurement, 1*(3), 385–401. https://doi.org/10.1177/014662167700100306

Rashid, A. T. (2016). Digital inclusion and social inequality: Gender differences in ICT access and use in five developing countries. *Gender, Technology and Development, 20*(3), 306–332.

Sarkisian, N., & Gerstel, N. (2004). Kin support among blacks and whites: Race and family organization. *American Sociological Review, 69*(6), 812–837. https://doi.org/10.1177/000312240406900604

Shaw, L., & Gant, L. (2002). Users divided? Exploring the gender gap in internet use. *Cyber Psychol Behav, 5*(6), 517–527.

Sims, T., Reed, A. E., & Carr, D. C. (2017). Information and communication technology use is related to higher well-being among the oldest-old. *The Journals of Gerontology: Series B, 72*(5), 761–770. https://doi.org/10.1093/geronb/gbw130

Singh, S. (2001). Gender and the use of the internet at home. *New Media & Society, 3*(4), 395–415.

Sriramatr, S., Berry, T. R., & Spence, J. C. (2014). An internet-based intervention for promoting and maintaining physical activity: A randomized controlled trial. *American Journal of Health Behavior, 38*(3), 430–439. https://doi.org/10.5993/AJHB.38.3.12

Wilson, G., Gates, J., Vijayakumar, S., & Morgan, D. (2021). Understanding older adults' use of social technology and the factors influencing use. *Ageing & Society, 43*(1), 222–245.

Xie, B. (2003). Older adults, computers, and the internet: Future directions. *Geron, 2*(4), 289–305. https://doi.org/10.4017/gt.2003.02.04.002.00

Yang, J., & Du, P. (2021). Gender, capital endowment and digital exclusion of older people in China. *Ageing & Society, 41*(11), 2502–2526.

Yoon, H., Jang, Y., Vaughan, P. W., et al. (2018). Older adults' internet use for health information: Digital divide by race/ethnicity and socioeconomic status. *Journal of Applied Gerontology, 39*(1), 105–110. https://doi.org/10.1177/0733464818770772

Yu, R. P., Ellison, N. B., McCammon, R. J., et al. (2016). Mapping the two levels of digital divide: Internet access and social network site adoption among older adults in the USA. *Information, Communication & Society, 19*(10), 1445–1464. https://doi.org/10.1080/1369118X.2015.1109695

Yu, K., Wu, S., & Chi, I. (2020). Internet use and loneliness of older adults over time: The mediating effect of social contact. *The Journals of Gerontology: Series B, 76*, 541–550. https://doi.org/10.1093/geronb/gbaa004

Chapter 6
Associates of Internet and Social Media Use Among Older Adults in China

Danan Gu, Qiushi Feng, Yan Mo, and Zuqi Cai

6.1 Introduction

The rapid proliferation of digital technologies has transformed how individuals interact, access information, and engage with society (van Deursen & Helsper, 2015; Hargittai et al., 2019). Among older adults, the adoption of the internet and social media has become increasingly significant, offering opportunities for social connection, access to healthcare, and participation in the digital economy (Lu & Wei, 2023; Nordin et al., 2021; Schulz et al., 2015). However, older adults often face unique barriers to digital engagement, including limited digital literacy, physical and cognitive challenges, and socioeconomic disparities (Charness & Boot, 2009; Bhattacharjee et al., 2021). Understanding the factors associated with internet and social media use among older adults is critical for addressing the digital divide and ensuring equitable access to the benefits of digital technologies (Hargittai et al., 2019; van Dijk, 2020).

D. Gu (✉)
Population Division, UN Department of Economic and Social Affairs, New York, NY, USA
e-mail: gudanan@yahoo.com

Q. Feng · Y. Mo
Centre for Family and Population Research/Department of Sociology and Anthropology, National University of Singapore, Singapore, Singapore
e-mail: socfq@nus.edu.sg; moyan@u.nus.edu

Z. Cai
Department of Sociology and Anthropology, National University of Singapore, Singapore, Singapore

Centre for Family and Population Research, National University of Singapore, Singapore, Singapore
e-mail: cai_zuqi@nus.edu.sg

K. Wang et al. (eds.), *ICT Use and Healthy Longevity*, Advances in Studies of Aging and Health 5, https://doi.org/10.1007/978-3-031-98964-3_6

This chapter examines the associates of internet and social media use among older adults in mainland China (hereafter China), using data from the China Longitudinal Aging Social Survey (CLASS). By exploring the interplay of demographic, socioeconomic, family, health, and attitudinal factors affecting the use of the internet and social media among older adults in China, this research contributes to the growing body of literature on aging and digital inclusion.

6.1.1 Literature Review

The adoption of digital technologies among older adults has been widely studied, with researchers identifying a range of factors that influence internet and social media use, such as demographic characteristics, socioeconomic status, family and social support, health conditions, and attitudinal factors. Several theoretical frameworks, such as the Technology Acceptance Model (TAM) (Davis, 1989), the Senior Technology Acceptance Model (STAM) (Chen & Chan, 2014; Renaud & van Biljon, 2008), the Unified Theory of Acceptance and Use of Technology (UTAUT) (Venkatesh et al., 2003), and the Socioemotional Selectivity Theory (SST) (Carstensen, 1991), as shown in Chap. 3, have provided useful lenses for understanding these dynamics.

Demographic factors, particularly age and sex, are consistently shown to be associated with digital engagement in the literature. Older age is a significant barrier to internet use, with studies showing a steady decline in adoption rates as individuals move into their 70s and 80s (Anderson & Perrin, 2017; Hu & Xu, 2024; König et al., 2018). This trend is often attributed to age-related declines in physical and cognitive abilities, as well as lower exposure to digital technologies earlier in life (Anderson & Perrin, 2017; Freese et al., 2006; Wang, 2020). Sex or gender differences are also evident, with older men more likely to use the internet than older women, possibly due to gender disparities in education and related socioeconomic opportunities (Hargittai & Dobransky, 2017).

Socioeconomic status, including education, income, and occupation, plays a critical role in shaping digital access and skills. Higher levels of education are strongly associated with greater internet use, as education enhances digital literacy and confidence in using technology (van Deursen & van Dijk, 2014; Sun et al., 2020; Hu & Xu, 2024). Similarly, individuals with higher incomes are more likely to afford digital devices and internet subscriptions, thus reducing barriers to access (Bertolazzi et al., 2024; Hu & Xu, 2024). Occupational background also plays a significant role, with white-collar workers generally exhibiting higher levels of digital engagement compared to blue-collar and agricultural workers. This disparity arises because blue-collar and agricultural occupations typically involve less digital integration, resulting in reduced exposure to technology and subsequently lower levels of digital access and proficiency (Mesch & Talmud, 2011; Pick et al., 2018; Research on Aging, Policies and Practice, 2017).

Family and social support are increasingly recognized as important facilitators of digital adoption. Older adults with larger social networks or close family members who use the internet are more likely to adopt digital technologies themselves (Chopik, 2016; Ding & Zhang, 2021; Kebede et al., 2022). Intergenerational support, in particular, plays a crucial role, as younger family members often provide technical assistance and encouragement (Freeman et al., 2020). Marital status is another relevant factor, with married individuals more likely to use the internet than their unmarried counterparts, possibly due to shared resources and social influence by spouse (Lu et al., 2022).

Health conditions, including chronic diseases and functional limitations, are significant barriers to digital engagement. Older adults with disabilities or poor self-rated health are less likely to use the internet, as physical and cognitive challenges can hinder device operation and navigation (Freese et al., 2006; Hunsaker & Hargittai, 2018). Poor cognition is associated with lower use of the internet (Sakaguchi-Tang et al., 2017; Wieczorek et al., 2024). However, some studies suggest that as the internet can serve as a valuable resource for managing health conditions (Li et al., 2023; Randine et al., 2022; Wildenbos et al., 2018; Zhou et al., 2024), it is possible that there are higher adoption rates among individuals with chronic diseases.

Attitudinal factors, including perceptions of technology and attitudes toward aging, also influence digital adoption. Older adults with positive views of the internet's benefits, such as improved communication and access to information, are more likely to use it (Vroman et al., 2015; Pan & Jordan-Marsh, 2010). Conversely, negative stereotypes about aging, such as the belief that older adults are incapable of learning new technologies, can deter adoption (Lei et al., 2024). In this regard, SST suggests that older adults may prioritize emotionally meaningful goals in later life, perceiving digital technologies as irrelevant to their needs (Carstensen et al., 1999).

Despite these insights, several gaps remain in the existing literature. First, most studies focus on Western contexts, with limited attention to developing countries like China, where cultural and institutional factors may shape older adults' digital adoption differently. Second, while demographic, socioeconomic and health factors have been extensively studied, relatively few studies have examined the role of family and social support and attitudinal factors in affecting digital engagement in later life. Third, the reliance on cross-sectional data in most studies in the field limits the ability to draw causal inferences or examine changes in digital adoption over time.

Motivated by the established literature and the current research gaps, this chapter examines the factors associated with internet and social media use among older adults in China, and specifically sees to answer the following research questions: (1) What are the demographic, socioeconomic, family, and health-related factors associated with internet and social media use among older adults in China? (2) How do attitudes toward aging and perceptions of the internet influence their digital engagement? (3) What are the key predictors of transitioning from non-use to use of the internet over time? This chapter aims to provide a comprehensive understanding on factors associated with digital engagement among older adults in China.

The significance of this study lies in its focus on China, a country undergoing both rapid population aging and digital transformation. With over 208 million adults aged 65 and older, China has one of the world's largest aging populations, a figure projected to reach 390 million by 2050 (United Nations, 2024). Simultaneously, the country has experienced exponential growth in internet penetration, with more than 1.1 billion internet users and a similar number of social media users by the end of 2024 (China internet Network Information Center [CNNIC], 2025). Despite this digital expansion, older adults remain one of the least connected demographics, raising concerns about social exclusion and digital divide. By identifying the factors that facilitate or hinder internet and social media use among older adults, this study offers valuable insights for policymakers, researchers, and practitioners striving to promote digital inclusion and enhance the well-being of aging populations.

6.2 Data and Methods

6.2.1 Data Sources

To achieve our research objectives, this chapter draws on data from the China Longitudinal Aging Social Survey (CLASS), a nationally representative longitudinal survey designed to examine the health, socioeconomic status, and psychosocial well-being of China's aging population. The survey covers all 31 provinces of mainland China except for Hainan, Xizang, and Xinjiang, accounting for more than 98% of the total older people aged 60 or older of mainland China in the 2020 census. CLASS employs a multi-stage, stratified sampling approach to ensure a representative sample, capturing regional and socioeconomic disparities by including participants from both urban and rural areas across various income and social strata (Dong et al., 2019; Jin & Zhao, 2019). This robust sampling framework enables researchers to analyze aging-related trends across diverse demographic contexts.

CLASS primarily targets adults aged 60 or older, employing a replenishment strategy to mitigate sample attrition due to mortality or loss to follow-up, thereby maintaining its statistical power over time. To better capture health conditions and care needs of the oldest-old, CLASS oversampled those older people aged 80 or older and those in Northeast provinces; as a result, the proportions of sampled older men, illiterate respondents, and individuals with poor health are slightly higher than the census estimates. Following two pilot surveys in 2011 and 2012, the baseline wave was officially launched in 2014 with 11,510 participants. Subsequent follow-up waves were conducted in 2016 (11,471 respondents), 2018 (11,419 respondents), and 2020 (11,398 respondents), underscoring the study's commitment to long-term monitoring of China's aging population.

CLASS utilizes a mixed-methods approach, combining face-to-face interviews with objective physical health assessments. The survey is one of the most comprehensive publicly available aging surveys in China, and covers a wide range of domains, including physical health (e.g., chronic diseases, functional limitations), mental health (e.g., depression, cognitive function), socioeconomic status (e.g., income, education, employment history), family dynamics (e.g., living arrangements, intergenerational support), healthcare utilization (e.g., access to medical services, insurance coverage), and digital engagement (e.g., internet use, smartphone adoption, and social media activity). With its rigorous methodology, broad thematic coverage, and longitudinal design, CLASS serves as a vital resource for policymakers and researchers seeking to understand and address the challenges of aging in China. Particularly, the rich data on older adults' digital engagement in CLASS offer valuable chances to investigate the digital divide and technology adoption among aging populations.

A more detailed module on digital engagement was introduced by CLASS in its 2020 wave than earlier waves, which explored social media use, purposes of use, and barriers to digital adoption, complementing the general internet use questions included in previous waves. Thus, we primarily utilize data from the 2020 wave, in addition to the information of the internet use from the 2018 wave. Due to the limited number of respondents under the age of 65 in this wave, our analytical sample is restricted to adults aged 65 and older, resulting in a total analytical sample of 11,228 participants.

6.2.2 Measures

Internet and Social Media Use

CLASS included more than a dozen questions on internet use, covering frequency, devices used, specific apps and platforms, social media engagement, purposes of use, barriers to use, and perceived benefits, among other aspects. We classified respondents as non-users if they reported never using the internet based on the question, "How often do you use the internet?" internet users were further categorized as smartphone users if they selected "smartphone" in response to the question, "If you use the internet, what device do you use?" Additionally, we identified social media users as those who reported using any of 12 apps or platforms, including *WeChat, Douyin (Chinese TikTok), Xigua Video or Bilibili (similar to YouTube), Taobao (similar to Amazon), and Didi (similar to Uber)*, among others.

Associated Factors with Internet and Social Media Use

Based on our literature review in the earlier section and the theories, and specially the STAM framework discussed in Chap. 3, along with the availability of relevant data in CLASS, we included the following variables in our analysis. Demographic variables include age, categorized into three groups (65–74, 75–84, and 85+), sex (men vs. women), ethnicity (Han vs. minority groups), and place of residence (urban vs. rural).

Socioeconomic status is measured by educational attainment (no education [0 years of schooling], primary school [1–6 years of schooling], and middle school or above [7+ years of schooling]), self-reported economic condition as compared to others in the community (poor vs. not poor), and primary lifetime occupation (white-collar, blue-collar, or agricultural work).

Family and social support are measured through marital status (currently married vs. not married) and the number of close family members and/or friends available to provide assistance in times of need. Engagement in leisure and social activities is also measured as a dichotomous variable. Respondents were classified as engaging in such activities and coded as 1 if they regularly participated in any of the following: religious activities, attending learning classes, watching TV, listening to the radio, reading books or newspapers, listening to operas, singing or playing musical instruments, playing mahjong or cards, dancing, or participating in neighborhood activities. Those who did not engage in any of these activities were coded as 0.

To measure views on the internet, we generated a variable based on eight questions asking the respondents to rate impacts of internet technology development on daily life, regarding aspects such as social contact and communication, shopping, access to news and information, entertainment, travel and tourism, healthcare services, financial activities, and learning and training. The response that the internet had "made things convenient" was coded as 1, while the response of inconvenience or "do not know" was coded as 0. The total score ranges from 0 to 8.

Views on aging were measured based on four negative and three positive statements on aging. Negative statements included "I feel I am already old," "In my view, aging is a process of loss," "Once I get old, it becomes difficult for me to make new friends," and "Because of my age, I feel isolated by others." Positive statements included "The older one gets, the greater their ability to cope with daily life," "Knowledge increases with age," and "Aging is a pleasant experience." Each item was rated on a five-point scale from strongly disagree to strongly agree. Responses to the three positive statements were reverse-coded. The reliability coefficient for these seven items was approximately 0.50. For the sake of convenience, we summed the responses, with the total score ranging from 7 to 35, to generate a variable of positive views on aging. Separate inclusion of these seven variables in models did not alter the conclusions in the sensitivity analyses.

We also created a variable to indicate perceived aging based on eight questions. Four statements are on social participation, including "If given the opportunity, I am willing to participate in Neighborhood Residential Committee/Village Committee work," "I often wish to contribute to society," "I enjoy learning new things," and "I feel I am still a useful member of society." Additional four statements are about challenges or difficulties in adapting to social change, including "It is difficult for me to adapt to the rapidly changing environment," "Nowadays, it is difficult for me to accept increasingly common viewpoints," "It is becoming harder for me to accept new social policies," and "Recent social changes have not been beneficial for older adults." The last four items were reversely coded, and all responses were summed, yielding a total score ranging from 8 to 40, for a variable of positive perceived aging. The reliability coefficient was 0.81, indicating its high internal consistency.

Health status was assessed through multiple measures, including the presence of chronic diseases (1+ disease vs. none), disability in Activities of Daily Living

(ADLs) and Instrumental Activities of Daily Living (IADLs), cognitive impaired (yes vs. no), and self-rated health (very good/good vs. other). ADL disability was determined based on whether respondents required assistance with six daily activities: bathing, dressing, indoor mobility, toileting, incontinence management, and eating. The ADL scale is widely used in aging research, with a reliability coefficient of 0.88 in the 2020 CLASS wave. IADL disability was measured with eight activities: climbing stairs, outdoor walking, shopping, lifting a 5 kg object, cooking, housekeeping, using transportation, and managing finances. The reliability coefficient for these items was 0.92, indicating strong internal consistency and high measurement validity.

The cognitive function was measured by a short version of the normal version of the Mini-Mental State Examination (MMSE) (Folstein et al., 1975), with only 16 items (or scores) designed in the CLASS questionnaire. The reliability coefficient is 0.85, indicating a good internal consistency. In the original MMSE scale, 24 out of the total 30 scores (the 20th percentile in scoring) was used as the threshold to define cognitive impairment (Folstein et al., 1975). Following the similar threshold, we applied the 13 score out of 16 as the cut point (the 19th percentile in scoring) to define cognitive impairment. Other options were also tested and the findings are very similar. The disease conditions were measured from more than 20 chronic disease conditions, vast majority of the reported conditions (97%) were diagnosed by doctors, indicating a good reliability of self-reported conditions.

Finally, a variable of region was included in our analysis to reflect regional contextual differences in levels of internet infrastructure and socioeconomic development. The region is classified into East, Central, West, and Northeast, following the definition given by the National Bureau of Statistics of China (2011).

Overall, these variables provide a comprehensive framework for analyzing major aspects of internet and social media use, including demographic and socioeconomic factors, family and social support, engagement in activities, views on aging, perceived aging, and health status.

6.2.3 Analytical Strategies

In addition to descriptive analyses, we utilized multiple logistic regression models to address our research objectives. To systematically identify factors associated with internet and social media adoption, we constructed a series of models, each incorporating distinct clusters of variables. Five models were developed to evaluate the individual effects of the following sets of factors: (1) demographic characteristics, (2) socioeconomic status, (3) family and social support, (4) engagement in leisure and social activities, perceptions of internet utility, self-perceived aging, and attitudes toward aging, and (5) health conditions. Finally, a comprehensive full model integrating all variables was created to provide a holistic assessment of their collective influence.

Given the substantial similarity in results between the individual models and the full model, with only minor discrepancies observed, we opted to present the full model exclusively in this chapter. This approach streamlines interpretation and ensures clarity by avoiding redundant discussion of near-identical findings across models.

To evaluate the robustness of our findings, we performed supplementary analyses focused on predictors of new internet adoption among individuals who reported no internet use during the 2018 wave. This longitudinal approach allowed us to isolate factors associated with their subsequent adoption of internet services during the 2-year study period. Parallel models were constructed to analyze smartphone and social media adoption patterns using the same methodological framework. Given the methodological and conceptual overlap with internet adoption patterns, these results have been omitted from the main presentation but remain available upon request.

Descriptive analyses incorporated sampling weights to ensure representativeness, while regression models were conducted without weighting. This approach was adopted because the variables used to calculate sampling weights were already accounted for in the regression specifications. Including weights in the regression framework would risk inflating standard errors without providing additional explanatory power (Winship & Radbill, 1994). All analyses were performed using Stata 18.0.

6.3 Results

Table 6.1 presents the weighted and unweighted percentage distributions of the analytical sample across study variables. The two sets of distributions are largely similar, with noticeable differences observed in distributions for age groups, regions, and health. Minor discrepancies exist in sex, education, and marital status. The weighted estimates indicate that 30% of Chinese adults aged 65 or older were internet users in 2020, with 28% engaging in social media. Among internet users, 97% accessed the internet via smartphones. These estimates closely align with the China's official statistics presented in Chap. 2, which are derived from registered data and large survey data (CNNIC, 2021), affirming the reliability of internet and social media use estimates in CLASS.

Table 6.2 presents both the weighted prevalence rates of internet and social media use for all study variables. The results reveal significant differences in internet use across various subgroups, with ethnicity being the only factor showing no noticeable variation between Han Chinese and the minorities. For example, only about 5% of the oldest-old Chinese adults (aged 85 or older) used the internet or social media in 2020, compared to 37.6% among those aged 65–74. Older men demonstrated a higher usage rate than older women by nearly 5 percentage points, while urban older adults used the internet (38.3%) at nearly double the rate of their rural counterparts (20.7%). Education also plays a crucial role: those with 7+ years

Table 6.1 Unweighted and Weighted percentage distribution of the analytical sample by study variables, 2020, CLASS (N = 11,228)

Variables in 2020	Weighted	Unweighted
% Use of the internet	30.0	27.0
% of which, via a smartphone	97.3	96.2
%Use of social media	28.2	25.0
%Ages 65–74	64.8	38.0
%Ages 75–85	27.1	44.7
%Ages 85+	8.1	17.3
%Men	47.5	50.5
%Han ethnicity	95.5	94.0
%Urban residents	52.7	54.9
%0 years of schooling	24.4	23.6
%1–6 years of schooling	39.1	41.2
%7+ years of schooling	36.5	35.2
%Economically poor	10.4	11.5
%White-collar workers	10.8	11.7
%Blue-collar workers	27.5	29.9
% Agricultural workers	61.7	58.4
%Currently married	78.1	75.3
%Having 2+ close family members	80.5	79.7
%Having 2+ close friends	71.4	70.6
%Frequent engagement in leisure activity	82.1	83.2
Positive views on internet impact (0–8)[a]	2.12	2.08
Positive views on aging (7–35)[a]	20.68	20.60
Positive perceived of aging (8–40)[a]	23.91	23.98
%Having 1+ diseases	79.6	80.4
%IADL disabled	18.7	24.2
%ADL disabled	11.3	15.1
%Cognitively impaired	24.5	30.4
%Good self-rated health	50.3	46.8
%East	38.5	36.1
%Central	27.1	25.7
%West	25.7	24.8
%Northeast	8.6	13.4

Note: [a] refer to the mean score of the variable. The number in parentheses is the score range. ADL: Activities of daily living. IADL: Instrumental ADL

Table 6.2 Weighted percentages of older adults who access the internet and use social media by study variables, 2020, CLASS (N = 11,228)

Variables in 2020	Internet use	Social media	Variables in 2020	Internet use	Social media
Total	30.0	28.2	Not frequent engagement in leisure activity	18.5	16.7
Ages 65–74	37.6	35.4	Frequent engagement in leisure activity	32.5	30.6
Ages 75–85	19.1	17.7	Positive views on internet impact (0–3)[a]	20.9	18.7
Ages 85+	5.1	4.7	Positive views on internet impact (4–8)[a]	48.3	47.2
Women	27.8	26.1	Positive views on aging (7–22)[a]	27.9	26.3
Men	32.4	30.4	Positive views on aging (23–35)[a]	34.5	32.4
Non-Han minorities	29.6	28.7	Positive perceived aging (8–25)[a]	27.0	25.2
Han ethnicity	30.0	28.1	Positive perceived aging (26–40)[a]	37.5	35.7
Rural residents	20.7	19.4	Having no chronic disease	34.9	32.1
Urban residents	38.3	36.0	Having 1+ diseases	28.7	27.2
0 years of schooling	11.9	11.2	IADL not diseased	33.3	31.4
1–6 years of schooling	23.7	22.5	IADL disabled	15.3	14.1
7+ years of schooling	48.8	45.5	ADL not disabled	31.1	29.2
Economically not poor	30.5	28.7	ADL disabled	20.8	19.6
Economically poor	25.0	23.5	Cognitively unimpaired	35.3	33.3
White-collar workers	60.7	57.9	Cognitively impaired	13.6	12.4
Blue-collar workers	44.8	41.7	Self-rated not good health	22.6	21.2
Agricultural workers	18.0	16.9	Self-rated good health	37.3	35.0
Currently not married	17.8	17.0	East	42.7	41.8
Currently married	33.4	31.3	Central	20.4	19.0
Having <2 close family members	22.2	21.2	West	18.0	16.1
Having 2+ close family members	31.8	29.8	Northeast	38.6	31.8
Having <2 close friends	22.5	21.4			
Having 2+ close friends	33.0	30.8			

Note: [a]referring to the score range of the variable. ADL: Activities of daily living. IADL: Instrumental ADL. The percentages were weighted using the frequency weight. The patterns for the use of smart phones are very similar to those of internet use and are not presented in the table. Except for ethnicity, the subgroup difference of a variable is all statistically significant at $p < 0.001$. Statistical differences are based on chi-square tests after applying with the analytical weight of schooling had a usage rate close to 50%, whereas only slightly than 10% of those without formal education engaged with digital technologies.

Regional disparities are also evident, with older adults in East and Northeast China reporting internet use rates around 40%, compared to only 20% in the Central and West regions. Occupational background further influences usage patterns, as white-collar workers (former professionals and administrators) had a usage rate over 60%, while agricultural workers reported less than 20%. Social factors such as marital status and social support also matter, with married individuals or those with a larger network of close family or friends usually having internet usage rates 60–100% higher than those with fewer social connections. Similarly, older adults with positive views on attitudes toward aging and active social engagement reported usage rates 60–100% higher than their less engaged peers. Health status is another key determinant, with individuals in good health generally having internet use rates 50–160% higher than those in poor health. Finally, economic conditions are strongly correlated with digital access, with those in poorer economic situations using the internet at a rate of five percentage points lower than their wealthier counterparts.

Table 6.3 presents odds ratios of internet use by clusters of variables, illustrating how bivariate relationships change when controlling for other covariates in multiple regression models. While the overall associational patterns remain largely consistent with the findings in Table 6.2, several noteworthy differences emerge. First, the significantly higher odds of internet use among urban older adults compared to their rural counterparts diminish when all study variables are controlled for. It seems that socioeconomic factors account for much of the urban-rural difference (not shown). Similarly, the observed sex disparity in internet use is largely attenuated after adjusting for socioeconomic variables. Second, the initially positive association between having more close family members and internet use becomes statistically not significant once other covariates are accounted for; similarly, the positive association between active views on aging and internet use also disappears in multivariate models. Third, interestingly, the presence of at least one disease condition is linked to higher odds of internet use when demographic factors are controlled for, which is primarily due to age adjustment (results not shown in the table but available upon request).

Table 6.3 further examines the factors associated with smartphone-based internet use and social media engagement. The findings in these tables mostly align with those in Table 6.3, reinforcing the robustness of the observed associations.

To further assess the robustness of these findings and mitigate potential endogeneity issues inherent in cross-sectional analyses, we conducted a longitudinal analysis focusing on individuals who were not internet users in the wave of 2018 in CLASS. We examined how study variables measured in 2018 were associated with the consequent transition to internet use in 2020. The results, presented in Table 6.4, reveal two notable differences compared to the cross-sectional findings. First, older adults in urban areas were less likely to become new internet users compared to their rural counterparts, likely due to the fact that the prevalence of internet use in urban settings is already higher than the rural settings. Second, while IADL and self-rated health are significantly associated with the new use of the internet when

Table 6.3 Odds ratios of internet access by study variables, 2020, CLASS

Variables in 2020	Internet use	Smartphone use	Social media use
Ages 75–85 (65–74)	0.56***	0.59***	0.55***
Ages 85+ (65–74)	0.15***	0.17***	0.15***
Men (women)	0.91+	0.90*	0.95
Han ethnicity (minor)	0.80+	0.93	0.74*
Urban (rural)	1.07	1.04	1.09
1–6 years of schooling (0)	1.52***	1.71***	1.57***
7+ years of schooling (0)	2.84***	3.12***	2.76***
Economically poor (no)	0.97	0.85+	0.96
Blue-collar workers (white-collar)	0.77**	0.83*	0.72***
Agricultural workers (white-collar)	0.38***	0.42***	0.37***
Currently married (no)	1.48***	1.47***	1.49***
Having 2+ close family members (<2)	0.99	1.03	0.96
Having 2+ close friends (<2)	1.08	1.08	1.01
Frequent leisure activity (no)	1.93***	1.96***	1.98***
Positive views on internet impact (0–8)	1.29***	1.30***	1.31***
Positive views on aging (7–35)	1.01	1.01*	1.01
Positive perceived aging (8–40)	1.05***	1.04***	1.05***
Having 1+ diseases (no)	1.25***	1.28***	1.32***
IADL disabled (no)	0.77**	0.72***	0.72***
ADL disabled (no)	0.78**	0.77**	0.72***
Cognitively impaired (no)	0.52***	0.49***	0.51***
Good self-rated health (no)	1.16**	1.18**	1.12*
Central (East)	0.44***	0.47***	0.38***
West (East)	0.45***	0.43***	0.39***
Northeast (East)	0.80**	0.85*	0.57***
-Log likelihood	4641.8	4572.0	4400.4
LR chi-square	3819.0	3723.9	3822.6
Degree of freedom	25	25	25
No. of individuals	11,228	11,228	11,228

Note: The results were obtained from logistic regression models. The category of a variable in the parentheses is the reference. ADL: Activities of daily living. IADL: Instrumental ADL
$+p < 0.1$, $*p < 0.05$, $**p < 0.01$, $***p < 0.001$

only demographic factors are controlled for, neither ADL/IADL disability nor self-rated health showed a significant association with internet adoption when all other factors are controlled. This indicates that the associations between these three health indicators and new internet use are partially explained by other variables. The relationships between other study variables and internet use remained largely consistent with those in Table 6.3. The patterns of social media use closely mirror those of internet use and are thus not detailed in the main text, but results are available upon request.

Table 6.4 Odds ratios of the new use of the internet from 2018 to 2020 by study variables, CLASS

Variables in 2018	Model 1	Model 2	Model 3	Model 4	Model 5	Model 6
Ages 75–85 (65–74)	0.20***	0.25***	0.26***	0.25***	0.27***	0.30***
Ages 85+ (65–74)	0.04***	0.15***	0.16***	0.15***	0.18***	0.23***
Men (women)	1.20**	1.02	1.11	1.17*	1.19*	0.96
Han ethnicity (minor	0.72*	1.51+	1.42+	1.56*	1.54*	1.64*
Urban (rural)	0.39***	0.82+	0.31***	0.34***	0.33***	0.84
1–6 years of schooling (0)		1.85***				1.58***
7+ years of schooling (0)		4.88***				3.86***
Blue-collar workers (white-collar)		0.99				0.99
Agricultural workers (white-collar)		0.33***				0.37***
Currently married (no)			1.64***			1.37**
Having 2+ close family members (<2)			1.31*			1.25*
Having 2+ close friends (< 2)			1.21*			1.05
Positive views on internet impact (0–8)				1.11***		1.07***
Positive views on aging (7–35)				0.99		0.99
Positive aging practice (8–40)				1.07***		1.05***
Having 1+ diseases (no)					1.71***	1.56***
IADL disabled (no)					0.71***	0.81+
ADL disabled (no)					0.92	0.87
Cognitively impaired (no)					0.45***	0.59***
Good self-rated health (no)					1.06	0.92
Central (East)	0.42***	0.36***	0.30***	0.34***	0.28***	0.37***
West (East)	0.34***	0.51***	0.37***	0.41***	0.32***	0.57***
Northeast (East)	0.68***	0.92	0.98	1.32**	0.96	1.15
-Log likelihood	3083.6	2357.3	2575.0	2545.1	2523.6	2288.4
LR chi-square	914.1	1373.1	937.7	997.3	1040.4	1510.9
Degree of freedom	8	12	11	11	13	23
No. of individuals	7245	7245	7245	7245	7245	7245

Note: The results were obtained from logistic regression models. The category of a variable in the parentheses is the reference. ADL: Activities of daily living. IADL: Instrumental ADL
$+p < 0.1$, $*p < 0.05$, $**p < 0.01$, $***p < 0.001$

6.4 Discussion

Drawing on a nationally representative survey on older adults in China, this chapter systematically investigated the factors associated with internet and social media use among this population. The findings of this study provide valuable insights into the factors associated with internet and social media use among older adults in China. Consistent with previous literature, demographic factors such as age and sex play a significant role in shaping digital engagement (Charness & Boot, 2009; Czaja et al., 2006; Selwyn et al. 2003). The decline in internet use with advancing age aligns with SST, which posits that older adults may prioritize emotionally meaningful activities over learning new technologies (Carstensen et al., 1999; Selwyn et al., 2003). The gender disparity in internet use, with older men more likely to be users than older women, reflects broader societal inequalities in education and economic opportunities (Hargittai & Dobransky, 2017; Helsper & van Deursen, 2017). This is confirmed by the attenuation of this disparity in multivariable models, in which socioeconomic factors, such as education and income, largely account for the observed differences (Zhang & Chen, 2013).

Socioeconomic status emerges as a critical determinant of digital adoption, consistent with TAM, STAM, and UTAUT (Scheerder et al., 2017). Higher levels of education and income are strongly associated with greater internet use, as these factors enhance digital literacy and reduce financial barriers to digital access (Choi & DiNitto, 2013; Hu & Xu, 2024; Porter & Donthu, 2006; van Deursen & van Dijk, 2014). The occupational background also matters, with former white-collar workers demonstrating higher rates of digital engagement compared to blue-collar or agricultural workers. This finding underscores the importance of addressing structural inequalities in digital access and skills.

One interesting finding is that self-rated economic conditions are less robust than education and occupation in associating with internet use and social media use (e.g., Blank & Lutz, 2016; van Deursen & Helsper, 2015). This is probably because education and occupation often serve as stronger predictors of digital engagement by shaping individuals' cognitive skills, technological literacy, and professional incentives for using digital tools. Higher levels of education are associated with greater digital skills and confidence in navigating online platforms, which in turn facilitate more frequent internet and social media use (Schradie, 2011; van Deursen & Helsper, 2015). Additionally, occupation influences digital engagement through workplace exposure, as certain professions require continuous internet use for communication, networking, or productivity (Helsper & Eynon, 2013). In contrast, self-rated economic conditions may be less predictive because individuals with similar income levels can have vastly different digital habits depending on their educational background and occupational requirements. Moreover, the role of income may matter more for undeveloped societies where digital access could still be an issue for the majority due to financial difficulties. Research also suggests that economic factors primarily affect access to devices and broadband services rather than patterns of online behavior, which are more strongly linked to education and professional roles (Blank & Lutz, 2016).

Family and social support play a nuanced role in shaping digital adoption (Francis et al., 2019). While bivariate analyses suggest that having more close family members or friends is associated with higher internet use, this relationship becomes not significant in multivariable regression models. This finding contrasts with previous studies emphasizing the importance of intergenerational support (Freeman et al., 2020) but may reflect the unique cultural context of China, where family dynamics and social networks differ from Western settings (e.g. Djundeva et al., 2019). It is possible that having close contact with digital skills may reduce, instead of increasing, the need for internet and social media use among older people, as contact could provide immediate help whenever needed. Further research is needed to explore these dynamics in greater depth (Yuan et al., 2016).

Attitudinal factors, including perceptions of the impacts of internet technology advancement on social development and attitudes toward aging, also influence digital engagement. The disappearance of the positive association between favorable attitudes toward aging and internet use in multivariate models suggests that these attitudes may be mediated by other factors, such as socioeconomic status or health conditions (Mitzner et al., 2019). This finding highlights the complexity of attitudinal influences and the need for further research to disentangle these relationships.

Health conditions, particularly cognitive functioning, chronic diseases, and functional limitations, are significant barriers to digital engagement (Hunsaker & Hargittai, 2018; Wieczorek et al., 2024; Wildenbos et al., 2018; Wilson et al., 2021). The positive association between having chronic diseases and internet use in multivariate models is intriguing and may reflect the use of digital technologies for health management (Chang & Im, 2014). However, the lack of a significant association between ADL disability and internet adoption in longitudinal analyses suggests that physical challenges may deter initial adoption but not necessarily sustained use.

In comparison to other regions, the East region shows a significantly higher prevalence of internet use, which reflects both the higher level of socioeconomic development and more advanced infrastructure in this area.

There are several strengths of this study: the use of nationally representative longitudinal data, comprehensive set of variables, and the focus on China, a context that has received limited attention in the literature. However, several limitations should be acknowledged. First, the reliance on self-reported data may introduce measurement bias, particularly for variables such as internet use and health status. Second, while the longitudinal design allows for examining transitions in digital adoption, the two-year interval between waves may not capture longer-term changes. Third, although this study focuses on a non-Western context, it does not explore the role of cultural factors within China, such as filial piety or collectivist values, which may shape digital adoption in unique ways.

Our findings have important policy implications. First, efforts to promote digital inclusion among older adults should address structural inequalities in education and income, as these factors are foundational determinants of digital access and skills. Second, related interventions should leverage family and social networks to provide technical assistance and encouragement, particularly for older adults with limited digital literacy. Third, healthcare providers can play a role in promoting the use of digital technologies for health management, particularly for individuals with chronic diseases.

Future research should explore the role of cultural and institutional factors in shaping digital adoption, particularly in non-Western contexts. Longitudinal studies with shorter and longer intervals between waves are warranted to provide deeper insights into the dynamics of digital adoption over time. Due to the complexity of these associative factors of internet and social media use, qualitative research should be encouraged to complement quantitative analyses by exploring the lived experiences of older adults and the barriers they face in adopting digital technologies.

Acknowledgement The authors would like to thank the Research Center for Population & Development and the Institute of Gerontology, Renmin University for providing access to the China Longitudinal Aging and Social Survey (CLASS) dataset used in this chapter.

Disclaimer Views expressed in the chapter are solely those of the authors and do not necessarily reflect those of the United Nations and the National University of Singapore.

References

Anderson, M., & Perrin, A. (2017). *Tech adoption climbs among older adults*. Pew Research Center. Retrieved from https://www.pewresearch.org/internet/wp-content/uploads/sites/9/2017/05/PI_2017.05.17_Older-Americans-Tech_FINAL.pdf

Bertolazzi, A., Quaglia, V., & Bongelli, R. (2024). Barriers and facilitators to health technology adoption by older adults with chronic diseases: An integrative systematic review. *BMC Public Health, 24*(1), 506.

Bhattacharjee, P., Baker, S., & Waycott, J. (2021). Older adults and their acquisition of digital skills: A review of current research evidence. In *Proceedings of the 32nd Australian Conference on Human-Computer Interaction* (pp. 437–443).

Blank, G., & Lutz, C. (2016). Benefits and harms from Internet use: A differentiated analysis of Great Britain. *New Media & Society, 20*(2), 618–640.

Carstensen, L. L. (1991). Selectivity theory: Social activity in life-span context. *Annual Review of Gerontology and Geriatrics, 11*, 195–217.

Carstensen, L. L., Isaacowitz, D. M., & Charles, S. T. (1999). Taking time seriously: A theory of socioemotional selectivity. *American Psychologist, 65*(3), 165–181.

Chang, S. J., & Im, E. O. (2014). A path analysis of internet health information seeking behaviors among older adults. *Geriatric Nursing, 35*(2), 137–141.

Charness, N., & Boot, W. R. (2009). Aging and information technology use: Potential and barriers. *Current Directions in Psychological Science, 18*(5), 253–258.

Chen, K., & Chan, A. H. (2014). Gerontechnology acceptance by elderly Hong Kong Chinese: A senior technology acceptance model (STAM). *Ergonomics, 57*(5), 635–652.

China Internet Network Information Center (CNNIC). (2021). *The 47th Statistical Report on China's Internet Development*. Retrieved from https://www.cnnic.cn/n4/2022/0401/c88-1125.html [in Chinese]

China Internet Network Information Center (CNNIC). (2025). *The 55th Statistical Report on China's Internet Development*. Retrieved from https://www.cnnic.net.cn/n4/2025/0117/c88-11229.html [in Chinese]

Choi, N. G., & DiNitto, D. M. (2013). Internet use among older adults: Association with health needs, psychological capital, and social capital. *Journal of Medical Internet Research, 15*(5), e93.

Chopik, W. J. (2016). The benefits of social technology use among older adults are mediated by reduced loneliness. *Cyberpsychology, Behavior, and Social Networking, 19*(9), 551–556.

Czaja, S. J., Charness, N., Fisk, A. D., Hertzog, C., Nair, S. N., Rogers, W. A., & Sharit, J. (2006). Factors predicting the use of technology: Findings from the Center for Research and Education on Aging and Technology Enhancement (CREATE). *Psychology and Aging, 21*(2), 333–352.

Davis, F. D. (1989). Perceived usefulness, perceived ease of use, and user acceptance of information technology. *MIS Quarterly, 13*(3), 319–340.

Ding, Z., & Zhang, X. (2021). Internet use among older adults in urban China and its influencing factors. *Population Research, 45*(2), 61–74. [In Chinese].

Djundeva, M., Dykstra, P. A., & Emery, T. (2019). Family dynamics in China and Europe in the last half-century. *Chinese Journal of Sociology, 5*(2), 143–172.

Dong, T., Zhu, Z., Guo, M., Du, P., & Wu, B. (2019). Association between dying experience and place of death: Urban–rural differences among older Chinese adults. *Journal of Palliative Medicine, 22*(11), 1386–1393.

Folstein, M. F., Folstein, S. E., & McHugh, P. R. (1975). "Mini-mental state". A practical method for grading the cognitive state of patients for the clinician. *Journal of Psychiatric Research, 12*(3), 189–198.

Francis, J., Ball, C., Kadylak, T., & Cotten, S. R. (2019). Aging in the digital age: Conceptualizing technology adoption and digital inequalities among older adults. In B. B. Neves & F. Vetere (Eds.), *Ageing and digital technology* (pp. 35–49). Springer.

Freeman, S., Xiong, B., Olynick, J., Marston, H. R., Genoe, R., Kulczycki, C., & Musselwhite, C. (2020). Intergenerational connections through technology: Insights from the Technology Use in Later Life multi-site study. *Innovation in Aging, 4*(Suppl 1), 928–929.

Freese, J., Rivas, S., & Hargittai, E. (2006). Cognitive ability and Internet use among older adults. *Poetics, 34*, 236–249.

Hargittai, E., & Dobransky, K. (2017). Old dogs, new clicks: Digital inequality in skills and uses among older adults. *Canadian Journal of Communication, 42*(2), 195–211.

Hargittai, E., Piper, A. M., & Morris, M. R. (2019). From internet access to internet skills: Digital inequality among older adults. *Universal Access in the Information Society, 18*(4), 881–890.

Helsper, E. J., & Eynon, R. (2013). Distinct skill pathways to digital engagement. *European Journal of Communication, 28*(6), 696–713.

Helsper, E. J., & Van Deursen, A. J. A. M. (2017). Do the rich get digitally richer? Quantity and quality of support for digital engagement. *Information, Communication & Society, 20*(5), 700–714.

Hu, H., & Xu, W. (2024). Socioeconomic differences in digital inequality among Chinese older adults: Results from a nationally representative sample. *PLoS One, 19*(4), e0300433.

Hunsaker, A., & Hargittai, E. (2018). A review of Internet use among older adults. *New Media & Society, 20*(10), 3937–3954.

Jin, Y., & Zhao, M. (2019). Internet access and the elderly's active aging in China—A study based on 2016 China Longitudinal Aging Social Survey. *Population Journal, 6*, 44–55. [in Chinese].

Kebede, A. S., Ozolins, L. L., Holst, H., & Galvin, K. (2022). Digital engagement of older adults: Scoping review. *Journal of Medical Internet Research, 24*(12), e40192.

König, R., Seifert, A., & Doh, M. (2018). Internet use among older Europeans: An analysis based on SHARE data. *Universal Access in the Information Society, 17*(2), 621–633.

Lei, X., Matovic, D., Leung, W.-Y., Viju, A., & Wuthrich, V. M. (2024). The relationship between social media use and psychosocial outcomes in older adults: A systematic review. *International Psychogeriatrics, 36*(9), 714–746.

Li, Z., Wang, Y., Li, X., & Luo, Y. (2023). The correlation between digital health literacy and physical health status in middle-aged and elderly adults: The mediating effect of physical exercise behavior. *China Sport Science and Technology, 59*(12), 44–51. [In Chinese].

Lu, J., & Wei, X. (2023). Relationship between online engagements and social trust: An empirical study based on the CGSS 2018 wave. *Population Journal, 45*(1), 54–67. [In Chinses].

Lu, X., Yao, Y., & Jin, Y. (2022). Digital exclusion and functional dependence in older people: Findings from five longitudinal cohort studies. *EClinicalMedicine, 54*, 101708.

Mesch, G. S., & Talmud, I. (2011). Ethnic differences in Internet access. *Information, Communication & Society, 14*, 445–471.

Mitzner, T. L., Savla, J., Boot, W. R., Sharit, J., Charness, N., Czaja, S. J., & Rogers, W. A. (2019). Technology adoption by older adults: Findings from the PRISM trial. *The Gerontologist, 59*(1), 34–44.

National Bureau of Statistics of China. (2011). *Definitions for Chinese Regions*. Retrieved from https://www.stats.gov.cn/zt_18555/zthd/sjtjr/dejtjkfr/tjkp/202302/t20230216_1909741.htm [in Chinese]

Nordin, S., Sturge, J., Ayoub, M., Jones, A., McKee, K., Dahlberg, et al. (2021). The role of information and communication technology (ICT) for older adults' decision-making related to health, and health and social care services in daily life—A scoping review. *International Journal of Environmental Research and Public Health, 19*(1), 151.

Pan, S., & Jordan-Marsh, M. (2010). Internet use intention and adoption among Chinese older adults: From the expanded technology acceptance model perspective. *Computers in Human Behavior, 26*(5), 1111–1119.

Pick, J., Sarkar, A., & Parrish, E. (2018). Internet use and online activities in US States: Geographic disparities and socio-economic influences. In *the 51st Hawaii International Conference on System Sciences (HICSS 2018) Proceedings*, IEEE (pp. 3853–3863).

Porter, C. E., & Donthu, N. (2006). Using the technology acceptance model to explain how attitudes determine internet usage: The role of perceived access barriers and demographics. *Journal of Business Research, 59*(9), 999–1007.

Randine, P., Sharma, A., Hartvigsen, G., Johansen, H. D., & Årsand, E. (2022). Information and communication technology-based interventions for chronic diseases consultation: Scoping review. *International Journal of Medical Informatics, 163*, 104784.

Renaud, K., & van Biljon, J. (2008). Predicting technology acceptance and adoption by the elderly: A qualitative study. In *Proceedings of the 2008 annual research conference of the South African Institute of Computer Scientists and Information Technologists* (pp. 210–219).

Research on Aging, Policies and Practice. (2017). *How deep is the digital divide? ICT literacy and the role of assistive technology in helping older workers*. Facts. Retrieved from https://rapp.ualberta.ca/wp-content/uploads/sites/49/2018/04/ICT-literacy-of-older-workers_2017May.pdf?utm_source=chatgpt.com

Sakaguchi-Tang, D. K., Bosold, A. L., Choi, Y. K., & Turner, A. M. (2017). Patient portal use and experience among older adults: Systematic review. *JMIR Medical Informatics, 5*(4), e38.

Scheerder, A., van Deursen, A. J., & van Dijk, J. A. (2017). Determinants of Internet skills, uses, and outcomes: A systematic review of the second- and third-level digital divide. *Telematics and Informatics, 34*(8), 1607–1624.

Schradie, J. (2011). The digital production gap: The digital divide and Web 2.0 collide. *Poetics, 39*(2), 145–168.

Schulz, R., Wahl, H.-W., Matthews, J. T., De Vito Dabbs, A., Beach, S. R., & Czaja, S. J. (2015). Advancing the aging and technology agenda in gerontology. *The Gerontologist, 55*(5), 724–734.

Selwyn, N., Gorard, S., Furlong, J., & Madden, L. (2003). Older adults' use of information and communications technology in everyday life. *Ageing and Society, 23*(5), 561–582.

Sun, X., Yan, W., Zhou, H., Wang, Z., Zhang, X., Huang, S., & Li, L. (2020). Internet use and need for digital health technology among the elderly: A cross-sectional survey in China. *BMC Public Health, 20*, 1386.

United Nations. (2024). *The world population prospects 2024*. The United Nations. Retrieved from https://population.un.org/wpp/

van Deursen, A. J., & Helsper, E. J. (2015). The third-level digital divide: Who benefits most from being online? *Communication and Information Technologies Annual, 10*, 29–52.

van Deursen, A. J., & van Dijk, J. A. (2014). The digital divide shifts to differences in usage. *New Media & Society, 16*(3), 507–526.

van Dijk, J. (2020). *The digital divide*. Polity Press.

Venkatesh, V., Morris, M. G., Davis, G. B., & Davis, F. D. (2003). User acceptance of information technology: Toward a unified view. *MIS Quarterly, 27*(3), 425–478.

Vroman, K. G., Arthanat, S., & Lysack, C. (2015). "Who over 65 is online?" Older adults' dispositions toward information and communication technology. *Computers in Human Behavior, 43*, 156–166.

Wang, B. (2020). The determinants of the Chinese elderly's internet use from a multidimensional perspective. *Population & Development, 26*(3), 98–106. [In Chinses].

Wieczorek, M., Reinecke, R., Borrat-Besson, C., et al. (2024). Cognitive functioning and sustained internet use amid the COVID-19 pandemic: Longitudinal evidence from older adults in Switzerland. *Scientific Reports, 14*, 18815.

Wildenbos, G. A., Peute, L., & Jaspers, M. (2018). Aging barriers influencing mobile health usability for older adults: A literature based framework (MOLD-US). *International Journal of Medical Informatics, 114*, 66–75.

Wilson, J., Heinsch, M., Betts, D., Booth, D., & Kay-Lambkin, F. (2021). Barriers and facilitators to the use of ehealth by older adults: A scoping review. *BMC Public Health, 21*(1556), 1–12.

Winship, C., & Radbill, L. (1994). Sampling weights and regression analysis. *Sociological Methods & Research, 23*, 230–257.

Yuan, S., Hussain, S. A., Hales, K. D., & Cotten, S. R. (2016). What do they like? Communication preferences and patterns of older adults in the United States: The role of technology. *Educational Gerontology, 42*(3), 163–174.

Zhang, S., & Chen, G. (2013). Associates of old people's new media use among urban Chinese: A survey in Chaoyang District of Beijing. *South China Population, 28*(4), 64–72. [In Chinese].

Zhou, Y., Bai, Y., & Wang, J. (2024). The impact of internet use on health among older adults in China: A nationally representative study. *BMC Public Health, 24*, 1065.

Chapter 7
The Role of Socio-Cultural Factors and the Intention to Use Welfare Technology Among Older Adults Living in the Community: Comparison Between Korea and U.S. During the COVID-19 Pandemic

Suk-Young Kang and Jeungkun Kim

7.1 Introduction

Recent innovations in novel technology for older people have the potential to enhance their quality of life (Schulz et al., 2015), a concept encapsulated by the term "welfare technology." Welfare technology refers to the knowledge and utilization of technology that fosters "the feeling of safety, activity, participation, and independence" across various age groups (Frennert & Baudin, 2021; Lee, 2018). Welfare technology incorporates a broad approach, particularly one of embracing information and communication technology (ICT), and encompasses various devices and tools (National Institute of Child Health and Human Development, 2018).

Northern European policymakers have introduced welfare technology into their societies, presenting it as a versatile tool beneficial for people of all ages (Kim, 2018; Nordic Welfare Center, 2020). In these countries, the integration of technology includes using smart speakers for remote family connections, employing companion robots, and implementing health-monitoring sensors to link individuals with healthcare systems. As these welfare technologies advance, several devices developed in different countries are being introduced to the world market. For example, there is US-originated technology such as virtual reality headsets, Israeli-originated technology such as ElliQ (elliq.com), Korean-originated technology such as Hyodol (hyodol.com), and Japanese-originated technology such as PARO (http://www.

S.-Y. Kang (✉)
Binghamton University, Binghamton, NY, USA
e-mail: sykang@binghamton.edu

J. Kim
Kangnam University, Yongin, South Korea
e-mail: jkkim@kangnam.ac.kr

K. Wang et al. (eds.), *ICT Use and Healthy Longevity*, Advances in Studies of Aging and Health 5, https://doi.org/10.1007/978-3-031-98964-3_7

parorobots.com/). The increasing prevalence of welfare technology brings advantages, but its novelty poses challenges to our understanding of the acceptance among older adults and their families in different cultures.

Current research lacks a clear identification of the socio-cultural factors influencing the adoption of these new technologies. The reasons older adults embrace or resist novel technology may be linked to their unique life experiences and perspectives (Molzahn et al., 2010; Wang et al., 2011). While cross-cultural studies have explored the relationship between individual factors and technology acceptance among younger populations (Merchant, 2007), such investigations among older adults remain limited. This study compares the socio-cultural factors found in qualitative studies of two groups of older adults and analyzes how the socio-cultural factors are associated with their adoption between two countries.

7.2 Methods

With support from the National Research Foundation of Korea (NRF-2019S1A5a2A03048377), we conducted the project in three parts using a sequential research method (Hooyman & Kiyak, 2018) of two Focus Group Interviews (FGI) and one cross-sectional survey for comparison. We completed two qualitative studies to identify socio-cultural factors in Korea and the US, and followed with one quantitative study in both countries.

We interviewed professionals from diverse disciplines who work with older people to include their expert perspectives in identifying the socio-cultural factors that can improve understanding of new technology use. Following these individual interviews with twenty (20) professionals (10 in Korea and 10 in the US), we conducted focus group interviews with 25 people, 65 and older, living in the community (15 in Korea and 10 in the US—5 people in the US were unable to attend due to COVID-19). In the US, we held these just before the lockdown in March 2020, while social distancing was used to meet with 15 people in Korea. Financial incentives were provided: $80 per in-depth interview with professionals and $40 per each focus group participant.

7.2.1 Qualitative Interviews in Korea and US

Qualitative data analysis was conducted based on the individual interviews with experts and the focus group interviews with older adults to explore and identify socio-cultural factors affecting the acceptance and utilization of welfare technology among older populations in Korea and the United States. The results were used to conceptualize and measure differences among those socio-cultural factors (Kang et al., 2021).

Seven (7) primary themes were identified from the qualitative data analysis coding results: (1) Self-determination or peer influence or social influence; (2) Same-family-oriented culture; (3) Benefit compared to cost - Pragmatism (cost); (4) Low context culture vs. high context culture; (5) Importance of privacy; (6) Improvement of individual's quality of life and a culture of pursuing more indulgence-Fun; and (7) A horizontal culture that does not easily conform to authority (less hierarchical) vs a vertical culture that conforms (Hoftstede Insights, 2021).

7.2.2 *Measurement Developed from Qualitative Study*

Family-oriented culture was reported as similar for both groups. For the remaining six (6) primary themes, we used a 5-point Likert scale (1 = strongly disagree to 5 = strongly agree) for the following questions in Table 7.1:

In addition, questions in Table 7.2 were used to gather their opinions on technology and robots.

7.3 Results from Cross-Sectional Quantitative Study

Quantitative data results suggest that there are differences in the intention to use welfare technology among older adults in these two countries. All participants were provided with $40 gift cards to incentivize individual participation in the quantitative survey. Due to the COVID-19 pandemic, these were provided by mail. In the US, cards were sent by first-class mail and over 90 percent of the participants acknowledged receipt, also by mail. In Korea, cards were sent via registered mail.

7.3.1 *Demographic Background of Participants in Korea and US*

A total of 334 people, 65 and over, received and responded to the survey, including 154 from Korea and 180 from the United States. The demographic characteristics of participants were reported in the study (Kim & Kang, 2022a, b) and are summarized below. Several demographics are similar for both groups: The average age is 72.7 from Korea and 73.7 from the US; women accounted for approximately 70% of respondents, and men approximately 30% for both Korea and the US; and the proportion of married people in both countries was the highest in the category, at 51.9% in Korea and 44.4% in the United States. The proportion of singles in the United States was 11.1%, which was higher than 3.2% in Korea (Kim & Kang, 2022a, b).

Table 7.1 Measurement questions with themes from two qualitative studies

Themes from qualitative studies	Questions used in quantitative survey
Self-determination or peer influence or social influence	When I see other people using welfare technology devices, I want to use them too
	Current newspaper, media, or internet makes me want to use welfare technology devices
Benefit compared to cost—Pragmatism (cost)	The benefit of using welfare technology devices is bigger than the cost
	The benefit of using welfare technology devices is bigger than the effort I put in to use them
Low context culture vs. high context culture	When I deliver my opinions, I tend to clarify my point first
	When I deliver my opinions, I am sensitive to the situation, atmosphere, and emotions of others
Importance of privacy	I feel uncomfortable with the possibility that my private and personal information may be leaked while using welfare technology devices
	I am worried that others may look at my private and personal information that I shared through welfare technology devices
Trust in government	Generally, I trust the government to keep my private and personal information gained from welfare technology devices
	Generally, I trust the government to use my private and personal information gained from welfare technology devices for public interests
Trust in private corporations	Generally, I trust private corporations to keep my private and personal information gained from welfare technology devices
	Generally, I trust private corporations to use my private and personal information gained from welfare technology devices for public interests
Improvement of individual's quality of life	I will use welfare technology devices to find new ways to manage my health
	I will use welfare technology devices to manage my health
Culture of pursuing more indulgence—Fun	I will use welfare technology devices to find new fun activities to do
	To have fun, I will use welfare technology devices
A horizontal culture that does not easily conform to authority (less hierarchical) vs vertical culture that conforms—Collectivism	Individuals should sacrifice self-interest for the group
	Group success is more important than individual success

The level of education showed the greatest difference between Korean and American respondents, and was statistically significant. The proportion of US respondents with a high school diploma or higher (including high school graduation and college graduation) was higher than expected at 100%, while in Korea it was 67.5% (Kim & Kang, 2022a, b).

Table 7.2 Measurement questions related to opinions on technology, science and robots

Themes	Questions used in quantitative survey
Technology and science	Technology makes our life healthier and more comfortable
	Technology solves more problems than it creates
	Technology performs more positive functions than negative ones
Opinions on robots	Robots are good for our society because they are helpful for human beings
	Robots are necessary because they can do dangerous or difficult tasks for humans
	Robots will take jobs away from humans
Technology support	I think I can get detailed explanations when I use welfare technology devices
	When I encounter a difficult issue while using welfare technology devices, I think I can get help from an expert or people around me
Future-oriented culture	Today's sacrifice will guarantee success in the future
	It is important to work hard today for future success

Table 7.3 Comparison of health conditions

	Korea	U.S.	*P* value
	N = 154	N = 180	
	M (SD)	M (SD)	
Self-rated physical health (1–5)	3.29 (0.98)	3.34 (0.79)	No sig
Aging anxiety (5–25)	**7.19 (4.06)**	**10.97 (3.61)**	**<0.001**
Feeling lonely (0–6)	**3.16 (1.75)**	**2.02 (1.68)**	**<0.001**
Depression (0–5)	**1.12 (1.32)**	**0.68 (1.10)**	**<0.001**

7.3.2 Comparison of Health Status

Table 7.3 shows comparison results of physical- and mental-health-related status.

There was no statistically significant difference between Korean and American respondents self-rated physical health. We used items related to psychological concerns from the 20-item Anxiety about Aging Scale (Lasher & Faulkender, 1993). The mean of the Aging Anxiety score was significantly higher for American respondents than for Korean respondents. The means of the DeJong Gierveld Loneliness Scores (De Jong Gierveld & Van Tilburg, 2006) and the 5-item GDS scores were significantly higher for Korean respondents than for American respondents.

To measure technology-related knowledge and experience (Table 7.4), participants were asked about their capacity to use a smartphone and computer compared to peers. There was no statistically significant difference between the two groups for smartphone use. For computer use, however, the reported scores among participants were statistically significant, with US respondents higher (Kim & Kang, 2022a, b).

In measuring technology-related usage ability (1–10 points) between Korean and American seniors, there was no significant difference in smartphone usage ability, but there was a slight difference in computer usage ability. The average smartphone

Table 7.4 Comparison of technology-related knowledge and experience

	Korea	U.S.	*P* value
	N = 154	N = 180	
Technology-related knowledge and experience (Range 1 = very low to 10 = very high)	M (SD)	M (SD)	
How would you rate your ability to use smartphone functions other than making phone calls compared to your peers?	5.69 (2.35)	5.36 (2.96)	No sig.
Compared to your peers, how would you rate your ability to use smartphone applications for such activities as sending text messages, watching videos, listening to radio, or playing games?	5.61 (2.50)	5.56 (3.19)	No sig.
Compared to your peers, how would you rate your ability to use a computer for internet search or email messages?	**4.59 (2.91)**	**6.89 (2.95)**	**<0.001**
How would you rate your ability to use computer software programs such as Microsoft Word or Excel compared to your peers?	**4.10 (2.71)**	**5.02 (3.07)**	**0.004**

use ability was located between 5 and 6 points, which is the middle level in both countries, but the computer use ability of the Korean participants was 4.59 points, lower than the 6.89 points of the American respondents, a statistically significant difference.

To learn their opinions about welfare technology, we used the definition of Technology for Older People (TOP) as welfare technology. TOP is defined as devices that can be helpful for older people to live independently. Some of these devices provide appointment notifications and/or schedule alarms for medications. They can also interact as conversation partners and even provide help in case of an emergency. For example, TOP can be a smartphone that allows a person who lives alone to have a video phone call with family members or friends. An Artificial Intelligence (AI) speaker can communicate with them and turn on the music that they would like to listen to. TOP can also be a device that senses users' movement in their home and calls 911 (119 in Korea) in case of an emergency such as a fall. Social robots (robots that can interact with you) or Virtual Reality (VR) headsets are other examples of TOP.

After the research team members provided participants with the definition of welfare technology and showed pictures of six (6) devices to offer a better and more tangible idea of what they are, respondents were asked to share their opinions on socio-cultural factors, thoughts about science and technology, and their views about robots, utilizing a 5-point Likert scale (1 = Strongly disagree to 5 = Strongly Agree).

7.3.3 Comparison of Socio-Cultural Factors

In the results summarized in Table 7.5, significant differences were observed between Korean and American respondents across various dimensions. Korean respondents demonstrated stronger agreement on questions related to

Table 7.5 Comparison of the socio-cultural themes

	Korea	U.S.	*P* value
	N = 154	N = 180	
Self-determination vs. peer influence or social influence			
When I see other people using welfare technology devices, I want to use them too	**3.71**	**3.00**	**<0.001**
Current newspaper, media, or internet makes me want to use welfare technology devices	**3.52**	**2.87**	**<0.001**
Benefit compared to cost			
The benefit of using welfare technology devices is bigger than the cost	**3.55**	**3.11**	**<0.001**
The benefit of using welfare technology devices is bigger than the effort I put in to use them	**3.65**	**3.28**	**0.002**
Low-context vs. high-context culture			
When I deliver my opinions, I tend to clarify my point first	**3.74**	3.49	**0.009**
When I deliver my opinions, I am sensitive to the situation, atmosphere, and emotions of others	3.68	**3.91**	**0.008**
Importance of privacy			
I feel uncomfortable with the possibility that my private and personal information may be leaked while using welfare technology devices	**2.96**	**3.7**	**<0.001**
I am worried that others may look at my private and personal information that I shared through welfare technology devices	**2.82**	**3.74**	**<0.001**
Trust in government			
Generally, I trust the government to keep my private and personal information gained from TOP devices	**3.09**	**2.60**	**<0.001**
Generally, I trust the government to use my private and personal information gained from TOP devices for public interests	**3.14**	**2.44**	**<0.001**
Trust in private corporations			
Generally, I trust private corporations to keep my private and personal information gained from TOP devices	2.23	2.25	n.s.
Generally, I trust private corporations to use my private and personal information gained from TOP devices for public interests	**2.48**	**2.16**	**0.008**
Motivation for health			
I will use welfare technology devices to find new ways to manage my health	**4.01**	**3.04**	**<0.001**
I will use welfare technology devices to manage my health	**3.99**	**2.97**	**<0.001**
Fun—Culture of pursuing more indulgence			
I will use welfare technology devices to find new fun activities to do	**3.52**	**2.87**	**<0.001**
To have fun, I will use welfare technology devices	**3.46**	**2.77**	**<0.001**
Collectivism			
Individuals should sacrifice self-interest for the group	**3.14**	**2.77**	**0.002**
Group success is more important than individual success	**3.36**	**2.91**	**<0.001**

self-determination, peer influence, and social influence compared to their American counterparts, with statistically significant differences (M = 3.71 vs. M = 3.00 and M = 3.52 vs. M = 2.87, $p < 0.001$). Similarly, Korean respondents agreed more on benefit vs. cost-related questions (M = 3.55 vs. M = 3.11, $p = 0.002$ and M = 3.65 vs. M = 3.28, $p < 0.001$). In the context of low-context vs. high-context culture, Korean respondents were more likely to clarify their points first (M = 3.74 vs. M = 3.49, $p = 0.009$), while American respondents showed greater sensitivity to situational and emotional cues when expressing opinions (M = 3.91 vs. M = 3.68, $p = 0.008$). Regarding privacy, American respondents placed higher importance on privacy-related issues (M = 3.70 vs. M = 2.96 and M = 3.74 vs. M = 2.82, $p < 0.001$), whereas Korean respondents expressed greater trust in the government (M = 3.09 vs. M = 2.60 and M = 3.14 vs. M = 2.44, $p < 0.001$) and slightly higher trust in private corporations on one of two questions (M = 2.48 vs. M = 2.16, $p = 0.008$). Korean respondents also reported stronger motivation for health-related behaviors (M = 4.01 vs. M = 3.04 and M = 3.99 vs. M = 2.97, $p < 0.001$) and greater agreement on fun-related questions (M = 3.52 vs. M = 2.87 and M = 3.46 vs. M = 2.77, $p < 0.001$). Finally, Korean respondents scored higher on collectivism-related measures (M = 3.14 vs. M = 2.77 and M = 3.36 vs. M = 2.91, $p < 0.001$), highlighting cultural differences in these domains.

7.3.4 Comparison of Opinions on Technologies and Future

In the results presented in Table 7.6, notable differences emerged between Korean and American respondents regarding their opinions on technology, robots, technology support, and future-oriented culture. Korean respondents expressed more positive views toward technology, agreeing significantly more on three related questions compared to American respondents (M = 4.25 vs. M = 3.74, M = 4.00 vs. M = 3.48, and M = 4.14 vs. M = 3.63, $p < 0.001$). Similarly, Korean respondents were more likely to agree that robots are good (M = 3.63 vs. M = 3.20, $p < 0.001$) and necessary (M = 4.08 vs. M = 3.66, $p < 0.001$), while American respondents were more concerned that robots would take jobs away from humans (M = 3.71 vs. M = 2.16, $p < 0.001$). Additionally, Korean respondents showed stronger agreement on questions related to technology support, indicating a greater reliance on or satisfaction with technological assistance (M = 3.72 vs. M = 2.96 and M = 3.91 vs. M = 3.31, $p < 0.001$). Finally, Korean respondents demonstrated a more future-oriented mindset, agreeing more on future-related questions compared to American respondents (M = 3.76 vs. M = 2.99 and M = 4.47 vs. M = 3.89, $p < 0.001$). These findings highlight distinct cultural perspectives on technology, robotics, and future orientation between the two groups.

Table 7.6 Comparison of the opinions on technology, science, robots, and future

	Korea	U.S.	*P* value
	N = 154	N = 180	
Trust in science or positivism toward technology			
Technology makes our life healthier and more comfortable	**4.25**	**3.74**	**<0.001**
Technology solves more problems than it creates.	**4.00**	**3.48**	**<0.001**
Technology performs more positive functions than negative ones.	**4.14**	**3.63**	**<0.001**
Robots			
Robots are good for our society because they are helpful for human beings	**3.63**	**3.20**	**<0.001**
Robots are necessary because they can do dangerous or difficult tasks for humans	**4.08**	**3.66**	**<0.001**
Robots will take away jobs from humans	**2.16**	**3.71**	**<0.001**
Technology support			
I think I can get detailed explanations when I use welfare technology devices	**3.72**	**2.96**	**<0.001**
When I encounter a difficult issue while using welfare technology devices, I think I can receive help from an expert or people around me	**3.91**	**3.31**	**<0.001**
Future-oriented culture			
Today's sacrifice will guarantee success in the future	**3.76**	**2.99**	**<0.001**
It is important to work hard today for future success	**4.47**	**3.89**	**<0.001**

7.4 Discussion

The findings of this study reveal significant differences in technology-related knowledge, experiences, and socio-cultural attitudes between older adults in Korea and the United States. These differences are shaped by cultural, economic, and societal factors, which influence how older adults perceive and adopt welfare technology. Below, we discuss the key themes and implications of the findings.

7.4.1 *Technology-Related Knowledge and Experience*

The results suggest that differences in smartphone and computer use may reflect variations in life experiences with technology. Smartphones are widely accepted and used by older adults in both countries, likely due to their accessibility and ease of use. However, computers may not be as necessary or commonly used after retirement, particularly among older adults. This disparity highlights the importance of considering the specific technological experiences and needs of older populations when designing and implementing welfare technology solutions.

7.4.2 Comparison of Socio-Cultural Themes

Cultural differences play a significant role in shaping attitudes toward welfare technology. In the United States, self-determination is a key factor in technology adoption, with older adults making decisions based on their own needs rather than external influences. In contrast, Korean respondents are more likely to adopt technology based on community decision-making or social necessity, reflecting the influence of their social networks. This aligns with the quantitative findings, which suggest that Koreans are more receptive to welfare technology when it is introduced or encouraged by others.

Another key finding relates to the balance between benefit and cost. While qualitative data suggested that Americans are more likely to weigh the pros and cons of technology adoption, the quantitative results indicated that Koreans are more willing to use welfare technology based on their own cost-benefit analysis. This discrepancy may be influenced by the Korean government's efforts to provide affordable technology devices for older adults, particularly given the high poverty rate in this demographic (OECD, 2023).

Cultural differences in communication styles also emerged as a significant factor. In the United States, a low-context culture (Hall, 1981), clear explanations and step-by-step manuals are critical for building trust and facilitating the use of welfare technology. In Korea, a high-context culture, older adults may prefer technology that does not require complex explanations, as they tend to prioritize understanding and expressing emotions over logical persuasion. However, the quantitative findings did not fully align with this cultural framework, suggesting that other factors, such as accessibility or prior experience, may also play a role.

Privacy and trust were additional areas of divergence. American respondents placed a higher value on privacy, while Koreans expressed greater trust in the government. This difference may explain the Korean government's success in implementing technology-driven initiatives, such as contact tracing during the COVID-19 pandemic. In contrast, trust in institutions and large corporations is notably low in the United States, as evidenced by recent Gallup surveys (Fleck, 2024). Interestingly, there was no significant difference in trust in private corporations between the two groups, though Koreans were more likely to believe that corporations would use their personal information for public benefit.

Finally, the study highlighted differences in motivation for health, pursuit of fun, and collectivism. Korean respondents demonstrated a stronger motivation to use welfare technology for health management, reflecting a desire to prevent age-related health risks. They also reported a greater inclination toward fun activities, contrary to the qualitative findings. Additionally, Korean respondents exhibited stronger collectivist tendencies, likely influenced by their experiences during Korea's group-centered economic development (Kim, 1998). In contrast, American culture's individualistic tendencies and resistance to authority, particularly in response to government-led initiatives, may hinder the adoption of welfare technology.

7.4.3 Comparison of Additional Opinions

Korean respondents reported greater access to support for using welfare technology and more favorable attitudes toward robots and new technology. This may be attributed to Korea's strong culture of respect for older adults and the availability of technological support systems. In contrast, American respondents exhibited lower expectations for the future, potentially due to the impact of COVID-19 or a lack of societal support for older adults. These findings highlight the importance of fostering a supportive environment for older adults to encourage technology adoption.

7.4.4 Conclusions and Recommendations for Future Actions

Older adults are a diverse group (Boot et al., 2021), and their willingness to adopt new technology is influenced by factors such as gender, culture, socio-economic status, and past experiences. Skill attainment, literacy, and numeracy are particularly important considerations when developing and introducing new technologies. Additionally, past traumatic experiences with technology, such as financial exploitation or identity theft, can create barriers to adoption and must be addressed through targeted interventions.

The role of messengers in delivering new technology is critical. Demonstrating technology with evidence-based engagement can help build trust and encourage adoption. Future studies should explore the impact of recent advancements in technology, such as Generative AI (e.g., Bard or ChatGPT), which have the potential to significantly impact older adults, particularly those with fixed incomes who may struggle to afford new technologies.

Finally, service providers should focus on disseminating information about policy changes, such as the Affordable Connectivity Program (ACP) in the United States, to ensure that eligible individuals can navigate and benefit from these initiatives. By addressing these factors, policymakers and technology developers can create more inclusive and effective solutions for older adults.

References

Boot, W. R., Charness, N., Czaja, S. J., & Rogers, W. A. (2021). *Designing for older adults: Case studies, methods, and tools*. CRC Press Taylor & Francis Group.

De Jong Gierveld, J., & Van Tilburg, T. (2006). A 6-item scale for overall, emotional, and social loneliness: Confirmatory tests on survey data. *Research on Aging, 28*(5), 582–598. https://doi.org/10.1177/0164027506289723

Fleck, A. (2024). *Confidence in Institutions: The institutions Americans trust most and least*. https://www.statista.com/chart/14514/the-institutions-americans-trust-most-and-least/?utm_source=Statista+Newsletters&utm_campaign=4ec4d7f33c-All_InfographTicker_daily_

COM_PM_KW37_2023_Th_COPY&utm_medium=email&utm_term=0_662f7ed75e-4ec4d7f33c-340328886

Frennert, S., & Baudin, K. (2021). The concept of welfare technology in Swedish municipal eldercare. *Disability and Rehabilitation, 43*(9), 1220–1227. https://doi.org/10.1080/09638288.2019.1661035

Hall, E. T. (1981). *Beyond culture*. Anchor Book.

Hofstede Insights. (2021). *Country comparison*. https://www.hofstede-insights.com/country-comparis on/south-korea/

Hooyman, N. R., & Kiyak, H. A. (2018). *Social gerontology: A multidisciplinary perspective* (10th ed.). Pearson.

Kang, S. Y., Kim, J. K., Winthal, J., & Lenz, R. (2021). An analysis of professionals' perspectives on the roles of socio-cultural factors and welfare technology among older adults in the US. *Korea Convergence Society, 12*(8), 215–228. https://doi.org/10.15207/JKCS.2021.12.8.215

Kim, W. B. (1998). Family, social relations, and Asian capitalism. *Journal of International and Area Studies, 5*(1), 65–79.

Kim, J. K. (2018). Study on welfare technology and welfare technology assessment for older adults. *Journal of Korea Contents Association, 5*, 156–166.

Kim, J. K., & Kang, S. Y. (2022a). Cross-national differences in the intention to use of welfare technology among older adults between Korea and the U.S.: Focusing on technology acceptance model (written in Korean language). *Journal of Korea Convergence Society, 13*(4), 421–432. https://doi.org/10.15207/JKCS.2022.13.04.421

Kim, J. K., & Kang, S. Y. (2022b). The effect of psychological aging anxiety on depression with mediating effect of ability to use a smart-phone (written in Korean language). *Korean Journal of Gerontological Social Welfare, 77*(4), 273–300. https://doi.org/10.21194/kjgsw.77.4.202212.273

Lasher, K. P., & Faulkender, P. J. (1993). Measurement of aging anxiety: Development of the anxiety about aging scale. *The International Journal of Aging and Human Development, 37*(4), 247–259.

Lee, J. A. (2018). Trend and challenges of using welfare technology in elderly care. *International Journal of Contents, 14*(2), 30–34. https://doi.org/10.5392/IJoC.2018.14.2.030

Merchant, S. (2007). Exploring the influence of cultural values on the acceptance of information technology: An application of the technology acceptance model. *Issues in Informing Science and Information Technology, 4*, 430–443.

Molzahn, A. E., Kalfoss, M., Schick, M. K., & Skevington, S. M. (2010). Comparing the importance of different aspects of quality of life to older adults across diverse culture. *Age and Ageing, 40*(2), 192–199.

National Institute of Child Health and Human Development. (2018). *What are some types of assistive devices and how are they used?* Retrieved from https://www.nichd.nih.gov/health/topics/rehabtech/conditioninfo/device

Nordic Welfare Center. (2020). *Welfare technology*. Retrieved from https://nordicwelfare.org/en/welfare-policy/welfare-technology/#:~:text=Welfare%20technology%20is%20all%20%20technology,a%20disability%20or%20the%20elderly

OECD. (2023). *Pensions at a glance 2023: OECD and G20 indicators*. OECD Publishing. https://doi.org/10.1787/678055dd-en

Schulz, R., Wahl, H. W., Matthews, J. T., Dabbs, A. D. V., Beach, S. R., & Czaja, S. (2015). Advancing the aging and technology agenda in gerontology. *The Gerontologist, 55*(5), 724–734. https://doi.org/10.1093/geront/gnu071

Wang, L., Rau, P. L. P., & Salvendy, G. (2011). A cross-culture study on older adults' information technology acceptance. *International Journal of Mobile Communications, 9*(5), 421–220.

Chapter 8
Multinational Comparisons of Factors Associated with Internet Use Among Older Adults

Danan Gu, Qiushi Feng, Kun Wang, Haiyan Zhu, and Summer Xiayu Chen

8.1 Introduction

The digital revolution has transformed global connectivity, with internet access emerging as a critical determinant of social, economic, and health outcomes in daily life. By February 2025, approximately 5.6 billion people, accounting for 68% of the global population, were using the internet (Kemp, 2025), yet internet access remains stratified across geographic, economic, and generational lines (ITU, 2024; Kemp, 2025; Petrosyan, 2024). While some more developed nations, such as the United States and Singapore, have boasted near-universal broadband penetration, many developing countries are confronting persistent infrastructural deficits, affordability

D. Gu (✉)
Population Division, UN Department of Economic and Social Affairs, New York, NY, USA
e-mail: gudanan@yahoo.com

Q. Feng
Centre for Family and Population Research/Department of Sociology and Anthropology, National University of Singapore, Singapore, Singapore
e-mail: socfq@nus.edu.sg

K. Wang
Department of Social Work, College of Arts and Sciences, University of Alabama at Birmingham, Birmingham, AL, USA
e-mail: kw2@uab.edu

H. Zhu
Department of Sociology, Virginia Tech, Blacksburg, VA, USA
e-mail: zhuh@vt.edu

S. X. Chen
School of Social Work, University of Illinois Urbana-Champaign, Champaign, IL, USA
e-mail: xiayuyc2@illinois.edu

K. Wang et al. (eds.), *ICT Use and Healthy Longevity*, Advances in Studies of Aging and Health 5, https://doi.org/10.1007/978-3-031-98964-3_8

challenges, and sociocultural barriers (GSMA, 2023; United Nations, 2023; World Bank, 2025; also see Chap. 2).

These disparities are particularly pronounced among older adults. While younger generations have largely grown up with these digital tools (see Chap. 2), a significant portion of the older population remains marginalized in an increasingly digital world, experiencing a digital divide, marked by disadvantages in access, skills, and usage patterns (Kemp, 2025; also see Chaps. 2 and 9). Nevertheless, they are increasingly turning to internet technologies for social connectivity, health management, information access, and daily tasks (Hunsaker & Hargittai, 2018; Kakulla, 2021; see Chaps. 2 and 14). Promoting digital inclusion for the older population is therefore crucial, not only to reduce social isolation and foster social participation, but also to support healthy aging, improve quality of life, and enhance access to essential services such as healthcare and social support (Mohan et al., 2024).

As population aging becomes a global phenomenon, understanding how older adults engage with technology has emerged as a critical issue of international significance. However, the digital experiences of older adults vary markedly across countries, influenced by differing levels of socioeconomic development, cultural norms, policy frameworks, and the availability of digital infrastructure (Chinn & Fairlie, 2007; ITU, 2021, 2023, 2024; Li et al., 2025; Renaud & van Biljon, 2008; van Dijk, 2005, 2020; Zhang, 2023; see also Chaps. 3 and 4). Although a growing number of studies have undertaken cross-national comparisons, these efforts remain narrow in scope. Most focus on only two countries (e.g., Xie & Jaeger, 2008), a small group of nations (e.g., Ono & Zavodny, 2007), specific regions (e.g., Alvarez-Galvez et al., 2020; Coley et al., 2022; Richard et al., 2019; Wang et al., 2022), or a particular economic context, either developing countries (Donner, 2008; Hilbert, 2011; Steyn & van Greunen, 2015) or developed ones (Büchi et al., 2016; Goodman-Deane et al., 2024). While several studies (e.g., Lei et al., 2024; Li, 2024; Lu et al., 2022; Wang et al., 2025) have used or reviewed multinational datasets that include both developed and developing countries across diverse cultures, they have primarily focused on the association between internet use and health outcomes, without examining the factors influencing internet use itself. Consequently, studies remain scarce, that offer truly comprehensive international perspectives on the associates of internet use while taking into account variations in national wealth, education systems, and digital policies across different geographic regions. This leaves substantial gaps in our understanding of how macro-level structures interact with individual-level characteristics to shape digital engagement in later life (Bhuiyan et al., 2025; Gulati & Yates, 2012).

A multinational approach that includes countries from different geographic regions and from different economic contexts is thus important for assessing whether patterns observed in Western contexts apply elsewhere in response to local cultural and structural conditions (Li et al., 2025). Comparative studies of this nature are essential for identifying both shared challenges and effective strategies that transcend national boundaries (Schroeder et al., 2023). Moreover, multinational comparisons provide critical insights to inform culturally sensitive, contextually appropriate policies aimed at fostering digital inclusion among aging populations worldwide (United Nations, 2023).

This chapter presents a multinational comparative study of internet use among older adults across 31 countries, which include Brazil, China, India, Singapore, the United States, and 26 European nations participating in the Survey of Health, Ageing and Retirement in Europe (SHARE). Drawing on these wide-ranging datasets, the study examines how individual-level factors associated with internet use vary across national contexts. In doing so, it offers profound insights into the structural and cultural roots of the digital divide between the Global South and the Global North. By addressing key gaps in the literature, this chapter contributes to both theoretical understandings of digital inclusion and practical strategies for achieving the Sustainable Development Goals (SDGs) and fostering inclusive, age-friendly digital futures across the globe.

8.1.1 Literature Review

Internet use among older adults is a complex, multifactorial phenomenon influenced by demographic, socioeconomic, family/social support, and health-related factors. Previous multinational studies in the current literature have revealed commonalities and differences in these factors across diverse contexts, highlighting the nuanced interplay between individual characteristics and broader structural and cultural conditions. Below, we summarize key findings in the existing literature.

Demographic Factors

Age emerges as a consistent demographic determinant shaping internet adoption within older populations globally. Young-old adults (typically those aged 60–74 years old) are more likely to use the internet than their old-old (those aged 75–84 years old) or oldest-old (those aged 85 years or older) counterparts. This gradient reflects cohort effects and differing levels of exposure to digital technologies over the life course (Chen et al., 2015; König et al., 2018), which is documented in both developed and developing countries, including the United States, Europe, China, and Brazil, underscoring a pervasive trend whereby advancing age correlates with lower digital engagement (Bhuiyan et al., 2025; da Silva et al., 2023; Li & Luximon, 2018; Pew Research Center, 2017; Xie & Jaeger, 2008). The variation is also partly explained by cognitive and physical declines that can limit usability and confidence with digital tools among the old-old populations (Benge & Scullin, 2025; Hunsaker & Hargittai, 2018). Encouragingly, increasing evidence has shown that internet adoption is increasing over time among the younger-old cohorts, potentially narrowing intergenerational digital divides (Kemp, 2025; Pew Research Center, 2022; also see Chap. 2).

Gender differences in internet use among older adults are more complex and context dependent. In some Western contexts, older women show lower internet use rates compared to men, attributed to historical disparities in education and occupational exposure to technology (Choi & DiNitto, 2013; Richard et al., 2019). The similar pattern has also been observed among developing Asian countries, such as China and India, where older women remain less likely to use the internet due to persistent educational and occupational disadvantages (Jena & Paltasingh, 2025; also see Chap. 6). However, recent studies in developed countries indicate that these gender gaps are narrowing, especially among younger cohorts of older adults (König et al., 2018; Wang et al., 2024a). In some contexts, older women are now more likely than men to use specific digital tools, such as social media (Schehl et al., 2019; Yu et al., 2016; Wang et al., 2024a). These shifts may reflect changing generational experiences and evolving social roles, as older women often report higher levels of social engagement than men, particularly in activities centered on communication and relationships (Choi et al., 2021; Wang et al., 2024b).

Urban-rural digital divides persist in many countries, where urban residents benefit from improved infrastructure and digital literacy programs, in contrast to their rural counterparts facing connectivity challenges and sparse technical support (Chen et al., 2015; ITU, 2024). In China, 37% of urban older adults used smartphones for internet access in 2020, whereas rural adoption lagged behind at 20%, reflecting disparities in infrastructural and social support (Li & Luximon, 2018). The urban-rural divide is also evident in Brazil and India, where regionally targeted digital inclusion initiatives have been proposed (Jena & Paltasingh, 2025; Nishijima et al., 2017).

Socioeconomic Factors

Socioeconomic status (SES) consistently ranks as the strongest predictor of internet adoption and use intensity among older adults across countries, cutting across diverse geopolitical and economic contexts (König et al., 2018; Pew Research Center, 2017). Education and income play pivotal roles by influencing both access to digital technology and the digital literacy and skills necessary for meaningful online engagements (Choi & DiNitto, 2013; da Silva et al., 2023). Longitudinal analyses further suggest that socioeconomic disparities accumulate over the life-course, with those experiencing persistent SES advantages exhibiting higher digital engagement into older age (Hu & Xu, 2024; Silver, 2013; Wang et al., 2024a).

In developed countries such as the United States and Europe, older adults with higher levels of education and income are substantially more likely to use the internet (Pew Research Center, 2014; OECD, 2021). For instance, 94% of American older adults earning $75,000 or more annually in 2016 reported regular internet use, compared to only 46% among those earning less than $30,000 (Pew Research Center, 2017). In these contexts, higher-income older adults often tend to use the internet for a wide range of activities, including health management, social networking, education, and financial tasks, whereas those with lower-income tend to focus narrowly on communication or entertainment (Choi & DiNitto, 2013; Pew Research Center, 2017).

In developing countries, similar SES gradients are observed, but additional barriers, such as inadequate infrastructure and limited access to quality education, exacerbate the digital divide. Cost considerations, such as device affordability and internet subscription fees, remain key barriers for older adults in these countries (da Silva et al., 2023; Jena & Paltasingh, 2025). In Brazil and India, for example, lower income levels and educational attainment combined with limited and unreliable internet access and high relative cost, further prevent older adults from digital engagement (Chan et al., 2023; da Silva et al., 2023; Gallo et al., 2024; Nishijima et al., 2017; William & Murugesh, 2018). In China, SES not only affects internet access but also shapes the scope of internet use and the availability of social and technical support for digital engagement (Chen et al., 2015; Li & Luximon, 2018; see Chap. 6).

Family and Social Support Factors

Family and social support networks are widely recognized as key enablers to internet use among older adults, with their influence varying across cultural and regional contexts. In general, family members and peers support older adults' digital engagement by offering emotional encouragement, instrumental assistance, and informal digital literacy training (Mo et al., 2025; Zhang, 2023). This support not only facilitates initial adoption but also builds confidence and competence in navigating online activities (Xiong & Zuo, 2019).

Evidence from China, Brazil, and the United States shows that older adults who receive support from younger family members or friends are more likely to become regular internet users, particularly for social communication and health-related purposes (Chen et al., 2015; William & Murugesh, 2018). In China, such family-based support networks have been found to reduce depression and loneliness by promoting online social participation, thereby enhancing older adults' mental well-being (Wang et al., 2023; Zhang et al., 2024). In the United States, support from family and peers similarly fosters internet use and social connection among older adults (Heo et al., 2015). Among low-income, homebound American older adults, lack of family support is frequently cited as a major barrier to digital inclusion, while those with regular assistance are more likely to use the internet consistently (Choi & DiNitto, 2013).

The nature of social support also varies by geographic context, especially between urban and rural areas. For example, in rural China, family support is often the primary facilitator of digital engagement, compensating for limited formal infrastructure or public digital literacy resources, while in urban areas where community services are more accessible, peer support from friends plays a more prominent role (Yiting et al., 2023).

Importantly, the relationship between internet use and social support is reciprocal. Internet use fosters social engagement, reduces loneliness, and enhances psychological well-being, while socially active older adults are more likely to adopt and sustain digital behaviors (Anderberg et al., 2021; Zhang & Li, 2022). This dynamic has been documented across Europe, North America, and Asia, reinforcing the broader psychosocial benefits of digital inclusion (Zhang, 2023; Wang et al., 2022). However, many digital literacy programs fail to account for disparities in social support availability, particularly among rural, low-income, or socially isolated older adults, potentially perpetuating usage gaps (OECD, 2021).

Health Factors

Health status, encompassing physical, cognitive, and sensory capabilities, plays a critical role in shaping internet use among older adults worldwide. Declining health can pose significant barriers to technology adoption by limiting fine motor skills, vision, hearing, and cognitive function, necessary for effective digital engagement (Chen et al., 2015; Hunsaker & Hargittai, 2018). Older adults with disabilities or chronic conditions consistently exhibit lower rates of internet use, underscoring the need for accessible technology design and health-sensitive digital literacy support (Czaja et al., 2006).

At the same time, internet use is positively associated with a range of health outcomes in the later life. Studies in China, Brazil, and Europe demonstrate that internet use is associated with improved self-rated health, reduced depression, enhanced cognitive functioning, and greater health literacy among older adults (Chen et al., 2015; da Silva et al., 2023; Heo et al., 2015; Mohan et al., 2024; Yiting et al., 2023). These benefits are often related to the functional use of the internet, such as actively seeking health information, accessing telehealth services, managing medications, and maintaining social connections—all contributing to independence and healthy aging (Wong et al., 2014; Zhang, 2023).

In sum, findings in the existing literature indicate that across countries, demographic and socioeconomic factors such as age, education, income, and urban residence consistently predict older adults' internet use. Family and social support can act as facilitators depending on cultural and geographic contexts. These social networks not only enable digital adoption but also mediate its broader benefits for health and well-being. Health status presents a dual influence: while physical, cognitive, and sensory limitations can hinder internet use, digital engagement can in turn promote better health outcomes, including improved mental health, cognitive functioning, and access to care. Differences in internet access and usage patterns are shaped by structural disparities between developed and developing countries, with infrastructure, affordability, and policy environments. Regional disparities within countries, such as the urban-rural divide, further complicate the access and usage patterns. These findings underscore the need for nuanced, culturally sensitive approaches to promote equitable digital inclusion among older populations worldwide.

8.1.2 Research Questions

Despite growing interest in aging and technology, existing research suffers from several critical limitations. Many studies are confined to specific geographic regions or single-country contexts, limiting their ability to offer a global perspective of internet use on how older adults engage with digital technologies. Moreover, much of the existing literature overlooks the complex interplay of demographic, socioeconomic, and health-related factors that shape internet adoption across different cultural and economic settings. These gaps hinder the comprehensive understanding of how various macro-level influences affect older adults' digital engagement, especially in diverse national and regional contexts.

Motivated by these gaps, this study is driven by the following core objectives: (1) to empirically compare the prevalence of internet use and its associated factors among older adults in economically and culturally diverse nations; (2) to provide actionable recommendations for policymakers to design inclusive digital strategies that align with regional realities. Guided by these objectives, the study addresses the following research questions: (1) How does the prevalence of internet use among older adults vary across study countries: Brazil, China, India, Europe, Singapore, and the Unite States? (2) What are similarities and differences in factors associated with internet use in terms of demographic factors, socioeconomic status, cultural factors (e.g., familial support), and health conditions?

8.2 Data and Methods

8.2.1 Data Sources

To achieve the research objectives of this study, we focused on Brazil, China, India, Singapore, most European countries, and the United States. This selection of countries encompasses both more developed and less developed nations, ensuring the robustness and diversity of our findings. This selection includes both high-income and lower-middle-income nations, allowing for meaningful comparisons across different levels of economic development. Importantly, these countries also represent a range of cultural orientations—from more individualistic societies, such as the United States. and most European countries, to more family- or group-oriented cultures, such as China, India, and Brazil. This diversity enables us to examine how cultural norms surrounding aging, family support, and social participation shape older adults' internet use in distinct ways across global contexts.

Brazilian Longitudinal Study of Aging (ELSI-Brazil)
The Brazilian dataset used in this study was derived from the Brazilian Longitudinal Study of Aging (ELSI-Brazil), a sister study to the Health Retirement Study (Lima-Costa et al., 2021). ELSI-Brazil is the first large-scale longitudinal study of older adults in Brazil (Lima-Costa et al., 2018). This nationally representative, population-based cohort study focuses on individuals aged 50 and older. The baseline survey, conducted between 2015 and 2016, included 9412 participants from 70 municipalities across five Brazilian regions. The second wave of data collection, conducted between 2019 and 2021, expanded to 9949 respondents (Lima-Costa et al., 2023). ELSI-Brazil aims to explore the aging process, including its health, psychosocial,

and economic determinants, as well as its societal consequences. A key goal of the study is to build a comprehensive understanding of aging in Brazil, and to provide scientific data that can inform policy changes affecting older adults. This chapter draws upon data from 5114 participants aged 65 years or older from Wave 2 of ELSI-Brazil.

China Longitudinal Aging Social Survey (CLASS)
For China, we relied on the China Longitudinal Aging Social Survey (CLASS), which is a nationally representative longitudinal survey designed to examine the health, socioeconomic status, and psychosocial well-being of China's aging population, with 11,395 participants aged 60 or older. The detailed description about CLASS can be found in Chap. 6 and some earlier publications (Dong et al., 2019; Jin & Zhao, 2019). As this chapter focuses on older adults aged 65 years or older, there are 11,228 participants in the final analytical sample of CLASS for this chapter.

Longitudinal Aging Study in India (LASI)
India's data were derived from the Longitudinal Aging Study in India (LASI), the country's first nationally representative longitudinal study focusing on health and retirement. Originally conceptualized in 2006, the study's first pilot was conducted in 2010–2011 (Bloom et al., 2021). LASI boasts the largest single-country sample size among health and retirement studies (HRS), with Wave 1 (2017–2019) including over 72,000 adults aged 45 and older (Perianayagam et al., 2021). In 2020–2021, more than 1000 additional participants from remote areas were included, further expanding the sample to represent all 30 states and 6 union territories of India (https://www.g2aging.org/home). The LASI sample includes community-dwelling individuals aged 45 and older, as well as their spouses, regardless of age. The primary goal of LASI is to provide policymakers with detailed, comprehensive, and longitudinal data on the key economic, social, and health characteristics of India's older population (Bloom et al., 2021; Perianayagam et al., 2021). For this study, we utilized the LASI data from 21,646 respondents aged 65 and older.

Singapore's Lifelong Education for Aging Productively (LEAP)
For Singapore, we used data from the Lifelong Education for Aging Productively (LEAP) project, a nationally representative, cross-sectional survey funded by the government of Singapore. LEAP aims to examine the learning and productive activities of older adults in Singapore, specifically those aged 65–80 years (Mo et al., 2025). A weight variable was created for prevalence statistics, based on the age-gender-race/ethnicity distribution from the most recent 2020 census. The Chinese sample was drawn from the Singapore 70 (SG70) study, a subsample of surviving participants aged 68–80 within the prospective cohort of the Singapore Chinese Health Study (SCHS) conducted between 2022 and 2024 (Mo et al., 2025). Malay and Indian participants were randomly selected from a list of households with at least one older Malay or Indian individual aged 65–80, provided by Singapore's Department of Statistics (Mo et al., 2025). The total sample used in this chapter consists of 2545 individuals, including 1694 Chinese, 428 Malays, and 423 Indians.

Survey of Health, Ageing and Retirement in Europe (SHARE)
For European countries, we utilized data from the Survey of Health, Ageing, and Retirement in Europe (SHARE). Established in 2004, SHARE aims to provide high-quality, comparable longitudinal data to support research on aging and inform evidence-based policymaking in Europe (Börsch-Supan et al., 2013; Börsch-Supan & Scherpenzeel, 2021). It is a multidisciplinary, cross-national panel database that collects microdata on health, socioeconomic status, and social and family networks of individuals aged 50 and older. The sample design is based on probability sampling of households with individuals aged 50 or older, and includes both the target individuals and their partners, regardless of age.

SHARE has conducted nine waves of data collection, with Wave 1 in 2004 and Wave 9 in 2021/2022 (https://share-eric.eu/). Since Wave 7 in 2017 (https://share-eric.eu/data/data-documentation/waves-overview/wave-7), SHARE has expanded to include 28 European countries and Israel, covering a broad geographic range from northern and western Europe (e.g., Sweden, Germany) to southern and eastern Europe (e.g., Italy, Greece, Poland). Its international scope and standardized methodology make it a vital resource for comparative aging research and policy development across Europe. For this chapter, we relied on data from Wave 8, conducted in 2019/2020, which included 34,205 respondents aged 65 or older from 26 European countries. The sample size varied by country, ranging from 409 respondents in Slovakia to 2348 in Germany.

National Health and Aging Trends Study (NHATS)
For the United States, we used data from the National Health and Aging Trends Study (NHATS), an annual survey of a nationally representative sample of Medicare beneficiaries aged 65 or older. The survey collects detailed information through in-person interviews on the disablement process and its consequences (https://www.nhats.org/researcher/nhats). NHATS was initiated in 2011 and replenished in 2015 and 2022 to ensure a nationally representative sample (Jiao & Freedman, 2024). The publicly available NHATS data used in this study categorizes age in five-year intervals. The final sample for the 2020 wave included 3985 respondents aged 65 or older.

8.2.2 *Measures*

Internet Use
Internet use was derived from the question of whether the respondent accessed the internet regularly (ELSI-Brazil, CLASS, LASI), ever used the internet (LEAP), used the internet in the last week (SHARE), or used the internet in the last month (NHATS).

Associated Factors
Guided primarily by the Senior Technology Acceptance Model (STAM) and the existing literature (Chen & Chan, 2014; Friemel, 2016; Hunsaker & Hargittai, 2018;

Wang et al., 2024a; Yang & Du, 2021), we explored the factors associated with internet use among older adults in different countries by including the following key sets of factors, encompassing demographic, socioeconomic, family and social support, and health-related variables.

Demographic factors include age (65–74 years old, 75–84 years old, 85 years or older), sex (men vs. women), ethnicity (Han vs. minorities for China; Chinese vs. others for Singapore) or race (Non-Hispanic White for the United States), as well as urban versus rural residence (urban vs. rural for Brazil, China, and India). Socioeconomic factors include education (years of schooling: 0, 1–6, 7+ for Brazil, China, India, and Singapore; proportion of education with high school or higher for Europe and the United States), income (low income [<US$30,000] vs. others for the United States; self-rated poor economic status [yes vs. no] for other countries), and occupation (referring to primary lifetime occupation for non-European countries and the last job occupation for European countries: white-collar worker, blue-collar worker, agricultural worker or others). For India, we also included a variable of caste status to measure social class (scheduled caste, scheduled tribes, other backward tribes vs. others), with the first three categories representing lower social classes.

Family and social support were measured by several proxies, including marital status (married vs. not married), number of close family members, number of close friends, and social networks (for Europe and the United States). Other measures include religious attendance (yes vs. no for Brazil and Singapore), social participation (yes vs. no for Singapore), regular exercise (yes vs. no for Brazil and Singapore), and leisure activities (yes vs. no for China and Singapore).

Health conditions were assessed through self-reported disease status (1+ disease condition vs. none; for all countries, most self-reported diseases were diagnosed by a doctor or medical professional), activities of daily living (ADL) and instrumental activities of daily living (IADL) disabilities (yes vs. no for both variables), and self-rated health (good/very good vs. fair/poor/very poor). Cognitive impairment was included for China, as it is readily available in the dataset.

Finally, we included a regional variable for China, India, and Europe, as geographic information was available in the dataset. For further details, please refer to Table 8.1.

8.2.3 Analytical Strategies

We primarily employed multiple logistic regression models, complemented by descriptive analyses, to examine the commonalities and differences in factors associated with internet use across the study countries. We developed two models: Model I, which includes only demographic variables along with each study variable (referred to as the partial model), and Model II, which incorporates all study variables (referred to as the full model).

Table 8.1 Weighted sample distribution of analytical variables for countries under study

	Brazil, 2019–2021	China, 2020	India, 2017–2021[a]	Singapore, 2022–2024	Europe, 2019–2020	United States, 2020
Total sample size	5114	11,228	21,646	2545	34,205	3985[b]
% internet use	11.5	30.0	4.1	89.7	44.6	94.6
% Ages 65–74	60.4	64.8	67.8	74.7[c]	52.0	59.3
% Ages 75–85	31.0	27.1	25.6	25.3[c]	35.0	29.3
% Ages 85+	8.6	8.1	6.9	–[c]	13.0	11.4
% Men	44.9	47.5	47.8	42.5	42.8	43.7
% Han ethnicity, China or Singapore	–	95.4	–	79.7	–	–
% Non-Hispanic White, USA	–	–	–	–	–	80.5
% Urban	84.8	52.7	30.1	–	–	–
% 0 years of schooling	19.8	24.4	58.4	9.0	–	–
% 1–6 years of schooling	53.8	39.1	19.2	30.7	–	–
% 7+ years of schooling	26.5	36.5	22.4	60.3	–	–
% Education: high school+	–	–	–		60.5	86.2
% Covered by pension	80.3	–	–	–	–	–
% Low income	–	–	–	–	–	30.9
% Economically poor	–	10.4	38.3	6.6	10.1	----
% White-collar worker	11.0	10.8	6.8	35.5	30.2[d]	43.8
% Blue-collar workers	32.1	28.5	9.3	64.5	54.3[d]	42.9
% Agricultural workers or others	57.0	61.7	83.9	0.0	15.5[d]	13.3
% Scheduled caste, India	–	–	19.9	–	–	–
% Scheduled tribes, India	–	–	7.8	–	–	–
% Other backward tribes, India	–	—	45.5	–	–	–
% Others, India	–	–	27.8	–	–	–
% Currently married	52.5	78.1	55.2	71.5	57.8	55.6
% Social network high	–	–	–	–	26.1	42.3
% Having 2+ close family members	–	80.4	33.0	–	–	–
% Having 2+ close friends	–	71.4	14.3	–	69.4	–
Frequent contact with friends	83.0	–	–	–	–	–
% Do regular exercise	12.7	–	–	62.5	–	–

(continued)

Table 8.1 (continued)

	Brazil, 2019–2021	China, 2020	India, 2017–2021[a]	Singapore, 2022–2024	Europe, 2019–2020	United States, 2020
% Social participation	–	–	–	70.0	–	–
Freq. leisure and social activity	–	82.0	–	–	81.2	–
% Being religious	82.3	–	–	20.7	–	–
% Hindu, India	–	–	82.0	–	–	–
% Muslin, India	–	–	11.4	–	–	–
% Others, India	–	–	6.6	–	–	–
% Having 1+ diseases	85.4	79.6	74.4	81.7	86.7	95.3
% IADL disabled	–	18.7	53.5	–	26.3	–
% ADL disabled	19.2	11.3	27.8	12.9	17.4	43.2
% Cognitively impaired	–	24.5	–	–	–	–
% Good self-rated health	39.4	50.3	27.3	25.9	15.4	45.3
% East China	–	38.5	–	–	–	–
% Central China	–	27.1	–	–	–	–
% West China	–	25.7	–	–	–	–
% Northeast China	–	8.7	–	–	–	–
% North India	–	–	12.3	–	–	–
% Northeast India	–	–	3.0	–	–	–
% Central India	–	–	20.8	–	–	–
% East India	–	–	22.8	–	–	–
% West India	–	–	17.2	–	–	–
% South India	–	–	23.9	–	–	–
% East Europe	–	–	–	–	19.5	–
% North Europe	–	–	–	–	6.5	–
% South Europe	–	–	–	–	27.9	–
% West Europe	–	–	–	–	46.1	–

(1) The results were based on the full logistic regression models that controlled for all factors available specifically for each country/survey
(2) The category of the variable in the parentheses is the reference group
(3) ADL: Activities of daily living; IADL: Instrumental ADLs
(4) [a] more than 98% of the respondents in India's survey were interviewed in 2017–2019; [b] the United States survey was re-weighted to match the age-sex-specific distribution of population in the 2020 census; [c] the Singapore's survey did not include individuals aged 85 or older; [d] referring to the latest occupation
(5) Low income for US older adults was defined as any annual incomes less than US$30,000
(6) "–", not applicable
(7) $+p < 0.1$, $^{*}p < 0.05$, $^{**}p < 0.01$, $^{***}p < 0.001$

To ensure the robustness of our results, we also recoded certain variables into alternative forms, such as transforming ordinal variables to categorical variables. In nearly all cases, the results were consistent, further supporting the robustness of our findings. For the descriptive analyses, sampling weights were applied, whereas in the regression analyses, sampling weights were not used, following the approach used in Chap. 6 and other chapters. All statistical analyses were conducted using Stata version 18.0.

8.3 Results

Table 8.1 presents the weighted sample distribution for internet use and all study variables across the study countries. Note that the data as used cover a range of periods from 2017–2021 in India to 2022–2024 in Singapore. The proportions of internet use among older adults aged 65 and older vary greatly across countries. The proportion of Internet users in the United States is as high as nearly 95%, closely aligns with figures published by the Pew Research Center in Chap. 2. In Singapore, the proportion of older adults using the internet is also high, reaching 90% in 2022–2024. Older adults in European countries and China fall into the middle tier, with 45% and 30% of aged individuals using the internet, respectively. Brazil and India represent the lower end of the spectrum, with 12% and 4% of older adults using the internet, respectively.

Table 8.1 also reveals that the population aged 65 and older in Europe and the United States tends to be older than their counterparts in Brazil, China, and India. The proportion of men in more developed countries (Europe, the United States, and Singapore) is generally lower than in less developed countries. Additionally, older adults in more developed countries have a higher proportion with high school education or above, as well as a greater share of individuals employed in white-collar sectors.

Older adults in China and Singapore are more likely to be married, and they also have a lower prevalence of ADL disability. In contrast, older adults in Brazil, Europe, and the United States report a higher proportion of chronic disease conditions compared to other countries in the study. For psychosocial characteristics, comparisons across countries are generally not possible due to inconsistencies in measurement.

Table 8.2 compares the odds ratios for internet use based on various associated factors when only demographic variables are included in the analysis. The results reveal several interesting patterns. Demographically, the older the respondents, the lower their odds of using the internet. For the oldest-old adults (aged 85 or older), the odds ratios for internet use ranged from 0.05 to 0.12 across most countries, indicating that their odds of using the internet are approximately 88–95% lower than those of young-old adults (aged 65–74 years). An exception was found in India, where both the old-old and oldest-old adults showed similarly lower odds of internet use, with odds ratios of 0.66–0.70—approximately 30% to 34% lower than the young-old adults. Men are more likely than women to use the internet, with the lowest odds ratio found in China (1.19) and the highest in India (2.15), indicating that men had approximately 19% increased odds of internet use than women in China and more than double the odds in India. In Singapore, the ethnic majority

Table 8.2 Comparisons of odds ratios of internet use for associated factors by countries under study, the partial models

	Brazil, 2019/2021	China, 2020	India, 2017–2021	Singapore, 2022–2024	Europe, 2019–2020	United States, 2020
Ages 75–85 (65–74)	0.39***	0.43***	0.70***	0.56*	0.31***	0.48*
Ages 85+ (65–74)	0.12***	0.05***	0.66***	–	0.09***	0.10***
Men (women)	1.30**	1.19*	2.15***	1.47**	1.38***	1.48***
Han ethnicity (minority)	–	0.62*	–	2.66***	–	–
Non-Hispanic White (others)	–	–	–	–	–	2.16***
Urban (rural)	5.26***	2.55*	3.32***	–	–	–
1–6 years of schooling (0)	5.23***	1.83***	1.09	1.84**	–	–
7+ years of schooling (0)	24.7***	3.85***	2.35***	5.04***	–	–
High school (< high school)	–	–	–	–	2.82***	1.77***
Having a pension (no)	1.19	–	–	–	–	–
Low income (no)	–	–	–	–	–	0.37***
Economically poor (no)	–	0.83*	0.92	0.94	0.36***	–
Blue-collar workers (white-collar)	0.45***	0.74**	0.54***	0.38***	0.56***	0.84
Agricultural workers (white-collar)	0.45***	0.34***	0.58***	–	0.37***	0.52***
Scheduled caste (others)	–	–	0.78*	–	–	–
Scheduled tribes (others)	–	–	0.94			–
Other backward tribes (others)	–	–	0.77**	–	–	–
Currently married (no)	1.38***	1.75***	1.61**	1.22	1.33***	2.50***
Social network high (no)	–	–	–	–	1.53***	3.52***
Having 2+ close family members (<2)	–	1.18*	0.99	–	–	–
Having 2+ close friends (< 2)	–	1.09	1.93***	–	1.37***	–
Frequent contact with friends (no)	2.69***	–	–	–	–	–
Doing regular exercise (no)	2.03***	–	–	1.48***	–	–

(continued)

Table 8.2 (continued)

	Brazil, 2019/2021	China, 2020	India, 2017–2021	Singapore, 2022–2024	Europe, 2019–2020	United States, 2020
Social participation (no)	–	–	–	1.72***	–	–
Freq. leisure and social activity (no)	–	1.67***	–	–	2.92***	–
Being religious (no)	1.54*	–	–	1.60**	–	–
Muslin (Hindu)	–	–	0.60***	–	–	–
Others (Hindu)	–	–	1.40**	–	–	–
Having 1+ diseases (no)	1.17	1.32***	1.41*	1.36*	1.00	5.39***
IADL disabled (no)	–	0.61**	0.53***	–	0.44***	–
ADL disabled (no)	0.73*	0.91	1.08	0.48***	0.75***	0.57**
Cognitively impaired (no)	–	0.40***	–	–	–	–
Good self-rated health (no)	2.36***	1.37**	1.52***	0.99	2.39***	1.87***
Central China (East China)	–	0.31***	–	–	–	–
West China (East China)	–	0.26***	–	–	–	–
Northeast China (East China)	–	0.55**	–	–	–	–
Northeast India (North India)	–	–	1.16	–	–	–
Central India (North India)	–	–	0.64**	–	–	–
East India (North India)	–	–	0.46***	–	–	–
West India (North India)	–	–	0.79*	–	–	–
South India (North India)	–	–	0.75**	–	–	–
North Europe (East Europe)	–	–	–	–	4.25***	–
South Europe (East Europe)	–	–	–	–	0.90***	–
West Europe (East Europe)	–	–	–	–	4.14***	–
No. of individuals	5114	11,228	21,646	2533	34,205	3985

(1) The results were based on partial logistic regression models that only controlled for demographic factors available specifically for each country/survey
(2) The category of the variable in the parentheses is the reference group
(3) ADL: Activities of daily living; IADL: Instrumental ADL
(4) "–", not applicable
(5) $+p < 0.1$, $*p < 0.05$, $**p < 0.01$, $***p < 0.001$

(Han Chinese) is associated with higher odds of internet use. Similarly, in the United States, non-Hispanic whites are more likely to use the internet than ethnic minorities. However, the pattern is reversed in China, where ethnic minorities have higher odds of being internet users compared to the ethnic majority. Additionally, in Brazil, China, and India, where data on urban-rural residence are available, respondents living in urban areas are 5.3, 2.6, and 3.3 times more likely to use the internet compared to their rural counterparts, respectively.

Socioeconomic factors play a significant role in internet use among older adults. In general, individuals with more years of education are more likely to use the internet. For instance, in Brazil, those with 1–6 years of schooling are 5.2 times more likely, and those with more than 7 years of schooling are nearly 25 times more likely to use the internet compared to those with no formal education. In Singapore, the corresponding figures are 1.8 and 5.0 times, respectively. In European countries and the United States, individuals with at least a high school education are up to 2.8 and 1.8 times more likely, respectively, to use the internet than those without a high school diploma.

Lower income or poor economic conditions are associated with reduced odds of internet use in China, Europe, and the United States, but this association is not significant in India and Singapore. Occupational background also play a significant role: older adults whose lifetime primary occupation or most recent occupation was in white-collar jobs are more likely to use the internet compared to those in other sectors or without formal employment. However, this pattern does not hold in the United States, where no significant difference is observed between white- and blue-collar workers. In India, caste status also influences internet use, with individuals from lower castes experiencing significantly lower odds of being online.

From the perspective of family and social support, married respondents are 1.3–2.5 times likely to use the internet compared to their unmarried counterparts, with the exception of Singapore. Despite the different variables used across countries, greater family/social support, regular exercise, religious participation, and social engagement are all associated with higher odds of internet use.

Regarding health conditions, the relationship between health and internet use is somewhat complex. When health status is measured by ADL/IADL disability and self-rated health, poor health is generally associated with lower odds of using the internet in most cases. However, when health is assessed based on chronic disease conditions, having one or more chronic conditions is associated with higher odds of internet use, except in Brazil and Europe.

Geographically, for countries with available data, there is considerable regional variation within each country, with more socioeconomically developed regions generally showing greater odds of internet use. For instance, compared to older adults in East China, the country's more developed region, older adults in Central China, West China, and Northeast China are 69%, 74%, and 45% less likely to use the internet, respectively. Similarly, older adults in Northern and Western Europe are 4.3 and 4.1 times more likely to use the internet, respectively, compared to their counterparts in Eastern Europe.

Table 8.3 presents the odds ratios for internet use after adjusting for all other variables. The results show that, with a few exceptions, most patterns observed in

Table 8.3 Comparisons of odds ratios of internet use for associated factors by countries under study, the full models

	Brazil, 2019–2021	China, 2020	India, 2017–2021	Singapore, 2022–2024	Europe, 2019–2020	United States, 2020
Ages 75–85 (65–74)	0.59***	0.53***	0.86+	0.66*	0.39***	0.57*
Ages 85+ (65–74)	0.22***	0.14***	1.02	–	0.17***	0.16***
Men (women)	1.18	0.92	1.14	0.95	1.31***	1.04
Han ethnicity (minority)	–	0.68*	–	2.31***	–	–
Other races (non-Hispanic White)	–	–	–	–	–	1.20
Urban (rural)	3.30***	1.18*	2.09***	–	–	–
1–6 years of schooling (0)	4.66***	1.58***	1.00	1.85***	–	–
7+ years of schooling (0)	20.4***	3.06***	2.73***	5.15***	–	–
High school (<high school)	–	–	–	–	2.68***	1.70***
Having a pension (no)	1.29+	–	–	–	–	–
Low income (no)	–	–	–	–	–	0.51***
Economically poor (no)	–	0.90	0.89	1.17	0.44***	–
Blue-collar workers (white-collar)	0.47***	0.71**	0.59***	0.40***	0.60***	0.90
Agricultural workers (white-collar)	0.45***	0.34***	0.59***	–	0.40***	0.60**
Scheduled caste (others)	–	–	0.76*	–	–	–
Scheduled tribes (others)	–	–	0.84	–	–	–
Other backward tribes (others)	–	–	0.78**	–	–	–
Currently married (no)	1.56***	1.48***	1.40**	1.12	1.23***	1.99***
Social network high (no)	–	–	–	–	1.45***	3.01***
Having 2+ close family members (<2)	–	1.05	0.98	–	–	–
Having 2+ close friends (< 2)	–	0.98	1.65***	–	1.35***	–
Frequent contact with friends (no)	2.05***	–	–	–	–	–
Doing regular exercise (no)	1.71***	–	–	1.25+	–	–
Social participation (no)	–	–	–	1.70***	–	–
Freq. leisure and social activity (no)	–	1.66***	–	–	1.82***	–

(continued)

Table 8.3 (continued)

	Brazil, 2019–2021	China, 2020	India, 2017–2021	Singapore, 2022–2024	Europe, 2019–2020	United States, 2020
Being religious (no)	1.46*	–	–	1.53**	–	–
Muslin (Hindu)	–	–	0.72***	–	–	–
Others (Hindu)	–	–	1.35**	–	–	–
Having 1+ diseases (no)	1.19	1.33***	1.21*	1.44*	0.97	4.09***
IADL disabled (no)	–	0.70**	0.63***	–	0.55***	–
ADL disabled (no)	0.88	0.77**	1.05	0.54***	0.87***	0.60**
Cognitively impaired (no)	–	0.46***	–	–	–	–
Good self-rated health (no)	1.77***	1.31**	1.39***	1.11	2.06***	1.60***
Central China (East China)	–	0.39***	–	–	–	–
West China (East China)	–	0.36***	–	–	–	–
Northeast China (East China)	–	0.56**	–	–	–	–
Northeast India (North India)	–	–	0.91	–	–	–
Central India (North India)	–	–	0.78+	–	–	–
East India (North India)	–	–	0.49***	–	–	–
West India (North India)	–	–	0.80*	–	–	–
South India (North India)	–	–	0.86	–	–	–
North Europe (East Europe)	–	–	–	–	3.81***	–
South Europe (East Europe)	–	–	–	–	1.15***	–
Western Europe (East Europe)	–	–	–	–	3.60***	–
- Log likelihood	1227.1	4879.7	3476.7	829.9	17586.0	1083.2
Degree of freedom	16	22	36	13	16	14
LR Chi square	784.7	3343.2	1161.4	254.3	12107.6	643.8
No. of individuals	5114	11,228	21,646	2533	34,205	3985

(1) The results were based on the full logistic regression models that controlled for all factors available specifically for each country/survey

(2) The category of the variable in the parentheses is the reference group

(3) ADL: Activities of daily living; IADL: Instrumental ADLs

(4) "–", not applicable

(5) $+p < 0.1$, $*p < 0.05$, $**p < 0.01$, $***p < 0.001$

Table 8.2 are attenuated but remain statistically significant. The few exceptions primarily involve demographic and socioeconomic variables. For instance, age becomes insignificant in India after adjustment. Gender differences, except in Europe, are no longer statistically significant, suggesting that men's advantages of using the internet are primarily explained by other factors, especially socioeconomic ones. Similarly, the racial differential in internet use becomes insignificant in the United States as well. While lower income and poor economic conditions remain significant in Europe and the United States, they are no longer significant in Brazil, China, and India. This indicates that income-related barriers to internet access in these developing countries are largely driven by other factors.

8.4 Discussion

This chapter provides a comprehensive cross-national examination of internet use among older adults aged 65 and above across countries with diverse socioeconomic and cultural contexts, including India, Brazil, China, Singapore, Europe (as a whole), and the United States. By analyzing data from multiple countries with varying levels of internet penetration, diversified demographic profiles, and different stages of socioeconomic development, this research sheds light on the multifaceted factors influencing digital engagement among older populations. Below, we interpret the key findings, discuss potential underlying mechanisms, and compare them with existing literature.

8.4.1 Interpretation of Key Findings

Variation in the Prevalence of Internet Use Across Countries

The wide variation in internet use among older adults, from 4% in India to nearly 95% in the United States, reflects disparities in digital infrastructure, socioeconomic development, and digital literacy across countries (van Deursen & Helsper, 2015). The high internet adoption in the United States and Singapore is consistent with their advanced technological environments, widespread internet access, and extensive digital inclusion policies targeting older adults (Friemel, 2016; Chen & Chan, 2014). Conversely, lower adoption rates in India and Brazil correspond with infrastructural limitations, digital divides, and socioeconomic constraints, typical of developing countries (Hilbert, 2011; Ragnedda & Muschert, 2013).Older adults in Europe and China fall in the mid-range in this regard, highlighting a transitional process where internet infrastructure and digital literacy programs are growing but have not yet reached saturation (Helsper & Reisdorf, 2017). Notably, China's relatively low internet use, despite its economic growth, may be attributable to urban-rural divides and generational disparities in education and digital access (Hu & Xu, 2024; ICMARA, 2023).

Age and Gender Difference in Internet Use

Consistent with prior research, advanced age is associated with decreased odds of internet use, particularly among the oldest-old (Choi & DiNitto, 2013). This likely results from age-related health declines in cognitive, sensory, and motor functions, as well as the low digital literacy due to limited exposure to technology during formative years throughout life course (Mitzner et al., 2010). The exception is India, where old-old and oldest-old adults show similar odds of use, as might be explained by its generally low baseline usage and more homogenous digital exclusion within older cohorts (Jena & Paltasingh, 2025; Mohan et al., 2024; William & Murugesh, 2018).

Gender disparities favoring men, as observed in this study, are also consistent with previous findings, though these differences diminish when socioeconomic variables are controlled. This finding confirms that structural factors such as education, income, and occupational history can indeed modify gender gaps in digital adoption (Hargittai & Shaw, 2015; van Deursen & van Dijk, 2019).

Most prior studies on Western populations show that ethnic majorities tend to have higher internet use, even after controlling for various factors (Chan et al., 2023; Mesch & Talmud, 2011; Mitchell et al., 2019; Suntai & Beltran, 2023; Wang et al., 2024a, 2024b). Our findings for the United States align with this pattern. However, in China, we observed a reversed trend among older adults, with ethnic minorities showing higher internet use in the presence of basic demographic factors. This may reflect the early introduction of bilingual smartphone interfaces, localized digital training programs (Ministry of Education, 2007), and recent IT infrastructure improvements in minority regions, driven by China's push for digital inclusion and regional development (CNNIC, 2025; Pick et al., 2024). These advances may have helped narrow the digital divide in China. However, it is also possible that the CLASS survey's exclusion of three remote provinces with large minority populations may have biased the results. Further research is essential to better understand ethnic digital inequality in China.

The strong urban advantage in internet use, particularly in Brazil, China, and India, reflects infrastructural disparities, including internet availability, network speed, and digital services, which are often concentrated in urban centers (Wang et al., 2025). Regional socioeconomic development within a country further influences internet use, as seen in China and Europe, where more developed regions show significantly higher odds of use. These findings align with studies that emphasize the role of digital infrastructure and regional inequality in shaping internet adoption (OECD, 2019).

Socioeconomic Factors: Education, Income, and Occupation

Education emerges as a robust predictor of internet use across countries, aligning with the concept of digital capital, where formal education enhances digital skills, access, and confidence (Bourdieu, 1986; DiMaggio & Hargittai, 2001). The exponential increase in odds of internet use with schooling levels in Brazil and Singapore underscores education's critical role in bridging digital divides.

Income-related barriers remained significant in developed countries (i.e., Europe and the United States) even after accounting for other variables, but not in developing contexts. This might be due to the relative cost burden of digital technologies being proportionally greater in wealthier contexts, or alternatively, to the limited availability or underdeveloped infrastructure for digital technology in developing countries (Bhuiyan et al., 2025; Chan et al., 2023; van Deursen et al., 2017; Wang et al., 2022).

Occupation history, especially doing white-collar work in life, correlates with greater digital engagement, likely reflecting both economic resources and prior online exposure in professional settings (Friemel, 2016). The comparable proportions of internet users between white- and blue-collar workers in the United States may reflect the broader adoption of mobile internet and social media platforms among working-class groups, a trend noted in recent digital behavior studies (Pew Research Center, 2017, 2022). This pattern is consistent with the Diffusion of Innovations Theory, which suggests that new technologies are typically adopted first by individuals from higher socioeconomic backgrounds and gradually spread to less advantaged groups as these technologies become more affordable, accessible, and integrated into daily life (Rogers et al., 2014). While this diffusion trajectory is well documented in high-income countries, its progression in lower-income or infrastructure-constrained settings tends to be slower or more uneven due to persistent structural barriers. Further research is needed to comprehensively understand the dynamics of technology diffusion across diverse socioeconomic and regional contexts.

Overall, our results suggest that self-rated economic conditions are less robust than education and occupation in associating with internet use, which confirmed previous literature (e.g., Blank & Lutz, 2018; van Deursen & Helsper, 2015; also see Chap. 6). This is probably because education and occupation often serve as stronger predictors of digital engagement by shaping individuals' cognitive skills, technological literacy, and professional incentives for using digital tools.

Family and Social Support Influences

Marriage and greater social engagement are associated with increased internet use in this study, and this is consistent with theories that social resources and networks facilitate technology adoption through social learning and support (Selwyn, 2004; Shapira et al., 2007). Married older adults may benefit from spousal encouragement or shared technology use, while social participation may expose individuals to peer norms favoring internet use (Chen & Schulz, 2016). The Singapore exception, where marriage did not significantly increase internet use, might be attributed to the good integration of spouseless older adults or the nearly universal internet rate (Leong et al., 2024).

Health Status and ICT Use

The complex relationship between health and internet use reflects divergent pathways. Poor self-rated health and ADL/IADL disability generally reduce internet use, likely due to functional limitations and lower motivation (Choi & Dinitto, 2013). However, the positive association between chronic disease presence and internet use in many countries (except Brazil and Europe) may come from the needs to use the internet for health information seeking, management, and social support by those managing chronic conditions (Mitzner et al., 2010; Leist, 2013). This is consistent with the "silver surfer" phenomenon, where health needs motivate the online management (Bitterman & Shalev, 2004; Zhang, 2023).

8.4.2 Strengths and Limitations

A major strength of this study lies in its cross-national comparative approach, including both major developed and developing countries, as well as individual- and group-oriented cultural norms. This design enhances the generalizability and policy relevance of the findings across diverse socioeconomic and cultural contexts. The inclusion of multiple factors, such as demographic, socioeconomic, health, relational, and geographic, provides a comprehensive understanding of the multifactorial determinants of older adults' internet use.

However, several limitations merit consideration. First, the cross-sectional design limits causal inferences regarding the relationships between variables and internet use. Longitudinal studies are needed to examine how changes in health, social support, and socioeconomic status affect digital engagement over time. Second, variations in variable measurements across countries, particularly psychosocial factors, limit direct comparability and the ability to conduct pooled analyses on these dimensions. Future research should aim for standardized measurement tools across international surveys. Third, a few important factors such as digital skills, attitudes toward technology, and availability of tailored digital literacy programs may also influence internet use, but were not consistently available in all datasets. Fourth, inconsistent definitions of internet use across surveys may introduce some possible biases. Finally, the exclusion of institutionalized older adults may lead to underestimation of digital inequalities, as those in long-term care settings often have lower digital access and engagement (Seifert et al., 2021).

8.4.3 Policy Implications

The findings in this chapter have important implications for policies aimed at narrowing the digital divide among older adults and fostering more inclusive digital societies. First, digital literacy and training programs should be age-appropriate and culturally sensitive, with a particular focus on the oldest-old and those with lower levels of education. These programs should aim to build both skills and confidence in using the internet (Heart & Kalderon, 2013). Incorporating health-related content into training can be especially effective, as older adults are often motivated to go online for health management.

Second, ensuring affordable access to digital devices and internet services, especially in low-income and rural areas, is essential for reducing access disparities. In developing countries, investments in infrastructure and partnerships between public and private sectors can help expand connectivity in underserved regions (Hilbert, 2011).

Third, strengthening family and community support can significantly boost internet adoption among older adults. Intergenerational initiatives, where younger family members or volunteers help older adults learn to use technology, have shown encouraging results (Mitzner et al., 2010).

Fourth, healthcare systems should integrate digital tools designed with older users in mind, acknowledging their increasing reliance on the internet for managing chronic conditions and maintaining social connections. Telehealth and e-health platforms must be accessible and user-friendly for older adults to reduce health inequities and support continuous care (Leist, 2013).

Finally, national digital inclusion strategies must address regional disparities by directing targeted investments and interventions toward less developed and rural areas. Solutions such as mobile internet services, community access hubs, and digital ambassador programs can play a critical role in engaging older adults and closing the digital gap (OECD, 2019).

8.5 Conclusions

This chapter highlights the complex, multidimensional landscape of internet use among older adults across varied national and cultural contexts. By employing a rigorous cross-national comparative approach encompassing both developed and developing countries, it reveals that digital engagement in later life is shaped by a confluence of individual-level characteristics, such as age, gender, educational attainment, occupational background, health status, and the strength of social networks, as well as broader societal factors. While education and prior exposure to technology through one's profession consistently emerge as strong predictors of internet use, the analysis also uncovers distinct contextual variations. These differences reflect the influence of cultural norms, regional development trajectories, and life course experiences on patterns of digital inclusion.

The findings underscore the need for tailored, context-sensitive strategies that move beyond one-size-fits-all approaches. Although limitations such as reliance on cross-sectional data and variation in survey instruments across countries must be acknowledged, the chapter offers valuable empirical evidence to inform inclusive digital policies and interventions. As the global population continues to age, a renewed commitment to ensuring that older adults are not left behind in the digital transformation is essential for building more equitable, resilient, and inclusive societies.

Acknowledgement The authors would like to thank the Research Center for Population and Development and the Institute of Gerontology at Renmin University for providing access to the China Longitudinal Aging and Social Survey (CLASS) dataset used in this chapter. We also gratefully acknowledge the Gateway to Global Aging Data for facilitating access to the harmonized datasets of the Brazilian Longitudinal Study of Aging (ELSI-Brazil) and the Longitudinal Aging Study in India (LASI). In addition, we thank the teams behind the Survey of Health, Ageing and Retirement in Europe (SHARE), the National Health and Aging Trends Study (NHATS), and the Lifelong Education for Aging Productively (LEAP) for providing access to their respective datasets.

Disclaimer Views expressed in the chapter are solely those of the authors and do not necessarily reflect those of the United Nations, the National University of Singapore, the University of Alabama at Birmingham, Vigirnia Tech, and the University of Illinois Urbana-Champaign.

References

Alvarez-Galvez, J., Salinas-Perez, J. A., Montagni, I., & Salvador-Carulla, L. (2020). The persistence of digital divides in the use of health information: A comparative study in 28 European countries. *International Journal of Public Health, 65*(3), 325–333.

Anderberg, P., Abrahamsson, L., & Berglund, J. S. (2021). An instrument for measuring social participation to examine older adults' use of the internet as a social platform: Development and validation study. *JMIR Aging, 4*(2), e23591.

Benge, J. F., & Scullin, M. K. (2025). A meta-analysis of technology use and cognitive aging. *Nature Human Behaviour.* Online first. https://doi.org/10.1038/s41562-025-01835-4

Bhuiyan, M. H. M., Varvello, M., Staicu, C.-A., & Zaki, Y. (2025). *Digital disparities: A comparative web measurement study across economic boundaries* [Conference contribution]. CISPA. Retrieved from https://doi.org/10.60882/cispa.28365449.v1

Bitterman, N., & Shalev, I. (2004). The silver surfer: Making the internet usable for seniors. *Ergonomics in Design, 12*(1), 24–28.

Bloom, D. E., Sekher, T. V., & Lee, J. (2021). Longitudinal Aging Study in India (LASI): New data resources for addressing aging in India. *Nature Aging, 1*, 1070–1072.

Börsch-Supan, A., & Scherpenzeel, A. (2021). The survey of health, ageing and retirement in Europe. In D. Gu & M. E. Dupre (Eds.), *Encyclopedia of gerontology and population aging* (pp. 5113–5119). Springer Nature.

Börsch-Supan, A., Brandt, M., Hunkler, C., Kneip, T., Korbmacher, J., Malter, F., Zuber, S., et al. (2013). Data resource profile: the Survey of Health, Ageing and Retirement in Europe (SHARE). *International Journal of Epidemiology, 42*(4), 992–1001.

Bourdieu, P. (1986). The forms of capital. In J. G. Richardson (Ed.), *Handbook of Theory and Research for the Sociology of Education* (pp. 241–258). Greenwood Press.

Büchi, M., Just, N., & Latzer, M. (2016). Modeling the second-level digital divide: A five-country study of social differences in Internet use. *New Media & Society, 18*(11), 2703–2722.

Chan, D. Y. L., Lee, S. W. H., & The, P. L. (2023). Factors influencing technology use among low-income older adults: A systematic review. *Heliyon, 9*(9), e20111.

Chen, K., & Chan, A. H. (2014). Gerontechnology acceptance by elderly Hong Kong Chinese: A senior technology acceptance model (STAM). *Ergonomics, 57*(5), 635–652.

Chen, Y. R., & Schulz, P. J. (2016). The effect of information communication technology interventions on reducing social isolation in the elderly: A systematic review. *Journal of Medical Internet Research., 18*(1), e18.

Chen, A. N., Downey, J. P., McGaughey, R. E., & Jin, K. (2015). Seniors and information technology in China. *International Journal of Human-Computer Interaction, 32*(2), 132–142.

China Internet Network Information Center (CNNIC). (2025). *The 55th Statistical Report on China's Internet Development*. Retrieved from https://www.cnnic.net.cn/n4/2025/0117/c88-11229.html [in Chinese].

Chinn, M. D., & Fairlie, R. W. (2007). The determinants of the global digital divide: A cross-country analysis of computer and internet penetration. *Oxford Economic Papers, 59*(1), 16–44.

Choi, N. G., & DiNitto, D. M. (2013). The digital divide among low-income homebound older adults: Internet use patterns, eHealth literacy, and attitudes toward computer/Internet use. *Journal of Medical Internet Research, 15*(5), e2645.

Choi, E., Han, K. M., Chang, J., Lee, Y. J., Choi, K. W., Han, C., & Ham, B. J. (2021). Social participation and depressive symptoms in community-dwelling older adults: Emotional social support as a mediator. *Journal of Psychiatric Research, 137*, 589–596.

Coley, N., Andre, L., Hoevenaar-Blom, M. P., Ngandu, T., Beishuizen, C., Barbera, M., et al. (2022). Factors predicting engagement of older adults with a coach-supported eHealth intervention promoting lifestyle change and associations between engagement and changes in cardiovascular and dementia risk: Secondary analysis of an 18-month multinational randomized controlled trial. *Journal of Medical Internet Research, 24*(5), e32006.

Czaja, S. J., Charness, N., Fisk, A. D., Hertzog, C., Nair, S. N., Rogers, W. A., & Sharit, J. (2006). Factors predicting the use of technology: Findings from the Center for Research and Education on Aging and Technology Enhancement (CREATE). *Psychology and Aging, 21*(2), 333–352.

da Silva, L. F., Zitkus, E., & Freire, A. P. (2023). An exploratory study of the use of the internet and e-government by older adults in the countryside of Brazil. *Information, 14*(4), 225.

DiMaggio, P., & Hargittai, E. (2001). From the 'digital divide' to 'digital inequality': Studying Internet use as penetration increases. Working Paper 15, Center for Arts and Cultural Policy Studies, Woodrow Wilson School, Princeton University. https://digitalinclusion.typepad.com/digital_inclusion/documentos/digitalinequality.pdf

Dong, T., Zhu, Z., Guo, M., Du, P., & Wu, B. (2019). Association between dying experience and place of death: Urban–rural differences among older Chinese adults. *Journal of Palliative Medicine, 22*(11), 1386–1393.

Donner, J. (2008). Research approaches to mobile use in the developing world: A review of the literature. *The Information Society, 24*(3), 140–159.

Gallo, A. M., Laranjeira, C., Araújo, J. P., Marques, F. R. D. M., Baccon, W. C., Carreira, L., et al. (2024). The experiences of daily smartphone use among older adults in Brazil: A grounded theory analysis. *Heliyon, 10*(15), e35120.

Goodman-Deane, J., Waller, S., Bradley, M., et al. (2024). User factors affecting the use of digital services in five European regions and countries. *Scientific Data, 11*, 468.

GSMA. (2023). *The state of mobile internet connectivity 2023*. Retrieved from https://www.gsma.com/r/wp-content/uploads/2023/10/The-State-of-Mobile-Internet-Connectivity-Report-2023.pdf

Gulati, G. J., & Yates, D. J. (2012). Different paths to universal access: The impact of policy and regulation on broadband diffusion in the developed and developing worlds. *Telecommunications Policy, 36*(9), 749–761.

Hargittai, E., & Shaw, A. (2015). Mind the skills gap: The role of Internet know-how and gender in differentiated contributions to Wikipedia. *Information, Communication & Society, 18*(4), 424–442.

Heart, T., & Kalderon, E. (2013). Older adults: Are they ready to adopt health-related ICT? *International Journal of Medical Informatics, 82*(11), e209–e231.

Helsper, E. J., & Reisdorf, B. C. (2017). The emergence of a "digital underclass" in Great Britain and Sweden: Changing reasons for digital exclusion. *New Media & Society, 19*(8), 1253–1270.

Heo, J., Chun, S., Lee, S., Lee, K. H., & Kim, J. (2015). Internet use and well-being in older adults. *Cyberpsychology Behavior, and Social Networking, 18*(5), 268–272.

Hilbert, M. (2011). Digital gender divide or technologically empowered women in developing countries? A typical case of lies, damned lies, and statistics. *Women's Studies International Forum, 34*(6), 479–489.

Hu, H., & Xu, W. (2024). Socioeconomic differences in digital inequality among Chinese older adults: Results from a nationally representative sample. *PLoS One, 19*(4), e0300433.

Hunsaker, A., & Hargittai, E. (2018). A review of Internet use among older adults. *New Media & Society, 20*(10), 3937–3954.

Information Center of the Ministry of Agriculture and Rural Affairs (ICMARA). (2023). *The report on the development of digital villages in China (2022).* [in Chinese]. Retrieved from https://www.cac.gov.cn/2023-03/01/c_1679309718486615.htm

International Telecommunication Union (ITU). (2021). *Ageing in a digital world—From vulnerable to valuable.* Retrieved from https://www.itu.int/en/ITU-D/Digital-Inclusion/Pages/ageing-in-a-digital-world/default.aspx

International Telecommunication Union (ITU). (2023). *Measuring digital development: Facts and figures—Focus on least developed countries.* Retrieved from https://www.itu.int/en/ITU-D/Statistics/pages/facts/default.aspx

International Telecommunication Union (ITU). (2024). *Measuring digital development: Facts and figures 2024.* Retrieved from https://www.itu.int/en/ITU-D/Statistics/pages/facts/default.aspx

Jena, B., & Paltasingh, T. (2025). Digital literacy among older adults: A systematic review in Indian context. *Educational Gerontology, 51*(4), 371–386.

Jiao, R., & Freedman, V. A. (2024). *National health and aging trends study round 13 sample design and selection.* NHATS Technical Paper #46. Johns Hopkins Bloomberg School of Public Health. Retrieved from https://www.nhats.org/sites/default/files/2024-12/NHATSTechnicalPaper46_12092024.pdf

Jin, Y., & Zhao, M. (2019). Internet access and the elderly's active aging in China—a study based on 2016 China Longitudinal Aging Social Survey. *Population Journal, 6*, 44–55. [in Chinese].

Kakulla, B. (2021). *Tech trends and the 50-plus: Top 10 biggest trends.* AARP Research. Retrieved from https://doi.org/10.26419/res.00420.001

Kemp, S. (2025). *Digital 2025: Global overview report.* Retrieved from https://datareportal.com/reports/digital-2025-global-overview-report

König, R., Seifert, A., & Doh, M. (2018). Internet use among older Europeans: An analysis based on SHARE data. *Universal Access in the Information Society, 17*(3), 621–633.

Lei, X., Matovic, D., Leung, W.-Y., Viju, A., & Wuthrich, V. M. (2024). The relationship between social media use and psychosocial outcomes in older adults: A systematic review. *International Psychogeriatrics, 36*(9), 714–746.

Leist, A. K. (2013). Social media use of older adults: A mini-review. *Gerontology, 59*(4), 378–384.

Leong, Q. Y., Lee, V. V., Ng, W. Y., Vijayakumar, S., Lau, N. Y., Mauritzon, I., Blasiak, A., & Ho, D. (2024). Older adults' perspectives and experiences with digital health in Singapore: Qualitative study. *JMIR Human Factors, 11*, e58641.

Li, L. (2024). Internet use and frailty in middle-aged and older adults: Findings from developed and developing countries. *Global Health, 20*(1), 53.

Li, Q., & Luximon, Y. (2018). Understanding older adults' post-adoption usage behavior and perceptions of mobile technology. *International Journal of Design, 12*(3), 93–110.

Li, S., Yunus, M. M., Hussain, R. B. B. M., & Lin, W. (2025). Cultural adaptation to aging: A study on digital cultural adaptation needs of Chinese older adults based on KANO model. *Frontiers in Public Health, 13*, 1554552.

Lima-Costa, M. F., de Andrade, F. B., de Souza, P. R. B., Neri, A. L., de Oliveira Duart, Y., Castro-Costa, E., & de Oliveirz, C. (2018). The Brazilian longitudinal study of aging (ELSI-Brazil): Objectives and design. *American Journal of Epidemiology, 187*(7), 1345–1353.

Lima-Costa, M. F., de Andrade, F. B., & de Oliveira, C. (2021). Brazilian longitudinal study of aging (ELSI-Brazil). In D. Gu & M. E. Dupre (Eds.), *Encyclopedia of gerontology and population aging* (pp. 708–712). Springer Nature.

Lima-Costa, M. R., de Melo Mambrini, J. V., de Andrade, F. B., de Souza, P. R. B., de Vasconcellos, M. T. L., et al. (2023). Cohort profile: The Brazilian Longitudinal Study of Ageing (ELSI-Brazil). *International Journal of Epidemiology*, e57–e65.

Lu, X., Yao, Y., & Jin, Y. (2022). Digital exclusion and functional dependence in older people: Findings from five longitudinal cohort studies. *EClinicalMedicine, 54*, 101708.

Mesch, G. S., & Talmud, I. (2011). Ethnic differences in Internet access. *Information, Communication & Society, 14*, 445–471.

Ministry of Education [China] (2007). *Report on the language situation in China (2007)*. Retrieved from http://www.moe.gov.cn/s78/A19/A19_ztzl/baogao/201202/t20120210_130364.html [in Chinese]

Mitchell, U. A., Chebli, P. G., Ruggiero, L., & Muramatsu, N. (2019). The digital divide in health-related technology use: The significance of race/ethnicity. *The Gerontologist, 59*(1), 6–14.

Mitzner, T. L., Boron, J. B., Fausset, C. B., Adams, A. E., Charness, N., Czaja, S. J., Dijkstra, K., Fisk, A. D., Rogers, W. A., & Sharit, J. (2010). Older adults talk technology: Technology usage and attitudes. *Computers in Human Behavior., 26*(6), 1710–1721.

Mo, Y., Liu, Y., Yeung, J., Koh, W-P., Gu, D., & Feng, Q. (2025). From digital divide to digital equality: The role of learning in older Singaporeans. *Journal of Gerontology: Social Sciences* (Forthcoming).

Mohan, R., Saleem, F., Voderhobli, K., & Sheikh-Akbari, A. (2024). Ensuring sustainable digital inclusion among the elderly: A comprehensive analysis. *Sustainability, 16*(17), 7485.

Nishijima, M., Ivanauskas, T. M., & Sarti, F. M. (2017). Evolution and determinants of digital divide in Brazil (2005–2013). *Telecommunications Policy, 41*(1), 12–24.

Ono, H., & Zavodny, M. (2007). Digital inequality: A five country comparison using microdata. *Social Science Research, 36*(3), 1135–1155.

Organization for Economic Cooperation and Development (OECD). (2019). *Going digital: Shaping policies, improving lives*. OECD Publishing. https://doi.org/10.1787/9789264312012-en

Organization for Economic Cooperation and Development (OECD). (2021). *Bridging digital divides in G20 Countries*. OECD Publishing. Retrieved from https://www.oecd.org/en/publications/bridging-digital-divides-in-g20-countries_35c1d850-en.html

Perianayagam, A., Bloom, D. E., Lee, J., Sekher, T. V., Mohanty, S. K., & Agarwal, A. (2021). Longitudinal aging study in India. In D. Gu & M. E. Dupre (Eds.), *Encyclopedia of gerontology and population aging* (pp. 3003–3007). Springer Nature.

Petrosyan, A. (2024). *Age distribution of internet users worldwide 2024*. Statista. Retrieved from https://www.statista.com/statistics/272365/age-distribution-of-internet-users-worldwide/

Pew Research Center. (2014). *Older adults and technology use*. Retrieved from https://www.pewresearch.org/internet/2014/04/03/older-adults-and-technology-use/

Pew Research Center. (2017). *Technology use among seniors*. Retrieved from https://www.pewresearch.org/internet/2017/05/17/technology-use-among-seniors/

Pew Research Center. (2022). *Share of those 65 and older who are tech users has grown in the past decade*. Retrieved from https://pewrsr.ch/3HZd2ao

Pick, J., Ren, F., & Sarkar, A. (2024). Digital inequalities in China in 2020: Spatial and multivariate analysis. *Applied Sciences, 14*(13), 5385.

Ragnedda, M., & Muschert, G. W. (Eds.). (2013). *The digital divide: The Internet and social inequality in international perspective* (1st ed.). Routledge.

Renaud, K., & van Biljon, J. (2008). Predicting technology acceptance and adoption by the elderly: A qualitative study. In *Proceedings of the 2008 Annual Research Conference of the South African Institute of Computer Scientists and Information Technologists* (pp. 210–219).

Richard, E., Moll van Charante, E. P., Hoevenaar-Blom, M. P., Coley, N., Barbera, M., van der Groep, A., et al. (2019). Healthy ageing through internet counselling in the elderly (HATICE): A multinational, randomised controlled trial. *The Lancet Digital Health, 1*(8), e424–e434.

Rogers, E. M., Singhal, A., & Quinlan, M. M. (2014). Diffusion of innovations. In *An integrated approach to communication theory and research* (pp. 432–448). Routledge.

Schehl, B., Leukel, J., & Sugumaran, V. (2019). Understanding differentiated internet use in older adults: A study of informational, social, and instrumental online activities. *Computers in Human Behavior, 97*, 222–230.

Schroeder, T., Dodds, L., Georgiou, A., Gewald, H., & Siette, J. (2023). Older adults and new technology: Mapping review of the factors associated with older adults' intention to adopt digital technologies. *JMIR Aging, 6*, e44564.

Seifert, A., Cotten, S. R., & Xie, B. (2021). A double burden of exclusion? Digital and social exclusion of older adults in times of COVID-19. *Journal of Gerontology: Social Sciences, 76*(3), e99–e103.

Selwyn, N. (2004). The information aged: A qualitative study of older adults' use of information and communications technology. *Journal of Aging Studies, 18*(4), 369–384.

Shapira, N., Barak, A., & Gal, I. (2007). Promoting older adults' well-being through Internet training and use. *Aging & Mental Health, 11*(5), 477–484.

Silver, M. P. (2013). Socio-economic status over the lifecourse and internet use in older adulthood. *Ageing and Society, 34*, 1019–1034.

Steyn, J., & van Greunen, D. (2015). *ICTs for inclusive communities in developing societies*. Cambridge Scholars Publishing.

Suntai, Z., & Beltran, S. J. (2023). The intersectional impact of race/ethnicity and sex on access to technology among older adults. *The Gerontologist, 63*(7), 1162–1171.

United Nation. (2023). *Science, technology and innovation for sustainable development: Report of the Secretary-General*. Retrieved from https://docs.un.org/en/A/78/232

van Deursen, A. J., & Helsper, E. J. (2015). The third-level digital divide: Who benefits most from being online? *Communication and Information Technologies Annual: Digital Distinctions and Inequalities Studies in Media and Communications, 10*, 29–52.

van Deursen, A. J., & van Dijk, J. (2019). The first-level digital divide shifts from inequalities in physical access to inequalities in material access. *New Media & Society, 21*(2), 354–375.

Van Deursen, A. J., Helsper, E., Eynon, R., & van Dijk, J. (2017). The compoundness and sequentiality of digital inequality. *International Journal Of Communication, 11*, 22.

van Dijk, J. (2005). *The deepening divide: Inequality in the information society*. Sage.

van Dijk, J. (2020). *The digital divide*. Polity.

Wang, X., Shi, J., & Lee, K. M. (2022). The digital divide and seeking health information on smartphones in Asia: Survey study of ten countries. *Journal of Medical Internet Research, 24*(1), e24086.

Wang, C., Zhu, Y., Ma, J., & Chu, J. (2023). The association between internet use and depression among older adults in China: The mediating role of social networks. *Digital Health, 9*, 20552076231207587.

Wang, K., Chen, X. S., Gu, D., Smith, B. D., Dong, Y., & Peet, J. Z. (2024a). Examining first- and second-level digital divide at the intersection of race/ethnicity, gender, and socioeconomic status: an analysis of the National Health and Aging trends Study. *The Gerontologist, 64*(9), gnae079.

Wang, K., Chen, X. S., Kang, S. Y., Smith, B. D., & Gu, D. (2024b). Older adults' online activities and cognition: Investigating the psychological mechanisms and age and gender differences. *Social Science & Medicine, 352*, 116988.

Wang, J., Lu, X., Ngai, S. B. C., Xie, L., Liu, X., Yao, Y., & Jin, Y. (2025). Digital exclusion and depressive symptoms among older people: Findings from five aging cohort studies across 24 countries. *Health Data Science, 5*, 0218.

William, J. A., & Murugesh, R. (2018). Senior citizens' usage towards and perception of modern technology in India. In J. Zhou & G. Salvendy (Eds.), *Human aspects of IT for the aged population: Acceptance, communication and participation. ITAP 2018* (pp. 179–193). Springer.

Wong, C. K., Yeung, D. Y., Ho, H. C., Tse, K., & Lam, C. (2014). Chinese older adults' internet use for health information. *Journal of Applied Gerontology, 33*, 316–335.

World Bank. (2025). *World development indicators*. Retrieved from https://databank.worldbank.org/source/world-development-indicators

Xie, B., & Jaeger, P. T. (2008). Older adults and political participation on the internet: A cross-cultural comparison of the USA and China. *Journal of Cross-Cultural Gerontology, 23*, 1–15.

Xiong, J., & Zuo, M. (2019). How does family support work when older adults obtain information from mobile internet? *Information Technology & People, 32*(6), 1496–1516.

Yang, J., & Du, P. (2021). Gender, capital endowment and digital exclusion of older people in China. *Ageing & Society, 41*(11), 2502–2526.

Yiting, E., Yang, J., Niu, L., & Lu, C. (2023). The impact of internet use on health status among older adults in China: The mediating role of social support. *Frontiers in Public Health, 11*, 1023763.

Yu, R. P., Ellison, N. B., McCammon, R. J., & Langa, K. M. (2016). Mapping the two levels of digital divide: Internet access and social network site adoption among older adults in the USA. *Information, Communication & Society, 19*(10), 1445–1464.

Zhang, M. (2023). Older people's attitudes towards emerging technologies: A systematic literature review. *Public Understanding of Science, 32*(8), 948–968.

Zhang, Q., & Li, Z. (2022). The impact of internet use on the social networks of the elderly in China—The mediating effect of social participation. *International Journal of Environmental Research and Public Health, 19*(15), 9576.

Zhang, K., Burr, J. A., Mutchler, J. E., & Lu, J. (2024). Internet use and loneliness among urban and non-urban Chinese older adults: The roles of family support, friend support, and social participation. *Journals of Gerontology: Social Sciences, 79*(7), gbae081.

Chapter 9
Digital Inequality and Barriers Among Older Adults in China

Danan Gu, Qiushi Feng, Kun Wang, and Haiyan Zhu

9.1 Introduction

As global internet usage continues to rise, its benefits are not equally distributed. This is particularly true among older adults, who face significant barriers in terms of digital access, skills, and usage as seen in earlier previous chapters and later chapters of this book. In China, where the population is aging rapidly (United Nations, 2024), the digital divide among older adults has become a pressing social issue. This divide has profound implications for older adults' ability to access essential services, stay connected with family and society, and engage in the digital economy (Ogbo et al., 2021; van Deursen & Helsper, 2015). Common barriers faced by older adults include a lack of appropriate digital devices, poor or restricted internet connectivity, limited digital knowledge or skills, and few opportunities to use the internet in meaningful ways (Chen et al., 2016; van Deursen & van Dijk, 2019; Yang & Du, 2021). Understanding and addressing these barriers is crucial for China's aging

D. Gu (✉)
Population Division, UN Department of Economic and Social Affairs, New York, NY, USA
e-mail: gudanan@yahoo.com

Q. Feng
Centre for Family and Population Research/Department of Sociology and Anthropology, National University of Singapore, Singapore, Singapore
e-mail: socfq@nus.edu.sg

K. Wang
Department of Social Work, College of Arts and Sciences, University of Alabama at Birmingham, Birmingham, AL, USA
e-mail: kw2@uab.edu

H. Zhu
Department of Sociology, Virginia Tech, Blacksburg, VA, USA
e-mail: zhuh@vt.edu

K. Wang et al. (eds.), *ICT Use and Healthy Longevity*, Advances in Studies of Aging and Health 5, https://doi.org/10.1007/978-3-031-98964-3_9

population to become more digitally integrated with the advancement of the digital society.

While there has been growing attention to digital inequality, research specifically focusing on older adults in China has been limited, with a few notable exceptions (e.g., Chen et al., 2016; Yang & Du, 2021; Zhang & He, 2022). Much of the existing literature on China is limited in its scope on of the digital divide, often examining digital divide such as access or skills without addressing how these factors intersect. This chapter seeks to provide a comprehensive analysis of the digital divide in China, considering not only access but also digital knowledge and skill patterns. By offering a more holistic view, the present study aims to contribute valuable insights into the specific barriers and different divides to digital engagement faced by older adults in China, framed through three core dimensions: access, knowledge, and skills.

Guided by van Dijk's theory of the deepening divide (van Dijk, 2005, 2017), the present study conceptualizes digital inequality as a multifaceted phenomenon that extends beyond disparities in physical access to encompass gaps in digital literacy and competence in usage. By identifying factors contributing to barriers to digital engagement and comparing patterns between internet users and non-users, the present analysis aims to inform targeted interventions to reduce digital exclusion among aging populations.

Notably, van Dijk's framework includes a third level of inequality—the usage/outcome divide. Though this chapter focuses solely on barriers related to access, knowledge, and digital skills in use, later chapters of the book will explore the broader consequences of differential technology use, including its impact on health, subjective well-being, and social or economic life. Addressing these first- and second-level divides is foundational for fostering digital inclusion among older adults, particularly as digital services become indispensable to healthcare, social participation, and government services. Reducing disparities in access and literacy can enhance older adults' autonomy, improve healthcare access, and mitigate social isolation, ultimately advancing their quality of life in an increasingly digitized society.

The following sections begin by reviewing the existing literature on digital divides in aging populations, followed by an explanation of the study's rationale and the potential contributions of this research to the broader field of digital inclusion for older adults. Next, the data sources, research design, and methodology, for the present study will be introduced, followed by a presentation of the key findings. Lastly, interpretations of the key findings will be offered in a discussion and, in closing, recommendations to address the challenges in bridging the digital divide among older populations will be made.

9.1.1 Literature Review

The concept of the digital divide has evolved dramatically since its inception, shifting from a focus on access to technology to a more nuanced understanding of how digital inequalities manifest in multiple dimensions of access, skills, and usage (see

Chap. 3). As technology becomes more deeply integrated into everyday life, the implications of these divides become increasingly important for older adults, who often face compounded barriers due to age-related factors (Wilson et al., 2021).

Van Dijk's foundational theory of the digital divide identifies three sequential levels of inequality: *access, skills/knowledge, and benefits* (van Dijk, 2005, 2017, 2020). The first level, *access*, encompasses disparities in the availability and affordability of devices, connectivity, and infrastructure (Hargittai, 2002; Scheerder et al., 2017). The second level, *knowledge/skills*, refers to inequalities in the ability to effectively use digital tools, including operational competencies (e.g., navigating interfaces) and critical skills (e.g., evaluating online information) (van Deursen & van Dijk, 2014). The third level, *benefits*, focuses on differential outcomes derived from technology use, such as improved health access, social inclusion, or economic opportunities (Helsper, 2021). These levels collectively highlight the multidimensional nature of digital inequality, particularly among older adults, who often face barriers across multiple domains.

To operationalize these disparities, scholars have turned these concepts into distinct and measurable gaps. *Access gaps* (first-level divide) reflect unequal distribution of devices, connectivity, and affordability (Scheerder et al., 2017). *Knowledge gaps* describe deficits in understanding how to operate devices or apps (Friemel, 2016), while *skill gaps* refer to the inability to perform tasks like information retrieval, privacy management, or content creation (Hargittai, 2002). Usage gaps, usually defined as differences in the frequency, diversity, or purpose of technology use (Wei et al., 2011), straddle the second and third levels of van Dijk's framework: they measure behavioral engagement but do not inherently address meaningful outcomes (Helsper, 2021). Therefore, there is a need to disentangle use from benefit when addressing digital exclusion.

Access Gaps

Access gaps, that is, disparities in device ownership and reliable internet connectivity, remain a significant barrier to digital inclusion for older adults worldwide, particularly in developing economies (Chinn & Fairlie, 2007; Kemp, 2025). These gaps are shaped by a combination of socio-economic and infrastructural, as outlined in van Dijk's (2005) multi-level framework. Disadvantaged socio-economic status (SES) is a critical factor limiting the ability to afford devices or subscriptions, especially in developing economies where technology costs may be beyond household budgets (Friemel, 2016; GSMA, 2023). Even in high-income countries, retirees often face financial trade-offs between essential needs and digital access (Vogels, 2021). These factors result in physical barriers such as device ownership and connectivity, which disproportionately affect older adults in low-income and rural areas (Chinn & Fairlie, 2007; Donner, 2008; also see Chaps. 2 and 6).

Infrastructural or contextual challenges compound these difficulties. For example, rural areas often lack reliable broadband, forcing older adults to rely on outdated or intermittent connections (Donner, 2008; van Deursen & van Dijk, 2019). Even in urban areas, though connectivity is generally better, older adults may still face "material access" barriers, such as incompatible devices or insufficient data plans, which hinder meaningful engagement (van Deursen & Helsper, 2015).

Moreover, cognitive and physical deterioration at older ages, including declining dexterity, vision impairments, and low digital literacy, further limit older adults' ability to navigate increasingly complex digital interfaces (Yusif et al., 2016; Hargittai & Dobransky, 2017).

In China, these challenges are particularly pronounced in rural and some remote areas where older adults often face systemic marginalization due to inadequate digital infrastructure investment and limited access to affordable devices, restricting their ability to engage with essential services like telehealth or online banking (Chen et al., 2016; Yang & Du, 2021; Zhang & He, 2022). These issues are exacerbated by socioeconomic factors, with many seniors in rural and inland remote areas living on fixed incomes and prioritizing basic needs over technology expenditures (Yang & Du, 2021; Zhang & He, 2022). Even in urban and coastal areas, where infrastructure is more robust, financial barriers such as the high cost of modern devices and broadband subscriptions still strain limited retirement budgets, leaving many older adults reliant on outdated, incompatible devices (Li & Luximon, 2018).

Knowledge Gaps

Knowledge gaps in the context of digital divide refer to disparities in individuals' understanding of how digital technologies function, including the ability to recognize basic operations of devices or applications (van Dijk, 2017, 2020). Distinct from skill gaps, which involve practical competencies like navigating interfaces, knowledge gaps reflect deficits in foundational awareness, such as knowing how to install software, differentiate between apps, or troubleshoot common errors (Friemel, 2016; Hargittai, 2002). Empirical studies highlight several factors contributing to these gaps.

Age is a critical determinant, as older adults often face steeper knowledge gaps due to limited exposure to digital technologies during their formative years and age-related cognitive declines that hinder the acquisition of new information (Freese et al., 2006; Hunsaker & Hargittai, 2018). SES further exacerbates disparities: individuals with lower education and income levels often lack the knowledge necessary to understand digital workflows. Those with limited formal education may struggle to grasp abstract digital concepts, such as distinguishing a web browser from a search engine (Helsper 2021); and those in lower-income groups may lack access to formal education and training programs, further widening the knowledge gap (van Dijk, 2005). It is also noteworthy that gender disparities in knowledge gaps may diminish when controlling for SES and age Helsper (2021). Geographic location also plays a role: rural populations, particularly in developing regions, often lack access to formal digital literacy programs or peer networks that facilitate knowledge exchange, perpetuating gaps (González et al., 2012; Yang & Du, 2021; Zhang & He, 2022).

Cultural and linguistic barriers compound these challenges. Non-native language speakers or individuals from non-Western cultural contexts may misinterpret interface terminologies or design conventions, leading to persistent misunderstandings (Scheerder et al., 2017). Cognitive factors, including low digital self-efficacy or cognitive impairments, further reduce motivation to engage with technology, creating cyclical knowledge deficits (Freese et al., 2006; Hunsaker & Hargittai, 2018). For example, older adults experiencing memory decline may avoid learning new digital tasks due to a fear of failure (Czaja et al., 2006). Studies also emphasize social networks in knowledge transmission. Older adults who are reliant on younger family members for technical support often develop fragmented, passive knowledge, as they depend on others to perform tasks rather than internalizing processes (Friemel, 2016).

Skills Gaps

Skill gaps represent disparities in individuals' practical ability to execute digital tasks, such as securing data privacy, discerning credible online content, or adapting to new platforms (Hargittai, 2018; van Deursen & van Dijk, 2014). These gaps are different from those based on knowledge. For instance, older adults may understand the importance of online security (knowledge) but lack the skill to implement two-factor authentication, a task which requires sequential problem-solving and interface familiarity (Czaja et al., 2006).

Factors associated with skill gaps largely overlap with those knowledge gaps such as age, SES, and geographical location. Socioeconomic disparities not only limit access to digital knowledge but also restrict opportunities for hands-on experimentation, hindering skill mastery (Hargittai, 2002). Rural populations, while aware of digital tools, may still lack skills to troubleshoot connectivity issues independently, relying instead on intermittent community support (González et al., 2012). However, skill gaps are uniquely shaped by procedural complexity (e.g., motor coordination, problem-solving adaptability) and experiential learning pathways (Friemel, 2016; Helsper, 2021). Cognitive-motor challenges uniquely compound skill gaps. Declining dexterity complicates precise interactions (e.g., touchscreen navigation), while reduced processing speed impedes real-time decision-making in dynamic interfaces (Czaja et al., 2006).

Learning pathways also play a distinct role in knowledge gaps. Dependence on family for technical assistance often substitutes skill-building with passive dependency, whereas self-directed experimentation fosters adaptability (Friemel, 2016; Helsper, 2021). For example, older adults who delegate tasks like online banking to relatives may stagnate in skill development, whereas those who engage independently gradually refine their competencies. In this sense, community context also matters. Individuals from communities with limited digital integration (e.g., agrarian economies) may recognize technology's utility but lack procedural fluency due to infrequent practice (Scheerder et al., 2017).

9.1.2 Research Questions

Despite the growing research on the digital divide among older adults, significant gaps remain. First, with few exceptions (e.g., Chung et al., 2010), many studies fail to distinguish between internet users and non-users, overlooking the unique barriers each group faces (Hargittai, 2018; van Deursen & Helsper, 2015; van Dijk, 2020). Barriers can vary due to factors such as education, income, and rural-urban residence. Understanding the differences between these two groups, particularly within the second-level digital divide, is essential (Hargittai, 2018). In China, some studies on internet use among older adults have examined urban-rural differences (Yu et al., 2024), yet research comparing users and non-users remains limited.

Second, research from a Western perspective often ignores cultural and infrastructural factors in developing nations. One example of salient factors that are often ignored by Western research on Chinese populations is the emphasis of filial piety in Chinese culture, which may discourage older adults from seeking technological help for fear of burdening younger family members (Chen & Chan, 2014). Moreover, factors like ethnicity and family structure that can exacerbate digital exclusion are often neglected (Zheng & Walsham, 2021). Motivated by the need to fill the research gap and deepen understanding of digital exclusion among internet users and non-users, the present study aims to address the following research questions:

1. What is the prevalence of access, knowledge, and skill gaps among Chinese older adults?
2. Which factors are associated with each gap?
3. How do barriers differ between current internet users and non-users, and what does this imply for targeted interventions?

Answering these questions could offer insights into effective interventions to promote digital inclusion among older populations in China and beyond, helping policymakers and practitioners design tailored strategies to bridge the digital divide and enhance digital equality for older adults.

9.2 Data and Methods

9.2.1 Data Sources

To achieve the current research objectives, this chapter utilizes data from the China Longitudinal Aging Social Survey (CLASS), a nationally representative longitudinal survey in China, to conduct its analysis. A detailed description of CLASS is available in Chap. 6 or in previous publications referenced in this book (Dong et al., 2019; Jin & Zhao, 2019). Given the specific research focus and the availability of specifically relevant data, the present study primarily used data from the 2020 wave. However, due to the limited number of respondents under the age of 65 in this wave, the analytical sample is restricted to adults aged 65 or older, resulting in a total sample of 11,228 participants.

9.2.2 *Measures*

Internet Use Barriers

CLASS included eight dichotomous questions which assess barriers or inconveniences in accessing and using the internet. These barriers encompass: (1) lack of a suitable device (e.g., desktop/laptop, tablet/iPad, smartphone), (2) poor internet connection, (3) lack of knowledge on how to operate a device, (4) difficulty using certain apps, (5) difficulty reading text on screens due to small font size, (6) inability to find necessary information, (7) concerns about the accuracy of news or information, and (8) concerns about the leakage of confidential information.

To systematically categorize these barriers in alignment with the three gaps discussed above, a dichotomous variable for access barriers (access gap), classifying respondents as having an access barrier if they answered "yes" to either of the first two questions. Likewise, those who reported difficulties in the third or fourth question were identified as having a knowledge barrier (knowledge gap) was constructed. Finally, respondents who indicated challenges in the last four questions from fifth to eighth were categorized as experiencing a skill barrier (skill gap), which can also be considered a part of usage gaps. The access gap is the first level of the digital divide, while both the knowledge and skill gaps fall into the second level of the digital divide (van Dijk, 2005, 2020).

In addition to these three dichotomous outcome variables, a composite dichotomous variable was constructed to reflect the prevalence of the digital divide using all eight items. Furthermore, a separate outcome variable that quantifies the number of barriers experienced, with a score ranging from 0 to 8, for supplementary analysis. Collectively, these CLASS barrier questions capture key dimensions of the first and second levels of the digital divide (van Dijk, 2005; van Deursen & van Dijk, 2014), providing valuable insights into the challenges older adults in China face as they engage with digital technologies.

Associated Factors with Barriers

Following the STAM and other digital divide frameworks detailed in Chap. 3, all five sets of variables were used to examine the associates of internet use in Chap. 6. These variables provide a comprehensive framework for analyzing key aspects of aging, including (1) demographic variables, (2) socioeconomic variables, (3) family and social support network, (4) views on aging, perceived aging, and advances in internet technology, and (5) health status. The region variable is always controlled for in all models. Please refer to detailed definition and coding in Chap. 6.

Analytical Strategies

We primarily employed multiple logistic regression models and linear regression models alongside descriptive analyses. Initially, following the analytical strategy outlined in Chap. 6, partial models were constructed to examine the independent associations between each set of variables and the five digital barrier outcomes. However, given that the coefficients in the full models, in which all control variables are included, are highly similar to those in the partial models, only the results from the full models are being presented for clarity and conciseness. Consistent with the approach in Chap. 6, sampling weights were applied in descriptive analyses but not in the regression models.

Unlike many previous studies on the digital divide, which have primarily focused on either internet users (van Deursen & Helsper, 2015; Hargittai & Dobransky, 2017) or the general population (Scheerder et al., 2017; Blank & Groselj, 2014), the present analysis distinguishes between users and non-users. Specifically, analyses were conducted among three groups: internet users, non-users, and the total population. This differentiation allows for the development of more tailored interventions aimed at addressing the specific digital barriers encountered by each group. All statistical analyses were conducted using Stata 18.0.

9.3 Results

Table 9.1 displays the weighted and unweighted distributions of the study variables, highlighting the prevalence of digital barriers among Chinese older adults. First, slightly more than one-third of older adults in China faced access barriers (the first-level digital divide) in 2020. These barriers included inadequate access to devices (e.g., smartphones, tablets, or computers), unreliable internet connectivity. Second, approximately two-thirds of respondents reported knowledge gaps (a part of the second-level digital divide), indicating insufficient understanding to operate devices or navigate applications. More than 70% of older adults experienced skill gaps (also part of the second-level divide), struggling with tasks such as locating information online, evaluating the credibility of digital content, managing data privacy concerns, or non-age-friendly technological designs, such as small font sizes that hindered readability, rendering internet use difficult or impossible.

Overall, the results demonstrate that 90% of older adults encountered at least one digital barrier, with individuals facing an average of 2.6 barriers out of the eight barriers measured. These findings underscore the significant digital divide existing among older adults in China, the multifaceted nature of digital exclusion among this population, and the overlapping challenges compounding accessibility and participation in the digital sphere.

Figure 9.1 presents the reported barriers to internet use among both users and non-users. Among internet users, concerns about the leakage of confidential information emerged as the most significant barrier, affecting over 42% of older adults. This was followed by non-user-friendly device and app designs, which made tasks such as reading and navigation difficult. Two knowledge-related barriers ranked third and fourth, reflecting a lack of sufficient understanding to use the internet or mobile devices efficiently or effectively. By contrast, access barriers, particularly the lack of a device, were reported less frequently, suggesting that technology availability is not the primary challenge for older adult users in contemporary China.

Among non-users, the most significant barrier was insufficient knowledge of how to use digital devices or apps. This aligns with 2020 data from CNNIC, which

Table 9.1 Unweighted and weighted percentage distribution of the analytical sample by study variable, 2020, CLASS (N = 11,228)

	Weighted	Unweighted
% Use the internet	30.0	27.0
% Having an access gap	34.4	36.0
% Having a knowledge gap	64.5	65.3
% Having a skill gap	70.5	71.4
% Having 1+ listed barriers in internet use	90.0	90.8
Number of reported barriers (0–8)[a]	2.63	2.70
%Ages 65–74	64.8	38.0
%Ages 75–85	27.1	44.7
%Ages 85+	8.1	17.3
%Men	47.5	50.5
%Han ethnicity	95.5	94.0
%Urban residents	52.7	54.9
%0 years of schooling	24.4	23.6
%1–6 years of schooling	39.1	41.2
%7+ years of schooling	36.5	35.2
%Economically poor	10.4	11.5
%White-collar occupation	10.8	11.7
%Blue-collar occupation	27.5	29.9
%Agricultural workers	61.7	58.4
%Currently Married	78.1	75.3
%Having 2+ close family members	80.5	79.7
%Having 2+ close friends	71.4	70.6
%Frequent engagement in leisure activity	82.1	83.2
Positive views on internet impact (0–8)[a]	2.12	2.08
Positive views on aging (7–35)[a]	20.68	20.60
Positive perceived aging (8–40)[a]	23.91	23.98
%Having 1+ diseases	79.6	80.4
%IADL disabled	18.7	24.2
%ADL disabled	11.3	15.1
%Cognitively impaired	24.5	30.4
%Good self-rated health	50.3	46.8
% East	38.5	36.1
% Central	27.1	25.7
% West	25.7	24.8
% Northeast	8.6	13.4

[a] The mean score of the variable. ADL: Activities of daily living. IADL: Instrumental ADL

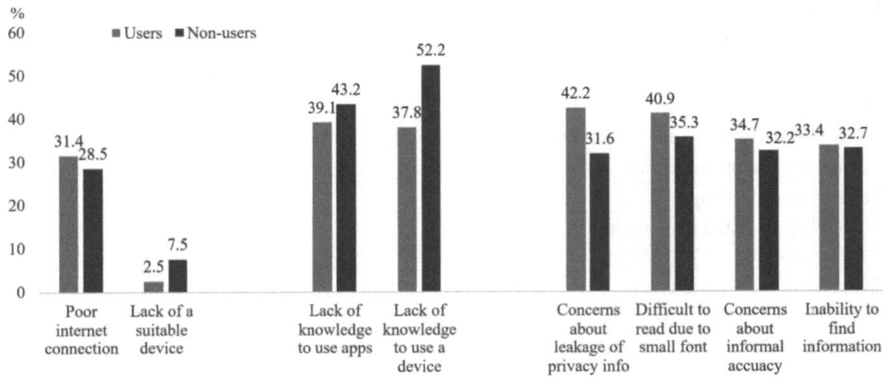

Fig. 9.1 Percentages of reported barriers among users and non-users, 2020, CLASS. Note: The percentages were weighted. Each respondent can report multiple barriers

reported that 49% of non-users cited a lack of digital skills as their reason for not using the internet (CNNIC, 2021). Among skill-related barriers, difficulty reading screens ranked the highest. The remaining three skill-related barriers were reported at similar levels. Although access barriers were generally lower among non-users, the lack of a device was notably more prevalent compared to users.

Table 9.2 compares the weighted percentages of older adults encountering barriers to internet access and use between internet users and non-users stratified by three groups: urban residents, rural residents, and the total sample, without taking into consideration of other study factors. While no differences in reported barriers were found between users and non-users in access gaps or the average number of barriers, notable disparities emerged in knowledge gaps, skill gaps, and the overall prevalence of experiencing at least one barrier. These differences show that compared to users, non-users faced greater knowledge gaps (68.3% vs. 55.5% in the total population, for example) and were more likely to report at least one barrier (91.3% vs. 87%). However, they reported a lower proportion of having a skill barrier than users (67.3% vs. 77.9%), possibly due to a lack of unawareness of the specific skills needed for digital engagement. This pattern remained consistent across urban, rural, and the total populations.

We further compared urban and rural differences in reported barriers. Among users, urban-rural disparity was only observed in the average number of barriers, with urban older adults having more barriers than their rural counterparts (see the significance levels in the table denoted by a, b, c). Among non-users, rural older adults had a higher proportion of access barriers than urban residents (36.4% vs. 33.5%), but they reported fewer skill barriers than their urban counterparts (65.9% vs. 71.1%) and more total number of barriers (2.58 vs. 2.70). This discrepancy may stem from rural individuals' comparatively limited exposure to digital technologies, potentially reducing their awareness of the skills required for effective digital engagement.

Table 9.2 Weighted proportion of the respondents who reported having different types of barriers in using the internet, 2020, CLASS

	Among internet users N = 3034	Among non-internet users N = 8194	Among the total sample N = 11,228
Total (n = 11,228)			
% Having an access gap	32.9	35.1	34.4
% Having a knowledge gap	55.5***	68.3***	64.5
% Having a skill gap	77.9***	67.3***	70.5
% Having 1+ listed barriers in internet use	87.0***	91.3***	90.0
Average of the number reported barriers (0–8)	2.62	2.64	2.63
Rural (n = 5061)			
% Having an access gap	34.2	36.4[b]	35.9[b]
% Having a knowledge gap	54.3***	65.9***[c]	63.5[a]
% Having a skill gap	76.6***	68.0***	69.8
% Having 1+ listed barriers in internet use	88.7***	91.0***	90.5
Average of the number reported barriers (0–8)	2.52[a]	2.58[c]	2.56[a]
Urban (n = 6167)			
% Having an access gap	32.4	33.5[b]	33.1[b]
% Having a knowledge gap	56.1***	71.1***[c]	65.4[a]
% Having a skill gap	78.5***	66.4***	71.1
% Having 1+ listed barriers in internet use	86.2***	91.7***	89.6
Average of the number reported barriers (0–8)	2.67[a]	2.70[c]	2.69[a]

Note: The tests are for differences between urban and rural areas for the total sample, internet users, and non-users, respectively, based on chi-square tests of all variables but the number of barriers that was based on T-tests

p values for users vs. non-users: $+p < 0.1$, $*p < 0.05$, $**p < 0.01$, $***p < 0.001$

p values for differences between urban and rural: a < 0.05, b < 0.01, c < 0.001

Tables 9.3, 9.4 and 9.5 present the results of multiple regression models analyzing factors associated with three aspects of the digital divide (access, knowledge, and skill gaps) as well as overall barriers and the number of reported barriers across three groups: internet users, non-users, and the total population. Several consistent patterns emerged across the models.

First, no gender difference was found across types of barriers and user status, indicating that older men and women encountered similar challenges in digital access, knowledge, and skills.

Second, Han ethnicity, economic disadvantage, cognitive impairment, and ADL disability were consistently associated with greater barriers in most cases, regardless of the specific divide dimension, number of barriers, or user status. Older adults facing financial constraints had significantly higher odds of reporting access,

Table 9.3 Odds ratios or coefficients of overall and specific barriers to internet use among users by study variables, 2020, CLASS

	Access gap	Knowledge gap	Skill gap	Having 1+ barrier	Number of barriers
Ages 75–85 (65–74)	0.88	0.86+	0.97	0.94	−0.13*
Ages 85+ (65–74)	0.66+	0.65*	0.78	0.55+	−0.47**
Men (women)	1.06	1.04	0.95	1.10	−0.00
Han ethnicity (minor	1.88**	2.28***	1.56*	2.52***	0.61***
Urban (rural)	0.82+	1.06	0.70*	0.53***	−0.07
1–6 years of schooling (0)	0.94	0.80	0.95	0.65	−0.38**
7+ years of schooling (0)	1.09	0.97	1.22	0.89	−0.16
Economically poor (no)	1.74***	1.63***	1.49*	1.93*	0.38***
Blue-collar occupation (white-collar)	1.06	1.04	1.15	1.31+	0.13+
Agricultural workers (white-collar)	0.97	1.05	0.81	0.92	−0.01
Currently married (no)	1.27*	1.11	1.08	1.00	0.20*
Having 2+ close family members (<2)	1.17	1.41**	1.33+	1.60*	0.23*
Having 2+ close friends (< 2)	1.03	0.90	0.95	0.73+	0.05
Leisure and social activity (no)	0.82	1.04	1.02	0.43***	0.16
Positive views on internet impact (0–8)	0.93***	0.83***	0.82***	0.76***	−0.15***
Positive views on aging (7–35)	0.99	0.98+	1.00	0.98	0.01
Positive perceived aging (8–40)	1.01	1.03**	0.99	1.01	0.01
Having 1+ diseases (no)	0.82+	1.01	0.95	1.12	−0.00
IADL disabled (no)	0.79+	0.92	0.92	1.41	−0.17+
ADL disabled (no)	0.89	1.92***	1.56*	4.43***	0.53***
Cognitively impaired (no)	1.15	1.45**	2.32***	3.78***	0.35***
Good self-rated health (no)	0.82*	0.81*	1.05	1.27+	−0.16*
Central (East)	0.88	0.76*	0.37***	0.30***	−0.49***
West (East)	1.56**	0.67**	0.42***	0.24***	−0.27**
Northeast (East)	2.18***	1.63***	1.70**	7.56***	0.47***
-LL	1816.8	1932.2	1380.8	907.8	–
LR chi-square	194/2	321.8	275.4	406.7	–
Adj. R-square	–	–	–	–	0.12
Chi-square	–	–	–	–	18.3

Note: The results for the first four dependent variables were based on logistic regression models, and the results for the fifth dependent variable (number of barriers) were based on linear regression models. The category of a variable in the parentheses is the reference. IADL: Instrumental activities of daily living. ADL: Activities of daily living. The degree of freedom is 25, and the sample size is N = 3034. "–" not applicable

+$p < 0.1$, *$p < 0.05$, **$p < 0.01$, ***$p < 0.001$

Table 9.4 Odds ratios or coefficients of overall and specific barriers to internet use among non-users by study variables, 2020, CLASS

	Access gap	Knowledge gap	Skill gap	Having 1+ barrier	Number of barriers
Ages 75–85 (65–74)	0.99	1.02	0.90*	1.03	−0.04
Ages 85+ (65–74)	0.92	0.96	0.68***	0.72**	−0.21***
Men (women)	0.97	1.04	1.00	1.14+	0.01
Han ethnicity (minor	1.88***	2.19***	4.72***	4.60***	1.25***
Urban (rural)	0.88*	1.18**	0.89*	0.75***	0.07+
1–6 years of schooling (0)	0.93	0.87*	1.13*	0.77**	−0.07+
7+ years of schooling (0)	1.05	0.94	1.48***	0.87	0.13**
Economically poor (no)	1.43***	1.27***	1.70***	1.81***	0.29***
Blue-collar occupation (white-collar)	0.99	1.20**	1.00	1.55***	0.06
Agricultural workers (white-collar)	0.96	1.39***	0.68***	1.34*	0.01
Currently married (no)	1.14**	0.99	1.16**	1.07	0.09*
Having 2+ close family members (<2)	1.21**	1.13*	1.02	1.57***	0.07
Having 2+ close friends (< 2)	1.00	1.03	0.97	0.88	0.05
Leisure and social activity (no)	0.91+	1.27***	1.19**	0.97	0.21***
Positive views on internet impact (0–8)	0.97*	0.92***	1.01	0.97+	−0.03***
Positive views on aging (7–35)	1.02**	0.98***	1.01*	1.01	0.01*
Positive perceived aging (8–40)	0.99	1.00	1.05***	1.01	0.01*
Having 1+ diseases (no)	0.81***	1.02	0.76***	1.18+	−0.13**
IADL disabled (no)	0.94	0.93	1.17*	1.05	−0.03
ADL disabled (no)	1.07	1.33***	1.01	1.72***	0.29***
Cognitively impaired (no)	1.00	1.35***	1.29***	1.77***	0.18***
Good self-rated health (no)	0.88**	1.00	1.04	1.45***	−0.03
Central (East)	1.19**	0.77***	1.05	0.42***	−0.12**
West (East)	2.01***	1.08	2.34***	1.14	0.47***
Northeast (East)	2.39***	1.59***	9.01***	14.45***	0.93***
-LL	5244.2	4896.5	4431.9	1936.8	–
LR chi-square	337.0	357.4	1385.0	750.8	–
Adj. R-square	–	–	–	–	0.12
Chi-square	–	–	–	–	44.9

Note: The results for the first four dependent variables were based on logistic regression models, and the results for the fifth dependent variable (number of barriers) were based on linear regression models. The category of a variable in the parentheses is the reference. IADL: Instrumental activities of daily living. ADL: Activities of daily living. The degree of freedom is 25, and the sample size is N = 8194. "–" not applicable

+$p < 0.1$, *$p < 0.05$, **$p < 0.01$, ***$p < 0.001$

Table 9.5 Odds ratios or coefficients of overall and specific barriers of use of the internet among the total sample by study variables, 2020, CLASS

	Access gap	Knowledge gap	Skill gap	Having 1+ barrier	Number of barriers
Ages 75–85 (65–74)	0.92+	1.02	0.93	1.03	−0.04
Ages 85+ (65–74)	0.78***	0.96	0.71***	0.72**	−0.21***
Men (women)	1.00	1.04	0.96	1.14+	0.01
Han ethnicity (minor	2.53***	2.19***	5.53***	4.60***	1.25***
Urban (rural)	0.89*	1.18**	0.94	0.75***	0.07+
1–6 years of schooling (0)	1.02	0.87*	0.96	0.77**	−0.07+
7+ years of schooling (0)	1.18**	0.94	1.30***	0.87	0.13**
Economically poor (no)	1.51***	1.27***	1.41***	1.81***	0.29***
Blue-collar occupation (white-collar)	0.91	1.20**	1.08	1.55***	0.06
Agricultural workers (white-collar)	0.78**	1.39***	0.77***	1.34*	0.01
Currently married (no)	1.16**	0.99	1.10+	1.07	0.09*
Having 2+ close family members (<2)	1.21**	1.13*	1.01	1.57***	0.07
Having 2+ close friends (<2)	1.06	1.03	1.05	0.88	0.05
Leisure and social activity (no)	0.86**	1.27***	1.41***	0.97	0.21***
Positive views on internet impact (0–8)	1.00	0.92***	1.01	0.97+	−0.03***
Positive views on aging (7–35)	1.02***	0.98***	1.02***	1.01	0.01*
Positive perceived aging (8–40)	1.00	1.00	1.04***	1.01	0.01*
Having 1+ diseases (no)	0.84**	1.02	0.82***	1.18+	−0.13**
IADL disabled (no)	0.97	0.93	1.09	1.05	−0.03
ADL disabled (no)	1.10	1.33***	0.99	1.72***	0.29***
Cognitively impaired (no)	1.31***	1.35***	1.06	1.77***	0.18***
Good self-rated health (no)	0.90**	1.00	1.00	1.45***	−0.03
Central (East)	1.04	0.77***	1.24***	0.42***	−0.12**
West (East)	1.98***	1.08	2.63***	1.14	0.47***
Northeast (East)	2.96***	1.59***	6.36***	14.45***	0.93***
-LL	7096.1	5981.3	6017.9	3056.7	–
LR chi-square	483.3	527.8	1408.1	770.2	–
Adj. R-square	–	–	–	–	0.10
Chi-square	–	–	–	–	52.0

Note: The results for the first four dependent variables were based on logistic regression models, and the results for the fifth dependent variable (number of barriers) were based on linear regression models. The category of a variable in the parentheses is the reference. IADL: Instrumental activities of daily living. ADL: Activities of daily living. The degree of freedom is 25, and the sample size is N = 11,228. "–" not applicable

$+p < 0.1$, $*p < 0.05$, $**p < 0.01$, $***p < 0.001$

knowledge, and skill barriers, likely because limited financial resources directly hinder their ability to acquire and effectively use digital technologies. Similarly, cognitive impairment exacerbated difficulties in learning digital skills and navigating internet use. With a few exceptions, older adults with ADL disabilities also faced greater odds of encountering barriers, possibly due to physical limitations that make interacting with digital devices more challenging, as well as a reduced capacity for sustained learning and engagement with technology.

Third, compared to older adults in East China, those in Northeast China exhibited significantly higher odds of reporting barriers across all types and user groups. This pattern is likely attributable to a combination of infrastructural limitations, economic disparities, reduced access to digital education, and limited exposure to advanced technology, as further elaborated in the Discussion section.

Fourth, counterintuitively, the oldest-old (aged 85+) often reported fewer barriers than young older adults (65–74), a trend consistent with bivariate analyses (not shown). This paradoxical finding may reflect their lower expectations regarding digital technology or reduced awareness of barriers, as discussed later.

Fifth, married older adults and those with larger family and social ties reported more access, knowledge, and skill barriers. This could be attributed to their greater reliance on digital tools for communication and daily tasks, despite their higher rates of internet use.

Finally, with few exceptions, older adults who held positive views on the impact of advancement of internet technology were significantly less likely to report barriers, regardless of their user status or the type of barrier. This suggests that a more optimistic outlook on digital technology may enhance motivation to learn and engage with online platforms.

The relationships between other factors and reported barriers varied by specific type of gap and user group. For instance, compared to users in East China, users in Central China reported fewer barriers across all models (Table 9.3). However, among non-users, those in Central China had higher odds of experiencing access barriers than their counterparts in East China, despite being less likely to report knowledge barriers (Table 9.4). In general, older adults in West China were more likely to face access barriers regardless of their user status. Yet, while users in West China reported lower odds of knowledge and skill barriers, non-users in the same region exhibited higher odds of skill barriers. This pattern suggests that non-users in Central and West China may underestimate the knowledge required to navigate digital technologies due to their limited exposure to digital ecosystems, as further discussed in the Discussion section.

Education and primary lifetime occupation were not significant predictors of reported barriers among users, however, these factors were significant predictors among non-users and their effects varied by the type of barriers. More years of schooling were associated with a greater likelihood of reporting skill barriers but a lower likelihood of knowledge barriers. Blue-collar and agricultural workers were more likely to report knowledge barriers, although agricultural workers had lower odds of reporting skill barriers.

Having at least one chronic disease was not associated with reported barriers among users, but among non-users, it was linked to lower odds of experiencing access and skill barriers. Urban older adults generally had lower odds of reporting barriers than their rural counterparts. However, urban non-users were more likely to report knowledge gaps than their rural counterparts, a pattern consistent with the bivariate findings in Table 9.2.

9.4 Discussion

Guided by van Dijk's (2005, 2020) three-level digital divide framework and drawing on data from the 2020 wave of CLASS, this chapter examines the barriers to digital engagement among older adults in China. The findings indicate that 90% of the sampled older adults reported experiencing at least one obstacle to internet use, with these barriers shaped by a complex interplay of socioeconomic, cognitive, cultural, and other contextual factors. The following discussion synthesizes the key findings, theoretical contributions, and policy implications, while also addressing the study's limitations and proposing directions for future research.

9.4.1 Key Findings and Interpretations

High Prevalence and Huge Barriers

One of the most striking findings is the high prevalence of digital barriers in China, with nearly 90% of older adults facing at least one form of digital exclusion and an average of 2.6 barriers per individual. Specifically, slightly more than one-third of older adults lacked reliable access to digital devices or the internet, and this issue was exacerbated in rural regions where infrastructural deficits (e.g., scarce broadband connectivity and limited availability of affordable devices) further compounded existing inequalities (Yang & Du, 2021; Zhang & He, 2022). These findings underscore the urgency of addressing material access gaps in China, particularly in underserved areas, to ensure equitable participation in digital communication, healthcare, and social services.

Beyond access barriers, the present findings reveal pervasive gaps in digital knowledge and skills. Nearly two-thirds of participants struggled with basic operation or app navigation, whereas more than 70% of them faced challenges in advanced tasks such as identifying credible information or safeguarding privacy. These findings align with the recommendations of existing literature that digital literacy programs must transcend rudimentary skills training (e.g. device usage to cultivate critical competencies) to include more advanced skills and education which address things such as cybersecurity awareness, information evaluation, and adaptive problem-solving (Helsper, 2021; van Deursen & van Dijk, 2014). Tailored interventions addressing these gaps are essential to empower older adults to navigate increasingly complex digital ecosystems safely and effectively (Hargittai et al., 2019).

Age and Ethnic Inequalities

Analysis indicated that the oldest-old (aged 85+) often reported fewer barriers than younger older adults (65–74). Though counterintuitive at a glance, this finding may reflect lower expectations of digital use in this age group and/or a lack of awareness about their own skill gaps, which reduces their perceptions of digital barriers. This aligns with the Unified Theory of Acceptance and Use of Technology (Venkatesh et al., 2003; see Chap. 3), which suggests that perceptions of usefulness and ease of use influence technology adoption. For older adults with technological incompetence who are hesitant or reluctant in digital adoption, often referred to as "digital resignation" (Schroeder et al., 2023), they are often discouraged from recognizing the barriers they face. Similarly, perceived relevance can also play a crucial role (Helsper, 2021). When older adults see little personal need for digital technology, they are less motivated to interact with it and thus may avoid acknowledging any barriers (Venkatesh et al., 2003). Though the present findings provide explanations for the lower barriers among the oldest-old group, the insights gleaned make observed patterns more worrisome. It is apparent that, based on these findings, efforts must be made to highlight the importance of tailoring digital literacy programs to different age groups. In tailoring digital literacy programs to different age groups, recognizing that the oldest-old may require distinct strategies compared to younger older adults to foster digital inclusion effectively will be paramount (Oswald & Wagner, 2023; Schlomann et al., 2020; von Humboldt & Leal 2015).

Analyses also reveal that Han Chinese older adults reported higher digital barriers, challenging assumptions about majority-group privilege in some Western contexts (Wang et al., 2025). Similar to the case of the age group as discussed, this may reflect a greater awareness of digital expectations and self-awareness of technological deficiencies among older Han Chinese than the other ethnicities in China (Chen & Chan, 2014; Zhang & He, 2022). Research suggests that individuals with greater exposure to digital technology are also more likely to recognize their own limitations (van Deursen & Helsper, 2015). In this sense, the disadvantaged exposure of Chinese minorities who tend to live in the borderline areas may help to explain this pattern as well. On the other hand, it is worth noting that ethnic minorities may have benefited from the introduction of bilingual smartphone interfaces in the early 2000s, localized digital training programs (Ministry of Education, 2007), and the rapid development of IT infrastructure in many minority provinces in recent years, driven by China's increasing focus on regional economic growth and digital inclusion (CNNIC, 2025; Pick et al., 2024). These technological and developmental advancements may have helped to narrow the digital divide for ethnic minorities in certain regions of China. Additionally, the exclusion of three remote provinces, where ethnic minorities constitute a relatively higher share of the population, from the CLASS survey may have introduced some bias into these findings. Given the limited research on ethnic digital inequality in China, further studies are needed.

This study found no significant gender differences in the digital divide, despite older women having a lower internet usage rate than men (31.5% vs. 26.6%; see Table 6.2). This suggests that gender may not be a key factor contributing to digital disparities among older adults in contemporary China. Several factors may explain this finding, including improvements in women's social status, shared generational experiences with technology exposure and adoption, and the Chinese government's ongoing efforts to promote gender equality and women's empowerment (CNNIC, 2025; Zou et al., 2024).

Urban-Rural Paradoxes and Regional Disparities

In most cases, urban older adults tended to report more barriers than their rural counterparts, which is expected due to similar reasons as discussed in the sessions on age and rural/urban disparities. However, there is a noteworthy pattern that urban non-users were more likely to report knowledge gaps than rural non-users. Surrounded by pervasive technology, urban non-users may internalize their lack of engagement as a personal failure, whereas those in rural areas may not yet fully recognize their needs on these knowledge and skills (Friemel, 2016; Yu et al., 2024; Zhang & He, 2022). Moreover, urban non-users, who tend to be better educated than their rural counterparts, may be skeptical of using digital technologies due to concerns about data privacy (Zheng & Walsham, 2021), yet their rural counterparts may instead perceive these technologies as irrelevant to later lives. These explanations are well in line with Hargittai's (2018) theory on the *second-level divide*, in which disparities in self-efficacy and autonomy shape digital engagement outcomes.

The finding that regional disparities significantly influenced digital inclusion in China is a key contribution of this study to the literature. Among users, older adults in Central and West China reported lower odds of knowledge and skill barriers compared to their counterparts in East China. Given the lower prevalence of internet use in these regions (see Chap. 6), this may stem from limited exposure to digital ecosystems or lower expectations for internet activities, leading them to underestimate the knowledge and skills required for technology use. Similarly, non-users in these regions also reported lower odds of knowledge barriers. They further reported higher odds of access and skill barriers than their East China counterparts, reflecting disadvantaged internet infrastructure in these areas.

Older adults in Northeast China, a region experiencing economic stagnation and out-migration in recent decades, consistently reported the most severe digital barriers across all types. Several factors which are significant to barriers must be considered. First, economic decline and population loss may have led to reduced investments in technological infrastructure and digital literacy programs in this region. At the same time, the high demand for digital communication to stay connected with out-migrated children exacerbates digital exclusion among older people. Second, norms and attitudes toward technology and aging may further hinder digital adoption among older adults in this region (Charness & Boot, 2009; Czaja et al., 2006). Lastly, Northeast China has the second-highest internet use among older adults (see Chap. 6), which may heighten awareness of digital challenges, leading to reporting of greater barriers.

These findings, alongside urban-rural paradoxes among non-users, highlight the need for region-specific policies of digital equity that address local infrastructure, education, and economic conditions. Context-specific interventions must improve digital literacy, expand infrastructure, and strengthen support networks to foster digital inclusion among older adults (Donner, 2008; Friemel, 2016; van Deursen & van Dijk, 2019).

Socioeconomic Disparities
Regarding socioeconomic disparities in the digital divide, our findings indicate that economic disadvantage remains a key predictor of digital exclusion, reinforcing van Dijk's (2005) argument that material access is foundational. Older adults with limited incomes struggle to afford devices or internet subscriptions, restricting access to essential services like telehealth and online banking (Chen et al., 2016). In China, rapid digitization has intensified socioeconomic disparities, particularly in rural areas with inadequate broadband infrastructure (GSMA, 2023). This is similar to the findings from developing societies which indicate low-income retirees prioritize basic needs over technology, further widening the digital divide (Vogels, 2021). Unlike in high-income nations, where digital adoption barriers may often arise from generational or psychological factors, affordability remains the primary obstacle in China, deepening digital inequities (Wang & Kubanga, 2021).

Interestingly, non-users with higher education levels report greater skill barriers. Educated older adults may have a heightened awareness of digital complexities, making them more conscious of their own skill gaps (van Deursen & van Dijk, 2011; Hargittai, 2002). Their self-expectations for proficiency and perceived societal standards may heighten anxiety about digital adoption (Czaja et al., 2006; Charness & Boot, 2009). Additionally, formal education does not guarantee digital competence, especially for those who completed their schooling before the digital era. While they may excel in knowledge and skills of the non-digital domains, they often struggle with hands-on digital navigation, reinforcing their perception of skill barriers (Friemel, 2016).

Older adults from agricultural backgrounds report fewer skill barriers, likely due to less awareness and/or a greater reliance on family members or community networks for digital assistance (Friemel, 2016). Compared with white-collar workers, blue-collar or agricultural workers faced greater knowledge barriers. This is likely because, unlike their white-collar counterparts who may have had some exposure to computers in professional settings, many blue-collar retirees had minimal contact with digital tools throughout their working lives (Research on Aging, Policies and Practice, 2017), reducing both their familiarity and motivation to engage with digital technology (Hargittai, 2002; van Deursen & Helsper, 2015).

Impact of Health Conditions
The present findings confirmed that declining health conditions, particularly cognitive decline and functional disability, were consistently associated with increased digital exclusion, as established by previous research (Wildenbos et al., 2018). Older adults with cognitive impairment experienced higher odds of digital barriers, which aligns with existing research suggesting that cognitive decline makes it more

difficult to learn and adapt to new technologies for navigation and information discernment, deepening second-level divides (Freese et al., 2006; Hunsaker & Hargittai, 2018). Functional disabilities, such as impaired vision, mobility, or dexterity, compound these challenges by limiting physical interactions with devices, further restricting access and usability (Heart & Kalderon, 2013; Oswald & Wagner, 2023). However, as observed in this study, individuals with chronic diseases, such as hypertension or diabetes, tended to report fewer access and skill barriers. This may be explained by people with chronic health conditions often relying on family members or caregivers for support, reducing their need to independently access or use digital tools (Wildenbos et al., 2018). In addition, these individuals may frequently use online consultancy and are thus proficient in using the internet services (Randine et al., 2022; Scalvini et al., 2014), which may lead to reporting fewer barriers.

Role of Family and Social Networks

The role of social and family support also emerged as a key factor influencing digital engagement. Interestingly, in the present study, married older adults and those with larger families reported more access barriers, particularly among non-users. This outcome contrasts with findings from Western studies, where familial support often helps mitigate digital exclusion (Friemel, 2016; Helsper, 2021; Seifert et al., 2021). In China, filial piety norms dictate that children should provide care and support to their elderly parents. However, research finds that many older adults are reluctant to seek assistance due to concerns of being a 'burden' on their children (Ang & Malhotra, 2022; Bai et al., 2020). For example, they may delegate tasks such as online banking to family members instead of handling these tasks themselves. While this reliance on others may provide convenience, it also discourages older adults from learning digital skills, reinforcing gaps in their knowledge and skills (Chen & Chan, 2014; Chen et al., 2016). At the same time, those with strong social and family networks may be more reliant on digital technology to maintain connections or receive care. This increased exposure may heighten their awareness of digital challenges, while higher expectations for digital competence could further emphasize their perceived limitations.

Impacts of Views About Technology and Aging

In the present study, older adults who positively viewed the advancement of digital technology were less likely to report barriers, regardless of their user status or the type of barrier. This finding suggests that a more favorable perception of digital technology may foster greater motivation to acquire digital knowledge and skills and actively engage with online platforms (Mazur et al., 2012). However, the relationship between views on aging and reporting barriers is complex. Older adults with more positive views of aging were more likely to report skill barriers, suggesting that those with an optimistic outlook on aging or involving in social activities are more willing to engage with technology and as they face challenges, they are more likely to recognize these difficulties (Vaportzis et al., 2017). Conversely, older adults who hold more negative views of aging may perceive the digital divide as less pressing, which could result in lower awareness of or concern about digital barriers (Köttl et al., 2021; Wang & Gu, 2023). This pattern also applies to access barriers.

These findings highlight the complex relationship between views on aging or perceived aging and digital engagement, where a more proactive attitude towards aging may lead to greater sensitivity to technological challenges.

Divergent Barriers Between Internet Users and Non-users
One uniqueness of the present study is to examine the digital divide between internet users and non-users. The study reveals critical differences in reporting barriers between internet users and non-users, presenting distinctive digital barriers for them. For users, barriers centered on skill gaps (e.g., privacy management, information discernment) may be most significant, reflecting van Dijk's (2017, 2020) third-level divide, where unequal outcomes stem from differential usage quality. Non-users, however, faced knowledge barriers, highlighting the second-level digital divides, where disparities arise from varying levels of digital literacy (Scheerder et al., 2017). These findings underscore the importance of tailored interventions that address the distinct challenges faced by each group. In short, intervention should focus on enhancing digital skills for users while fostering foundational digital awareness for non-users.

9.4.2 Theoretical and Practical Implications

Theoretical Implications
The present study reinforces van Dijk's (2005) deepening divide framework, while also highlighting its limitations in non-Western contexts. The first-level divide (access) remains a critical issue in rural China, where infrastructural deficits and negative impacts reflect patterns observed in developing economies (Chinn & Fairlie, 2007). However, the prominence of second-level divides (knowledge/skills) among urban populations challenges implicit assumptions that material access guarantees meaningful engagement. For instance, urban non-users with device access still lacked operational knowledge, suggesting that cognitive and attitudinal factors, such as technophobia or low self-efficacy, may mediate the effect from access to engagement (Friemel, 2016; Hargittai & Dobransky, 2017).

Along this line, the conceptual separation of knowledge and skills also seems necessary to address these issues. For example, critical literacy (i.e., an understanding of online safety) must accompany skill development. This is a challenge that is often overlooked in traditional digital divide remediation models. Furthermore, Hargittai's (2018) *second-level divide* does not adequately capture intersectional factors like ethnicity, which uniquely shape digital exclusion in China's collectivist context. Although this chapter did not examine the intersectionality of ethnicity in relation to internet use barriers, the significant difference in internet use between Han Chinese and minorities demands for the integration of intersectionality theory (Wang et al., 2024; Zheng & Walsham, 2021) into digital divide frameworks to account for the ways in which ethnicity, gender, and SES interact to shape exclusion.

The present study's counterintuitive findings (e.g. educated non-users reporting more barriers) challenge the universality of the Technology Acceptance Model (TAM) (Venkatesh et al., 2003). In China, higher education may heighten awareness of risks, such as data privacy concerns, without equipping individuals with the necessary tools to mitigate them. This can lead to undesirable outcomes, fostering skepticism rather than adoption. This aligns with Yang and Du's (2021) argument that cultural capital (e.g., *Hukou* status) interacts with technology differently in non-Western contexts, necessitating culturally grounded models like the Senior Technology Acceptance Model (STAM) proposed by Renaud and van Biljon (2008) and Chen and Chan (2014). STAM prioritizes perceived need and social influence over ease of use, reflecting collectivist values where family expectations strongly shape adoption of use behaviors. Similarly, we also found that the oldest-old group, rural residents, minority groups, people with agriculture background, and people with less family connections tended to report fewer barriers than their counterparts. These counterintuitive patterns could be explained through multiple perspectives as discussed above, suggesting the complexity of factors to shape digital barriers in the non-Western context.

The findings of this study highlight the importance of distinguishing between *perceived* and *objective* digital divides. To more effectively measure the latter, researchers should consider employing the anchoring vignette approach, a method increasingly used to measure objective disability and other health indicators (e.g., King et al., 2004; Yin & Heiland, 2017). By calibrating self-reported data against standardized benchmarks, this approach can enhance the measurement of the objective digital divide, facilitating more accurate cross-cultural and cross-national comparisons while minimizing measurement biases.

Practical Implications

Findings of the present study highlight key considerations for policymakers and digital designers in fostering digital inclusion for older adults. Beyond further promoting device access, interventions must emphasize digital literacy, particularly in rural and disadvantaged areas in China. Digital strategies should also account for regional and demographic differences, with rural populations needing better access and urban older adults benefiting from advanced training in privacy and security. Additionally, addressing intersectional barriers, such as ethnicity, cognitive impairment, and financial constraints, through tailored programs is crucial. A holistic approach that combines accessibility, education, and inclusive design can create a more equitable digital environment for older adults.

9.4.3 Strengths and Limitations

The present study advances digital divide research in three keyways. First, its use of the CLASS 2020 dataset, a nationally representative sample of 11,228 older adults, offers unprecedented granularity into barriers across urban-rural and user/non-user divides in China. Unlike smaller-scale studies, this dataset captures regional variations, such as the heightened access barriers in rural areas, which are often overlooked by urban-centric research in Western literature. Second, differentiating between users and non-users addresses a critical gap in prior studies, which often conflate these groups (van Deursen & Helsper, 2015). For example, non-users' lower reporting of usage barriers, which is rooted in limited exposure, highlights the need for distinct intervention strategies. Third, urban-rural disparities in digital inequality were examined in relation to a wide set of factors that are typically overlooked in existing literature (e.g. filial piety). The present findings provide a nuanced understanding of how factors, such as urban-rural, region, ethnicity, family structure, and economic status, contribute to the digital exclusion of older adults. This study supports the call by Zheng and Walsham's (2021) for "contextualized intersectionality" in research on digital inequality.

Despite its strengths, the present study has several limitations. First, its cross-sectional design precludes causal inferences; longitudinal data are needed to track barrier evolution as China's digital policies unfold. Second, self-reported barriers may underestimate challenges among non-users lacking awareness of digital possibilities. For example, a non-user unaware of telehealth services cannot report their inaccessibility, creating a "blind spot" in data (Friemel, 2016). Third, the lack of qualitative data limits insight into cultural mechanisms (e.g., why Han ethnicity correlates with barriers), necessitating mixed method approaches in future work. Finally, the present study only focused on internet use barriers, while overlooking enablers (e.g., community support or successful aging practices) that could inform strengths-based interventions.

Future research should explore how digital barriers among Chinese older adults have evolved with policy interventions, leveraging longitudinal data to assess whether infrastructure investments reduce access gaps or shift disparities, in addition to previous trend analyses (Cui, 2019; Yan et al., 2022; Zhao & Kuang, 2025). Ethnographic studies can uncover cultural narratives influencing Han seniors' reluctance to seek digital help. Understanding non-user perceptions, elucidating whether their non-use is due to exclusion or disinterest, requires mixed-method approaches. Comparative studies with collectivist societies like Japan and South Korea could reveal universal trends in digital exclusion. Additionally, intersectional models integrating socio-economic, ethnic, and generational factors can provide deeper insights, adapting frameworks like Wang et al.'s (2024) U.S. study to China's context.

9.4.4 Conclusions

In conclusion, the present study reveals the high prevalence of the digital gap among Chinese older adults. More importantly, it highlights the multifaceted nature of digital inequality among older adults in China, where barriers extend beyond access to include skills, socioeconomic status, and cultural perceptions. Bridging the digital divide requires comprehensive interventions that address infrastructure, provide digital literacy training, and challenge age-related stereotypes. Factors such as cognitive impairment, financial constraints, and regional disparities must be considered when designing inclusive policies. As China advances its "Digital Silk Road," ensuring equitable participation for older adults is both a technological and ethical imperative. Digital inclusion of older adults is essential for fostering a society where aging and innovation coexist in alignment with global healthy aging goals.

Acknowledgement The authors would like to thank the Research Center for Population & Development and the Institute of Gerontology, Renmin University for providing access to the China Longitudinal Aging and Social Survey (CLASS) dataset used in this chapter.

Disclaimer Views expressed in the chapter are solely those of the authors and do not necessarily reflect those of the United Nations, the National University of Singapore, the University of Alabama at Birmingham, and Virginia Tech.

References

Ang, S., & Malhotra, R. (2022). The filial piety paradox: Receiving social support from children can be negatively associated with quality of life. *Social Science & Medicine, 303*, 115835.

Bai, X., Lai, D. W. L., & Liu, C. (2020). Personal care expectations: Photovoices of Chinese ageing adults in Hong Kong. *Health and Social Care in the Community, 28*(3), 1071–1081.

Blank, G., & Groselj, D. (2014). Dimensions of Internet use: Amount, variety, and types. *Information, Communication & Society, 17*(4), 417–435.

Charness, N., & Boot, W. (2009). Aging and information technology use: Potential and barriers. *Current Directions in Psychological Science, 18*(5), 253–258.

Chen, K., & Chan, A. H. (2014). Gerontechnology acceptance by elderly Hong Kong Chinese: A senior technology acceptance model (STAM). *Ergonomics, 57*(5), 635–652.

Chen, A. N., Downey, J. P., McGaughey, R. E., & Jin, K. (2016). Seniors and information technology in China. *International Journal of Human-Computer Interaction, 32*(2), 132–142.

China Internet Network Information Center (CNNIC). (2021). *The 47th statistical report on China's Internet development*. Retrieved from https://www.cnnic.cn/n4/2022/0401/c88-1125.html [in Chinese]

China Internet Network Information Center (CNNIC). (2025). *The 55th Statistical Report on China's Internet Development*. Retrieved from https://www.cnnic.net.cn/n4/2025/0117/c88-11229.html [in Chinese]

Chinn, M. D., & Fairlie, R. W. (2007). The determinants of the global digital divide: A cross-country analysis of computer and internet penetration. *Oxford Economic Papers, 59*(1), 16–44.

Chung, J. E., Park, N., Wang, H., Fulk, J., & McLaughlin, M. (2010). Age differences in perceptions of online community participation among non-users: An extension of the technology acceptance model. *Computers in Human Behavior, 26*, 1674–1684.

Cui, K. (2019). Metaphorical culture and dual lag: A decade of Internet diffusion in China (2005–2015): Analysis using the APC model based on four sets of CGSS. *Modern Communication, 41*(2), 159–166.

Czaja, S. J., Charness, N., Fisk, A. D., Hertzog, C., Nair, S. N., Rogers, W. A., & Sharit, J. (2006). Factors predicting the use of technology: Findings from the Center for Research and Education on Aging and Technology Enhancement (CREATE). *Psychology and Aging, 21*(2), 333–352.

Dong, T., Zhu, Z., Guo, M., Du, P., & Wu, B. (2019). Association between dying experience and place of death: Urban–rural differences among older Chinese adults. *Journal of Palliative Medicine, 22*(11), 1386–1393.

Donner, J. (2008). Research approaches to mobile use in the developing world: A review of the literature. *The Information Society, 24*(3), 140–159.

Freese, J., Rivas, S., & Hargittai, E. (2006). Cognitive ability and Internet use among older adults. *Poetics, 34*, 236–249.

Friemel, T. N. (2016). The digital divide has grown old: Determinants of a digital divide among seniors. *New Media & Society, 18*(2), 313–331.

González, A., Ramírez, M. P., & Viadel, V. (2012). Attitudes of the elderly toward information and communications technologies. *Educational Gerontology, 38*(9), 585–594.

GSMA. (2023). *The state of mobile internet connectivity 2023*. Retrieved from https://www.gsma.com/r/wp-content/uploads/2023/10/The-State-of-Mobile-Internet-Connectivity-Report-2023.pdf

Hargittai, E. (2002). Second-level digital divide: Mapping differences in people's online skills. *First Monday, 7*(4). https://doi.org/10.5210/fm.v7i4.942

Hargittai, E. (2018). A review of internet use among older adults. *New Media & Society, 20*(10), 3937–3954.

Hargittai, E., & Dobransky, K. (2017). Old dogs, new clicks: Digital inequality in skills and uses among older adults. *Canadian Journal of Communication, 42*(2), 195–212.

Hargittai, E., Piper, A. M., & Morris, M. R. (2019). From internet access to internet skills: Digital inequality among older adults. *Universal Access in the Information Society, 18*(4), 881–890.

Heart, T., & Kalderon, E. (2013). Older adults: Are they ready to adopt health-related ICT? *International Journal of Medical Informatics, 82*(11), e209–e231.

Helsper, E. (2021). *The digital disconnect: The social causes and consequences of digital inequalities*. Sage.

Hunsaker, A., & Hargittai, E. (2018). A review of internet use among older adults. *New Media & Society, 20*(10), 3937–3954.

Jin, Y., & Zhao, M. (2019). Internet access and the elderly's active aging in China—A study based on 2016 China longitudinal aging social survey. *Population Journal, 6*, 44–55. [in Chinese].

Kemp, S. (2025). *Digital 2025: Global overview report*. Retrieved from https://datareportal.com/reports/digital-2025-global-overview-report

King, G., Murray, C. J. L., Salomon, J., & Tandon, A. (2004). Enhancing the validity and cross-cultural comparability of measurement in survey research. *American Political Science Review, 98*, 184–191.

Köttl, H., Gallistl, V., Rohner, R., & Ayalon, L. (2021). "But at the age of 85? Forget it!": Internalized ageism, a barrier to technology use. *Frontiers in Psychology, 12*, 737485.

Li, Q., & Luximon, Y. (2018). Understanding older adults' post-adoption usage behavior and perceptions of mobile technology. *International Journal of Design, 12*(3), 93–110.

Mazur, E., Signorella, M., & Hough, M. (2012). Older adults and their internet behaviors. In Z. Yan (Ed.), *Encyclopedia of cyber behavior* (Vol. 1, pp. 608–618). IGI Global.

Ministry of Education [China]. (2007). *Report on the language situation in China (2007)*. Retrieved from http://www.moe.gov.cn/s78/A19/A19_ztzl/baogao/201202/t20120210_130364.html [in Chinese]

Ogbo, E., Brown, T., Gant, J., & Sicker, D. (2021). When being connected is not enough: An analysis of the second and third levels of the digital divide in a developing country. *Journal of Information Policy, 11*, 104–146.

Oswald, V., & Wagner, M. (2023). Internet usage among the oldest-old: Does functional health moderate the relationship between internet usage and autonomy? *European Journal of Ageing, 20*(1), 3.

Pick, J., Ren, F., & Sarkar, A. (2024). Digital inequalities in China in 2020: Spatial and multivariate analysis. *Applied Sciences, 14*(13), 5385.

Randine, P., Sharma, A., Hartvigsen, G., Johansen, H. D., & Årsand, E. (2022). Information and communication technology-based interventions for chronic diseases consultation: Scoping review. *International Journal of Medical Informatics, 163*, 104784.
Renaud, K., & van Biljon, J. (2008). Predicting technology acceptance and adoption by the elderly: A qualitative study. In *Proceedings of the 2008 Annual Research Conference of the South African Institute of Computer Scientists and Information Technologists* (pp. 210–219).
Research on Aging, Policies and Practice. (2017). *How deep is the digital divide? ICT literacy and the role of assistive technology in helping older workers*. Facts. Retrieved from https://rapp.ualberta.ca/wp-content/uploads/sites/49/2018/04/ICT-literacy-of-older-workers_2017May.pdf?utm_source=chatgpt.com
Scalvini, S., Baratti, D., Assoni, G., et al. (2014). Information and communication technology in chronic diseases: A patient's opportunity. *Journal of Medical Perspectives, 12*, 91–95.
Scheerder, A., van Deursen, A., & van Dijk, J. (2017). Determinants of Internet skills, use, and outcomes: A systematic review of the second- and third-level digital divide. *Telematics and Informatics, 34*(8), 1607–1624.
Schlomann, A., Seifert, A., Zank, S., Woopen, C., & Rietz, C. (2020). Use of information and communication technology (ICT) devices among the oldest-old: Loneliness, anomie, and autonomy. *Innovation in Aging, 4*(2), igz050.
Schroeder, T., Dodds, L., Georgiou, A., Gewald, H., & Siette, J. (2023). Older adults and new technology: Mapping review of the factors associated with older adults' intention to adopt digital technologies. *JMIR Aging, 6*, e44564.
Seifert, A., Cotten, S. R., & Xie, B. (2021). A double burden of exclusion? Digital and social exclusion of older adults in times of COVID-19. *Journals of Gerontology: Social Sciences, 76*(3), e99–e103.
United Nations. (2024). *World population prospects 2024*. Retrieved from https://population.un.org/wpp/
van Deursen, A. J., & Helsper, E. J. (2015). The third-level digital divide: Who benefits most from being online? *Communication and Information Technologies Annual: Digital Distinctions and Inequalities Studies in Media and Communications, 10*, 29–52.
van Deursen, A. J. & van Dijk, J. (2011). Internet skills and the digital divide. *New Media & Society, 13*(6), 893–911.
van Deursen, A. J., & van Dijk, J. (2014). The digital divide shifts to differences in usage. *New Media & Society, 16*(3), 507–526.
van Deursen, A. J., & van Dijk, J. (2019). The first-level digital divide shifts from inequalities in physical access to inequalities in material access. *New Media & Society, 21*(2), 354–375.
van Dijk, J. (2005). *The deepening divide: Inequality in the information society*. Sage.
van Dijk, J. (2017). Afterword: The state of digital divide theory. In M. Ragnedda & G. W. Muschert (Eds.), *Theorizing digital divides* (pp. 199–206). Routledge.
van Dijk, J. (2020). *The digital divide*. Polity.
Vaportzis, E., Giatsi Clausen, M., & Gow, A. J. (2017). Older adults' perceptions of technology and barriers to interacting with tablet computers: A focus group study. *Frontiers in Psychology, 8*, 1687.
Venkatesh, V., Morris, M. G., Davis, G. B., & Davis, F. D. (2003). User acceptance of information technology: Toward a unified view. *MIS Quarterly, 27*(3), 425–478.
Vogels, E. (2021). *Digital divide persists even as Americans with lower incomes make gains in tech adoption*. Pew Research Center. Retrieved from https://www.pewresearch.org/short-reads/2021/06/22/digital-divide-persists-even-as-americans-with-lower-incomes-make-gains-in-tech-adoption
von Humboldt, S., & Leal, I. (2015). The old and the oldest-old: Do they have different perspectives on adjustment to aging? *International Journal of Gerontology, 9*(3), 156–160.
Wang, K., & Gu, D. (2023). Reciprocal associations between social media use and self-perception of aging among older adults: Do men and women differ? *Social Science & Medicine, 321*, 115786.

Wang, K., & Kubanga, K. (2021). Correlates of Internet use among African American older adults: Gender and age differences. *International Journal of Population Studies, 6*(2), 26–38.

Wang, K., Chen, X. S., Gu, D., Smith, B. D., Dong, Y., & Peet, J. Z. (2024). Examining first and second-level digital divide at the intersection of race/ethnicity, gender, and socioeconomic status: An analysis of the National Health and Aging Trends Study. *The Gerontologist, 64*(3), gnae079.

Wang, K., Chen, X. S., Dong, Y., Sanabria Véaz, K., & Gu, D. (2025). Bridging the access gap: A decade of narrowing the digital divide for Hispanic older adults in the United States. *Journal of Aging and Health, 37*(3/4), 182–191.

Wei, K., Teo, H., Chan, H., & Tan, B. (2011). Conceptualizing and testing a social cognitive model of the digital divide. *Information Systems Research, 22*, 170–187.

Wildenbos, G. A., Peute, L., & Jaspers, M. (2018). Aging barriers influencing mobile health usability for older adults: A literature based framework (MOLD-US). *International Journal of Medical Informatics, 114*, 66–75.

Wilson, J., Heinsch, M., Betts, D., Booth, D., & Kay-Lambkin, F. (2021). Barriers and facilitators to the use of e-health by older adults: A scoping review. *BMC Public Health, 21*(1556), 1–12.

Yan, P., Lin, W., & Zhou, W. (2022). Digital divides in China: A comparative study between 2012 and 2020. *Library and Information Service, 66*(20), 180–189.

Yang, J., & Du, P. (2021). Gender, capital endowment and digital exclusion of older people in China. *Ageing & Society, 41*(11), 2502–2526.

Yin, N., & Heiland, F. (2017). Disability policies and public views on work disability: A comparative analysis using anchoring vignette data. *International Journal of Population Studies, 3*(1), 42–63.

Yu, X., Ang, S., & Zhang, Y. (2024). Exploring rural-urban differences in the association between internet use and cognitive functioning among older adults in China. *Journal of Gerontology. Social Sciences, 79*(4), gbad195.

Yusif, S., Soar, J., & Hafeez-Baig, A. (2016). Older people, assistive technologies, and the barriers to adoption: A systematic review. *International Journal of Medical Informatics, 94*, 112–116.

Zhang, H., & He, R. (2022). A study on digital inclusion of Chinese rural older adults from a life course perspective. *Frontiers in Public Health, 10*, 974998.

Zhao, Y., & Kuang, M. (2025). Digital divides in China: Evidence from CGSS2005-2021. *Chinese Sociological Review*, online first, 1–62. https://doi.org/10.1080/21620555.2025.2475430

Zheng, Y., & Walsham, G. (2021). Inequality of what? An intersectional approach to digital inequality under Covid-19. *Information and Organization, 31*(1), 100341.

Zou, Y., Wang, H., Chen, W., Shen, K., Huang, K., Gui, J. F., Zhang, G., Feng, Q. S., & Liu, H. Y. (2024). Embrace the past and forge ahead: The China report on the 30th anniversary of the International Conference on Population and Development (ICPD). *China Population and Development Studies, 8*, 239–286.

Chapter 10
Examining First and Second-Level Digital Divide at the Intersection of Race/Ethnicity, Gender, and Socioeconomic Status: An Analysis of the National Health and Aging Trends Study

Kun Wang, Xiayu Summer Chen, Danan Gu, Brenda D. Smith, Yanjun Dong, and Jared Zak Peet

---

Note on Reuse of Published Materials
This chapter incorporates a revised and expanded version of material originally published in the article *"Examining First- and Second-Level Digital Divide at the Intersection of Race/Ethnicity, Gender, and Socioeconomic Status: An Analysis of the National Health and Aging Trends Study"* by Wang, K., Chen, X. S., Gu, D., Smith, B. D., Dong, Y., & Peet, J. Z. (2024), published in *The Gerontologist, 64*(9), gnae079. The original work has been adapted and updated, in accordance with the publisher's policies.

K. Wang (✉)
Department of Social Work, College of Arts and Sciences, University of Alabama at Birmingham, Birmingham, AL, USA
e-mail: kw2@uab.edu

X. S. Chen
University of Illinois Urbana-Champaign, Champaign, IL, USA
e-mail: xiayuyc2@illinois.edu

D. Gu
Population Division, UN Department of Economic and Social Affairs, New York, NY, USA
e-mail: gudanan@yahoo.com

B. D. Smith
University of Alabama, Tuscaloosa, AL, USA
e-mail: bsmith2@sw.ua.edu

Y. Dong
University at Albany, State University of New York, Albany, NY, USA
e-mail: ydong2@albany.edu

J. Z. Peet
Binghamton University, Binghamton, NY, USA

K. Wang et al. (eds.), *ICT Use and Healthy Longevity*, Advances in Studies of Aging and Health 5, https://doi.org/10.1007/978-3-031-98964-3_10

10.1 Introduction

The 2010s witnessed a spiking increase in internet use among older adults in the United States (U.S.), from 46% in 2010 (Perrin & Duggan, 2019) to 75% in 2021 (Faviero, 2022). Recent studies highlight age as a primary determinant of digital exclusion, with the digital divide widening across generations as individuals grow older (Mubarak & Suomi, 2022). Older adults, particularly those born before the digital era, face greater barriers to technology adoption due to limited digital literacy, lower confidence in using online services, and accessibility challenges (Bertolazzi et al., 2024).With healthy aging becoming a critical societal issue in recent decades, previous studies indicate that digital technology, including the internet, may help to mitigate aging challenges (Lindeman, 2017; Szabo et al., 2019). Transcending geographic distance, internet use facilitates older adults' social connections and communication and provides easy access to enormous online resources (Szabo et al., 2019; Vassli & Farshchian, 2018). Older community dwellers commonly can use the internet to meet social (e.g., accessing social networking sites), personal tasks-related (e.g., online shopping and banking), and health-related needs (e.g., online health information seeking). Growing evidence suggests that internet use may diversify older community dwellers' social engagement (Szabo et al., 2019), increase positive self-perception of aging (Wang & Gu, 2023), maintain independence (Lindeman, 2017; Vassli & Farshchian, 2018), and promote well-being (Szabo et al., 2019).

10.1.1 Race/Ethnicity and the Digital Divide in the U.S.

Despite the essential increase in internet use, the digital divide, described as inequalities in digital technology use, mainly from three levels—material access (first-level), capability and skills in use (second-level), and consequences and beneficial outcomes (third-level)—still exists among older community dwellers (Castells, 2002; Hargittai, 2001). Marginalized social identities relevant to age, gender, race/ethnicity, education, income, disability status, and urban/rural residency are consistently linked to the digital divide (Choi & DiNitto, 2013; Scheerder et al., 2017). Most importantly, reflecting the racialized structural disparities in the U.S., older community dwellers who are Black, indigenous, and other people of color (BIPOC) are less likely to access the internet and use it than their non-Hispanic white counterparts.

Prior research points to the significance of race/ethnicity in explaining the first-level digital divide among older community dwellers in the U.S. over the past decade. Studies using nationally representative data around the earlier years of the 2010s, such as the 2011 National Health and Aging Trends Study (NHATS) (Choi & DiNitto, 2013) and 2012 Health and Retirement Study (HRS) (Yu et al., 2016), and more recent data, such as the 2016 HRS (Choi et al., 2020, 2022a), 2018

National Health Interview Survey (NHIS) (He et al., 2022), and 2018 NHATS (Bell et al., 2013), found that older BIPOC community dwellers were less likely to have access to the internet than their counterparts of non-Hispanic white.

Regarding the second-level digital divide, consistent evidence over the past decade indicates disparities in health-related internet use between older BIPOC and non-Hispanic white community dwellers. Older BIPOC community dwellers were less likely to use the internet for health-related purposes in the 2011 NHATS (Choi & DiNitto, 2013), 2012 California Health Interview Survey (CHIS) (Yoon et al., 2018), 2014 HRS (Liu et al., 2020; Mitchell et al., 2019), and 2018 NHIS (He et al., 2022; Hung et al., 2020). In terms of social and personal-task use, contradictory evidence is reported in the literature. Racial/ethnic disparity in the social use of the internet, favoring older non-Hispanic white community dwellers, was identified in the 2012 HRS (Yu et al., 2016), whereas no significant differences were found in the 2016 HRS (Byrne et al., 2021) or online convenient samples in the early 2010s (Bell et al., 2013; Hutto et al., 2015). As for using the internet for personal tasks, some studies indicated no racial/ethnic differences in online shopping and banking (Choi & DiNitto, 2013) and searching news and other information online (Li et al., 2021; Tsetsi & Rains, 2017). Other studies found that older BIPOC dwellers were less likely to use e-shopping (Li et al., 2021; Li, 2023) and other personal tasks (Li et al., 2021), such as taking classes or webinars, getting directions or traffic information, downloading or purchasing apps, and using a voice-activated assistant. Given the importance of internet use, these inconsistent findings warrant more future studies to have a better understanding of the racial/ethnic digital divide to promote older community dwellers' health outcomes (Lindeman, 2017; Shapira et al., 2007) and reduce health disparities (Byrne et al., 2021; Du & Xu, 2016).

10.1.2 Societal and Technological Environments in the 2010s

In the 2010s in the U.S., internet and smartphone device use increased sharply and pervaded many aspects of people's lives (Faviero, 2022). However, household income and wealth inequalities continued a widening trend (Horowitz et al., 2020). The incomes of the top 10% of households in 2018 were 12.6 times that of the other 90%, with a steady 10% increase per decade since 1980 (Horowitz et al., 2020). Reflecting historical and enduring structural racism in the U.S., the median wealth gaps based on race/ethnicity have remained large: in 2019, 80% of non-Hispanic Black and Hispanic families had less wealth than the typical white family (Kent & Ricketts, 2020). The absolute wealth gaps by educational attainment have further enlarged, continuing to favor college-educated families (Kent & Ricketts, 2020).

Given changes in societal and technological environments in the past decade, the impact of race/ethnicity on the digital divide needs to be viewed from an evolving perspective. Despite several studies examining trends of the racial/ethnic impact on the digital divide in the 2010s, most focused on internet access and a health-related digital divide (Hung et al., 2020; Yoon et al., 2020). Using data from CHIS between

2011 and 2016, researchers found that internet users among older white community dwellers increased significantly by more than 9%, while no significant changes were observed among subgroups of BIPOC community dwellers (Yoon et al., 2020). Hung et al. (2020) found that Black, Hispanic, and Asian older adults were consistently less likely to use health information technology than white older adults in the 2009 and 2018 NHIS. To our knowledge, no studies have investigated the trend of racial/ethnic disparities in internet use for social and personal-tasks.

10.1.3 Theoretical Background

The digital divide is not just a technological issue but is deeply rooted in social determinants that shape individuals' access to and use of digital technologies. A fundamental factor influencing the digital divide is socioeconomic status (SES), usually encompassing income, education, and occupation. Recent studies have underscored the persistence of income-related disparities, with lower-income individuals facing challenges in acquiring necessary devices and internet connectivity (Van Deursen & Helsper, 2015). Educational attainment remains a critical factor, and research highlights a positive correlation between higher levels of education and digital proficiency (Leukel et al., 2021). Occupational roles also contribute significantly, as individuals in certain professions may benefit from greater exposure and familiarity with digital tools (Hecker et al., 2021).

However, these inequalities in digital access are inextricably associated with race and ethnicity (Hamilton, 2020; Masullo Chen, 2016). The intersectionality framework, developed by Crenshaw (2013), highlights the complex interplay between multi-dimensional and co-occurrence identities, such as race/ ethnicity, gender, and socioeconomic status, in influencing people's experience (Crenshaw, 2017). In the context of the digital divide, this framework recognizes that older adults occupy multiple social positions simultaneously, and the combination of these positions may impact their digital technology usage (Suntai & Beltran, 2022; Zheng & Walsham, 2021). Applying this conceptual framework offers us a powerful lens for understanding the complexities of the digital divide by examining how multiple social identities intersect to shape individuals' access to and use of digital technologies (Suntai & Beltran, 2022; van Dijk, 2005). Hence, for BIPOC older adults, racial/ethnic identity may further interact with other marginalized social identities, causing increased hardships and diminishing opportunities to access and use the internet (Nakamura & Chow-White, 2010; Suntai & Beltran, 2022; Zheng & Walsham, 2021). Accordingly, in the field of digital divide study, it is essential to consider how intersecting phenomena disproportionately affect BIPOC older adults.

Few studies have investigated the effects of race/ethnicity intersecting with other marginalized identities on the digital divide (Suntai & Beltran, 2022; Yoon et al., 2018). Using the 2012 CHIS, Yoon et al. (2018) found that BIPOC older adults with the lowest levels of SES had reduced odds of using the internet for health information. Suntai and Beltran (2022) indicated that compared to non-Hispanic white men, other intersectional groups by race/ethnicity and gender were less likely to have a working cellphone or a working laptop/computer in the 2018 NHATS. Nevertheless, several limitations exist in the current literature. First, most of these studies have focused on onetime point. No studies have investigated the trend of the impact of race/ethnicity intersecting with other marginalized social identities on the digital divide over the past decade. Second, most studies have focused on internet access or health-related digital divides, with few investigations on a digital divide in social or personal-tasks.

Recent literature continues to highlight racial/ethnic disparities in digital technology access and usage among older adults. Recent research suggests nuanced differences between Black and Hispanic older adults regarding internet access and use patterns. Specifically, Black older adults are more likely to rely on mobile devices rather than home computers, partly due to affordability and accessibility factors, whereas Hispanic older adults may experience additional barriers such as language and culturally specific content gaps (Medero et al., 2022). Furthermore, the association between age and decreased internet use via home computers was notably stronger among Hispanic older adults, suggesting that Hispanic older adults might face compounded challenges due to both linguistic barriers and age-related accessibility issues (Medero et al., 2022). These distinct patterns highlight the importance of differentiating within BIPOC categories to design more precise and effective interventions that address the unique needs of each racial/ethnic subgroup. Given that Black older adults represent the largest subgroup within the BIPOC older adults, it is essential to clarify whether significant internal differences exist between Black and other racial/ethnic minorities in terms of digital technology access and specific internet usage activities.

10.1.4 Current Study

Using nationally representative data among older community dwellers from 2011/2013, 2015, and 2019 NHATS, this study aimed to fill these research gaps by answering two questions: (1) What were the trends regarding the effect of race/ethnicity on the first- and second-level digital divide (i.e., social, personal-task, and health-related use) among older community dwellers in the 2010s? (2) What were the trends regarding the intersecting effects of race/ethnicity and other marginalized social identities related to gender, education, income, and occupation on the digital divide? Findings in this study may deepen our understanding of the race/ethnicity-related evolvement of the digital divide and inform future policies to facilitate digital technology use among older BIPOC community dwellers in promoting health and well-being, extending independent living in their communities, and reducing health disparities.

10.2 Methods

10.2.1 Data Source and Study Sample

The present study utilized data from the 2011/2013, 2015, and 2019 National Health and Ageing Trend Study (NHATS), an annual survey of nationally representative sample of Medicare beneficiaries aged 65 or older in the U.S. The initial sample was first interviewed in 2011 and replenished in 2015 to maintain national representative. A total of 8245 older adults participated in the 2011 NHATS. Due to the focus on community dwellers in this study, participants in nursing homes or residential care facilities ($n = 1048$) were excluded. Also, participants who may lack the capacity to use the internet due to physical health or cognitive function limitations were excluded from this study. These included participants utilizing a proxy to answer the questionnaire ($n = 517$), those with a diagnosis of dementia or Alzheimer's disease ($n = 177$), and those with possible or probable dementia ($n = 1289$) (Kasper et al., 2013). In all, 5214 older adults were included in our final analytic sample for 2011. The question relevant to the social use of the internet was first asked in the 2013 NHATS. Applying the same inclusion and exclusion criteria, 3469 participants were included in the final analytic sample of the 2013 NHATS. Similarly, the final analytical sample sizes in 2015 and 2019 were 5543 and 3242, respectively. The NHATS has been reviewed and approved by the Institutional Review Board at the Johns Hopkins Bloomberg School of Public Health. The public available NHATS data used in this study can be retrieved at www.nhats.org.

10.2.2 Measures

Digital Divide The first- and second-level digital divide were measured by two sets of variables. First, all participants were asked to indicate whether they had access to a working cellphone or computer and knew how to use a computer. Participants were considered as having the first-level digital divide if they answered "no" to all these questions. Second, those who did not have the first-level digital divide (i.e., answered "yes" to at least one of the previous questions) were asked to indicate their second-level digital divide. More specifically, they were asked whether they had used the internet for reasons other than email or text within the last month, including "shopping for groceries or personal items," "paying bills or doing banking," "ordering or refilling prescription," "visiting social networking site," "contacting any of your or your spouse's medical providers," "handling Medicare or other health insurance matter," and "getting information about your or your spouse's health condition." All seven internet use activities were measured dichotomously (0 = no, 1 = yes). The first three activities were defined as personal tasks, and the last three were considered as health-related use (Choi & DiNitto, 2013).

Social Identities Social identities in this study included race/ethnicity (0 = non-Hispanic white, 1 = Black, indigenous, and people of color), gender (0 = male,

1 = female), and SES. SES was measured by low education (0 = some college, vocational education, college graduate or higher, 1 = high school graduate or lower), low income (0 = medium and high income, >=$30,000, 1 = low income, <$30,000, 2 = missing), and blue-collar jobs (0 = no, 1 = yes).

Covariates Based on the literature (Hunsaker & Hargittai, 2018; Yu et al., 2016), age (1 = 65–74, 2 = 75–84, and 3 = 85 and older), living arrangement (0 = living with others, 1 = living alone), and health-related factors such as self-rated health status (1 = poor, 2 = fair, 3 = good, 4 = very good, 5 = excellent), self-rated memory (1 = poor, 2 = fair, 3 = good, 4 = very good, 5 = excellent), pain (0 = no, 1 = yes), and chronic illness (0–9, including heart attack, any other heart disease, high blood pressure, arthritis, osteoporosis, diabetes, lung disease, stroke, and cancer) were included as covariates.

10.2.3 Analytic Strategy

A preliminary study that combined all 2011–2019 rounds of data was conducted to examine the general trend of the effect of race/ethnicity on internet use. Results showed a significant interaction between survey round, measured yearly, and BIPOC status (*OR* = 1.04, *CI* = [1.00, 1.08], $p < 0.05$). As shown in Fig. 10.1, as

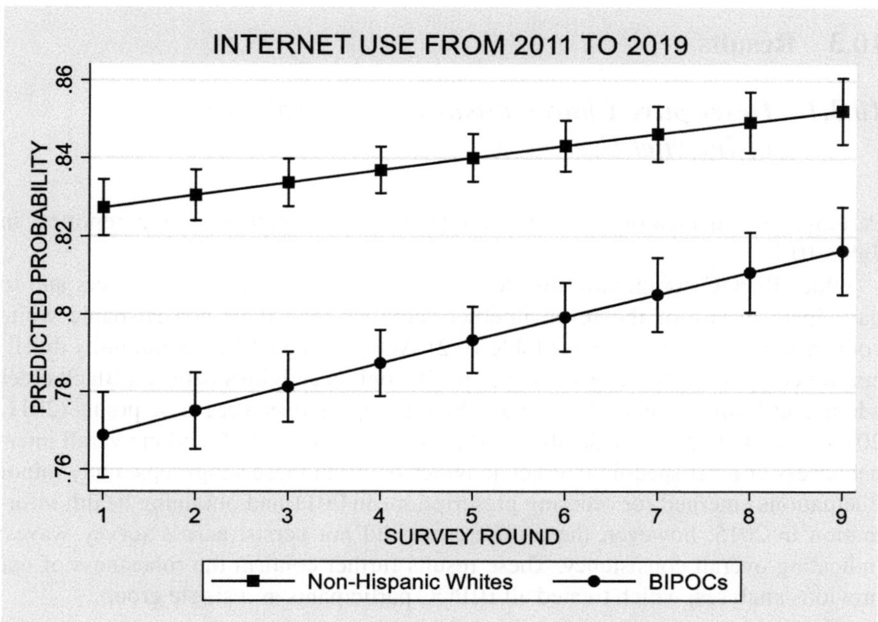

Fig. 10.1 Internet use trajectory (2011–2019) by BIPOC status. Note. BIPOC stands for Black, indigenous, and other people of color

time passed, the differences in the predicted probability of using the internet between older BIPOC and non-Hispanic white adults decreased, indicating reduced racial/ethnic disparities with time. To better understand the trend of the racial/ethnic digital divide among the general older community dwellers in the U.S., we chose three time points (2011/2013, 2015, and 2019) and applied the sample weights in the analyses. Below are the specific procedures.

First, descriptive statistics were calculated to understand participants' characteristics. Then, bivariate analyses were utilized to assess associations between race/ethnicity and the digital divides in 2011/2013, 2015, and 2019. To confirm the robustness of our findings, we conducted subgroup analyses comparing internet access and specific internet usage (personal, social, and health-related activities) among BIPOC groups. Next, logistic regression models were conducted to examine the effects of race/ethnicity on the digital divides, with covariates included in the models. Lastly, interactions (BIPOC × female; BIPOC × low education; BIPOC × low income; BIPOC × blue-collar jobs) were included in the full models. Sample weights were applied to bivariate and logistic regression analyses to adjust for differential selection probabilities and nonresponse (Freedman et al., 2020). Income had significant portions of missing values. To fully use the data, we treated the missing value as a category and compared it to the reference group, medium and high income category. Given our interest, we focused on comparing the low-income to the medium and high income category. All analyses were performed using Stata 17 software (StataCorp, 2021).

10.3 Results

10.3.1 Descriptive Characteristics and Prevalence of Internet Use

Participants' characteristics, both weighted and unweighted, were reported in Table 10.1.

Older BIPOC community dwellers were less likely to be internet users and to participate in any of the seven internet activities than their non-Hispanic white counterparts across the 3 years (Table 10.2). Also, among BIPOC community dwellers, we compared internet access and specific online activities between Black older adults and Hispanic and other racial/ethnic groups across three time points (2011, 2015, and 2019). No statistically significant differences were found in overall internet access or most specific internet activities between these subgroups. Only minor fluctuations emerged for ordering prescriptions in 2011 and obtaining health information in 2015; however, these differences did not persist across survey waves, indicating overall consistency. These results further confirm the robustness of our previous analyses, which treated all BIPOC participants as a single group.

Table 10.1 Descriptive characteristics (Unweighted and Weighted) in 2011 (n = 5214)/2013 (n = 3469), 2015 (n = 5543), and 2019 (n = 3242)

	Unweighted			Weighted		
	2011/2013	2015	2019	2011/2013	2015	2019
BIPOC (yes)	26.69%/25.19%	26.39%	25.70%	15.49%/15.75%	17.26%	17.06%
Female (yes)	57.86%/57.51%	57.35%	57.06%	56.38%/55.51%	55.29%	55.03%
Low education (yes)	48.35%/46.53%	43.13%	39.63%	44.14%/43.61%	38.40%	35.33%
Income						
Low	26.41%/25.66%	23.27%	23.84%	23.86%/23.62%	19.94%	21.24%
Medium and high	31.65%/37.88%	36.06%	48.98%	35.85%42.37%	41.01%	54.57%
Missing	41.94%/36.47%	40.66%	27.17%	40.29%34.01%	39.05%	24.19%
Occupation (blue collar)	41.56%/41.56%	41.56%	41.56%	30.01%/30.03%	31.85%	29.71%
Age						
65–74	47.81%/39.61%	44.56%	26.87%	60.55%/52.58%	62.55%	45.89%
75–84	39.01%/42.46%	40.25%	52.22%	31.73%/36.96%	29.7%	43.43%
85 and older	13.18%/17.93%	15.19%	20.91%	7.72%/10.46%	7.75%	10.69%
Living alone (yes)	30.48%/31.88%	31.70%	32.63%	27.07%/28.06%	27.57%	29.01%
Self-rated health (1–5)	3 [3–4]/3 [3–4]	3 [3–4]	3 [3–4]	3 [3–4]/3 [3–4]	3 [3–4]	3 [3–4]
Self-rated memory (1–5)	3 [3–4]/3 [3–4]	3 [3–4]	3 [3–4]	4 [3–4]/3 [3–4]	3 [3–4]	3 [3–4]
Bothered by pain (yes)	52.80%/53.17%	54.90%	58.80%	52.00%/53.38%	53.57%	57.10%
# Chronic illnesses (0–9)	2 [1–3]/0 [0–2]	1 [0–2]	0 [0–0]	2 [1–3]/1 [0–2]	1 [0–3]	0 [0–0]

For self-rated health, self-rated memory, and number of chronic illnesses, medians, and interquartile ranges were reported

BIPOC stands for Black, indigenous, and other people of color

10.3.2 Effects of Race/Ethnicity on the Digital Divide

As shown in Table 10.3, older BIPOC community dwellers were less likely to use the internet than their non-Hispanic white counterparts in 2011 and 2015 but not in 2019. However, they were consistently less likely to use the internet for all three personal tasks, visiting social networking sites, and getting health information than their non-Hispanic white counterparts across the 3 years. Regarding the other two types of health-related internet use, although not significant in 2011, BIPOC participants had significantly lower odds in 2015 and 2019.

In addition, low education and low income were consistently associated with lower odds of engaging in all seven internet activities across the 3 years. People with blue-collar jobs were less likely to use the internet for all seven types of online activities except for online shopping in 2019. Female gender was consistently associated with higher odds of visiting social networking sites across 3 years. Although females were less likely to use the internet for other activities in 2011 and 2015, the effects were not significant in 2019, except for ordering/refilling prescriptions and handling health insurance.

Table 10.2 Prevalence of ICT Use by BIPOC Status in 2011/2013, 2015, and 2019 (Weighted)

	2011			2015			2019		
	White	BIPOC	ρ	White	BIPOC	ρ	White	BIPOC	ρ
Among total participants									
Internet users	91.78%	85.75%	***	96.13%	91.04%	***	97.35%	95.19%	*
Among internet users									
1. Shop for groceries or personal items	19.99%	11.38%	***	29.31%	14.46%	***	38.70%	16.65%	***
2. Pay bills or do banking	27.26%	17.88%	***	40.61%	22.73%	***	46.31%	24.63%	***
3. Order or refill prescriptions	11.53%	5.05%	***	17.03%	8.93%	***	25.45%	14.56%	***
4. Visit social networking sites	26.74% (2013)	12.14% (2013)	***	36.83%	19.77%	***	43.95%	19.75%	***
5. Contact any of medical providers	9.96%	6.08%	***	22.28%	10.56%	***	32.70%	11.69%	***
6. Handle Medicare or other health insurance matters	7.42%	4.67%	*	13.94%	7.47%	***	16.69%	7.76%	***
7. Get information about health conditions	23.00%	11.21%	***	30.67%	16.17%	***	37.29%	14.54%	***
	2011			2015			2019		
	Black	Hispanic and others	ρ	Black	Hispanic and others	ρ	Black	Hispanic and others	ρ
Among all BIPOC participants									
Internet users	0.85	0.87		0.92	0.90		0.93	0.97	**
Among BIPOC internet users	0.11	0.12		0.16	0.14		0.19	0.15	
1. Shop for groceries or personal items	0.17	0.19		0.22	0.24		0.23	0.26	
2. Pay bills or do banking	0.06	0.04	**	0.08	0.10		0.13	0.16	
3. Order or refill prescriptions	0.11 (2013)	0.13 (2013)							

(continued)

Table 10.2 (continued)

4. Visit social networking sites	0.06	0.06		0.10	0.11		0.12	0.11	
5. Contact any of medical providers	0.04	0.05		0.08	0.07		0.10	0.06	
6. Handle Medicare or other health insurance matters	0.10	0.13		0.14	0.18	**	0.15	0.14	
7. Get information about health conditions	0.85	0.87		0.92	0.90		0.93	0.97	**

White refers to non-Hispanic white people; BIPOC stands for Black, indigenous, and other people of color

Regarding significance, * $p < 0.05$; ** $p < 0.01$; and *** $p < 0.001$

10.3.3 Intersecting Effects with Other Marginalized Identities on the Digital Divide

Results relevant to the intersecting effects of race/ethnicity with gender, education, income, and occupation were reported in Table 10.4. In terms of online shopping, significant interactions were found with low education in 2011 ($OR = 0.39$, $CI = [0.18, 0.81]$, $p < 0.05$) and low income in 2015 ($OR = 0.44$, $CI = [0.29, 0.94]$, $p < 0.05$) but nothing in 2019. That is, the racial/ethnic gaps in the probability of online shopping, favoring non-Hispanic white dwellers, were significantly larger at the low education level in 2011 and low-income level in 2015 compared to their respective high levels. The good thing is that the exacerbated racial/ethnic gaps due to low education or income became non-significant in 2019. Similarly, for online banking, significant interactions were found with low income in 2011 ($OR = 0.51$, $CI = [0.27, 0.97]$, $p < 0.05$) and female gender ($OR = 0.59$, $CI = [0.37, 0.95]$, $p < 0.05$), low education ($OR = 0.45$, $CI = [0.27, 0.76]$, $p < 0.01$), and low income ($OR = 0.37$, $CI = [0.20, 0.67]$, $p < 0.01$) in 2015 but nothing in 2019. For ordering/refilling prescriptions online, significant interactions were found with female gender in 2011 ($OR = .39$, $CI = [0.17, 0.89]$, $p < 0.05$) and low education in 2015 ($OR = 0.34$, $CI = [0.15, 0.76]$, $p < 0.01$), but nothing in 2019.

As for visiting social networking sites, significant interactions were found with low education in 2013 ($OR = 0.33$, $CI = [0.15, 0.74]$, $p < 0.01$) and low income in 2015 ($OR = 0.44$, $CI = [0.25, 0.76]$, $p < 0.01$) and low education in 2019 ($OR = 0.52$, $CI = [0.27, 0.98]$, $p < 0.05$), indicating that the racial/ethnic gaps in the social use of the internet, favoring non-Hispanic white participants, were significantly larger for the low SES group. Regarding health-related use, several significant interactions were found in 2015 and/or 2019. The interaction between BIPOC status and low education was significant in predicting contacting medical providers online in 2019

Table 10.3 Odds ratios from weighted logistic regressions on the digital divide in 2011/2013, 2015, and 2019

	2011	2015	2019	2011	2015	2019	2011	2015	2019
First-level	Using the internet								
BIPOC	0.62^{***}	0.58^{**}	0.93						
Female	0.92	0.90	1.29						
Low education	0.31^{***}	0.41^{***}	0.57^{*}						
Low-income[a]	0.36^{***}	0.31^{***}	0.24^{***}						
Blue collar	0.72^{**}	0.71^{*}	0.74						
Second-level	Shopping			Banking			Ordering/refilling prescriptions		
BIPOC	0.67^{**}	0.55^{***}	0.44^{***}	0.73^{**}	0.57^{***}	0.53^{***}	0.52^{***}	0.61^{**}	0.65^{*}
Female	0.67^{***}	0.93	1.10	0.79^{**}	0.83^{*}	0.82	0.72^{**}	0.66^{***}	0.76^{*}
Low education	0.41^{***}	0.43^{***}	0.35^{***}	0.31^{***}	0.39^{***}	0.41^{***}	0.39^{***}	0.57^{***}	0.51^{***}
Low-income[a]	0.54^{***}	0.50^{***}	0.43^{***}	0.61^{***}	0.51^{***}	0.45^{***}	0.47^{***}	0.46^{***}	0.51^{***}
Blue collar	0.54^{***}	0.59^{***}	0.80	0.62^{***}	0.50^{***}	0.61^{***}	0.60^{**}	0.63^{**}	0.71^{*}
Second-level	Visiting social networking sites (2013)								
BIPOC	0.51^{***}	0.48^{***}	0.39^{***}						
Female	1.36^{**}	1.54^{***}	1.62^{***}						
Low education	0.61^{***}	0.54^{***}	0.62^{***}						
Low-income[a]	0.59^{**}	0.76^{*}	0.60^{***}						
Blue collar	0.79	0.73^{**}	0.69^{**}						
Second-level	Contacting medical providers			Handling health insurance			Getting health information		
BIPOC	0.81	0.59^{**}	0.39^{***}	0.83	0.72^{*}	0.57^{**}	0.49^{***}	0.57^{***}	0.37^{***}
Female	0.76^{*}	0.80^{*}	0.86	0.75	0.70^{**}	0.65^{**}	0.92	0.94	1.01
Low education	0.30^{***}	0.39^{***}	0.36^{***}	0.31^{***}	0.33^{***}	0.48^{***}	0.39^{***}	0.34^{***}	0.43^{***}
Low-income[a]	0.49^{**}	0.43^{***}	0.47^{***}	0.53^{**}	0.42^{***}	0.65	0.65^{**}	0.50^{***}	0.53^{***}
Blue collar	0.52^{**}	0.55^{***}	0.60^{**}	0.50^{**}	0.51^{***}	0.58^{**}	0.52^{***}	0.53^{***}	0.51^{***}

Age, living alone or not, self-rated health, self-rated memory, bothered by pain, and number of chronic illnesses were included as covariates. BIPOC stands for Black, indigenous, and other people of color. Regarding significance, $^{*}p < 0.05$; $^{**}p < 0.01$; and $^{***}p < 0.001$

[a] Income included three categories, that is, low income, income missing, and medium and high income (reference group). Only the comparisons between low income and medium and high income were reported due to our research interest in this study

($OR = 0.38$, $CI = [0.16, 0.90]$, $p < 0.05$). A significant interaction was also found with low education in predicting handling health insurance online 2015 ($OR = 0.37$, $CI = [0.14, 0.95]$, $p < 0.05$). For getting health information online, significant interactions with female gender in 2015 ($OR = .60$, $CI = [0.36, 0.98]$, $p < 0.05$) and low income in 2019 ($OR = 0.39$, $CI = [0.17, 0.89]$, $p < 0.05$) were also found.

Table 10.4 Odds ratios from weighted logistic regressions on the digital divide in 2011/2013, 2015, and 2019 (interactions)

	2011	2015	2019	2011	2015	2019	2011	2015	2019
	Shopping			Banking			Ordering/refilling prescriptions		
BIPOC	1.06	0.93	0.69	1.04	1.15	0.74	0.98	0.99	1.23
Female	0.68***	0.94	1.15	0.77**	0.88	0.84	0.76*	0.68**	0.79
Low education	0.44***	0.46***	0.36***	0.32***	0.43***	0.43***	0.41***	0.64**	0.56***
Low-income[a]	0.59**	0.56***	0.49***	0.68**	0.61***	0.49***	0.48***	0.51***	0.56**
Blue collar	0.52***	0.56***	0.79	0.67**	0.49***	0.59***	0.62**	0.61**	0.73
BIPOC × Female	0.68	0.91	0.60	1.07	0.59*	0.82	0.39*	0.68	0.62
BIPOC ×Low education	0.39*	0.52	0.70	0.75	0.45**	0.86	0.45	0.34**	0.46
BIPOC × Low-income	0.50	0.44*	0.52	0.51*	0.37**	0.63	0.81	0.51	0.72
BIPOC × Blue collar	1.37	1.49	1.00	0.54	1.22	1.19	0.68	1.15	0.77
	Visiting social networking sites (2013)								
BIPOC	1.31	0.95	0.69						
Female	1.42**	1.61***	1.68***						
Low education	0.66**	0.55***	0.67**						
Low-income[a]	0.63**	0.86	0.63**						
Blue collar	0.42*	0.73**	0.66**						
BIPOC × Female	0.49	0.70	0.67						
BIPOC ×Low education	0.33**	0.95	0.52						
BIPOC × Low-income	0.63	0.44**	0.73						
BIPOC × Blue collar	1.00	1.04	1.33						
	Contacting medical providers			Handling health insurance			Getting health information		
BIPOC	0.79	0.71	0.65	0.76	1.14	0.55*	0.70	0.95	0.76
Female	0.75*	0.82	0.89	0.73*	0.73*	0.62**	0.93	0.99	1.03
Low education	0.31***	0.39***	0.39***	0.32***	0.36***	0.52**	0.41***	0.36***	0.46***
Low-income[a]	0.49**	0.46***	0.54**	0.53**	0.47**	0.74	0.65**	0.52***	0.61**
Blue collar	0.50**	0.53***	0.55***	0.54*	0.49***	0.55	0.53***	0.56***	0.52***
BIPOC × Female	1.15	0.83	0.61	1.36	0.60	1.82	0.90	0.60*	0.73

(continued)

Table 10.4 (continued)

	2011	2015	2019	2011	2015	2019	2011	2015	2019
BIPOC ×Low education	0.82	0.84	0.38*	0.89	0.37*	0.54	0.65	0.67	0.57
BIPOC × Low-income	0.93	0.64	0.41	1.11	0.50	0.49	0.87	0.79	0.39*
BIPOC × Blue collar	1.44	1.42	2.00	0.46	1.26	1.64	0.90	0.98	0.81

Note. Age, living alone or not, self-rated health, self-rated memory, bothered by pain, number of chronic illnesses were included as covariates. BIPOC stands for Black, indigenous, and other people of color. Regarding significance, * $p < 0.05$; ** $p < 0.01$; and *** $p < 0.001$

[a] Income included three categories, that is, low income, income missing, and medium and high income (reference group). Only the comparisons between low income and (medium and high) income were reported, due to our research interest in this study

10.4 Discussion

This study aims to examine the trends regarding the first and second levels of the digital divide among older community dwellers in the U.S., focusing on the impact of race/ethnicity and its intersecting effects with other marginalized social identities related to gender, education, income, and occupation. Findings in this study showed a high prevalence of internet access among both non-Hispanic white and BIPOC older community dwellers. The first-level digital divide, which pertains to material access, showed a positive trend as the disparities between non-Hispanic white and BIPOC older adults became non-significant in 2019, consistent with a recent survey indicating no significant difference in internet use by race and ethnicity (Perrin & Atske, 2021). This indicates progress in bridging the racial/ethnic gap in internet access among older adults. However, concerning the second-level digital divide, which refers to internet use for various purposes, racial/ethnic disparities still exist. BIPOC older adults consistently exhibited lower internet usage than non-Hispanic white older adults for personal tasks, social networking sites, and health-related purposes. This result aligns with prior studies highlighting racial/ethnic disparities in older adults' internet usage (Scheerder et al., 2017; Suntai & Beltran, 2022). By employing a trend study and intersectionality lens, the present research adds nuanced insights to the existing findings.

Interesting trends regarding the intersecting effects of race/ethnicity with other marginalized social identities were revealed in this study. For personal-task internet use, including shopping, banking, and ordering/refilling prescription online, the interactions with female gender and low SES variables became non-significant in 2019 compared to the significant status in 2011 or 2015. This suggests an encouraging trend, indicating that female gender and low SES did not further exacerbate the racial/ethnic disparities in personal-task use of the internet. This positive change aligns with the notion that as digital technology becomes more widespread and user-friendly (Vassilakopoulou & Hustad, 2023), it can effectively bridge the gap between individuals with different socioeconomic backgrounds (Scheerder et al.,

2017). For instance, technological advancements have improved user interfaces, making it easier for individuals with limited digital literacy to navigate online platforms (Fisk et al., 2020). Targeted efforts by governments and organizations to promote digital inclusion and provide digital literacy training to marginalized populations may have contributed to the positive change. Additionally, the growing ubiquity of smartphones and mobile internet access among older adults might have enhanced accessibility to these internet activities (Faviero, 2022).

Interesting patterns emerged when comparing Black older adults with Hispanic and other racial/ethnic minority groups regarding internet access and specific online activities. Overall, no significant differences were observed between these groups across most internet use domains, reinforcing the robustness of prior findings that treated BIPOC older adults as a single category. This suggests that shared structural barriers, such as socioeconomic disadvantages, digital literacy gaps, and historical marginalization may have a more pronounced role in shaping digital inclusion than racial/ethnic subgroup differences alone. However, some variations were observed in specific internet activities between Black older adults and Hispanic and other racial/ethnic groups, particularly in online health-related tasks such as ordering prescriptions and obtaining health information. Although these differences did not remain consistent across time, they suggest that factors beyond racial/ethnic identity, such as cultural norms, health literacy, and trust in digital health services, may influence engagement in online health activities. Prior research indicates that Hispanic older adults, in particular, may face additional barriers related to language accessibility and culturally relevant digital content, which could contribute to their lower engagement in online health management tools compared to Black older adults (Medero et al., 2022). Conversely, Black older adults may be more likely to access mobile-based health resources, a trend linked to higher smartphone dependency within this population (Chen et al., 2021). These patterns highlight the need to examine not only broad digital disparities but also the specific sociocultural and systemic factors that may drive subgroup differences in technology use.

However, regarding social and health-related internet use, the interactions with low SES indicators turned significant in 2015 or 2019, indicating racial/ethnic gaps for low SES older adults deepened. Our findings confirmed prior evidence that the intersection of lower income and education level would shape the experience of BIPOC older adults in utilizing the internet for health management and information-seeking purposes (Hung et al., 2020; Liu et al., 2020; Mitchell et al., 2019). While online health management has become more prevalent in recent years (Choi et al., 2022b), older community dwellers of color may have educational and economic barriers to access and navigate internet platforms for health-related purposes due to limited access to education, economic opportunities, and resources earlier in life (Farrell et al., 2022; Lyles et al., 2023; Zheng & Walsham, 2021). These challenges may lead to decreased involvement in crucial health-related tasks and hinder the ability to make informed decisions about their health, further creating a cycle of disadvantage and exclusion in the digital realm and enlarged health disparities. Thus, initiatives focusing on enhancing digital literacy, providing targeted training programs, and developing user-friendly health-related internet platforms may help mitigate the disparities observed in this study (Busse et al., 2022). By promoting digital inclusion and equitable access to health information online, policymakers and healthcare providers can improve older adults' overall health and well-being.

The findings in this study suggest that the gender-related digital divide is less clear (Hunsaker & Hargittai, 2018), but the results point to a positive trend. The effects of gender on personal-task and health-related internet activities were not significant in 2015 or 2019 in most cases. This is consistent with previous studies suggesting a closing digital divide or movement toward an even more advantaged position for women (Cotten et al., 2016; Perrin & Atske, 2021). Regarding visiting social networking sites, female gender was consistently associated with higher odds across the 3 years. Existing research has also found females to be more active users of social media platforms (Fleming & Agnew-Brune, 2015; Kuss & Griffiths, 2011; Tufekci, 2008), as they may prioritize maintaining social connections and seeking emotional support through online networks (Kuss & Griffiths, 2011).

It is also worth noting that even after adding the interactions, low SES variables, including low education, low income, and blue-collar jobs were consistently associated with lower odds of accessing the internet and engaging in most of the seven internet activities across all 3 years. The findings of this study align with previous research highlighting the significance of income and education as predictors of the digital divide (Hargittai & Dobransky, 2017) and a recent Pew Research Center survey indicating the persistent digital divide despite gains in technology adoption among the low-income population (Vogels, 2021). More importantly, it also indicates that the racial/ethnic disparities in the second-level digital divide may be due to socioeconomic disparities, consistent with racial/ethnic disparities research in other areas, such as health and mental health (Do et al., 2012; Jackson et al., 2016; Kahng, 2010), child maltreatment (Kim & Drake, 2018), and criminal justice (Jackson et al., 2016; Stringer & Holland, 2016). Thus, in reducing racial/ethnic disparities in the digital divide, multisectoral efforts should focus on alleviating the underlying socioeconomic disparities.

10.4.1 Theoretical and Practical Implications

In this study, the use of intersectionality provides a powerful framework for examining the digital divide, shedding light on the complex interplay between race, gender, socioeconomic status, and internet use. It helps clarify how systemic racism perpetuates disparities and how race-related social constructs influence access and use of digital technology among BIPOC older adults, especially when intersecting with other marginalized social categories and identities (Crenshaw, 2017). It's also worth mentioning that the underrepresentation of diverse voices in technology development can perpetuate digital inequities. When technology and online platforms are designed without considering the specific needs of diverse communities, they may inadvertently create barriers to access and limit digital literacy development (Fisk et al., 2020). Lack of inclusivity in the technology sector can hinder the creation of user-friendly platforms that are accessible and relevant to marginalized populations. Without incorporating culturally relevant and specific needs into practice, marginalized communities will likely continue to face barriers and challenges.

Drawing from the Intersectionality perspective, we recognize that the digital divide is not simply a matter of individual choices but is deeply rooted in historical and systemic inequalities (Delgado, 2001; Veenstra, 2011). Aiming to address the digital divide among older community dwellers, particularly BIPOC older adults, our findings have important implications for policymakers and stakeholders such as industry partners and service organizations. First, to effectively bridge the existing disparities in health-related internet use, targeted digital literacy initiatives tailored to members of marginalized older groups are crucial. These initiatives should not only provide basic digital skills but also focus on equipping BIPOC older adults with the necessary competencies to confidently use health-related internet platforms. Additionally, there is a need for collaboration between industry partners, aging service organizations, and healthcare providers to develop internet platforms that are tailored to the unique needs of this population. Such platforms should be user-friendly and designed with a focus on language inclusivity, cultural relevance, and accessibility, ensuring that they are easily navigable for BIPOC older adults (Fisk et al., 2020). Additionally, expanding community-based digital literacy programs that provide hands-on training in both English and Spanish may further bridge the gap, ensuring that Hispanic older adults can fully engage with online health resources. These findings emphasize the importance of culturally responsive digital inclusion efforts that recognize subgroup-specific needs rather than assuming a one-size-fits-all approach to digital adoption. Furthermore, a broader approach to improving internet infrastructure and accessibility is crucial. This includes advocating for equitable access to high-speed internet and affordable digital devices in marginalized communities. By expanding internet access and offering cost-effective solutions, we can help level the playing field, allowing older adults from diverse backgrounds to fully engage in the digital world.

10.4.2 Limitations

The limitations of the study should also be noted. One limitation is the missing data on income in the original NHATS study, which can potentially introduce uncertainties and bias in the analysis. To mitigate this concern, the study handled missing income values by treating them as a separate category, and we also performed multiple imputations as a sensitivity analysis, and the results showed robustness. Another limitation is the potential impact of the post-COVID era on internet use among older community dwellers. The COVID-19 pandemic led to a significant shift in internet usage patterns worldwide, with many individuals, including older adults, relying heavily on digital platforms for various tasks due to lockdowns and social distancing measures (Choi et al., 2022b). The study uses data before 2019, which cannot capture the potential changes in internet use behaviors during and after the pandemic. Future studies should consider incorporating the latest data for a more comprehensive understanding of digital use trends and patterns. Next, many other variables, such as rural/urban residence and neighborhood−/ community-level characteristics, may also affect the digital divide among older adults. However, due to the limitations of archival data from NHATS, we were not able to include these geographic variables in this study. Future studies may consider examining the impact of these variables on older adults' technology use. Lastly, in this study, we selected a relatively healthy sample of older adults living in their communities. Findings from this study may not be generalizable to older adults with different characteristics, such as those living in nursing homes, with cognitive impairment, and others with substantial health challenges. Also, BIPOC older adults are not a homogeneous population. However, due to the small sample size of some racial/ethnic groups, we combined them together. Future studies may examine and compare digital technology use among different racial/ethnic groups.

10.4.3 Conclusions

In conclusion, this trend study examines the first- and second-level digital divide among older community dwellers in the U.S. through an intersectionality framework. The findings highlight persistent disparities in internet use, particularly among BIPOC older adults with lower education and income. Moreover, interactions with marginalized social identities also influence the digital technology experience. A unique aspect of this study is the expansion on existing research to investigate the trend of the digital divide, with a specific focus on detailed usage purposes. As technological integration becomes increasingly prevalent in society, understanding and actively addressing digital disparities is crucial for promoting equitable access to digital technology among older community dwellers. Attention also needs to be directed toward addressing the second-level digital divide, especially regarding health-related internet use. To achieve this goal, efforts to enhance digital literacy, develop user-friendly platforms, and improve internet infrastructure and accessibility are essential. By fostering a more equitable digital landscape, policymakers and stakeholders can contribute to improved health outcomes, enhanced social engagement, and greater overall well-being for older community dwellers of all backgrounds.

Acknowledgments NHATS is supported by the National Institute on Aging under a cooperative agreement with the Johns Hopkins University Bloomberg School of Public Health (U01AG032947), with data collection by Westat.

Disclaimer The views expressed in this chapter are solely those of the authors and do not necessarily reflect those of the University of Alabama at Birmingham, the University of Illinois Urbana-Champaign, the United Nations, the University of Alabama, the University at Albany, or Binghamton University.

Conflict of Interest We have no conflict of interest to declare.

Funding None reported.

References

Bell, C., Fausset, C., Farmer, S., Nguyen, J., Harley, L., & Fain, W. B. (2013). Examining social media use among older adults. In *Proceedings of the 24th ACM conference on hypertext and social media.*

Bertolazzi, A., Quaglia, V., & Bongelli, R. (2024). Barriers and facilitators to health technology adoption by older adults with chronic diseases: An integrative systematic review. *BMC Public Health, 24*(1), 506. https://doi.org/10.1186/s12889-024-18036-5

Busse, T. S., Nitsche, J., Kernebeck, S., Jux, C., Weitz, J., Ehlers, J. P., & Bork, U. (2022). Approaches to improvement of digital health literacy (eHL) in the context of person-centered care. *International Journal of Environmental Research and Public Health, 19*(14). https://doi.org/10.3390/ijerph19148309

Byrne, K. A., Anaraky, R. G., Dye, C., Ross, L. A., Chalil Madathil, K., Knijnenburg, B., & Levkoff, S. (2021). Examining rural and racial disparities in the relationship between loneliness and social technology use among older adults. *Frontiers in Public Health, 9*, 723925.

Castells, M. (2002). *The Internet galaxy: Reflections on the internet, business, and society*. Oxford University Press on Demand.

Chen, J., Li, K. Y., Andino, J., Hill, C. E., Ng, S., Steppe, E., & Ellimoottil, C. (2021). Predictors of audio-only versus video telehealth visits during the COVID-19 pandemic. *Journal of General Internal Medicine, 37*(5), 1138–1144. https://doi.org/10.1007/s11606-021-07172-y

Choi, N., & DiNitto, D. (2013). Internet use among older adults: Association with health needs, psychological capital, and social capital. *Journal of Medical Internet Research, 15*(5), e97. https://doi.org/10.2196/jmir.2333

Choi, E. Y., Kim, Y., Chipalo, E., & Lee, H. Y. (2020). Does perceived ageism widen the digital divide? And does it vary by gender? *The Gerontologist, 60*(7), 1213–1223. https://doi.org/10.1093/geront/gnaa066

Choi, E. Y., Wisniewski, K. M., & Zelinski, E. M. (2021). Information and communication technology use in older adults: A unidirectional or Bi-directional association with cognitive function? *Computers in Human Behavior, 121, 106813.* https://doi.org/https://doi.org/10.1016/j.chb.2021.106813

Choi, E. Y., Kanthawala, S., Kim, Y. S., & Lee, H. Y. (2022a). Urban/rural digital divide exists in older adults: Does it vary by racial/ethnic groups? *Journal of Applied Gerontology, 41*(5), 1348–1356. https://doi.org/10.1177/07334648211073605

Choi, N. G., DiNitto, D. M., Marti, C. N., & Choi, B. Y. (2022b). Telehealth use among older adults during COVID-19: Associations with sociodemographic and health characteristics, technology device ownership, and technology learning. *Journal of Applied Gerontology, 41*(3), 600–609. https://doi.org/10.1177/07334648211047347

Cotten, S. R., Francis, J., Kadylak, T., Rikard, R. V., Huang, T., Ball, C., & DeCook, J. (2016). *A tale of two divides: Technology experiences among racially and socioeconomically diverse older adults. Human aspects of IT for the aged population*. Design for Aging.

Crenshaw, K. W. (2013). Mapping the margins: Intersectionality, identity politics, and violence against women of color. In *The public nature of private violence* (pp. 93–118). Routledge.

Crenshaw, K. (2017). *On intersectionality essential writings*. The New Press.

Delgado, R. S. J (2001). *Critical race theory: An introduction*. NYU Press. http://www.jstor.org/stable/j.ctt9qg26k

Do, D. P., Frank, R., & Finch, B. K. (2012). Does SES explain more of the black/white health gap than we thought? Revisiting our approach toward understanding racial disparities in health. *Social Science & Medicine, 74*(9), 1385–1393.

Du, Y., & Xu, Q. (2016). Health disparities and delayed health care among older adults in California: A perspective from race, ethnicity, and immigration. *Public Health Nursing, 33*(5), 383–394.

Farrell, T. W., Hung, W. W., Unroe, K. T., Brown, T. R., Furman, C. D., Jih, J., Karani, R., Mulhausen, P., Napoles, A. M., Nnodim, J. O., Upchurch, G., Whittaker, C. F., Kim, A.,

Lundebjerg, N. E., & Rhodes, R. L. (2022). Exploring the intersection of structural racism and ageism in healthcare. *Journal of the American Geriatrics Society, 70*(12), 3366–3377. https://doi.org/10.1111/jgs.18105

Faviero, M. (2022). Share of those 65 and older who are tech users has grown in the past decade. *Pew Research Center, January, 13.*

Fisk, A. D., Czaja, S. J., Rogers, W. A., Charness, N., & Sharit, J. (2020). *Designing for older adults: Principles and creative human factors approaches*. CRC Press.

Fleming, P. J., & Agnew-Brune, C. (2015). Current trends in the study of gender norms and health behaviors. *Current Opinion in Psychology, 5*, 72–77. https://doi.org/10.1016/j.copsyc.2015.05.001

Freedman, V. A., Hu, M., DeMatteis, J., & Kasper, J. (2020). *Accounting for sample design in NHATS and NSOC analyses: Frequently asked questions*.

Hamilton, A. M. (2020). A genealogy of critical race and digital studies: Past, present, and future. *Sociology of Race and Ethnicity, 6*(3), 292–301. https://doi.org/10.1177/2332649220922577

Hargittai, E. (2001). Second-level digital divide: Mapping differences in people's online skills. *arXiv preprint cs/0109068*.

Hargittai, E., & Dobransky, K. (2017). Old dogs, new clicks: Digital inequality in skills and uses among older adults. *Canadian Journal of Communication, 42*(2), 195–212. https://doi.org/10.22230/cjc2017v42n2a3176

He, W., Cao, L., Liu, R., Wu, Y., & Zhang, W. (2022). Factors associated with internet use and health information technology use among older people with multi-morbidity in the United States: Findings from the National Health Interview Survey 2018. *BMC Geriatrics, 22*(1), 733. https://doi.org/10.1186/s12877-022-03410-y

Hecker, I., Spaulding, S., & Kuehn, D. (2021). Digital skills and older workers. Urban Institute, 2021, 1–24. https://www.urban.org/sites/default/files/publication/104771/digital-skills-and-older-work-ers_0.pdf

Horowitz, J. M., Igielnik, R., & Kochhar, R. (2020). *Trends in income and wealth inequality*. https://www.pewresearch.org/social-trends/2020/01/09/trends-in-income-and-wealth-inequality/

Hung, L.-Y., Lyons, J. G., & Wu, C.-H. (2020). Health information technology use among older adults in the United States, 2009–2018. *Current Medical Research and Opinion, 36*(5), 789–797. https://doi.org/10.1080/03007995.2020.1734782

Hunsaker, A., & Hargittai, E. (2018). A review of internet use among older adults. *New Media & Society, 20*(10), 3937–3954. https://doi.org/10.1177/1461444818787348

Hutto, C. J., Bell, C., Farmer, S., Fausset, C., Harley, L., Nguyen, J., & Fain, B. (2015). *Social media gerontology: Understanding social media usage among older adults*. Web intelligence.

Gatto, S. L., & Tak, S. H. (2008). Computer, Internet, and e-mail use among older adults: Benefits and barriers. *Educational Gerontology, 34*(9), 800–811.

Jackson, J. W., Williams, D. R., & VanderWeele, T. J. (2016). Disparities at the intersection of marginalized groups. *Social Psychiatry and Psychiatric Epidemiology, 51*(10), 1349–1359. https://doi.org/10.1007/s00127-016-1276-6

Kahng, S. K. (2010). Can racial disparity in health between black and white Americans be attributed to racial disparities in body weight and socioeconomic status? *Health & Social Work, 35*(4), 257–266.

Kasper, J. D., Freedman, V. A., & Spillman, B. C. (2013). *Classification of persons by dementia status in the National Health and Aging Trends Study*.

Kent, A. H., & Ricketts, L. R. (2020). Has wealth inequality in America changed over time? *Here are key statistics*.

Kim, H., & Drake, B. (2018). Child maltreatment risk as a function of poverty and race/ethnicity in the USA. *International Journal of Epidemiology, 47*(3), 780–787. https://doi.org/10.1093/ije/dyx280

Kuss, D. J., & Griffiths, M. D. (2011). Online social networking and addiction--a review of the psychological literature. *International Journal of Environmental Research and Public Health, 8*(9), 3528–3552. https://doi.org/10.3390/ijerph8093528

Leukel, J., Schehl, B., & Sugumaran, V. (2021). Digital inequality among older adults: Explaining differences in the breadth of Internet use. *Information, Communication & Society, 26*(1), 139–154. https://doi.org/10.1080/1369118x.2021.1942951

Li, S. (2023). Revisiting the relationship between information and communication technologies and travel behavior: An investigation of older Americans. *Transportation Research Part A: Policy and Practice, 172*, 103689. https://doi.org/10.1016/j.tra.2023.103689

Li, C., Zeng, X., Wang, K., Neugroschl, J. A., Aloysi, A., Cai, D., Martin, J., Sewell, M., Greenberg, J., Xu, M., Evans, K., Pun, K., Tocco, C., Ardolino, A., Meuser, C., Sheppard, F., Gamino, J., Velasco, N., Sano, M., Zhu, C. W., et al. (2021). Smartphone ownership and usage in Chinese- and English-speaking older adults. *Alzheimer's & Dementia, 17*(S11), e054680. https://doi.org/10.1002/alz.054680

Lindeman, D. A. (2017). Improving the independence of older adults through technology: Directions for public policy. *Public Policy & Aging Report, 27*(2), 49–52. https://doi.org/10.1093/ppar/prx011

Liu, D., Yamashita, T., Burston, B., & Keene, J. R. (2020). The use of online health-management tools and health care utilization among older Americans. *The Gerontologist, 60*(7), 1224–1232. https://doi.org/10.1093/geront/gnaa068

Lyles, C. R., Nguyen, O. K., Khoong, E. C., Aguilera, A., & Sarkar, U. (2023). Multilevel determinants of digital health equity: A literature synthesis to advance the field. *Annual Review of Public Health, 44*, 383–405. https://doi.org/10.1146/annurev-publhealth-071521-023913

Masullo Chen, G. (2016). Social media: From digital divide to empowerment. In *The Routledge companion to media and race*. Taylor & Francis.

Medero, K., Merrill, K., Jr., & Ross, M. Q. (2022). Access across the digital divide for intersectional groups seeking online health information: A national survey (preprint). *Journal of Medical Internet Research*. https://doi.org/10.2196/32678

Mitchell, U. A., Chebli, P. G., Ruggiero, L., & Muramatsu, N. (2019). The digital divide in health-related technology use: The significance of race/ethnicity. *The Gerontologist, 59*(1), 6–14. https://doi.org/10.1093/geront/gny138

Mubarak, F., & Suomi, R. (2022). Elderly forgotten? Digital exclusion in the information age and the rising Grey digital divide. *INQUIRY: The Journal of Health Care Organization, Provision, and Financing, 59*(1), 004695802210962. https://doi.org/10.1177/00469580221096272

Nakamura, L., & Chow-White, P. (2010). *Race after the Internet*. Routledge.

Perrin, A., & Atske, S. (2021). *7% of Americans don't use the internet. Who are they*. Retrieved April 14th from

Perrin, A., & Duggan, M. (2019). Americans' internet access: 2000-2015: As internet use nears saturation for some groups, a look at patterns of adoption. 2015. *Pew Internet project data memo*.

Scheerder, A., van Deursen, A., & van Dijk, J. (2017). Determinants of Internet skills, uses and outcomes. A systematic review of the second- and third-level digital divide. *Telematics and Informatics, 34*(8), 1607–1624. https://doi.org/10.1016/j.tele.2017.07.007

Shapira, N., Barak, A., & Gal, I. (2007). Promoting older adults' well-being through Internet training and use. *Aging & Mental Health, 11*(5), 477–484. https://doi.org/10.1080/13607860601086546

StataCorp. 2021. Stata Statistical Software: Release 17. StataCorp LLC.

Stringer, R. J., & Holland, M. M. (2016). It's not all black and white: A propensity score matched, multilevel examination of racial drug sentencing disparities. *Journal of Ethnicity In Criminal Justice, 14*(4), 327–347.

Suntai, Z., & Beltran, S. J. (2022). The intersectional impact of race/ethnicity and sex on access to technology among older adults. *Gerontologist, 63*(7), 1162–1171. https://doi.org/10.1093/geront/gnac178

Szabo, A., Allen, J., Stephens, C., & Alpass, F. (2019). Longitudinal analysis of the relationship between purposes of Internet use and well-being among older adults. *The Gerontologist, 59*(1), 58–68. https://doi.org/10.1093/geront/gny036

Tsetsi, E., & Rains, S. A. (2017). Smartphone Internet access and use: Extending the digital divide and usage gap. *Mobile Media & Communication, 5*(3), 239–255. https://doi.org/10.1177/2050157917708329

Tufekci, Z. (2008). Grooming, gossip, Facebook and Myspace. *Information, Communication & Society, 11*(4), 544–564. https://doi.org/10.1080/13691180801999050

Van Deursen, A. J. A. M., & Helsper, E. J. (2015). The third-level digital divide: Who benefits most from being online? *Communication and Information Technologies Annual, 10*, 29–52.

van Dijk, J. (2005). *The deepening divide: Inequality in the information society*. Sage.

Vassilakopoulou, P., & Hustad, E. (2023). Bridging digital divides: A literature review and research agenda for information systems research. *Information Systems Frontiers, 25*(3), 955–969. https://doi.org/10.1007/s10796-020-10096-3

Vassli, L. T., & Farshchian, B. A. (2018). Acceptance of health-related ICT among elderly people living in the community: A systematic review of qualitative evidence. *International Journal of Human–Computer Interaction, 34*(2), 99–116. https://doi.org/10.1080/10447318.2017.1328024

Veenstra, G. (2011). Race, gender, class, and sexual orientation: Intersecting axes of inequality and self-rated health in Canada. *International Journal for Equity in Health, 10*(1), 3. https://doi.org/10.1186/1475-9276-10-3

Vogels, E. A. (2021). Digital divide persists even as Americans with lower incomes make gains in tech adoption. *Pew Research Center, 22*.

Wang, K., & Gu, D. (2023). Reciprocal associations between social media use and self-perception of aging among older adults: Do men and women differ? *Social Science & Medicine, 321*, 115786.

Yoon, H., Jang, Y., Vaughan, P. W., & Garcia, M. (2018). Older adults' internet use for health information: Digital divide by race/ethnicity and socioeconomic status. *Journal of Applied Gerontology, 39*(1), 105–110. https://doi.org/10.1177/0733464818770772

Yoon, H., Jang, Y., Kim, S., Speasmaker, A., & Nam, I. (2020). Trends in internet use among older adults in the United States, 2011–2016. *Journal of Applied Gerontology, 40*(5), 466–470. https://doi.org/10.1177/0733464820908427

Yu, R. P., Ellison, N. B., McCammon, R. J., & Langa, K. M. (2016). Mapping the two levels of digital divide: Internet access and social network site adoption among older adults in the USA. *Information, Communication & Society, 19*(10), 1445–1464. https://doi.org/10.1080/1369118X.2015.1109695

Zheng, Y., & Walsham, G. (2021). Inequality of what? An intersectional approach to digital inequality under Covid-19. *Information and Organization., 31*(1), 100341. https://doi.org/10.1016/j.infoandorg.2021.100341

Chapter 11
Bridging the Access Gap: A Decade of Narrowing the Digital Divide for Hispanic Older Adults in the United States

Kun Wang, Xiayu Summer Chen, Yanjun Dong, Karla G. Sanabria Véaz, and Danan Gu

11.1 Introduction

The older Hispanic population holds importance and complexity within the dynamic framework of the United States (U.S.) demographics. As the country undergoes a significant demographic transition, the older population is projected to outnumber children by 2034 (U.S. Census Bureau, 2018). Within this evolving landscape, the

---

Note on Reuse of Published Materials
This chapter incorporates a revised and expanded version of material originally published in the article *"Bridging the access gap: A decade of narrowing the digital divide for Hispanic older adults in the United States."* by Wang, K., Chen, X. S., Dong, Y., Sanabria Véaz, K. G., & Gu, D. (2025), published in *Journal of Aging and Health, 37*(3–4), 182–191. The original work has been adapted and updated, in accordance with the publisher's policies.

K. Wang (✉)
Department of Social Work, College of Arts and Sciences, University of Alabama at Birmingham, Birmingham, AL, USA
e-mail: kw2@uab.edu

X. S. Chen · K. G. Sanabria Véaz
University of Illinois Urbana-Champaign, Champaign, IL, USA
e-mail: xiayuyc2@illinois.edu; karlags2@illinois.edu

Y. Dong
University at Albany, State University of New York, Albany, NY, USA
e-mail: ydong2@albany.edu

D. Gu
Population Division, UN Department of Economic and Social Affairs, New York, NY, USA
e-mail: gudanan@yahoo.com

K. Wang et al. (eds.), *ICT Use and Healthy Longevity*, Advances in Studies of Aging and Health 5, https://doi.org/10.1007/978-3-031-98964-3_11

older Hispanic population is emerging as an influential subset, representing 9% of the overall older population in 2020 (Administration for Community Living, 2021). This population is anticipated to experience a substantial increase of 148% from 2020 to 2040, accounting for 21% of the country's older population by 2060 (Administration for Community Living, 2021). Along with the growing presence, Hispanic older adults are still encountering enduring obstacles from linguistic barriers, socioeconomic disparities, and distinctive cultural factors in their daily lives.

Along with the rapidly increasing number of Hispanic older adults, the past decades also witnessed a significant increase in internet use among U.S. older adults from 46% in 2010 (Perrin & Duggan, 2015) to 75% in 2021 (Faverio, 2022). While the internet has been suggested to mitigate various aging challenges (Erickson & Johnson, 2011; Szabo et al., 2019), the digital divide still exists among older adults (Hargittai & Dobransky, 2017). The digital divide refers to the inequalities in digital technology use, from technology access and fundamental internet connectivity to the capability and skills in use (Van Deursen & Van Dijk, 2019). Older adults are vulnerable to digital inequality as they are often the last to adopt emerging digital innovation (Hong & Cho, 2017). Moreover, marginalized social identities relevant to race/ethnicity, gender, education, and income are consistently linked to the digital divide (Choi & DiNitto, 2013; Ihm & Hsieh, 2015; Tappen et al., 2022). Compared to their non-Hispanic White counterparts, Hispanic older adults are less likely to access the internet and use the internet for different activities (Lopez et al., 2013; Mitchell et al., 2019; Perrin & Duggan, 2015).

11.1.1 Is the Digital Gap Narrowing Across Time Within the Hispanic Community?

The digital access disparity between Hispanic and non-Hispanic White people has shown signs of a reduced digital divide than before the COVID-19 pandemic (Brown et al., 2016). The onset of the pandemic in 2020 has catalyzed a shift to virtual platforms for various aspects of daily life, including employment, education, healthcare, and social engagements, accelerating digital device adoption across diverse demographic groups. According to the 2021 Pew Research Center Survey, 80% of Hispanic adults reported owning smartphones and 50% owning tablets, with no significant difference compared to non-Hispanic White and Black adults (Perrin & Atske, 2021). Moreover, Hispanic and Black communities exhibited significant increases in home broadband adoption during the pandemic (Perrin & Atske, 2021).

Despite certain technological advancements, a persistent digital gap remains, particularly among people with lower socioeconomic status. The percentages of internet users across various income categories, either through home broadband or a smartphone, remained the same between 2019 and 2021 (Vogels, 2021). Moreover, Early and Hernandez (2021) suggested that digital inequality was exacerbated due to the increasing income disparities and poverty issues in communities of Black, indigenous, and other people of color (BIPOC). Another report from the National League of Cities (2021) also indicated the diverse challenges concerning broadband affordability and accessibility among the Hispanic communities during the COVID-19 pandemic. Thus, it remains unclear whether the digital divide between Hispanic and non-Hispanic White older adults has alleviated or escalated during the past decade, especially after the pandemic. Furthermore, most research on digital disparities focuses on the differences between non-Hispanic White and Black populations (Rodriguez-Elliott & Vachuska, 2023), which fails to adequately explain the complexities of the disparities experienced by Hispanic communities. Thus, more studies are needed to focus on the older Hispanic communities to better understand their technology access and usage and meet their needs.

Moreover, having general internet access does not necessarily translate into equitable use of digital technology across different purposes. There is limited research on the digital engagement of Hispanic older adults, particularly in the domains of personal and social use. In the health domain, lower usage of online health services among Hispanic older adults has been documented, which may be attributed to distrust in digital health systems, limited health literacy, and economic constraints (Chavarria et al., 2022). Examining disparities in these specific internet usage domains (personal, health-related, and social use) is crucial, as they directly impact older adults' quality of life, healthcare outcomes, and social connectedness. Therefore, beyond measuring general digital access, this study also investigates whether racial/ethnic disparities persist in these particular areas of digital technology use over the past decade.

11.1.2 Digital Divide Through an Intersectional Lens

Intersectionality offers a profound lens for understanding the dynamic interplay between systems of oppression, privilege, and identity (Cho et al., 2013; Crenshaw, 1988, 2011). The theory is underpinned by two principles. Firstly, it recognizes that systems of oppression, such as classism, racism, and ableism, represent complex and intersecting axes of subordination that interact and transform each other. Secondly, it suggests that these systems foster identities that embody both oppressive and privileged characteristics and that these identities can coexist (Delgado & Stefancic, 2023). When applying the intersectional lens, it is necessary to consider individuals' identities through various dimensions, encompassing race, ethnicity, gender, socioeconomic status, geographic location, immigrant status, medical issues, and language proficiency (Ford & Airhihenbuwa, 2010).

Research exploring the digital divide from an intersectional perspective reveals the multifaceted nature of marginalization in technology access and usage (Suntai & Beltran, 2023). Studies on digital usage and innovation during COVID-19 (Zheng & Walsham, 2021) indicated that technological developments and utilizations were deeply embedded within social and power structures, highlighting how economic instability, gender inequality, and racial discrimination contribute to digital inequality.

An intersectional analysis of the disparities in digital device accessibility between Hispanic and non-Hispanic White older adults will provide nuanced insights into how digital inequalities are perpetuated by power systems that reinforce marginalization and privilege across gender, educational attainment, and income levels. Importantly, Hispanic older adults are not a homogeneous group. The intersection of gender norms with racial discrimination uniquely impacts digital access and usage beyond the effects of race or gender in isolation. Furthermore, given that 17.1% of Hispanic older adults live in poverty and 63% possess only a high school diploma (Administration for Community Living, 2021), socioeconomic factors are expected to significantly influence the ability of Hispanic older adults to acquire digital technologies.

Guided by the intersectionality lens, this study aims to bridge gaps in the literature by analyzing 11 waves of data from the National Health and Aging Trend Study (NHATS). The major research questions include: (1) Is the disparity in digital device access between Hispanic and non-Hispanic White older adults in the U.S. narrowing down or deepening from 2011 to 2021? (2) Does the change of disparity in digital device access differ by gender, education, and income from 2011 to 2021?

11.2 Methods

11.2.1 Data Source and Study Sample

Data used in this study were extracted from the 2011–2021 National Health and Aging Trend Study, an annual survey of a nationally representative sample of Medicare beneficiaries aged 65 and older in the U.S. NHATS was initiated in 2011 and replenished in 2015 to maintain a nationally representative sample. During these 11 survey waves, 12,427 older adults participated, with a total of 66,508 observations. The publicly available NHATS data in this study measured age by 5-year categories. The youngest age group was between 65 and 69. A group of participants had missing values in age and contributed 4118 observations over the study period. Furthermore, to ensure the comparable age structure of the participants over time, only observations made by participants aged 70 and older at each wave were included, excluding 5423 observations. In addition, due to the physical and cognitive capacities required to use digital devices, only participants who lived in their communities without missing values on study variables and who did not have possible, probable, or diagnosed dementia and had no missing values on these questions were included in the analysis, which excluded 7842 and 10,866 observations, respectively. Possible and probable dementia was defined based on previous studies (Kasper et al., 2013). Finally, two participants without information on digital device use were excluded, who contributed six observations. In sum, 38,253 observations from 8503 participants were included in this study (see Fig. 11.1). NHATS has been reviewed and approved by the Institutional Review Board at the Johns Hopkins Bloomberg School of Public Health. The publicly available NHATS data used in this study can be retrieved at www.nhats.org.

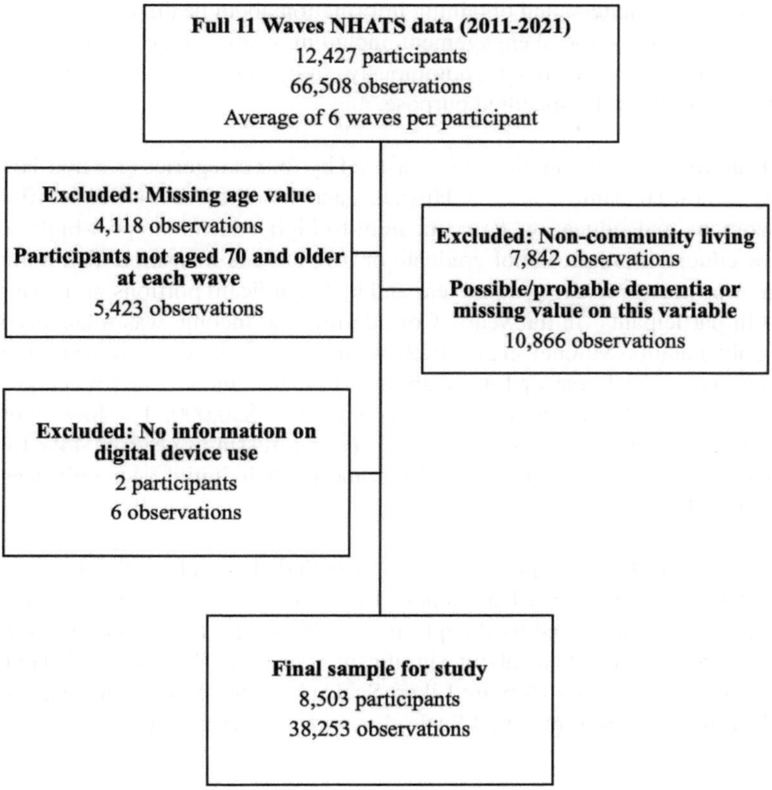

Fig. 11.1 Sample selection flowcha

11.2.2 Measures

The Digital Divide Participants were asked at each wave whether they had a working cellphone, any other phones, or a computer and whether they used a computer at locations outside the home. This question measures the prevalence of access to a digital device. In the present study, if they answered ("yes" to at least one of these questions), they were considered having digital access (or having no digital divide); otherwise ("no" to all these questions), they were considered not having digital access or having digital divide.

Digital Technology Use Purpose In addition to general digital access, we categorized internet usage into three specific domains: personal, health, and social use. Personal use encompassed activities such as shopping for groceries or personal items and managing financial transactions, including paying bills or banking online. Health use involved engaging in online health-related activities, such as ordering or refilling prescriptions, contacting medical providers, handling Medicare or other health insurance matters, and obtaining information about health conditions. Social use referred to online social engagement, including visiting social networking sites. Each domain was measured dichotomously, indicating whether individuals had used the internet for the specified purpose.

Social Identity Race/ethnicity was measured by four categories (1 = non-Hispanic White, 2 = non-Hispanic Black, 3 = Hispanic, and 4 = other races). Gender (0 = men, 1 = women) and education (0 = medium-to-high education, post-high school, 1 = low education, high school graduate or lower) were measured dichotomously. Income was measured every other year and had significant portions of missing data (44%) in participants' initial years. Considering that income was relatively stable among older adults (Mitchell et al., 2022), we used the first income value participants ever reported (initial year or follow-up years) as their income and recoded it into three categories (0 = medium-to-high income, > = $30,000, 1 = low income, < $30,000, and 2 = income missing). It reduced the missing rate from 44% to 24%. Sensitivity analysis with participants' income in their initial year only was conducted to test the robustness.

Other Covariates Time-varying covariates included age (1 = 70–74, 2 = 75–79, 3 = 80–84, 4 = 85–89, 5 = 90 and older), living alone (0 = no, 1 = yes), social networking size was measured by the question of "naming a maximum of five people a participant would talk to about significant issues" (0–5) (Marin & Hampton, 2007), self-rated memory (5-point Likert Scale, 1 = poor, 5 = Excellent), and self-rated health status (5-point Likert Scale, 1 = poor, 5 = Excellent).

11.2.3 Analytic Strategy

First, descriptive statistics in the initial and replenishing years (2011 and 2015) were calculated to better understand participant characteristics. Then, multilevel logistic regressions were conducted to examine the digital divide between older Hispanic and non-Hispanic White participants and how this racial/ethnic digital divide changed over time, including interactions (survey wave × race/ethnicity). Third, stratified analyses by gender, education level, and income level were conducted to investigate whether the digital divide changes differed across subgroups. Lastly, to further examine the digital divide by specific internet use purposes, we also conducted multilevel logistic regression models separately predicting personal use, health use, and social use of digital technology. These analyses controlled demographic variables (age, gender, and race/ethnicity) and tested interactions between survey waves and racial groups (Wave × Black, Wave × N-HB, Wave × Other races) to explore trends in usage disparities across specific digital domains. All analyses were completed using Stata 17 software.

11.3 Results

11.3.1 Descriptive Characteristics

Participants' characteristics in the initial and replenishing years are reported in Table 11.1. Overall, the proportion of digital access among non-Hispanic Whites was the highest compared to other races. Hispanics had the lowest level of digital access or the highest digital divide among all race categories. However, the digital

Table 11.1 Descriptive characteristics in the initial and replenishing years: 2011 and 2015

	Sample distribution		Percentages of digital access	
	2011	2015	2011	2015
Total sample size, #	4068	4720	4068	4720
Total, %	100.0	100.0	84.4	92.4
Race/ethnicity				
% Non-Hispanic White	74.4	74.6	86.7	93.8
% Non-Hispanic Black	19.0	18.3	83.0	88.5
% Hispanic	4.5	4.7	75.6	87.6
% Others	2.2	2.4	78.7	89.3
Gender				
% Men	41.4	42.3	89.0	94.4
% Women	58.6	57.7	82.9	91.1
Educational attainment				
% High school or lower	50.7	45.1	78.3	87.2
% Higher than high school	49.3	54.9	92.7	96.7
Income group				
% Low	29.5	32.4	78.0	86.7
% Medium and high	26.9	39.0	94.1	97.6
% Missing	43.5	28.6	85.1	92.2
Age				
% 70–74	31.5	32.9	92.7	97.1
% 75–79	27.6	27.6	89.6	93.1
% 80–84	23.6	20.9	80.3	91.9
% 85–89	11.7	12.5	76.4	87.0
% 90 and older	5.6	6.1	64.8	78.5
Living alone				
% No	94.4	93.9	88.1	94.3
% Yes	33.0	33.4	80.3	89.0
Mean (SD), social network size (0–5)	1.95 (1.29)	2.25 (1.35)	–	–
Mean (SD), self-rated health (1–5)	3.25 (1.08)	3.28 (1.03)	–	–
Mean (SD), self-rated memory (1–5)	3.38 (0.99)	3.27 (0.95)	–	–

Note. SD refers to standard deviation. All percentages or means were not weighted. The weighted outcomes are very similar. Participants replenished in 2015 had more education, less poverty, larger social networks, and lower self-rated memory gap between these two races/ethnicities was narrowed in the survey replenishing year 2015 compared to the initial year 2011.

11.3.2 The Digital Divide Changes Between Hispanic and Non-Hispanic White Participants

In Table 11.2, multilevel logistic regression showed that, compared to non-Hispanic White participants, those who were Hispanic (*OR* = 0.42, 95% *CI* = 0.25–0.70) had significantly lower odds of having digital device access (Model 0). Moderation analyses showed that the interaction between the survey wave and Hispanic ethnicity was significant regardless of whether some key covariates were not adjusted (*OR* = 1.17, 95%*CI* = 1.05–1.29) (Model 1 in Table 11.2) or were adjusted (*OR* = 1.17, 95%*CI* = 1.06–1.30) (Model 2 in Table 11.2), indicating that the digital divide between Hispanic and non-Hispanic White participants was reducing with time, and that Hispanic even caught up with non-Hispanic White after 2020 when education, income, social network, and self-rated memory and overall health conditions were further controlled (Fig. 11.2).

11.3.3 The Digital Divide Changes by Gender, Education, and Income

As presented in Table 11.3 when all study covariates were controlled, the interaction between the survey wave and Hispanic ethnicity was significant among older men (*OR* = 1.23, 95% *CI* = 1.03–1.46) and older women (*OR* = 1.15, 95% *CI* = 1.00–1.31).

Table 11.2 Odds ratio and 95% confidence interval of multilevel logistic regressions on digital access

	Model 0	Model 1	Model 2
Survey wave	**1.29** (1.25, 1.34)	**1.31** (1.27, 1.35)	**1.29** (1.24, 1.33)
Non-Hispanic Black (N-HB)	**0.41** (0.31, 0.56)	**0.27** (0.19, 0.40)	**0.48** (0.32, 0.71)
Hispanic	**0.42** (0.25, 0.70)	**0.07** (0.04, 0.15)	**0.18** (0.09, 0.36)
Other races	**0.40** (0.18, 0.88)	**0.21** (0.07, 0.58)	**0.29** (0.10, 0.89)
Women	**0.65** (0.50, 0.85)	**0.40** (0.31, 0.51)	**0.61** (0.47, 0.80)
Low education	**0.12** (0.09, 0.16)		**0.11** (0.08, 0.15)
Wave × N-HB		0.95 (0.90, 1.01)	0.96 (0.90, 1.01)
Wave × Hispanic		**1.17** (1.05, 1.29)	**1.17** (1.06, 1.30)
Wave × Other races		1.03 (0.88, 1/21)	1.03 (0.87, 1.22)

Note. Models 0 and 2 controlled age, income, living alone, social network size, self-rated memory, and self-rated health status as time-varying covariates, while Model I did not include these covariates Odds ratios in boldface are significant at the level of 0.05. The reference group for race is non-Hispanic White

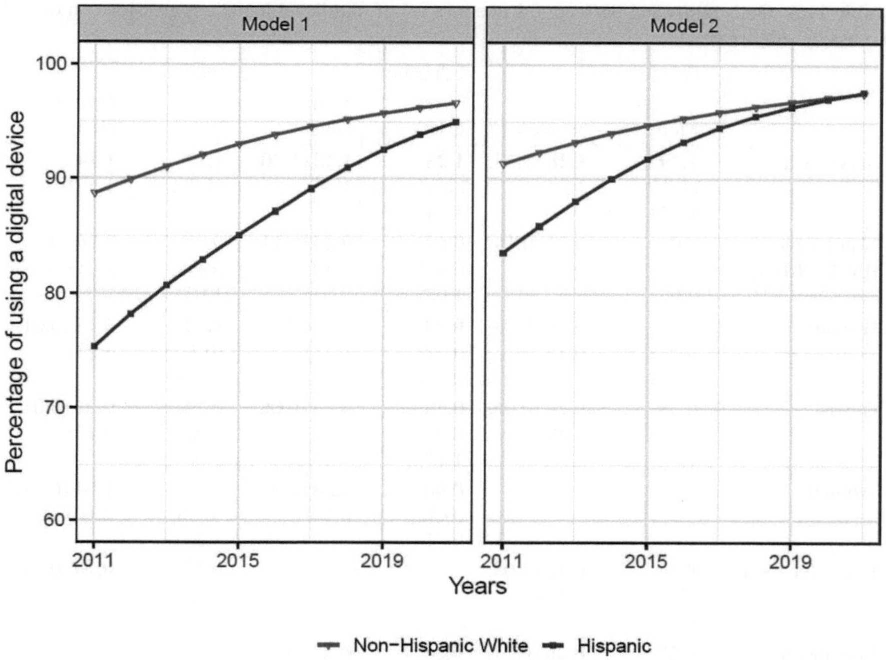

Fig. 11.2 Model-predicted percentages of digital access between Hispanic and non-Hispanic White participants from 2011 to 2021. Note: Results were derived from regression Models 1 and 2. In estimating the predicted percentages, all covariates were set at their means. Model 1 included survey year, race/ethnicity, gender, and age groups, whereas Model 2 additionally controlled education, income, living alone, social network size, self-rated memory, and self-rated health status at each wave

This indicated that the digital divide between Hispanic and non-Hispanic White participants was reduced significantly with time among older men and women (see Fig. 11.3). The by-education stratified analyses showed that the interaction between survey wave and Hispanic ethnicity was only significant among participants with low education level ($OR = 1.20$, 95% $CI = 1.06–1.35$) but not among those with medium-to-high level ($OR = 1.00$, 95% $CI = 0.77–1.30$). That is, the digital divide between Hispanic and non-Hispanic White participants reduced with time only among those with low education (see Fig. 11.3). Similarly, the by-income stratified analyses showed that the interaction between survey wave and Hispanic ethnicity was significant among those with low income ($OR = 1.24$, 95% $CI = 1.08–1.42$) but not among those with medium-to-high income ($OR = 1.11$, 95% $CI = 0.71–1.73$). This means that, among those with low income, the digital divide was reducing with time (see Fig. 11.3).

It is worth noting that the narrowing trend in the racial digital divide between Hispanic and non-Hispanic White older adults was less dramatic when only demographics were controlled in modeling (see Fig. 11.4). This indicates that factors

Table 11.3 Odds ratios and 95% confidence interval of multilevel logistic regressions on digital access by subgroup

	Gender		Education		Income	
	Men	Women	Low	Medium/ High	Low	Medium/ High
Survey wave	**1.29** (1.22, 1.37)	**1.28** (1.22, 1.34)	**1.28** (1.23, 1.34)	**1.28** (1.20, 1.36)	**1.27** (1.21, 1.34)	**1.44** (1.33, 1.57)
Non-Hispanic Black (N-HB)	1.03 (0.51, 2.06)	**0.32** (0.19, 0.53)	0.67 (0.42, 1.08)	**0.24** (0.11, 0.49)	0.57 (0.31, 1.03)	0.96 (0.24, 3.91)
Hispanic	**0.17** (0.06, 0.47)	**0.20** (0.08, 0.49)	**0.20** (0.09, 0.42)	0.25 (0.05, 1.21)	**0.24** (0.10, 0.59)	0.18 (0.01, 3.23)
Others	0.35 (0.07, 1.71)	0.29 (0.06, 1.40)	0.28 (0.07, 1.17)	0.33 (0.06, 1.95)	0.24 (0.05, 1.08)	0.22 (0.01, 9.45)
Women			**0.66** (0.48, 0.91)	**0.54** (0.35, 0.86)	0.85 (0.58, 1.24)	1.04 (0.51, 2.10)
Low education	**0.10** (0.06, 0.15)	**0.12** (0.08, 0.17)			**0.12** (0.08, 0.18)	**0.10** (0.05, 0.19)
Low income	**0.29** (0.20, 0.42)	**0.26** (0.17, 0.38)	**0.28** (0.19, 0.39)	**0.27** (0.18, 0.42)		
Income missing	**0.44** (0.29, 0.67)	**0.34** (0.23, 0.51)	**0.38** (0.26, 0.55)	**0.38** (0.25, 0.60)		
Wave × (N-HB)	0.91 (0.82, 1.02)	0.98 (0.91, 1.05)	0.94 (0.88, 1.01)	0.98 (0.88, 1.09)	0.97 (0.89, 1.06)	0.87 (0.72, 1.04)
Wave × Hispanic	**1.23** (1.03, 1.46)	**1.15** (1.00, 1.31)	**1.20** (1.06, 1.35)	1.00 (.77, 1.30)	**1.24** (1.08, 1.42)	1.11 (0.71, 1.73)
Wave × Other races	0.95 (0.74, 1.22)	1.09 (0.86, 1.38)	1.07 (0.86, 1.34)	0.95 (0.72, 1.26)	1.11 (0.88, 1.41)	0.90 (0.54, 1.50)

Note: Age, income, living alone, social network size, self-rated memory, and self-rated health status were included as time-varying covariates. Odds ratios in boldface are significant at the level of 0.05. The reference group for race is non-Hispanic White

such as socioeconomic status, living arrangements, and health played a certain role in influencing the trend in the racial digital divide between these two races/ethnicities. In sum, our analysis suggests that the digital divide is narrowing over time between these two racial/ethnic groups, especially those socioeconomically disadvantaged.

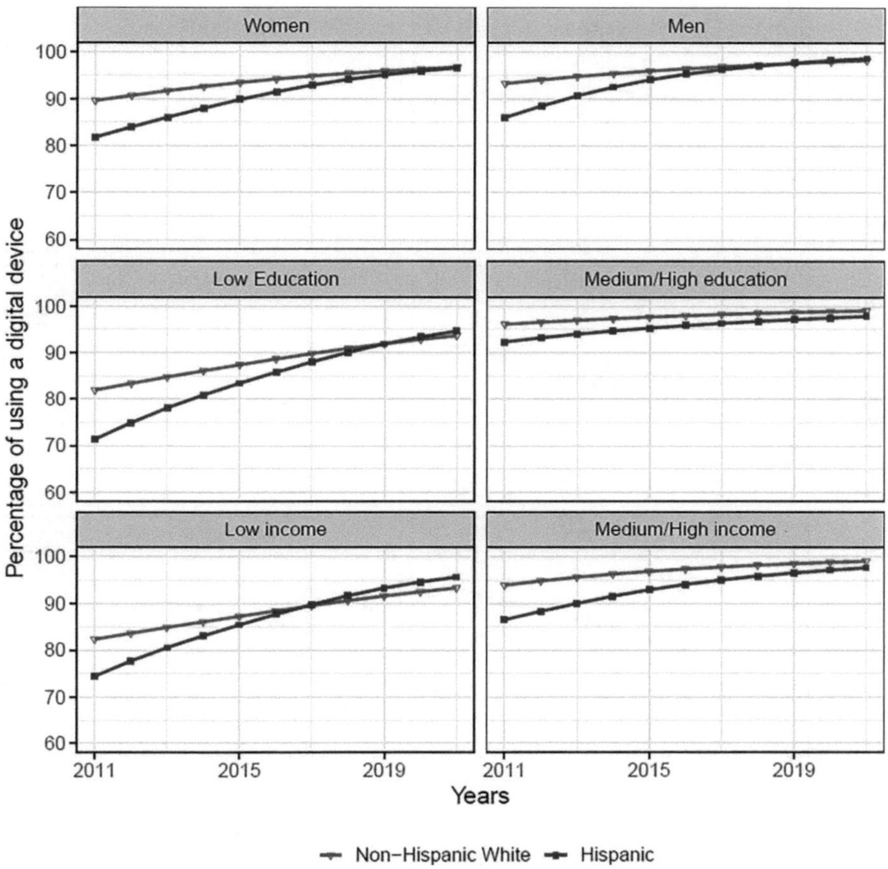

Fig. 11.3 Model-predicted percentages of digital access between Hispanic and non-Hispanic White participants from 2011 to 2021 by gender, education, and income. Note: The results were derived from Model 2 that included survey year, age, gender, education, income, living alone, social network size, self-rated memory, and self-rated health status at each wave. In estimating the predicted percentages, all covariates were set at their means

Table 11.4 further examined whether the digital usage gap narrowed over time across three specific types of internet use (personal, health, and social use) by testing interactions between survey wave and Hispanic ethnicity. Although overall internet usage significantly increased across survey waves for personal (OR = 1.37, 95% CI: 1.34–1.40), health (OR = 1.26, 95% CI = 1.23–1.28), and social use (OR = 1.24, 95% CI = 1.21–1.28), none of the wave-by-Hispanic ethnicity interactions were statistically significant. These findings suggest that, despite overall improvements in digital technology usage, the specific gaps between Hispanic and non-Hispanic White older adults in these three domains remained stable over

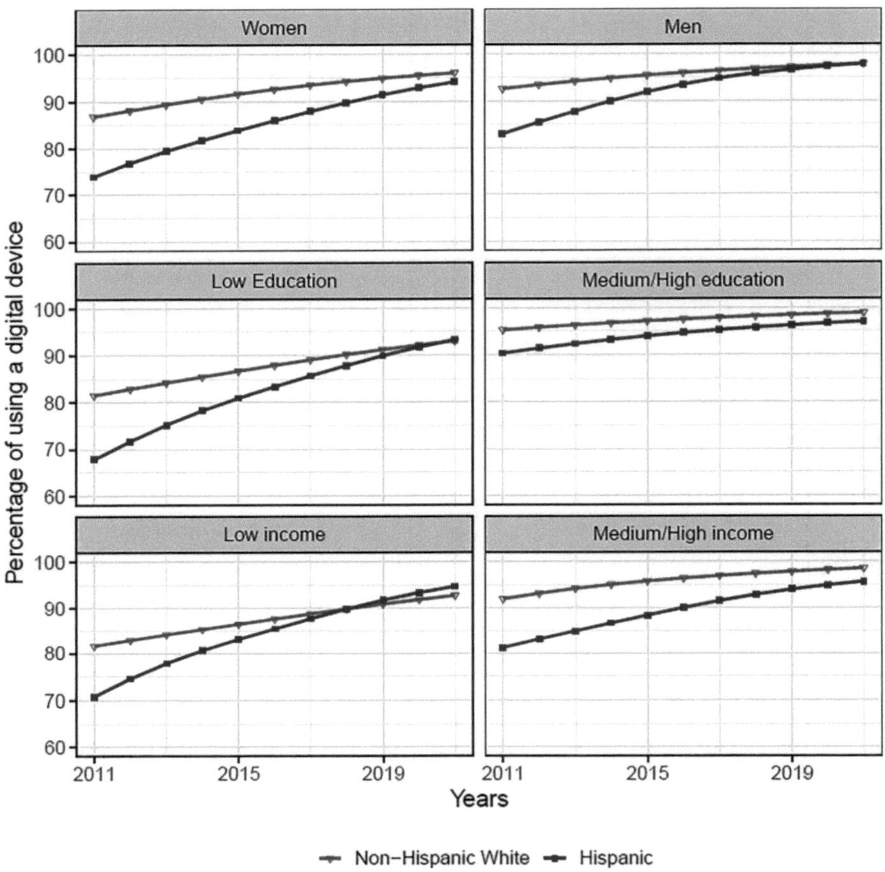

Fig. 11.4 Model-predicted percentages of digital access between Hispanic and non-Hispanic White participants from 2011 to 2021 by gender, education, and income. Note: The results were obtained from the models that included race, wave, age and gender at each wave. In estimating the predicted percentages, all covariates were set at their means

time. Additional subgroup analyses by gender, education, and income, controlling only demographic variables, revealed no significant interactions (results not reported).

11.3.4 Sensitivity Analysis

In sensitivity analysis, participants' income was measured only by the income in their initial year. With this measurement, 44% of participants had missing values, 30% reported low, and 26% reported medium-to-high income. The same result patterns were identified with this measure of income, indicating the robustness of our findings.

Table 11.4 Odds ratios and 95% confidence intervals from multilevel logistic regression predicting digital access by personal, health, and social use

	Personal use		Health use		Social use	
Survey wave	**1.37**	(1.34, 1.40)	**1.26**	(1.23, 1.28)	**1.24**	(1.21, 1.28)
Race/Ethnicity						
Non-Hispanic Black (N-HB)	**0.05**	(0.03, 0.08)	**0.09**	(0.07, 0.14)	**0.05**	(0.03, 0.09)
Hispanic	**0.03**	(0.01, 0.07)	**0.06**	(0.03, 0.14)	**0.06**	(0.02, 0.17)
Other races	0.49	(0.18, 1.30)	**0.36**	(0.15, 0.86)	0.33	(0.09, 1.18)
Wave × N-HB	0.97	(0.92, 1.02)	1.01	(0.97, 1.05)	1.03	(0.97, 1.10)
Wave × Hispanic	0.92	(0.82, 1.04)	0.97	(0.87, 1.08)	0.98	(0.87, 1.12)
Wave × Other races	**0.87**	(0.78, 0.98)	1.00	(0.90, 1.11)	0.95	(0.82, 1.11)
Age						
75–79	**0.35**	(0.30, 0.40)	**0.60**	(0.53, 0.68)	**0.44**	(0.38, 0.51)
80–84	**0.13**	(0.10, 0.15)	**0.32**	(0.27, 0.38)	**0.18**	(0.15, 0.22)
85–89	**0.05**	(0.04, 0.06)	**0.14**	(0.11, 0.18)	**0.07**	(0.05, 0.09)
90+	**0.01**	(0.01, 0.02)	**0.05**	(0.04, 0.08)	**0.02**	(0.01, 0.03)
Women	**0.42**	(0.33, 0.53)	**0.58**	(0.48, 0.70)	**1.76**	(1.39, 2.23)

Odds ratio and 95% confidence interval of multilevel logistic regressions on digital access
Note. Odds ratios in boldface are significant at the level of 0.05. The reference group for race is non-Hispanic White

11.4 Discussion

This study investigated the digital access divide between Hispanic and non-Hispanic White older adults in the U.S. from 2011 to 2021 from the intersectionality perspective. Despite the persistent gap, the divide in digital device access between Hispanic and Hispanic and non-Hispanic White older adults has been significantly narrowed over the decade. In particular, the divide was reduced significantly with time among both older Hispanic men and women, those with low education and with low income, when compared to their non-Hispanic White counterparts. Our finding presented a positive trend despite the enduring presence of digital access gaps. This progression is noteworthy, as It reflects the gradual bridging of the digital divide that has historically marginalized race/ethnicity groups across the pandemic period (Perrin & Atske, 2021). Our finding is generally consistent with a previous study that reported a narrowing gap in using the internet between Latinos and non-Hispanic White adults from 2009 to 2015 (Brown et al., 2016). Such narrowing of the digital divide is not just a matter of equitable access to technology but has far-reaching implications for the well-being, social inclusion, and digital empowerment of Hispanic older adults. Access to digital devices and the internet opens up a potential approach for enhanced communication, access to information, healthcare services, and lifelong learning and engagement opportunities.

We applied the intersectionality theory to better examine how race/ethnicity interacted with gender, education, and income to affect digital device access. The observed narrowing of the digital divide in the past decade between Hispanic and non-Hispanic White older adults, both men and women and those with lower education and income levels, suggests there have been improvements in digital inclusivity for these subgroups.

The improvement observed among the Hispanic older population may be attributed to the prevalent family-centered culture among Hispanic older adults, given their greater need for contact with their families. Additionally, a contributing factor could be that many Hispanic older adults are immigrants who need to stay connected with family in their home countries. About 65.5% of older Hispanics in this sample were non-US-born. Another plausible explanation is the significant improvement in nationwide digital access since 2010 for almost all Caribbean and Latin American countries (World Bank, 2023), including older adults (Pew Research Center, 2019), the primary origin of most American Hispanics (United Nations, 2020). This surge in digital access in their home countries has, in turn, bolstered the digital connectivity of many Hispanic immigrants in the United States regardless of their socioeconomic status, facilitating contact with family members in their countries of origin.

Our findings resonate with the core principle of intersectionality, which proposes that oppression and privileged experiences can coexist within an individual's interactions with digital inequities (Cho et al., 2013; Crenshaw, 2011; Zheng & Walsham, 2021). Moreover, this progress reflects broader efforts to address inequalities and enhance digital accessibility in the U.S. At the federal level, according to the U.S. Government Accountability Office (GAO) (2022), more than 100 federal programs administered by 15 agencies were provided to expand broadband access in recent years. However, these programs are fragmented and overlapping. As suggested by GAO, endorsing a unified national broadband strategy is needed to guide federal efforts to reduce the digital divide more efficiently. Also, institutional and community initiatives have been instrumental, including those from community senior centers, local libraries, and outreach programs by technology companies. These efforts have provided digital devices and training specifically tailored to improve the digital literacy of older adults. Many resources have also been offered in Spanish, eliminating the language barriers among older Hispanic groups.

It is essential to note that despite the progress, disparities still exist among Hispanic older adults. A cross-sectional study examining the combined impact of intersectional identities on technology access and usage suggested that Hispanic older adults of both genders are still less likely to have a working cellphone or computer device than White male older adults (Suntai & Beltran, 2023). Another study focusing on low-income, homebound older adults in the U.S. suggested that internet nonusers were associated with older age, being Black or Hispanic, and having lower incomes (Choi & DiNitto, 2013). During the COVID-19 pandemic, Hispanic communities faced challenges regarding internet affordability, accessibility, and digital literacy skills (National League of Cities, 2021). The existing evidence emphasizes the need for continued efforts at the policy and community level to bridge the digital divide among older Hispanic adults.

Our findings emphasize that while digital access disparities have narrowed in general, significant and persistent gaps remain in internet usage across personal, health, and social domains between Hispanic and non-Hispanic White older adults over the past decade. This persistence underscores the complexity of digital inequality—having digital access alone does not guarantee equitable digital participation across specific purposes. Prior research has similarly found that even when digital tools become accessible, Hispanic older adults may still experience barriers such as insufficient digital literacy, concerns about privacy, or limited culturally relevant content (National League of Cities, 2021; Rodriguez-Elliott & Vachuska, 2023). Thus, policy interventions must extend beyond basic access and address these deeper, culturally-specific barriers, ensuring Hispanic older adults can fully benefit from digital technologies across all life domains.

However, several key factors complicate the efforts to bridge the digital divide within the Hispanic community. On the one hand, a pervasive mistrust in governmental entities, intensified by the recurrent experiences of discrimination, has inhibited the communities' engagement with initiatives or programs designed to foster digital equity for older adults (Bazargan et al., 2021; National League of Cities, 2021). Additionally, concerns about privacy within this community have made it challenging for authorities to connect them with beneficial services, as many programs require sharing personal information with adults (National League of Cities, 2021). On the other hand, a considerable segment of the Hispanic population in the U.S., predominantly older, female, less-educated, and foreign-born individuals, navigate their daily lives in languages other than English (Morales et al., 2002). Yet many governmental programs predominantly operate in English for their public program enrollment or digital information service, restricting access to digital resources (National League of Cities, 2021). In addition to language barriers, Hispanics in the U.S. may face challenges due to poor generational wealth and limited access to capital, complicating their ability to afford costly internet subscriptions and the necessary devices for online access (National League of Cities, 2021). All these barriers underscore the importance of recognizing the unique challenges of the Hispanic older adult population. Customized strategies that consider these individuals' cultural experiences and circumstances are crucial for effectively addressing the digital divide and promoting equitable access to digital technologies.

Based on our findings and discussions, we present the following policy recommendations. First, it is essential to establish an agenda that identifies the digital divide as a core policy problem, considering the impact of various social structures (e.g., race, class, gender) on the Hispanic community and other minority communities while acknowledging different identity constructions and symbolic representations. Integral to this is the need to ensure transparency in how personal data is used in government programs and establish clear privacy policies to build trust. Second, we suggest formulating policies that offer diverse alternatives and recommendations specifically tailored to the unique social realities of groups with varying levels of education, income, and immigration backgrounds within the Hispanic community. It is also vital to ensure that government programs are accessible in multiple languages and staffed with bilingual representatives to maintain cultural relevance. Third, implementing and monitoring these policies should be inclusive and responsive, actively involving Hispanic older adults in decision-making processes to address structural power imbalances. This also involves continuous engagement with the Hispanic community to understand their evolving needs and to receive feedback on existing programs. Finally, the effectiveness of these policies should be assessed by comparing them to the baseline conditions of Hispanic older adults, focusing on whether the digital divide has narrowed in terms of education, income, and gender.

11.4.1 Limitations

This study has several limitations. First, the reliance on self-reported data might introduce bias, particularly among older adults with memory or comprehension challenges. Second, while the research primarily emphasizes material access to digital devices, it does not explore the disparities in digital skills and usage across time. Additionally, the study does not provide an in-depth analysis of the reasons behind the narrowing of the digital divide or the specific interventions that might have contributed to this development. Further study should investigate the comprehensive digital skills and usage disparities among Hispanic older adults. In addition, the small sample size of Hispanics, especially those in low-income or low-education groups, may introduce some biases in estimation. Lastly, although our analysis expands across the past decade, encompassing data from the COVID-19 era, a more exhaustive exploration of the post-pandemic is essential to provide a holistic understanding of digital utilization among this population.

11.4.2 Conclusions

Despite its limitations, this study provides the most current analysis of the digital access gap between Hispanic and non-Hispanic White older adults in the U.S. from 2011 to 2021. We observed notable progress in digital inclusivity for those with lower education and income levels. This trend underscores the effectiveness of efforts to enhance digital accessibility, aligning with intersectionality principles that recognize complex interplays of oppression and privilege. Persistent disparities, however, highlight the need for continued, targeted efforts. Policies must focus on the nuanced needs of the Hispanic older adult community, addressing structural challenges such as mistrust in government, privacy concerns, and language barriers. Active engagement of Hispanic older adults in decision-making processes is crucial for developing responsive and inclusive strategies. Moving forward, it is essential to focus on bridging the digital divide, not only in terms of access but also in the effective use of digital technologies. Ensuring an inclusive and empowering digital environment is vital for the well-being and social inclusion of the aging Hispanic population.

Disclaimer The views expressed in this chapter are solely those of the authors and do not necessarily reflect the views of the University of Alabama at Birmingham, the University of Illinois Urbana-Champaign, the University at Albany, or the United Nations.

References

Administration for Community Living. (2021). *2020 profile of older Americans*. https://acl.gov/sites/default/files/aging%20and%20Disability%20In%20America/2020Profileolderamericans.final_.pdf

Bazargan, M., Cobb, S., & Assari, S. (2021). Discrimination and medical mistrust in a racially and ethnically diverse sample of California adults. *Annals of Family Medicine, 19*(1), 4–15. https://doi.org/10.1370/afm.2632

Brown, A., López, G., & López, M. H. (2016). *Digital divide narrows for Latinos as more Spanish speakers and immigrants go online*. https://www.pewresearch.org/hispanic/2016/07/20/digital-divide-narrows-for-latinos-as-more-spanish-speakers-and-immigrants-go-online/

Chavarria, E. A., Christy, S. M., Feng, H., Miao, H., Abdulla, R., Gutierrez, L., Lopez, D., Sanchez, J., Gwede, C. K., & Meade, C. D. (2022). Online health information seeking and eHealth literacy among Spanish language–Dominant Latino adults receiving care in a community clinic: Secondary analysis of pilot randomized controlled trial data. *JMIR Formative Research, 6*(10), e37687. https://doi.org/10.2196/37687

Cho, S., Crenshaw, K. W., & McCall, L. (2013). Toward a field of intersectionality studies: Theory, applications, and praxis. *Signs: Journal of Women in Culture and Society, 38*(4), 785–810.

Choi, N. G., & DiNitto, D. M. (2013). The digital divide among low-income homebound older adults: Internet use patterns, eHealth literacy, and attitudes toward computer/internet use. *Journal of Medical Internet Research, 15*(5), e2645. https://doi.org/10.2196/jmir.2645

Crenshaw, K. W. (1988). Toward a race-conscious pedagogy in legal education. *National Black Law Journal, 11*, 1.

Crenshaw, K. W. (2011). From private violence to mass incarceration: Thinking intersectionally about women, race, and social control. *UCLA Law Review, 59*, 1418.

Delgado, R., & Stefancic, J. (2023). *Critical race theory: An introduction* (Vol. 87). NyU Press.

Early, J., & Hernandez, A. (2021). Digital disenfranchisement and COVID-19: Broadband internet access as a social determinant of health. *Health Promotion Practice, 22*(5), 605–610. https://doi.org/10.1177/15248399211014490

Erickson, J., & Johnson, G. M. (2011). Internet use and psychological wellness during late adulthood. *Canadian Journal on Aging/La Revue Canadienne Du Vieillissement, 30*(2), 197–209.

Faverio, M. (2022, January 13). *Share of those 65 and older who are tech users has grown in the past decade*. Pew Research Center. https://www.pewresearch.org/short-reads/2022/01/13/share-of-those-65-and-older-who-are-tech-users-has-grown-in-the-past-decade/

Ford, C. L., & Airhihenbuwa, C. O. (2010). Critical race theory, race equity, and public health: Toward antiracism praxis. *American Journal of Public Health, 100*(S1), S30–S35.

Hargittai, E., & Dobransky, K. (2017). Old dogs, new clicks: Digital inequality in skills and uses among older adults. *Canadian Journal of Communication, 42*(2), 195–212.

Hong, Y. A., & Cho, J. (2017). Has the digital health divide widened? Trends of health-related internet use among older adults from 2003 to 2011. *The Journals of Gerontology: Series B, 72*(5), 856–863. https://doi.org/10.1093/geronb/gbw100

Ihm, J., & Hsieh, Y. P. (2015). The implications of information and communication technology use for the social Well-being of older adults. *Information, Communication & Society, 18*(10), 1123–1138.

Kasper, J. D., Freedman, V. A., & Spillman, B. C. (2013). Classification of persons by dementia status in the National Health and Aging Trends Study. *Technical Paper, 5*, 1–4.

Lopez, M. H., Gonzalez-Barrera, A., & Patten, E. (2013). *Closing the digital divide*. Latinos and Technology Adoption.
Marin, A., & Hampton, K. N. (2007). Simplifying the personal network name generator: Alternatives to traditional multiple and single name generators. *Field Methods, 19*(2), 163–193. https://doi.org/10.1177/1525822X06298588
Mitchell, U. A., Chebli, P. G., Ruggiero, L., & Muramatsu, N. (2019). The digital divide in health-related technology use: The significance of race/ethnicity. *The Gerontologist, 59*(1), 6–14. https://doi.org/10.1093/geront/gny138
Mitchell, O. S., Clark, R. L., & Lusardi, A. (2022). Income trajectories in later life: Longitudinal evidence from the Health and Retirement Study. *The Journal of the Economics of Ageing, 22*, 100371. https://doi.org/10.1016/j.jeoa.2022.100371
Morales, L. S., Lara, M., Kington, R. S., Valdez, R. O., & Escarce, J. J. (2002). Socioeconomic, cultural, and behavioral factors affecting Hispanic health outcomes. *Journal of Health Care for the Poor and Underserved, 13*(4), 477–503.
National League of Cities. (2021). *State of the digital divide in the Hispanic community*. https://www.nlc.org/wp-content/uploads/2021/11/HELO-POLICY-BRIEF-1.pdf
Perrin, A., & Atske, S. (2021). *7% of Americans don't use the internet. Who are they?* https://www.pewresearch.org/short-reads/2021/04/02/7-of-americans-dont-use-the-internet-who-are-they/
Perrin, A., & Duggan, M. (2015, June 26). *Americans' internet access: 2000–2015*. Pew Research Center: internet, Science & Tech. https://www.pewresearch.org/internet/2015/06/26/americans-internet-access-2000-2015/
Pew Research Center. (2019). *Smartphone ownership is growing rapidly around the world, but not always equally*. Accessed January 18, 2024, from https://www.pewresearch.org/global/2019/02/05/smartphone-ownership-is-growing-rapidly-around-the-world-but-not-always-equally/
Rodriguez-Elliott, S., & Vachuska, K. (2023). Measuring the digital divide: A neighborhood-level analysis of racial inequality in internet speed during the COVID-19 pandemic. *Societies, 13*(4), 92.
Suntai, Z., & Beltran, S. J. (2023). The intersectional impact of race/ethnicity and sex on access to technology among older adults. *The Gerontologist, 63*(7), 1162–1171. https://doi.org/10.1093/geront/gnac178
Szabo, A., Allen, J., Stephens, C., & Alpass, F. (2019). Longitudinal analysis of the relationship between purposes of internet use and well-being among older adults. *The Gerontologist, 59*(1), 58–68.
Tappen, R. M., Cooley, M. E., Luckmann, R., & Panday, S. (2022). Digital health information disparities in older adults: A mixed methods study. *Journal of Racial and Ethnic Health Disparities, 9*(1), 82–92. https://doi.org/10.1007/s40615-020-00931-3
U. S. Government Accountability Office. (2022, August 11). *Broadband: National strategy needed to guide federal efforts to reduce digital divide* | U.S. GAO. https://www.gao.gov/products/gao-22-104611
U.S. Census Bureau. (2018). *Older people projected to outnumber children for first time in U.S. history*. https://www.census.gov/newsroom/press-releases/2018/cb18-41-population-projections.html
United Nations. (2020). *International migration stock database*. Accessed January 20, 2024, from https://www.un.org/development/desa/pd/content/international-migrant-stock
Van Deursen, A. J., & Van Dijk, J. A. (2019). The first-level digital divide shifts from inequalities in physical access to inequalities in material access. *New Media & Society, 21*(2), 354–375. https://doi.org/10.1177/1461444818797082
Vogels, E. (2021). *Digital divide persists even as Americans with lower incomes make gains in tech adoption*. https://www.pewresearch.org/short-reads/2021/06/22/digital-divide-persists-even-as-americans-with-lower-incomes-make-gains-in-tech-adoption/

World Bank. (2023). *International Telecommunication Union (ITU) World Telecommunication/ICT Indicators Database*. Accessed January 18, 2024, from https://data.worldbank.org/indicator/IT.NET.USER.ZS

Zheng, Y., & Walsham, G. (2021). Inequality of what? An intersectional approach to digital inequality under Covid-19. *Information and Organization, 31*(1), 100341. https://doi.org/10.1016/j.infoandorg.2021.100341

Section III
ICT Use and Health Behaviors and Perception of Aging

Chapter 12
Does the Use of Social Media Affect Online Health Information-Seeking Behaviors Among Underserved African Americans in Rural Alabama?

Hee Yun Lee, Kun Wang, Karen Johnson, Kefentse P. Malele, Areum Han, Eunyoung Choi, and Maxwell Sleep-Frankel

12.1 Introduction

United States (U.S.) households have increasingly turned to the Internet (e.g. via Google, Yahoo, Web page searches) as a whole, and social media platforms (e.g. Facebook, Twitter) specifically, to seek information regarding their health and to access concrete health supports (Calixte et al., 2020; Nikoloudakis et al., 2018; Sinjini & Rema, 2012; Smailhodzic et al., 2016). In a study using four administrations of the Health Information National Trends Survey (HINTS) from 2008 through 2017, more than 61% of American adults reported turning to the internet for health advice in 2008; this number increased to nearly 75% in 2017 (Finney Rutten et al., 2019). In a separate survey in 2012, close to 50% of U.S. individuals indicated that

Note: This chapter is adapted from a previously published article:
Lee, H. Y., Wang, K., Johnson, K., Kubanga, K., Han, A., & Choi, E. (2022). Does the Use of Social Media Affect Online Health Information-Seeking Behaviors among Underserved African Americans in Rural Alabama?. *Journal of health care for the poor and underserved, 33*(4), 1949–1964. https://doi.org/10.1353/hpu.2022.0147

H. Y. Lee (✉)
School of Social Work, University of Georgia, Athens, GA, USA
e-mail: heeyunlee@uga.edu

K. Wang
Department of Social Work, College of Arts and Sciences, University of Alabama at Birmingham, Birmingham, AL, USA
e-mail: kw2@uab.edu

K. Johnson · M. Sleep-Frankel
School of Social Work, University of Alabama, Tuscaloosa, AL, USA
e-mail: kjohnson38@ua.edu; mdsleepfrankel@crimson.ua.edu

K. Wang et al. (eds.), *ICT Use and Healthy Longevity*, Advances in Studies of Aging and Health 5, https://doi.org/10.1007/978-3-031-98964-3_12

they were more likely to search the web than to seek out support from treatment providers when making health care decisions ($n = 1060$) (PricewaterhouseCoopers Health Research Institute, 2012). Respondents also indicated that health information sought out through social media platforms directly influenced their decisions to seek a second opinion from a medical doctor, helped them cope with chronic health conditions, and realize health-related goals (PricewaterhouseCoopers Health Research Institute, 2012).

The existing literature underscores the internet's and social media's viability as online vehicles through which patients and their relatives can access useful health-related information, ask for advice, and share experiences (Smailhodzic et al., 2016; Zhao & Zhang, 2017). Among those who turn to social media for information about primary prevention of diseases, their symptoms, and medication are individuals with chronic and/or life-threatening health conditions such as diabetes, cancer, and mental health (Nikoloudakis et al., 2018; Shaw & Johnson, 2011; Zhao & Zhang, 2017). Also among these individuals are people younger than 40 (Bhaskaran, Kumar, & Manthan, 2017; Nikoloudakis et al., 2018; Powell et al., 2011), women (Bhaskaran et al., 2017; Nikoloudakis et al., 2018; Powell et al., 2011; Rowley et al., 2016; Thackeray et al., 2013), and those with high educational attainment (Kontos et al., 2014). Younger individuals are also more likely to use social media because they adopt new technologies more quickly than older people and desire connections to start or maintain relationships (Andreassen et al., 2017). Generally, women tend to be more expressive than men (Fischer & LaFrance, 2015). As a result, they tend to use these platforms more frequently to connect with others, express their emotions, and seek information related to their health conditions (Ihm & Hsieh, 2015; Parkins, 2012; van Deursen & Helsper, 2015). Furthermore, a study in England indicated that women were also more likely to look for online health information on behalf of a loved one, or for themselves and their loved ones, in comparison with men (Powell et al., 2011). People with higher educational status are more likely to understand the information they read online about their medical conditions and are thus better equipped to seek additional information (Bouclaous et al., 2023; Jeong & Kim, 2016; Lee et al., 2015). Literature also demonstrates that social media is increasingly utilized for health promotion activities (Alsuyayfi et al., 2025; Jeong & Kim, 2016; Sinjini & Rema, 2012), for finding and sharing

K. P. Malele
Department of Social Work, University of Botswana, Gaborone, Botswana
e-mail: malelek@ub.ac.bw

A. Han
College of Nursing, University of South Florida, Tampa, FL, USA
e-mail: areumhan@usf.edu

E. Choi
Leonard Davis School of Gerontology, University of Southern California, Los Angeles, CA, USA
e-mail: choieuny@usc.edu

health-related information regarding newborn infants (Dzubaty, 2016; Ruggiero et al., 2011), and for staying abreast of the latest safety precautions during the COVID-19 pandemic (Ebrahim et al., 2020; Fenta et al., 2024).

However, significant gaps remain regarding the use of the internet and social media for online health information-seeking purposes in rural America (Fischer & LaFrance, 2015; Ebrahim et al., 2020; Greenberg et al., 2018). There are no peer-reviewed manuscripts regarding African Americans' use in these regions. The absence of scholarly evidence regarding the internet's potential utility in rural areas as a whole and among African Americans residing in rural regions, in particular, represents a significant gap given well-established associations between technological and other structural inequities and poorer health outcomes (Benda et al., 2020; Glied & Lleras-Muney, 2008; Lopez et al., 2018). Although there are no scholarly manuscripts regarding this issue among African Americans to date, the literature points to the importance of better understanding (1) structural inequities that are technological in nature; and (2) the ways in which broadband may be better used by treatment professions themselves and/or by rural citizens engaged in self-initiated efforts to navigate these challenges (Benda et al., 2020; Glied & Lleras-Muney, 2008; Lopez et al., 2018). This need is particularly acute among African Americans due to racialized structural disparities limiting access to health care in the Southeast (Bailey et al., 2017; Gee & Ford, 2011; Kuzawa & Sweet, 2009; Volpe et al., 2021).

Available evidence does, however, confirm that the percentage of U.S. adults in rural America who endorse using different forms of social media is significantly lower than the percentages in urban and suburban areas (Smith & Anderson, 2018). A study in 2017 found that only 18% of those who reported using social media for health-seeking purposes ($n = 156$) resided in rural regions of the county (Bhaskaran et al., 2017). This discrepancy has been attributed to poorly developed infrastructure in the U.S. and lagging internet connectivity in areas of the country with the highest percentages of rurality (Gilbert et al., 2010).

Deep South states such as Alabama, with rural regions in 100% of its 67 counties, follow this pattern (Alabama Rural Health Association [ARHA], 2021). While research regarding the intersection between social media and health information-seeking behaviors in Alabama is scant, a smattering of peer- reviewed studies underscores the deficits in Alabama's technological and infrastructure (Jain et al., 2019; Lee et al., 2023). Key observations include Alabama's inadequate broadband (Jain et al., 2019), internet capabilities (Vaughn et al., 2015), and the lack of access to smartphones among Alabama's poorest citizens (Park et al., 2020), particularly those living in rural portions of the state. Exacerbating these challenges are numerous intersecting structural barriers that place those living in rural regions at increased risk for poor health and lagging health indicators (Ormond et al., 2000; United Health Foundation, 2022). Barriers include widespread hospital and clinic closures (Kempf et al., 2010; Miller et al., 2021) and long distances that must be traversed to access medical services (Kempf et al., 2010; Miller et al., 2020; Moneyham et al., 2010; Troske & Davis, 2019). For impoverished men and women in Alabama's Black Belt counties specifically, and predominantly for African Americans, these structural barriers are even more concentrated and acutely felt, leading to even higher physical and mental health morbidity and mortality rates (Barry-Jester, 2017; Kempf et al., 2010; Maron, 2017).

These regions are also marked by a scarcity of public transportation, and poverty rates double or triple the national average (Chi et al., 2019; Cogbill et al., 2014). Due largely to these intersecting socio- structural determinants of health, Alabama consistently ranked among the top ten least healthy states in the nation for the past two decades and 46th specifically in 2022 (Barry-Jester, 2017; Maron, 2017; United Health Foundation, 2022). Combined, these micro and macro-level challenges underscore the need for efficient and effective access to medical and mental health-related support, facilitated by technology. To date, however, this represents a significant unmet and understudied need in Alabama.

In addition to the urban-rural disparities already mentioned, the internet and social media's use for health purposes varies by race. African Americans have had low eHealth literacy and limited internet access, again in part attributed to racialized barriers that are systemic in nature and are believed to depress online health information-seeking behaviors (Chi et al., 2019; Cogbill et al., 2014; Mitchell et al., 2014). For example, 59% of Black neighborhoods had broadband access from 2017–2021, which is much lower than the 75% reported for White and Asian American majority neighborhoods (Li et al., 2023). Moreover, in a 2020 study using data collected in 2013 from a national sample in the U.S., only 35% of African Americans sought online health information (Hills & Shah, 2020). Similarly, in a 2019 study using data collected between 2015 and 2016 (n = 42,087; weighted sample of 29,236,426), African Americans were significantly less likely to use the internet for health-seeking purposes (OR: 0.2, 95% CI 0.2–0.4 for African Americans) than non- Hispanic Whites (Din et al., 2019). There is a strong need to promote internet use and web-based searching for health in this population and increase access to digital media. Few studies, however, have investigated the levels and predictors of online health information-seeking behaviors among African Americans (Mitchell et al., 2014; Sherman et al., 2021).

As the first-ever study to use data collected with African Americans residing in rural Alabama to examine how the use of social media affects online health-seeking behaviors, this study fills a significant gap. We sought to answer four questions: (1) What are the levels of technology device access among African Americans in rural Alabama? (2) What are the levels of social media use among African Americans in rural Alabama? (3) What is the profile of rural African American online health information-seeking behaviors? and (4) What is the relationship between technology device access and social media use, and online health information-seeking behaviors? These findings serve to advance understanding of ways to make use of social media and other web-based technology to facilitate access to life-saving medical information and care among African Americans living in rural regions of America.

12.2 Methods

12.2.1 Research Design and Study Sample

A cross-sectional research design was applied to examine factors related to online health information-seeking behaviors. A convenience sampling strategy was used to recruit research participants through African American community organizations in rural counties in Alabama. African American community organizations were identified and contacted via phone and emails. Two organizations agreed to participate in this study. Our research team held information sessions for these two organizations. Data collection was conducted in two sites: a local health care agency and a recreational community center. A series of data collection events was held from July 2019 to February 2020. A sample of 185 African Americans aged 18 years and older was recruited. Data were collected through self-administered questionnaires. Participants provided written informed consent before starting the questionnaire. The questionnaires took about 30–60 minutes; participants were compensated with a $15 gift card for their participation. This study has been approved by the authors' university's institutional review board.

12.2.2 Measures

12.2.2.1 Online Health Information-Seeking Behavior

Online health information-seeking behavior was measured by an 11-item scale drawn from the Health Information National Trends Survey (HINTS), specifically, HINTS 4 Cycle 1 (Cantor et al., 2009). Participants were asked to indicate whether they "looked for information about quitting smoking," "bought medicine or vitamins," "participated in an online support group for people with a similar health or medical issue," "used email or the internet to communicate with a doctor or doctor's office," "used a website to help you with your diet, weight, or physical activity," "looked for a healthcare provider," "downloaded health-related information to a mobile device," "visited a social networking site to read and share about medical topics," "wrote in an online diary or blog about any type of health topic," "kept track of personal health information," and "looked for health or medical information for someone else" in the last 12 months. The online health information-seeking behaviors score was the sum of the 11 binary questions, ranging from 0 to 11, with a higher score indicating more online health information-seeking behaviors. The internal reliability in the current sample was high (Kuder-Richardson 20 = .82).

12.2.2.2 Health Status

This study's health status variables included the number of chronic diseases, whether the person was bothered by pain, and self-rated health and mental health status. The number of chronic diseases was measured continuously, ranging from 0 to 6. Bothered by pain was an ordinal variable, with 1 indicating not bothered at all, 2 indicating somewhat bothered, and 3 indicating strongly bothered by pain. Self-rated health and mental health status were both measured by five-point Likert scales (1 = poor, 5 = excellent).

12.2.2.3 Health Service Access

Health service access variables included health insurance, primary physician, and annual checkup. All these three variables were measured dichotomously (0 = No, 1 = Yes).

12.2.2.4 Technology Device Access and Social Media Use

Technology device access variables included home internet access, smartphone, and tablet/computer. Participants were asked to indicate if they had internet access in their home, a smartphone, and a tablet/ computer (0 = No, 1 = Yes). Participants were also asked to indicate whether they were currently actively using the major social networking sites (Facebook, Twitter, and Instagram). The three apps chosen were selected due to their popularity. As of September 2019, the top four social networking apps among mobile users in the U.S. were Facebook (90.90%), Instagram (64.92%), Facebook Messenger (56.97%), and Twitter (43.62%) (Statista, 2022). Social networking site use was coded as 1 if they use at least one social networking site; otherwise, social networking sites use was coded as 0.

12.2.2.5 Control Variables

Age, gender, marital status, education, and employment were control variables in this study. Age was a continuous variable. Gender (0 = female, 1 = male), marital status (0 = others, 1 = married or partnered), education (0 = less than bachelors' degree, 1 = bachelor's degree or higher), and employment status (0 = not employed, 1 = employed) were all categorical variables.

12.2.3 *Analysis Strategy*

Univariate analysis was conducted to better understand the characteristics of participants and their online health information-seeking behaviors. Multilinear regression was performed to identify factors that were associated with online health information-seeking behaviors. The variance inflation (VIF) factor was 2.09, indicating that the degree of multicollinearity was low. All the analyses were completed in Stata 14 (StataCorp, 2015).

12.3 Results

12.3.1 *Sample Characteristics*

Table 12.1 presents the characteristics of the participants. The mean age was 55.86 (SD = 15.85). About 20% of participants were male, 34% were married or partnered, 17% had a bachelor's degree or higher, and 22% were employed. Concerning health status, the average number of chronic diseases was 1.83 (SD = 1.14), and the medians of self-rated health status and mental health status were both 4 (health: IQR 3–4; mental health: IQR 4–5). Nearly one-quarter of participants were not bothered by pain, nearly half were somewhat bothered by pain, and another one-quarter were strongly bothered by pain. Approximately 88% of participants had health insurance and primary care physicians, and 86% had annual checkups. About 60% of participants had home internet; 58% had a smartphone, and 55% had a tablet or computer. Nearly 55% of participants were currently actively using social networking sites: 53% used Facebook, 8% used Twitter, and 18% used Instagram.

12.3.2 *Online Health Information-Seeking Behaviors*

Descriptive analyses of participants' online health information-seeking behaviors are summarized in Table 12.2. The most frequent behavior among this sample was keeping track of personal health information such as care received, test results, or upcoming medical appointments, which was endorsed by 36.8%. Approximately one-third of participants looked for health or medical information for someone else (34.1%) and visited a social networking site to read and share about medical topics (31.4%). More than one-fourth of participants used a website to help you with your diet, weight, or physical activity (27.6%) and downloaded health-related information to a mobile device, such as an MP3 player, cell phone, tablet computer or electronic book device (ex. Download mobile apps)" (27.6%). Less than 20% of

Table 12.1 Sample characteristics ($N = 185$)

Variables	Means (SD)	N(%)
Demographic characteristics		
Age	55.86 (15.85)	
Gender (1 = male)		37 (20.0%)
Marital status (1 = married or partnered)		63 (34.1%)
Bachelor's degree (1 = yes)		32 (17.3%)
Employment (1 = yes)		41 (22.2%)
Health status		
Number of chronic diseases (0–6)	1.83 (1.14)	
Bothered by pain		
Not bothered at all (1 = yes)		45 (24.9%)
Somewhat bothered (1 = yes)		90 (48.1%)
Strongly bothered (1 = yes)		44 (23.8%)
Self-rated health status (1–5)	4 (3–4)[a]	
Self-rated mental health status (1–5)	4 (4–5)[a]	
Health service access		
Health insurance (1 = yes)		162 (87.6%)
Primary physician (1 = yes)		162 (87.6%)
Annual checkup (1 = yes)		159 (85.9%)
Technology device access		
Home Internet access (1 = yes)		111 (60.0%)
Having a smartphone (1 = yes)		108 (58.4%)
Having tablets or computers (1 = yes)		102 (55.1%)
Using social networking site (1 = yes)		101 (54.6%)
Facebook		99 (53.3%)
Twitter		15 (8.1%)
Instagram		33 (17.8%)

[a]Represents median and interquartile range

Table 12.2 Descriptive analysis on online health information- seeking behaviors ($N = 185$)

Variables	*n*	%
Looked for information about quitting smoking	14	7.6
Bought medicine or vitamins online	26	14.1
Participated in an online support group for people with a similar health or medical issue	11	5.9
Used e-mail or the Internet to communicate with a doctor or doctor's office	36	19.5
Used a website to help you with your diet, weight, or physical activity	51	27.6
Looked for a health care provider	32	17.3
Downloaded health-related information to a mobile device, such as an MP3 player, cell phone, table computer or electronic book device (ex. Download mobile apps)	51	27.6
Visited a "social networking" site, such as "Facebook" or "LinkedIn" to read and share about medical topics	58	31.4
Wrote in an online diary or "blog" (i.e. Web log) about any type of health topic	14	7.6
Kept track of personal health information such as care received, test results or upcoming medical appointments	68	36.8
Looked for health or medical information for someone else	63	34.1

participants used e-mail or the internet to communicate with a doctor or doctor's office (19.5%), looked for a health care provider (17.3%), bought medicine or vitamins online (14.1%). Less than 10% of participants looked for information about quitting smoking (7.6%), wrote in an online diary or "blog" (i.e., web log) about any health topic" (7.6%), and participated in an online support group for people with a similar health or medical issue (5.4%).

12.3.3 Multilinear Regression of Online Health Information-Seeking Behaviors

Multilinear regression results are presented in Table 12.3. Using social networking sites was positively associated with the number of online health information-seeking behaviors ($B = 1.37, p < .01$). Participants who were currently active users of social networking sites tended to have 1.37 online health information-seeking behaviors more than their counterparts who were not active users. Compared with participants without smartphones, those who had smartphones had more online health information-seeking behaviors ($B = .96, p < .05$). No other technology device access variables were significant. Two health service access variables, having health insurance ($B = 1.66, p < .01$) and having a primary care physician ($B = 1.52, p < .05$), were also associated with more online health information-seeking behaviors. Compared with those who were not bothered by pain at all, participants strongly bothered by pain had more online health information- seeking behaviors ($B = 1.41, p < .01$). Age was negatively associated with the number of online health information-seeking behaviors ($B = -.04$, $p < .05$). No other demographic variables were significant in this model.

Table 12.3 Multiple linear regression of online health information-seeking behaviors ($N = 185$)

Variables	*B*	S.E.	t
Demographic characteristics			
Age	−.04	.01	**−2.74***
Gender (1 = male)	.30	.49	.61
Marital status (1 = married or partnered)	.15	.37	.41
Bachelor's degree (1 = yes)	.54	.46	1.18
Employment (1 = yes)	−.02	.45	−.03
Health status			
Number of chronic diseases (0–6)	−.09	.17	−.53
Somewhat bothered by pain (1 = yes)	.53	.45	1.17
Strongly bothered by pain (1 = yes)	1.41	.53	**2.65****
Self-rated health status (1–5)	−.11	.26	−.41
Self-rated mental health status (1–5)	.25	.21	1.18
Health service access			
Health insurance (1 = yes)	1.66	.58	**2.89****
Primary physician (1 = yes)	1.52	.63	**2.40***
Annual checkup (1 = yes)	−.96	.64	−1.50
Technology device access and social media use			
Home Internet access (1 = yes)	.52	.44	1.20
Having a smartphone (1 = yes)	.96	.44	**2.19***
Having tablets or computers (1 = yes)	.18	.47	.38
Using social networking sites (1 = yes)	1.37	.24	**3.09****

Note: B represents unstandardized regression coefficient; * $p < .05$; ** $p < .001$

12.4 Discussion

Online health information-seeking behavior leads to improved health knowledge, positive attitudes, and better communication with health providers (Alruwailli et al., 2025; Tan & Goonawardene, 2017; Walsh et al., 2010), and the importance of it may be greater for the rural and marginalized groups given their systemic health care challenges (i.e., health care provider shortages and fewer resources) (Rosenblatt et al., 2006). The present study sought a better understanding of the challenges that linked to online health information-seeking behaviors among African Americans in rural Alabama. Specifically, we examined levels of technology device access and social media use among African Americans in rural Alabama, investigated the profiles of their online health information-seeking behaviors, and identified the relationship between technology device access and social media use, and online health information-seeking behaviors. We found that just more than half of the participants had access to the internet (60%) and one or more technology devices (58% for a smartphone and 55% for a tablet/computer). As for social media use, nearly 55% of participants used social networking sites, with 53% using Facebook. Our African American sample showed low overall levels of online health information-seeking behaviors (mostly <30%), with some of the activities (i.e., participating in an online support group) being very limited (<10%). In addition, this study found positive associations of online health information-seeking behaviors with smartphone ownership, social media use, health insurance, having a primary care physician, being bothered by pain, and younger age. However, online health information-seeking behaviors were not associated with the other demographic, health, and other technology access factors.

Findings of the present study are supported by the previous literature to some extent, including the positive associations of online health information-seeking behaviors with social media use (Feng & Xie, 2015; Nikoloudakis et al., 2018), having a primary care physician (Thackeray et al., 2013), having health insurance (Arora et al., 2008), and younger age (Ghweeba et al., 2017; Lee et al., 2014; Nikoloudakis et al., 2018; Thackeray et al., 2013). We also found that those who reported being bothered by pain were more likely to engage in online health information-seeking behaviors. This finding is in line with a few prior studies suggesting that individuals with pain may go online for help with pain and self-management (Henderson et al., 2013; Nath et al., 2016). However, given that they used the internet only when all other forms of pain information were not available and were not generally satisfied with online content (Henderson et al., 2013), the value of online pain information-seeking should be carefully considered.

Mixed results exist for the associations of online health information-seeking behaviors with other indicators of health status. Like the present study, some studies including data for both genders found no associations between online health information-seeking behaviors and the number of chronic diseases and self-rated health status (Nikoloudakis et al., 2018). In Nikoloudakis et al. (2018), the associations were positive for women only. Other studies showed that online health information-seeking behaviors were related to having a chronic disease and the number of chronic diseases (Bansil et al., 2006; Feng & Xie, 2015; Popovac & Roomaney, 2022). The conflicting results from the present study warrant further studies investigating if gender and geographic community type (e.g., rural vs. urban/suburban) differently affect the association between online health information-seeking behaviors and health status.

It was notable that in our sample, online health information-seeking was associated only with smartphone ownership but not with other types of digital technology access. This finding may relate to the different patterns of the digital divide by devices. A survey in 2021 showed that the racial/ethnic digital divide persists in using a traditional computer and home broadband access, whereas people who were Black or Hispanic had similar rates of smartphone use compared with people who were non-Hispanic White (Atske & Perrin, 2021). Smartphones may play a critical role in accessing the internet for racial/ethnic minorities who would not be online otherwise (Atske & Perrin, 2021). This may explain why our respondents who had a smartphone were more likely to search health information online compared with those without a smartphone.

12.4.1 Limitation of the Study

Limitations of the present study should be considered when interpreting the findings. We used a convenience sampling strategy, limiting the generalizability of the study findings. Future research with a larger and more representative sample is needed for replication. Since this study was a cross-sectional study involving data collection at a single point in time, the causal patterns of the correlates of online health information-seeking behaviors cannot be determined. Longitudinal studies are needed to determine if social media use affected online health information-seeking behaviors or vice versa. Additionally, more future studies are needed to further investigate other factors that may also affect African Americans' online health information-seeking behaviors Because all the outcomes were self-reported, there is a possibility of recall and response bias. Finally, in the 11-item scale measuring the online health information-seeking behaviors, the option of "non-applicable" is not available. Participants without some specific needs, such as quitting smoking, might choose the answer not fitting them, which may cause conservative estimations in this study.

12.4.2 Conclusions

The present study contributes to the literature as it is the first to focus on African Americans living in rural areas. The findings from the present study may indicate that social media can be a platform that facilitates access to health information and health promotion behaviors for African American adults living in rural areas. Age- and culturally-appropriate designs and information and further support for older adults should be considered.

12.4.3 Implications for Health Practice and Policy

Our research showed that African Americans in rural Alabama report low levels of online health information-seeking, even compared with another racial/ethnic minority group in rural Alabama (Lee et al., 2022). Given that 75% of American adults used the internet as a primary source of health information (Finney Rutten et al., 2019; Lee et al., 2022), these findings provide further evidence for rural-urban and racial disparities (Hills & Shah, 2020; Prestin et al., 2015). It is also notable that participants' use of the internet for some activities (e.g., looking for health professionals) was more limited than for others (e.g., tracking personal health information). The findings underscore the importance of promoting internet use for health purposes among rural African Americans, with particular attention to specific geographic areas for change. Furthermore, we found subgroups of the sample (e.g., older and those without health insurance or primary care physician) had more challenges in obtaining online health information and, thus, were likely to be excluded from the benefits of digital health. Public health interventions such as education programs for technology use should target these groups to narrow the access gap. At the same time, it should be noted that heavy reliance on online health information carries the risk of reproducing or exacerbating health inequities (Jacobs et al., 2017). With heavy or even sole reliance on digital health, the subpopulation with limited access to digital health will be excluded from this powerful health information source and further disadvantaged. Thus, offline health information services should be provided in parallel for those who lack internet access and support.

The current study speaks to the structural inequality surrounding technology use and health care that African Americans in rural Alabama experience. Beyond individual- level factors, myriad social factors, including uneven socioeconomic opportunities, discrimination, and lack of access to a digital device, contribute to lower chances to lead healthy lives among this population. Macro-level responses are needed to properly address the key barriers to meet health care needs in this population. Those efforts would include the expansion of public health insurance coverage and improved access to community-based providers, as well as increased digital connectivity (Taylor, 2019).

Acknowledgement This study was funded by the Endowed Academic Chair Research Fund of the University of Alabama School of Social Work awarded to Dr. Hee Yun Lee.

References

Alabama Rural Health Association. (2021). What is rural? Retrieved July 12, 2025, from https://arhaonline.org/what-is-rural/

Alruwailli, A. N., Abuyabis, R. G., & Kofi, M. (2025). Online health information-seeking behavior among attendants to lifestyle clinics, PHCs, Riyadh, Saudi Arabia. *Scientia. Technology, Science and Society, 2*(1), 68–79. https://doi.org/10.59324/stss.2025.2(1).06

Alsuyayfi, S., Alsulimani, N., Aldhergham, A., Alahmary, A., & Alkhateeb, A. (2025). Social media and health promotion. *Nursing & Healthcare International Journal*. https://doi.org/10.23880/nhij-16000337

Andreassen, C. S., Pallesen, S., & Griffiths, M. D. (2017). The relationship between addictive use of social media, narcissism, and self-esteem: Findings from a large national survey. *Addictive Behaviors, 64*, 287–293. https://doi.org/10.1016/j.addbeh.2016.03.006

Arora, N. K., Hesse, B. W., Rimer, B. K., Viswanath, K., Clayman, M. L., & Croyle, R. T. (2008). Frustrated and confused: The American public rates its cancer-related information-seeking experiences. *Journal of General Internal Medicine, 23*(3), 223–228. https://doi.org/10.1007/s11606-007-0406-y

Atske, S., & Perrin, A. (2021). *Home broadband adoption, computer ownership vary by race, ethnicity in the US*. Pew Research Center. https://www.pewresearch.org/fact-tank/2021/07/16/home-broadband-adoption-computer-ownership-vary-by-race-ethnicity-in-the-u-s/

Bailey, Z. D., Krieger, N., Agénor, M., Graves, J., Linos, N., & Bassett, M. T. (2017). Structural racism and health inequities in the USA: Evidence and interventions. *The Lancet, 389*(10077), 1453–1463. https://doi.org/10.1016/S0140-6736(17)30569-X

Bansil, P., Keenan, N. L., Zlot, A. I., et al. (2006). Health-related information on the web: Results from the HealthStyles survey, 2002–2003. *Preventing Chronic Disease, 3*(2), A36.

Barry-Jester, A. M. (2017). *The health care system is leaving the Southern Black Belt behind.* FiveThirtyEight. https://fivethirtyeight.com/features/the-health-care-system-is-leaving-the-southern-black-belt-behind/

Benda, N. C., Veinot, T. C., Sieck, C. J., & Ancker, J. S. (2020). Broadband internet access is a social determinant of health! *American Journal of Public Health, 110*(8), 1123–1125. https://doi.org/10.2105/AJPH.2020.305784

Bhaskaran, N., Kumar, M., & Manthan, D. J. (2017). Use of social media for seeking health related information—An exploratory study. *Journal of Young Pharmacists, 9*(2), 267–271. https://doi.org/10.5530/jyp.2017.9.52

Bouclaous, C., Al Kamand, A., Daher, R., Alrazim, A., & Kaedbey, H. D. (2023). Digital health literacy and online information-seeking behavior of Lebanese university students in the time of the COVID-19 pandemic and infodemic. *Nordic Journal of Digital Literacy, 18*(1), 60–77. https://doi.org/10.18261/njdl.18.1.6

Calixte, R., Rivera, A., Oridota, O., Beauchamp, W., & Camacho-Rivera, M. (2020). Social and demographic patterns of health-related internet use among adults in the United States. *International Journal of Environmental Research and Public Health, 17*(18), 6856. https://doi.org/10.3390/ijerph17186856

Cantor, D., Coa, K., Crystal-Mansour, S., Davis, T., Dipko, S., & Sigman, R. (2009). *Health Information National Trends Survey (HINTS) 4: Cycle 1 methodology report.* Westat.

Chi, G., Shapley, D., Yang, T.-C., & Matthews, S. A. (2019). Lost in the Black Belt South: Health outcomes and transportation infrastructure. *Environmental Monitoring and Assessment, 191*(Suppl 2), 297. https://doi.org/10.1007/s10661-019-7416-1

Cogbill, S., Francis, B., & Thompson, V. L. S. (2014). Factors affecting African American men's use of online colorectal cancer education. *Journal of Cancer Education, 29*(1), 25–29. https://doi.org/10.1007/s13187-013-0532-7

Din, H. N., McDaniels-Davidson, C., Nodora, J., & Madanat, H. (2019). Profiles of a health information–seeking population and the current digital divide: Cross-sectional analysis of the 2015–2016 California Health Interview Survey. *Journal of Medical Internet Research, 21*(5), e11931. https://doi.org/10.2196/11931

Dzubaty, D. R. (2016). Supporting neonatal intensive care unit parents through social media. *The Journal of Perinatal & Neonatal Nursing, 30*(3), 214–217. https://doi.org/10.1097/JPN.0000000000000199

Ebrahim, A., Saif, Z., & Buheji, M. (2020). COVID-19 information-seeking behavior and anxiety symptoms among parents. *OSP Journal of Health Care and Medicine, 1*(1), 1–9.

Feng, Y., & Xie, W. (2015). Digital divide 2.0: The role of social networking sites in seeking health information online from a longitudinal perspective. *Journal of Health Communication, 20*(1), 60–68. https://doi.org/10.1080/10810730.2014.906522

Fenta, E. T., Bogale, E. K., & Anagaw, T. F. (2024). The role of social media on COVID-19 preventive behaviors worldwide: Systematic review. *PLoS One, 19*, e0306284. https://doi.org/10.1371/journal.pone.0306284

Finney Rutten, L. J., Blake, K. D., Greenberg-Worisek, A. J., et al. (2019). Online health information seeking among US adults: Measuring progress toward a Healthy People 2020 objective. *Public Health Reports, 134*(6), 617–625. https://doi.org/10.1177/0033354919874074

Fischer, A., & LaFrance, M. (2015). What drives the smile and the tear: Why women are more emotionally expressive than men. *Emotion Review, 7*(1), 22–29. https://doi.org/10.1177/1754073914544406

Gee, G. C., & Ford, C. L. (2011). Structural racism and health inequities: Old issues, new directions. *Du Bois Review: Social Science Research on Race, 8*(1), 115–132. https://doi.org/10.1017/S1742058X11000130

Ghweeba, M., Lindenmeyer, A., Shishi, S., et al. (2017). What predicts online health information-seeking behavior among Egyptian adults? A cross-sectional study. *Journal of Medical Internet Research, 19*(6), e216. https://doi.org/10.2196/jmir.6855

Gilbert, E., Karahalios, K., & Sandvig, C. (2010). The network in the garden: Designing social media for rural life. *American Behavioral Scientist, 53*(9), 1367–1388. https://doi.org/10.1177/0002764210361690

Glied, S., & Lleras-Muney, A. (2008). Technological innovation and inequality in health. *Demography, 45*(3), 741–761. https://doi.org/10.1353/dem.0.0017

Greenberg, A. J., Haney, D., Blake, K. D., Moser, R. P., & Hesse, B. W. (2018). Differences in access to and use of electronic personal health information between rural and urban residents in the United States. *The Journal of Rural Health, 34*(s1), s30–s38. https://doi.org/10.1111/jrh.12228

Henderson, E. M., Keogh, E., Rosser, B. A., et al. (2013). Searching the Internet for help with pain: Adolescent search, coping, and medication behaviour. *British Journal of Health Psychology, 18*(1), 218–232. https://doi.org/10.1111/bjhp.12005

Hills, O., & Shah, D. (2020). Online health information seeking, medical care beliefs and timeliness of medical check-ups among African Americans. *Patient Education and Counseling, 103*(12), 2468–2476. https://doi.org/10.1016/j.pec.2020.06.006

Ihm, J., & Hsieh, Y. P. (2015). The implications of information and communication technology use for the social well-being of older adults. *Information, Communication & Society, 18*(10), 1123–1138. https://doi.org/10.1080/1369118X.2015.1019912

Jacobs, W., Amuta, A. O., & Jeon, K. C. (2017). Health information seeking in the digital age: An analysis of health information seeking behavior among US adults. *Cogent Social Science, 3*(1). https://doi.org/10.1080/23311886.2017.1302785

Jain, K. M., Bhat, P., Maulsby, C., et al. (2019). Extending access to care across the rural US South: Preliminary results from the Alabama eHealth programme. *Journal of Telemedicine and Telecare, 25*(5), 301–309. https://doi.org/10.1177/1357633X18755227

Jeong, S. H., & Kim, H. K. (2016). Health literacy and barriers to health information seeking: A nationwide survey in South Korea. *Patient Education and Counseling, 99*(11), 1880–1887. https://doi.org/10.1016/j.pec.2016.06.015

Kempf, M.-C., McLeod, J., Boehme, A. K., et al. (2010). A qualitative study of the barriers and facilitators to retention-in-care among HIV-positive women in the rural southeastern United States: Implications for targeted interventions. *AIDS Patient Care and STDs, 24*(8), 515–520. https://doi.org/10.1089/apc.2010.0065

Kontos, E., Blake, K. D., Chou, W.-Y. S., & Prestin, A. (2014). Predictors of eHealth usage: Insights on the digital divide from the Health Information National Trends Survey 2012. *Journal of Medical Internet Research, 16*(7), e172. https://doi.org/10.2196/jmir.3117

Kuzawa, C. W., & Sweet, E. (2009). Epigenetics and the embodiment of race: Developmental origins of US racial disparities in cardiovascular health. *American Journal of Human Biology, 21*(1), 2–15. https://doi.org/10.1002/ajhb.20822

Lee, Y. J., Boden-Albala, B., Larson, E., et al. (2014). Online health information seeking behaviors of Hispanics in New York City: A community-based cross-sectional study. *Journal of Medical Internet Research, 16*(7), e176. https://doi.org/10.2196/jmir.3499

Lee, H. Y., Lee, J., & Kim, N. K. (2015). Gender differences in health literacy among Korean Adults: Do women have a higher level of health literacy than men? *American Journal of Men's Health, 9*(5), 370–379. https://doi.org/10.1177/1557988314545485

Lee, H. Y., Hao, Z., & Choi, E. Y. (2022). Online health information-seeking behavior among Korean American immigrants in rural Alabama: Does discrimination matter? *Journal of Immigrant and Minority Health, 24*(4), 996–1004. https://doi.org/10.1007/s10903-021-01317-1

Lee, H., Kois, L. E., Wang, K., Won, C., Han, A., & Allen, R. (2023). Correlations between social determinants of health and technology access among rural African American Alabamians. *Journal of Health Care for the Poor and Underserved, 34*(1), 21–34. https://doi.org/10.1353/hpu.2023.0003

Li, Y., Spoer, B. R., Lampe, T. M., Hsieh, P. Y., Nelson, I. S., Vierse, A., Thorpe, L. E., & Gourevitch, M. N. (2023). Racial/ethnic and income disparities in neighborhood-level

broadband access in 905 US cities, 2017–2021. *Public Health, 217*, 205–211. https://doi.org/10.1016/j.puhe.2023.02.001
López, C. M., Qanungo, S., Jenkins, C. M., et al. (2018). Technology as a means to address disparities in mental health research: A guide to "tele-tailoring" your research methods. *Professional Psychology: Research and Practice, 49*(1), 57–64. https://doi.org/10.1037/pro0000176
Maron, D. (2017). *Maternal health care is disappearing in rural America*. Scientific American. Retrieved from https://www.scientificamerican.com/article/maternal-health-care-is-disappearing-in-rural-america/
Miller, K. E. M., James, H. J., Holmes, G. M., & Van Houtven, C. H. (2020). The effect of rural hospital closures on emergency medical service response and transport times. *Health Services Research, 55*(2), 288–300. https://doi.org/10.1111/1475-6773.13254
Miller, K. E. M., Miller, K. L., Knocke, K., Pink, G. H., Holmes, G. M., & Kaufman, B. G. (2021). Access to outpatient services in rural communities changes after hospital closure. *Health Services Research, 56*(5), 788–801. https://doi.org/10.1111/1475-6773.13694
Mitchell, J. A., Thompson, H. S., Watkins, D. C., et al. (2014). Disparities in health-related Internet use among African American men, 2010. *Preventing Chronic Disease, 11*, E43. https://doi.org/10.5888/pcd11.130217
Moneyham, L., McLeod, J., Boehme, A., et al. (2010). Perceived barriers to HIV care among HIV-infected women in the Deep South. *Journal of the Association of Nurses in AIDS Care, 21*(6), 467–477. https://doi.org/10.1016/j.jana.2010.03.003
Nath, C., Huh, J., Adupa, A. K., et al. (2016). Website sharing in online health communities: A descriptive analysis. *Journal of Medical Internet Research, 18*(1), e11. https://doi.org/10.2196/jmir.5237
Nikoloudakis, I. A., Vandelanotte, C., Rebar, A. L., et al. (2018). Examining the correlates of online health information–seeking behavior among men compared with women. *American Journal of Men's Health, 12*(5), 1358–1367. https://doi.org/10.1177/1557988316650625
Ormond, B. A., Wallin, S., Goldenson, S. M., & Urban Institute & Assessing the New Federalism (Program). (2000). *Supporting the rural health care safety net*. Urban Institute.
Park, M. S., Oh, H., & You, S. (2020). Health information seeking among people with multiple chronic conditions: Contextual factors and their associations mined from questions in social media. *Library & Information Science Research, 42*(3), 101030. https://doi.org/10.1016/j.lisr.2020.101030
Parkins, R. (2012). Gender and emotional expressiveness: An analysis of prosodic features in emotional expression. *Griffith Working Papers in Pragmatics and Intercultural Communication, 5*(1), 46–54.
Popovac, M., & Roomaney, R. (2022). Measuring online health-seeking behaviour: Construction and initial validation of a new scale. *British Journal of Health Psychology, 27*(3), 756–776. https://doi.org/10.1111/bjhp.12571
Powell, J., Inglis, N., Ronnie, J., & Large, S. (2011). The characteristics and motivations of online health information seekers: Cross-sectional survey and qualitative interview study. *Journal of Medical Internet Research, 13*(1), e20. https://doi.org/10.2196/jmir.1600
Prestin, A., Vieux, S. N., & Chou, W.-y. S. (2015). Is online health activity alive and well or flatlining? Findings from 10 years of the Health Information National Trends Survey. *Journal of Health Communication, 20*(7), 790–798. https://doi.org/10.1080/10810730.2015.1018590
PricewaterhouseCoopers (PwC) Health Research Institute. (2012). *Social media "likes" healthcare: From marketing to social business*. PwC.
Rosenblatt, R. A., Andrilla, C. H., Curtin, T., & Hart, L. G. (2006). Shortages of medical personnel at community health centers: Implications for planned expansion. *JAMA, 295*(9), 1042–1049. https://doi.org/10.1001/jama.295.9.1042
Rowley, J., Johnson, F., & Sbaffi, L. (2016). Gender as an influencer of online health information-seeking and evaluation behavior. *Journal of the Association for Information Science and Technology, 68*(1), 36–47. https://doi.org/10.1002/asi.23597
Ruggiero, K. J., Gros, D. F., McCauley, J., et al. (2011). Rural adults' use of health-related information online: Data from a 2006 National Online Health Survey. *Telemedicine and e-Health, 17*(5), 329–334. https://doi.org/10.1089/tmj.2010.0195

Shaw, R. J., & Johnson, C. M. (2011). Health information seeking and social media use on the internet among people with diabetes. *Online Journal of Public Health Informatics, 3*(1), ojphi.v3i1.3561. https://doi.org/10.5210/ojphi.v3i1.3561

Sherman, L. D., Goidel, K., Bergeron, C. D., & Smith, M. L. (2021). Web-based health information seeking among African American and hispanic men living with chronic conditions: Cross-sectional survey study. *Journal of Medical Internet Research, 23*(7), e26180. https://doi.org/10.2196/26180

Sinjini, M., & Rema, P. (2012). Exploring social media for health and wellness: A health plan case study. *Journal of Cases on Information Technology (JCIT), 14*(2), 42–64. https://doi.org/10.4018/jcit.2012040104

Smailhodzic, E., Hooijsma, W., Boonstra, A., & Langley, D. J. (2016). Social media use in healthcare: A systematic review of effects on patients and on their relationship with healthcare professionals. *BMC Health Services Research, 16*(1), 442. https://doi.org/10.1186/s12913-016-1691-0

Smith, A., & Anderson, M. (2018). *Social media use in 2018*. Pew Research Center. https://www.pewresearch.org/internet/2018/03/01/social-media-use-in-2018/

StataCorp. (2015). *Stata statistical software: Release 14*. StataCorp LP.

Statista. (2022). *Most popular mobile social networking apps in the United States as of September 2019, by reach*. Statista Inc. https://www.statista.com/statistics/579334/most-popular-us-social-networking-apps-ranked-by-reach/

Tan, S. S.-L., & Goonawardene, N. (2017). Internet health information seeking and the patient–physician relationship: A systematic review. *Journal of Medical Internet Research, 19*(1), e9. https://doi.org/10.2196/jmir.5729

Taylor, J. (2019). *Racism, inequality, and health care for African Americans*. The Century Foundation. https://tcf.org/content/report/racism-inequality-health-care-african-americans/

Thackeray, R., Crookston, B. T., & West, J. H. (2013). Correlates of health-related social media use among adults. *Journal of Medical Internet Research, 15*(1), e21. https://doi.org/10.2196/jmir.2297

Troske, S., & Davis, A. (2019). *Do hospital closures affect patient time in an ambulance?* Rural & Underserved Health Research Center, University of Kentucky. https://uknowledge.uky.edu/ruhrc_reports/8

United Health Foundation. (2022). *America's health rankings annual report 2022*. UnitedHealth Group. https://www.americashealthrankings.org/learn/reports/2022-annual-report/state-rankings?utm_source=chatgpt

van Deursen, A. J. A. M., & Helsper, E. J. (2015). A nuanced understanding of Internet use and non-use among the elderly. *European Journal of Communication, 30*(2), 171–187. https://doi.org/10.1177/0267323115578059

Vaughn, J., Harrell, A., & Dayton, A. E. (2015). Digital literacy in rural women's lives. *Community Literacy Journal, 9*(2), 26–47. https://doi.org/10.1353/clj.2015.0010

Volpe, V. V., Hoggard, L. S., Willis, H. A., & Tynes, B. M. (2021). Anti-Black structural racism goes online: A conceptual model for racial health disparities research. *Ethnicity & Disease, 31*(Suppl 1), 311–318. https://doi.org/10.18865/ed.31.S1.311

Walsh, M. C., Trentham-Dietz, A., Schroepfer, T. A., et al. (2010). Cancer information sources used by patients to inform and influence treatment decisions. *Journal of Health Communication, 15*(4), 445–463. https://doi.org/10.1080/10810731003753109

Zhao, Y., & Zhang, J. (2017). Consumer health information seeking in social media: A literature review. *Health Information and Libraries Journal, 34*(4), 268–283. https://doi.org/10.1111/hir.12192

Chapter 13
Information and Communication Technology Use for Seeking Health Information in Vietnamese Living in Rural Areas

Hee Yun Lee, Kun Wang, Danielle F. Deavours, Jiyoung Lee, Tanya Ott-Fulmore, Jongwook Lee, Sangchul Yoon, and Maxwell Sleep-Frankel

13.1 Introduction

Vietnam's economy has experienced dramatic growth over the past 35 years, becoming a middle-income country from one of the poorest nations in the world (Tran et al., 2020a). GDP per capita in Vietnam increased by 5.5 times between 1986 and 2020, lifting millions out of poverty (Nguyen & Pincus, 2021; Nguyen & Poczta-Wajda, 2024). Despite fast economic development, Vietnam is still a high endemic

Note: This chapter is adapted from a previously published article:
Hee Yun Lee, Kun Wang, Danielle F. Deavours, Jiyoung Lee, Tanya-Fulmore Ott, Jongwook Lee & Sangchul Yoon (2023) Information and communication technology use for seeking health information in Vietnamese living in rural areas, International Journal of Health Promotion and Education, 61:6, 307–316, DOI: https://doi.org/10.1080/14635240.2022.2059694

H. Y. Lee (✉)
School of Social Work, University of Georgia, Athens, GA, USA
e-mail: heeyunlee@uga.edu

K. Wang
Department of Social Work, College of Arts and Sciences, University of Alabama at Birmingham, Birmingham, AL, USA
e-mail: kw2@uab.edu

D. F. Deavours
Department of Communications and Media, Howard College of Arts and Sciences, Samford University, Homewood, AL, USA
e-mail: ddeavour@samford.edu

K. Wang et al. (eds.), *ICT Use and Healthy Longevity*, Advances in Studies of Aging and Health 5, https://doi.org/10.1007/978-3-031-98964-3_13

country of many infectious diseases, such as Dengue (Hung et al., 2018), hepatitis B virus (Flower et al., 2022), hepatitis C virus (Son Huy 2015), cysticercosis (Rajshekhar et al., 2003; Willingham et al., 2003) and also a country with high maternal and children health problems (Målqvist et al., 2012; Målqvist, 2011). These diseases have influenced Vietnamese quality of life and well-being and imposed many economic burdens on Vietnam's health care system (Giang et al., 2020; Shepard et al., 2016). Particularly, for Vietnamese living in rural areas, inadequate health care system capacity and a lack of access to health information and health care services further increased their risks of vulnerability (Tran et al., 2020b). McBride et al. (2024) found that ethnic minority women who lived in remote rural areas had four times the risk of maternal mortality than Khin women, and children living in rural areas were almost twice as likely to be stunted (Tan et al., 2024).

The WorldWideWeb was first introduced in 1990 (Berners-Lee). Vietnam joined the global internet network in 1997 (Pham, 2017). Fueled by a rapidly expanding economy and the younger generation, the number of Vietnamese internet users has increased dramatically to 80 million people, more than half of the country's population (Statista Research Department, 2025). About 74% of Vietnamese internet users had daily internet access, mainly through smartphones (Think With Google). In 2020, Vietnam announced a national digital transformation plan that prioritizes eight sectors, including healthcare (Samuel, n.d.). The COVID-19 pandemic has also accelerated the push for enhanced use of information and communication technology (ICT) in Vietnam (PwC Vietnam, 2021).

Education and access to information are crucial factors for improving residents' lives in rural communities. The Internet offers an expansive source of health-related information. People can search for health information, download eHealthCare Apps, join patient clubs, and communicate with physicians online through the Internet. Previous studies showed that online health information was an essential source for patients' self-diagnosis and management, and it also promoted effective

J. Lee
College of Social Sciences, Sungkyunkwan University, Seoul, South Korea
e-mail: jiyoung.lee@skku.edu

T. Ott-Fulmore
Department of Journalism and Media Studies, College of Liberal Arts and Sciences, Mercer University, Macon, GA, USA
e-mail: ott-fulmore_tl@mercer.edu

J. Lee
Department of Agricultural Economics and Rural Development, Seoul National University, Seoul, South Korea
e-mail: jongwooklee@snu.ac.kr

S. Yoon
Graduate School of Public Health, Catholic University of Korea, Seoul, South Korea
e-mail: syoon22@catholic.ac.kr

M. Sleep-Frankel
School of Social Work, University of Alabama, Tuscaloosa, AL, USA
e-mail: mdsleepfrankel@crimson.ua.edu

communications and shared decision making between patients and physicians (Waterworth & Honey, 2018; Susannah & Health Duggan, 2013; Ayers & Jacobs Kronenfeld, 2007; Nettleton et al., 2005). There have been systematic reviews of residents' online health-seeking behaviors in western developed countries (Zhao & Zhang, 2017), but little is known about lower-middle-income countries like Vietnam. What is clear is that the COVID-19 pandemic pushed Vietnam to experiment with telehealth strategies to connect larger, more urban hospitals with health care providers in more rural areas (Nguyen et al., 2021). Although this was a doctor-to-doctor connection, there are calls for expanding the telehealth model to connect doctors in more centralized locations with patients in rural areas.

Previous studies showed that long distance to the closest health facility, discriminatory behaviors from health staff, lack of primacy, and lack of female health staff attributed to the inequality in maternal and children health in Vietnam (Målqvist et al., 2012; Nielsen et al., 2016; Tran et al., 2016). Therefore, promoting online health information-seeking behaviors might be a good choice to reduce health inequality in Vietnam. However, studies on online health-seeking behaviors in Vietnam are very sparse. A recently published study reported promising findings that among the high-risk HIV group in Vietnam, 75% of participants had searched HIV/STI or other sexual health-related information online (Nguyen et al., 2018). Another study found that participants who spent 50–70% of their online time reading health-related information were less likely to smoke (Tran et al., 2018). However, studies on factors related to Vietnamese' general online health information-seeking behaviors are still missing. Therefore, this study will investigate the ICT use among rural Vietnamese and examine factors associated with online health information-seeking behaviors.

13.2 Methods

13.2.1 Research Design

13.2.1.1 Study Sample and Data Collection

This cross-sectional study is a part of a large research project examining rural Vietnamese's health and cancer screening literacy conducted in 2017. Given our interest in ICT use in rural Vietnamese, this study used purposive sampling to recruit participants living in a rural area. A convenient sample of 226 Vietnamese aged 25–70 years old was recruited from a rural town in Quang Tri Province, Vietnam. Data was collected in person from local public areas, such as local farmers' markets, schools, and community gatherings. Considering the low educational levels among the local rural population, we hired and trained college students to help collect data. The questionnaires were read to participants and filled out by trained college students based on participants' answers. This paper-and-pencil survey took about 20–30 min to be completed. Informed consent was obtained before the start of the survey. This study was approved by the Institutional Research Board (IRB) at the authors' institutions.

13.2.2 Measures

13.2.2.1 Dependent Variable

The dependent variable, online health information-seeking behavior, was measured by one single question, that is, 'In the past 12 months, have you used the Internet to look for health or medical information for yourself?' (0 = No, 1 = Yes).

13.2.2.2 Independent Variables

In this study, Andersen's Behavioral Model of Health Service Utilization was used as a framework to investigate factors relevant to Vietnamese's online health-seeking behaviors (Andersen, 1995). Based on Andersen's model, determinants of health service utilization could be categorized into three dimensions: predisposing factors, enabling factors, and need factors (Andersen, 1995).

Predisposing Variables

Age, gender, marital status, and education level are predisposing variables in this study. Age was a continuous variable. Education was measured continuously through years in school, ranging from 0 to 15. Gender (0 = Male, 1 = Female) and marital status (0 = Not married/ partnered, 1 = Married/ partnered) were both measured dichotomously.

Enabling Variables

Employment status, health insurance, annual checkups, information and communication technology (ICT) use, and health literacy are enabling variables. Employment status (0 = No, 1 = Yes), having health insurance (0 = No, 1 = Yes), and having annual checkups (0 = No, 1 = Yes) were all measured dichotomously.

ICT use was measured by the sum of 6 binary questions, including 'Do you ever go online to access the Internet or World Wide Web, or to send and receive e-mail?' 'Do you have a mobile phone?', 'Do you use text messages using your mobile phone?', 'Is your mobile phone a Smartphone?', 'Do you have a computer or a tablet PC (ex. iPad, Galaxy Tab) at home?', 'Do you use mobile applications (mobile apps) with your Smartphone or tablet?' (0 = No, 1 = Yes). ICT use ranged from 0 to 6, with a higher score indicating more use of ICT.

Health literacy was measured by the Health Literacy Scale in Behavioral Risk Factor Surveillance System (BRFSS) (Centers for Disease Control and Prevention, 2019). It included three items, specifically, 'How difficult is it for you to get advice or information about health or medical topics if you needed it?', 'How difficult is it for you to understand information that doctors, nurses and other health professionals tell you?', and 'You can find written information about health on the Internet, in newspapers and magazines, and brochures in the doctor's office and clinic. In general, how difficult is it for you to understand written health information?' A 5-point Likert scale measured each item (0 = Not at all, 4 = Always). Health literacy in this study was the sum of the three items, ranging from 0 to 12, with a higher score indicating a higher level of health literacy.

Need Variables

Family cancer history and self-rated health status were two need variables in this study. Both were measured dichotomously – family cancer history (0 = No, 1 = Yes), and self-rated health status (0 = Very poor/poor, 1 = Good/very good/excellent).

13.2.3 Data Analysis

Univariate analysis was firstly conducted to examine participants' sociodemographic characteristics and descriptively analyze their ICT use. Bivariate statistics, such as *t*-test, and Chi-square test, were used to test the associations between having online health information-seeking behavior and participants' characteristics. Finally, binary logistic regression was conducted to identify significant online health information-seeking behavior variables. 'One in ten' rule was followed to ensure the statistical power. All the analyses in this study were completed in SPSS version 25.0.

13.3 Results

13.3.1 Sociodemographic Characteristics of the Sample

As shown in Table 13.1, a total of 226 participants were analyzed in this study: the average age was 41.6 (SD = 5.88); the mean education level was 9.57 years in school (SD = 3.30); average health literacy was 4.32 (SD = 2.93); mean ICT use score was 3.66 (SD = 1.88). Among the 226 participants, the majority were female (85.4%), married/ partnered (92.5%), employed (90.3%), and in good/ very good/ excellent health status (90.3%). More than three-fourths of the participants had health insurance (80.5%) and did not have a family cancer history (76.1%). Only slightly higher than half of the sample had annual checkups (54.0%). People who had online health information-seeking behaviors tended to be younger ($p < .05$), more educated ($p < .001$), employed ($p < .001$), having health insurance ($p < .05$), having annual checkups ($p < .001$), and having more ICT use ($p < .001$).

Table 13.1 Sociodemographic characteristics of the samples ($N = 226$).

Characteristics	n (%)	ICT use (0 ~ 6)		Online Health Information Seeking Behavior (1 = Yes)	
		M(SD)	t	n (%)	x^2
Gender					
Male	33 (14.6%)	3.72 (1.998)	.84	17 (51.5%)	.33
Female	193 (85.4%)	3.65 (1.864)		89 (46.1%)	
Marital status					
Married/ partnered	209 (92.5%)	3.64 (1.865)	.655	95 (45.5%)	2.34
Other	17 (7.5%)	3.87 (2.100)		11 (64.7%)	
Employment status					
Yes	204 (90.3%)	3.84 (1.835)	−6.80***	103 (50.5%)	10.83***
No	22 (9.7%)	1.79 (1.182)		3 (13.6%)	
Having health insurance					
Yes	182 (80.5%)	3.79 (1.911)	−2.43*	92 (50.5%)	4.99*
No	44 (19.5%)	3.08 (1.623)		14 (31.8%)	
Having annual checkup					
Yes	122 (54.0%)	4.14 (1.798)	−4.46***	75 (61.5%)	22.61***
No	104 (46.0%)	3.03 (1.802)		31 (29.8%)	
Having a family cancer history					
Yes	54 (23.9%)	3.736 (1.882)	−.351	29 (53.7%)	1.32
No	172 (76.1%)	3.631 (1.882)		77 (44.8%)	
Self-rated health status					
Very poor/Poor	22 (9.7%)	2.83 (1.886)	−1.96	7 (31.8%)	2.23
Good/Very good/ Excellent	204 (90.3%)	3.73 (1.864)		99 (48.5%)	

Characteristics	M(SD)	ICT use (0 ~ 6)		Online Health Information-Seeking Behavior (1 = Yes)	
		R	p	M(SD)	t
Age	41.60 (5.88)	−.24	.00***	40.64 (4.923)	2.37*
Education	9.57 (3.30)	.71	.00***	11.54 (2.645)	−10.23***
Health literacy	4.32 (2.93)	−.05	.44	4.25 (2.835)	.33
ICT use	3.66 (1.88)			4.98 (1.302)	−14.36***

Note. *$p < .05$, *** $p < .001$

13.3.2 Descriptive Analysis on ICT Use

As Table 13.2 indicated, most participants had 'a mobile phone' (94.2%), and about three-fourths had 'texted message using their mobile phone' (75.2%). However, less than half of participants gave 'Yes' answers to questions such as 'Do you ever go online to access the Internet or World Wide Web, or to send and receive e-mail' (42.0%), 'Is your mobile phone a Smartphone' (45.6%), 'Do you have a computer or tablet PC (EX. I-Pad, Galaxy Tab)' (46.0%), and 'Do you use mobile applications (mobile apps) with your Smartphone or tablet' (42%).

13.3.3 Binary Logistic regression Analysis on Online Health Information-Seeking Behavior

Table 13.3 shows that this model fit the data well (Hosmer-Lemeshow goodness-of-fit $\chi^2(8) = 5.786$, $p > .05$), and could explain almost 65% of the total variance of online health information-seeking behavior. Among predisposing variables, gender

Table 13.2 Descriptive analysis on ICT use

Questions on ICT use	Yes	%
1. Do you ever go online to access the Internet or World Wide Web, or to send and receive e-mail?	95	42.0%
2. Do you have a mobile phone?	213	94.2%
3. Do you use text messages using your mobile phone?	170	75.2%
4. Is your mobile phone a Smartphone?	103	45.6%
5. Do you have a computer or a tablet PC (ex. iPad, Galaxy Tab) at home?	104	46.0%
6. Do you use mobile applications (mobile apps) with your Smartphone or tablet?	95	42.0%

Table 13.3 Binary logistic regression analysis on online health information-seeking behavior ($N = 226$)

		Online Health Information-Seeking Behavior			
				(1 = Yes)	
Factors	Variables	OR	SE	95% CI	
Predisposing	Age (29 ~ 67)	.95	.041	.881	1.034
	Gender (Ref = male)	.22*	.758	.050	.967
	Marital status (Ref = not married/partnered)	.09*	.966	.013	.589
	Education level (0 ~ 15)	1.21	.097	1.000	1.460
Enabling	Employment status (Ref = no)	.58	.831	.113	2.941
	Having health insurance (Ref = no)	.85	.554	.287	2.516
	Having annual checkup (Ref = no)	2.89*	.480	1.129	7.409

(continued)

Table 13.3 (continued)

Factors	Variables	Online Health Information-Seeking Behavior			
				(1 = Yes)	
		OR	SE	95% CI	
	ICT use (0 ~ 6)	2.58***	.166	1.865	3.571
	Health literacy (0 ~ 12)	1.07	.071	.927	1.226
Need	Family cancer history (Ref = no)	1.14	.523	.409	3.185
	Self-rated health status (Ref = very poor/poor)	.83	.816	.167	4.085
Constant		1.17	2.550		
Pseudo R^2		.65			
x^2		5.786 (p > .05)			
−2 Log likelihood		153.43			

Note. Pseudo R^2 is Nagelkerke's R^2; B = coefficient, OR = odds ratio; *$p < .05$, ***$p < .001$

(OR = .22, SE = .758, CI = [.050, .967]) and marital status (OR = .09, SE = .966, CI = [.013, .589]) were significant predictors of online health information-seeking behavior. The odds of having online health information-seeking behavior for females is .22 times that of males, while the odds for married or partnered individuals were .09 times that of those who were not. With respect to enabling factors, having annual checkups (OR = 2.89, SE = .480, CI = [1.129, 7.409]) and higher ICT use (OR = 2.58, SE = .166, CI = [1.865, 3.571]) were associated with online health information-seeking behavior. People who had annual checkups were 2.89 times as likely as those who did not to have online health information-seeking behavior. For a one-unit increase in ICT use, the odds of having online health information-seeking behavior would be 2.58 times higher. There were no significant need variables in this model.

13.4 Discussion

The primary aim of this study was to investigate ICT use among rural Vietnamese and examine the correlates of their online health information-seeking behaviors. This study provides unique insights into the existing literature through the findings below.

Results showed that most rural Vietnamese had access to technology devices, such as mobile phones (94.2%); however, less than half of them used technology devices for the Internet (42%) or mobile apps (42%) use. There could be various reasons for this, drawn from previous research in this area, such as a lack of access to a reliable, affordable Internet connection, limited knowledge about the benefits of

Internet use, or lack of education on how to use the technology for these purposes (Amante et al., 2015; Kosowicz et al., 2022; Vong & Song, 2015). The hesitancy does not seem to stem from the technology itself since over 75% of survey participants used their mobile phones for text messaging; this suggests connectivity, education, or awareness issues specific to Internet use instead. This is a significant finding that needs further investigation since over half of the surveyed participants are not using the Internet regularly for any purpose, let alone to access health information. It also provides applicable information for health officials who need to consider the digital divide when planning initiatives in or around rural communities.

This study also suggests factors associated with online health information-seeking behavior among rural Vietnamese. Males and married people were more likely to use the Internet for health information in the rural Vietnamese population, which aligned with previous studies (Amante et al., 2015; Hoang, 2020). In addition, consistent with previous studies (Lee et al., 2021; Aida et al., 2020; Vong & Song, 2015), those who had annual checkups and had more technology devices were also more likely to seek health information online. This finding suggests that those with access to healthcare and technical information will continue to use these advantages when seeking further health information.

Contrary to a prior study (Hoang, 2020), the current study findings showed that age was not a significant predictor for online health information-seeking behavior among rural Vietnamese. This aligned with findings from studies in other countries, which suggested that those who were middle-aged (approximately ages 35–60) tend to be the most frequent users of health information technology, as older people were not using digital technology, and younger people were not as interested in health information (Amante et al., 2015).

13.4.1 Study Limitations

Because this study utilized a convenient purposive sampling and collected data from one rural town, findings in this study may not be generalizable to the general rural population in Vietnam. Future studies can use randomized sampling techniques. Also, the population was limited to ages 25 to 70, and the researchers recognize that the findings may not generalize to either younger or older members of the rural Vietnamese communities. Future studies should consider using a more comprehensive age range to capture these populations' user habits. In addition, the survey was delivered in-person using a paper-and-pencil survey, limiting the sample size; however, because of the focus on digital practices of rural Vietnamese populations, this approach was necessary to capture non-computer user responses. Finally, the survey relied on self-reporting methods, and questions were asked by and filled out by research assistants. Participants may not have accurately reported all responses due to social desirability bias. Future researchers could use other methods, like in-depth interviews and observations, for additional insight into ICT use among rural Vietnamese populations.

13.4.2 Implications for Health Practice and Policy

This study hopes to provide practical applicability for health practitioners and policymakers. First, health practitioners and policymakers need to consider initiatives that encourage Internet use in rural Vietnamese communities to increase digital health-seeking practices. Our findings suggest that over half the population is not connecting to the Internet, and if a person is not willing or able to access the Internet, digital health-seeking practices would likewise be hindered. While practitioners may be eager to get patients to incorporate digital health-seeking practices in their healthcare routines, providers must ensure that they have regular Internet access and know how to use digital technology. Then they can educate patients on the specific resources available for online health information. Second, having annual checkups is a significant predictor for health-seeking practices online. Campaigns that focus on the importance of annual checkups may increase the number of patients seeking health information online. Finally, the non-significant findings can serve as a roadmap for policymakers and providers about what populations may need more assistance accessing online health information, such as the elderly or less educated. Overall, the study suggests that health practitioners and policymakers need more work to connect the areas of digital access, healthcare, and online health-seeking behavior in rural Vietnamese populations.

Acknowledgement This study was funded by the Endowed Academic Chair Research Fund of the University of Alabama School of Social Work awarded to Dr. Hee Yun Lee.

Disclosure Statement No potential conflict of interest was reported by the author(s).

References

Aida, A., Svensson, T., Kishi Svensson, A., Urushiyama, H., Okushin, K., Oguri, G., Kubota, N., et al. (2020). Using mHealth to provide mobile app users with visualization of health checkup data and educational videos on lifestyle-related diseases: Methodological framework for content development. *JMIR mHealth and uHealth, 8*(10), e20982. https://doi.org/10.2196/20982

Amante, D. J., Timothy, P., Hogan, S. L., Pagoto, T. M. E., & Lapane, K. L. (2015). Access to care and use of the Internet to search for health information: Results from the US National Health Interview Survey. *Journal of Medical Internet Research, 17*(4), e106. https://doi.org/10.2196/jmir.4126

Andersen, R. M. (1995). Revisiting the behavioral model and access to medical care: Does it matter? *Journal of Health and Social Behavior, 36*(1), 1–10. https://doi.org/10.2307/2137284

Ayers, S. L., & Jacobs Kronenfeld, J. (2007). Chronic illness and health-seeking information on the Internet. *Health, 11*(3), 327–347. https://doi.org/10.1177/1363459307077547

Centers for Disease Control and Prevention. (2019). 2019 Behavioral Risk Factor Surveillance System (BRFSS) overview. U.S. Department of Health and Human Services. Retrieved from https://www.cdc.gov/brfss/annual_data/annual_2019.html

Flower, B., Hong, D. D., Vu, H. T. K., Pham, K. M., Geskus, R., Day, J., & Cooke, G. (2022). Seroprevalence of hepatitis B, C, and D in Vietnam: A systematic review and meta-analysis.

The Lancet Regional Health – Western Pacific, 24, 100468. https://doi.org/10.1016/j.lanwpc.2022.100468

Giang, N. H., Thi Mai Oanh, T., Anh Tuan, K., Hong Van, P., & Jayasuriya, R. (2020). Is health insurance associated with health service utilization and economic burden of non-communicable diseases on households in Vietnam? *Health Systems & Reform, 6*(1), e1619065. https://doi.org/10.1080/23288604.2019.1619065

Hoang, H. G. (2020). Use of information and communication technologies by Vietnamese smallholders: Implications for extension strategies. *Information Development, 37*(2), 221–230. https://doi.org/10.1177/0266666920906603

Hung, T. M., Clapham, H. E., Bettis, A. A., Cuong, H. Q., Thwaites, G. E., Wills, B. A., Boni, M. F., & Turner, H. C. (2018). The estimates of the health and economic burden of dengue in Vietnam. *Trends in Parasitology, 34*(10), 904–918. https://doi.org/10.1016/j.pt.2018.07.007

Kosowicz, L., Tran, K., Tran Khanh, T., Dang, T., Pham, V. A., Ta Thi Kim, H., Duong, H. T. B., Nguyen, T. D., Phuong, A. T., Le, T. H., Ta, V. A., Wickramasinghe, N., Schofield, P., Zelcer, J., Pham Le, T., & Nguyen, T. A. (2022). Lessons for Vietnam on the use of digital technologies to support patient-centered care in low- and middle-income countries in the Asia-Pacific region: Scoping review. *Journal of Medical Internet Research, 25*. https://doi.org/10.2196/43224

Lee, H. Y., Won Jin, S., Henning-Smith, C., Lee, J., & Lee, J. (2021). Role of health literacy in health-related information-seeking behavior online: Cross-sectional study. *Journal of Medical Internet Research, 23*(1), e14088. https://doi.org/10.2196/14088

Målqvist, M. (2011). Neonatal mortality: An invisible and marginalized trauma. *Global Health Action, 4*(1), 5724. https://doi.org/10.3402/gha.v4i0.5724

Målqvist, M., Hoa, D. T., & Thomsen, S. (2012). Causes and determinants of inequity in maternal and child health in Vietnam. *BMC Public Health, 12*(1), 641. https://doi.org/10.1186/1471-2458-12-641

McBride, B., Kane, S., O'Neil, J., & Nguyen, L. T. (2024). The best healthcare (commodity) available (for purchase): provider-induced demand for obstetric ultrasonography among ethnic minority women in rural northern Vietnam. *AJOG global reports, 4*(3), 100375. https://doi.org/10.1016/j.xagr.2024.100375

Nettleton, S., Burrows, R., & O'Malley, L. (2005). The mundane realities of the everyday lay use of the Internet for health, and their consequences for media convergence. *Sociology of Health & Illness, 27*(7), 972–992. https://doi.org/10.1111/j.1467-9566.2005.00466.x

Nguyen, M. X., Krishnan, A., Le, G. M., Nguyen, Q. T., Bhadra, N. M., Nguyen, S. M., Miller, W. C., & Go, V. F. (2018). The use of technology to find sexual health information online among men who have sex with men in Hanoi, Vietnam, 2016. *International Journal of STD & AIDS, 29*(5), 505–510. https://doi.org/10.1177/0956462417738680

Nguyen, T., & Pincus, J. (2021). *Economic recovery and progress toward the SDGs: Viet Nam in multiple transformations*. United Nations Development Programme (UNDP). https://www.undp.org/vietnam/publications/economic-recovery-and-progress-toward-sdgs-viet-nam-multiple-transformations

Nguyen, A. T., & Poczta-Wajda, A. (2024). The relationship between Foreign Direct Investment, trade openness, exchange rate, and Gross Domestic Product per capita in Vietnam. *Journal of Economics & Management, 46*, 189–212. https://doi.org/10.22367/jem.2024.46.08

Nguyen, N. H., Quang Nguyen, A., Thi Bich Ha, V., Duong, P. X., & Van Nguyen, T. (2021). Using emerging telehealth technology as a future model in Vietnam during the COVID-19 pandemic: Practical experience from Phutho General Hospital. *JMIR Formative Research, 5*(6), e27968. https://doi.org/10.2196/27968

Nielsen, A., Thi Lan, P., Marrone, G., Dang Phuc, H., Thi Kim Chuc, N., & Stålsby Lundborg, C. (2016). Reproductive tract infections in rural Vietnam, women's knowledge, and health-seeking behavior: A cross-sectional study. *Health Care for Women International, 37*(4), 392–411. https://doi.org/10.1080/07399332.2014.920021

Partnership for Action in Health Equity. (2011). *Health equity in Vietnam: A civil society perspective.*

Pham, K. (2017). A brief history of the Internet in Vietnam on its 20th birthday. *Saigoneer.*

PwC Vietnam. (2021). *Vietnam digital readiness report: PwC Vietnam's survey on technology, jobs and skills*. https://www.pwc.com/vn/en/publications/2021/pwc-vietnam-digital-readiness-report-en.pdf

Rajshekhar, V., Joshi, D. D., Doanh, N. Q., van De, N., & Xiaonong, Z. (2003). Taenia solium taeniosis/cysticercosis in Asia: Epidemiology, impact and issues. *Acta Tropica, 87*(1), 53–60. https://doi.org/10.1016/s0001-706x(03)00055-x

Samuel, P. (n.d.). *Vietnam's digital transformation plan through 2025.*

Shepard, D. S., Undurraga, E. A., Halasa, Y. A., & Stanaway, J. D. (2016). The global economic burden of dengue: A systematic analysis. *The Lancet Infectious Diseases, 16*(8), 935–941. https://doi.org/10.1016/S1473-3099(16)00146-8

Son Huy, D. (2015). Epidemiology of hepatitis B and C virus infections and liver cancer in Vietnam. *Euroasian Journal of Hepatogastroenterology, 5*(1), 49–51. https://doi.org/10.5005/jp-journals-10018-1130

Statista. (2025, March 19). *Internet usage in Vietnam – Statistics & facts*. Statista. https://www.statista.com/topics/6231/internet-usage-in-vietnam/

Susannah, F., & Health Duggan, M. J. (2013). *Health online 2013*. Pew Research Center. https://www.pewresearch.org/internet/2013/01/15/health-online-2013/

Tan, P., Som, V., Nguyen, S., Tan, X., Tran, D. T., Tran, T. N., Tran, V. K., Dye, L., Moore, J. B., Caton, S., Ensaff, H., Lin, X., Smith, G., & Gong, Y. (2024). Triple burden of malnutrition and its key demographic and socioeconomic determinants among Vietnamese children: Insights from the General Nutrition Survey 2020. *Proceedings of the Nutrition Society*. https://doi.org/10.1017/s0029665124005433

Tran, D. T., Doan, M. H., & Do, N. T. (2020a). Vietnam after 2020: Toward a prosperous economy, social inclusion, and environmental sustainability. *International Journal of Economic Policy Studies, 14*, 313–326. https://doi.org/10.1007/s42495-020-00046-x

Tran, B. X., Hoang Nguyen, L., Minh Nong, V., & Tat Nguyen, C. (2016). Health status and health service utilization in remote and mountainous areas in Vietnam. *Health and Quality of Life Outcomes, 14*(1), 85. https://doi.org/10.1186/s12955-016-0485-8

Tran, B., Hoang, M. T., Pham, H., Hoang, C. L., Le, H., Latkin, C., Ho, C. S. H., & Ho, R. (2020b). The operational readiness capacities of the grassroots health system in responses to epidemics: Implications for COVID-19 control in Vietnam. *Journal of Global Health, 10*. https://doi.org/10.7189/jogh.10.011006

Tran, B. X., Xuan Thanh Thi, L., Phuong Ngoc, N., Quynh Ngoc Hoang, L., Hue Thi, M., Huong Lan Thi, N., Huong Thi, L., et al. (2018). Feasibility of e-health interventions on smoking cessation among Vietnamese active Internet users. *International Journal of Environmental Research and Public Health, 15*(1), 165. https://doi.org/10.3390/ijerph15010165

Vong, J., & Song, I. (2015). Application of ICT to improve rural livelihood in Vietnam. In J. Fodor & I. J. Rudas (Eds.), *Emerging technologies for emerging markets* (pp. 179–204). Springer.

Waterworth, S., & Honey, M. (2018). On-line health seeking activity of older adults: An integrative review of the literature. *Geriatric Nursing, 39*(3), 310–317. https://doi.org/10.1016/j.gerinurse.2017.10.016

Willingham, A. L., III, De, N. V., Doanh, N. Q., Cong Le, D., Dung, T. V., Dorny, P., Cam, P. D., & Dalsgaard, A. (2003). Current status of cysticercosis in Vietnam. *The Southeast Asian Journal of Tropical Medicine and Public Health, 34*(1), 35–50.

Zhao, Y., & Zhang, J. (2017). Consumer health information seeking in social media: A literature review. *Health Information and Libraries Journal, 34*(4), 268–283. https://doi.org/10.1111/hir.12192

Chapter 14
Purposes of Using Social Media Among Older Adults in China

Danan Gu, Qiushi Feng, Haiyan Zhu, Siyao Lu, and Yuanying Liu

14.1 Introduction

The rapid development of information and communication technology (ICT) has significantly transformed how individuals interact, access information, and participate in social and economic activities. In China, where digital infrastructure has been expanding at an unprecedented pace (CNNIC, 2025), older adults are increasingly becoming part of the digital landscape. As of December 2024, the internet penetration rate among older Chinese adults aged 60 or older had reached 52.7%, representing over 150 million old-age internet users, a sharp increase from 9 million in 2010 (CNNIC, 2011, 2025). A significant portion of their online activity involves engagement with social media platforms such as *WeChat, Douyin (TikTok), Xiaohongshu*

D. Gu (✉)
Population Division, UN Department of Economic and Social Affairs, New York, NY, USA
e-mail: gudanan@yahoo.com

Q. Feng
Centre for Family and Population Research/Department of Sociology and Anthropology, National University of Singapore, Singapore, Singapore
e-mail: socfq@nus.edu.sg

H. Zhu
Department of Sociology, Virginia Tech, Blacksburg, VA, USA
e-mail: zhuh@vt.edu

S. Lu
Department of Sociology, Yale University, New Haven, CT, USA
e-mail: siyao.lu@yale.edu

Y. Liu
Department of Sociology and Anthropology, National University of Singapore, Singapore, Singapore
e-mail: e1154500@u.nus.edu

K. Wang et al. (eds.), *ICT Use and Healthy Longevity*, Advances in Studies of Aging and Health 5, https://doi.org/10.1007/978-3-031-98964-3_14

(RedNote, similar to Instagram), Youku, Xigua Video, and Bilibili (akin to YouTube), as well as e-commerce platforms like *Taobao and Jingdong* (Amazon equivalent). These platforms serve multiple functions for their later lives, including communication, information seeking, entertainment, and social participation.

Despite the increasing use of social media among older Chinese adults, limited research has been done to systematically examine their specific purposes of this online engagement and how these purposes vary across different demographic and socioeconomic groups. Understanding the motivations of using social media amongst older adults is crucial in the context of China's rapidly aging population and broader societal shifts toward digitalization. Insights into older adults' social media use can inform the development of age-friendly digital policies and targeted interventions that enhance digital inclusion and social connectedness. This chapter addresses this research gap by exploring the major purposes of social media use among older Chinese adults and identifying key factors that influence these purposes.

14.1.1 Literature Review

Among numerous theories and frameworks on the purposes of social media use, the Uses and Gratifications Theory (UGT; Katz et al., 1973), the Theory of Planned Behavior (TPB; Ajzen, 1991), and the Senior Technology Acceptance Model (STAM; Chen & Chan, 2014; Renaud & van Biljon, 2008) are widely used to understand why and how older adults engage with social media. For details, please refer to Chap. 3.

Empirical research has consistently revealed that older adults engage with social media for multiple purposes (see Chaps. 2 and 3). Communication remains one of the primary purposes, as social media facilitate connections with family members, friends, and social ties (see Chap. 2), mitigating feelings of isolation and loneliness (Cotten et al., 2013). Information seeking is another major motivation (see Chap. 2), with older adults utilizing social media to access news, health-related content, and notices of government services (Choi & DiNitto, 2013; Seifert et al., 2021). Entertainment, including video streaming, short-form videos, and interactive content, is also a prevalent purpose (Büchi, 2024). Additionally, digital commerce and financial transactions have become increasingly popular among older adults when using social media, allowing them to engage in online shopping, banking, and digital payments (Wu & Song, 2021).

While these findings provide valuable insights, existing studies have several limitations. First, much of the research has focused on Western contexts, with limited empirical studies examining social media engagement among older Chinese adults. Given China's distinctive sociocultural and institutional environment, findings from Western studies may not fully apply. Second, most studies from the literature are committed to analyzing the use of ICT, the internet, or social media but paid less attention on specific purposes behind the use (for a few exceptions, see Szabo et al., 2019; Wang et al., 2024). Third, research on how demographic and socioeconomic factors, such as age, gender, education, health status, and urban-rural residence, shape social media use among older adults remains scarce, and even fewer studies have explored on cultural and other characteristics of the old-age respondents. Finally, policy-relevant discussions on how digital interventions can be tailored to different older adult subgroups are largely absent from the existing literature. These research gaps underscore the need for a more systematic and context-specific investigation into the purposes of using social media among Chinese seniors.

14.1.2 Research Objectives

Given the increasing digital engagement of older Chinese adults, understanding the motivations of social media use is crucial for designing inclusive digital policies. This study thus seeks to address the following research questions:

1. What are the major purposes of using social media among older Chinese adults?
2. Do these purposes vary by groups of older adults with different characteristics (e.g., age, gender, education, health status, urban-rural residence)?
3. How could patterns of purposes among older adults in using social media inform targeted interventions to promote digital inclusion?

This study is driven by both theoretical and practical concerns. Theoretically, while frameworks such as the three-level digital divide have provided valuable insights into digital inequalities (see Chap. 3), how cultural and contextual factors may shape social media use among older adults are not fully explored. Unlike Western countries, where individualism prevails, China's Confucian norms and collectivist culture emphasize family connectivity and social harmony (Yang & Du, 2021; Zhang & He, 2022), which may lead to different patterns of social media use in later life. This study thus aims to expand the applicability of existing digital inclusion theories by incorporating the case of China.

From a policy perspective, the Chinese government has recognized the importance of digital empowerment for older adults, launching initiatives such as the "Bridging the Digital Divide for the Elderly" (2020) to improve national digital literacy (State Council, 2020). However, without a clear understanding of why older adults use social media, interventions may be poorly developed. This study is committed to providing empirical evidence to support the development of policies tailored to different social and demographic groups, ensuring that digital inclusion strategies could comprehensively and effectively accommodate the needs of China's aging population. Moreover, addressing digital disparities has far-reaching implications for health, social engagement, and economic participation among older adults. It is well evidenced that active social media use can mitigate loneliness, improve cognitive function, and facilitate access to healthcare resources among older adults (Chopik, 2016; Khoo & Yang, 2020; Myhre et al., 2017). By examining why older Chinese adults use social media, this study contributes to the ongoing discourses on healthy aging in the digital era, a major theme on the United Nations' agenda (2015, 2020).

14.2 Data and Methods

14.2.1 Data Sources

We utilized data from the China Longitudinal Aging Social Survey (CLASS), a nationally representative longitudinal survey in China. A comprehensive description of CLASS can be found in Chap. 6 or previous studies (Dong et al., 2019; Jin & Zhao, 2019). Consistent with Chaps. 6 and 9, our analysis is entirely based on the 2020 wave of CLASS. Given the research objectives of this chapter, we focused exclusively on respondents aged 65 and older who regularly used social media in their daily lives at the time of the survey. This selection resulted in a final analytical sample of 2,805 participants.

14.2.2 Measures

14.2.2.1 Purposes of Using Social Media

Twelve dichotomous questions were included in the questionnaire of the 2020 wave of CLASS to assess respondents' purposes for using social media: (1) chatting or contacting family and friends (via voice or video), (2) texting with family and friends, (3) shopping, (4) reading news, (5) seeking information or reading articles, (6) listening to music or radio, or watching videos/shows or TV, (7) playing games, (8) travel, (9) managing health, (10) investment/financing, (11) learning or training, and (12) other activities. For analytical purposes, we combined (1) and (2) under "chatting" (i.e., contact family and friends), and merged (6) and (7) into "entertainment." Due to the low prevalence, "investment/financing" and "learning/training" were excluded from our modeling. Consequently, our analysis focused on seven key purposes: chatting, reading news, accessing general information, entertainment, shopping, travel, and health management. These categories capture the primary domains of purposes of social media use, helpful for understanding user motivations and behaviors under the frameworks reviewed above.

14.2.2.2 Associated Factors with Purposes of Social Media Use

Following the STAM and other digital divide frameworks detailed in Chap. 3, we employed all five sets of variables used for examining the associates of internet use in Chap. 6. These variables provide a comprehensive list for analyzing aging-related issues, including (1) demographics, (2) socioeconomics, (3) family and social support networks, (4) views on aging, perceived aging, and views on advances in internet technology, and (5) health status. The region variable is always controlled for in all models. Please refer to the detailed definition and coding of these variables above in Chap. 6.

14.2.3 Analytical Strategies

We primarily employed multiple logistic regression models alongside descriptive analyses. Following the analytical strategy outlined in Chap. 6, we initially constructed partial models to examine the independent associations between each set of variables and the seven purposes of using social media. However, given that the coefficients in the full models where all variables are included were highly similar to those in the partial models, we presented only the results from the full models for clarity and conciseness. Consistent with the approach in Chap. 6, sampling weights were applied in descriptive analyses but not in the regression models. All statistical analyses were conducted using Stata 18.0.

14.3 Results

14.3.1 Descriptive Analysis

Table 14.1 presents the sample distribution of social media users ($N = 2{,}805$) compared to the overall sample. The most common purpose for using social media was chatting/communication (93.1%), followed by reading news (72.1%), entertainment (63.2%), seeking general information (44.4%), online shopping (29.4%), travel (18.0%), and health management (8.9%). This distribution aligns with global patterns discussed in Chap. 2. Table 14.1 also describes the profile of these users in comparison with the total sample. Demographically, social media users were mostly younger than 75 years old, more likely to be male, urban residents, and better educated. They were also more likely to be white-collar or blue-collar workers but less likely to be agricultural workers, had stronger family and social ties, held more positive attitudes toward ICT advancements and aging, reported better health, and resided in East and Northeast China.

Table 14.2 presents the weighted proportions of purposes using social media across different study variables. Older adults reported lower engagement in reading news, entertainment, information-seeking, shopping, travel, and health management. However, they were not significantly less likely to use social media for chatting/communication. Men had lower proportions of using social media for chatting/communication, entertainment, and shopping but were more likely to be motivated by reading news and information-seeking. Han Chinese reported higher proportions of using social media for entertainment and general information than ethnic minorities.

Urban residents and those with higher education levels consistently exhibited greater proportion of having all seven purposes of social media use than their respective counterparts. Economically disadvantaged individuals were less likely to use social media for chatting/communication, reading news, shopping, and travel. Blue-collar workers and agricultural workers had lower proportions for most

Table 14.1 Unweighted and weighted percentage distribution of the analytical sample by study variable, 2020, CLASS

	Social media users		Overall sample	
	Weighted	Unweighted	Weighted	Unweighted
N	2,805	2,805	11,228	11,228
% Use social media	–	–	28.2	25.0
Purposes of using social media				
% Chatting/communication	93.1	93.2	–	–
% Reading news	72.1	69.1	–	–
% Entertainments	63.2	65.3	–	–
% General information	44.4	44.3	–	–
% Shopping	29.4	26.8	–	–
% Travel	18.0	18.7	–	–
% Health	8.9	7.7	–	–
% Ages 65–74	81.6	58.4	64.8	38.0
% Ages 75–85	17.0	38.0	27.1	44.7
% Ages 85+	1.4	3.5	8.1	17.3
% Men	51.3	53.0	47.5	50.5
% Han ethnicity	95.4	94.9	95.5	94.0
% Urban residents	67.4	74.3	52.7	54.9
% 0 years of schooling	9.7	7.6	24.4	23.6
% 1–6 years of schooling	31.3	30.1	39.1	41.2
% 7+ years of schooling	59.0	62.4	36.5	35.2
% Economically poor	8.7	10.0	10.4	11.5
% White-collar occupation	22.3	23.1	10.8	11.7
% Blue-collar occupation	40.7	45.8	27.5	29.9
% Agricultural workers	37.0	31.1	61.7	58.4
% Currently Married	86.8	85.8	78.1	75.3
% Having 2+ close family members	85.3	83.6	80.5	79.7
% Having 2+ close friends	78.2	77.3	71.4	70.6
% Frequent engagement in leisure activity	89.4	91.9	82.1	83.2
Positive views on internet impact (0–8)[a]	3.33	3.33	2.12	2.08
Positive views on aging (7–35)[a]	21.24	21.01	20.68	20.60
Positive perceived aging (8–40)[a]	24.75	25.12	23.91	23.98
%Having 1+ diseases	76.8	81.2	79.6	80.4
% IADL disabled	9.4	11.5	18.7	24.2
% ADL disabled	7.9	9.3	11.3	15.1
% Cognitively impaired	10.8	13	24.5	30.4
% Good self-rated health	62.6	59.4	50.3	46.8
% East China	57.2	58.5	38.5	36.1
% Central China	18.3	15.2	27.1	25.7
% West China	14.7	12.5	25.7	24.8
% Northeast China	9.7	13.7	8.6	13.4

ADL activities of daily living, *IADL* instrumental ADL
[a]The mean score of the variable

Table 14.2 Weighted proportions of purposes for social media use among older adults in China, 2020, CLASS ($N = 2,805$)

	Chatting/communication	News	Entertainments	General info.	Shopping	Travel	Health
Total	93.1	72.1	63.2	44.4	29.4	18.0	8.9
Ages 65–74	93.3	73.5***	65.6***	46.5***	31.4***	19.4***	9.8***
Ages 75–85	92.3	67.1***	54.4***	36.5***	21.3***	12.6***	4.8***
Ages 85+	91.0	52.3***	28.5***	17.7***	9.2***	3.8***	1.6***
Women	94.3*	68.1***	68.0***	42.8+	31.7**	17.0	7.9+
Men	91.9*	75.9***	58.6***	46.0+	27.1**	19.0	9.8+
Non-Han minorities	96.7+	66.4	45.5***	28.1***	35.9+	20.0	6.1
Han ethnicity	92.9+	72.4	64.0***	45.2***	29.0+	17.9	9.0
Rural residents	90.5***	64.9***	58.2***	29.8***	25.1***	13.4***	3.9***
Urban residents	94.3***	75.6***	65.6***	51.5***	31.4***	20.3***	11.3***
0 years of schooling	87.2***	52.3***	59.0***	24.7***	17.9***	5.2***	3.7***
1–6 years of schooling	92.3***	65.4***	55.0***	32.6***	21.3***	9.5***	2.3***
7+ years of schooling	94.5***	78.9***	68.2***	53.9***	35.5***	24.6***	13.2***
Economically not poor	93.6**	73.1***	62.8	44.7	30.5***	18.6**	9.0
Economically poor	88.2**	61.9***	66.8	41.7	17.4***	11.6**	7.0
White-collar occupation	92.9***	83.6***	66.5***	58.2***	43.4***	27.6***	17.6***
Blue-collar occupation	95.2***	70.4***	68.6***	51.0***	31.4***	20.9***	10.6***
Agricultural workers	90.9***	67.1***	55.2***	28.9***	18.7***	9.1***	1.7***
Currently not married	93.7	68.8	54.2***	41.6	26.2	15.3	5.9*
Currently married	93.0	72.6	64.5***	44.8	29.8	18.4	9.3*
Having <2 close family members	87.1***	65.3***	59.9	42.7	23.8**	17.9	4.9**
Having 2+ close family members	94.1***	73.3***	63.7	44.7	30.3**	18.1	9.5**
Having < 2 close friends	89.4***	68.4*	60.2+	34.0***	20.1***	18.0	4.9***
Having 2+ close friends	94.1***	73.1*	64.0+	47.3***	31.9***	18.0	10.0***

(continued)

Table 14.2 (continued)

	Chatting/communication	News	Entertainments	General info.	Shopping	Travel	Health
Not freq. engagement in leisure activity	86.5***	65.7**	43.1***	17.0***	22.9*	10.4***	0.8***
Frequent engagement in leisure activity	93.9***	72.9**	65.6***	47.7***	30.1*	18.9***	9.8***
Positive views on internet impact (0–3)[a]	87.6***	66.5***	54.7***	34.0***	10.4***	8.0***	4.0***
Positive views on internet impact (4–8)[a]	97.5***	76.6***	69.9***	52.8***	44.5***	26.0***	12.8***
Positive views on aging (7–22)[a]	92.5^{+}	74.6***	60.4***	42.9*	28.8	18.4	9.7*
Positive views on aging (23–35)[a]	94.2^{+}	67.6***	68.2***	47.1*	30.5	17.5	7.4*
Positive perceived aging (8–25)[a]	93.9*	70.5*	59.5***	40.8***	30.3	15.8***	7.8**
Positive perceived aging (26–40)[a]	91.6*	75.0*	69.8***	51.1***	27.7	22.1***	10.8**
Having no chronic disease	89.0***	77.7***	61.0	40.2*	30.1	21.4*	11.0*
Having 1+ diseases	94.3***	70.4***	63.8	45.7*	29.1	17.0*	8.2*
IADL not diseased	94.1***	73.3***	64.8***	46.3***	30.5***	19.2***	9.7***
IADL disabled	83.4***	60.6***	47.3***	25.8***	18.6***	6.4***	0.9***
ADL not disabled	93.6***	73.5***	63.0	44.4	28.0***	17.0***	7.5***
ADL disabled	87.0***	56.2***	64.9	44.5	45.2***	29.6***	24.4***
Cognitively unimpaired	94.7***	72.9**	62.8	44.3	30.4***	18.4	9.5***
Cognitively impaired	79.8***	65.2**	65.9	45.5	20.6***	15.1	3.9***
Not good self-rated health	90.7***	70.9	59.7**	38.8***	29.3	17.2	10.2^{+}
Good Self-rated health	94.5***	72.8	65.2**	47.8***	29.4	18.5	8.1^{+}
East China	97.0***	71.0***	68.2***	58.1***	39.9***	23.9***	12.8***
Central China	89.7***	75.7***	52.3***	27.9***	13.6***	9.3***	0.3***
West China	83.8***	67.2***	51.4***	21.9***	23.0***	12.5***	7.6***
Northeast China	90.5***	79.0***	72.1***	29.2***	6.6***	8.0***	3.6***

ADL activities of daily living, IADL instrumental ADL

The percentages were weighted using the frequency weight. Statistical differences are based on chi-square tests after applying with the analytical weight

[a]Referring to the score range of the variable

$+p < 0.1$, $*p < 0.05$, $**p < 0.01$, $***p < 0.001$

purposes, except for chatting/communication and entertainment, compared to white-collar workers.

Married older adults were more likely to use social media for entertainment and health management than their unmarried counterparts. Individuals with larger family networks had a higher proportion of purposes for chatting/communication, reading news, shopping, and health management, whereas those with a greater number of close friends had higher proportions in almost all purposes, except for travel. Frequent participation in leisure activities and positive views and perceptions on internet technology were consistently associated with higher proportions in all seven purposes.

Regarding health status, individuals with at least one chronic condition were more likely to use social media for chatting and information-seeking but less likely to use it for reading news, travel, and health management. IADL disability was associated with lower proportions in all seven purposes, while ADL disability was linked to lower proportions for chatting or communication and reading news but higher proportions for shopping, travel, and health management. Individuals with cognitive impairment had lower proportions in most purposes except for entertainment, information-seeking, and travel. Those with good self-rated health reported higher proportions of purpose for chatting/communication, entertainment, and information-seeking.

Regional differences were also evident. Older adults in East China had the highest engagement in chatting, information-seeking, shopping, travel, and health management. Northeast residents reported greater engagement in reading news and entertainment but had the lowest engagement in shopping and travel. Participants from West China had the lowest proportions of chatting, reading news, entertainment, and information-seeking, while residents in Central China had the lowest engagement in health management.

14.3.2 Multivariable Regression Model Results

Table 14.3 presents the findings from multivariable regression models, which reveal several key patterns. After controlling for other factors, age differences were not significant for chatting/communication and reading news, whereas age was associated with lower odds of using social media for all other purposes. Gender patterns remained largely consistent with the results of bivariate analyses above: men were more likely to use social media for reading news and information-seeking, while women were more likely to use it for chatting/communication, entertainment, and shopping. Han Chinese were more likely to use social media for reading news and entertainment but less likely for chatting/communication. No statistically significant ethnic differences were observed for remaining purposes. Contrary to the findings of bivariate analyses above, differences between urban and rural residents were no longer significant after adjusting for socioeconomic status (SES), suggesting that disparities observed earlier were primarily due to differences in education, occupation, and income levels.

Table 14.3 Odds ratios of purposes for using social media by study variables, 2020, CLASS

	Chatting/communication	News	Entertainments	General info.	Shopping	Travel	Health
Ages 75–85 (65–74)	1.00	1.02	0.78**	0.72***	0.72**	0.67***	0.75+
Ages 85+ (65–74)	1.33	0.80	0.34***	0.37***	0.36**	0.50	0.61
Men (women)	0.66*	1.64***	0.73***	1.29**	0.82*	1.23+	1.24
Han ethnicity (minority)	0.35*	1.59*	2.46***	1.26	0.88	1.10	0.58+
Urban (rural)	1.46+	0.94	0.93	1.19	0.90	1.02	1.33
1–6 years of schooling (0)	3.26***	1.25	0.70*	1.59*	1.45	1.57	0.51
7+ years of schooling (0)	3.29***	1.68**	0.90	1.75**	1.68*	3.23***	1.22
Economically poor (no)	0.66	0.81	1.18	0.77+	0.79	0.68+	0.88
Blue-collar occupation (white-collar)	1.48	0.58***	1.36**	0.88	0.62***	0.95	0.77
Agricultural workers (white-collar)	1.93*	0.66**	1.23	0.71*	0.44***	0.56**	0.47*
Currently married (no)	0.88	1.07	1.30*	1.05	0.99	1.02	0.98
Having 2+ close family members (<2)	1.09	0.97	0.98	0.58***	0.59***	0.96	1.33
Having 2+ close friends (<2)	1.26	0.91	1.04	1.45**	1.14	0.70*	1.43
Freq. leisure and social activity (no)	1.84*	1.43*	1.49*	2.07***	0.93	1.12	1.75
Positive views on internet impact (0–8)	1.42***	1.18***	1.08***	1.12***	1.33***	1.30***	1.20***

Positive views on aging (7–35)	1.06**	0.96***	1.06***	0.99	1.02^{+}	0.99	1.02
Positive perceived aging (8–40)	0.94**	1.01	1.02*	1.10***	1.03**	1.08***	1.10***
Having 1+ diseases (no)	3.59***	0.81^{+}	1.00	1.29*	0.66***	0.61***	0.58**
IADL disabled (no)	0.51*	0.80	0.48***	0.55***	0.71^{+}	0.36***	0.15***
ADL disabled (no)	0.72	0.32***	1.03	0.82	0.92	1.58*	2.37***
Cognitively impaired (no)	0.33***	0.93	1.26^{+}	1.44**	0.88	1.25	1.20
Good self-rated health (no)	1.02	1.13	1.13	1.29**	0.95	0.85	0.69*
Central China (East China)	0.19***	1.82***	0.65***	0.40***	0.37***	0.39***	0.11***
West China (East China)	0.10***	1.29^{+}	0.81	0.33***	1.07	0.88	1.24
Northeast China (East China)	0.27***	2.31***	1.82***	0.70**	0.26***	0.46***	0.67
-LL	456.2	1584.4	1673.6	1627.1	1316.8	1086.2	618.1
LR chi-square	482.7	300.2	275.2	597.6	629.8	529.2	291.3

ADL activities of daily living, *IADL* instrumental ADL
The degree of freedom for all models is 25
$+p < 0.1$, $*p < 0.05$, $**p < 0.01$, $***p < 0.001$

Education remained a strong predictor for purposes using social media: with the exception of entertainment and health management, more years of schooling were associated with higher odds of having all other purposes. However, economic status was no longer a significant factor after controlling for other variables, differing from the bivariate findings that showed significant disparities across five of the seven purposes. Occupational differences remained consistent: blue-collar and agricultural workers were more likely to use social media for chatting/communication or entertainment, while white-collar workers were more likely to have the other five purposes.

Marital status also played a role: married older adults had higher odds of using social media for entertainment than their unmarried counterparts. The effect of social ties was mixed. Having a greater number of close family members was associated with lower odds of using social media for information-seeking and shopping, while having more close friends was linked to greater odds of using social media for information-seeking but lower odds of using it for travel, differing from results of bivariate analyses. Engagement in leisure activities and positive views on internet technology were generally associated with higher odds of using social media for all purposes, aligning with the findings of bivariate analyses. Positive perceived aging was associated with higher odds of using social media for most purposes, except for reading news and chatting/communication. Similarly, holding positive views on aging showed comparable patterns when positive behaviors were not controlled for (results not shown). However, after accounting for the practice of positive aging behaviors, holding positive views on aging was associated only with higher odds of using social media for chatting/communication and entertainment, and lower odds for reading news.

The results of health-related variables were mixed. IADL disability was the most consistent predictor, showing lower engagements across all seven purposes. Older adults with one or more chronic conditions had lower odds of using social media for shopping, travel, and health management, but higher odds for chatting/communication and information-seeking. ADL disability was associated with higher odds of having purposes for travel and health-related use but lower odds of having the purpose for reading news. Cognitive impairment, unlike in bivariate analyses, was associated with higher odds of having the purpose for information-seeking but lower odds of having the purpose for chatting/communication, possibly due to interactions with other health factors. Good self-rated health was linked to higher odds of having the purpose for information-seeking but lower odds of having the purpose for health management, again differing from the results of bivariate analyses due to confounding effects.

Regional differences are consistent with those in bivariate associations in Table 14.2. Specifically, compared to older adults in East China, individuals in Northeast China had higher odds of using social media for reading news and entertainment but lower odds for other purposes, after taking other factors into account. Older adults in Central China had lower odds across all seven purposes, while those in West China were less likely to use social media for chatting and information-seeking.

14.4 Discussion

Using the latest publicly available wave of CLASS, we examined the purposes of using social media among older adults aged 65 or older in China. Our findings reveal that chatting and/or contacting family and friends are the most prevalent purposes, reported by 93.1% of users. This finding underscores the primary role of social media as a communication tool, aligning with global patterns reported in Chap. 2. Reading news was the second prevalent purpose, reported by 72.1%, followed by entertainment (63.2%) and general information-seeking (44.4%). In contrast, more specialized purposes such as online shopping (29.4%), travelling (18.0%), and health management (8.9%) are less prevalent.

These patterns highlight a strong preference for interpersonal communication and information access among older adults in China, indicating the social media's centrality in later lives for maintaining social connections and staying informed. Entertainment and information-seeking further illustrate the role of social media as a multifaceted platform to serve various needs at older ages. However, the relatively less prevalence in purposes for more specialized tasks, such as health management and travel planning, suggests that social media has not been stepped into all corners of later lives of older Chinese adults. Overall, these patterns mirror global and regional patterns that social media function primarily as a tool for communication and content consumption rather than task-specific applications (Kemp, 2025). The findings confirm the dual utility of social media in contemporary aging societies, both as a platform for social interaction and a gateway to information, while its potential for more specialized uses remains underutilized among older populations.

The multivariable regression analyses presented in this chapter reveal intricate patterns in the purposes of social media use among older adults in China, shaped by demographic, socioeconomic, social, lifestyle, health, and regional factors. These findings underscore the complexity of digital engagement in later life and highlight the interplay between structural inequalities, individual resources, and sociocultural contexts. Below, we interpret these results variable by variable, contextualizing empirical evidence and elucidating potential mechanisms based on prior studies.

14.4.1 Key Findings and Interpretations

14.4.1.1 Demographic Factors

The absence of significant age differences in social media use for chatting/communication and reading news aligns with prior research, indicating the universal adoption of social media to stay connected with family and access news (Cotten et al., 2013; Hunsaker & Hargittai, 2018). These activities fulfill fundamental social and cognitive needs, consistent with UGT (Katz et al., 1973), which posits that individuals actively seek media to satisfy needs on social interaction and information acquisition (Yuan et al., 2016). However, older adults exhibited lower odds of using social media for more complex or leisure-oriented purposes (e.g., shopping and travel). This is likely due to age-related declines in digital literacy or perceived relevance (Czaja et al., 2019; Friemel, 2016). This aligns with STAM (Chen & Chan, 2014; Renaud & van Biljon, 2008), which highlights perceived usefulness and ease of use as critical determinants of older adults' technology adoption.

Men's higher engagement in news consumption and information-seeking reflects gendered patterns of socialization, wherein men have traditionally prioritized instrumental and knowledge-based activities (Knobloch-Westerwick & Alter, 2007; Gao & Martin-Kratzer, 2011). Conversely, women's more frequent use of social media for chatting/communication, entertainment, and shopping aligns with studies emphasizing their role in maintaining kinship networks and managing household responsibilities (Gao & Martin-Kratzer, 2011), which is also consistent with the global data shown in Chap. 2 as well as studies in other countries (e.g., Omar & Hirst, 2006; Tutar et al., 2024). These gendered patterns may also stem from gender differences in perceiving the utility of social media; for instance, online shopping could be perceived by women as a convenient approach in household management (Peng, 2022).

The higher engagement of Han Chinese individuals in news and entertainment is in line with the broader trends of their higher digital engagement, likely due to their greater socioeconomic resources and more urbanized living environments (Yang & Du, 2021). Their lower likelihood of using social media for chatting/communication may reflect a preference for face-to-face interactions within Han-dominant communities. Alternatively, it may indicate a strong reliance on traditional communication methods among ethnic minorities, who maintain close-knit social structures (Zhang & He, 2022). The lack of ethnic differences in other purposes is possibly because rapid ICT development in ethnic minority regions and/or the CLASS sampling issue as noted in Chap. 9 may contribute to such ethnic differences. We welcome more research on ethnic differences in social media use.

The disappearance of urban-rural differences after adjusting for SES underscores the central role of education, occupation, and income in shaping digital access and use. Rural older adults' lower SES may restrict their ability to acquire devices, afford data plans, or develop advanced skills, thereby perpetuating digital inequalities (Zhao & Kuang, 2025). This finding aligns with the established literature that the digital divide between urban and rural older adults is primarily mediated by socioeconomic resources rather than geographic location alone (Hu & Xu, 2024), also consistent with van Deursen and Helsper's (2015) argument that material resources and digital skills, not mere physical access, determine meaningful digital participation.

14.4.1.2 Socioeconomic Factors

The strong association between education and most purposes of using social media (excluding entertainment and health management) highlights the role of education as a form of resource capital that enables older adults to use social media for complex purposes such as information-seeking effectively and confidently (Bhattacharjee et al., 2021; Helsper & Van Deursen, 2017). According to TPB (Ajzen, 1991), education enhances perceived behavioral control, making individuals more likely to engage with digital tools (Khoo & Yang, 2020). The non-significant association between SES and entertainment and health management suggests that these activities may rely less on formal education but more on intrinsic motivation or immediate needs; for example, health-related use of social media may be driven by health urgency rather than skills (Heponiemi et al., 2020). The non-significance of economic status in multivariable model, despite its significance in bivariate analyses, implies that income disparities in the purpose of using social media are mediated by education and occupation. This supports with Calderón Gómez's (2021) bidirectional capital conversion theory: while economic capital can facilitate social media access (e.g., device ownership), its impact diminishes without complementary human capital (e.g., digital skills).

Blue-collar and agricultural workers' preference for chatting/communication and entertainment mirrors their limited exposure to advanced digital tools, which constrains their usage to socially oriented activities. By contrast, white-collar workers' broader engagement patterns align with their routine exposure to digital technologies in work settings, where diverse applications are normalized and integrated into daily task (Büchi et al., 2016). These occupational divides reflect entrenched class-based inequalities in digital capital accumulation (Hargittai, 2002).

14.4.1.3 Social and Lifestyle Factors

The higher odds of using social media for entertainment among married older adults may stem from spousal companionship, which encourages shared leisure activities, facilitated by social media (Szabo et al., 2019). Conversely, unmarried individuals may prioritize functional uses of social media (e.g., health management) due to reduced social support (Heponiemi et al., 2020). The mixed effects of family members and friends underscore the dual role of social networks: while family ties may reduce the need for information-seeking (e.g., seeking advice for relative), close friends, which are often sources of novel information, may encourage exploratory behaviors online (Myhre et al., 2017). The negative association between friends and the purpose of social media for travel may reflect a trade-off in which maintaining expansive online friendships online could limit opportunities for travel.

Positive views and perceived aging were linked to having most purposes of using social media, except for news reading and chatting/communication. This supports Levy et al.'s (2002) assertion that proactive aging attitudes motivate health-promoting behaviors, including the adoption of related technologies. Considering UGT (Katz et al., 1973) that people use media based on personal needs, older adults with positive perceived aging may be more inclined to use digital platforms for entertainment, health management, and shopping, viewing social media as tools that enhance their autonomy and well-being. Conversely, news consumption and chatting/communication may be perceived as habitual activities, thus less influenced by one's self-perceptions.

14.4.1.4 Health Factors

The consistent negative associated between IADL disability and all purposes highlights the cascading effects of physical decline on digital engagement. Older adults with IADL disability may struggle with manipulating devices, suffering digital exclusion (Yusif et al., 2016). Conversely, the positive association between ADL disability and social media use for travel and health-related purposes may reflect compensatory strategies. For example, individuals with mobility limitations may turn to social media to access telehealth services or participate in virtual tours (Zaman et al., 2022). This is consistent with previous research showing that physically limited older adults often use technology as a compensatory tool to access the outside world (Bertolazzi, et al., 2024).

The dual effects of chronic diseases, reducing shopping, travel, and health management but increasing chatting/communication and information-seeking, suggests that health status reshapes behavioral priorities. Individuals with chronic conditions may withdraw from resource-intensive activities (e.g., travel) to intensify online communication to seek health information and support (Yuan, 2021). The reversal of cognitive impairment's effects in multivariable models, where information-seeking increased while chatting/communication decreased, may stem from compensatory mechanisms (Baltes & Baltes, 1993; Kraut et al., 1998, 2002). Cognitively impaired older adults, for example, might prioritize information-seeking to manage health, while avoiding complex social interactions (Wang et al., 2024). This aligns with Lachman and Andreoletti's (2006) finding that strategic use of social media mediates impact of cognitive decline on behaviors. Additionally, caregivers may facilitate online engagement by assisting individuals with cognitive difficulties in navigating online for health information (Zaman et al., 2022).

14.4.1.5 Regional Differences

Persistent regional disparities reflect uneven economic development and infrastructural investment in China. Older adults from Northeast China had higher odds of using social media for news reading and entertainment, but lower engagement in other purposes, may stem from industrial legacies. The dominance of state-owned enterprises in the region has historically fostered media consumption habits while limiting exposure to diverse digital services (Zhang & He, 2022). Central China's uniformly lower odds of all purposes can be attributed to its agrarian economy and lower SES of the local residents, while West China's deficits in chatting and information-seeking mirror its underdeveloped economy, limited digital infrastructure, ethnic diversity, and lower digital literacy (Zhao, 2015).

14.4.1.6 Strengths and Limitations

This study's strengths include its comprehensive consideration of variables across sociodemographic, psychosocial, and health domains and its use of nationally representative data. The integration of health and psychosocial factors advances beyond traditional digital divide frameworks focused solely on access (van Deursen & van Dijk, 2019). However, limitations include the cross-sectional design, which precludes causal inferences. Self-reported measures may introduce recall bias, and unobserved variables (e.g., platform-specific affordances) could influence usage patterns. Additionally, cultural dynamics not captured in the data could influence the findings, necessitating qualitative research for deeper insights.

14.4.2 Policy Implications

Tailored interventions are needed to address digital skill gaps among rural, less-educated, and older-old populations. Expanding broadband access in rural and western regions is critical. Although China's State Council (2020) has outlined plans to improve the accessibility of smart technology, effective implementation must prioritize marginalized communities. Policymakers should promote telehealth platforms that accommodate functional limitations, in line with the UN *Decade of Healthy Ageing* (United Nations, 2020). Moreover, platforms should cater to women's preferences (e.g., integrating shopping tools with family management features) and men's informational needs (e.g., curated news feeds).

14.4.3 Future Research Directions

Longitudinal studies are needed to unravel temporal dynamics between health declines and digital engagement. Qualitative approaches are also essential to elucidate how cultural norms shape usage preferences, for instance, by exploring ethnic minorities' platform experiences. Additionally, experimental studies could test interventions designed to convert economic capital into digital capital among low-SES older adults. Finally, cross-national comparative studies are needed to identify which determinants of digital inclusion are universal and which are context-specific, strengthening the generalizability of findings across different aging societies.

14.4.4 Conclusions

This chapter examined the complex factors shaping purposes of social media use among older adults in China, highlighting the role of structural inequalities, individual resources, and sociocultural contexts. Understanding the purposes of social media use is key to promoting digital inclusion. By identifying older adults' motivations, whether for social connection, information access, or civic participation when using social media, researchers can pinpoint barriers to effective digital engagement. These insights thus can inform targeted policies and interventions that enhance the relevance, accessibility, and usability of digital tools and training for older populations. Moreover, uncovering the goals of social media use helps advance our understanding of digital literacy, and thus helps bridge generational divides and foster a more inclusive digital society where older adults can fully participate in social and economic life in the digital era.

Acknowledgement The authors would like to thank the Research Center for Population & Development and the Institute of Gerontology, Renmin University for providing access to the China Longitudinal Aging and Social Survey (CLASS) dataset used in this chapter.

Disclaimer Views expressed in the chapter are solely those of the authors and do not necessarily reflect those of the United Nations, the National University of Singapore, Virginia Tech, and Yale University.

References

Ajzen, I. (1991). The theory of planned behavior. *Organizational Behavior and Human Decision Processes, 50*(2), 179–211.
Baltes, P. B., & Baltes, M. M. (1993). *Successful aging: Perspectives from the behavioral sciences* (Vol. 4). Cambridge University Press.
Bertolazzi, A., Quaglia, V., & Bongelli, R. (2024). Barriers and facilitators to health technology adoption by older adults with chronic diseases: An integrative systematic review. *BMC Public Health, 24*(1), 506.
Bhattacharjee, P., Baker, S., & Waycott, J. (2021). Older adults and their acquisition of digital skills: A review of current research evidence. In *Proceedings of the 32nd Australian conference on human-computer interaction* (pp. 437–443).
Büchi, M. (2024). Digital well-being theory and research. *New Media & Society, 26*(1), 172–189.
Büchi, M., Just, N., & Latzer, M. (2016). Modeling the second-level digital divide: A five-country study of social differences in Internet use. *New Media & Society, 18*(11), 2703–2722.
Calderón Gómez, D. (2021). The third digital divide and Bourdieu: Bidirectional conversion of economic, cultural, and social capital to (and from) digital capital among young people in Madrid. *New Media & Society, 23*(9), 2534–2553.
Chen, K., & Chan, A. H. (2014). Gerontechnology acceptance by elderly Hong Kong Chinese: A senior technology acceptance model (STAM). *Ergonomics, 57*(5), 635–652.
China Internet Network Information Center (CNNIC). (2011). *The 27th statistical report on China's Internet development*. https://www.cac.gov.cn/files/pdf/hlwtjbg/hlwlfzzkdctjbg027.pdf [in Chinese].
China Internet Network Information Center (CNNIC). (2025). *The 55th statistical report on China's Internet development*. https://www.cnnic.net.cn/n4/2025/0117/c88-11229.html [in Chinese].

Choi, N. G., & DiNitto, D. M. (2013). Internet use among older adults: Association with health needs, psychological capital, and social capital. *Journal of Medical Internet Research, 15*(5), e93.

Chopik, W. J. (2016). The benefits of social technology use among older adults are mediated by reduced loneliness. *Cyberpsychology, Behavior, and Social Networking, 19*(9), 551–556.

Cotten, S. R., Anderson, W. A., & McCullough, B. M. (2013). Impact of Internet use on loneliness and contact with others among older adults: Cross-sectional analysis. *Journal of Medical Internet Research, 15*(2), e39.

Czaja, S. J., Boot, W. R., Charness, N., & Rogers, W. A. (2019). *Designing for older adults: Principles and creative human factors approaches*. CRC Press.

Dong, T., Zhu, Z., Guo, M., Du, P., & Wu, B. (2019). Association between dying experience and place of death: Urban–rural differences among older Chinese adults. *Journal of Palliative Medicine, 22*(11), 1386–1393.

Friemel, T. N. (2016). The digital divide has grown old: Determinants of a digital divide among seniors. *New Media & Society, 18*(2), 313–331.

Gao, F., & Martin-Kratzer, R. (2011). Gender differences in Chinese journalists' blogs. *Chinese Journal of Communication, 4*(02), 167–181.

Hargittai, E. (2002). Second-level digital divide: Mapping differences in people's online skills. *First Monday, 7*(4). https://doi.org/10.5210/fm.v7i4.942

Helsper, E. J., & Van Deursen, A. J. A. M. (2017). Do the rich get digitally richer? Quantity and quality of support for digital engagement. *Information, Communication & Society, 20*(5), 700–714.

Heponiemi, T., Jormanainen, V., Leemann, L., Manderbacka, K., Aalto, A.-M., & Hyppönen, H. (2020). Digital divide in perceived benefits of online health care and social welfare services: National cross-sectional survey study. *Journal of Medical Internet Research, 22*(7), e17616.

Hu, H., & Xu, W. (2024). Socioeconomic differences in digital inequality among older Chinese adults: Results from a nationally representative sample. *PLoS One, 19*(4), e0300433.

Hunsaker, A., & Hargittai, E. (2018). A review of Internet use among older adults. *New Media & Society, 20*(10), 3937–3954.

Jin, Y., & Zhao, M. (2019). Internet access and the elderly's active aging in China—A study based on 2016 China Longitudinal Aging Social Survey. *Population Journal, 6*, 44–55. [in Chinese].

Katz, E., Blumler, J. G., & Gurevitch, M. (1973). Uses and gratifications research. *Public Opinion Quarterly, 37*(4), 509–523.

Kemp, S. (2025). Digital 2025: Global Overview Report. https://datareportal.com/reports/digital-2025-global-overview-report

Khoo, S. S., & Yang, H. (2020). Social media use improves executive functions in middle-aged and older adults: A structural equation modeling analysis. *Computers in Human Behavior, 111*, 106388.

Knobloch-Westerwick, S., & Alter, S. (2007). The gender news use divide: Americans' sex-typed selective exposure to online news topics. *Journal of Communication, 57*(4), 739–758.

Kraut, R., Kiesler, S., Boneva, B., Cummings, J., Helgeson, V., & Crawford, A. (2002). Internet paradox revisited. *Journal of Social Issues, 58*(1), 49–74.

Kraut, R., Patterson, M., Lundmark, V., Kiesler, S., Mukopadhyay, T., & Scherlis, W. (1998). Internet paradox: A social technology that reduces social involvement and psychological well-being? *American Psychologist, 53*(9), 1017–1031.

Lachman, M. E., & Andreoletti, C. (2006). Strategy use mediates the relationship between control beliefs and memory performance for middle-aged and older adults. *Journal of Gerontology: Psychological Sciences, 61*(2), 88–94.

Levy, B. R., Slade, M. D., & Kasl, S. V. (2002). Longitudinal benefit of positive self-perceptions of aging on functional health. *Journal of Gerontology: Psychological Sciences, 57*(5), 409–417.

Myhre, J. W., Mehl, M. R., & Glisky, E. L. (2017). Cognitive benefits of online social networking for healthy older adults. *Journal of Gerontology: Psychological Sciences, 72*(5), 752–760.

Omar, O. E., & Hirst, A. (2006). Apparel shopping: A focus on the attitudes of women towards online shopping. *International Journal of Electronic Marketing and Retailing, 1*(2), 169–182.

Peng, Y. (2022). Gendered division of digital labor in parenting: A qualitative study in urban China. *Sex Roles, 86*(5–6), 283–304.

Renaud, K., & van Biljon, J. (2008). Predicting technology acceptance and adoption by the elderly: A qualitative study. In *Proceedings of the 2008 annual research conference of the South African Institute of Computer Scientists and Information Technologists* (pp. 210–219).

Seifert, A., Cotten, S. R., & Xie, B. (2021). A double burden of exclusion? Digital and social exclusion of older adults in times of COVID-19. *The Journals of Gerontology: Series B, 76*(3), e99–e103.

State Council. (2020). *Implementation plan for effectively addressing the difficulties faced by older adults in using smart technology.* https://www.gov.cn/zhengce/zhengceku/2020-11/24/content_5563804.htm [in Chinese].

Szabo, A., Allen, J., Stephens, C., & Alpass, F. (2019). Longitudinal analysis of the relationship between purposes of internet use and well-being among older adults. *The Gerontologist, 59*(1), 58–68.

Tutar, G., Küçükoğlu, H., Özdemir, A., Alkan, Ö., & Ipekten, O. B. (2024). An investigation of gender differences in e-commerce shopping frequency during COVID-19: Evidence from Türkiye. *SAGE Open, 14*(4). https://doi.org/10.1177/21582440241287

United Nations. (2015). *Transforming our world: The 2030 agenda for sustainable development.* https://sdgs.un.org/2030agenda

United Nations. (2020). *Decade of healthy aging (2021–2030).* https://www.who.int/initiatives/decade-of-healthy-ageing

van Deursen, A. J. A. M., & Helsper, E. J. (2015). The third-level digital divide: Who benefits most from being online? In L. Robinson, S. R. Cotten, J. Schulz, T. M. Hale, & A. Williams (Eds.), *Communication and information technologies annual: Digital distinctions and inequalities* (Vol. 10, pp. 29–52). Emerald Group Publishing.

van Deursen, A. J., & van Dijk, J. (2019). The first-level digital divide shifts from inequalities in physical access to inequalities in material access. *New Media & Society, 21*(2), 354–375.

Wang, K., Chen, X. S., Kang, S. Y., Smith, B. D., & Gu, D. (2024). Older adults' online activities and cognition: Investigating the psychological mechanisms and age and gender differences. *Social Science & Medicine, 352*, 116988.

Wu, J., & Song, S. (2021). Older adults' online shopping continuance intentions: Applying the Technology Acceptance Model and the Theory of Planned Behavior. *International Journal of Human Computer Interaction, 37*(10), 938–948.

Yang, J., & Du, P. (2021). Gender, capital endowment and digital exclusion of older people in China. *Ageing and Society, 41*(11), 2502–2526.

Yuan, H. (2021). Internet use and mental health problems among older people in Shanghai, China: The moderating roles of chronic diseases and household income. *Aging & Mental Health, 25*(4), 657–663.

Yuan, S., Hussain, S. A., Hales, K. D., & Cotten, S. R. (2016). What do they like? Communication preferences and patterns of older adults in the United States: The role of technology. *Educational Gerontology, 42*(3), 163–174.

Yusif, S., Soar, J., & Hafeez-Baig, A. (2016). Older people, assistive technologies, and the barriers to adoption: A systematic review. *International Journal of Medical Informatics, 94*, 112–116.

Zaman, S. B., Khan, R. K., Evans, R. G., Thrift, A. G., Maddison, R., & Islam, S. M. S. (2022). Exploring barriers to and enablers of the adoption of information and communication technology for the care of older adults with chronic diseases: Scoping review. *JMIR Aging, 5*(1), e25251.

Zhang, H., & He, R. (2022). A study on digital inclusion of Chinese rural older adults from a life course perspective. *Frontiers in Public Health, 10*, 974998.

Zhao, L. (2015). The digital divides among undergraduates in China: An analysis based on the survey data from 12 universities and colleges. *Sociological Studies, 30*(06), 145–168.

Zhao, Y., & Kuang, M. (2025). Digital divides in China: Evidence from CGSS2005-2021. *Chinese Sociological Review*, 1–62.

Chapter 15
Reciprocal Associations Between Self-perception of Aging and Social Media Use Among Older Adults: Exploring Gender and Age Differences

Kun Wang and Danan Gu

15.1 Introduction

Despite the fast growth of social media use in the past two decades, more than half of older adults in the United States (U.S.) did not report any social media use in 2020 (Pew Research Center, 2021). Previous studies indicate that older adults' self-perception of aging (SPA) may be an important factor in their technology adoption and usage (Chen & Chan, 2014; Choi et al., 2020). SPA, older adults' attitudes toward their own aging (Levy et al., 2002), comprises both positive and negative dimensions (Barker et al., 2007; Brown et al., 2021). The positive dimension includes positive attitudes and perceptions in terms of self-control and the consequences of aging, while the negative dimension incorporates an awareness of aging, a negative perception of self-control, and negative emotions attached to the process of aging (Brown et al., 2021). Research has shown that the elevation of one dimension does not necessarily imply that the other cannot be elevated, as individuals can

Note on Reuse of Published Materials
This chapter incorporates a revised and expanded version of material originally published in the article *"Reciprocal associations between social media use and self-perception of aging among older adults: Do men and women differ?"* by Wang, K. & Gu, D. (2023), published in *Social Science & Medicine, 321,* 115786. The original work has been adapted and updated, in accordance with the publisher's policies.

K. Wang (✉)
Department of Social Work, College of Arts and Sciences, University of Alabama at Birmingham, Birmingham, AL, USA
e-mail: kw2@uab.edu

D. Gu
Population Division, UN Department of Economic and Social Affairs, New York, NY, USA
e-mail: gudanan@yahoo.com

K. Wang et al. (eds.), *ICT Use and Healthy Longevity*, Advances in Studies of Aging and Health 5, https://doi.org/10.1007/978-3-031-98964-3_15

endorse both positive and negative SPA simultaneously, and their SPA can change over time (Blawert & Wurm, 2021; Sargent-Cox et al., 2014)

Older adults' internalized negative stereotypes about aging, that is, the negative dimension of SPA, may cause them to devalue their competencies and feel too old to learn and use social media (Choi et al., 2020; Lagacé et al., 2015). On the other hand, in the era of modern technology, being excluded from networking in a virtual world may reduce their sources of social support (Yu et al., 2021; Zhang et al., 2021), increase social isolation and loneliness (Szabo et al., 2019; Yu et al., 2021), lower their life satisfaction and well-being (Gaia et al., 2021; Szabo et al., 2019), and ultimately contribute to negative attitudes towards aging. Although less common than negative SPA, positive SPA has also been reported among older adults (Barker et al., 2007; Brown et al., 2021). With higher endorsements of positive SPA, older adults may have more confidence and willingness to learn and use social media (Chen & Chan, 2014). Meanwhile, social interactions and social support gained via social media may reduce social isolation and loneliness (Yu et al., 2021; Zhang et al., 2021) and promote more positive SPA (Köttl et al., 2021).

However, no studies have examined reciprocal associations between SPA and social media use among older adults. Despite a few longitudinal studies investigating associations between SPA and digital technology use, contradictory results have been reported. In a recently published paper based on the 2014 and 2017 waves of the German Ageing Survey, researchers found that more use of everyday information and communication technology (ICT) demonstrated a recursive, negative relationship with the personal competence aspect of negative SPA (Köttl et al., 2021). By contrast, using the same datasets, Mariano et al. (2021a) found that the associations between internet use and the competence aspect of SPA were reciprocal. Another recent study by the same researchers indicated reciprocal associations between computer use and SPA among middle-aged and older adults from the US and Germany, despite a stronger impact of SPA on computer use (Mariano et al., 2021b). Thus, more studies are needed to further examine the reciprocal associations between SPA and social media use among older adults. Moreover, gender differences have been widely noted in social media use. Older women are more likely to use social media than older men (Ihm & Hsieh, 2015; Newman et al., 2021). In terms of use purpose, women are more likely to use social media to maintain their close social ties, while men are more interested in broadening their social circle (Baumeister & Sommer, 1997; Krasnova et al., 2017). These gender differences in social media use may lead to different impacts on SPA for men and women that deserve further exploration.

Thus, in this study, we aim to investigate the reciprocal associations between SPA (positive and negative) and social media use and examine whether the reciprocal associations differ by gender. This study's findings may deepen our understanding of these associations and provide more empirical evidence for future interventions to increase older adults' social media use and reduce their negative SPA or promote positive SPA.

15.1.1 The Impact of SPA on Social Media Use

Older adults' unique characteristics and capacities need to be considered in understanding their technology acceptance and usage behaviors (Chen & Chan, 2014). Incorporating aging-related factors, such as physical and cognitive capacities, psychological well-being, and life course events, Chen and Chan (2014) proposed the Senior Technology Adoption Model (STAM) (Chen & Chan, 2014). Along with life satisfaction, attitude toward aging (positive SPA) was included to compose the psychological well-being construct in STAM, a positive predictor of technology use found in a sample of older adults in Hong Kong (Chen & Chan, 2014). Older adults with high positive SPA may have high perceived control (Levy et al., 2002), defined as the "belief that one has a choice among responses that are differentially effective in achieving the desired outcome" (Langer & Abelson, 1983, p. 20). Consistent with several studies indicating a positive relationship between perceived control and acceptance of new technologies in the general population (Huang et al., 2011; Le et al., 2022), high perceived self-control may reduce technophobia and bring older adults the confidence to learn and use new technology.

On the other hand, negative SPA, also known as internalized ageism or self-directed ageism, is the negative attitude that older adults perceive about the aging process. Self-fulfilling prophecies may be relevant to negative SPA to the extent that older adults high in negative SPA unintentionally engage in behaviors that reify their negative SPA (Allport, 1954; Merton, 1957). For example, Levy et al. (2002) indicated that the development of SPA happens at two life stages: first, prior to late adulthood, individuals collect and internalize expectations about aging based on how they observe others' attributes changing at different life stages; second, these expectations about aging are consolidated with daily encounters at older ages. The negative expectations, such as the inability to learn in old age (van Deursen & Helsper, 2015), may unconsciously affect older adults' thoughts and behaviors (Levy et al., 2002). It may intensify their technophobia (Hogan, 2009), lower their motivation and self-efficacy to learn new technology (Lagacé et al., 2015), and eventually fulfill their expectations by leading them to believe that they are too old to learn or use social media. Emerging evidence supports the association between negative SPA and older adults' lower ICT use (Choi et al., 2020; Lagacé et al., 2015). Among a convenience sample of Canadian older adults, Lagacé et al. (2015) found that endorsement of ageist stereotypes was negatively associated with ICT use competency. Using a nationally representative sample in the U.S., researchers revealed that older women with more self-directed ageism used the internet less frequently (Choi et al., 2020).

Based on these reviews, we thus propose our first hypothesis:

H1a: Higher positive SPA predicts more frequent social media use among older adults.

H1b: Higher negative SPA predicts less frequent social media use among older adults.

15.1.2 The Impact of Social Media Use on SPA

Growing evidence has linked social media and other forms of ICT use to various positive health and well-being outcomes, such as reduced social isolation and loneliness (Cotten et al., 2013), reduced depression (Jeon et al., 2020), better physical and cognitive functioning (Dasgupta et al., 2016; Myhre et al., 2017), and increased well-being (Szabo et al., 2019). Thus, it is plausible that social media use may also benefit older adults' SPA. The benefits may be derived from two parts: new technology use in general and social media use specifically.

With the fast advancement and wide adoption of new technologies, society is gradually moving to the Fourth Industrial Revolution, characterized by various new technologies fusing the physical, digital, and biological worlds and changing individuals' lives and minds (Schwab, 2017). However, for older adults who did not grow up with these new technologies, joining the Fourth Industrial Revolution or not becomes a critical challenge. The lifespan theory of control posits that individuals actively shape their lives across their lifespan and endeavor to exert control over their immediate environment through primary and secondary control (Heckhausen & Schulz, 1995). Primary control reflects direct outward strategies to change the external environment to achieve desired goals; secondary control reflects inward strategies to adjust one's own mind to align with the current situation (Heckhausen & Schulz, 1995). Although primary control has primacy over secondary control, physiological and cognitive decline in late adulthood may make it very difficult for older adults to take primary control strategies to learn and use new technologies (Heckhausen, 1999; Schulz & Heckhausen, 1996). If they can learn and use new technologies, this goal achievement may serve as a "sally port" to break the vicious self-fulfilling prophecy and reduce negative SPA. As shown in a qualitative study, older adults indicated that technology use made them feel young and modern, perhaps changing negative preconceived ideas that they possessed about technology and aging (Juárez et al., 2016). In a study among a large sample of older Americans, Steward and Hasche (2021) found that computer use increased older adults' positive SPA directly and indirectly through increased self-efficacy. However, if older adults cannot learn and use new technologies, they may implement secondary control strategies to disengage from the goal or think in a self-protective manner (Heckhausen & Schulz, 1995). For example, they may devalue the importance of new technology or perseverate upon negative age stereotypes such as "too old to learn". Although it may reach a final balance, stress caused by the process of inwardly adjusting their cognition (Haynes et al., 2009) may evoke older adults' negative thoughts about aging and reduce their positive SPA. Köttl et al. (2021) found that low engagement in everyday ICT use predicted increased negative SPA in personal competence among older adults.

Besides the general benefits of new technology use, social media, as an important online communication tool, may affect older adults' SPA through its unique attribute—social networking. Previous theories and studies indicate positive associations between social interactions and older adults' well-being (Baumeister &

Leary, 1995; Havighurst, 1961; Luo et al., 2022). However, due to physiological decline and social role changes, such as muscle mass loss (Makizako et al., 2019), functioning disability (Schneider et al., 2011), retirement (Oliffe et al., 2013), and widowhood (Yang & Gu, 2021), many older adults have reduced social network sizes and interactions and may have falsely believed that late adulthood is a time of loneliness. Social media use breaks the restrictions of distance and mobility and increases older adults' opportunities to enhance their social interactions. Thus, increased interactions via social media may reduce older adults' loneliness (Cotten et al., 2013; Szabo et al., 2019) and depression (Jeon et al., 2020) and promote well-being (Dasgupta et al., 2016; Szabo et al., 2019), which may reduce negative stereotypes of old age and facilitate positive attitudes about aging. Thus, we propose our second hypothesis:

H2a: More frequent use of social media predicts increased positive SPA.
H2b: More frequent use of social media predicts reduced negative SPA.

15.1.3 Gender Differences

The "double standard of aging" (Sontag, 1972) suggests that older women are more harshly judged than older men. Due to the intersection of ageism and sexism, older women not only experience stereotypes against their old age, including "weak", "forgetful", and "old-fashioned" (Richeson & Shelton, 2006) but also are stigmatized as "weak" and/or "not interested in science and technology" because of their female gender (Koenig, 2018). However, several studies have argued that the gender difference regarding ageism is domain-specific (Kornadt et al., 2013; Rothermund & Kornadt, 2015). For example, Kornadt et al. (2013) found that, despite the reverse effect in domains relevant to agency (e.g., work, finance), older women were rated more positively than older men in domains pertaining to social contacts, such as friends, religion, and leisure. Although social media can be used to maintain and promote social contacts, it is a form of digital technology, which is stereotyped as a masculine domain: women are believed to be less proficient than men in using digital technology across age groups (Bausch et al., 2014; Franz et al., 2019). Thus, societal expectations may be internalized by older women in the form of negative SPA, resulting in a more pronounced negative impact on internet and social media use (Choi et al., 2020).

Thus, we propose our third hypothesis:

H3: The negative impact of negative SPA on social media use is stronger among older women than older men.

Compared to older women, older men tend to have smaller social network sizes and are less likely to maintain social interactions with people out of the household (Cornwell, 2011). At the same time, masculine values may discourage them from opening up to their family and friends about their loneliness and depression to seek support (Oliffe et al., 2013; Tudiver & Talbot, 1999). Using social media to send updates, share daily life events, and check and comment on others' posts may be a more casual and less stigmatizing way for older men to increase communications with family and friends. Thus, social media use may be more critical for older men to maintain social interactions, reduce social isolation and loneliness, and benefit their SPA. As a result, compared to older women, older men may benefit more from using social media to meet their social interaction needs.

Thus, we propose our fourth hypothesis:

H4a: The impact of social media use on positive SPA is stronger among older men than older women.

H4b: The impact of social media use on negative SPA is stronger among older men than older women.

15.1.4 Age Differences

Older adults are not a homogeneous population; individuals at younger and older ages within this group differ significantly in various ways. For younger older adults, the official transition to older adulthood, often marked by retirement, represents a major life change (Choi et al., 2020; Helson et al., 2006). This shift from regular employment to increased free time can pose psychological challenges, potentially triggering negative self-perceptions of aging (SPA) (Wang et al., 2022). In contrast, older adults at more advanced ages, having successfully navigated this transition, may have adapted to their retirement lifestyle and developed more positive attitudes toward aging and retirement (Olesen et al., 2015). Furthermore, while younger older adults tend to exhibit more frequent use of information and communication technologies (ICT) and possess higher digital skills (Anderson & Perrin, 2017; König et al., 2018), older adults at more advanced ages often face greater functional limitations and smaller social network sizes (Charles & Carstensen, 2010; Vidovićová, 2018). As a result, ICT use may hold greater value and provide more significant benefits for older adults at older ages, as they may rely more heavily on these technologies to maintain social connections and compensate for reduced offline engagement. Consequently, the positive influence of ICT use on SPA may be more pronounced among older adults at older ages compared to their younger counterparts.

Based on these observations, we propose the following hypothesis:

H5: The impact of social media use on positive SPA is stronger among older adults at older ages than among those at younger ages.

15.1.5 *Current Study*

To address the abovementioned research gaps in the literature, we aim to (1) investigate the reciprocal associations between SPA (positive and negative) and social media use and (2) examine whether reciprocal associations differ by gender and age subgroups using a national survey of older adults in the U.S. by testing above four hypotheses.

15.2 Materials and Methods

15.2.1 *Study Participants*

Data used in this study were drawn from the 2014 and 2018 Health and Retirement Study (HRS), a national longitudinal panel survey of U.S. adults aged 50 and older and their spouses focused on health, cognition, healthcare utilization, health insurance, retirement, and economic well-being. First launched in 1992 (Wave 1) and administered every other year, the HRS had finished 14 waves by 2018. Aiming to assess psychosocial issues in aging, HRS piloted a new feature for data collection in 2004. The "Leave Behind Questionnaire (LBQ)", a self-administered questionnaire regarding psychosocial and lifestyle factors, was added for those who completed enhanced in-person interviews. Participants could complete the LBQ in their own time and return it by mail. A $20 incentive was provided for the LBQ. Officially starting from 2006, a random half of the participants in the core survey were selected to participate in the 2006 LBQ and follow-ups in 2010, 2014, and 2018. The other half received the LBQ in 2008, 2012, and 2016. Thus, older participants reported on psychological well-being-related questions every 4 years. In the current study, the HRS 2014 and 2018 data were selected because one of our focal variables, social media use, was first collected in the 2014 LBQ and followed in 2018. This study merged the 2014 and 2018 LBQ with the 1996–2018 RAND file (Bugliari et al., 2022). Social media use, SPA, and social relationship variables were drawn from the LBQ; health status and other sociodemographic variables were drawn from the 1996–2018 RAND file.

The 2014 HRS survey response rate was 87.1%. Among the total participants in 2014 (n = 18,747), 9,549 were eligible for the LBQ, and 7,435 completed and returned their questionnaires. In this study, older adults were defined as participants aged 65 and older, so after excluding those under 65 years old, we had 4,334 older participants. Considering the cognitive capacity requirement for using social media, we only included participants with normal cognitive functioning. In HRS, cognitive functioning was measured by a modified version of the Telephone Interview Cognitive Screen (TIC-S), ranging from 0 to 35. This study applied the same cutoff point as a previous study (Reuser et al., 2011) indicating that older adults with cognitive scores higher than 10 points were considered to have normal cognitive functioning. Thus, 4,101 older participants with normal cognitive functioning in 2014 (T1) were included in the final analytic sample, among whom in 2018 (T2), 2,969 still participated, 528 deceased, and 608 chose to not continue participating. Sampling weights were not applied in this study. HRS data were publicly available and exempt from IRB oversight of the authors' institutes.

15.2.2 Measures

Self-Perception of Aging (SPA) SPA was measured by eight items derived from the Philadelphia Geriatric Center Morale Scale (Lawton, 1975) and the Berlin Aging Study (Baltes et al., 1993). Based on the recommendation of HRS, two latent variables, positive and negative SPA, were generated separately. Positive SPA was measured by four manifest indicators, including "I have as much as pep as I did last year", "I am as happy now as I was when I was younger", "As I get older, things are better than I thought they would be", and "So far, I am satisfied with the way that I am aging". Negative SPA was measured by the other four manifest indicators, including "Things keep getting worse as I get older", "The older I get, the more useless I feel", "The older I get, the more I have had to stop doing things that I liked", and "Getting older has brought with it many things that I do not like". Response options ranged from 1 = strongly disagree to 6 = strongly agree. Cronbach's alphas for positive SPA were $\alpha_{T1} = .75$, $\alpha_{T2} = .76$ (negative SPA: $\alpha_{T1} = .78$, $\alpha_{T2} = .77$).

Social Media Use Social media use was measured by three manifest indicators—"communicate by Skype, Facebook, or other social media" with children, other family members, and friends. Response options ranged from 1 = three or more times a week to 6 = less than once a year or never. Response options were all reverse-coded, with higher scores indicating more frequent social media use. Cronbach's alphas were $\alpha_{T1} = .86$, $\alpha_{T2} = .86$.

Social Relationship Social relationship was measured through three variables: social network composition, the number of close relationships, and loneliness. Social network composition was measured by three binary questions asking whether participants had living children, family members, and friends. The unweighted sum was created to measure social network composition, ranging from 0 to 3. The number of close relationships was measured by three questions inquiring about close relationships with living children, family members, and friends. Responses were re-coded to range from 0 to 10 or more (Ailshire & Crimmins, 2011). The unweighted mean of the three types of close relationships was created, with higher scores indicating more close relationships. Loneliness was measured by 11 items derived from the 20-item Revised UCLA Loneliness Scale (Russell, 1996). Response options included 1 = often, 2 = some of the time, and 3 = hardly ever or never. Four items, "you lack companionship", "left out", "isolated from others", and "alone", were reverse coded, and the unweighted mean of the 11 items was calculated as the total score, ranging from 1 to 3, with a higher score representing a higher level of loneliness (Cronbach's alphas: $\alpha_{T1} = .87$, $\alpha_{T2} = .87$).

Health and Functioning Health and functioning-related variables in this study included self-rated health status, limitations in activities of daily living (ADLs), and limitations in instrumental activities of daily living (IADLs). Self-rated health status was measured by a 5-point Likert Scale and was reverse coded as 1 = poor, 2 = fair, 3 = good, 4 = very good, and 5 = excellent. Limitations in ADLs were measured by activities, including bathing, dressing, walking across a room, and getting in and out of bed. Limitations in IADLs were measured by instrumental activities, including using a phone, using money, taking medications, shopping for groceries, and preparing hot meals. Unweighted sums were created for limitations in ADLs and IADLs separately, ranging from 0 to 5, with higher scores indicating more limitations.

Other Covariates Age (0 = less than 75, 1 = 75 or older), race (0 = Black, Hispanic or others, 1 = non-Hispanic white), gender (0 = men, 1 = women), marital status (0 = divorced, separated, widowed, or never married, 1 = married or partnered), education (0 = less than bachelor's degree, 1 = bachelor's degree or higher), poverty (0 = above the poverty line, 1 = below the poverty line), and living alone (0 = no, 1 = yes) were all measured dichotomously. Covariates were included based on previous studies (Choi et al., 2020; Kim et al., 2017). Age and gender were also used as moderators for subgroup analyses.

15.2.3 Analytic Strategies

For the first and second hypotheses, to examine reciprocal relationships between ICT use and SPA (both positive and negative), autoregressive cross-lagged models within the structural equation modeling (SEM) framework were performed (Bollen & Curran, 2006). SEM, a combination of factor analysis and path analysis, allows for simultaneously testing different paths in a model while accounting for measurement error (Fan et al., 2016). The cross-lagged model is a specific model that estimates the directional influence that variables have on each other over time (Kearney, 2017). Before testing the proposed model, we started with assessing measurement models. With acceptable measurement model fit indices, we tested the structural models. Specifically, after controlling for the social relationship, health status, and other covariates at T1, we investigated (1) whether higher positive SPA or lower negative SPA at T1 predicted more frequent social media use at T2 and (2) whether more frequent use of social media at T1 predicts higher positive SPA or lower negative SPA at T2.

Multiple group analyses were planned to test the third, fourth, and fifth hypotheses regarding whether the associations between ICT use and SPA (positive and negative) differ by gender and age subgroups (Anderson & Gerbing, 1988). Before that, measurement invariance between subgroups was tested, including configural invariance (same factor structures), metric invariance (same factor loadings), and scalar invariance (same intercepts) (Anderson & Gerbing, 1988; Vandenberg & Lance, 2000). Nested models were compared through chi-square difference tests to identify the best level of measurement invariance. If measurement invariance was met, multigroup cross-lagged models would be conducted, and z-statistics would be created to test gender differences. If measurement invariance was not met, then cross-lagged models would be conducted separately by gender and age subgroups, and the associations between SPA (positive and negative) and social media use would be checked separately among subgroups.

Analyses were conducted under the maximum likelihood (ML) estimator. Missing data were handled by the full information maximum likelihood (FIML) criterion. Measurement and structural model fit indices adopted in this study included the root mean square error of approximation (RMSEA) less than .06, the comparative fit index (CFI) and Tucker-Lewis index (TLI) greater than .90, and standardized root mean square residual (SRMR) less than .08 (Hu & Bentler, 1999). Descriptive and bivariate analyses were conducted in SPSS version 25 (IBMCorp Ibm, 2017), and SEM analyses were completed in Mplus 8.4 (Muthén & Muthén, 2017).

15.3 Results

15.3.1 Baseline Demographic Characteristics of the Sample

Participants' characteristics are presented in Table 15.1. Bivariate analysis showed that older women had significantly lower rates of being married/partnered (χ^2 = 362.33, $p < .001$) and having a bachelor's degree or higher ($\chi^2 = 63.34$, $p < .001$), and had higher rates of living in poverty ($\chi^2 = 21.20$, $p < .001$) and alone (χ^2 = 152.62, $p < .001$) than older men. Also, older women tended to have significantly larger social network composition ($t = -2.12$, $p < .05$), more close relationships (t = -2.74, $p < .01$), and lower levels of loneliness ($t = 3.26$, $p < .01$) but more limitations in IADLs ($t = -2.00$, $p < .05$). Bivariate analysis revealed that young-old adults were significantly more likely to be married or partnered ($\chi^2 = 137.90$, $p <$ .001), less likely to live alone ($\chi^2 = 111.61$, $p < .001$), and reported fewer close relationships ($t = -6.46$, $p < .001$). Additionally, they exhibited lower levels of IADL limitations ($t = -4.51$, $p < .001$) and ADL limitations ($t = -6.40$, $p < .001$). However, young-old adults also reported poorer self-rated health compared to their older counterparts ($t = -6.78$, $p < .001$). Descriptive statistics and correlations for focal variables are summarized in Table 15.2. All focal variables correlated to each other.

Table 15.1 Participants' characteristics

Variables	All (N = 4,101)		Men (n = 1,674)	Women (n = 2,427)		Young-old (n = 2,028)	Old-old (n = 2,073)	
	% (M)	n (SD)	% (M)	% (M)	χ^2 (t)	% (M)	% (M)	χ^2 (t)
Age (≥ *75*)	50.55	2,069	49.28	51.26	1.54	–	–	–
Race (*non-Hispanic white*)	77.86	3,193	78.38	77.50	.44	73.47	82.17	1.54
Gender (*female*)	59.18	2,427	–	–	–	58.22	60.13	1.54
Marital status (*married/ partnered*)	60.06	2,463	77.64	48.02	362.33^{***}	69.18	51.21	137.90^{***}
Education (≥ *Bachelor*)	23.31	956	29.65	18.95	63.34^{***}	24.32	22.33	2.28
In poverty (*yes*)	7.22	296	5.03	8.84	21.20^{***}	6.81	7.73	1.27
Living alone (*yes*)	28.80	1,181	18.28	36.05	152.62^{***}	21.26	36.20	111.61^{***}
Social network composition (*0–3*)	(2.74)	(.51)	(2.72)	(2.75)	(-2.12^{*})	(2.75)	(2.73)	(1.05)
Close relationship (*0–10*)	(3.34)	(1.91)	(3.24)	(3.41)	(-2.74^{**})	(3.15)	(3.53)	(-6.46^{***})
Loneliness (*1–3*)	(1.51)	(.42)	(1.54)	(1.49)	(3.26^{**})	(1.51)	(1.52)	(−.75)
Self-rated health (*1–5*)	(3.12)	(1.00)	(3.11)	(3.13)	(−.72)	(2.80)	(2.94)	(-4.51^{***})
IADLs Limitations (*0–5*)	(.23)	(.67)	(.20)	(.25)	(-2.00^{*})	(.16)	(.30)	(-6.40^{***})
ADLs Limitations (*0–5*)	(.30)	(.82)	(.28)	(.32)	(−.12)	(.22)	(.38)	(-6.78^{***})

ADLs activities of daily living, *IADLs* instrumental activities of daily living
$^{*}p < .05$, $^{**}p < .01$, $^{***}p < .001$

15.3.2 Associations Between SPA (Positive and Negative) and Social Media Use

Both the positive and negative SPA models showed good or acceptable measurement model fit (Positive: *RMSEA* = .04, *CFI* = .97, *TLI* = .96, *SRMR* = .03; Negative: *RMSEA* = .05, *CFI* = .95, *TLI* = .94, *SRMR* = .03). The structural model examining

Table 15.2 Correlation matrix for focal variables

	M	SD	1	2	3	4	5
1. Positive SPA T1	3.99	1.20					
2. Positive SPA T2	4.04	1.17	.53**				
3. Negative SPA T1	3.42	1.18	−.42**	−.38**			
4. Negative SPA T2	3.45	1.17	−.38**	−.42**	.62**		
5. Social media use T1	1.85	1.38	.07**	.06**	−.14**	−.09**	
6. Social media use T2	2.20	1.57	.06**	.09**	−.08**	−.11**	.55**

SPA self-perception of aging
$^{**}p < .01$, $^{***}p < .001$

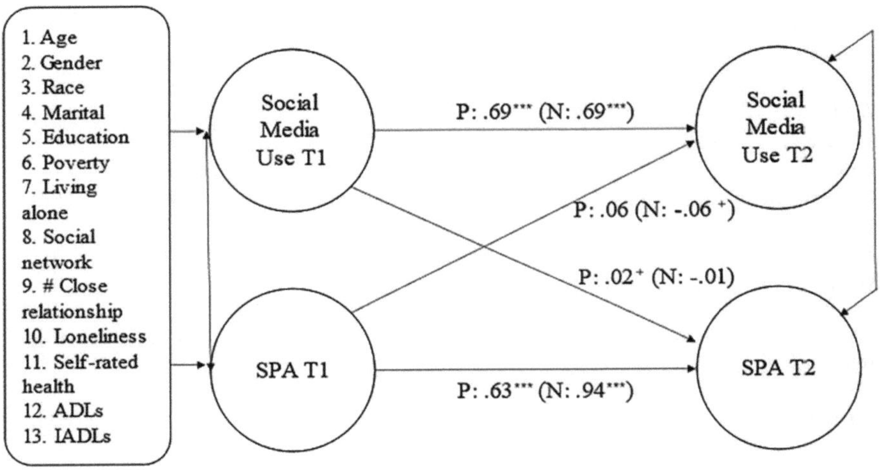

Fig. 15.1 Associations between social media use and SPA among total sample. *SPA* positive self-perception of aging, *T1* time 1, *T2* time 2, *P* positive SPA model, *N* negative SPA model. $^{+}p < .10$, $^{***}p < .001$

associations between positive SPA and social media use had acceptable model fit (*RMSEA* = .04, *CFI* = .94, *TLI* = .93, *SRMR* = .03). As shown in Fig. 15.1, a marginally significant path from social media use at T1 to positive SPA at T2 ($B = .02$, $p = .071$) was identified. Specifically, a one-unit increase in social media use frequency at T1 was associated with a marginally significant .02-unit increase in older adults' positive SPA at T2. However, the path from positive SPA at T1 to social media use at T2 was not significant. The structural model with negative SPA also had acceptable model fit (*RMSEA* = .04, *CFI* = .94, *TLI* = .92, *SRMR* = .03). In Fig. 15.1, the path from negative SPA at T1 to social media use at T2 was marginally significant ($B = -.06$, $p = .082$), indicating that every unit increase in negative SPA at T1 was associated with a marginally significant .06-unit decrease in social media use at T2. However, the path from social media use at T1 to negative SPA at T2 was not statistically significant.

15.3.3 Associations Between SPA and Social Media Use by Subgroups

The results of the measurement invariance tests are presented in Table 15.3. Nested model comparisons for positive and negative SPA revealed that the configural model demonstrated significantly better fit than models with higher levels of measurement invariance. This indicates that while the factor structure of SPA was consistent across gender and age subgroups, the factor loadings and intercepts differed significantly. Given these findings, it was not appropriate to directly compare parameter differences by gender or age in the structural models. Consequently, the structural models were tested separately for men and women, as well as for young-old and old-old adults.

Associations between SPA (both positive and negative) and social media use by gender groups are presented in Table 15.4. All models have acceptable structural model fit (see note for Table 15.4). Results showed that the effect of social media use at T1 on positive SPA at T2 was significant only among older men ($B = .04, p < .05$) but not older women ($B = .01, p > .05$). For a one-unit increase in social media

Table 15.3 Tests of measurement invariance across gender and age

Gender	Positive SPA			Negative SPA		
Model fit index	Configural	Metric	Scalar	Configural	Metric	Scalar
RMSEA	.05	.04	.04	.05	.05	.05
CFI	.97	.96	.96	.95	.95	.95
TLI	.96	.96	.96	.94	.94	.94
SRMR	.03	.04	.04	.03	.04	.04
χ^2	732.04	763.10	776.50	920.70	949.57	989.09
df	142	152	162	142	152	162
$\Delta\chi^2$		31.06	44.46		28.87	68.39
Δdf		10	20		10	20
$\Delta\chi^2$/ Δdf (ref: configural)		$p < .001$	$p < .01$		$p < .01$	$p < .001$
Age	**Positive SPA**			**Negative SPA**		
Model fit index	Configural	Metric	Scalar	Configural	Metric	Scalar
RMSEA	.04	.04	.05	.05	.05	.05
CFI	.97	.97	.96	.95	.95	.94
TLI	.96	.96	.95	.94	.94	.93
SRMR	.03	.03	.04	.04	.04	.04
χ^2	691.23	737.70	888.53	925.14	972.03	1094.24
df	148	152	162	148	152	162
$\Delta\chi^2$		46.47	197.3		46.89	169.10
Δdf		4	14		4	14
$\Delta\chi^2$/ Δdf (ref: configural)		$p < .001$	$p < .001$		$p < .001$	$p < .001$

SPA self-perception of aging

Table 15.4 Associations between social media use and SPA by gender and age

	Men		Women	
Paths	B	SE	B	SE
Social Media Use T1→ Positive SPA T2	.04*	.02	.01	.01
Social Media Use T1→ Negative SPA T2	−.04	.03	−.01	.02
Positive SPA T1 → Social Media Use T2	.02	.06	.09	.06
Negative SPA T1 → Social Media Use T2	.02	.05	−.13*	.05
	Young-old		**Old-old**	
Paths	B	SE	B	SE
Social Media Use T1→ Positive SPA T2	.02	.01	.01	.02
Social Media Use T1→ Negative SPA T2	−.01	.02	−.01	.03
Positive SPA T1 → Social Media Use T2	.09	.06	.00	.07
Negative SPA T1 → Social Media Use T2	−.04	.05	−.03	.05

SPA: self-perception of aging, *T1* time 1, *T2* time 2
Positive SPA Model (gender): *RMSEA* = .04, *CFI* = .94, *TLI* = .92, *SRMR* = .04 (men); *RMSEA* = .04, *CFI* = .94, *TLI* = .93, *SRMR* = .04 (women)
Negative SPA Model (gender): *RMSEA* = .04, *CFI* = .94, *TLI* = .92, *SRMR* = .03 (men); *RMSEA* = .04, *CFI* = .94, *TLI* = .92, *SRMR* = .03 (women)
Positive SPA Model (age): *RMSEA* = .04, *CFI* = .94, *TLI* = .93, *SRMR* = .03 (young-old); *RMSEA* = .03, *CFI* = .95, *TLI* = .94, *SRMR* = .03 (old-old)
Negative SPA Model (age): *RMSEA* = .04, *CFI* = .93, *TLI* = .92, *SRMR* = .03 (young-old); *RMSEA* = .03, *CFI* = .94, *TLI* = .92, *SRMR* = .03 (old-old)
$^{*}p < .05$, $^{**}p < .01$

use frequency at T1, there would be a .04-unit increase in older men's positive SPA at T2. By contrast, the path from negative SPA at T1 to social media use at T2 was significant only among older women ($B = -.13, p < .01$) but not older men ($B = .02$, $p > .05$). For every unit increase in negative SPA at T1, there would be a .13-unit decrease in older women's social media use at T2. None of the cross-lagged effect in the age subgroup analyses was significant, indicating that age may not play a meaningful moderating role.

15.4 Discussion

Using two waves of data (2014 and 2018) from the Health and Retirement Study (HRS), this study examined the reciprocal associations between self-perceptions of aging (SPA), both positive and negative, and social media use among older adults in the U.S., as well as potential gender and age differences in these relationships. The results showed that, among the total sample, baseline social media use marginally predicted increased positive SPA 4 years later, while baseline negative SPA marginally predicted reduced social media use 4 years later. However, gender-stratified analyses revealed that the positive effect of social media use on SPA was significant only among older men, and the negative effect of SPA on social media use was significant only among older women. These findings suggest notable gender differences in the associations between SPA and social media use. In contrast, subgroup analyses by age (young-old vs. old-old) did not reveal any significant cross-lagged effects, indicating that age may not play a significant moderating role in these relationships.

15.4.1 Findings About SPA's Impacts on Social Media Use

Partially supporting H1b and H3, this study found that negative SPA marginally predicted reduced social media use 4 years later, with this effect being significant only among older women, not older men. This finding contradicts a recent study by Köttl et al. (2021), which found that negative SPA did not predict lower everyday ICT use among older adults. The discrepancy may stem from differences in measurement: Köttl et al. (2021) examined SPA across domains (physical loss, social loss, and personal competence) rather than from the perspective of positive or negative valence. Nevertheless, the current finding aligns with a prior study using a nationally representative sample of older adults in the U.S., which found that self-directed ageism (negative SPA) was associated with less internet use among older women but not older men (Choi et al., 2020). Similarly, Venkatesh and colleagues (2000, 2003) suggested that social influence, including stereotypes, may have a stronger impact on women than men, particularly in the context of technology acceptance. Thus, negative stereotypes about older adults' technology use may disproportionately reduce older women's engagement with social media.

In contrast to H1a and two previous studies linking positive SPA to digital technology use (Mariano et al., 2021a, b), our results showed that higher levels of positive SPA did not significantly predict more frequent social media use among men or women. Combined with the findings for H1b, this suggests that positive and negative SPA are distinct constructs, underscoring the importance of examining them separately. The concept of "negativity bias" may help explain this difference: people tend to remember and weigh negative events more heavily than positive ones (Kanouse, 1984), and negative experiences often have a stronger impact on thoughts and behaviors than positive ones of the same magnitude (Baumeister et al., 2001). This notion is supported by the finding that the lagged effect of negative SPA from T1 to T2 was significantly larger than that of positive SPA (Positive: $B = .63$, $p < .001$; Negative: $B = .93$, $p < .001$), indicating that negative SPA may have a more enduring influence. Thus, internalized negative age stereotypes may persistently discourage older adults, particularly older women, from using social media, whereas the effects of positive SPA may not be strong or lasting enough to promote social media use. Future studies are needed to further explore this phenomenon.

15.4.2 Findings About Social Media Use's Impact on SPA

Partially supporting H2a and H4a, more frequent social media use was marginally predictive of increased positive SPA 4 years later. This finding aligns with a recent study showing that frequent computer use was associated with more positive SPA over 3 years among middle-aged and older Germans (Mariano et al., 2021b). Further gender-stratified analyses revealed that this positive association was significant only among older men, not older women. Similarly, a previous study found a significant negative association between social networking site use and depression among older Korean men but not women (Jeon et al., 2020).

The lack of a significant impact of social media use on SPA among older women may be explained by gendered ageism, which makes changes in SPA more challenging for older women. Due to the intersection of gender and age, older women are often exposed to more stigmatizing attitudes than older men (Choi et al., 2020; McGann et al., 2016). Stereotypes portraying older women as more vulnerable or less capable may be internalized (McGann et al., 2016), leading to greater concerns and fewer positive feelings about aging (Berger, 2017). Given that these internalized attitudes develop over the lifespan (Levy et al., 2002), existing negative perceptions of aging among older women may be difficult to reduce, and positive perceptions may be harder to enhance. Additionally, Baumeister and Leary (1995) suggested that individuals with sufficient social bonds may be less motivated to seek social interactions to fulfill their belongingness needs. Correspondingly, older adults with robust social networks may be less sensitive to the benefits of social interaction (Luo et al., 2022). This explanation is supported by the finding that older women reported larger social networks ($t = -2.12$, $p < .05$), more close relationships ($t = -2.74$, $p < .01$), and lower levels of loneliness ($t = 3.26$, $p < .01$) compared to older men.

Contradicting H5, we found no significant cross-lagged effects of social media use on positive SPA among either young-old or old-old adults, despite the large sample sizes in both subgroups. This suggests that age does not meaningfully moderate the relationship between social media use and SPA, challenging the assumption that young-old and old-old adults differ significantly in how social media use shapes their perceptions of aging. Instead, other factors, such as individual differences in social media engagement, the type of content consumed, or the purpose of use, may play a more critical role. Future research should explore these factors to better understand the conditions under which social media use might influence SPA.

Contrary to H2b and H4b, frequent social media use did not significantly reduce negative SPA among older men or women. A possible explanation for these findings can be drawn from the work of Köttl et al. (2021), who found that SPA significantly impacts personal competence but not physical or social domains. This suggests that measures of SPA should consider not only the valence (positive or negative) but also the specific life domains, such as physical, social, and personal competence. It is possible that social media use may reduce negative SPA in certain domains not captured by the measure used in this study. Additionally, negative SPA may be more resistant to change due to negativity bias, which is supported by the finding that negative SPA had a stronger lagged effect from T1 to T2 (Positive: $B = .63$, $p < .001$; Negative: $B = .93$, $p < .001$). Furthermore, emerging evidence highlights potential adverse effects of social media use, such as promoting less healthy behaviors (Duplaga, 2021), increasing emotional loneliness (Lagacé et al., 2015), and exposing users to online discrimination (Meisner, 2021). These negative effects may counteract the potential benefits of social media use, resulting in no significant reduction in negative SPA. Future longitudinal mediation studies are needed to explore these mechanisms in greater depth.

15.4.3 Limitations

This study has several limitations that should be acknowledged. First, the findings may be influenced by sample selection bias. Due to the cognitive demands of social media use, only participants with normal cognitive function were included, potentially excluding those with cognitive impairments. Additionally, the poverty rate in the study sample (7.2%) was lower than the national poverty rate for adults aged 65 and older in 2014 (10.0%) (Fontenot & Renwick, 2016). Furthermore, the HRS grouped "less than once a year" and "never" social media use together, making it impossible to exclude non-users from the sample. These factors limit the generalizability of the findings to the broader older adult population.

Second, attrition bias may have affected the results. Of the 4,104 older adults included in 2014, only 2,969 (72%) participated in the 2018 survey. The remaining 28% either refused to participate or were deceased. Attrition analyses revealed significant differences in socio-demographic characteristics among these groups, which may have introduced bias into the findings.

Third, the reciprocal associations between social media use and SPA may not be directly comparable between older men and women due to differences in factor loadings. The observed differences in significant paths could be attributed to measurement invariance issues. Future studies should validate these findings using more robust measures of social media use.

Fourth, while social media use may have detrimental effects on older adults' health and well-being, which could indirectly influence their SPA (both positive and negative), the availability of only two waves of social media use data in the HRS limited our ability to explore potential underlying mechanisms. Future research should investigate mediators, such as mental health or social support, that may explain the relationship between social media use and SPA.

Finally, beyond gender identity, other demographic characteristics (e.g., socioeconomic status, education, or cultural background) may moderate the associations between SPA and social media use. Future studies are encouraged to examine these potential moderating factors to provide a more comprehensive understanding of these relationships.

15.4.4 Implications

Despite these limitations, this study holds broad implications for aging research, particularly in an era where online social interactions have become increasingly popular and integral to lifelong learning, especially in the context of the global pandemic (Gu et al., 2021). The findings suggest that promoting older adults' social media use requires consideration of not only individual-level characteristics but also macro-level factors. SPA are not merely personal views; they are shaped by societal attitudes and internalized over the lifespan. Addressing negative SPA and fostering positive SPA demand integrated societal efforts.

The United Nations General Assembly's *Decade of Healthy Ageing* (2021–2030) emphasizes the need to change how we think (stereotypes), feel (prejudices), and act (discrimination) toward age and aging (United Nations, 2020). Building an age-friendly society offers a promising solution. The World Health Organization's (WHO) Age-Friendly Cities Framework outlines eight interconnected domains: "community and health care," "transportation," "housing," "social participation," "outdoor spaces and buildings," "respect and social inclusion," "civic participation and employment," and "communication and information". By addressing societal stereotypes, prejudices, and discrimination, an age-friendly society can help remove barriers to learning and using social media. Simultaneously, increased use of ICT among older adults can further support the development of such a society.

Cognitive and individual growth, though slower, continues into late adulthood (Baltes, 1987; Hertzog et al., 2008). Older adults remain capable of learning, developing, and thriving (Baltes, 1987). Lifelong learning not only stimulates cognitive function but also enhances well-being (Gu et al., 2021), fostering positive perspectives on aging. The findings of this study highlight the need for digital technology training programs to consider gender differences and adopt gender-specific approaches. Additionally, gender-tailored interventions to promote positive SPA and reduce negative SPA are essential to overcoming psychological barriers to older adults' adoption of digital technology.

15.4.5 Conclusions

This study examined the reciprocal associations between SPA and social media use among older adults and explored potential gender and age differences in these relationships. The results indicate that social media use enhances positive SPA for older men, while negative SPA reduces social media use frequency among older women. These findings underscore the need for societal efforts to combat stereotypes, prejudices, and discrimination against aging and to build an age-friendly society where older adults can learn, grow, and age successfully.

Disclaimer The views expressed in this chapter are solely those of the authors and do not necessarily reflect the views of the University of Alabama at Birmingham, or the United Nations.

References

Ailshire, J. A., & Crimmins, E. M. (2011). Psychosocial factors associated with longevity in the United States: Age differences between the old and oldest-old in the health and retirement study. *Journal of Aging Research, 2011*, 530534. https://doi.org/10.4061/2011/530534

Allport, G. W. (1954). *The nature of prejudice*. Addison-Wesley.

Anderson, J. C., & Gerbing, D. W. (1988). Structural equation modeling in practice: A review and recommended two-step approach. *Psychological Bulletin, 103*(3), 411–423. https://doi.org/10.1037/0033-2909.103.3.411

Anderson, M., & Perrin, A. (2017). *Technology use among seniors*. chrome-extension://efaidnbmnnnibpcajpcglclefindmkaj/https://www.pewresearch.org/internet/wp-content/uploads/sites/9/2017/05/PI_2017.05.17_Older-Americans-Tech_FINAL.pdf

Baltes, P. B. (1987). Theoretical propositions of life-span developmental psychology: On the dynamics between growth and decline. *Developmental Psychology, 23*(5), 611. https://doi.org/10.1037/0012-1649.23.5.611

Baltes, P. B., Mayer, K. U., Helmchen, H., & Steinhagen-Thiessen, E. (1993). The Berlin Aging Study (BASE): Overview and design. *Ageing and Society, 13*(4), 483–515. https://doi.org/10.1017/S0144686X00001343

Barker, M., O'Hanlon, A., McGee, H. M., Hickey, A., & Conroy, R. M. (2007). Cross-sectional validation of the Aging Perceptions Questionnaire: A multidimensional instrument for assessing self-perceptions of aging. *BMC Geriatrics, 7*(1), 9. https://doi.org/10.1186/1471-2318-7-9

Baumeister, R. F., Bratslavsky, E., Finkenauer, C., & Vohs, K. D. (2001). Bad is stronger than good. *Review of General Psychology, 5*(4), 323–370. https://doi.org/10.1037/1089-2680.5.4.323

Baumeister, R. F., & Leary, M. R. (1995). The need to belong: Desire for interpersonal attachments as a fundamental human motivation. *Psychological Bulletin, 117(3)*, 497–529. https://doi.org/10.1037/0033-2909.117.3.497

Baumeister, R. F., & Sommer, K. L. (1997). What do men want? Gender differences and two spheres of belongingness: Comment on Cross and Madson (1997). *Psychological Bulletin, 122*(1), 38–44.; discussion 51–35. https://doi.org/10.1037/0033-2909.122.1.38

Bausch, S., Michel, A., & Sonntag, K. (2014). How gender influences the effect of age on self-efficacy and training success. *International Journal of Training and Development, 18*(3), 171–187. https://doi.org/10.1111/ijtd.12027

Berger, R. (2017). Aging in America: Ageism and general attitudes toward growing old and the elderly. *Open Journal of Social Sciences, 5*(08), 16., Article 78445. https://doi.org/10.4236/jss.2017.58015

Blawert, A., & Wurm, S. (2021). Shifting self-perceptions of ageing: Differential effects of value priorities on self-perceptions of ageing beyond age stereotypes. *European Journal of Ageing, 18*(2), 257–267. https://doi.org/10.1007/s10433-020-00578-3

Bollen, K. A., & Curran, P. J. (2006). *Latent curve models: A structural equation perspective* (Vol. 467). John Wiley & Sons. https://doi.org/10.1353/sof.0.0084

Brown, K. E., Kim, J., Stewart, T., Fulton, E., & McCarrey, A. C. (2021). Positive, but not negative, self-perceptions of aging predict cognitive function among older adults. *International Journal of Aging & Human Development, 93*(1), 543–561. https://doi.org/10.1177/0091415020917681

Bugliari, D., Carroll, J., Hayden, O., Hayes, J., Hurd, M. D., Karabatakis, A., Main, R., McCullough, C. M., Meijer, E., Moldoff, M. B., Pantoja, P., Rohwedder, S., & St. Clair, P. A. (2022). *RAND HRS longitudinal file 2018 (V2) documentation: Includes 1992–2018 (final release)*. RAND Corporation. https://doi.org/10.7249/TLA2097-1

Charles, S. T., & Carstensen, L. L. (2010). Social and emotional aging. *Annual Review of Psychology, 61*, 383–409. https://doi.org/10.1146/annurev.psych.093008.100448

Chen, K., & Chan, A. H. S. (2014). Gerontechnology acceptance by elderly Hong Kong Chinese: A senior technology acceptance model (STAM). *Ergonomics, 57*(5), 635–652. https://doi.org/10.1080/00140139.2014.895855

Choi, E. Y., Kim, Y., Chipalo, E., & Lee, H. Y. (2020). Does perceived ageism widen the digital divide? And does it vary by gender? *The Gerontologist, 60*(7), 1213–1223. https://doi.org/10.1093/geront/gnaa066

Cornwell, B. (2011). Independence through social networks: Bridging potential among older women and men. *The Journals of Gerontology: Series B, 66B*(6), 782–794. https://doi.org/10.1093/geronb/gbr111

Cotten, S. R., Anderson, W. A., & McCullough, B. M. (2013). Impact of internet use on loneliness and contact with others among older adults: Cross-sectional analysis. *Journal of Medical Internet Research, 15*(2), e39. https://doi.org/10.2196/jmir.2306

Dasgupta, D., Chaudhry, B., Koh, E., & Chawla, N. V. (2016). A survey of tablet applications for promoting successful aging in older adults. *IEEE Access, 4*, 9005–9017. https://doi.org/10.1109/access.2016.2632818

Duplaga, M. (2021). The association between internet use and health-related outcomes in older adults and the elderly: A cross-sectional study. *BMC Medical Informatics and Decision Making, 21*(1), 150. https://doi.org/10.1186/s12911-021-01500-2

Fan, Y., Chen, J., Shirkey, G., John, R., Wu, S. R., Park, H., & Shao, C. (2016). Applications of structural equation modeling (SEM) in ecological studies: An updated review. *Ecological Processes, 5*(1), 19. https://doi.org/10.1186/s13717-016-0063-3

Fontenot, K. R., & Renwick, T. J. (2016, April). Poverty by Age and Sex: An Examination of the Distribution in Poverty between 1966 and 2014. In US Census Bureau. Poster Presented at the Annual Meeting of the Population Association of America.

Franz, R. L., Findlater, L., Neves, B. B., & Wobbrock, J. O. (2019). *Gender and help seeking by older adults when learning new technologies*. In *The 21st international ACM SIGACCESS conference on computers and accessibility*. https://doi.org/10.1145/3308561.3353807

Gaia, A., Sala, E., & Cerati, G. (2021). Social networking sites use and life satisfaction. A quantitative study on older people living in Europe. *European Societies, 23*(1), 98–118. https://doi.org/10.1080/14616696.2020.1762910

Gu Hoh, J., Lu, S., & Feng, Q. (2021). Senior learning. In D. Gu & M. E. Dupre (Eds.), *Encyclopedia of gerontology and population aging* (pp. 4475–4487). Cham AG.

Havighurst, R. J. (1961). Successful aging. *The Gerontologist, 1*, 8–13. https://doi.org/10.1093/geront/1.1.8

Haynes, T. L., Heckhausen, J., Chipperfield, J. G., Perry, R. P., & Newall, N. E. (2009). Primary and secondary control strategies: Implications for health and well-being among older adults. *Journal of Social and Clinical Psychology, 28*(2), 165–197. https://doi.org/10.1521/jscp.2009.28.2.165

Heckhausen, J. (1999). *Developmental regulation in adulthood: Age-normative and sociostructural constraints as adaptive challenges*. Cambridge University Press.

Heckhausen, J., & Schulz, R. (1995). A life-span theory of control. *Psychological Review, 102*(2), 284–304. https://doi.org/10.1037/0033-295x.102.2.284

Helson, R., Soto, C. J., & Cate, R. A. (2006). From young adulthood through the middle ages. In *Handbook of personality development* (pp. 337–352).

Hertzog, C., Kramer, A. F., Wilson, R. S., & Lindenberger, U. (2008). Enrichment effects on adult cognitive development: Can the functional capacity of older adults be preserved and enhanced? *Psychological Science in the Public Interest, 9*(1), 1–65. https://doi.org/10.1111/j.1539-6053.2009.01034.x

Hogan, M. (2009). Age differences in technophobia: An Irish study. In W. Wojtkowski, G. Wojtkowski, M. Lang, K. Conboy, & C. Barry (Eds.), *Information systems development: Challenges in practice, theory, and education* (Vol. 1, pp. 117–130). Springer US. https://doi.org/10.1007/978-0-387-68772-8_10

Hu, L., & Bentler, P. M. (1999). Cutoff criteria for fit indexes in covariance structure analysis: Conventional criteria versus new alternatives. *Structural Equation Modeling: A Multidisciplinary Journal, 6*(1), 1–55. https://doi.org/10.1080/10705519909540118

Huang, D.-L., Patrick Rau, P.-L., Salvendy, G., Gao, F., & Zhou, J. (2011). Factors affecting perception of information security and their impacts on IT adoption and security practices. *International Journal of Human-Computer Studies, 69*(12), 870–883. https://doi.org/10.1016/j.ijhcs.2011.07.007

IBMCorp Ibm, S. (2017). *Statistics for windows, version 25.0.* IBM Corp.

Ihm, J., & Hsieh, Y. P. (2015). The implications of information and communication technology use for the social well-being of older adults. *Information, Communication & Society, 18*(10), 1123–1138. https://doi.org/10.1080/1369118X.2015.1019912

Jeon, G.-S., Choi, K.-W., & Jang, K.-S. (2020). Social networking site usage and its impact on depressive symptoms among older men and women in South Korea. *International Journal of Environmental Research and Public Health, 17*(8), 2670. https://doi.org/10.3390/ijerph17082670

Juárez, M. A. R., González, V. M., & Favela, J. (2016). Effect of technology on aging perception. *Health Informatics Journal, 24*(2), 171–181. https://doi.org/10.1177/1460458216661863

Kanouse, D. E. (1984). Explaining negativity biases in evaluation and choice behavior: Theory and research. In T. C. Kinnear (Ed.), *Advances in consumer research* (Vol. 11, pp. 703–708). Association for Consumer Research.

Kearney, M. W. (2017). Cross lagged panel analysis. In *The SAGE encyclopedia of communication research methods* (pp. 312–314).

Kim, J., Lee, H. Y., Christensen, M. C., & Merighi, J. R. (2017). Technology access and use, and their associations with social engagement among older adults: Do women and men differ? *The Journals of Gerontology: Series B, 72*(5), 836–845. https://doi.org/10.1093/geronb/gbw123

Koenig, A. M. (2018). Comparing prescriptive and descriptive gender stereotypes about children, adults, and the elderly. *Frontiers in Psychology, 9*(1086), 1–13. https://doi.org/10.3389/fpsyg.2018.01086

König, R., Seifert, A., & Doh, M. (2018). Internet use among older Europeans: An analysis based on SHARE data. *Universal Access in the Information Society, 17*(3), 621–633. https://doi.org/10.1007/s10209-018-0609-5

Kornadt, A. E., Voss, P., & Rothermund, K. (2013). Multiple standards of aging: Gender-specific age stereotypes in different life domains. *European Journal of Ageing, 10*(4), 335–344. https://doi.org/10.1007/s10433-013-0281-9

Köttl, H., Cohn-Schwartz, E., & Ayalon, L. (2021). Self-perceptions of aging and everyday ICT engagement: A test of reciprocal associations. *The Journals of Gerontology. Series B, Psychological Sciences and Social Sciences, 76*(9), 1913–1922. https://doi.org/10.1093/geronb/gbaa168

Krasnova, H., Veltri, N. F., Eling, N., & Buxmann, P. (2017). Why men and women continue to use social networking sites: The role of gender differences. *The Journal of Strategic Information Systems, 26*(4), 261–284. https://doi.org/10.1016/j.jsis.2017.01.004

Lagacé, M., Charmarkeh, H., Laplante, J., & Tanguay, A. (2015). How ageism contributes to the second-level digital divide: The case of Canadian seniors. *Journal of Technologies and Human Usability, 11*(3), 1–13. https://doi.org/10.18848/2381-9227/cgp/v11i04/56439

Langer, E. J., & Abelson, R. P. (1983). *The psychology of control*. SAGE Publications, Incorporated.

Lawton, M. P. (1975). The Philadelphia geriatric center morale scale: A revision. *Journal of Gerontology, 30*(1), 85–89. https://doi.org/10.1093/geronj/30.1.85

Le, N. T., Rao Hill, S., & Troshani, I. (2022). Perceived control and perceived risk in self-service technology recovery. *Journal of Computer Information Systems, 62*(1), 164–173. https://doi.org/10.1080/08874417.2020.1756533

Levy, B. R., Slade, M. D., & Kasl, S. V. (2002). Longitudinal benefit of positive self-perceptions of aging on functional health. *The Journals of Gerontology: Series B, 57*(5), P409–P417. https://doi.org/10.1093/geronb/57.5.P409

Luo, M., Macdonald, B., & Hülür, G. (2022). Not "The More The Merrier": Diminishing returns to daily face-to-face social interaction frequency for well-being in older age. *The Journals of Gerontology: Series B*, gbac010. https://doi.org/10.1093/geronb/gbac010

Makizako, H., Kubozono, T., Kiyama, R., Takenaka, T., Kuwahata, S., Tabira, T., Kanoya, T., Horinouchi, K., Shimada, H., & Ohishi, M. (2019). Associations of social frailty with loss of muscle mass and muscle weakness among community-dwelling older adults. *Geriatrics & Gerontology International, 19*(1), 76–80. https://doi.org/10.1111/ggi.13571

Mariano, J., Marques, S., Ramos, M. R., & de Vries, H. (2021a). Internet use by middle-aged and older adults: Longitudinal relationships with functional ability, social support, and self-perceptions of aging. *Psychology and Aging, 36*, 983–995. https://doi.org/10.1037/pag0000643

Mariano, J., Marques, S., Ramos, M. R., & de Vries, H. (2021b). Cognitive functioning mediates the relationship between self-perceptions of aging and computer use behavior in late adulthood: Evidence from two longitudinal studies. *Computers in Human Behavior, 121*, 106807. https://doi.org/10.1016/j.chb.2021.106807

McGann, M., Ong, R., Bowman, D., Duncan, A., Kimberley, H., & Biggs, S. (2016). Gendered ageism in Australia: Changing perceptions of age discrimination among older men and women. *Economic Papers: A Journal of Applied Economics and Policy, 35*(4), 375–388. https://doi.org/10.1111/1759-3441.12155

Meisner, B. A. (2021). Are you OK, boomer? Intensification of ageism and intergenerational tensions on social media amid COVID-19. *Leisure Sciences, 43*(1–2), 56–61. https://doi.org/10.1080/01490400.2020.1773983

Merton, R. (1957). *Social theory and social structure In*. The Free Press.

Muthén, L., & Muthén, B. (2017). *Mplus user's guide: Statistical analysis with latent variables.*

Myhre, J. W., Mehl, M. R., & Glisky, E. L. (2017). Cognitive benefits of online social networking for healthy older adults. *The Journals of Gerontology: Series B, 72*(5), 752–760. https://doi.org/10.1093/geronb/gbw025

Newman, L., Stoner, C., & Spector, A. (2021). Social networking sites and the experience of older adult users: A systematic review. *Ageing and Society, 41*(2), 377–402. https://doi.org/10.1017/S0144686X19001144

Olesen, K., Rod, N. H., Madsen, I. E. H., Bonde, J. P., & Rugulies, R. (2015). Does retirement reduce the risk of mental disorders? A national registry-linkage study of treatment for mental disorders before and after retirement of 245 082 Danish residents, *72*(5), 366–372. https://doi.org/10.1136/oemed-2014-102228

Oliffe, J. L., Rasmussen, B., Bottorff, J. L., Kelly, M. T., Galdas, P. M., Phinney, A., & Ogrodniczuk, J. S. (2013). Masculinities, work, and retirement among older men who experience depression. *Qualitative Health Research, 23*(12), 1626–1637. https://doi.org/10.1177/1049732313509408

Pew Research Center. (2021). *Social media fact sheet.* Retrieved May 15, from https://www.pewresearch.org/internet/fact-sheet/social-media/

Reuser, M., Willekens, F. J., & Bonneux, L. (2011). Higher education delays and shortens cognitive impairment. A multistate life table analysis of the US Health and Retirement Study. *European Journal of Epidemiology, 26*(5), 395–403. https://doi.org/10.1007/s10654-011-9553-x

Richeson, J. A., & Shelton, J. N. (2006). A social psychological perspective on the stigmatization of older adults. In *When I'm 64* (pp. 174–208). The National Academies Press.

Rothermund, K., & Kornadt, A. E. (2015). Views on aging: Domain-specific approaches and implications for developmental regulation. *Annual Review of Gerontology and Geriatrics, 35*(1), 121–144. https://doi.org/10.1891/0198-8794.35.121

Russell, D. W. (1996). UCLA loneliness scale (version 3): Reliability, validity, and factor structure. *Journal of Personality Assessment, 66*(1), 20–40. https://doi.org/10.1207/s15327752jpa6601_2

Sargent-Cox, K. A., Anstey, K. J., & Luszcz, M. A. (2014). Longitudinal change of self-perceptions of aging and mortality. *The Journals of Gerontology: Series B, 69*(2), 168–173. https://doi.org/10.1093/geronb/gbt005

Schneider, J. M., Gopinath, B., McMahon, C. M., Leeder, S. R., Mitchell, P., & Wang, J. J. (2011). Dual sensory impairment in older age. *Journal of Aging and Health, 23*(8), 1309–1324. https://doi.org/10.1177/0898264311408418

Schulz, R., & Heckhausen, J. (1996). A life span model of successful aging. *The American Psychologist, 51*(7), 702–714. https://doi.org/10.1037/0003-066x.51.7.702

Schwab, K. (2017). *The fourth industrial revolution*. Currency.

Sontag, S. (1972). The double standard of aging. *Saturday Review of Literature, 39*, 29–38.

Steward, A., & Hasche, L. (2021). Exploring lifestyle activities to reduce internalized ageism: Self-efficacy as a mediator between exercise, volunteering, computer use, and self-perceptions of aging. *The International Journal of Aging and Human Development*, 00914150211024175. https://doi.org/10.1177/00914150211024175

Szabo, A., Allen, J., Stephens, C., & Alpass, F. (2019). Longitudinal analysis of the relationship between purposes of internet use and well-being among older adults. *The Gerontologist, 59*(1), 58–68. https://doi.org/10.1093/geront/gny036

Tudiver, F., & Talbot, Y. (1999). Why don't men seek help? Family physicians' perspectives on help-seeking behavior in men. *Journal of Family Practice, 48*, 47–52.

United Nations. (2020). *Dacade of healthy ageing 2020*. Retrieved May 25, from https://www.who.int/docs/default-source/decade-of-healthy-ageing/final-decade-proposal/decade-proposal-final-apr2020-en.pdf?sfvrsn=73137ef_4

van Deursen, A. J. A. M., & Helsper, E. J. (2015). A nuanced understanding of internet use and non-use among the elderly. *European Journal of Communication, 30*(2), 171–187. https://doi.org/10.1177/0267323115578059

Vandenberg, R. J., & Lance, C. E. (2000). A review and synthesis of the measurement invariance literature: Suggestions, practices, and recommendations for organizational research. *Organizational Research Methods, 3*(1), 4–70.

Venkatesh, V., & Morris, M. G. (2000). Why don't men ever stop to ask for directions? Gender, social influence, and their role in technology acceptance and usage behavior. *MIS Quarterly, 24*(1), 115–139. https://doi.org/10.2307/3250981

Venkatesh, V., Morris, M. G., Davis, G. B., & Davis, F. D. (2003). User acceptance of information technology: Toward a unified view. *MIS Quarterly, 27*(3), 425–478. https://doi.org/10.2307/30036540

Vidovićová, L. (2018). New roles for older people. *Journal of Population Ageing, 11*(1), 1–6. https://doi.org/10.1007/s12062-017-9217-z

Wang, K., Marbut, A. R., Suntai, Z., Zheng, D., & Chen, X. (2022). Patterns in older adults' perceived chronic stressor types and cognitive functioning trajectories: Are perceived chronic stressors always bad? *Social Science & Medicine, 311*, 115297.

Yang, F., & Gu, D. (2021). Widowhood, widowhood duration, and loneliness among older adults in China. *Social Science & Medicine, 283*, 114179. https://doi.org/10.1016/j.socscimed.2021.114179

Yu, K., Wu, S., & Chi, I. (2021). internet use and loneliness of older adults over time: The mediating effect of social contact. *The Journals of Gerontology: Series B, 76*(3), 541–550. https://doi.org/10.1093/geronb/gbaa004

Zhang, K., Kim, K., Silverstein, N. M., Song, Q., & Burr, J. A. (2021). Social media communication and loneliness among older adults: The mediating roles of social support and social contact. *The Gerontologist, 61*(6), 888–896. https://doi.org/10.1093/geront/gnaa197

Section IV
ICT Use and Healthy Aging

Chapter 16
Exploring the Associations Between ICT Access, Frequency, Breadth, and Cognitive Functioning in Older Adults

Yanjun Dong, Charles Johnson, and Kun Wang

16.1 Introduction

Technological advancements have increased human lifespans. While prolonged lifespans are highly desirable, the risk of cognitive impairment, dementia, and other health consequences increase with age (Abbott, 2011; Livingston et al., 2017). Cognitive functioning, defined as individuals' abilities to perform different mental activities relevant to thinking, learning, memory, and problem-solving, serves a critical role in people's daily life (National Institute on Aging, 2020). Although slight forgetfulness and age-related cognitive decline are common aspects of normal aging, a significant proportion of older adults experience more severe memory issues, developing mild cognitive impairment (MCI) or dementia (National Institute on Aging, 2020).

Dementia, first described in 1906 by German psychiatrist Alois Alzheimer, is defined by the 10th version of the International Statistical Classification of Diseases and Related Health Problems (ICD-10) as "*a syndrome due to disease of the brain, usually of a chronic or progressive nature, characterized by disturbances in multiple higher cortical functions, including memory, thinking, orientation, comprehension, calculation, learning capacity, language, and judgment*." Dementia represents a broad category of severe cognitive impairments, including Alzheimer's disease (the most common cause), vascular dementia, Lewy body dementia, and

Y. Dong
University at Albany, State University of New York, Albany, NY, USA
e-mail: ydong2@albany.edu

C. Johnson · K. Wang (✉)
Department of Social Work, College of Arts and Sciences, University of Alabama at Birmingham, Birmingham, AL, USA
e-mail: cwjohnso@uab.edu; kw2@uab.edu

K. Wang et al. (eds.), *ICT Use and Healthy Longevity*, Advances in Studies of Aging and Health 5, https://doi.org/10.1007/978-3-031-98964-3_16

frontotemporal dementia (Centers for Disease Control and Prevention, 2019). Alzheimer's disease, a neurodegenerative disorder, accounts for 60–80% of dementia cases and often leads to dementia as it progresses (Mayo Clinic, 2024). While Alzheimer's disease and dementia are distinct conditions, they are frequently studied together due to their overlapping symptoms and treatment approaches. Dementia is chronic and progressive, and although treatments such as behavioral therapy and pharmacological interventions can help manage its symptoms, there are currently no known cures. While recent advances in disease-modifying therapies offer some promise for slowing progression—particularly in the early stages of Alzheimer's disease—the overall impact remains limited. In 2020, approximately 6.07 million older adults in the United States were living with Alzheimer's disease and related dementias (ADRD). Without the development of a cure, this number is projected to rise to 13.85 million by 2060 (Rajan et al., 2021; Alzheimer's Association, 2021). Given the growing public health burden and the absence of curative treatments, ADRD is posing an urgent and escalating public health crisis.

Memory loss is the hallmark characteristic of ADRD. As a result, ADRD has been linked to psychological death, the experience of forgetting personal life history and having difficulty in retaining even fragmentary reminiscences of life (Yang et al., 2016). However, the complexity of ADRD extends beyond memory issues. Many older adults living with ADRD have problems with attention, communication, thinking, and decision-making (Abbott, 2011; Centers for Disease Control and Prevention, 2019, p. 201; Livingston et al., 2020). The impairment or loss of cognitive abilities significantly affects older adults' activities of daily living (ADL) and instrumental activities of daily living (IADL) (Cipriani et al., 2020; Lee et al., 2019). Also, this condition places a substantial burden on caregivers and the U.S. public healthcare system, with the cost of medical care related to ADRD estimated to exceed $355 billion in 2021 (Alzheimer's Association, 2021).

In response to these challenges posed by ADRD, researchers have increasingly explored the potential of information and communication technology (ICT) to support cognitive health in older adults. However, the definition of ICT use remains varied, encompassing dimensions such as access, frequency, and breadth of use, which raises questions about which aspects are most critical for cognitive health (Choudrie et al., 2021; van Deursen & van Dijk, 2014). While prior studies have primarily focused on ICT access, this study expands the scope by examining multiple dimensions of ICT engagement, offering a more nuanced understanding of its relationship with cognitive functioning in older adults. Specifically, this study employs a multifaceted approach to systematically investigate the positive associations between ICT use and cognitive functioning. It measures ICT use through three distinct variables: ICT access/use, ICT use frequency, and ICT use breadth. This comprehensive perspective represents a novel contribution to the field, moving beyond conventional access-based approaches. By doing so, it aims to inform the development of targeted interventions and more effective strategies to promote cognitive health in aging populations.

16.1.1 Conceptual Framework

Over the past few decades, several interrelated concepts and theories have emerged to explain how cognitive functioning can be preserved and promoted in older adults. The "use it or lose it" hypothesis suggests that age-related cognitive decline may result from the disuse of cognitive skills over time (Hultsch et al., 1999; Salthouse, 2016). Conversely, engaging in cognitively demanding activities, referred to as "cognitive exercise", can help preserve cognitive functioning by maintaining or enhancing cognitive skills and compensatory mechanisms (Ericsson & Charness, 1994; Schaie & Willis, 1986).

Building on this idea, Cognitive Enrichment Theory expands the concept of cognitive exercise to include a broader range of behaviors, such as physical exercise, social interactions, and other health-related activities, that may promote cognitive functioning (Hertzog et al., 2008). Informed by the life-span development perspective (Baltes & Baltes, 1993), this theory posits that cognitive functioning remains malleable and open to enhancement throughout life. Even in older age, individuals can preserve or improve cognitive functioning through engagement in intellectual, physical, and social activities (Hertzog et al., 2008).

Further supporting this framework is the concept of cognitive plasticity, which refers to an individual's potential to acquire new cognitive skills and adapt to changing contexts (Willis & Schaie, 2009). While cognitive plasticity declines with age, significant neural plasticity remains, allowing older adults to improve cognitive functioning through targeted activities (Hertzog et al., 2008; Willis & Schaie, 2009). However, the extent to which individuals approach their maximum cognitive potential is influenced by environmental factors and cognitive-relevant behaviors (Denney, 1984; Kramer et al., 2004).

The concept of "digital nativity" adds another layer to this discussion. Digital natives—individuals from generations such as Millennials, Generation Z, and Generation Alpha—have grown up with widespread access to digital technologies, making them more proficient and adaptable to ICT use (Wang et al., 2019). In contrast, older adults often perceive digital technology as intellectually challenging and may lack the same level of proficiency (Kim & Choudhury, 2020). However, this perceived challenge also highlights the potential cognitive benefits of ICT use for older adults. Learning to use ICT requires intensive cognitive engagement, as users must navigate novel tasks, solve problems, and adapt to new interfaces. For older adults, particularly those living with dementia, this interaction with novel and engaging stimuli may create a protective effect against further cognitive decline.

By drawing on these theories and concepts, this study contributes to a broader understanding of how ICT use may support cognitive health in later life, uniquely capturing ICT engagement through measures of access, frequency, and breadth.

16.1.2 Literature Review

16.1.2.1 Cognitive Functioning Among Older Adults

Cognitive change is a natural part of aging, but the patterns and extent of these changes vary across different cognitive domains. Cognitive abilities are often categorized into crystallized intelligence and fluid intelligence (Harada et al., 2013). Crystallized intelligence, which reflects accumulated knowledge and skills from lifelong experiences, remains stable or even improves with age. In contrast, fluid intelligence, which involves problem-solving, reasoning, and processing unfamiliar information, declines significantly after peaking in one's 30s. This domain includes abilities such as memory, processing speed, executive function, and psychomotor skills (Harada et al., 2013).

While cognitive changes are a normal part of aging, they do not inevitably lead to cognitive impairment. The rate and severity of cognitive decline vary widely among older adults, influenced by sociodemographic factors (e.g., education, socioeconomic status) and lifestyle behaviors (e.g., physical activity, social engagement) (Berner et al., 2019; Livingston et al., 2020). Importantly, current research suggests that cognitive impairment is not an inevitable outcome of aging but rather a condition that can be prevented or managed through targeted interventions (Livingston et al., 2020). A key concept supporting this perspective is neuroplasticity, the brain's ability to adapt in response to new stimuli, even in the face of age-related decline. This adaptability can be enhanced through cognitively stimulating activities and social interactions, offering a pathway to prevent or manage cognitive decline (Berner et al., 2019; Calhoun & Lee, 2019). These findings underscore the potential for ICT interventions that promote cognitive health and resilience in older adults.

16.1.2.2 ICT Use and Older Adults' Cognitive Functioning

Longitudinal studies have reported consistent bi-directional associations between ICT use and older adults' cognitive functioning (Choi et al., 2021; Yu & Fiebig, 2020). For instance, research using national representative samples from China and the U.S. found reciprocal relationships between ICT use and cognitive functioning. Notably, the impact of ICT use on cognitive functioning was significantly stronger than the reverse effect (Choi et al., 2021; Yu & Fiebig, 2020). Additionally, ICT use was found to predict executive function, but not vice versa (Choi et al., 2021). Given the present study's goal of examining whether ICT use can promote cognitive functioning and prevent cognitive decline, this paper will focus on the direction from ICT use to cognitive functioning.

ICT use encompasses multiple dimensions, including access/use, frequency of use, and breadth of use (Moxley & Czaja, 2019; van Deursen & van Dijk, 2014). The first-level digital divide focuses on access to ICT devices and the , as well as whether individuals have ever used ICT (Gómez, 2018). However, with the widespread adoption of the internet and ICT devices, the traditional access divide has been criticized for oversimplifying a complex social phenomenon as merely a technological or economic issue (Gómez, 2018). Consequently, the second-level digital divide, which emphasizes disparities in ICT usage, including frequency and breadth, has gained attention (Gómez, 2018). This study reviews previous research on older adults' ICT use and cognitive functioning, considering these distinct dimensions of ICT use.

ICT Access/Use and Cognitive Functioning A 2021 report by the Pew Research Center revealed that while 99% of U.S. adults aged 18–29, 98% of those aged 30–49, and 96% of those aged 50–64 are users, only 75% of adults aged 65 or older use the internet. This means that one in four older adults does not use the internet, highlighting a significant disparity in ICT access/use. As the first-level digital divide, ICT access/use primarily examines the gap between those who have access to ICT and those who do not (Choudrie et al., 2021). For older adults, gaining access to and using ICT often involves a novel learning experience that requires significant cognitive effort, including executive function, episodic memory, and reasoning (Choi et al., 2021; Vaportzis et al., 2017). Consequently, older adults with ICT access/use may exhibit better cognitive functioning compared to those without such experience. This positive association between ICT access/use and global cognitive functioning has been consistently demonstrated across diverse populations, including European, Brazilian, and Chinese older adults (Berner et al., 2019; Kamin & Lang, 2020; Krug et al., 2019; Lin, 2017; Yu & Fiebig, 2020).

ICT Use Frequency and Cognitive Functioning The concept of "use it or lose it", derived from animal experiments, suggests that activating neurons within a physiological range during aging can benefit neuronal function and preserve cognitive abilities (Swaab, 1991). Extending this logic, more frequent activation of neurons (within the physiological range) may correlate with better cognitive functioning. Although findings vary across specific cognitive domains, studies have consistently shown that ICT use frequency is positively associated with global cognitive functioning in older adults across cultures (Tun & Lachman, 2010; Wu et al., 2019). Older adults who use ICT more frequently tend to have better cognitive functioning than those who use it less often.

ICT Use Breadth and Cognitive Functioning ICT provides older adults with access to a wide range of online activities, such as social networking, information searching, shopping, banking, self-learning, and entertainment. Emerging evidence suggests that different ICT activities may have varying cognitive benefits. For example, using social media to connect with family or friends has been linked to better executive function (Khoo & Yang, 2020), while engaging in digital games is associated with improved executive function and processing speed (Zhang & Kaufman, 2016). A study using data from the National Health and Aging Trends Study (NHATS, 2011–2015) found that activities like emailing, texting, and searching for medical information significantly reduced the odds of cognitive impairment, whereas online banking, grocery shopping, and prescription refilling did not show the same protective effect (Amini et al., 2019). More recent NHATS data (2013, 2015, and 2017) further support the idea that greater breadth of ICT use—engaging in more types of ICT activities—is associated with better episodic memory and executive function (Choi et al., 2021).

Despite the generally positive associations between ICT use and cognitive functioning, some studies report inconsistent results. For example, a 6-year longitudinal study of older Dutch adults (aged 50 or older) found that new computer users showed small but significant improvements in selective attention and memory compared to non-users. However, consistent computer users did not demonstrate significantly better cognitive functioning than non-users in other domains (Slegers et al., 2012). One possible explanation is that different measures of ICT use reflect distinct aspects of ICT engagement, which may have varying effects on cognitive functioning. However, few studies have systematically examined these differences. To address this gap, the present study investigates the associations between ICT use and cognitive functioning through three distinct measures: ICT access/use, use frequency, and use breadth.

16.2 Methodology

16.2.1 Data Source

This study used data from the Health and Retirement Study (HRS), a nationally representative panel study funded by the National Institute on Aging (NIA, U01AG009740) and conducted by the University of Michigan. Since 1992, the HRS has surveyed approximately 20,000 Americans aged 50+ and their spouses on health, cognitive functioning, retirement, and economic well-being. To assess psychological issues, the HRS introduced the Leave-Behind Questionnaire (LBQ) in 2004, a self-administered survey added to the core HRS in 2006. The LBQ collected data on life circumstances, subjective well-being, and lifestyle. Participants were randomly divided into two groups, completing the LBQ every 4 years (2006/2010/2014/2018 or 2008/2012/2016). While psychological well-being measures, including ICT use frequency, were collected every 4 years, other data (e.g., health status, cognitive functioning) were collected biennially.

The Internet Survey, an off-year study of the HRS, was conducted biennially from 2003 to 2013. Funded by the NIA (R01 AG020638) and developed by the University of Michigan and the RAND Corporation, it covered topics such as and computer use. The 2013 Internet Survey, which included prior participants and those who newly gained access, had a peak sample size of 7,744 eligible participants, with 5,813 completing the survey (response rate: 75%) (Health and Retirement Study, 2015).

16.2.2 Study Sample

To account for the delayed impact of ICT use, only older adults with consistent ICT use status (consistent users or non-users) over a 4-year period were included. Participants with changes in ICT access status during this interval were excluded. Detailed questions on ICT use breadth were only available in the 2013 Internet Survey, so this measure was assessed once in 2013. The 2013 Internet Survey sampled participants from the 2011 Internet Survey with ongoing access, an 80% random subsample of new cohort respondents (Middle Baby Boomers), and an 80% random subsample of panel respondents who newly gained access in 2012.

The study used HRS 2012 as the baseline (T1) and 2016 as the follow-up (T2), aligning with the 4-year LBQ intervals. Of the 20,554 participants in HRS 2012, 10,079 were randomly selected for the LBQ, with 7,330 completing it. Among these, 5,951 were eligible for the 2016 LBQ, and 4,600 completed it. After excluding participants under 65 ($N = 2{,}219$), those without ICT use data in 2012 and 2016 ($n = 70$), and those with dementia or dementia onset in 2012 ($n = 57$), 2,254 participants remained. Further exclusions were made for inconsistent ICT use status ($n = 224$) and missing ICT use breadth data ($n = 521$), resulting in a final analytic sample of 1,509 participants. This study used publicly available HRS data and received an "exempt" IRB designation from the authors' institution.

16.2.3 Measures

Data for this study were drawn from the HRS 2012 and 2016 surveys and the 2013 Internet Survey. Independent variables included ICT access/use and ICT use frequency, extracted from the Leave-Behind Questionnaire (LBQ) of 2012 HRS, and ICT use breadth, drawn from the 2013 Internet Survey. The outcome variable, cognitive functioning, was measured using data from HRS 2016. Socio-demographic characteristics and baseline cognitive functioning were obtained from HRS 2012. A summary of the variables used is provided in Table 16.1.

Information & Communication Technology (ICT) Use ICT use was measured using three variables: ICT access/use, ICT use frequency, and ICT use breadth.

ICT Access/Use ICT access/use was measured in HRS 2012 with the question, "How often do you use a computer for email, , or other tasks?" Responses ranged from 1 (daily) to 7 (never/not relevant). Participants who responded "never/not relevant" were classified as non-users, while others were classified as ICT users.

ICT Use Frequency Based on the same question as ICT access/use, responses were recoded as 0 (never/not relevant) to 6 (daily), with higher scores indicating more frequent ICT use.

Table 16.1 Descriptive analyses of participants' characteristics

	Mean ± SD	Minimum	Maximum	%	*N*
Variables at T1					
Age	74.40 ± 5.95	65	94		
Younger				53.48%	807
Older				46.52%	702
Gender					
Men				40.09%	605
Women				59.91%	904
Race/ethnicity					
White				85.42%	1,289
People of color				14.58%	220
Education	3.25 ± 1.33	1	5	Median = 3	IQR = 1
Less than high school				17.97%	271
GED				4.24%	64
High school graduate				34.48%	520
Some college				21.88%	330
College and above				21.42%	323
ICT access/use					
ICT non-user				49.64%	749
ICT user				50.36%	760
ICT use frequency	2.85 ± 2.89	0	6	Median = 2	IQR = 6
Never/not relevant				49.64%	749
Not in the last month				.27%	4
Once a month				.80%	12
Several times a month				.99%	15
Once a week				1.26%	19
Several times a week				6.96%	105
Daily				40.09%	605
ICT use breadth	1.57 ± 1.68	0	4	Median = 1	IQR = 3
Not use				49.83%	752
One category				2.92%	44
Two categories				7.49%	113
Three categories				20.41%	308
Four categories				19.35%	292
ICT use category					
Financial use				36.05%	544
Online shopping				44.73%	675
Social use				26.64%	402
General use				50.30%	759
Cognition (T1)	22.41 ± 4.27	0	35		

GED general educational development, *IQR* interquartile range
$^{*}p < .05$; $^{**}p < .01$; $^{***}p < .001$

Breadth of ICT Use Measured in the 2013 Internet Survey, this variable assessed the diversity of ICT use across four categories: financial use, online shopping, social use, and general use. Participants without ICT access/use were coded as 0, while scores ranged from 0 to 4 based on the number of categories in which they engaged.

Cognitive Functioning Cognitive functioning was measured using a reduced version of the Telephone Interview for Cognitive Status (TICS), a validated multidimensional tool for assessing cognitive abilities, including episodic memory, knowledge, language, and orientation (Breitner et al., 1995). The total score (range: 0–35) included immediate word recall (0–10), delayed word recall (0–10), Serial 7s (0–5), backward counting (0–2), date naming (0–4), object naming (0–2), and naming the President and Vice President of the U.S. (0–1 each). The outcome, cognitive functioning at T2, was extracted from HRS 2016.

Covariates Age, gender, race/ethnicity, education, and baseline cognitive functioning were added as covariates in this study. To compare different age groups, age was coded as a dichotomous variable: 0 for younger adults (65–74); 1 for older adults (75 or older) (Fang et al., 2018). Gender was measured dichotomously (0 = male, 1 = female). Considering the small sample size of non-Hispanic Blacks, Hispanics and participants of other races, race/ethnicity was measured dichotomously (0 = non-Hispanic White, 1 = people of color). Education was assessed in five categories (1 = less than high school, 2 = general educational development, 3 = high school graduate, 4 = some college, 5 = college and above). Cognitive functioning at T1 was extracted from HRS 2012, ranging from 0 to 35, with higher scores indicating better cognitive functioning.

16.2.4 Statistical Analyses

This study used HRS data to examine the associations between ICT use and cognitive functioning among older adults. Prior to the main analyses, univariate and bivariate statistics were conducted to understand the data and assess whether basic assumptions were met. Univariate statistics, including frequencies and measures of central tendency, were used to describe the data. For bivariate analyses, Pearson's correlation tests were conducted to examine the relationships between continuous independent variables and the outcome (cognitive functioning). For categorical independent variables, t-tests were used to assess their associations with the outcome. Although normality tests were initially considered, the large sample size (N = 1,509) allowed reliance on the central limit theorem, which states that parameter estimates will approximate a normal distribution regardless of the population's shape, provided the sample is sufficiently large (Field, 2013, p. 170). Thus, normality tests were deemed unnecessary. Additional bivariate analyses were conducted to test differences in participant characteristics by ICT use status.

To address the research question, three multiple linear regression models were conducted using maximum likelihood-based parameter estimation (ML). Each model assessed the association between a specific ICT use measure (ICT access/use, ICT use frequency, or ICT use breadth) and cognitive functioning, while controlling for age, gender, race/ethnicity, education, and baseline cognitive functioning.

16.3 Results

16.3.1 Participants' Characteristics and Bivariate Analyses

Participants' characteristics are summarized in Table 16.1. Among the 1,509 older adults in the study, nearly 57% were aged 75 or older, 60% were women, and 15% identified as people of color. Regarding education, approximately 18% had less than a high school education, 4% held a GED, 34% were high school graduates, 22% had some college experience, and 21% had a college degree or higher. The median education level was 3, with an interquartile range (IQR) of 1. In terms of ICT use, 50% of participants were non-users, while the remaining 50% reported varying levels of engagement. Less than 1% used ICT once a month, 1% used it several times a month, 1% used it once a week, 7% used it several times a week, and 40% used it daily. The median ICT use frequency was 2 (IQR = 6). For ICT use breadth, 50% were non-users, while 3% used ICT for one category of activities, 7% for two categories, 20% for three categories, and 19% for all four categories. The median ICT use breadth was 1 (IQR = 3). Specifically, 36% used ICT for financial purposes, 45% for online shopping, 27% for social purposes, and 50% for general purposes.

Bivariate analyses, presented in Table 16.2, revealed that all independent variables and covariates were significantly associated with cognitive functioning at T2. Specifically, older age, male gender, and people of color were associated with lower cognitive functioning at T2, while education, T1 cognitive functioning, ICT access/use, ICT use frequency, and ICT use breadth were positively associated with cognitive functioning at T2. Additionally, compared to ICT non-users, ICT users were more likely to be younger, male, and non-Hispanic White users also tended to have higher educational attainment and better baseline cognitive functioning than non-users.

16.3.2 Multiple Linear Regressions of ICT Use on Cognitive Functioning

The results of multiple linear regressions on cognitive functioning at T2 are presented in Table 16.3. In Model 1, ICT access/use at T1 was significantly associated with cognitive functioning at T2 ($B = 1.31, p < .001$), after controlling for cognitive functioning at T1 and other variables. This indicates that, compared to older adults

Table 16.2 Bivariate analyses of participants' characteristics with cognitive function at T2 and ICT use

	Cognition T2		ICT Use		
	Mean	*t*/*r*	No	Yes	χ^2/t
Variables at T1					
Age		10.28***			70.88***
Younger	22.38		39.53%	60.47%	
Older	19.98		61.25%	38.75%	
Gender		−2.45*			4.11*
Men	20.90		46.45%	53.55%	
Women	21.50		51.77%	48.23%	
Race/ethnicity		7.69***			42.73***
White	21.64		46.16%	53.84%	
People of color	19.06		70.00%	30.00%	
Education		.43**	2.55	3.93	−23.51***
ICT access/use		−20.49***			
ICT non-user	19.06				
ICT user	23.43				
ICT use frequency		.47**			
ICT use breadth		.46**			
Cognition (T1)		.71**	20.46	24.32	−19.66***

*$p < .05$; **$p < .01$; ***$p < .001$

Table 16.3 Unstandardized coefficients of ICT use on cognitive function at T2

	Model 1	Model 2	Model 3
ICT access/use	1.31***		
ICT use frequency		.24***	
ICT use breadth			.36***
Cognitive function (T1)	.63***	.63***	.64***
Older	−1.08***	−1.06***	−1.06***
Women	.19	.19	.17
People of color	−.59*	−.56*	−.58*
Education (1–5)	.23**	.22**	.26***
R square explained	.54	.54	.54

*$p < .05$; **$p < .01$; ***$p < .001$

without ICT access or use, ICT users had cognitive functioning scores at T2 that were 1.31 units higher. Similar results were observed in Model 2 and Model 3. ICT use frequency ($B = 0.24$, $p < .001$) and ICT use breadth ($B = 0.36$, $p < .001$) were also significantly associated with higher cognitive functioning at T2, after controlling for cognitive functioning at T1 and other variables. Across all three models, higher cognitive functioning at T1, younger age, non-Hispanic White race, and higher education levels were associated with better cognitive functioning at T2. Collectively, the three models explained 54% of the variance in cognitive functioning at T2.

16.4 Discussion

As the use of ICT among older adults continues to grow, increasing attention has been devoted to understanding its cognitive impacts. While numerous studies across different cultures have highlighted the cognitive benefits of ICT use in this demographic, there remains limited understanding of how various aspects of ICT engagement influence cognitive functioning. To address this gap, the present study examined the relationships between three key aspects of ICT use—ICT access/use, use frequency, and use breadth—and cognitive functioning in older adults. This investigation provides valuable insights into the complex relationship between ICT engagement and cognitive well-being in this population.

The findings of this study indicate that ICT use, encompassing ICT access/use, use frequency, and use breadth, is positively associated with cognitive functioning in older adults, supporting the hypothesis. This aligns with previous research (Berner et al., 2019; Choi et al., 2021; Kamin & Lang, 2020), which found a positive relationship between ICT access/use and higher cognitive function scores. ICT is often novel to older adults and requires learning new skills to navigate devices, apps, and techniques (Choi et al., 2021). According to Cognitive Enrichment Theory, engaging in intellectually stimulating learning activities can help older adults preserve or even enhance their cognitive functioning (Hertzog et al., 2008). Thus, the process of learning ICT may directly improve cognitive function by providing intellectual challenges. Intervention studies have consistently shown that learning ICT can enhance various cognitive domains, such as episodic memory, processing speed, executive function, and inhibitory control (Abduljalil, 2019; Quinn, 2018; Vaportzis et al., 2017).

Once older adults become proficient in ICT use, continued engagement with technology can further enhance their cognitive abilities. The clinical potential of ICT for cognitive health is vast and warrants further exploration. Even after acquiring basic ICT skills, some older adults may still face challenges using technology (Betts et al., 2019; Gitlow, 2014). They may need to spend time troubleshooting independently or learning from others. Additionally, some may seek to expand their ICT skills beyond the basics (Betts et al., 2019). These ongoing intellectual challenges can provide sustained cognitive stimulation, acting as an additional protective factor. Even for older adults using ICT for familiar activities, such as accessing new information online or staying connected with others, cognitive benefits may arise. This supports the notion of maintaining an active and productive lifestyle in later adulthood, as highlighted in previous studies (Ekerdt, 1986; Ruggiano et al., 2017). Ultimately, the active use of ICT offers older adults a daily opportunity for continuous learning and cognitive engagement (Quinn, 2018).

The univariate analysis revealed that, in 2012, 50.36% of participants were ICT users, a finding consistent with several prior surveys. For example, the Current Population Survey (US Census Bureau, 2014) indicated that 51.4% of adults aged 65 and older had access to the either at home or elsewhere. Similarly, the Pew Research Center (2017) reported that 54% of older adults in this age group used these technologies. These figures align with existing literature (Choi et al., 2021; Hänninen et al., 2021; Hargittai & Dobransky, 2017), which consistently finds that

ICT users tend to be younger, male, non-Hispanic White, more highly educated, and in better baseline cognitive health.

The bivariate analysis further highlighted that older age, male gender, and being a person of color are associated with lower cognitive functioning, underscoring these as potential risk factors for cognitive decline. These findings are consistent with prior research suggesting that older age (Han et al., 2022) and being a person of color (Zuelsdorff et al., 2020) can negatively influence cognitive health. However, the observed negative association with male gender deviates from some earlier studies (Levine et al., 2021), suggesting that contextual or methodological differences, such as population characteristics, measurement tools, or unaccounted environmental factors, may have influenced these results. Given this negative association, it is crucial to develop male-specific cognitive health strategies. These could involve increasing male participation in community and mental health services, where engagement tends to be lower, and addressing the stigma surrounding mental health support (Chatmon, 2020). Additionally, culturally sensitive interventions for people of color should consider language accessibility, cultural relevance in health communication, and the involvement of community leaders to improve engagement and program effectiveness.

16.4.1 Implication

The present study demonstrates a positive association between three aspects of ICT use—access/use, use frequency, and use breadth—and cognitive functioning among older adults. These findings offer timely and valuable insights that can inform strategies to promote successful cognitive aging. The implications can be translated into practice in promoting ICT access/use and delivering ICT-based cognitive interventions.

At the individual level, efforts are needed to raise older adults' awareness of the cognitive benefits of ICT use. This can be achieved through community talks, educational programs, and informational brochures. For older adults facing financial barriers to ICT access, practitioners can connect them to available resources, such as senior centers or public agencies offering free computer and access. Advocacy for additional resources, such as partnerships with local governments or companies to provide discounts on technology devices or services for older adults, is also critical.

At the macro level, governmental support is essential to promote ICT access among older adults, particularly those with low socioeconomic status. Subsidies for digital devices and connections, as well as collaborations with public libraries and senior centers to provide low-cost or rentable technology, could help bridge the digital divide. Additionally, expanding broadband and high-speed coverage in rural areas is crucial to ensure equitable access for older adults living in underserved regions. To address knowledge barriers, federal and state policies should include funding for ICT training programs tailored to older adults. These programs could be integrated into existing initiatives, such as the Older Americans Act, to ensure widespread access to ICT education and support.

16.4.2 Limitations

While this study provides valuable insights into the positive effects of ICT use on cognitive functioning, several limitations must be considered. First, the study focused on the unidirectional association from ICT use to cognitive functioning, although prior research suggests bidirectional relationships (Choi et al., 2021; Yu & Fiebig, 2020). Second, participants with dementia or severe cognitive impairment were excluded due to the cognitive demands of ICT use, limiting the generalizability of the findings to this population. Third, the overlap in the distributions of the three ICT use measures, due to the sampling strategy of the archival data, may have obscured nuanced effects. Future studies should develop more refined measures to better understand the distinct impacts of different aspects of ICT use.

16.4.3 Conclusions

This study contributes valuable insights into the relationship between ICT use and cognitive functioning among older adults. The findings reveal robust positive associations between ICT access, use frequency, use breadth, and cognitive functioning, even after controlling for demographic factors and baseline cognitive functioning. These results highlight the potential of ICT use as a tool to preserve cognitive health in aging populations. The study underscores the importance of implementing ICT training programs tailored for older adults, which can not only prevent cognitive decline but also enhance overall well-being in the context of a rapidly aging population.

Disclaimer The views expressed in this chapter are solely those of the authors and do not necessarily reflect the views of the University of Alabama at Birmingham or the University at Albany.

References

Abbott, A. (2011). Dementia: A problem for our age. *Nature, 475*(7355), S2–S4. https://doi.org/10.1038/475S2a

Abduljalil, S. (2019). *Effect of learning tablet applications on episodic memory in cognitively healthy older adults* (2295419681) [M.S., California State University, Fullerton]. ProQuest Dissertations & Theses Global.

Alzheimer's Association. (2021). 2021 Alzheimer's disease facts and figures. *Alzheimers Dement, 17*(3), 327–406. https://doi.org/10.1002/alz.12328

Amini, R., Chee, K. H., Mendieta, M., & Parker, S. (2019). Online engagement and cognitive function among older adults. *Geriatrics & Gerontology International, 19*(9), 918–923. https://doi.org/10.1111/ggi.13749

Baltes, P. B., & Baltes, M. M. (1993). *Successful aging: Perspectives from the behavioral sciences* (Vol. 4). Cambridge University Press.

Berner, J., Comijs, H., Elmståhl, S., Welmer, A.-K., Sanmartin Berglund, J., Anderberg, P., & Deeg, D. (2019). Maintaining cognitive function with use: A two-country, six-year longitudinal study. *International Psychogeriatrics, 31*(7), 929–936. Cambridge Core. https://doi.org/10.1017/S1041610219000668

Betts, L. R., Hill, R., & Gardner, S. E. (2019). "There's Not Enough Knowledge Out There": Examining older adults' perceptions of digital technology use and digital inclusion classes. *Journal of Applied Gerontology, 38*(8), 1147–1166. https://doi.org/10.1177/0733464817737621

Breitner, J. C. S., Welsh, K. A., Gau, B. A., McDonald, W. M., Steffens, D. C., Saunders, A. M., Magruder, K. M., Helms, M. J., Plassman, B. L., Folstein, M. F., Brandt, J., Robinette, C. D., & Page, W. F. (1995). Alzheimer's disease in the National Academy of Sciences—National Research Council Registry of aging twin veterans: III. Detection of cases, longitudinal results, and observations on twin concordance. *Archives of Neurology, 52*(8), 763–771. https://doi.org/10.1001/archneur.1995.00540320035011

Calhoun, D., & Lee, S. B. (2019). Computer usage and cognitive capability of older adults: Analysis of data from the Health and Retirement Study. *Educational Gerontology, 45*(1), 22–33. https://doi.org/10.1080/03601277.2019.1575026

Centers for Disease Control and Prevention. (2019). *What is dementia?* https://www.cdc.gov/aging/dementia/index.html

Chatmon, B. N. (2020). Males and mental health stigma. *American Journal of Men's Health, 14*(4). https://doi.org/10.1177/1557988320949322

Choi, E. Y., Wisniewski, K. M., & Zelinski, E. M. (2021). Information and communication technology use in older adults: A unidirectional or Bi-directional association with cognitive function? *Computers in Human Behavior, 121*, 106813. https://doi.org/10.1016/j.chb.2021.106813

Choudrie, J., Zamani, E., & Obuekwe, C. (2021). Bridging the digital divide in ethnic minority older adults: An organisational qualitative study. *Information Systems Frontiers*. https://doi.org/10.1007/s10796-021-10126-8

Cipriani, G., Danti, S., Picchi, L., Nuti, A., & Fiorino, M. D. (2020). Daily functioning and dementia. *Dementia Neuropsychologia, 14*, 93–102. https://doi.org/10.1590/1980-57642020dn14-020001

Denney, N. W. (1984). A model of cognitive development across the life span. *Developmental Review, 4*(2), 171–191. https://doi.org/10.1016/0273-2297(84)90006-6

Ekerdt, D. J. (1986). The busy ethic: Moral continuity between work and retirement. *The Gerontologist, 26*(3), 239–244. https://doi.org/10.1093/geront/26.3.239

Ericsson, K. A., & Charness, N. (1994). Expert performance: Its structure and acquisition. *American Psychologist, 49*(8), 725–747. APA PsycArticles. https://doi.org/10.1037/0003-066X.49.8.725

Fang, Y., Chau, A. K. C., Wong, A., Fung, H. H., & Woo, J. (2018). Information and communicative technology use enhances psychological well-being of older adults: The roles of age, social connectedness, and frailty status. *Aging & Mental Health, 22*(11), 1516–1524. https://doi.org/10.1080/13607863.2017.1358354

Field, A. (2013). *Discovering statistics using IBM SPSS statistics* (4th ed.). SAGE.

Gitlow, L. (2014). Technology use by older adults and barriers to using technology. *Physical & Occupational Therapy in Geriatrics, 32*(3), 271–280. https://doi.org/10.3109/02703181.2014.946640

Gómez, D. C. (2018). *The three levels of the digital divide: Barriers in access, use and utility of among young people in Spain*. https://doi.org/10.31211/interacoes.n34.2018.a4

Han, F., Luo, C., Lv, D., Tian, L., & Qu, C. (2022). Risk factors affecting cognitive impairment of the elderly aged 65 and over: A cross-sectional study. *Frontiers in Aging Neuroscience, 14*. https://doi.org/10.3389/fnagi.2022.903794

Hänninen, R., Taipale, S., & Luostari, R. (2021). Exploring heterogeneous ICT use among older adults: The warm experts' perspective. *New Media & Society, 23*(6), 1584–1601. https://doi.org/10.1177/1461444820917353

Harada, C. N., Natelson Love, M. C., & Triebel, K. L. (2013). Normal cognitive aging. *Clinics in Geriatric Medicine, 29*(4), 737–752. https://doi.org/10.1016/j.cger.2013.07.002

Hargittai, E., & Dobransky, K. (2017). Old dogs, new clicks: Digital inequality in skills and uses among older adults. *Canadian Journal of Communication, 42*(2), 195–212. Academic Search Premier. https://doi.org/10.22230/cjc.2017v42n2a3176

Health and Retirement Study. (2015). *Health and retirement study 2013 survey (final, version 1.0).*

Hertzog, C., Kramer, A. F., Wilson, R. S., & Lindenberger, U. (2008). Enrichment effects on adult cognitive development: Can the functional capacity of older adults be preserved and enhanced? *Psychological Science in the Public Interest, 9*(1), 1–65. https://doi.org/10.1111/j.1539-6053.2009.01034.x

Hultsch, D. F., Hertzog, C., Small, B. J., & Dixon, R. A. (1999). Use it or lose it: Engaged lifestyle as a buffer of cognitive decline in aging? *Psychology and Aging, 14*(2), 245–263. https://doi.org/10.1037/0882-7974.14.2.245

Kamin, S. T., & Lang, F. R. (2020). Use and cognitive functioning in late adulthood: Longitudinal findings from the Survey of Health, Ageing and Retirement in Europe (SHARE). *The Journals of Gerontology: Series B, 75*(3), 534–539. https://doi.org/10.1093/geronb/gby123

Khoo, S. S., & Yang, H. (2020). Social media use improves executive functions in middle-aged and older adults: A structural equation modeling analysis. *Computers in Human Behavior, 111*, 106388. https://doi.org/10.1016/j.chb.2020.106388

Kim, S., & Choudhury, A. (2020). Comparison of older and younger adults' attitudes toward the adoption and use of activity trackers. *JMIR mHealth and uHealth, 8*(10), e18312. https://doi.org/10.2196/18312

Kramer, A. F., Bherer, L., Colcombe, S. J., Dong, W., & Greenough, W. T. (2004). Environmental influences on cognitive and brain plasticity during aging. *The Journals of Gerontology: Series A, 59*(9), M940–M957. https://doi.org/10.1093/gerona/59.9.M940

Krug, R. R., d'Orsi, E., & Xavier, A. J. (2019). Association between use of and the cognitive function in older adults, populational longitudinal study EpiFloripa Idoso. *Revista Brasileira de Epidemiologia, 22*, e190012. https://doi.org/10.1590/1980-549720190012

Lee, M.-T., Jang, Y., & Chang, W.-Y. (2019). How do impairments in cognitive functions affect activities of daily living functions in older adults? *PLoS One, 14*(6), e0218112. https://doi.org/10.1371/journal.pone.0218112

Levine, D. A., Gross, A. L., Briceño, E. M., Tilton, N., Giordani, B. J., Sussman, J. B., Hayward, R. A., Burke, J. F., Hingtgen, S., Elkind, M. S. V., Manly, J. J., Gottesman, R. F., Gaskin, D. J., Sidney, S., Sacco, R. L., Tom, S. E., Wright, C. B., Yaffe, K., & Galecki, A. T. (2021). Sex differences in cognitive decline among US adults. *JAMA Network Open, 4*(2), e210169. https://doi.org/10.1001/jamanetworkopen.2021.0169

Lin, S.-Y. (2017). 'Dementia-friendly communities' and being dementia friendly in healthcare settings. *Current Opinion in Psychiatry, 30*(2), 145–150. https://doi.org/10.1097/YCO.0000000000000304

Livingston, G., Huntley, J., Sommerlad, A., Ames, D., Ballard, C., Banerjee, S., Brayne, C., Burns, A., Cohen-Mansfield, J., Cooper, C., Costafreda, S. G., Dias, A., Fox, N., Gitlin, L. N., Howard, R., Kales, H. C., Kivimäki, M., Larson, E. B., Ogunniyi, A., et al. (2020). Dementia prevention, intervention, and care: 2020 report of the Lancet Commission. *Lancet (London, England), 396*(10248), 413–446. https://doi.org/10.1016/S0140-6736(20)30367-6

Livingston, G., Sommerlad, A., Orgeta, V., Costafreda, S. G., Huntley, J., Ames, D., Ballard, C., Banerjee, S., Burns, A., Cohen-Mansfield, J., Cooper, C., Fox, N., Gitlin, L. N., Howard, R., Kales, H. C., Larson, E. B., Ritchie, K., Rockwood, K., Sampson, E. L., et al. (2017). Dementia prevention, intervention, and care. *The Lancet, 390*(10113), 2673–2734. https://doi.org/10.1016/S0140-6736(17)31363-6

Mayo Foundation for Medical Education and Research. (2024, March 13). *Alzheimer's and dementia: What's the difference?* Mayo Clinic. https://www.mayoclinic.org/diseases-conditions/alzheimers-disease/expert-answers/alzheimers-and-dementia-whats-the-difference/faq-20396861

Moxley, J. H., & Czaja, S. J. (2019). Potential mediators of the relationship between usage and cognition. *International Psychogeriatrics, 31*(7), 917–919. Cambridge Core. https://doi.org/10.1017/S1041610219001054

National Institute on Aging. (2020). *Cognitive health and older adults*. https://www.nia.nih.gov/health/cognitive-health-and-older-adults

Quinn, K. (2018). Cognitive effects of social media use: A case of older adults. *Social Media + Society, 4*(3), 2056305118787203. https://doi.org/10.1177/2056305118787203

Rajan, K. B., Weuve, J., Barnes, L. L., McAninch, E. A., Wilson, R. S., & Evans, D. A. (2021). Population estimate of people with clinical Alzheimer's disease and mild cognitive impairment in the United States (2020–2060). *Alzheimer's & Dementia, n/a*(n/a). https://doi.org/10.1002/alz.12362

Ruggiano, N., O'Driscoll, J., Lukic, A., & Schotthoefer, L. (2017). "Work Is Like a Therapy That Prevents Aging": Perceptions of retirement, productivity, and health among minorities and immigrants. *SAGE Open, 7*(1), 2158244016687234. https://doi.org/10.1177/2158244016687234

Salthouse, T. A. (2016). *Theoretical perspectives on cognitive aging*. Psychology Press.

Schaie, K. W., & Willis, S. L. (1986). Can decline in adult intellectual functioning be reversed? *Developmental Psychology, 22*(2), 223–232. https://doi.org/10.1037/0012-1649.22.2.223

Shearer, E. (2017, September 7). News use across social media platforms 2017. Pew Research Center. https://www.pewresearch.org/journalism/2017/09/07/news-use-across-social-media-platforms-2017/

Slegers, K., van Boxtel, M. P. J., & Jolles, J. (2012). Computer use in older adults: Determinants and the relationship with cognitive change over a 6year episode. *Computers in Human Behavior, 28*(1), 1–10. https://doi.org/10.1016/j.chb.2011.08.003

Swaab, D. F. (1991). Brain aging and Alzheimer's disease, "Wear and tear" versus "Use it or lose it". *Neurobiology of Aging, 12*(4), 317–324. https://doi.org/10.1016/0197-4580(91)90008-8

Tun, P. A., & Lachman, M. E. (2010). The association between computer use and cognition across adulthood: Use it so you won't lose it? *Psychology and Aging, 25*(3), 560–568. https://doi.org/10.1037/a0019543

US Census Bureau. (2014). *Computer and access in the United States: 2012*.

van Deursen, A. J. A. M., & van Dijk, J. A. G. M. (2014). The digital divide shifts to differences in usage. *New Media & Society, 16*(3), 507–526. https://doi.org/10.1177/1461444813487959

Vaportzis, E., Martin, M., & Gow, A. J. (2017). A tablet for healthy ageing: The effect of a tablet computer training intervention on cognitive abilities in older adults. *The American Journal of Geriatric Psychiatry, 25*(8), 841–851. https://doi.org/10.1016/j.jagp.2016.11.015

Wang, H.-Y., Sigerson, L., & Cheng, C. (2019). Digital Nativity and information technology addiction: Age cohort versus individual difference approaches. *Computers in Human Behavior, 90*, 1–9. https://doi.org/10.1016/j.chb.2018.08.031

Willis, S. L., & Schaie, K. W. (2009). Cognitive training and plasticity: Theoretical perspective and methodological consequences. *Restorative Neurology and Neuroscience, 27*(5), 375–389. https://doi.org/10.3233/rnn-2009-0527

Wu, Y.-H., Lewis, M., & Rigaud, A.-S. (2019). Cognitive function and digital device use in older adults attending a memory clinic. *Gerontology and Geriatric Medicine, 5*, 2333721419844886. https://doi.org/10.1177/2333721419844886

Yang, H. D., Kim, D. H., Lee, S. B., & Young, L. D. (2016). History of Alzheimer's disease. *Dementia and Neurocognitive Disorders, 15*(4), 115–121. https://doi.org/10.12779/dnd.2016.15.4.115

Yu, D., & Fiebig, D. G. (2020). Use and cognition among middle-aged and older adults in China: A cross-lagged panel analysis. *The Journal of the Economics of Ageing, 17*, 100262. https://doi.org/10.1016/j.jeoa.2020.100262

Zhang, F., & Kaufman, D. (2016). Physical and cognitive impacts of digital games on older adults: A meta-analytic review. *Journal of Applied Gerontology, 35*(11), 1189–1210. https://doi.org/10.1177/0733464814566678

Zuelsdorff, M., Okonkwo, O. C., Norton, D., Barnes, L. L., Graham, K. L., Clark, L. R., Wyman, M. F., Benton, S. F., Gee, A., Lambrou, N., Johnson, S. C., & Gleason, C. E. (2020). Stressful life events and racial disparities in cognition among middle-aged and older adults. *Journal of Alzheimer's Disease, 73*(2), 671–682. https://doi.org/10.3233/jad-190439

Chapter 17
Exploring the Impact of ICT Use on Cognitive Decline in Older Adults: Mediating Effects of Perceived Control and Depression

Yanjun Dong, Charles Johnson, and Kun Wang

17.1 Introduction

The specter of dementia looms large over the aging population, extending beyond memory loss to encompass profound challenges in daily activities (H. D. Yang et al., 2016). Cognitive decline significantly affects older adults' abilities to perform basic tasks, leading to increased difficulties in activities of daily living (ADL) and instrumental activities of daily living (IADL) (Dodge et al., 2005). Older dementia patients tend to have more chronic illnesses, more hospital stays, higher levels of fragility, and reduced quality of life and well-being than their counterparts without dementia (Amjad et al., 2018; Harvey et al., 2016; LaMantia et al., 2016). Between 2000 and 2019, the number of deaths caused by Alzheimer's disease, a common type of dementia, had increased by 145.2% in the United States (U.S.), while the number one leading cause of death (heart disease) had decreased by 7.3% (Alzheimer's Association, 2021). Taking care of dementia patients also causes a burden to their caregivers, to both family members and formal healthcare workers, and negatively impact their health and mental health (Bangerter et al., 2019; Brown et al., 2019; Ruggiano et al., 2019). The repercussions ripple through the healthcare system, with dementia-related medical expenditures projected to skyrocket, reaching over $1.1 trillion in 2050 (Alzheimer's Association, 2020). Together, these statistics underscore the urgent need for proactive efforts to prevent Alzheimer's

Y. Dong
University at Albany, State University of New York, Albany, NY, USA
e-mail: ydong2@albany.edu

C. Johnson · K. Wang (✉)
Department of Social Work, College of Arts and Sciences, University of Alabama at Birmingham, Birmingham, AL, USA
e-mail: cwjohnso@uab.edu; kw2@uab.edu

K. Wang et al. (eds.), *ICT Use and Healthy Longevity*, Advances in Studies of Aging and Health 5, https://doi.org/10.1007/978-3-031-98964-3_17

disease and related dementias (ADRD) and to mitigate their far-reaching impacts on individuals, families, and the healthcare system.

As the digital era continues to unfold, researchers and practitioners are exploring innovative ways to integrate information and communication technology (ICT) into interventions tailored to promote cognitive health and reduce cognitive decline among older adults. This shift not only reflects a response to the urgent need for effective strategies but also aligns with the broader societal evolution into the Fourth Industrial Revolution, where technology intertwines with the physical, digital, and biological realms (Schwab, 2017). Digitalized cognitive training, ranging from virtual reality-based interventions to computerized cognitive programs, has demonstrated efficacy despite barriers like cost and accessibility (Garrett et al., 2018). In contrast, the general use of ICT, encompassing various online activities, has become increasingly prevalent among older adults, particularly during the COVID-19 pandemic (Pew Research Center, 2021a).

Amidst the optimism surrounding ICT use, gaps persist in understanding the intricate associations and mechanisms underpinning its impact on older adults' cognitive functioning. Emerging evidence has shown the effectiveness of ICT use in stimulating, preserving, or reversing older adults' cognitive functioning (Calhoun & Lee, 2019; Wu et al., 2019; Yu & Fiebig, 2020). Nevertheless, the mechanisms regarding the associations between ICT use and older adults' cognitive functioning remain understudied. Existing literature lacks clarity on whether ICT use directly influences cognitive functioning or operates through indirect factors. In addition, most studies have focused on cognitive functioning as a static outcome, which limits the ability to capture individual cognitive changes and assess the potential causal impact of ICT use. Thus, this study aimed to examine the association between ICT use and cognitive decline and investigate the underlying psychological mechanisms.

17.1.1 Mechanisms Underlying the Association Between ICT Use and Cognitive Decline

Despite increasing studies on ICT use and older adults' cognitive functioning, few have examined the underlying mechanisms. Moreover, most of these studies addressing mechanisms have mainly focused on the mediation effect of social relationships, such as social connectivity, social isolation, and social support (Khoo & Yang, 2020; Moxley & Czaja, 2019). Thus, more studies are needed to explore other potential mediators and better understand how ICT use stimulates older adults' cognitive functioning (Moxley & Czaja, 2019). In a recently published review paper by *The Lancet Commission*, a life-course model with 12 modifiable risk factors was proposed to prevent or delay up to 40% of dementias (Livingston et al., 2020), including later-life depression, social isolation/loneliness. Building on this framework, the present study explores the potential mediating effects of social isolation/loneliness and depression. Additionally, drawing on previous research (Hertzog et al., 2008), the study investigates perceived control as a possible mediator, offering a more comprehensive understanding of the pathways through which ICT use may influence cognitive functioning.

ICT Use, Social Isolation/Loneliness, and Cognitive Decline Social isolation and loneliness are increasing public health issues in the U.S. Based on a recent study, nearly one-fourth of community dwellers aged 65 or older are considered to be socially isolated, and more than 40% of adults aged 60 or older reported feeling lonely in the U.S. (National Academies of Sciences & Medicine, 2020). It should be noted that, in the literature, social isolation and loneliness are closely associated but distinct. Social isolation refers to the objective status of having minimal social contact with others, while loneliness is defined as the subjective status of negative feelings associated with having a lower level of social contact than desired (Wenger et al., 1996). However, given the similarities of these two concepts and their close associations with cognitive functioning, the present study will not differentiate them.

The detrimental effects of social isolation/loneliness on older adults' cognitive functioning have been well-established in the literature (Evans et al., 2019; Livingston et al., 2020; Saito et al., 2018; Sommerlad et al., 2019). In a previous meta-analysis of 19 longitudinal cohort studies, the pooled estimates showed that dementia risk for older adults with less frequent social contact was 57% higher than those with more frequent social contact (Kuiper et al., 2015). In the 12 modifiable risk factor life-course model (Livingston et al., 2020), social isolation/loneliness accounted for 3.5% of the population attributable fraction of dementia, suggesting that preventing social isolation/loneliness could prevent or delay about 3.5% of dementia cases. In a recent meta-analysis of 51 longitudinal cohort studies among 102,035 adults aged 50 or older, researchers found that lower levels of social isolation were associated with better late-life cognitive functioning ($r = .054$, 95% CI: .043–.065), including global cognitive functioning, memory, and executive function (Evans et al., 2019).

Numerous studies have shown that ICT use increases older adults' social contact and reduces their social isolation and loneliness (Chopik, 2016; Ma et al., 2020; Rezvani & Wiewiora, 2016). In a systematic review of ICT intervention studies published between 2000 and 2015, researchers assessed the effect of eight categories of ICT use and concluded that technology use reduces social isolation among older adults (Rezvani & Wiewiora, 2016). Overall, ICT use may reduce social isolation in at least two ways. First, by overcoming limitations of geographical location and transportation (Evans et al., 2019, p. 73), ICT may help older adults, especially those with mobility limitations, connect with their children, family, and friends anytime and anywhere and provide them with virtual platforms to build up new friendships. Second, easily accessible and enormous resources online also engage older adults in multiple activities, which keeps them busy and enhances the feeling of mattering (Moxley & Czaja, 2019).

Thus, it is reasonable to assume that reduced social isolation/loneliness due to ICT use will promote older adults' cognitive functioning and delay the process of cognitive decline. Using a national representative cohort of adults in their 40s to 70s from the MIDUS refreshers Survey and Cognitive Project, Khoo and Yang (2020) tested the underlying path of social support and sense of control (personal mastery and perceived constraints). They found that perceived social support and constraints fully and serially mediated the relationship between social media use and executive function among middle-aged and older adults. However, to better understand whether ICT use can slow cognitive decline, more studies are needed that explicitly examine cognitive change over time and test the mediating role of social isolation/loneliness in this process.

ICT Use, Perceived Control, and Cognitive Decline Perceived control refers to individuals' beliefs about their ability to influence or manage important outcomes in their lives (Lachman & Weaver, 1998), which often overlaps and highly correlated with self-efficacy (Bandura, 1997). Previous studies have indicated that perceived control or self-efficacy is positively associated with older adults' cognitive functioning (Groeppel-Klein et al., 2017; Hertzog et al., 2008; Korten et al., 2017; Seeman et al., 1993). Analyzing a sample of 1,099 older adults from the Longitudinal Aging Study Amsterdam, researchers found that older adults with higher levels of perceived self-efficacy had significantly better cognitive functioning, including processing speed, episodic memory, semantic fluency, and digit span backward (Korten et al., 2017).

Perceived control's or self-efficacy's effects on cognitive functioning may be manifested in multiple ways (Hertzog et al., 2008). For example, older adults with higher perceived control or self-efficacy are more likely to engage in healthy behaviors, such as staying active in daily life and conducting physical activities, indirectly promoting their cognitive functioning (Schwarzer, 2008). Another manifestation of this effect is that older adults with higher perceived control or self-efficacy are less likely to experience depression and anxiety in achieving their goals, indirectly affecting their cognitive functioning (Bandura, 1997). Further, previous research indicates that negative beliefs about aging, including low self-efficacy, might directly affect older adults' cognitive functioning by activating and internalizing stereotypes about aging (Hess, 2005).

Previous studies have indicated that ICT use may increase older adults' perceived control or self-efficacy (Blok et al., 2020; Wang & Gu, 2021). According to the Model of Selection, Optimization, and Compensation, ICT can compensate for age-related functional limitations, helping older adults maintain their self-efficacy (Blok et al., 2020). Another explanation for the positive effect of ICT use on older adults' perceived control or self-efficacy is social comparison. Based on the Social Comparison Theory, individuals strive to evaluate their opinions and abilities and are more likely to compare themselves with others with similar opinions or abilities (Festinger, 1954). Despite the increasing popularity among older adults, a recent report by the Pew Research Center (2021b) showed that one in four older adults was still not an ICT user. ICT use is still seen as a novelty and something belonging to younger generations by many older adults (Knowles & Hanson, 2018; Neves et al., 2018). Thus, when older internet users compare themselves to their peers who are not internet users, they feel more capable and more confident in themselves, directly increasing their perceived control or self-efficacy and indirectly stimulating their cognitive functioning and slowing cognitive decline.

ICT Use, Depression, and Cognitive Decline Depression is one of the most common mental health issues among older adults (Gill & Moore, 2013; Haigh et al., 2018). Empirical studies have demonstrated that older adults' levels of depression are predictive of their cognitive functioning (Dotson et al., 2010; Sachs-Ericsson et al., 2005; Wilson et al., 2002). Based on biological studies, depression may affect older adults' levels of stress hormones, neuronal growth factors, and hippocampal volume and increase the risks of cognitive decline and dementia (Alexopoulos, 2003). In the 12 modifiable risk factor life-course model, depression accounted for 3.9% of the population attributable fraction of dementia cases (Livingston et al., 2020). Thus, reducing older adults' levels of depression may help reduce their levels of cognitive decline.

Previous studies have summarized multiple risk factors for depression in late adulthood, such as low socioeconomic status, chronic illness, functioning disabilities, loss of family or friends, and others (McDonnall, 2009; Park & Reynolds, 2015). As discussed earlier, ICT use provides older adults more opportunities to engage in online social activities. For example, older adults can use ICT to surf the internet, acquire new knowledge, skills, and hobbies, watch videos or movies, or even run small businesses online. These online activities may keep older adults active, increase their social interactions, maintain their independence, and reduce their levels of depression (Cotten et al., 2014; Lin et al., 2020). Analyzing data from four waves (2002–2008) of the Health and Retirement Study, Cotten et al. (2014) found that internet use reduced the probability of depression by 33%, especially for older adults living alone. In a recent study of Chinese adults, researchers found that mobile device users were less likely to have depressive symptoms than non-users (Lin et al., 2020). Consequentially, it is plausible to believe that ICT use may prevent older adults from cognitive decline through reduced levels of depression.

17.1.2 Current Study

Building on the reviewed theories and literature, this study proposes a series of mediation models to examine the psychological mechanisms underlying the association between ICT use and cognitive decline among older adults. Three separate mediation models are used to explore the roles of loneliness, perceived control, and depression as mediators. This approach provides a comprehensive understanding of how ICT use influence cognitive decline through specific psychological pathways, offering clear insights into the underlying mechanisms. More specifically, this study hypothesizes:

Hypothesis 1: ICT use slows cognitive decline through reduced loneliness.
Hypothesis 2: ICT use slows cognitive decline through reduced depression.
Hypothesis 3: ICT use slows cognitive decline through increased perceived-control.

17.2 Methods

17.2.1 Data Source and Sample

This study utilized data from the Health and Retirement Study (HRS), a nationally representative panel study funded by the National Institute on Aging (NIA, grant number U01AG009740) and conducted by the University of Michigan. The HRS, conducted biennially from 1992 to 2018, surveyed approximately 20,000 American adults aged 50 and older, along with their spouses. Since 2006, the inclusion of the Leave-Behind Questionnaire (LBQ) has provided additional insights into psychological well-being and internet usage. For this study, data from HRS 2012 and 2016 were used, with 2012 set as the baseline. Similar to our sample selection process in Chapter 16, after applying the following criteria: (1) eligible and completed 2012 LBQ, (2) aged 65 and older, (3) no diagnosis of Alzheimer's disease or related dementia, and (4) reported ICT use status, we has a sample of 2,022 participants for analyses. This study obtained an "exempt" non-medical IRB from the researchers' institute.

17.2.2 Measures

Information and Communication Technology (ICT) Use ICT use was measured in HRS 2012 using a single question: "How often do you use a computer for email, internet, or other tasks?" Responses were coded as 1 = daily, 2 = several times a week, 3 = once a week, 4 = several times a month, 5 = at least once a month, 6 = not in the last month, and 7 = never/not relevant. Responses were reverse-coded, with higher numbers indicating more frequent ICT use.

Cognitive Decline Cognitive functioning in HRS was assessed using a reduced version of the Telephone Interview for Cognitive Status (TICS), a validated multidimensional measure that includes episodic memory, knowledge, language, and orientation (Breitner et al., 1995). Cognitive functioning was scored on a scale of 0 to 35. To assess cognitive decline, we subtracted the 2016 cognitive functioning score from the 2012 score, with higher values indicating greater decline.

Mediators Mediators were sourced from HRS 2016. **Loneliness** was measured using 11 items (e.g., "lack of companionship"), scored as 1 = often, 2 = sometimes, and 3 = hardly or never, with four items reverse-coded. The total loneliness score ranged from 1 to 3, with higher scores indicating greater loneliness. **Perceived control** was assessed through participants' perceived control over health, social life, and financial situations, scored from 0 (no control) to 10 (very much control). The perceived control score was the mean of these three items, with higher scores indicating greater perceived control. **Depression** was measured using the Center for Epidemiologic Studies Depression (CES-D) scale, an eight-item instrument (e.g., "Much of the time during the past week, you felt depressed"), scored as 0 = no and 1 = yes, with two items reverse-coded. The total depression score ranged from 0 to 8, with higher scores indicating more severe depression.

Covariates included age (measured continuously from 65 to 94 years), marital status (0 = divorced, separated, widowed, or never married; 1 = married or partnered), education (0 = non-bachelor's degree; 1 = bachelor's degree or higher), gender (0 = male; 1 = female), and race/ethnicity (0 = non-Hispanic White; 1 = minority, including non-Hispanic Black, Hispanic, and other races). Additionally, the abilities to perform activities of daily living (ADL) and instrumental activities of daily living (IADL) were controlled for, each coded dichotomously (0 = no difficulty; 1 = difficulty). These covariates were included to account for potential confounding factors in the relationship between ICT use and cognitive decline.

17.2.3 Analytical Plan

To address the research question, a series of simple mediation analyses were conducted to examine the impact of ICT use on cognitive decline among older adults, with a focus on three mediating factors: loneliness, perceived control, and depression.

First, descriptive analyses were performed to understand the demographic and baseline health characteristics of the study population. Variables such as age, education, gender, minority status, marital status, and difficulties in ADL and IADL were assessed to provide a comprehensive overview of the sample.

Second, bivariate correlations were calculated to identify preliminary associations between predictor variables (ICT use in 2012), mediator variables (loneliness, self-efficacy, and depression in 2016), and the outcome variable (cognitive decline between 2012 and 2016). These correlations established the foundational relationships necessary for mediation analysis.

Third, mediation analyses were conducted using the PROCESS macro by Andrew F. Hayes in SPSS 21.0 (Hayes, 2022). Three separate mediation models were tested, one for each mediator. Each model estimated the direct effect of ICT use on cognitive decline and the indirect effect through the respective mediator. To ensure robust estimation of the mediation effects, the analysis used 5,000 bootstrapped samples to generate bias-corrected and accelerated 95% confidence intervals (CIs).

Baseline cognitive functioning was not included as a covariate in the mediation models because the outcome variable, cognitive decline, already accounts for baseline levels (Allison, 1990). This approach focuses on the effect of ICT use and mediators on cognitive decline, independent of baseline cognitive ability.

17.3 Results

17.3.1 Univariate and Bivariate Analyses

As shown in Table 17.1, the average age of participants was approximately 74 years (SD = 5.87, range: 65–94). About 23.12% of participants held a bachelor's degree, 60.40% were female, 64.80% were married, and 14.90% identified as racial/ethnic minorities. A small proportion of participants reported difficulties in ADL (8.67%) and IADL (11.44%), indicating a relatively independent and capable cohort of older adults. The mean score of cognitive functioning at baseline was 22.67 (SD = 4.17). The mean score of cognitive decline between 2012 and 2016 is 1.16 (SD = 3.52), indicating that participants' average cognitive functioning declined by 1.16 unit per 4 years.

Table 17.2 presents the means, standard deviations, and bivariate correlations. ICT use was negatively correlated with cognitive decline ($r = -.08$, $p < .01$). More frequent ICT use was associated with lower levels of loneliness ($r = -.12$, $p < .01$) and depression ($r = -.18$, $p < .01$). Higher levels of loneliness ($r = .05$, $p < .05$) and depression ($r = .06$, $p < .05$) were associated with more cognitive decline. Additionally, ICT use was positively correlated with perceived control ($r = .07$, $p < .01$), and higher levels of perceived control were associated with less cognitive decline ($r = -.09$, $p < .01$).

Table 17.1 Descriptive analyses of participants' characteristics

Variables	Mean ± SD	Minimum	Maximum	%	*N*
Age in 2012	74.08 ± 5.87	65	94		2202
Bachelor		0.00	1.00	23.12%	2202
Female		0.00	1.00	60.40%	2202
Minority		0.00	1.00	14.90%	2202
Married in 2012		0.00	1.00	64.80%	2202
ADL in 2012		0.00	1.00	8.67%	2202
IADL in 2012		0.00	1.00	11.44%	2202
Cognition in 2012	22.67 ± 4.17	2	35		2195
Cognitive decline	1.16 ± 3.52	−12	17		2195

Table 17.2 Means, standard deviations, and correlations of variables

Variables	Mean	SD	1	2	3	4	5
1. ICT use	3.32	2.76	–				
2. Loneliness	1.51	.42	−.12**	–			
3. Perceived control	7.60	1.91	.07**	−.38**	–		
4. Depression	1.21	1.76	−.18**	.39**	−.34**	–	
5. Cognitive decline	1.16	3.52	−.08**	.05*	−.09**	.06*	–

Note: $N = 2022$; $^{*}p < .05$; $^{**}p < .01$

Table 17.3 Mediation analysis results on cognitive functioning among total participants

	Model 1		Model 2		Model 3	
	Mediator	Outcome	Mediator	Outcome	Mediator	Outcome
Variables	Loneliness	Cognitive decline	Perceived control	Cognitive decline	Depression	Cognitive decline
ICT use	−0.01**	−0.06	0.03*	−0.05*	−0.08***	−0.05
Loneliness	–	0.32	–	–	–	–
Perceived control	–	–	–	−0.16***	–	–
Depression	–	–	–	–	–	0.09*
Age	.001	0.07***	−0.01	0.07***	−0.01	0.07***
Female	−0.03	0.25	−.001	0.24	0.42***	0.20
Minority	−0.03	−0.13	0.37**	−0.08	0.20*	−0.16
Bachelor	−0.08***	0.05	−0.03	0.02	−0.15	0.04
Married	−0.06**	−0.02	−0.26**	−0.08	−0.10	−0.03
ADL	0.08*	0.46	−0.90***	0.34	0.49***	0.44
IADL	0.15***	−0.36	−0.98***	−0.47	1.13***	0.42

*Note: *p < .05; **p < .01; ***p < .001*

17.3.2 Mediation Analysis

Table 17.3 shows the mediation analysis results examining the impact of ICT use on cognitive decline, while controlling for covariates such as age, gender, minority status, education, marital status, difficulties in ADL and IADL. ICT use at baseline was significantly associated with lower loneliness ($B = -0.01$, $p < 0.01$), higher perceived control ($B = 0.03$, $p < 0.05$), and lower depressive scores ($B = -0.08$, $p < 0.001$) at T2. Among these mediators, perceived control ($B = -0.16$, $p < 0.001$) and depressive scores ($B = 0.09$, $p < 0.05$) were significantly associated with cognitive decline, while the effect of loneliness was not significant. The effects of the covariates are also summarized in Table 17.3.

Table 17.4 Unstandardized coefficients of bootstrapping results from ICT use to cognitive decline

Mediator	Model	Effect	Lower LTCI	Upper LTCI
	Total Effects	**–0.06**	**–0.12**	**–0.001**
Loneliness	Direct Effect	–0.06	–0.12	0.002
	ICT Use → Loneliness → Cognitive decline	–0.003	–0.01	0.005
Perceived control	Direct Effect	–0.05	–0.11	0.004
	ICT Use → Perceived control → Cognitive decline	**–0.01**	**–0.01**	**–0.0001**
Depression	Direct Effect	–0.05	–0.11	0.01
	ICT Use → Depression → Cognitive decline	**–0.01**	**–0.02**	**–0.0001**

Note: Indirect effects whose bootstrapped 95% confidence intervals do not include zero are considered statistically significant and are shown in boldface in the tables

The results of the mediation analyses, including direct and indirect effects, are reported in Table 17.4. The total effect of ICT use on cognitive decline was negative and significant (B_total = –0.06, 95% CI [–0.12, –0.001]). The indirect effect through perceived control was significant (B_indirect = –0.01, 95% CI [–0.01, –0.0001]), while the direct effect was not significant, indicating that the impact of ICT use on reduced cognitive decline was fully mediated by perceived control. Similarly, the indirect effect through depression was significant (B_indirect = –0.01, 95% CI [–0.02, –0.0001]), while the direct effect was not significant, suggesting that ICT use reduced cognitive decline fully through reduced depression. In contrast, neither the direct nor the indirect effect through loneliness was significant.

17.4 Discussion

The present study examined the pathways through which ICT use affects cognitive decline in older adults, utilizing three separate mediators: loneliness, perceived control, and depression. The findings help fill a theoretical gap by explaining how ICT use impacts cognitive decline in older adults and provide practical guidelines for future intervention design and implementation.

17.4.1 Mechanisms Underlying the Associations of ICT Use and Cognitive Decline

Mediation analysis revealed that ICT use slowed cognitive decline through increased perceived control, supporting Hypothesis 2. This finding aligns with the Model of Selection, Optimization, and Compensation (Baltes & Baltes, 1993), which posits that older adults optimize their resources to adapt to age-related changes. ICT use provides older adults with tools to manage their health, social connections, and daily activities, enhancing their sense of control and self-efficacy. This increase in perceived control, in turn, promotes better cognitive functioning and slows the process of cognitive decline. Future ICT training and interventions may consider incorporating content or sessions that not only build digital skills but also teach older adults how to use technology to compensate for age-related losses and enhance their sense of agency in managing daily life.

Similarly, the mediation effect of reduced depression supports Hypothesis 3. ICT use was associated with lower levels of depression, which subsequently reduced the pace of cognitive decline. This pathway highlights the role of emotional well-being in cognitive health, as reducing depressive symptoms through active ICT engagement can lead to better cognitive outcomes. ICT-based mental health interventions, such as web-based therapies, mobile applications, and virtual reality systems, have been shown to be effective, feasible, and widely accepted by older adults (Castilla et al., 2020; Fonseca & Osma, 2021). These tools can complement traditional face-to-face services or serve as standalone treatments, offering accessible and scalable solutions for addressing depression in older adults.

In contrast, the mediation effect of loneliness was not significant, despite ICT use being associated with lower loneliness at T2, contradicting our Hypothesis 1. This suggests that while ICT use may reduce feelings of loneliness, this reduction does not translate into significant cognitive changes. This finding contrasts with some prior studies (e.g., Chopik, 2016; Penninkilampi et al., 2018) that emphasize the importance of social connectivity in mitigating cognitive decline. However, it is possible that the benefits of reduced loneliness on cognitive functioning are more subtle, accumulate over a longer period, or depend on the quality and depth of social interactions rather than their mere presence.

17.4.2 Implication

This study underscores the significant role of ICT in fostering cognitive decline among older adults, mediated by enhanced perceived control and reduced depression. These findings advance Cognitive Enrichment Theory by illustrating how ICT use supports cognitive health, offering a modern perspective on traditional cognitive frameworks. Digital engagement emerges as a potent form of cognitive stimulation, with benefits akin to conventional cognitive exercises (Gonçalves & da Silva, 2023), highlighting ICT's potential to promote cognitive well-being in aging populations. From a practical perspective, the study calls for policies and programs that integrate ICT tools into older adults' daily lives. Policymakers should prioritize subsidizing technology access and providing tailored ICT training as part of elder care initiatives. Such efforts could help curb cognitive decline and bridge disparities in technology access among older adults (Vassilakopoulou & Hustad, 2021). Moreover, ICT-based interventions should be designed to enhance perceived control and alleviate depression. For instance, training programs could empower older adults to use ICT for health management, social interaction, and daily tasks, fostering confidence and independence. Similarly, ICT-driven mental health solutions, such as online therapy or depression management apps, should be customized to older adults' unique needs and preferences to ensure effectiveness and accessibility. Academically, this study enriches gerontological and cognitive science literature by mapping the pathways through which ICT use influences cognitive health. It emphasizes the importance of examining multiple mediators, such as perceived control and depression, and lays the groundwork for future research to explore additional factors, including lifelong learning and social support, which may further clarify the relationship between ICT use and cognitive well-being.

17.4.3 Limitations

The present study has several limitations that should be considered when interpreting the results. First, the use of archival data limits the ability to establish causal inferences. Future studies should employ longitudinal or experimental designs to test the causal relationships between ICT use, mediators, and cognitive changes. Second, the reliance on self-reported measures for ICT use and mediators (e.g., loneliness, self-efficacy) may introduce bias and affect the accuracy of the findings. Objective measures of ICT engagement and cognitive changes could provide more reliable data. Third, the nonsignificant mediation effect of loneliness suggests that other factors may play a more critical role in linking ICT use to cognitive changes. Future research should explore additional mediators, such as physical activity or cognitive engagement, to better understand the mechanisms underlying this relationship.

17.4.4 Conclusions

In conclusion, this study elucidates the mechanisms through which ICT use influences cognitive decline in older adults. Mediation analysis revealed a robust positive association between ICT use and cognitive decline, with significant indirect effects through enhanced perceived control and reduced depression. These results are crucial for the development and optimization of ICT-based cognitive interventions. The study underscores the significance of integrating strategies that bolster older adults' perceived control and reduce depressive symptoms in interventions designed to promote cognitive changes. By focusing on these mediatory pathways, future interventions can be tailored to maximally leverage the therapeutic potential of ICT in sustaining and enhancing cognitive changes in aging populations.

Disclaimer The views expressed in this chapter are solely those of the authors and do not necessarily reflect the views of the University of Alabama at Birmingham or the University at Albany.

References

Alexopoulos, G. S. (2003). Vascular disease, depression, and dementia. *Journal of the American Geriatrics Society, 51*(8), 1178–1180. https://doi.org/10.1046/j.1532-5415.2003.51373.x

Allison, P. D. (1990). Change scores as dependent variables in regression analysis. *Sociological Methodology, 20*, 93–114. https://doi.org/10.2307/271083

Alzheimer's Association. (2020). 2020 Alzheimer's disease facts and figures. *Alzheimer's & Dementia, 16*(3), 391–460. https://doi.org/10.1002/alz.12068

Alzheimer's Association. (2021). 2021 Alzheimer's disease facts and figures. *Alzheimers Dement, 17*(3), 327–406. https://doi.org/10.1002/alz.12328

Amjad, H., Wong, S. K., Roth, D. L., Huang, J., Willink, A., Black, B. S., Johnston, D., Rabins, P. V., Gitlin, L. N., Lyketsos, C. G., & Samus, Q. M. (2018). Health services utilization in older adults with dementia receiving care coordination: The MIND at home trial. *Health Services Research, 53*(1), 556–579. https://doi.org/10.1111/1475-6773.12647

Baltes, P. B., & Baltes, M. M. (1993). *Successful aging: Perspectives from the behavioral sciences* (Vol. 4). Cambridge University Press.

Bandura, A. (1997). *Self-efficacy: The exercise of control*. W H Freeman/Times Books/ Henry Holt & Co.

Bangerter, L. R., Ruggiano, N., Griffin, J. M., & Malley, K. A. O. (2019). Federal policy efforts to support family caregivers: Past, present, and future. *Innovation in Aging, 3*(Suppl 1), S135–S136. https://doi.org/10.1093/geroni/igz038.493

Blok, M., van Ingen, E., de Boer, A. H., & Slootman, M. (2020). The use of information and communication technologies by older people with cognitive impairments: From barriers to benefits. *Computers in Human Behavior, 104*, 106173. https://doi.org/10.1016/j.chb.2019.106173

Breitner, J. C. S., & Welsh, K. A. (1995). Diagnosis and management of memory loss and cognitive disorders among elderly persons. *Psychiatric Services, 46*(1), 29–35. https://doi.org/10.1176/ps.46.1.29

Brown, E. L., Ruggiano, N., Li, J., Clarke, P. J., Kay, E. S., & Hristidis, V. (2019). Smartphone-based health technologies for dementia care: Opportunities, challenges, and current practices. *Journal of Applied Gerontology: The Official Journal of the Southern Gerontological Society, 38*(1), 73–91. https://doi.org/10.1177/0733464817723088

Calhoun, D., & Lee, S. B. (2019). Computer usage and cognitive capability of older adults: Analysis of data from the Health and Retirement Study. *Educational Gerontology, 45*(1), 22–33. https://doi.org/10.1080/03601277.2019.1575026

Castilla, D., Suso-Ribera, C., Zaragoza, I., Garcia-Palacios, A., & Botella, C. (2020). Designing ICTs for users with mild cognitive impairment: A usability study. *International Journal of Environmental Research and Public Health, 17*(14), 5153. https://doi.org/10.3390/ijerph17145153

Chopik, W. J. (2016). The benefits of social technology use among older adults are mediated by reduced loneliness. *Cyberpsychology, Behavior, and Social Networking, 19*(9), 551–556. https://doi.org/10.1089/cyber.2016.0151

Cotten, S. R., Ford, G., Ford, S., & Hale, T. M. (2014). Internet use and depression among retired older adults in the United States: A longitudinal analysis. *The Journals of Gerontology: Series B, 69*(5), 763–771. https://doi.org/10.1093/geronb/gbu018

Dodge, H. H., Kadowaki, T., Hayakawa, T., Yamakawa, M., Sekikawa, A., & Ueshima, H. (2005). Cognitive impairment as a strong predictor of incident disability in specific ADL–IADL tasks among community-dwelling elders: The Azuchi study. *The Gerontologist, 45*(2), 222–230. https://doi.org/10.1093/geront/45.2.222

Dotson, V. M., Beydoun, M. A., & Zonderman, A. B. (2010). Recurrent depressive symptoms and the incidence of dementia and mild cognitive impairment. *Neurology, 75*(1), 27. https://doi.org/10.1212/WNL.0b013e3181e62124

Evans, I. E. M., Martyr, A., Collins, R., Brayne, C., & Clare, L. (2019). Social isolation and cognitive function in later life: A systematic review and meta-analysis. *Journal of Alzheimer's Disease, 70*, S119–S144. https://doi.org/10.3233/JAD-180501

Festinger, L. (1954). A theory of social comparison processes. *Human Relations, 7*(2), 117–140. https://doi.org/10.1177/001872675400700202

Fonseca, A., & Osma, J. (2021). Using Information and Communication Technologies (ICT) for mental health prevention and treatment. *International Journal of Environmental Research and Public Health, 18*(2), 461. https://doi.org/10.3390/ijerph18020461

Garrett, B., Taverner, T., Gromala, D., Tao, G., Cordingley, E., & Sun, C. (2018). Virtual reality clinical research: Promises and challenges. *JMIR Serious Games, 6*(4), e10839. https://doi.org/10.2196/10839

Gill, J., & Moore, M. J. (2013). *The state of aging & health in America 2013.*

Gonçalves, H. I. M., & da Silva, F. O. (2023). Cognitive rehabilitation: A comparison model of a digital environment based on serious games and the traditional methods. *Procedia Computer Science, 219*, 1333–1340. https://doi.org/10.1016/j.procs.2023.01.418

Groeppel-Klein, A., Helfgen, J., Spilski, A., & Schreiber, L. (2017). The impact of age stereotypes on elderly consumers' self-efficacy and cognitive performance. *Journal of Strategic Marketing, 25*(3), 211–225. https://doi.org/10.1080/0965254X.2017.1299787

Haigh, E. A. P., Bogucki, O. E., Sigmon, S. T., & Blazer, D. G. (2018). Depression among older adults: A 20-year update on five common myths and misconceptions. *The American Journal of Geriatric Psychiatry, 26*(1), 107–122. https://doi.org/10.1016/j.jagp.2017.06.011

Harvey, L., Mitchell, R., Brodaty, H., Draper, B., & Close, J. (2016). The influence of dementia on injury-related hospitalisations and outcomes in older adults. *Injury, 47*(1), 226–234. https://doi.org/10.1016/j.injury.2015.09.021

Hayes, A. F. (2022). *Introduction to mediation, moderation, and conditional process analysis: A regression-based approach* (3rd ed.). Guilford Publications.

Hertzog, C., Kramer, A. F., Wilson, R. S., & Lindenberger, U. (2008). Enrichment effects on adult cognitive development: Can the functional capacity of older adults be preserved and enhanced? *Psychological Science in the Public Interest, 9*(1), 1–65. https://doi.org/10.1111/j.1539-6053.2009.01034.x

Hess, T. M. (2005). Memory and aging in context. *Psychological Bulletin, 131*(3), 383–406. https://doi.org/10.1037/0033-2909.131.3.383

Khoo, S. S., & Yang, H. (2020). Social media use improves executive functions in middle-aged and older adults: A structural equation modeling analysis. *Computers in Human Behavior, 111*, 106388. https://doi.org/10.1016/j.chb.2020.106388

Knowles, B., & Hanson, V. L. (2018). The wisdom of older technology (non)users. *Communications of the ACM, 61*(3), 72–77. https://doi.org/10.1145/3179995

Korten, N. C. M., Comijs, H. C., Penninx, B. W. J. H., & Deeg, D. J. H. (2017). Perceived stress and cognitive function in older adults: Which aspect of perceived stress is important? *International Journal of Geriatric Psychiatry, 32*(4), 439–445. https://doi.org/10.1002/gps.4486

Kuiper, J. S., Zuidersma, M., Oude Voshaar, R. C., Zuidema, S. U., van den Heuvel, E. R., Stolk, R. P., & Smidt, N. (2015). Social relationships and risk of dementia: A systematic review and meta-analysis of longitudinal cohort studies. *Ageing Research Reviews, 22*, 39–57. https://doi.org/10.1016/j.arr.2015.04.006

Lachman, M. E., & Weaver, S. L. (1998). The sense of control as a moderator of social class differences in health and well-being. *Journal of Personality and Social Psychology, 74*(3), 763.

LaMantia, M. A., Stump, T. E., Messina, F. C., Miller, D. K., & Callahan, C. M. (2016). Emergency department use among older adults with dementia. *Alzheimer Disease and Associated Disorders, 30*(1), 35–40. https://doi.org/10.1097/WAD.0000000000000118

Lin, L., Jing, X.-C., Lv, S.-J., Liang, J.-H., Tian, L., Li, H.-L., Puts, M., & Xu, Y. (2020). Mobile device use and the cognitive function and depressive symptoms of older adults living in residential care homes. *BMC Geriatrics, 20*(1), 41. https://doi.org/10.1186/s12877-020-1427-1

Livingston, G., Huntley, J., Sommerlad, A., Ames, D., Ballard, C., Banerjee, S., Brayne, C., Burns, A., Cohen-Mansfield, J., Cooper, C., Costafreda, S. G., Dias, A., Fox, N., Gitlin, L. N., Howard, R., Kales, H. C., Kivimäki, M., Larson, E. B., Ogunniyi, A., et al. (2020). Dementia prevention, intervention, and care: 2020 report of the Lancet Commission. *Lancet (London, England), 396*(10248), 413–446. https://doi.org/10.1016/S0140-6736(20)30367-6

Ma, R., Mann, F., Wang, J., Lloyd-Evans, B., Terhune, J., Al-Shihabi, A., & Johnson, S. (2020). The effectiveness of interventions for reducing subjective and objective social isolation among people with mental health problems: A systematic review. *Social Psychiatry and Psychiatric Epidemiology, 55*(7), 839–876. https://doi.org/10.1007/s00127-019-01800-z

McDonnall, M. C. (2009). Risk factors for depression among older adults with dual sensory loss. *Aging & Mental Health, 13*(4), 569–576. https://doi.org/10.1080/13607860902774410

Moxley, J. H., & Czaja, S. J. (2019). Potential mediators of the relationship between internet usage and cognition. *International Psychogeriatrics, 31*(7), 917–919. Cambridge Core. https://doi.org/10.1017/S1041610219001054

National Academies of Sciences, E. & Medicine. (2020). *Social isolation and loneliness in older adults: Opportunities for the health care system*. National Academies Press.

Neves, B. B., Waycott, J., & Malta, S. (2018). Old and afraid of new communication technologies? Reconceptualising and contesting the 'age-based digital divide'. *Journal of Sociology, 54*(2), 236–248. https://doi.org/10.1177/1440783318766119

Park, M., & Reynolds, C. F., III. (2015). Depression among older adults with diabetes mellitus. *Clinics in Geriatric Medicine, 31*(1), 117–137., ix. https://doi.org/10.1016/j.cger.2014.08.022

Penninkilampi, R., Casey, A.-N., Singh, M. F., & Brodaty, H. (2018). The association between social engagement, loneliness, and risk of dementia: A systematic review and meta-analysis. *Journal of Alzheimer's Disease, 66*, 1619–1633. https://doi.org/10.3233/JAD-180439

Pew Research Center. (2021a). *Internet/broadband fact sheet*.

Pew Research Center. (2021b). *Social media fact sheet*.

Rezvani, A., & Wiewiora, A. (2016). The impact of technology on older adults' social isolation. *Computers in Human Behavior, 63*, 594–603. https://doi.org/10.1016/j.chb.2016.05.092

Ruggiano, N., Brown, E. L., Shaw, S., Geldmacher, D., Clarke, P., Hristidis, V., & Bertram, J. (2019). The potential of information technology to navigate caregiving systems: Perspectives from dementia caregivers. *Journal of Gerontological Social Work, 62*(4), 432–450. https://doi.org/10.1080/01634372.2018.1546786

Sachs-Ericsson, N., Joiner, T., Plant, E. A., & Blazer, D. G. (2005). The influence of depression on cognitive decline in community-dwelling elderly persons. *The American Journal of Geriatric Psychiatry, 13*(5), 402–408. https://doi.org/10.1097/00019442-200505000-00009

Saito, T., Murata, C., Saito, M., Takeda, T., & Kondo, K. (2018). Influence of social relationship domains and their combinations on incident dementia: A prospective cohort study. *Journal of Epidemiology and Community Health, 72*(1), 7. https://doi.org/10.1136/jech-2017-209811

Schwab, K. (2017). *The fourth industrial revolution*. Brown Business.

Schwarzer, R. (2008). Modeling health behavior change: How to predict and modify the adoption and maintenance of health behaviors. *Applied Psychology, 57*(1), 1–29. https://doi.org/10.1111/j.1464-0597.2007.00325.x

Seeman, T. E., Rodin, J., & Albert, M. (1993). Self-efficacy and cognitive performance in high-functioning older individuals: MacArthur studies of successful aging. *Journal of Aging and Health, 5*(4), 455–474. https://doi.org/10.1177/089826439300500403

Sommerlad, A., Sabia, S., Singh-Manoux, A., Lewis, G., & Livingston, G. (2019). Association of social contact with dementia and cognition: 28-year follow-up of the Whitehall II cohort study. *PLoS Medicine, 16*(8), e1002862. https://doi.org/10.1371/journal.pmed.1002862

Vassilakopoulou, P., & Hustad, E. (2021). Bridging digital divides: A literature review and research agenda for information systems research. *Information Systems Frontiers, 25*(3), 955–969. Springer. https://doi.org/10.1007/s10796-020-10096-3

Wang, K., & Gu, D. (2021). *Reciprocal associations between information and communication technology use and self-perception of aging: Is older women different from men?*

Wenger, G. C., Davies, R., Shahtahmasebi, S., & Scott, A. (1996). Social isolation and loneliness in old age: Review and model refinement. *Ageing and Society, 16*(3), 333–358. Cambridge Core. https://doi.org/10.1017/S0144686X00003457

Wilson, R. S., Barnes, L. L., Mendes de Leon, C. F., Aggarwal, N. T., Schneider, J. S., Bach, J., Pilat, J., Beckett, L. A., Arnold, S. E., Evans, D. A., & Bennett, D. A. (2002). Depressive symptoms, cognitive decline, and risk of AD in older persons. *Neurology, 59*(3), 364. https://doi.org/10.1212/WNL.59.3.364

Wu, Y.-H., Lewis, M., & Rigaud, A.-S. (2019). Cognitive function and digital device use in older adults attending a memory clinic. *Gerontology and Geriatric Medicine, 5*, 2333721419844886. https://doi.org/10.1177/2333721419844886

Yang, H. D., Kim, D. H., Lee, S. B., & Young, L. D. (2016). History of Alzheimer's disease. *Dementia and Neurocognitive Disorders, 15*(4), 115–121. https://doi.org/10.12779/dnd.2016.15.4.115

Yu, D., & Fiebig, D. G. (2020). Internet use and cognition among middle-aged and older adults in China: A cross-lagged panel analysis. *The Journal of the Economics of Ageing, 17*, 100262. https://doi.org/10.1016/j.jeoa.2020.100262

Chapter 18
Older Adults' Online Activities and Cognition: Investigating the Psychological Mechanisms and Age and Gender Differences

Kun Wang, Xiayu Summer Chen, Sukyoung Kang, Brenda D. Smith, and Danan Gu

18.1 Introduction

Despite emerging evidence suggesting that internet use may have the potential to promote older adults' cognition (Choi et al., 2021; Yu & Fiebig, 2020), the underlying psychological mechanisms remain unknown. Limited studies on older adults'

Note on Reuse of Published Materials
This chapter incorporates a revised and expanded version of material originally published in the article *"Older adults' online activities and cognition: Investigating the psychological mechanisms and age and gender differences"* by Wang, K., Chen, X. S., Kang, S. Y., Smith, B. D., & Gu, D. (2024), published in *Social Science & Medicine, 352,* 116988. The original work has been adapted and updated, in accordance with the publisher's policies.

K. Wang (✉)
Department of Social Work, College of Arts and Sciences, University of Alabama at Birmingham, Birmingham, AL, USA
e-mail: kw2@uab.edu

X. S. Chen
University of Illinois Urbana-Champaign, Champaign, IL, USA
e-mail: xiayuyc2@illinois.edu

S. Kang
Binghamton University, Binghamton, NY, USA
e-mail: sykang@binghamton.edu

B. D. Smith
University of Alabama, Tuscaloosa, AL, USA
e-mail: bsmith2@sw.ua.edu

D. Gu
Population Division, UN Department of Economic and Social Affairs, New York, NY, USA
e-mail: gudanan@yahoo.com

K. Wang et al. (eds.), *ICT Use and Healthy Longevity*, Advances in Studies of Aging and Health 5, https://doi.org/10.1007/978-3-031-98964-3_18

social media use propose enhanced social engagement, social support, and reduced loneliness as potential mechanisms (Chopik, 2016; Khoo & Yang, 2020). However, as an effective tool with increasing popularity and importance, the internet covers more aspects of everyday life than social connections. Older adults can access the internet for many other activities, such as information searching, instrumental use, and entertainment. The underlying psychological mechanisms linking these online activities to cognition may differ from that of social media use. In addition, gender and age differences in older adults' internet usage have been reported in previous studies (Choi et al., 2021; Wang & Kubanga, 2021), which may also impact the mechanisms. Thus, in this study, we proposed a framework to systematically explain the psychological mechanisms linking different types of online activities and cognition among older adults. Findings from this study may bring an in-depth understanding of the internet use-cognition association among older adults and better inform internet-based interventions to promote successful cognitive aging.

18.1.1 Theoretical Framework

Over the past few decades, several interrelated concepts, such as "use it or lose it" or cognitive plasticity, have been developed to support interventions for preserving and promoting cognition in old age (Hultsch et al., 1999; Schaie & Willis, 1986). Building on these concepts and the life-span perspective on development (Baltes, 1987), Hertzog et al. (2008) proposed the cognitive enrichment hypothesis, positing that cognition is malleable and open to enhancement despite age-related constraints on maximum cognitive potential. According to this hypothesis, individuals can preserve their cognition by engaging in intellectually, physically, and socially challenging activities, even in old age (Hertzog et al., 2008). Regarding internet use, while most older adults may not be technology-savvy, they perceive it as intellectually challenging (Ivan & Cutler, 2021). Learning to use and actively engage with the internet may directly benefit older adults' cognition. Thus, we proposed our first hypothesis:

H1: Internet use has a positive direct effect on older adults' cognition.

Besides cognitive stimulation, internet use is positively associated with older adults' psychological well-being, such as reduced loneliness and depression, increased self-perception of aging, and increased social support and sense of control (Chopik, 2016; Khoo & Yang, 2020). Meanwhile, prior studies also suggest that high levels of loneliness and depression are associated with lower cognitive functioning among older adults (Cardona & Andrés, 2023; Livingston et al., 2020). In the 2020 report of the Lancet Commission (Livingston et al., 2020), a life-course model with 12 modifiable risk factors was proposed, accounting for around 40% of worldwide dementias. Based on this model, depression and social isolation could explain 3.9% and 3.5% of dementia incidence (Livingston et al., 2020). In addition, previous studies have found that older adults' control beliefs are positively associated with their cognitive performance (Infurna & Gerstorf, 2013; Lachman & Andreoletti,

2006). Given these well-established associations between psychological well-being and cognition, internet use may also influence cognition indirectly via these psychological factors. A limited number of studies have investigated the psychological mechanisms with a predominant focus on social media use and the mediating effect of social relationship factors, such as social support and loneliness (Chopik, 2016; Khoo & Yang, 2020). Less attention has been paid to other types of online activities and other potential psychological mediators. Thus, in this study, based on the activity theory of aging and the life-span theory of control, we proposed a more comprehensive model to better understand how internet use, considering four types of activities, affects older adults' cognition.

18.1.1.1 Activity Theory of Aging

As one of the three main psychosocial theories focusing on human development in old age, the activity theory of aging indicates a positive association between levels of activities, especially social interactions, and life satisfaction among older adults (Havighurst, 1961). This theory is based on the belief that older adults' psychological and social needs are essentially the same as middle-aged adults (Havighurst, 1968). However, due to declines in their physiological capacity (e.g., increased number of chronic illnesses, more mobility limitations, and hearing loss) and the reduction of social roles (e.g., retirement or loss of family members and friends), older adults' need to connect with others and engage in social activities may not be satisfied (Knapp, 1977) and produce a crisis in self-evaluation for older adults. As the number of limitations and disengaged activities increases with age, the crisis may worsen and cause late-life loneliness and depression (Hawkley & Kocherginsky, 2017; Li et al., 2021).

By overcoming some physical limitations, the internet provides older adults with an easily accessible platform to engage in activities that are otherwise impossible, such as social networking, shopping and banking, information searching, learning, and entertainment. These online activities can help older adults stay busy and maintain active relationships, ultimately reducing their loneliness and depression (Chopik, 2016; Gatto & Tak, 2008) and benefiting their cognition (Livingston et al., 2020; Yu & Fiebig, 2020). Thus, we hypothesized:

H2-a: Loneliness and depressive symptoms mediate the effect of internet use on cognition independently and sequentially.

18.1.1.2 Life-Span Theory of Control

Perceived control is essential for personal development across the lifespan, including late adulthood (Heckhausen & Schulz, 1995). As indicated by the life-span theory of control, individuals strive to maximize their primary control capacity throughout the life course to exert influence on their immediate external environment to meet their needs (Heckhausen & Schulz, 1995). Secondary control, which focuses on the internal adaptive process of making peace with one's needs, capacities, and environment, also assists in maximizing one's primary control capacity (Heckhausen & Schulz, 1995). Consistent evidence suggests that higher levels of perceived control are associated with better cognition outcomes (Infurna & Gerstorf, 2013; Khoo & Yang, 2020; Lachman & Andreoletti, 2006). Using a nationally representative sample of middle-aged and older Americans from the Health and Retirement Study (2006, 2008, 2010), Infurna and Gerstorf (2013) found that a higher level of perceived control over life was associated with a slower memory decline 4 years later both in middle-aged and older participants. Given the importance of perceived control in mitigating older adults' cognitive decline, training aimed at enhancing older adults' beliefs about controllability over the aging process is of great meaning (Lachman, 2006). Internet use may promote older adults' perceived control in two ways.

First, being able to learn and use the internet may be evidence of owning primary control over their life (Gatto & Tak, 2008). With the popularity of the internet, online options have been added to many aspects of daily life. Many people run errands online instead of going to stores, banks, hospitals, movie theaters, and libraries in person. However, unlike younger people, older people may continue to adhere to their traditional habits and may not have adopted online options into their daily lives. With significant societal change due to technological advances, many older adults are motivated to learn the internet to maintain primary control over their environments. As modern technologies are stereotyped as younger people's domain (Ivan & Cutler, 2021), learning and using the internet may be perceived as important evidence of capability by older adults (Gatto & Tak, 2008).

Second, online services may be good alternatives for older adults to maintain their primary control, especially for those with physical or functional limitations (Bernardo et al., 2022; Wu & Song, 2021). In late adulthood, physiological declines may hinder older adults' perceived control (Lachman, 2006) and cause depression, anxiety, and loneliness (Hawkley & Kocherginsky, 2017; Li et al., 2021). The secondary control process may assist older adults in adjusting their expectations and looking for alternatives within their capacities to meet their needs and maintain primary control. Thus, internet use, especially the instrumental use of the internet, may help older adults compensate for their declining functionality to maintain primary control. Therefore, we hypothesized that:

H2-b: Perceived control mediates the effect of internet use on cognition independently and sequentially via reduced loneliness and depressive symptoms.

18.1.2 Potential Group Differences by Age and Gender

Age Older adults of different age groups are not homogeneous. Young-old (<75 years) and old-old adults (75 + years) have different characteristics and face different stressors (Palgi, 2013; Wang et al., 2022a). Unlike old-old adults who may have already adjusted to late adulthood, young-old adults, many of whom are still in the process of transitioning from late-middle to later adulthood, may be stressed by associated changes, such as retirement, reduced social networking sizes, and the emergence of physiological declines and new health conditions and experience high psychological distress or depressive symptoms (Li et al., 2021; Wang et al., 2022b). A qualitative study revealed that regarding adjusting to aging, young-old adults focus more on occupation and achievement to "maintain busy and stay away from getting depressed" and social embeddedness to "enjoy being part of children's lives" (von Humboldt & Leal, 2015). As a commonly adopted and effective tool in daily life, internet use may assist young-old adults in engaging in activities, staying active, and mitigating psychological distress caused by the transition to later adulthood. Thus, the reduction in depression due to internet use becomes especially essential for young-old adults in promoting cognition.

In comparison, old-old adults may have adopted better regulation strategies to normalize these transitions (Palgi, 2013; Ramsey et al., 2016). However, they also tend to have worse health status and more functional limitations, restricting their social networking and daily activities (Hawkley & Kocherginsky, 2017; Shlisky et al., 2017). These restrictions will not only cause depression and loneliness but also pose huge threats to their autonomy, including self-control. Autonomy, a core value in Western societies, plays an essential role in the life of old-old adults (Patrão et al., 2019). Previous qualitative studies have revealed different perceptions of life focus between young-old and old-old adults (Patrão et al., 2019; von Humboldt & Leal, 2015). More specifically, old-old adults center more on attaining a life philosophy and self-enhancement, while young-old adults focus more on achievement and proximity with others (Patrão et al., 2019; von Humboldt & Leal, 2015). Quantitative studies have found that perceived control, such as perceived usefulness in daily life, played a similar or greater role among old-old adults than young-old adults in associating with different outcomes such as successful aging and mortality (Gu et al., 2017). Thus, given the importance of perceived control for old-old adults, utilizing the internet to compensate for their declined functionality and meet their needs may be especially crucial for them, consequently mitigating their loneliness and depression and promoting their cognition. Thus, we hypothesized:

H3-a: For young-old adults, the indirect effect of internet use on cognition was mainly via depressive symptoms, while for old-old adults, the indirect effect was mainly via perceived control.

Gender Stereotypical gender role beliefs have been historically widespread across societies (Charlesworth & Banaji, 2022). With the increase in high education and employment among women in recent years, gender stereotypes have decreased over time (Charlesworth & Banaji, 2022). Nevertheless, older adults who grew up and lived with these beliefs may have internalized these concepts across their lifespan (Levy, 2009), leading older men and women to have different self-expectations and psychological needs (Russell, 2007). According to gender stereotypes, men are often perceived as more agentic, task-oriented, and instrumental than women

(Bakan, 1966). However, as men age, physiological declines, role disruption, and loss of social status after retirement may cause more self-crisis, reduced self-esteem, and diminished control than older women (Specht et al., 2013). A trajectory analysis among German adults showed that despite men reporting higher perceived control than women across the lifespan, they tended to experience a decline after 60, while women had a slight increase (Specht et al., 2013). A previous study among older adults in China found that the association between perceived usefulness and mortality risk was stronger among men than women (Gu et al., 2017). Thus, as an effective tool to compensate for declined functionalities, internet use may be especially essential to promote older men's perceived control, consequently benefiting their cognitive functioning.

In comparison, women are commonly perceived as more communal, relationship-oriented, and expressive (Bakan, 1966). Social participation activities promote psychological well-being more for older women than older men (Cheung & Mui, 2023; Choi et al., 2021), as these activities are perceived as female-oriented (Russell, 2007). Considering the inclusion of social interactions in many online activities, older women may experience greater benefits than older men in terms of reduced loneliness and depressive symptoms that indirectly promote cognition. Thus, we hypothesized that:

H3-b: For older men, the indirect effect of internet use on cognition was mainly via perceived control, while for older women, the indirect effect was mainly via loneliness and depressive symptoms.

18.2 Methods

18.2.1 Data Source and Study Sample

Data used in this study were drawn from the 2012 and 2016 waves of the Health and Retirement Study (HRS) and the 2013 Internet Survey of the HRS, a nationally representative biennial panel study among U.S. adults over 50 and their spouses. A total of 20,554 individuals participated at baseline in 2012 (the HRS 2012). Given this study's focus on psychosocial mechanisms, individuals not eligible for psychological questions in the Leave-Behind Questionnaire (LBQ) module in the HRS 2012 were excluded (n = 10,475). After removing participants who did not complete or return the LBQ (n = 2,749), who aged under 65 years old (n = 3,249), who reported doctor-diagnosed Alzheimer's disease and related dementias and the onset of dementias (n = 168), and who did not report their internet use status (n = 67), we had a sample of 3,846 participants. Given this study's interest in the cognitive and psychological effects of different measures of internet use activities, participants who identified as internet users but did not report detailed internet use activities in the 2013 Internet Survey (n = 1,031) and those who completely missed on all mediator and outcome variables (n = 751) were excluded from this study. Thus, the final sample size was 2,064, including 1,137 internet users and 927 non-users. The detailed sample selection process is depicted in Figure 18.1. An "exempt" review was received from the IRB at the authors' institute. Bivariate analyses showed that compared to those included in this study, participants excluded due to missing values in internet use or all the psychological and cognitive measures had significantly higher proportions of old-old adults (aged ≥ 75), women, and older adults with limitations in activities in daily living (ADL) and instrumental activities in daily living (IADL), more chronic health conditions, and lower baseline cognition scores. However, these two groups were not significantly different in race/ethnicity, education, marital status, and poverty.

18.2.2 Measures

Detailed definitions for the focal variables are presented in Table 18.1. To ensure the robustness of our results, we controlled for a range of covariates. Race/ethnicity (0 = non-Hispanic White, 1 = racial/ethnic minorities), education (0 = less than a bachelor's degree, 1 = bachelor's degree or higher), marital status (0 = divorced, separated, or unmarried, 1 = married or partnered), and poverty status (0 = household income above the poverty line, 1 = household income below the poverty line) were dichotomized. ADL limitations were assessed across five activities: bathing, dressing, walking across a room, and getting in and out of bed. IADL limitations were measured across five activities: using a phone, managing money, taking medications, shopping for groceries, and preparing hot meals. Due to skewness in the data distribution, both ADL and IADL limitations were recoded dichotomously (0 = no limitations, 1 = having limitations). Chronic health conditions were measured as a sum (0–8) of conditions, including high blood pressure, diabetes, cancer, lung disease, heart problems, stroke, psychiatric problems, and arthritis. Baseline cognition was also included as a covariate, and the measurement was reported in Table 18.1.

18.2.3 Statistical Analyses

We used path analyses to examine the underlying mechanisms linking older adults' internet use and cognition. Internet access was measured in wave 2012, whereas detailed online activities were measured in 2013. Due to the special survey design of HRS, for our interest in analyzing different online activities, we only have independent variables in 2013, mediators and dependent variables in 2016. Given that only two waves of survey data have been made publicly available thus far, we adhered to a standard procedure in the field by utilizing baseline values for covariates while retaining mediators and the outcome variable from the follow-up wave (Hayes, 2022, pp. 570–571). We aimed to conduct five path analysis models, with the first model investigating the effect of internet access and the other four

Table 18.1 Summary of focal variables

Variables[a]	Source	Measures	Coding
IV: ICT access	HRS 2012	*How often do you use a computer for email, the internet, or other tasks?* 1=daily, 2=several times a week, 3=once a week, 4=several times a month, 5= at least once a month, 6=not in the last month, 7=never/not relevant.	Responses were re-coded into two categories (0 = no, 1 = yes). For those reported "never/not relevant", internet access was coded as 0; all others were coded as 1.
IV: Informational use	2013 Internet Survey	*Using the internet for any of the following activities in the past year:* send or read email; phone others using Skype, Facetime, or other such services; get recommendations on restaurants; get recommendations on service providers such plumbers or electricians; get news online; follow financial markets; get information about health and healthcare; watch movies or TV shows; research (ancestry, dictionary, Wiki); Hobbies or interests; get directions and maps; use the internet for work.	Participants using any of the specific activities within these four types of online activities were considered users of that type of online activity. Two other categories were non-internet users and internet users who were not users of that type of online activity. Dummy variables were created compared to non-internet users. Regarding informational use, the percentage of internet users but not users of that online activity was 0%; thus, only one dummy variable was created.
IV: Social use	2013 Internet Survey	*Do you use any of the following social networking sites for communication with other people?* MySpace, Facebook, Twitter, LinkedIn, and others.	
IV: Online shopping	2013 Internet Survey	*Using the internet for any of the following activities in the past year:* Buy an item online; Pay bills online; Book travel online; Buy tickets online; Make a reservation at a restaurant; Get a discount coupon; Buy or sell something using an online marketplace such as eBay; Buy or sell something using an online classified site such as Craigslist.	
IV: Online banking	2013 Internet Survey	*Using the internet for any of the following activities in the past year:* View bank balance or transaction; Make a banking transaction; View credit card balance or activity; View a brokerage, retirement, or mutual fund account; File a tax return; View a utility or other bill.	

(continued)

Table 18.1 (continued)

Variables[a]	Source	Measures	Coding
Covariate/DV: Cognition	HRS 2012/2016	Cognition was measured by a reduced version of Telephone Interview for Cognitive Status (TIC), composed of immediate word recall, delayed word recall, Serial 7s, backward counting, date naming (month, day, year, day of the week), object naming (scissors & cactus); naming the President, and Vice President of the United States.	The total cognition score ranged from 0 to 35, with higher scores indicating better cognition. Cognition in 2016 was the dependent variable, and cognition in 2012 was covariate.
M: Loneliness	HRS 2016	Loneliness was measured by 11 questions, including "lack of companionship", "feel left out", "feel isolated from others", "in tune with others", "alone", "have people to talk to", "have people to turn to", "have people understanding you", "have people that you are close to", "feel part of a group", "a lot in common with friends" (1 = often, 2 = some of the time, 3 = hardly or never).	Four items, including "lack companionship", "feel left out", "feel isolated from others", and "alone" were reversely coded. Loneliness was measured by the unweighted mean of the 11 items, ranging from 1 to 3, with high scores indicating higher levels of loneliness.
M: Depressive symptoms	HRS 2016	Depressive symptoms were measured by the Center for Epidemiologic Studies Depression (CESD) as a mediator. Participants were asked to answer whether during much of the time of the past week, "you felt depressed", "you felt that everything you did was an effort", "your sleep was restless", "you were happy", "you felt lonely", "you enjoyed life", "you felt sad", and "you could not get going" (0 = no, 1 = yes).	Responses for "you were happy" and "you enjoyed life" were reversely coded. Depressive symptoms were measured by the unweighted sum of the eight items, ranging from 0 to 8, with higher scores indicating higher levels of depressive symptoms.
M: Perceived control	HRS 2016	Participants were asked to rate the amount of control they had over their health, social life, and financial situation these days (0 = no control at all, 10 = very much control).	Perceived control was measured by the unweighted mean, ranging from 0 to 10, with higher scores indicating higher perceived control.

Note: [a]*IV* independent variable, *DV* dependent variable, *M* mediator. Age and gender were included as covariates in the total participant model. Age was measured in chronological years, and for subgroup analyses, it was recoded dichotomously (0 = aged 65–74, or young-old; 1 = aged 75 and older, or old-old). Gender was measured dichotomously (0 = male, 1 = female) investigating four online activities (i.e., informational use, social use, online shopping, and online banking). However, due to the very close percentages between informational use (44.77%) and internet access (44.91%), we only tested the model of informational use but not both. Also, given our interest in different online activities, only the results of dummy variables comparing different online activity users to non-internet users were reported. In addition, sensitivity analyses were conducted to examine the mechanisms underlying the associations between online activities and cognitive functioning only among internet users.

Multi-group path analyses were used to test potential age and gender group differences, as we had reviewed earlier. We conducted chi-square difference tests for nested models, commonly used to examine group differences in path analysis (Garson, 2013; Mazzer & Rickwood, 2015). We compared the constrained model (coefficients set to be equal between subgroups) and the unconstrained model (coefficients set to be free between subgroups) for age as well as gender groups. The results showed that the unconstrained models were significantly better than the constrained models for both age and gender groups, indicating significant model differences between young-old and old-old participants and between men and women. Such a subgroup analysis has some advantages and is widely used in the literature (Wang et al., 2022a; Wang & Ware, 2013; Wang et al., 2021).

To ensure the models' robustness, all covariates were controlled for the outcome variable and all mediators. Such a design is well documented in the literature (e.g., Albert, 2012; Mackinnon & Pirlott, 2015). In addition, following common practice in the literature (Hu & Bentler, 1999), path analyses were estimated by the maximum likelihood (ML) with bootstrapping (n = 5,000) using Mplus 8.4 (Muthen & Muthen, 2017) and bias-corrected bootstrap confidence intervals were applied for estimates of indirect effects. Full information maximum likelihood (FIML) was used to handle the missing values in our selected sample. Acceptable/good model fit indices cutoff points adopted in this study were the root mean square error of approximation (RMSEA) less than .06, the comparative fit index (CFI) and Tucker-Lewis index (TLI) no less than .90, and the standardized root mean square residual (SRMR) less than .08 (Hu & Bentler, 1999).

18.3 Results

18.3.1 Participants Characteristics

Participants' demographic characteristics are summarized in Table 18.2. Among the 2,064 older participants, about 45% were internet users. More specifically, about 45% of the participants reported using the internet for informational activities, 23% for social activities, 39% for online shopping, and 32% for online banking. Bivariate analysis showed significant internet use differences by age and gender. Young-old adults and men were more likely than their old-old and women counterparts, respectively, to be internet users and use the internet for information searching, shopping,

Table 18.2 Descriptive statistics ($n = 2,064$)

	Total	Young-old ($n = 1,093$)	Old-old ($n = 971$)	Men ($n = 811$)	Women ($n = 1,253$)
Variables in 2016					
Loneliness (1–3)	1.5 ± .4	1.5 ± .4	1.5 ± .4	1.5 ± .4	1.5 ± .4
Depressive symptoms (0–8)	1.3 ± 1.8	1.3 ± 1.8	1.4 ± 1.8	1.0 ± 1.5***	1.5 ± 2.0***
Perceived control (0–10)	7.6 ± 1.9	7.7 ± 1.8	7.5 ± 2.1	7.6 ± 1.9	7.6 ± 2.0
Cognition (2016, 0–35)	20.6 ± 5.1	21.9 ± 4.8***	19.2 ± 5.1***	20.4 ± 4.9	20.8 ± 5.3
Variables in 2012/2013					
Age (≥ 65)	74.7 ± 6.2	69.9 ± 2.9	80.0 ± 4.2	74.7 ± 6.0	74.6 ± 6.3
%Young-old (65–74)	53.0	100.0	0.0	52.2	53.5
%Old-old (75 and older)	47.0	0.0	100.0	47.8	46.5
%Women	60.7	61.3	60.0	0.0	100.0
%Racial/ethnic minorities	16.2	18.6**	13.6**	13.9*	17.7*
Education years (0–17)	12.5 ± 3.1	12.7 ± 3.0*	12.4 ± 3.2*	12.8 ± 3.3 **	12.4 ± 3.0 **
%Poverty	9.1	9.2	9.1	6.5	10.8
%ADL	14.3	12.2	16.7	13.2	15.0
%IADL	11.4	8.4	14.7	9.4	12.7
Chronic diseases (0–8)	2.4 ± 1.4	2.4 ± 1.4	2.5 ± 1.3	2.4 ± 1.4	2.5 ± 1.4
Cognition (2012, 0–35)	22.0 ± 4.5	22.8 ± 4.3***	21.2 ± 4.5***	21.7 ± 4.3 *	22.2 ± 4.6 *
%Internet user	44.9	54.4***	34.3***	49.0**	42.3**
Informational use[a]		***	***	**	**
%Yes	44.8	54.1	34.4	48.8	42.2
%No	1.1	0.9	1.2	1.6	0.7
%Non-internet user	54.1	45.0	64.3	49.6	57.0
Social use[a]		***	***		
%Yes	23.2	31.1	14.8	21.3	24.8
%No	21.9	23.5	20.3	28.6	17.8
%Non-internet user	54.1	45.4	64.9	50.1	57.4
Online shopping[a]		***	***	**	**
%Yes	39.1	48.9	28.2	43.0	36.8
%No	6.6	6.0	7.2	7.3	6.2
%Non-internet user	54.1	45.1	64.5	49.2	57.0
Online banking[a]		***	***	**	**
%Yes	31.8	39.9	23.0	36.7	28.9
%No	13.6	14.9	12.3	13.5	13.8
%Non-internet user	54.1	45.2	64.7	49.8	57.3

Note: $^{*}p < .05$, $^{**}p < .01$, $^{***}p < .001$

[a]The sum of total percentages was less than 100% because very few internet users (<1%) did not indicate the usage of online activities. Chi-square tests (for categorical variables) and t tests (for continuous variables) were performed between two age groups and between two gender groups

and banking. Additionally, a significant difference in social use was found by age group, favoring young-old adults. Correlations among focal variables were reported in Table 18.3.

18.3.2 Path Analysis Models Among Total Participants

All path analysis models showed acceptable/good model fit. As shown in Table 18.4, the direct and total indirect effects of informational use (direct: $\beta = .220$, $CI = [.143, .290]$; indirect: $\beta = .024$, $CI = [.012, .039]$), social use (direct: $\beta = .195$, $CI = [.118, .273]$; indirect: $\beta = .027$, $CI = [.013, .044]$), online shopping (direct: $\beta = .251$, $CI = [.176, .323]$; indirect: $\beta = .025$, $CI = [.013, .040]$), and online banking (direct: $\beta = .261$, $CI = [.186, .339]$; indirect: $\beta = .025$, $CI = [.011, .041]$) on cognition were all significant. The total indirect effects accounted for 9.58%–13.85% of the total effect across all the internet use models.

Regarding the significant indirect paths, depressive symptoms were found to partially mediate the effects of informational use ($\beta = .010$, $CI = [.003, .021]$), social use ($\beta = .013$, $CI = [.004, .025]$), online shopping ($\beta = .010$, $CI = [.003, .022]$), and online banking ($\beta = .009$, $CI = [.0021, .020]$) on cognition. Perceived control was found to partially mediate the effects of informational use ($\beta = .008$, $CI = [.002, .021]$), social use ($\beta = .008$, $CI = [.002, .022]$), online shopping ($\beta = .009$, $CI = [.002, .023]$) and online banking ($\beta = .009$, $CI = [.001, .023]$) on cognition. However, perceived control was not found to mediate the association sequentially via loneliness or depressive symptoms. In addition, loneliness did not mediate the association independently or sequentially via depression, except for online banking (loneliness→depressive symptoms: $\beta = .002$, $CI = [.001, .005]$). See Figs. 18.1, 18.2–18.5.

18.3.3 Path Analysis Models Among Internet Users

All path analysis models among internet users showed acceptable/good model fit. The coefficients of the relationships among online activities, psychological mediators, and cognition are summarized in Figs. 18.6, 18.7, and 18.8. Regarding the effects of social use on cognition, none of the total ($\beta = -.058$, $CI = [-.167, .045]$), direct ($\beta = -.065$, $CI = [-.166, .041]$) and total indirect ($\beta = .006$, $CI = [-.008, .025]$) effects was significant. These results indicated that social users of the internet did not have significantly different cognition compared to those who used the internet but not for social connection purposes. Regarding the effects of online shopping and banking on cognition, the total effects (online shopping: $\beta = .217$, $CI = [.054, .371]$; online banking: $\beta = .197$, $CI = [.081, .315]$) and direct effects (online shopping: $\beta = .207$, $CI = [.044, .362]$; online banking: $\beta = .195$, $CI = [.079, .315]$) were significant, but not the total indirect effects or any indirect paths. These findings

Table 18.3 Correlations among focal variables

	1	2	3	4	5	6	7	8
1.Cognition (2016)								
2.Internet use (yes vs. no)	.46**							
3.Informational use (yes vs. not internet user)	.45**	.97**						
4.Social use (yes vs. not internet user)	.29**	.60**	.60**					
5.Shopping use (yes vs. not internet user)	.44**	.87**	.88**	.57**				
6.Banking use (yes vs. not internet user)	.39**	.74**	.751*	.53**	.78**			
7.Loneliness	−.18**	−.14**	−.14**	−.08**	−.15**	−.14**		
8.Depression	−.24**	−.22**	−.22**	−.13**	−.20**	−.16**	.39**	
9.Perceived control	.18**	.10**	.09**	.05*	.09**	.07**	−.39**	−.33**

Note: $^{*}p < .05$, $^{**}p < .01$, $^{***}p < .001$

Table 18.4 Standardized coefficients of effects of internet use on cognition

	Total	Young-old (<5)	Old-old (≥75)	Men	Women
Model 1 (informational use[a])					
Total effects	**.220**	**.274**	**.223**	**.240**	**.232**
Direct effect	**.196**	**.240**	**.198**	**.157**	**.216**
Total indirect effects[b]	**.024**	**.033**	**.025**	**.046**	**.016**
Depressive symptoms	**.010**	**.021**	.003 (ns)	**.014**	**.010**
Perceived control	**.008**	.004 (ns)	**.020**	**.023**	.004 (ns)
Loneliness ➔ Depressive symptoms	.001 (ns)	.002 (ns)	.000 (ns)	.001 (ns)	.002 (ns)
Model 2 (social use[a])					
Total effects	**.195**	**.267**	**.168**	**.177**	**.208**
Direct effect	**.168**	**.229**	**.140**	**.142**	**.187**
Total indirect effects[b]	**.027**	**.038**	**.028**	.035 (ns)	**.021**
Depressive symptoms	**.013**	**.025**	.003 (ns)	**.015**	**.012**
Perceived control	**.008**	.004 (ns)	**.023**	.018 (ns)	.005 (ns)
Loneliness ➔ Depressive symptoms	.001 (ns)	.002 (ns)	.001 (ns)	−.001 (ns)	.002 (ns)
Model 3 (online shopping[a])					
Total effects	**.251**	**.310**	**.252**	**.253**	**.252**
Direct effect	**.226**	**.275**	**.222**	**.203**	**.235**
Total indirect effects[b]	**.025**	**.035**	**.029**	**.050**	**.017**
Depressive symptoms	**.010**	**.021**	.003 (ns)	**.013**	**.011**
Perceived control	**.009**	.004 (ns)	**.024**	**.026**	.004 (ns)
Loneliness ➔ Depressive symptoms	.002 (ns)	.003 (ns)	.001 (ns)	.001 (ns)	.002 (ns)
Model 4 (online banking[a])					
Total effects	**.261**	**.326**	**.251**	**.235**	**.282**
Direct effect	**.236**	**.290**	**.227**	**.182**	**.266**
Total indirect effects[b]	**.025**	**.036**	.024 (ns)	**.053**	**.016**
Depressive symptoms	**.009**	**.022**	.000 (ns)	.010 (ns)	**.010**
Perceived control	**.009**	.004 (ns)	**.022**	**.027**	.004 (ns)
Loneliness ➔ Depressive symptoms	**.002**	.003 (ns)	.002 (ns)	.002 (ns)	.002 (ns)

Note: Standardized coefficients in boldface were statistically significant. ns stands for non-significant. Age, gender, race/ethnicity, marital status, poverty, limitations in ADL and IADL, number of chronic health conditions, and baseline cognition were included as covariates in all four models

[a]In all the models, users of different types of online activities were compared to non-internet users

[b]Other indirect paths through (1) loneliness, (2) perceived control and loneliness, (3) perceived control and depressive symptoms, and (4) perceived control, loneliness, and depressive symptoms were also tested but were not significant in any model; thus, they are not presented in the table

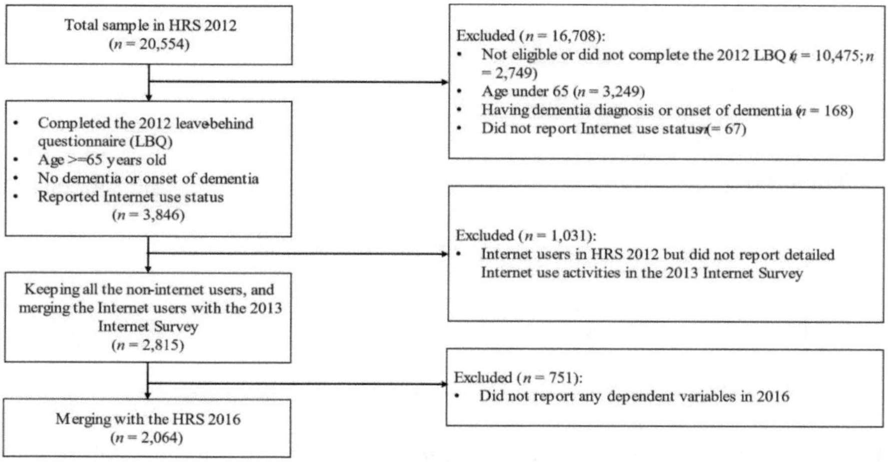

Fig. 18.1 Sample Selection Process

suggest that among internet users, those who engaged in online shopping or banking had better overall cognitive scores than those who did not use the internet for these specific activities. However, these cognitive benefits were not explained by the mediators tested in this study. Given the lack of significant indirect effects in the analyses, subgroup analyses by age and gender subgroups among internet users were not performed).

18.3.4 Multi-Group Path Analysis Models by Age and Gender

All the multi-group path analysis models had acceptable/good model fit. As summarized in Table 18.4, among young-old adults, the direct and indirect effects of all types of online activities were significant, and the total indirect effects accounted for 11.04%–14.23% of the total effects. The result indicated that there is a partial mediation by depressive symptoms on the effects of informational use (β = .021, *CI* = [.006, .040]), social use (β = .025, *CI* = [.007, .046]), online shopping (β = .021, *CI* = [.006, .041]), and online banking (β = .022, *CI* = [.006, .042]) among young-old adults. Among old-old adults, the direct effect of all types of online activities and the total indirect effects of all online activities except for online banking were significant, and the total indirect effects accounted for 11.21%–16.67% of the total effects. Perceived control partially mediated the effects of informational use (β = .020, *CI* = [.003, .049]), social use (β = .023, *CI* = [.003, .058]), online shopping (β = .024, *CI* = [.005, .055]), and online banking (β = .022, *CI* = [.004, .052]) among old-old adults.

Among older men, all the direct and total indirect effects, except for social use, were significant. The significant total indirect effects accounted for 19.17%–22.55%

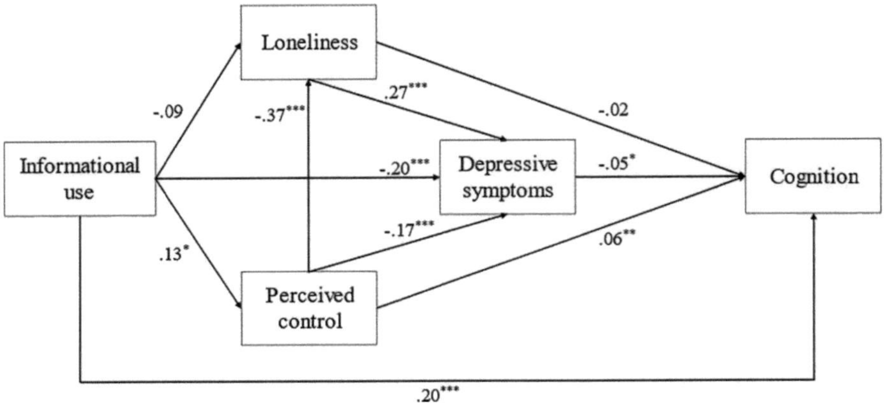

Fig. 18.2 Psychological mechanisms underlying the association between informational use of the internet and cognition, entire sample. *Note*: The coefficients are standardized. Age, gender, race/ethnicity, marital status, poverty, limitations in ADL and IADL, number of chronic health conditions, and baseline cognition were included as covariates in the model. $^{*}p < .05$, $^{**}p < .01$, $^{***}p < .001$

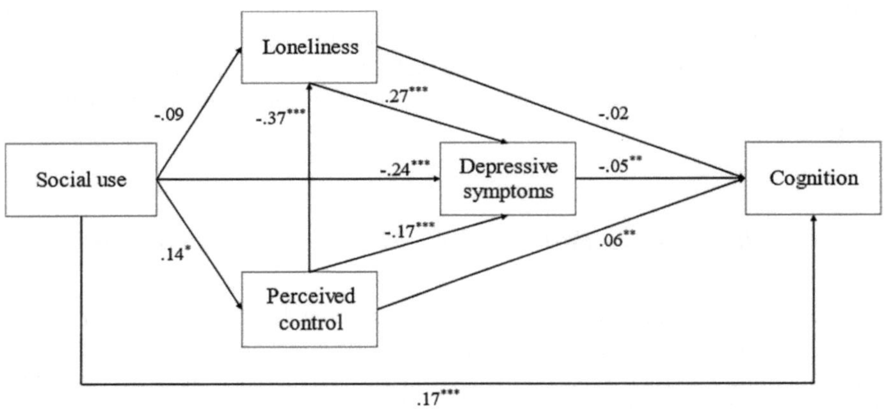

Fig. 18.3 Psychological mechanisms underlying the association between social use of the internet and cognition, entire sample. *Note*: The coefficients are standardized. Age, gender, race/ethnicity, marital status, poverty, limitations in ADL and IADL, number of chronic health conditions, and baseline cognition were included as covariates in the full models. $^{*}p < .05$, $^{**}p < .01$, $^{***}p < .001$

of the total effects among older men. Depressive symptoms partially mediated the effects of informational use (β = .014, *CI* = [.001, .035]), social use (β = .015, *CI* = [.001, .038]), and online shopping (β = .013, *CI* = [.001, .031]). Perceived control partially mediated the effects of informational use (β = .023, *CI* = [.005, .064]), online shopping (β = .026, *CI* = [.006, .067]), and online banking (β = .027, *CI* = [.006, .067]). Among older women, both the direct and total indirect effects

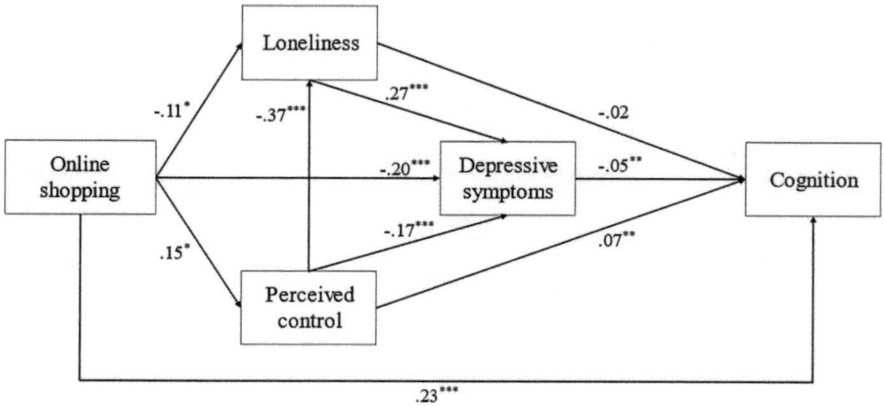

Fig. 18.4 Psychological mechanisms underlying the association between online shopping and cognition, entire sample. *Note*: The coefficients are standardized. Age, gender, race/ethnicity, marital status, poverty, limitations in ADL and IADL, number of chronic health conditions, and baseline cognition were included as covariates in the full models. $^{*}p < .05$, $^{**}p < .01$, $^{***}p < .001$

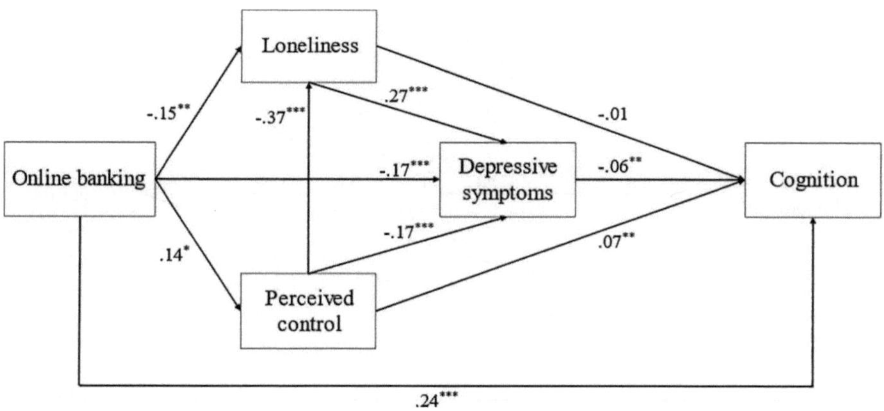

Fig. 18.5 Psychological mechanisms underlying the association between online banking and cognition, entire sample. *Note*: The coefficients are standardized. Age, gender, race/ethnicity, marital status, poverty, limitations in ADL and IADL, number of chronic health conditions, and baseline cognition were included as covariates in the full models. $^{*}p < .05$, $^{**}p < .01$, $^{***}p < .001$

of all online activities were significant. The total indirect effects accounted for 5.67%–10.10% of the total effects. Depressive symptoms partially mediated the effects of informational use ($\beta = .010$, $CI = [.001, .024]$), social use ($\beta = .012$, $CI = [.002, .030]$), online shopping ($\beta = .011$, $CI = [.001, .026]$), and online banking ($\beta = .010$, $CI = [.001, .025]$) on cognition among older women. However, loneliness did not mediate the effect of any online activities on cognition among older women.

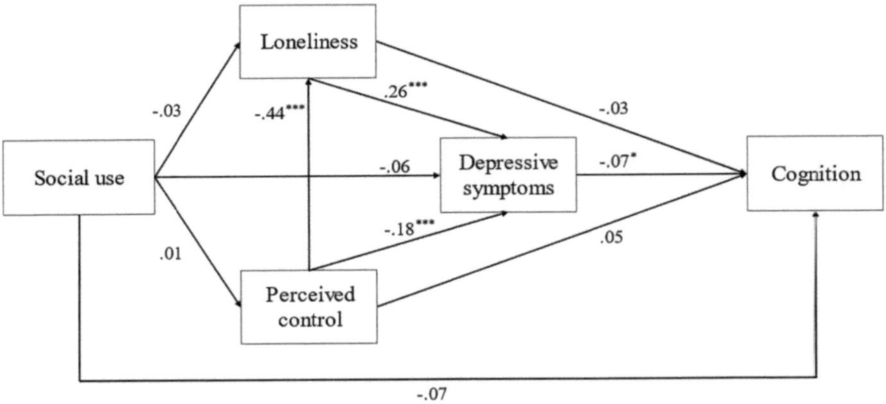

Fig. 18.6 Psychological mechanisms underlying the association between social use of the internet and cognition, internet user sample. *Note*: The coefficients are standardized. Age, gender, race/ethnicity, marital status, poverty, limitations in ADL and IADL, number of chronic health conditions, and baseline cognition were included as covariates in the full models. $^{*}p < .05$, $^{**}p < .01$, $^{***}p < .001$

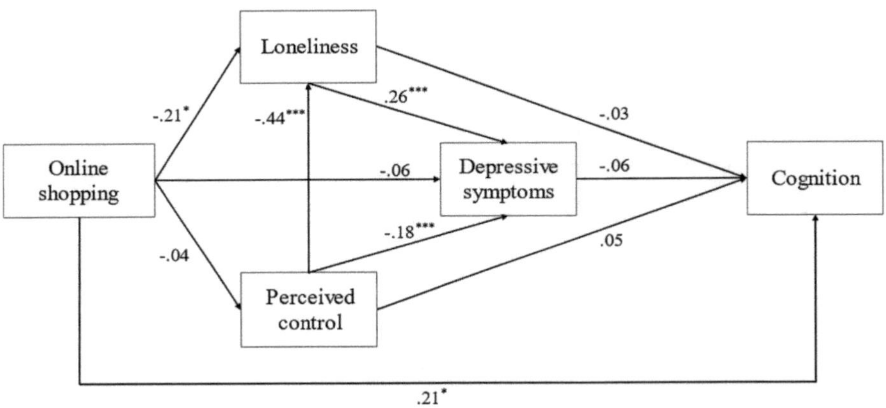

Fig. 18.7 Psychological mechanisms underlying the association between online shopping and cognition, internet user sample. *Note*: The coefficients are standardized. Age, gender, race/ethnicity, marital status, poverty, limitations in ADL and IADL, number of chronic health conditions, and baseline cognition were included as covariates in the full models. $^{*}p < .05$, $^{**}p < .01$, $^{***}p < .001$

18.4 Discussion

Using a large sample of older adults from the U.S., this study aimed to examine the psychological mechanism underlying the association between older adults' internet use and cognition and investigate potential age and gender differences. We found a significant positive direct effect of internet use on cognition across all online

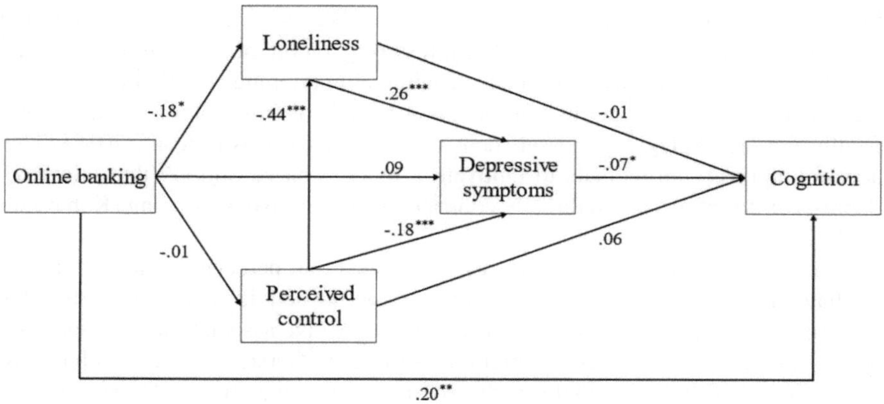

Fig. 18.8 Psychological mechanisms underlying the association between online banking and cognition, internet user sample. *Note*: The coefficients are standardized. Age, gender, race/ethnicity, marital status, poverty, limitations in ADL and IADL, number of chronic health conditions, and baseline cognition were included as covariates in the full models. $^{*}p < .05$, $^{**}p < .01$, $^{***}p < .001$

activities, thus supporting H1. This aligns with previous studies indicating the cognitive stimulating impacts of internet use among older adults (Choi et al., 2021; Yu & Fiebig, 2020) and echoes the activity theory of aging in its application to all types of online activities under study. The primary mechanism is that regularly engaging in various online activities can provide continuous cognitive stimulation that contributes to maintaining cognitive functioning or delaying cognitive decline at older ages. Thus, more internet training and internet-based cognitive interventions should be provided to older adults.

18.4.1 Psychological Mechanisms Among All Participants

Our study also reveals that engaging in online activities, irrespective of the specific purposes, appears to have a small yet statistically significant positive influence on cognition through alleviating depressive symptoms. This finding confirms parts of our hypothesis (H2-a), that is, depressive symptoms partially mediate the effect of internet use on cognition. This finding aligns with the activity theory of aging, emphasizing the importance of social interactions and maintaining an active lifestyle in later adulthood (Havighurst, 1968). The following interpretations may provide some insights into our findings. First, engaging in online activities, particularly those with a social focus, can serve as a valuable source of digital social connection, interactions, and support that contributes to a reduction in feelings of loneliness and social isolation, potentially acting as a buffer against depressive symptoms (Chopik, 2016; Khoo & Yang, 2020). Second, engaging in enjoyable and absorbing activities online, even those non-social activities, can serve as a coping mechanism to help individuals temporarily shift their focus away from stressors, negative thoughts, and loneliness (von Humboldt & Leal, 2015), fostering a more positive emotional state, which may, in turn, positively influence cognitive functioning. Third, through informal internet use, older adults can access a wealth of information about mental health, coping strategies, and self-help resources (Kobayashi et al., 2015). This access empowers individuals to cultivate a more positive outlook that alleviates depressive symptoms and indirectly contributes to cognitive well-being (Kobayashi et al., 2015).

Corroborating half of H2-b, our results showed that perceived control partially mediated the associations between all types of online activities and cognition. This finding supports previous studies indicating the positive association between older adults' perceived control and cognition (Infurna & Gerstorf, 2013; Lachman & Andreoletti, 2006). It also confirms that online services may be good alternatives to compensate for older adults' declined functionalities and help them maintain good control over their lives (Bernardo et al., 2022; Wu & Song, 2021). For example, Wu and Song (2021) found that older adults with lower perceived shopping mobilities tended to find online shopping more useful and have more positive attitudes and intentions to continue online shopping; at the same time, online shopping attitudes and intentions were positively associated with perceived behavioral control. The possible mechanisms may be as follows. First, online activities may reduce anxiety and uncertainty associated with specific tasks and empower them by providing a sense of autonomy and control over their daily activities (Oswald & Wagner, 2023; Schlomann et al., 2020). This may further contribute to an enhanced perception of control, leading to positive cognitive effects. Second, engagement in various online activities may involve acquiring digital skills. Mastering these skills might increase competence and control over the online environment (Gatto & Tak, 2008), positively influencing cognition. Third, online activities, especially instrumental ones, may introduce routine and structure into individuals' lives. Establishing a routine can contribute to a sense of predictability and control, potentially influencing cognitive well-being (Bergua et al., 2006).

18.4.2 Psychological Mechanisms by Subgroups

Supporting H3-a, our results showed that depressive symptoms partially mediated the effects of all types of online activities on cognition among young-old adults, while perceived control partially mediated all the effects among old-old adults. This finding aligns with the previous indications regarding the heterogeneous characteristics and stressors among older adults of different age groups (Palgi, 2013; Wang et al., 2022b). Young-old adults are in a period of significant life transitions, including retirement, changes in social networks, children leaving home, and potential lifestyle and health changes (Li et al., 2021; Wang et al., 2022b). These transitions are usually accompanied by increased stressors and a higher likelihood of experiencing depressive symptoms (Li et al., 2021; Wang et al., 2022b). By providing access to different social, practical, or instrumental activities, the internet plays a crucial role in keeping young-old adults busy, fostering social connectedness, and alleviating loneliness and depression, which benefits their cognition (Chopik, 2016; Khoo & Yang, 2020).

For old-old adults, due to their worse health conditions and more functional limitations (Hawkley & Kocherginsky, 2017; Shlisky et al., 2017), they are concerned the most about the threat of losing autonomy (Patrão et al., 2019; von Humboldt & Leal, 2015). By compensating old-old adults' declined functionalities to meet their needs for information seeking, social networking, shopping, and banking, the internet helps them maintain control over their lives, which may reduce loneliness and depressive symptoms and yield positive effects on cognitive outcomes, echoing the life course theory of control. This finding is also consistent with a recent study indicating the positive association between internet use and autonomy was greater for those with more functional disabilities among a large sample of older adults aged 80 and older in Germany (Oswald & Wagner, 2023). Thus, future cognitive interventions should consider older participants' age group and the needs and stressors faced by that group and provide more tailored interventions. More specifically, future cognitive interventions for young-old adults may consider incorporating more components to reduce their psychological distress, whereas, for old-old adults, cognitive interventions with a focus on enhancing perceived control may be more effective in promoting their cognition.

Confirming with most of H3-b, our findings showed that perceived control partially mediated the associations between internet use and cognition among older men, while depressive symptoms partially mediated the associations among older women. This finding is consistent with older adults' psychological needs informed by gender role expectations. Men tend to have more perceived control than women; however, as they age, men report a decline in perceived control, while women show an increase (Specht et al., 2013). The reduced perceived control is more detrimental for older men than women (Gu et al., 2017). Thus, enhanced perceived control via online activities may be more important for older men to better promote their cognition. Additionally, depressive symptoms partially mediated most online activities among older men. When the internet is used for practical, goal-oriented tasks, engaging in these tasks may provide older men a sense of accomplishment, alleviating depressive symptoms and promoting cognition. Meanwhile, given the essence of engagement in social activities for older women (Cheung & Mui, 2023; Choi et al., 2021), the social aspects embedded within various online activities could offer older women great value in reducing loneliness and depressive symptoms, and consequently, mitigating their cognitive decline. Therefore, gender roles should be considered in internet-based cognitive interventions. Specifically, online activities enhancing perceived control may be more cognitively effective for older men, while strengthening social interactions may benefit older women more in their cognition. Furthermore, incorporating elements to reduce older adults' depressive symptoms may be beneficial for their cognitive functioning for both older men and women.

However, we found that the indirect paths via loneliness diminished their significance across all online activities in the presence of depressive symptoms and perceived control. This suggests that the presence of depressive symptoms and perceived control alters the dynamics of how loneliness affects the relationship between internet use and cognitive outcomes. Although this contradicts the established association between loneliness and cognition among older adults (Livingston et al., 2020), it aligns with some prior findings showing the diminishing association between loneliness and cognition in the presence of depression and other psychological factors (Cardona & Andrés, 2023; Yang et al., 2021). Our finding suggests the interplay between loneliness, depressive symptoms, and perceived control and their impact on the mediation process. Depressive symptoms may independently influence cognition and interact with loneliness, affecting how loneliness mediates the relationship between internet use and cognition. The perception of control over one's life could mitigate the negative impact of loneliness on cognition, reducing its mediating significance. In addition, it may also stem from the inclusion of a psychologically healthy sample. More studies from different populations are needed to disentangle the mechanisms of loneliness in mediating the relationship between internet use and cognition in the presence of other mediators and covariates.

18.4.3 Sensitivity Analysis Among Internet Users

Sensitivity analyses restricted to internet users revealed that none of the total indirect effects or individual indirect paths of online activities were significant in predicting older adults' cognition. This lack of significant indirect effects suggests that the psychological mechanisms linking internet use to cognition may operate differently between users and non-users. As discussed earlier, for non-users, engaging in online activities may offer a novel and enriching experience that facilitates psychological change—such as increased perceived control or reduced loneliness—which, in turn, supports cognitive functioning (Gatto & Tak, 2008). In contrast, for existing internet users, these initial psychological benefits may no longer exert a strong influence, possibly because users have already adapted to the emotional or social aspects of digital engagement. For this group, cognitive benefits may be driven more by ongoing cognitive stimulation and task complexity rather than by changes in emotional well-being (Choi et al., 2021; Yu & Fiebig, 2020). This distinction suggests that the mechanisms linking ICT use to cognition may vary by one's prior experience or intensity of engagement. Future research should examine whether digital novelty, engagement quality, or specific activity types influence the cognitive benefits of ICT use among older adults with different usage histories.

18.4.4 Limitations and Future Directions

Several limitations need to be considered when interpreting the findings from this study. First, despite the bi-directional associations between internet use and cognition (Choi et al., 2021; Yu & Fiebig, 2020), this study only examined the direction from internet use to cognition. This is due to our interest in examining whether internet use could be a modifiable factor to help older adults preserve cognition and delay or prevent cognitive impairment. Considering the cognitive impact on older adults' internet use, we excluded participants with doctor-diagnosed ADRD and onsets of ADRD and included participants' baseline cognition as a covariate. Also, due to the limitation of archival data, mediators and cognition outcome were measured at the same time in this study. Future longitudinal studies with more waves are needed to better examine the mediation effection and the potential bi-directional association between internet use and cognition. Second, detailed internet use data were extracted from the 2013 internet Survey. Given the dramatic increase in older adults' internet adoption and usage in recent years (Pew Research Center, 2021), findings in this study may not reflect the association or mechanism among current older adults who likely have more internet experience. Third, given this study's focus on different types of online activities and psychological mechanisms, internet users who did not report their detailed use activities and older participants who missed all mediators and cognitive outcomes were excluded from the analyses. Bivariate analysis showed that those excluded had significantly worse health and functioning status. Thus, this study's results may only apply to a sample of relatively healthy older adults. Future studies are needed to examine the robustness of the results with samples of older adults with different levels of health and functioning status. In addition, most of the older participants in this study were non-Hispanic White (84%). Generalizations of findings from this study to racial/ethnic minorities may not be applicable, given the different racial profiles in internet use (Wang & Kubanga, 2021). Fourth, while how internet use (and with different purposive uses) is associated with cognition by age group and gender, and how depressive symptoms and perceived control mediate these associations have been tested in this research, the underly mechanisms are still unclear. Our abovementioned speculations deserve further empirical tests with more sophiscated design as well as availability data. Nevertheless, our study provides a foundation for future research to explore these avenues more thoroughly. Fifth, findings from this study indicate that most of the association between internet use and cognition is direct, and the mediating effects through depressive symptoms, loneliness, and perceived control only accounted for a very small proportion. However, this does not mean that the impact of internet use on cognition was truly mainly through the direct effect. The impacts of other potential mediators, such as lifelong learning, health literacy, and health behaviors, may not be captured in this study. Future research may consider examining the mediating effects of these potential factors.

18.4.5 Conclusions

This study contributes to the literature by investigating psychological pathways of depressive symptoms, perceived control, and loneliness of how internet use affects cognition by assessing engagement in four online activities and testing effects among age and gender subgroups. Findings in this study indicate that the cognitive benefit of internet use is via a large direct effect and small but statistically significant indirect effects via depressive symptoms and perceived control. In addition, the psychological mechanisms differ by age and gender. Future internet-based cognitive interventions should focus more on the direct stimulative effect and be more tailored to the characteristics and needs of participants' age and gender. Collaborations among researchers, practitioners, and policymakers are needed to learn more about the cognitive benefits of internet use among older adults, remove barriers, and promote internet access and usage among older adults.

Disclaimer The views expressed in this chapter are solely those of the authors and do not necessarily reflect those of the University of Alabama at Birmingham, the University of Illinois Urbana-Champaign, Binghamton University, the University of Alabama, or the United Nations.

References

Albert, J. M. (2012). Distribution-free mediation analysis for nonlinear models with confounding. *Epidemiology, 46*(6), 879–888. https://doi.org/10.1097/EDE.0b013e31826c2bb9

Bakan, D. (1966). *The duality of human existence: An essay on psychology and religion*. Rand Mcnally.

Baltes, P. B. (1987). Theoretical propositions of life-span developmental psychology: On the dynamics between growth and decline. *Developmental Psychology, 23*(5), 611.

Bergua, V., Fabrigoule, C., Barberger-Gateau, P., Dartigues, J.-F., Swendsen, J., & Bouisson, J. (2006, October 1). Preferences for routines in older people: Associations with cognitive and psychological vulnerability. *International Journal of Geriatric Psychiatry, 21*(10), 990–998. https://doi.org/10.1002/gps.1597

Bernardo, J., Apóstolo, J., Loureiro, R., Santana, E., Yaylagul, N. K., Dantas, C., Ventura, F., Duque, F. M., Jøranson, N., Zechner, M., Staalduinen, W. V., De Luca, V., Illario, M., & Silva, R. (2022). eHealth platforms to promote autonomous life and active aging: A scoping review. *International Journal of Environmental Research and Public Health, 19*(23).

Cardona, M., & Andrés, P. (2023). Are social isolation and loneliness associated with cognitive decline in ageing? *Frontiers in Aging Neuroscience, 15*, 1075563.

Charlesworth, T. E., & Banaji, M. R. (2022). Patterns of implicit and explicit stereotypes III: Long-term change in gender stereotypes. *Social Psychological and Personality Science, 13*(1), 14–26.

Cheung, E. S. L., & Mui, A. C. (2023). Gender variation and late-life depression: Findings from a national survey in the USA. *Ageing International, 48*(1), 263–280. https://doi.org/10.1007/s12126-021-09471-5

Choi, E. Y., Wisniewski, K. M., & Zelinski, E. M. (2021). Information and communication technology use in older adults: A unidirectional or Bi-directional association with cognitive function? Computers in Human Behavior, 121, 106813. https://doi.org/10.1016/j.chb.2021.106813

Chopik, W. J. (2016). The benefits of social technology use among older adults are mediated by reduced loneliness. *Cyberpsychology, Behavior, and Social Networking, 19*(9), 551–556.

Garson, G. D. (2013). *Path analysis*. Statistical Associates Publishing.

Gatto, S. L., & Tak, S. H. (2008). Computer, Internet, and e-mail use among older adults: Benefits and barriers. *Educational Gerontology, 34*(9), 800–811.

Gu, D., Dupre, M. E., & Qiu, L. (2017, January–February). Self-perception of uselessness and mortality among older adults in China. *Archives of Gerontology and Geriatrics, 68*,186–194.https://doi.org/10.1016/j.archger.2016.10.015

Havighurst, R. J. (1961). Successful aging. *The Gerontologist, 1*, 8–13. https://doi.org/10.1093/geront/1.1.8

Havighurst, R. J. (1968). A social-psychological perspective on aging. *The Gerontologist, 8*(2), 67–71. https://doi.org/10.1093/geront/8.2.67

Hawkley, L. C., & Kocherginsky, M. (2017, 2018, April 1). Transitions in loneliness among older adults: A 5-year follow-up in the national social life, health, and aging project. *Research on Aging, 40*(4), 365–387. https://doi.org/10.1177/0164027517698965

Hayes, A. F. (2022). *Introduction to mediation, moderation, and conditional process analysis* (3rd ed.). The Guilford Press.

Heckhausen, J., & Schulz, R. (1995, April). A life-span theory of control. *Psychological Review, 102*(2), 284–304. https://doi.org/10.1037/0033-295x.102.2.284

Hertzog, C., Kramer, A. F., Wilson, R. S., & Lindenberger, U. (2008, October 1). Enrichment effects on adult cognitive development: Can the functional capacity of older adults be preserved and enhanced? *Psychological Science in the Public Interest, 9*(1), 1–65. https://doi.org/10.1111/j.1539-6053.2009.01034.x

Hu, L. t., & Bentler, P. M. (1999, January 1). Cutoff criteria for fit indexes in covariance structure analysis: Conventional criteria versus new alternatives. *Structural Equation Modeling: A Multidisciplinary Journal, 6*(1), 1–55. https://doi.org/10.1080/10705519909540118

Hultsch, D. F., Hertzog, C., Small, B. J., & Dixon, R. A. (1999, June). Use it or lose it: Engaged lifestyle as a buffer of cognitive decline in aging? *Psychology and Aging, 14*(2), 245–263. https://doi.org/10.1037/0882-7974.14.2.245

Infurna, F. J., & Gerstorf, D. (2013, Dec). Linking perceived control, physical activity, and biological health to memory change. *Psychology and Aging, 28*(4), 1147–1163. https://doi.org/10.1037/a0033327

Ivan, L., & Cutler, S. J. (2021). Ageism and technology: The role of internalized stereotypes. *University of Toronto Quarterly, 90*(2), 127–139.

Khoo, S. S., & Yang, H. (2020, October 1). Social media use improves executive functions in middle-aged and older adults: A structural equation modeling analysis. *Computers in Human Behavior, 111*, 106388. https://doi.org/10.1016/j.chb.2020.106388

Knapp, M. R. J. (1977). The activity theory of aging an examination in the English context. *The Gerontologist, 17*(6), 553–559. https://doi.org/10.1093/geront/17.6.553

Kobayashi, L. C., Wardle, J., & von Wagner, C. (2015). Internet use, social engagement and health literacy decline during ageing in a longitudinal cohort of older English adults. *Journal of Epidemiology and Community Health, 69*(3), 278–283.

Lachman, M. E. (2006). Perceived control over aging-related declines: Adaptive beliefs and behaviors. *Current Directions in Psychological Science, 15*(6), 282–286.

Lachman, M. E., & Andreoletti, C. (2006, March). Strategy use mediates the relationship between control beliefs and memory performance for middle-aged and older adults. *The Journals of Gerontology. Series B, Psychological Sciences and Social Sciences, 61*(2), P88–P94. https://doi.org/10.1093/geronb/61.2.p88

Levy, B. (2009). Stereotype embodiment: A psychosocial approach to aging. *Current Directions in Psychological Science, 18*(6), 332–336.

Li, W., Ye, X., Zhu, D., & He, P. (2021). The longitudinal association between retirement and depression: A systematic review and meta-analysis. *American Journal of Epidemiology, 190*(10), 2220–2230. https://doi.org/10.1093/aje/kwab125

Livingston, G., Huntley, J., Sommerlad, A., Ames, D., Ballard, C., Banerjee, S., Brayne, C., Burns, A., Cohen-Mansfield, J., Cooper, C., Costafreda, S. G., Dias, A., Fox, N., Gitlin, L. N., Howard, R., Kales, H. C., Kivimäki, M., Larson, E. B., Ogunniyi, A., Orgeta, V., Ritchie, K., Rockwood, K., Sampson, E. L., Samus, Q., Schneider, L. S., Selbæk, G., Teri, L., & Mukadam, N. (2020). Dementia prevention, intervention, and care: 2020 report of the Lancet Commission. *The Lancet, 396*(10248), 413–446. https://doi.org/10.1016/S0140-6736(20)30367-6

MacKinnon, D. P., & Pirlott, A. G. (2015). Statistical approaches for enhancing causal interpretation of the M to Y relation in mediation analysis. *Personality and Social Psychology Review, 19*(1), 30–43. https://doi.org/10.1177/1088868314542878

Mazzer, K. R., & Rickwood, D. J. (2015). Teachers' and coaches' role perceptions for supporting young people's mental health: Multiple group path analyses. *Australian Journal of Psychology, 67*(1), 10–19.

Muthen, L., & Muthen, B. (2017). *Mplus user's guide* (8th ed.). Muthen & Muthen.

Oswald, V., & Wagner, M. (2023, February 21). Internet usage among the oldest-old: Does functional health moderate the relationship between internet usage and autonomy? *European Journal of Ageing, 20*(1), 3. https://doi.org/10.1007/s10433-023-00748-z

Palgi, Y. (2013, August 1). Ongoing cumulative chronic stressors as predictors of well-being in the second half of life. *Journal of Happiness Studies, 14*(4), 1127–1144. https://doi.org/10.1007/s10902-012-9371-1

Patrão, M., Oliveira, C. R., & Sousa, L. (2019, April 3). Autobiographical narratives of oldest-old persons: What matters at that age? *Journal of Constructivist Psychology, 32*(2), 199–212. https://doi.org/10.1080/10720537.2018.1456381

Pew Research Center. (2021). *Social media fact sheet.*

Ramsey, J. L., Neupert, S. D., Mroczek, D. K., & Spiro, A., III. (2016). The effects of daily co-occurrence of affect on older adults' reactivity to health stressors. *Psychology & Health, 31*(3), 364–378. https://doi.org/10.1080/08870446.2015.1111368

Russell, C. (2007). What do older women and men want? Gender differences in the 'lived experience'of ageing. *Current Sociology, 55*(2), 173–192.

Schaie, K. W., & Willis, S. L. (1986). Can decline in adult intellectual functioning be reversed? *Developmental Psychology, 22*(2), 223–232. https://doi.org/10.1037/0012-1649.22.2.223

Schlomann, A., Seifert, A., Zank, S., Woopen, C., & Rietz, C. (2020). Use of information and communication technology (ICT) devices among the oldest-old: Loneliness, anomie, and autonomy. *Innovation in Aging, 4*(2), igz050. https://doi.org/10.1093/geroni/igz050

Shlisky, J., Bloom, D. E., Beaudreault, A. R., Tucker, K. L., Keller, H. H., Freund-Levi, Y., Fielding, R. A., Cheng, F. W., Jensen, G. L., Wu, D., & Meydani, S. N. (2017). Nutritional considerations for healthy aging and reduction in age-related chronic disease. *Advances in nutrition (Bethesda, Md.), 8*(1), 17–26. https://doi.org/10.3945/an.116.013474

Specht, J., Egloff, B., & Schmukle, S. C. (2013). Everything under control? The effects of age, gender, and education on trajectories of perceived control in a nationally representative German sample. *Developmental Psychology, 49*(2), 353.

von Humboldt, S., & Leal, I. (2015, September 1). The old and the oldest-old: Do they have different perspectives on adjustment to aging? *International Journal of Gerontology, 9*(3), 156–160. https://doi.org/10.1016/j.ijge.2015.04.002

Wang, H., Wang, B., Tu, X.M., et al. (2022a). Inconsistency between overall and subgroup analyses. *General Psychiatry, 35*, e100732. https://doi.org/10.1136/gpsych-2021-100732

Wang, K., Marbut, A. R., Zheng, D., & Peet, J. Z. (2022b). Stressor appraisals among adults in late middle age and late adulthood in the United States: Applying the intersectionality framework. *International Journal of Stress Management*. https://doi.org/10.1037/str0000283

Wang, K., & Kubanga, K. (2021). Correlates of internet use among African American older adults: Gender and age differences. *International Journal of Population Studies, 6*(2), 26–38.

Wang, X., Piantadosi, S., Le-Rademacher, J., et al. (2021). Statistical considerations for subgroup analyses. *Journal of Thoracic Oncology, 16*(3), 375–380. https://doi.org/10.1016/j.jtho.2020.12.008

Wang, R., & Ware, J. H. (2013). Detecting moderator effects using subgroup analyses. *Prevention Science, 14*(2), 111–120. https://doi.org/10.1007/s11121-011-0221-x

Wu, J., & Song, S. (2021, June 15). Older adults' online shopping continuance intentions: Applying the technology acceptance model and the theory of planned behavior. *International Journal of Human Computer Interaction, 37*(10), 938–948. https://doi.org/10.1080/10447318.2020.1861419

Yang, H., Tng, G. Y. Q., Ng, W. Q., & Yang, S. (2021, July–September). Loneliness, sense of control, and risk of dementia in healthy older adults: A moderated mediation analysis. *Clinical Gerontologist, 44*(4), 392–405. https://doi.org/10.1080/07317115.2020.1799891

Yu, D., & Fiebig, D. G. (2020, October 1). Internet use and cognition among middle-aged and older adults in China: A cross-lagged panel analysis. *The Journal of the Economics of Ageing, 17*, 100262. https://doi.org/10.1016/j.jeoa.2020.100262

Chapter 19
Social Media Use and Self-rated Health Among Older Adults in China

Danan Gu, Haiyan Zhu, and Qushi Feng

19.1 Introduction

The importance of examining social media use in relation to older adults' self-rated health (SRH) stems from a constellation of interrelated demographic, technological, and social dynamics. First, population aging raises concerns around social isolation, chronic illness, and healthcare resource distribution. Second, older adults are increasingly present in digital spaces; although still lagging behind younger populations in overall usage rates, their rate of digital adoption has grown markedly in recent years. Third, SRH remains one of the most robust predictors of morbidity and mortality in epidemiological research and provides a valuable subjective lens through which the multifaceted experiences of aging can be understood (Duplaga, 2021; Kim et al., 2020).

In the context of China, these issues are intensified by distinctive social, cultural, and economic structures. The traditional practice of filial piety and intergenerational co-residence is weakening due to urbanization and migration. As a result, many older adults, especially those in rural or peri-urban areas, are becoming socially and emotionally vulnerable (Li et al., 2023; Liu et al., 2022). In this regard, social media platforms such as *WeChat, Douyin (akin to TikTok), and QQ* are emerging as virtual

D. Gu (✉)
Population Division, UN Department of Economic and Social Affairs, New York, NY, USA
e-mail: gudanan@yahoo.com

H. Zhu
Department of Sociology, Virginia Tech, Blacksburg, VA, USA
e-mail: zhuh@vt.edu

Q. Feng
Centre for Family and Population Research/Department of Sociology and Anthropology, National University of Singapore, Singapore, Singapore
e-mail: socfq@nus.edu.sg

K. Wang et al. (eds.), *ICT Use and Healthy Longevity*, Advances in Studies of Aging and Health 5, https://doi.org/10.1007/978-3-031-98964-3_19

lifelines, offering older adults novel forms of social participation, emotional expression, and access to health-related information (see Chaps. 2, 6, 9 and 14). However, the relationship between such engagement and health outcomes, particularly SRH, is complex and remains largely underexplored.

This chapter aims to investigate how social media use shapes older adults' perceptions of their health using a nationally representative survey, with particular attention to how factors, such as social support, social engagement, and psychological well-being, moderate the relationship between social media use and SRH. By reviewing the existing literature and situating the current study within theoretical frameworks, we hope to shed light on the mechanisms through which digital participation influences health in later life.

19.1.1 Literature Review

An increasing number of studies across disciplines have investigated the relationship between internet use and health outcomes of older adults. The emerging consensus suggests that internet use, particularly social media engagement, is associated with improved mental health, reduced loneliness, enhanced social connectedness, and better physical health outcomes (Duplaga, 2021; Richards et al., 2025; Wei et al., 2025). However, these relationships are not always straightforward and can vary based on socioeconomic status, psychosocial factors, and health conditions (Fu et al., 2024; Hajek & König, 2022; Li et al., 2023).

Research on internet use and SRH has shown significant evidence of the positive role of internet use in various countries. Studies by Duplaga (2021) in Poland and Falk Erhag et al. (2019) in Sweden found strong associations between internet use and SRH, particularly when the use was tied to social communication and information-seeking behaviors. These findings contribute to cross-cultural validations, reinforcing the robustness of the positive association while emphasizing the importance of contextual factors such as infrastructure, digital literacy, and cultural attitudes toward aging and technology. However, not all findings are uniformly optimistic. Seckin and Hughes (2021) cautioned that not all forms of internet use are beneficial, especially when digital engagement is passive or restricted by low digital literacy.

Studies conducted in China have reinforced these insights, revealing the positive effects of internet use. Wu et al. (2025) explored how digital disparities contribute to health inequalities among older adults in China and found that those with limited access to or knowledge of digital tools were less likely to report favorable health. More importantly, increasing studies from China suggest that internet use does not improve health outcomes in a vacuum; rather, it does so by fostering connectedness, reducing isolation, and providing access to health information and services (also see Chap. 4). Lyu and Sun (2021), for example, found that internet use was significantly associated with higher SRH among Chinese older adults, with social capital serving as a key mediating factor. Liu et al. (2022) confirmed the importance of social support as a mediating variable in the relationship between internet use and subjective health status.

Platform-specific studies provide a more detailed understanding of digital health implications. For instance, Luo et al. (2024) examined how *Douyin (akin to TikTok)* use impacted SRH among older adults in China during the pandemic, identifying entertainment and informational engagement as two pathways through which benefits were accrued. Similarly, Wei et al. (2022) explored the effect of *WeChat* and found that its use was positively correlated with subjective health among older users, emphasizing the role of online communication and group participation.

One emerging theme in literature is the importance of information access. Fu et al. (2024) highlighted that older adults who used the internet not only had better SRH but also enjoyed improved multidimensional health outcomes, physical, mental, and social, largely due to their increased ability to access and process health-related information. This is in line with the finding of Wen et al. (2023) that the purpose of internet use significantly influenced perceived physical and mental health among middle-aged and older Chinese adults.

Social engagement and community connectedness also feature prominently in this discourse. Li et al. (2023) demonstrated that both internet use and offline social activities independently and jointly contribute to better SRH. Similarly, Li et al. (2025) found that the positive effect of internet use on SRH was largely mediated by increased social engagement and perceived social support, affirming the importance of sociability in the digital age.

Several studies have also drawn attention to mental health as an intermediary between digital use and SRH. Wei et al. (2025) found that active social media use among older adults significantly reduced depressive symptoms, thereby improving overall mental health and self-rated well-being. Lin and He (2024) went further to propose a chain mediation model, in which internet use influenced depressive symptoms through increased physical activity and improved SRH, offering a multi-layered perspective to introduce behavioral and psychological pathways.

Moreover, digital engagement may also influence older adults' interactions with the healthcare system. Wang et al. (2024) showed that internet use significantly influenced older adults' preferences for medical institutions, suggesting that digital tools are reshaping health-seeking behavior and medical decision-making processes. Likewise, Ma et al. (2024) highlighted the relationship between internet use, health service utilization, and SRH, emphasizing that digitally active older adults are more likely to engage with preventative care and self-management strategies.

In sum, studies in the current literature, especially those from China, reveal a multifaceted and increasingly coherent narrative: internet and social media use among older adults are positively associated with SRH, mediated by a series of factors such as social support, social engagement, information access, mental well-being, and health-seeking behavior. However, these benefits also depend on individual characteristics (e.g., education, income, digital literacy), social environments, and how older people use the internet.

One important framework for understanding these findings is the Senior Technology Acceptance Model (STAM). This model posits that older adults' adoption and use of technology are determined by perceived usefulness and ease of use (Renaud & van Biljon, 2008), as well as health (Chen & Chan, 2014). STAM highlights the critical role of health in older adults' motivation to use digital technologies, especially among marginalized populations (DeLange Martinez et al., 2024; see Chap. 3). Theoretical frameworks such as Social Capital Theory and models of health behavior also provide valuable lenses. Together, these theoretical frameworks suggest that internet and social media use function not merely as technological artifacts but also as socio-behavioral tools that mediate access to emotional, cognitive, and instrumental resources critical for healthy aging.

The present study builds upon these theoretical and empirical foundations to examine how social media use influences SRH among Chinese older adults. It aims to explore (1) whether the relationship between social media use and SRH is still robust when different sets of confounding factors are presented, such as socioeconomic factors, family/social networks, and health conditions; (2) whether this relationship varies across different subgroups; and (3) whether the relationship differs by media types and usage purposes. Answering these questions will advance the current studies from China by providing a more rigorous examination of the association between social media use and SRH and a better understanding of the complex interplay between digital engagement and health in later life. It will also help identify specific subgroups of older adults who may benefit most or least from social media engagement, thus informing policies and interventions aimed at promoting digital inclusion and healthy aging in China and beyond.

19.2 Data and Methods

19.2.1 Data Sources

We utilized data from the China Longitudinal Aging Social Survey (CLASS), a nationally representative longitudinal survey in China. A comprehensive description of CLASS can be found in Chap. 6 and previous studies (Dong et al., 2019; Jin & Zhao, 2019). Consistent with Chaps. 6, 9, and 14, our analysis is entirely based on the 2020 wave of CLASS. Given the research objectives of this chapter, we focused exclusively on respondents aged 65 and older. This selection resulted in a final analytical sample of 11, 228 participants.

19.2.2 Measures

19.2.2.1 Self-rated Health

SRH is measured using a five-point Likert scale question that asks participants to evaluate their overall health condition at the time of the survey. Respondents select one of five options: very good, good, fair, poor, or very poor. This simple yet effective measure has been widely used in gerontological research and is considered a valid indicator of an individual's general health status. Numerous studies have demonstrated its reliability and predictive power for various health outcomes, including morbidity and mortality (Feng et al., 2016; Idler et al., 1999; Jylhä, 2009). For analytical purposes, we combined "very good" and "good" to represent good health and grouped the remaining three responses to indicate poor health.

19.2.2.2 Use of Social Media

Consistent with the approach in Chap. 14, respondents were dichotomized as users versus non-users. Participants were classified as non-users if they reported never using any of the 12 listed apps or platforms. These included *WeChat, Douyin (akin to TikTok), Xiguan Videos (similar to YouTube), Taobao (similar to Amazon), Didi (similar to Uber)*, among others.

19.2.2.3 Covariates

Building on the STAM framework and other digital divide models introduced in Chap. 3, we applied the same five sets of variables used in Chap. 6 that examines internet and social media use correlates. These variables offer a comprehensive foundation for analyzing aging-related issues and include: (1) demographic characteristics, (2) socioeconomic status, (3) family and social support networks, (4) engagement in leisure activities, as well as views, attitudes, and perceptions related to aging and technological advancement, and (5) health status. The variable region is consistently controlled for across all models. For detailed definitions and coding of these variables, please refer to Chap. 6.

19.2.3 Analytical strategies

We primarily employed multiple logistic regression models, supplemented by descriptive analyses. In line with the analytical strategy detailed in Chap. 6, we constructed a series of partial models to explore how the association between social media use and SRH was affected by the inclusion of different sets of covariates.

Consistent with the approaches used in Chaps. 6, 9, and 14, the sampling weight was applied in the descriptive analyses but not in the regression models. As part of our sensitivity analysis, we also estimated ordinal logistic and multinomial logistic regression models for SRH. The results remained generally consistent across all model specifications.

To assess the moderating effects of covariates on the relationship between social media use and SRH, we conducted subgroup analyses, an approach that differs from the more commonly used interaction modeling strategy. While both methods have their respective strengths and limitations, interaction analysis is often constrained by its inability to account for all possible two-way interactions, as including every potential interaction term in the model is generally impractical. Moreover, when the distribution or level of a covariate varies substantially across subgroups, the interpretability and utility of interaction terms may be limited. In addition, interaction models, particularly those based on linear regression, also assume homoscedastic residual variance, an assumption that is frequently violated in practice (Bobko & Russell, 1990; Kim & Seltzer, 2011).

By contrast, subgroup analysis stratifies the data and thus inherently considers all two-way interactions, enabling the detection of heterogeneous effects that might be overlooked in interaction models. Importantly, the absence of a statistically significant interaction effect in the overall model does not preclude the presence of meaningful subgroup variation (Corraini et al., 2017; Vanderweel, 2009; Wang & Ware, 2013; Wang et al., 2021, 2022). When sample sizes are sufficiently large, subgroup analysis is often preferable for exploring effect modification. In this study, there are 40 subgroups classified by 19 different covariates. All statistical analyses were performed using Stata version 18.0.

19.3 Results

Table 19.1 shows that in 2020, half of Chinese older adults aged 65 or older rated their overall health as good (weighted). Among social media users, nearly 63% rated their overall health as good (weighted) in comparison to 45% among non-users.

Table 19.2 presents the odds ratios of reporting good SRH for social media use across models with varying covariate adjustments. In the base model (Model I), which controls only for demographic characteristics, social media users have 56% higher odds of reporting good health compared to non-users (odds ratio = 1.56, $p<0.001$). The odds ratio declines to 1.44, indicating social media users have 44% increased odds of reporting good health, when socioeconomic factors are added (Model II). However, when marital status and close family ties are included in the base model (Model III), the odds ratio increases to 1.52 ($p<0.001$). When additional controls are introduced for internet attitudes, views on aging, and aging-related experiences, the odds ratio further decreases to 1.23 ($p<0.001$) (Model IV). After adjusting for health conditions in the base model, the odds ratio remains at 1.34 ($p<0.001$) (Model V). However, once all covariates are jointly accounted for,

Table 19.1 Unweighted and weighted percentage distribution of the analytical sample, 2020, CLASS

	Overall sample		User groups (weighted)	
	Weighted	Unweighted	Social media users	Non-users
N	11,228	11,228	2,806	8,422
% Good self-rated health	50.3	46.8	62.6	45.5
% Ages 65–74	64.8	38.0	81.6	58.3
% Ages 75–85	27.1	44.7	17.0	31.0
% Ages 85+	8.1	17.3	1.4	10.7
% Men	47.5	50.5	51.3	49.8
% Han ethnicity	95.5	94.0	95.4	20.7
% Urban residents	52.7	54.9	67.4	49.9
% 0 years of schooling	24.4	23.6	9.7	30.2
% 1–6 years of schooling	39.1	41.2	31.3	42.1
% 7+ years of schooling	36.5	35.2	59.0	27.7
% Economically poor	10.4	11.5	8.7	31.4
% White-collar occupation	10.8	11.7	22.3	6.4
% Blue-collar occupation	27.5	29.9	40.7	22.3
% Agricultural workers	61.7	58.4	37.0	71.3
% Currently Married	78.1	75.3	86.8	43.4
% Having 2+ close family members	80.5	79.7	85.3	41.0
% Having 2+ close friends	71.4	70.6	78.2	46.4
% Frequent engagement in leisure activity	82.1	83.2	89.4	40.6
Positive views on internet impact (0–8)[a]	2.12	2.08	3.33	1.64
Negative views on aging (7–35)[a]	21.32	21.41	20.76	21.54
Negative perceptions on aging (8–40)[a]	24.09	24.02	23.25	24.42
%Having 1+ diseases	79.6	80.4	76.8	80.8
% IADL disabled	18.7	24.2	9.4	22.3
% ADL disabled	11.3	15.1	7.9	12.7
% Cognitively impaired	24.5	30.4	10.8	29.9
% East China	38.5	36.1	57.2	31.2
% Central China	27.1	25.7	18.3	30.6
% West China	25.7	24.8	14.7	30.0
% Northeast China	8.6	13.4	9.7	8.2

ADL activities of daily living, *IADL* instrumental ADL
[a]The mean score of the variable

the association is no longer statistically significant, indicating that the observed positive relationship between social media use and good SRH is largely attributable to confounding factors considered in the analysis.

To further investigate the longitudinal association, Table 19.3 presents odds ratios for reporting good self-rated health (SRH) at time *T* (i.e., the 2020 wave) based on internet use at time *T*–1 (i.e., the 2018 wave), controlling for all covariates

Table 19.2 Odds ratios of reporting good self-rated health by social media use and covariates, 2020, CLASS

	Models for good self-rated health					
	Model I	Model II	Model III	Model IV	Model V	Model VI
Overall use of media (no)	1.56***	1.44***	1.52***	1.23***	1.34***	1.07
Ages 75–85 (65–74)	0.73***	0.74***	0.73***	0.75***	0.86***	0.88**
Ages 85+ (65–74)	0.48***	0.50***	0.51***	0.51***	0.81**	0.84**
Men (women)	1.20***	1.16***	1.16***	1.19***	1.09*	1.06
Han ethnicity (minority)	0.60***	0.60***	0.61***	0.63***	0.59***	0.64***
Urban (rural)	1.14**	0.98	1.15***	1.08^{+}	1.13**	0.99
1–6 years of schooling (0)		1.11^{+}				0.98
7+ years of schooling (0)		1.35***				1.10
Economically poor (no)		0.77***				0.83**
Blue-collar occupation (white-collar)		1.27***				1.22**
Agricultural workers (white-collar)		0.99				0.98
Currently married (no)			1.28***			1.13*
Having 2+ close family members (<2)			1.59***			1.53***
Having 2+ close friends (<2)			0.80***			0.79***
Freq. leisure and social activity (no)				0.91^{+}		0.89*
Positive views on internet impact (0–8)				1.11***		1.10***
Positive views on aging (7–35)				1.04***		1.03***
Positive perceptions of aging (8–40)				1.07***		1.06***
Having 1+ diseases (no)					0.44***	0.43***
IADL disabled (no)					0.54***	0.57***
ADL disabled (no)					0.45***	0.47***
Cognitively impaired (no)					0.68***	0.75***
Good self-rated health (no)	0.80***	0.83***	0.77***	0.75***	0.61***	0.60***
Central China (East China)	0.90^{+}	0.98	0.93	0.90^{+}	0.73***	0.79***
West China (East China)	1.04	1.05	1.05	1.18*	0.77***	0.91
Northeast China (East China)	1.53***	1.35*	1.01	0.13***	4.69***	0.47**
- Log likelihood	7518.4	7479.4	7471.7	7328.3	7064.1	6885.1
Degree of freedom	9	14	12	13	13	25
LR Chi square	482.9	560.9	576.2	863,1	1391.5	1749.3
No. of individuals	11,228	11,228	11,228	11,228	11,228	11,228

Note: (1) The results were based on the logistic regression models. (2). Numbers in the six right columns refer to odds ratio. The category of a variable in the parentheses is the reference. (3) *ADL* activities of daily living, IADL instrumental ADL; (4) The results for *WeChat, Douyin, Xigua Video*, and the number of media use are similar and thus not presented. (5) $+p < 0.1$, $*p < 0.05$, $**p < 0.01$, $***p < 0.001$

Table 19.3 Odds ratios of internet use in predicting good self-rated health (SRH), 2018–2020, CLASS

	Models of reporting good SRH in 2020					
	Model I	Model II	Model III	Model IV	Model V	Model VI
Internet use vs. no in 2018	1.14*	1.01	1.12*	1.01	1.08	0.92
Internet use vs. no in 2020	1.59***	1.47***	1.56***	1.28***	1.39***	1.12*

Note: (1) The results were based on the logistic regression models. (2). Numbers in the six right columns refer to odds ratios of reporting good SRH in 2020. Please refer to Table 19.2 for models' specifications. Controls in models refer to the status measured in the 2020 wave. (3) Because the 2018 wave of CLASS did not collect information on social media use, we employed internet use as the independent variable. Please refer to Chaps. 6 and 9 for more details regarding internet use and social media use among older adults in China. (4) $+p < 0.1$, $*p < 0.05$, $**p < 0.01$, $***p < 0.001$

measured at time *T*. Internet use is employed as the independent variable due to the unavailability of social media use data in the 2018 wave. The results indicate that, while the cross-sectional association is robust, the longitudinal association reaches statistical significance only when controlling for demographic factors (Model I) or when additional controls for family and social support are included (Model III).

Table 19.4 reports odds ratios for the association between social media use and good SRH across 40 subgroups, based on Model I (adjusting for demographic factors only) and Model VI (adjusting for all covariates). Additional results are presented for versions of Model VI that exclude either the set of factors related to perceptions of internet-driven social development, views on aging, and aging-related experiences (Model VI-x), or health conditions (Model VI-h).

The findings show that when only demographic factors are controlled for (Model I), social media use is significantly associated with higher odds of good SRH in 35 out of 40 subgroups ($p < 0.05$), with only five exceptions. This positive relationship remains largely robust in 28 subgroups ($p < 0.05$) when all covariates are controlled for, except for the sets of factors related to perceptions of internet advancement, aging views, and aging experiences (Model VI-x). However, when all covariates except health conditions are controlled for, the number of subgroups showing a significant positive association drops to 21 (Model VI-h). The association between social media use and good SRH largely disappears when all covariates are included (Model VI): only three subgroups retain a statistically significant relationship ($p < 0.05$).

Overall, without full adjustment for all covariates, the positive association between social media use and good SRH tends to be more consistent or stronger among specific subgroups. This includes older adults aged 75 years or older, women, rural residents, individuals of Han ethnicity, those with lower educational attainment, the economically non-poor, white-collar workers, individuals with greater family and social support, and those in relatively good health. Interestingly, among economically poor individuals, social media use is often associated with lower odds of reporting good SRH.

Table 19.5 presents odds ratios for reporting good SRH by different types of social media use. When controlling for demographic factors only (Model I), all

Table 19.4 Odds ratios of social media use in predicting good self-rated health (SRH) among different subgroups, 2020, CLASS

	Models of reporting good SRH			
Subgroups	Model I	Model VI-x	Model VI-h	Model VI
Ages 65–74 (*N* = 4,264)	1.39***	1.21*	1.08	1.07
Ages 75+ (*N* = 6,964)	1.63***	1.27***	1.22**	1.07
Women (*N* = 5,554)	1.79***	1.39***	1.27**	1.15+
Men (*N* = 5,674)	1.37***	1.14+	1.07	1.00
Rural (*N* = 5,061)	1.63***	1.31**	1.17+	1.09
Urban (*N* = 6,167)	1.55***	1.21**	1.17*	1.07
Ethnic minorities (*N* = 672)	1.45	0.91	0.83	0.72
Han majority (*N* = 10,556)	1.57***	1.28***	1.21***	1.11+
0–6 years of schooling (*N* = 7,271)	1.60***	1.38***	1.22**	1.14+
7+ years of schooling (*N* = 3,957)	1.38***	1.13	1.16+	1.00
Economically not poor (*N* = 9,937)	1.64***	1.36***	1.24***	1.15*
Economically poor (*N* = 1, 291)	0.97	0.62**	0.65*	0.58**
Blue-collar /agriculture job (*N* = 9,919)	1.50***	1.22***	1.14*	1.06
White-collar job (*N* = 1,309)	2.19***	1.57**	1.36*	1.21
Not married (*N* = 2,778)	1.61***	1.25+	1.21	1.00
Married (*N* = 8,450)	1.51***	1.27***	1.16*	1.09
Having <2 close family members (*N* = 2,279)	1.45***	1.02	1.00	0.87
Having 2+ close family members (*N* = 8,949)	1.57***	1.31***	1.22**	1.13+
Having <2 close friends (*N* = 3,300)	1.54***	1.14	1.08	0.98
Having 2+ close friends (*N* = 7,928)	1.56***	1.31***	1.29***	1.20**
Not freq. engage. in leisure activities (*N* = 1,889)	1.88***	1.52*	1.27	1.17
Freq. engagement in leisure activities (*N* = 9,339)	1.52***	1.23***	1.18**	1.09
Less positive views on internet tech. (*N* = 3,058)	1.56***	1.30*	1.32*	1.23
More positive views on internet tech. (*N* = 8,170)	1.50***	1.24***	1.23**	1.14*
Less positive views on aging (7–22)[a] (*N* = 7,752)	1.56***	1.17*	1.21**	1.05
More positive views on aging (23–35)[a] (*N* = 3,476)	1.43***	1.40***	1.10	1.12
Less positive perceptions of aging (8–25)[a] (*N* = 7,939)	1.52***	1.23***	1.26**	1.10
More positive perceptions of aging (26–40)[a] (*N* = 3,289)	1.48***	1.29**	1.10	1.06
Having no disease condition (*N* = 2,200)	1.88***	1.68***	1.62**	1.50**
Having 1+ disease condition (*N* = 9,028)	1.64***	1.23**	1.20**	1.04
IADL not disabled (*N* = 8,510)	1.32***	1.22**	1.02	1.03
IADL disabled (*N* = 2,718)	1.59***	1.31+	1.27+	1.14
ADL not disabled (*N* = 9,531)	1.41***	1.24***	1.06	1.05
ADL disabled (*N* = 1,697)	1.18	0.88	1.02	0.94
Cognitively unimpaired (*N* = 7,816)	1.41***	1.28***	1.11+	1.10
Cognitively impaired (*N* = 3,412)	1.21	0.99	0.98	0.85

(continued)

Table 19.4 (continued)

	Models of reporting good SRH			
Subgroups	Model I	Model VI-x	Model VI-h	Model VI
East China (N = 4,055)	1.70***	1.21*	1.40***	1.12
Central China (N = 2,883)	2.17***	2.02***	1.72***	1.73
West China (N = 2,783)	1.50***	1.17	1.15	1.05
Northeast China (N = 1,507)	0.77*	0.80	0.67**	0.85

Note: (1) The results were based on logistic regression models. (2) Numbers in the three right columns refer to odds ratios. (3) Model I controls for demographic factors and region; Model VI controls for all factors in the table, Model VI-x controls for all factors except views on internet progress, views on aging, and aging experience; and Model VI-h controls for all factors except health indicators. (4) *ADL* activities of daily living; *IADL* instrumental ADL. (5) $+p < 0.1$, $*p < 0.05$, $**p < 0.01$, $***p < 0.001$

Table 19.5 Odds ratios of social media use in predicting good self-rated health (SRH) by types of social media, 2020, CLASS

	Models of reporting good SRH			
Types of social media	Model I	Model VI-x	Model VI-h	Model VI
Any type of social media use vs. no	1.56***	1.25***	1.16**	1.07
Use of Wechat vs. no	1.55***	1.26***	1.11+	1.03
Use of Douyin (akin to TikTok) vs. no	1.81***	1.46***	1.33***	1.22**
Use of Kuaishou video vs. no	1.73***	1.43***	1.30***	1.21**
Use of Xigua video vs. no	2.66***	2.24***	1.98***	1.87***
Use of News apps vs. no	1.73***	1.36***	1.32**	1.17*
Use of Shopping apps vs. no	1.75***	1.28**	1.08	0.91
Use of Transportation apps vs. no	1.77***	1.26*	1.12	0.94
Use Beautification apps vs. no	1.48***	1.05	0.84	0.71*
Use of Game apps vs. no	1.14	0.94	0.93	0.85+
Use of online payment apps vs. no	1.75***	1.38***	1.19*	1.06

Note: (1) The results were based on logistic regression models. (2) Numbers in the three right columns refer to odds ratios. (3) Model I controls for demographic factors and region; Model VI controls for all factors in the table, Model VI-x controls for all factors except views on internet progress, views on aging, and aging experience; and Model VI-h controls for all factors except health indicators. (4) $+p < 0.1$, $*p < 0.05$, $**p < 0.01$, $***p < 0.001$

types of social media use, except one (use of game apps), are significantly associated with higher odds of reporting good SRH, ranging from 48 to 166%. After further adjusting for socioeconomic status, family and social support, and health conditions (Model VI-x), these associations are moderately attenuated, with odds ratios ranging from 1.26 to 2.24; notably, the use of photo apps is no longer associated with better SRH.

When all covariates except health conditions are controlled for (Model VI-h), significant positive associations persist only for the use of video apps, news apps, and online payment apps. In the fully adjusted model (Model VI), only the use of video app and news app remains significantly associated with higher odds of good

Table 19.6 Odds ratios of social media use in predicting good self-rated health (SRH) by types of purposes, 2020, CLASS

	Models of reporting good SRH			
Purposes of social media use	Model I	Model VI-x	Model VI-h	Model VI
Overall use of social media (no)	1.56***	1.25***	1.16**	1.07
For contacting with family members/friends (no)	1.60***	1.29***	1.20**	1.11+
For reading /following-up news (no)	1.66***	1.30***	1.27***	1.13*
For entertainment (no)	1.62***	1.30***	1.19**	1.10
For seeking information (no)	1.80***	1.47***	1.24**	1.15+
For online shopping (no)	1.65***	1.26**	1.08	0.93
For travel (no)	1.48***	1.09	0.89	0.79*
For health management (no)	1.17	0.90	0.70*	0.64***

Note: (1) The results were based on logistic regression models. (2) Numbers in the three right columns refer to odds ratios. (3) Model I controls for demographic factors and region; Model VI controls for all factors in the table, Model VI-x controls for all factors except views on internet progress, views on aging, and aging experience; and Model VI-h controls for all factors except health indicators. (4) The category in the parentheses is the reference group, which includes non-users. (5) $+p < 0.1$, $*p < 0.05$, $**p < 0.01$, $***p < 0.001$

SRH, while the use of beautification apps is linked to lower odds of reporting good SRH.

Table 19.6 presents odds ratios for reporting good SRH based on different purposes of social media use. The results show that, with the exception of using social media for health management, all other purposes are associated with 48–80% increased odds of reporting good SRH when only demographic factors are controlled for (Model I). These odds were moderately reduced to 26–47% when socio-economic status, family and social support, and health conditions are further adjusted for, with the association for travel-related use becoming statistically not significant.

When controlling for all covariates except health conditions, using social media for communication, reading news, entertainment, and information-seeking remains significantly associated with 19–27% higher odds of reporting good SRH. Social media use for shopping does not show a significant association with SRH. In the fully adjusted model, only using social media for reading news remains positively associated with good SRH. By contrast, using social media for travel or health management is associated with lower odds of reporting good SRH, while using it for other purposes shows no statistically significant relationship.

19.4 Discussion

The relationship between social media use and SRH among older adults presents a complex interplay of technological, social, and psychological factors. Using CLASS, a nationally representative sample survey focusing on older adults in

China, with a sample of 11,228 participants aged 65 years or older, this chapter examined the relationship between social media use and SRH. Our findings reveal that while social media use is initially associated with higher odds of reporting good SRH, this relationship is largely attenuated when accounting for a wide set of confounding variables. These findings suggest that the observed benefits may stem from underlying resources (e.g., social support, economic stability, digital literacy) rather than digital engagement alone. In addition, this relationship varies significantly for different subgroups, presenting the heterogeneity of the impacts of social media use on SRH.

19.4.1 The Role of Confounding Factors

Our cross-sectional analysis demonstrates that the positive association between social media use and SRH diminishes significantly after adjusting for covariates, such as socioeconomic status, social support, and health conditions, particularly views on social impact of internet technology progress, views on aging, and experiences of aging. This aligns with prior research emphasizing that internet use often reflects broader advantages (e.g., education, income, social support) rather than directly causing health improvements (Chen et al., 2022; Fu et al., 2024; Wang & Chen, 2024). For instance, economically well-off individuals, who are more likely to afford devices and data plans, reported better SRH, whereas economically disadvantaged groups showed no benefits or even negative health consequences (Table 19.4). This echoes the findings by Wu et al. (2025) on how digital disparities could exacerbate health inequalities, particularly in rural areas where internet infrastructure may be lacking.

Our longitudinal analysis shows a further weakened association, as baseline internet use in 2018 only weakly predicted SRH in 2020. This suggests that social media's impact may be contingent on contemporaneous factors (e.g., changes in health status, social networks, or digital literacy) rather than sustained over time. Similar nuances were noted by Kim et al. (2020), who found that technology use correlated with better health only among older adults with preexisting social resources. Moreover, the lack of a robust longitudinal effect may reflect the dynamic nature of digital engagement,older adults who initially adopt social media may discontinue the use if they find it irrelevant or difficult to navigate (DeLange Martinez et al., 2024).

19.4.2 Subgroup Heterogeneity

One distinctive strength of this study lies in its extensive subgroup analyses, which illuminate how the association between social media use and SRH varies across different population segments. Our subgroup analyses (Table 19.4) reveal striking variations in the association between social media use and SRH. Stronger associations were found among rural residents, women, and older adults with lower education, who are groups traditionally marginalized in digital access (CNNIC, 2025; Zhao & Kuang, 2025). For these populations, social media may compensate for limited offline resources by fostering connections (Liu et al., 2022), providing health information (Fu et al., 2024), or enabling participation in virtual communities (Luo et al., 2024). This aligns with the "resource substitution" hypothesis, which posits that technology can mitigate disadvantages for underserved groups (Neves & Vetere, 2019).

Conversely, the lack of benefit among economically poor older adults underscores the limitations of digital tools in overcoming structural barriers. Those struggling with basic needs may even find social media use stressful or irrelevant, particularly if they lack digital literacy (Seckin & Hughes, 2021). This finding resonates with studies highlighting the "double burden" faced by low-income older adults, who may experience both material deprivation and digital exclusion (Wu et al., 2025).

19.4.3 Platform-Specific and Purpose-Driven Effects

Another notable contribution of this study is its focus on the platform-specific and purpose-driven dimensions of social media use in relation to SRH. Our results highlight that social media activities are not equally associated with SRH. Video and news apps retained significant positive associations with SRH even after adjustments, likely due to their roles in information access (Luo et al., 2024), cognitive engagement (Wei et al., 2025), and entertainment (Lyu & Sun, 2021). These platforms may provide older adults with opportunities for lifelong learning, social interaction, and mental stimulation, all of which are linked to better self-perceived health (Richards et al., 2025).

By contrast, beautification and travel-related uses were linked to poorer SRH, possibly reflecting financial strain (e.g., unrealistic beauty standards) or stress from navigating unfamiliar platforms (Seckin & Hughes, 2021; Wei et al., 2022). The lack of significant or negative association for health-management purposes aligns with the findings of Jeon & Choi's (2024), which indicate that passive health-information seeking, if without professional guidance, may not lead to improved self-perceived health. This suggests that simply accessing health content online is not enough; older adults may need support to interpret and apply this information effectively (Ma et al., 2024).

This study has important theoretical implications. Our findings support STAM (Chen & Chan, 2014; Renaud & van Biljon, 2008), which posits that older adults adopt technology when they perceive its utility and ease of use. Our results suggest that perceived utility, such as news apps for information or video apps for entertainment, may indirectly bolster SRH by enhancing social capital (Lyu & Sun, 2021) or reducing loneliness (Richards et al., 2025). However, STAM's emphasis on individual agency must be tempered by structural realities; for example, as revealed by our study, socioeconomically disadvantaged older adults may lack digital literacy to leverage platforms effectively (DeLange Martinez et al., 2024).

Social capital theory also provides a lens for understanding why family/social support moderates the relationship between social media use and SRH (Table 19.4). Platforms like *WeChat* may amplify existing strong ties (Wei et al., 2022), but they cannot replace deficient offline networks (Li et al., 2023). This duality mirrors Wang et al.'s (2024) argument that internet use reshapes health behaviors only when it is integrated into supportive environments.

Moreover, the stress process model (Idler et al., 1999) provides insights into why certain social media uses (e.g., travel-related) may negatively impact SRH. For older adults with limited resources, navigating complex platforms or comparing lifestyles online may induce stress, undermining perceived health (Seckin & Hughes, 2021). This is consistent with Kemp and Erades Pérez's (2023) findings on how digital fraud exacerbates vulnerability among older adults.

19.4.4 Strengths and Limitations

This study has several strengths, including the use of a nationally representative sample, rigorous adjustment for confounding factors, and detailed subgroup analyses that address gaps identified in prior work (e.g., Vanderweele, 2009; Wang & Chen, 2024). While the use of longitudinal data is limited, it provides preliminary insights into temporal dynamics (Lin & He, 2024).

However, several limitations should be acknowledged. First, the reliance on self-reported measures may introduce biases (Jylhä, 2009), though SRH's predictive validity for mortality is well-established (Feng et al., 2016). Second, the lack of detailed social media data (e.g., duration, frequency) in our study precludes disentangling active vs. passive use, which is an important distinction. This limitation may not fully unearth the role of internet use, given passive use's ties to poorer mental health (Kim et al., 2020). Third, while we conducted comprehensive subgroup analyses, there may still be residual confounding factors (e.g., unmeasured digital literacy) that could affect the outcomes (Corraini et al., 2017). Finally, the focus of the study on China limits the generalizability of findings to other cultural contexts, where aging policies and digital landscapes may differ (Falk Erhag et al., 2019).

19.4.5 Policy Implications and Future Research Directions

Our study has important policy implications. First, initiatives to improve social media use should prioritize rural, low-income, and less-educated older adults by providing subsidized devices, internet access, and tailored training to close the digital gap (see Chap. 9). Community-based programs, such as peer-led workshops, could enhance digital literacy and thus promote the health benefits of social media use (Renaud & van Biljon, 2008). Second, developers of social media platforms should optimize intuitive interfaces for news and video apps, which showed the strongest associations with SRH in this study. Features like voice commands, larger text, and offline functionality could reduce adoption barriers among older adults (Hu et al., 2024; see Chap. 9). Third, clinicians and policymakers could collaborate to promote credible health information online, leveraging platforms like *WeChat* for public health campaigns (Ma et al., 2024). Telemedicine initiatives could also bridge gaps in rural healthcare access (Wang et al., 2024). Fourth, digital policies must address the root causes of disparities, such as income inequality and urban-rural divides (Wu et al., 2025). Public-private partnerships could expand broadband infrastructure in underserved areas (Zhao & Kuang, 2025).

Our study also has implications for future research. First, to establish causality, future studies should track social media use and SRH over longer periods and employ methods like propensity score matching (Wang et al., 2021). Randomized trials are also recommended to test related interventions (e.g., digital literacy training) on SRH (Kim et al., 2023). Second, qualitative insights could clarify why certain types of uses (e.g., beautification apps) correlate with poorer SRH (Brainin & Neter, 2023). Ethnographic studies might be used to explore how older adults perceive and adapt to digital tools. Third, replicating this study in other aging societies (e.g., Japan, Sweden) could test the universality of these findings (Falk Erhag et al., 2019). Comparative research is recommended to further identify cultural moderators (e.g., filial piety norms). Fourth, future work can adopt more advanced statistical models (Lin & He, 2024) to examine mediating pathways (e.g., loneliness, physical activity) and apply biomarker data, which could complement self-reported measurements to assess physiological impacts (Niccodemi et al., 2025).

19.4.6 Conclusions

The relationship between social media use and SRH among Chinese older adults is shaped significantly by disparities in socioeconomic status, education, and psychosocial support. While certain forms of engagement, such as reading news or watching videos, have been shown to promote mental stimulation and emotional well-being, these benefits are not equitably distributed. The persistent digital divide continues to marginalize vulnerable groups, particularly those in rural areas or with limited financial means. To maximize the advantages of digital technologies for healthy aging, an equity-focused and context-sensitive approach is essential. Policymakers must address structural barriers to digital access, such as affordability and infrastructure, while technology developers should design age-friendly platforms that accommodate cognitive and physical changes associated with aging. Researchers can contribute by identifying which types of digital engagement most benefit well-being of older adults. Together, these efforts can transform social media into a powerful tool for inclusion, social connection, and empowerment in later life.

Acknowledgement The authors would like to thank the Research Center for Population & Development and the Institute of Gerontology, Renmin University for providing access to the China Longitudinal Aging and Social Survey (CLASS) dataset used in this chapter.

Disclaimer Views expressed in the chapter are solely those of the authors and do not necessarily reflect those of the United Nations, Virginia Tech, and the National University of Singapore.

References

Bobko, P., & Russell, C. (1990). Variance homogeneity in interactive regression: A clarifying note about data transformations. *Journal of Applied Psychology, 75*(1), 95–96.

Brainin, E., & Neter, E. (2023). Refined analysis of older eHealth users from an agency perspective: Quantitative telephone interview study. *JMIR Aging, 6*, e40004.

Chen, K., & Chan, A. H. (2014). Gerontechnology acceptance by elderly Hong Kong Chinese: A senior technology acceptance model (STAM). *Ergonomics, 57*(5), 635–652.

Chen, W. C., Yang, L., & Wang, X. Y. (2022). Internet use, cultural engagement, and multidimensional health of older adults: A cross-sectional study in China. *Frontiers in Public Health, 10*, 887840.

China Internet Network Information Center [CNNIC]. (2025). *The 55th statistical report on the development of China's Internet*. China Internet Network Information Center. [in Chinese].

Corraini, P., Olsen, M., Pedersen, L., Dekkers, O. M., & Vandenbroucke, J. P. (2017). Effect modification, interaction and mediation: an overview of theoretical insights for clinical investigators. *Clinical Epidemiology, 9*, 331–338.

DeLange Martinez, P., Tancredi, D., Pavel, M., Garcia, L., & Young, H. M. (2024). The role of health in the technology acceptance model among low-income Asian American older adults: Cross-sectional survey analysis. *JMIR Formative Research, 8*, e57009.

Dong, T., Zhu, Z., Guo, M., Du, P., & Wu, B. (2019). Association between dying experience and place of death: Urban–rural differences among older Chinese adults. *Journal of Palliative Medicine, 22*(11), 1386–1393.

Duplaga, M. (2021). The association between Internet use and health-related outcomes in older adults and the elderly: A cross-sectional study. *BMC Medical Informatics and Decision Making, 21*(1), 150.

Falk Erhag, H., Ahlner, F., Rydberg Sterner, T., Skoog, I., & Bergström, A. (2019). Internet use and self-rated health among Swedish 70-year-olds: A cross-sectional study. *BMC Geriatrics, 19*(1), 365.

Feng, Q., Zhu, H., Zhen, Z., & Gu, D. (2016). Self-rated health, interviewer-rated health, and their predictive powers on mortality in old age. *Journal of Gerontology: Social Sciences, 71*(3), 538–550.

Fu, L., Liu, C., Dong, Y., Ma, X., Cai, Q., Li, D., & Di, K. (2024). Mediating effects of information access on internet use and multidimensional health among middle-aged and older adults: Nationwide cross-sectional study. *Journal of Medical Internet Research, 26*, e49688.

Hajek, A., & König, H. H. (2022). Frequency of contact with friends and relatives via internet and psychosocial factors in middle-aged and older adults during the COVID-19 pandemic. *International Journal of Geriatric Psychiatry, 37*(1), 10–1002.

Hu, M., Han, S., Ghorbany, S., & Zhang, K. (2024). Healthy aging in place with the aid of smart technologies: A systematic review. *Encyclopedia, 4*(4), 1918–1932.

Idler, E. L., Hudson, S. V., & Leventhal, H. (1999). The meanings of self-ratings of health: A qualitative and quantitative approach. *Research on Aging, 21*, 458–476.

Jeon, G. S., & Choi, K. (2024). Purposes of internet use and its impacts on physical and psychological health of Korean older adults. *Healthcare (Basel), 12*(2), 244.

Jin, Y., & Zhao, M. (2019). Internet access and the elderly's active aging in China—A study based on 2016 China Longitudinal Aging Social Survey. *Population Journal, 6*, 44–55. [in Chinese].

Jylhä, M. (2009). What is self-rated health and why does it predict mortality? Towards a unified conceptual model. *Social Science & Medicine, 69*, 307–316.

Kemp, S., & Erades Pérez, N. (2023). Consumer fraud against older adults in digital society: Examining victimization and its impact. *International Journal of Environmental Research and Public Health, 20*(7), 5404.

Kim, H., Choi, H., Jung, Y. I., Kim, E., Lee, W., & Yi, J. Y. (2023). Evaluation of a technology-enhanced, integrated community health and wellness program for seniors (HWePS): Protocol of a non-randomized comparison trial. *BMC Public Health, 23*(1), 25.

Kim, J., Lee, H. Y., Won, C. R., Barr, T., & Merighi, J. R. (2020). Older adults' technology use and its association with health and depressive symptoms: Findings from the 2011 National Health and Aging Trends Study. *Nursing Outlook, 68*(5), 560–572.

Kim, J., & Seltzer, M. (2011). Examining heterogeneity in residual variance to detect differential response to treatments. *Psychological Methods, 16*(2), 192–208.

Li, C., Mo, W., & Wei, Q. (2023). The role of internet use and offline social engagement in the health of Chinese older adults: Evidence from nationally representative samples. *Healthcare (Basel), 11*(5), 653.

Li, P. Q., Sun, G. Y., Zhao, X. X., Hu, Z. X., & Gan, K. P. (2025). Internet use and self-rated health among Chinese older adults: The role of social engagement and social support. *Frontiers in Public Health, 12*, 1504940.

Lin, L., & He, P. (2024). The effect of internet use on depressive symptoms in older adults: Based on the chain mediating role ofphysical exercise and self-rated health. *Frontiers in Public Health, 12*, 1472445.

Liu, N., He, Y., & Li, Z. (2022). The relationship between internet use and self-rated health among older adults in China: The mediating role of social support. *International Journal of Environmental Research and Public Health, 19*(22), 14785.

Luo, Y., Yu, H., & Kuang, Y. (2024). Effects and mechanisms of TikTok use on self-rated health of older adults in China during the COVID-19 pandemic: A mediation analysis. *Healthcare (Basel), 12*(22), 2209.

Lyu, S., & Sun, J. (2021). Internet use and self-rated health among Chinese older adults: The mediating role of social capital. *Geriatrics & Gerontology International, 21*(1), 34–38.

Ma, X., Hu, Q., He, J., Wang, W., Chen, K., & Qiao, H. (2024). Association of internet use and health service utilization with self-rated health in middle-aged and older adults: Findings from a nationally representative longitudinal survey. *Frontiers in Public Health, 12*, 1429983.

Neves, B. B., & Vetere, F. (2019). *Ageing and digital technology: Designing and evaluating emerging technologies for older adults*. Springer Natural.

Niccodemi, G., Gaia, A., Novello, M., & Consolazio, D. (2025). Internet use and physical and mental health in old age during the COVID-19 pandemic: Evidence from partners in SHARE. *Economics and Human Biology, 57*, 101487.

Renaud, K., & van Biljon, J. (2008). Predicting technology acceptance and adoption by the elderly: A qualitative study. In *Proceedings of the 2008 annual research conference of the South African Institute of Computer Scientists and Information Technologists* (pp. 210–219).

Richards, T. A., Oman, D., DiMartino, A., & Kotwal, A. A. (2025). A technology-based intervention impacts quality of life for low-income older adults by reducing loneliness and improving healthcare self-efficacy and self-rated health. *Journal of Applied Gerontology, 44*(5), 825–837.

Seckin, G., & Hughes, S. (2021). Patient-reported outcomes in a nationally representative sample of older internet users: Cross-sectional survey. *JMIR Aging, 4*(4), e16006.

Vanderweele, T. J. (2009). On the distinction between interaction and effect modification. *Epidemiology, 20*(6), 863–871.

Wang, Y., & Chen, H. (2024). Effects of mobile internet use on the health of middle-aged and older adults: Evidences from China Health and Retirement Longitudinal Study. *BMC Public Health, 24*(1), 1490.

Wang, L., Cheng, Z., Ye, L., Rong, L., Chien, C. W., & Tung, T. H. (2024). The association between internet use and the choice of medical institution among Chinese older adults. *BMC Geriatrics, 24*(1), 537.

Wang, X., Piantadosi, S., Le-Rademacher, J., et al. (2021). Statistical considerations for subgroup analyses. *Journal of Thoracic Oncology, 16*(3), 375–380.

Wang, H., Wang, B., Tu, X. M., et al. (2022). Inconsistency between overall and subgroup analyses. *General Psychiatry, 35*, e100732.

Wang, R., & Ware, J. H. (2013). Detecting moderator effects using subgroup analyses. *Prevention Science, 14*(2), 111–120.

Wei, N., Sun, D., & Huang, W. (2022). Effects of WeChat use on the subjective health of older adults. *Frontiers in Psychology, 13*, 919889.

Wei, N., Sun, D., & Li, J. (2025). The impact of active social media use on the mental health of older adults. *BMC Psychology, 13*(1), 434.

Wen, W., Zhang, Y., Shi, W., & Li, J. (2023). Association between internet use and physical health, mental health, and subjective health in middle-aged and older adults: Nationally representative cross-sectional survey in China. *Journal of Medical Internet Research, 25*, e40956.

Wu, M., Xue, Y., & Ma, C. (2025). The association between the digital divide and health inequalities among older adults in China: Nationally representative cross-sectional survey. *Journal of Medical Internet Research, 27*, e62645.

Zhao, Y., & Kuang, M. (2025). Digital divides in China: Evidence from CGSS 2005–2021. *Chinese Sociological Review*, 1–62.

Chapter 20
Social Media Use and Subjective Well-Being Among Older Adults in China

Danan Gu, Qiushi Feng, Fang Yang, and Kun Wang

20.1 Introduction

China is undergoing a profound demographic transformation characterized by a rapidly aging population. According to the United Nations (2024), by the end of 2024, individuals aged 65 and above accounted for approximately 15% of the total population in China, a proportion projected to nearly double to 30% by 2050. This demographic shift is largely driven by sustained fertility decline, rising life expectancy, and the long-term effects of past birth control policies (Zou et al., 2024). As the population ages, China faces complex social, economic, and healthcare challenges. Among the most pressing is the need to safeguard and enhance the health, well-being, and quality of life of older adults, many of whom are increasingly vulnerable to chronic illness, social isolation, and financial insecurity.

Concurrently, China has been experiencing a remarkable expansion in digital connectivity. According to the China Internet Network Information Center (CNNIC, 2025), the number of internet users in China reached 1.11 billion by the end of

D. Gu (✉)
Population Division, UN Department of Economic and Social Affairs, New York, NY, USA
e-mail: gudanan@yahoo.com

Q. Feng
Centre for Family and Population Research/Department of Sociology and Anthropology, National University of Singapore, Singapore, Singapore
e-mail: socfq@nus.edu.sg

F. Yang
School of Sociology, Shanghai University, Shanghai, China

K. Wang
Department of Social Work, College of Arts and Sciences, University of Alabama at Birmingham, Birmingham, AL, USA
e-mail: kw2@uab.edu

K. Wang et al. (eds.), *ICT Use and Healthy Longevity*, Advances in Studies of Aging and Health 5, https://doi.org/10.1007/978-3-031-98964-3_20

2024, indicating the near-universal adoption of information and computer information (ICT) among younger and middle-aged populations and growing uptake among older adults. Notably, nearly 155 million Chinese aged 60 and above were internet users by the end of 2024, accounting for 53% of the total older population, a tenfold increase compared to 2010 (see Chap. 2). Although digital inclusion among older adults still lags behind that of younger groups, this trend marks a significant shift in how aging and digitalization are converging in contemporary China.

This convergence of population aging and expanding digital access raises critical questions about how internet use influences the subjective well-being (SWB) of older adults. As a multidimensional concept encompassing self-reported life satisfaction and emotional status, SWB is closely linked to physical health, longevity, and overall quality of life (House et al., 1988; Di Martino & Prilleltensky, 2020). Understanding this relationship between social media use and SWB is crucial for informing policy interventions that promote healthy and active aging in China, providing the key motivation for this chapter. The following sections present a review of relevant literature, outline the study's objectives, describe the data and analytical methods employed, and highlight the main findings. We conclude by interpreting these findings and offering recommendations to inform future research and policymaking.

20.1.1 Literature Review

The relationship between internet use, social media engagement, and SWB among older adults has been widely studied, yet findings remain complex and context dependent (Lei et al., 2024). Research generally indicates that internet use can enhance SWB by fostering social connections, providing access to information, and enabling participation in meaningful activities, whereas the extent of these benefits depends on factors such as usage patterns, digital literacy, and sociocultural context.

Several studies highlight the positive effects of internet use on SWB. Cotten et al. (2013) found that older adults who used the internet experienced reduced loneliness and increased social contact, suggesting that digital connectivity compensates for declining offline interactions. Similarly, Benvenuti et al. (2020) demonstrated that internet use enhances quality of life by facilitating communication with family and friends, particularly for those with limited mobility. In China, Dong et al. (2022) reported that internet use improved life satisfaction among older adults by strengthening social networks and increasing health insurance participation, illustrating how digital access can support SWB. Social media platforms, such as *WeChat*, which is popular in China, have been proven to play a particularly significant role in enhancing SWB among older Chinese adults. Song et al. (2021) found that *WeChat* use was positively associated with life satisfaction, mediated by increased intergenerational support and social engagement. Additionally, Li et al. (2015) observed that active engagement on social media (e.g., sharing content, messaging) was linked to greater perceived social support, which in turn boosted well-being.

However, some studies have observed that such positive impact may not be linear. In a longitudinal study, Zhang et al. (2024) analyzed five waves of CGSS data (2012–2018) and found a persistent positive link between internet use and SWB, but the effect weakened among the oldest-old. Szabo et al. (2019) similarly noted that long-term internet users reported stable well-being, whereas new adopters experienced initial boosts followed by plateaus.

Moreover, not all studies uniformly report positive outcomes, and the empirical findings suggest that the usage type, individual capabilities, and societal context of internet use can moderate the relationship between internet use and SWB. Yang et al. (2021), for example, found that internet use was negatively associated with life satisfaction among Chinese older adults, partly due to perceived social inequities exacerbated by online exposure. Similarly, Sagong and Yoon (2022) noted that excessive smartphone use could reduce SWB of older Koreans by increasing depressive symptoms, particularly among those with lower digital literacy. Research by Schehl et al. (2019) and Sims et al. (2017) further underscores that passive consumption of social media (e.g., scrolling through feeds) may diminish well-being, while active engagement in social media (e.g., direct communication with others) is often associated with more positive outcomes. And Lyu et al. (2022) found that internet use improved health outcomes by enabling access to telemedicine in rural China, whereas urban seniors benefited more from social networking.

The inconsistent findings above are supported by established theoretical frameworks (see Chaps. 3 and 4). For example, the Socioemotional Selectivity Theory (Carstensen et al., 1999) posits that older adults prioritize emotionally meaningful interactions, which the internet can facilitate (Antonucci et al., 2017), whereas the Activity Theory (Havighurst, 1961) further suggests that well-being depends on sustained engagement, whether online or offline (Nimrod, 2020). Empirical studies support these perspectives. Lifshitz et al. (2018), for example, found that older adults who used the internet for meaningful activities (e.g., learning, volunteering) reported higher SWB than passive users.

Overall, while internet and social media use generally promote SWB among older adults, outcomes vary by usage type, individual capabilities, and societal context. Future research should further explore mediating mechanisms (e.g., digital literacy, social support) and disparities (e.g., rural-urban divides) to understand this relationship better and optimize digital interventions for aging populations.

Despite growing interest in the relationship between internet use and well-being among older adults, several methodological and conceptual limitations persist in the literature. First, much of the existing research is centered on Western populations, often overlooking the unique sociocultural and institutional dynamics of China. Factors such as the enduring tradition of filial piety, pronounced rural–urban disparities in digital access, and a regulated digital environment profoundly influence how older Chinese adults engage with ICT (Lyu et al., 2022; Zhang et al., 2024; see Chap. 8). Without accounting for these contextual factors, findings from Western studies may not be directly applicable to the Chinese context.

Second, although prior research generally reports a positive association between internet use and subjective well-being, few studies rigorously examine whether this relationship is confounded or moderated by other factors, such as health conditions, levels of digital literacy, or availability of social support. Unpacking these moderating mechanisms is critical for identifying the specific conditions under which internet use contributes to, or potentially undermines, SWB among older adults.

Third, many studies treat "internet use" as a monolithic activity, overlooking the diversity of online behaviors such as communication, information seeking, entertainment, and access to digital health services. This lack of granularity limits our ability to discern which types of digital engagement are beneficial or detrimental. Therefore, greater specificity in defining and measuring digital behaviors is essential to developing effective, evidence-based digital interventions for aging populations.

This chapter aims to address these gaps by examining the association between social media use and subjective well-being among older adults in China. Specifically, we investigate (1) the robustness of this relationship, (2) the extent to which it is confounded or moderated by factors such as health status, socioeconomic status, social support, among others, and (3) whether different purposes of social media use, such as maintaining social ties, accessing health information, or seeking entertainment, result in differential effects on SWB. Through this analysis, we seek to generate insights that inform both theoretical understanding and practical strategies to promote healthy and inclusive digital aging in China.

20.2 Data and Methods

20.2.1 Data Sources

We utilized data from the China Longitudinal Aging Social Survey (CLASS), a nationally representative longitudinal survey in China. A comprehensive description of CLASS can be found in Chap. 6 and previous studies (Dong et al., 2019; Jin & Zhao, 2019). Consistent with Chaps. 6, 9, 14, and 19, our analysis is entirely based on the 2020 wave of CLASS. Given the research objectives of this chapter, we focused exclusively on respondents aged 65 and older. This selection resulted in a final analytical sample of 11, 228 participants.

20.2.2 Measures

20.2.2.1 Subjective Well-Being

SWB is assessed using three widely recognized indicators to reflect SWB's different dimensions: life satisfaction, feelings of loneliness, and feelings of uselessness. Life satisfaction is the core component of SWB (Diener et al., 2018); feelings of loneliness is a affective factor negative correlated with emotional well-being

(Hawkley & Cacioppo, 2010), and feelings of uselessness is related to older adults' psychological well-being (Windsor et al., 2015).

Life satisfaction was measured by the question, "Are you satisfied with your current life?", using a five-point Likert scale: very satisfied, satisfied, fair, not satisfied, and not satisfied at all. For analysis, responses of fair, not satisfied, and not satisfied at all were grouped as poor life satisfaction and coded as 1, while very satisfied and satisfied were coded as 0. Feelings of Loneliness were assessed by asking, "Did you feel lonely in the past week?", with three response options: no, sometimes, and often. This variable was dichotomized, with often coded as 1 and the other two responses as 0. Similarly, feelings of uselessness were measured with the question, "Did you feel useless in the past week?", using the same three response categories above. Responses of "often" were coded as 1, and no or sometimes as 0.

20.2.2.2 Use of Social Media

Consistent with the approach in Chaps. 14 and 19, respondents were classified as non-users of social media if they reported never using any of the 12 listed apps or platforms. These included *WeChat, Douyin (akin to TikTok), Xiguan Videos (similar to YouTube), Taobao (similar to Amazon), Didi (similar to Uber)*, among others.

20.2.2.3 Covariates

Building on the STAM framework and other digital divide models introduced in Chap. 3, we applied the same five sets of variables used in Chap. 6 that examines internet and social media use correlates. These variables offer a comprehensive foundation for analyzing aging-related issues and include: (1) demographic characteristics, (2) socioeconomic status, (3) family and social support networks, (4) engagement in leisure activities, as well as views, attitudes, and perceptions related to aging and technological advancement, and (5) health status. The regional variable is consistently controlled for across all models. For detailed definitions and coding of these variables, please refer to Chap. 6.

20.2.3 Analytical Strategies

We primarily employed multiple logistic regression models, supplemented by descriptive analyses. In line with the analytical strategy detailed in Chap. 6, we constructed a series of partial models to explore how the associations between social media use and the three indicators of SWB were affected by the inclusion of different sets of covariates. Consistent with the approaches used in Chaps. 6, 9, 14, and 19, the sampling weight was applied in the descriptive analyses but not in the regression models. As part of our sensitivity analysis, we also estimated ordinal logistic and multinomial logistic regression models for the three SWB indicators. The results remained generally consistent across all model specifications.

To assess the moderating effects of covariates on the relationship between social media use and SWB, we conducted subgroup analyses, similarly to those used in Chap. 19. In total, there are 42 subgroups classified by 20 different covariates. All statistical analyses were performed using Stata version 18.0.

20.3 Results

Table 20.1 presents both the weighted and unweighted distributions of study variables for the overall sample, as well as the weighted distributions for social media users and non-users. The differences between weighted and unweighted percentages for the three SWB indicators are minimal, particularly for feelings of loneliness and uselessness. The table also indicates that the proportions of individuals reporting poor life satisfaction, feelings of loneliness, and feelings of uselessness are consistently lower among social media users compared to non-users.

Table 20.2 shows that social media use is associated with a 31% reduction in the odds of reporting poor life satisfaction ($p < 0.001$) when only demographic variables are controlled for (Model I). When separately controlling for socioeconomic factors (Model II), family and social support (Model III), engagement in leisure activities, attitudes toward internet technology, views on aging, and perceived aging (Model IV), and health conditions (Model V), the association remains significant, with social media use linked to 21% ($p < 0.001$), 29% ($p < 0.001$), 10% ($p < 0.1$), and 18% ($p < 0.001$) lower odds of reporting poor life satisfaction, respectively. These results suggest that views on the internet advances, views on aging, perceived aging, captured in Model IV, played the most significant role in modifying the association between social media use and poor life satisfaction. However, when all covariates are included simultaneously, the association between social media use and poor life satisfaction is no longer statistically significant.

Tables 20.3 and 20.4 present the odds ratios of feelings of loneliness and uselessness in relation to social media use under different controls. The patterns observed for social media use are broadly consistent with those reported in Table 20.2, although the reductions in the odds of feeling lonely and useless are slightly greater than those associated with poor life satisfaction. When all covariates are included in the models, the associations between social media use and reduced feelings of loneliness and uselessness remain marginally significant. These results suggest that engagement in leisure activities, attitudes toward internet development, views on aging, and perceived aging are the most influential factors in shaping the relationship between social media use and these two indicators of subjective well-being.

Table 20.5 presents odds ratios for reporting poor life satisfaction, feelings of loneliness, and feelings of uselessness associated with social media use across subgroups. Results are shown for Model I (adjusted for demographic factors only) and Model VI (adjusted for all covariates in Table 20.1). When only demographic

Table 20.1 Unweighted and weighted percentage distribution of the analytical sample by study variable, 2020, CLASS

	Overall sample		Selected (weighted)	
	Weighted	Unweighted	Media users	Non-media users
N	11,228	11,228	2,806	8,422
Subjective well-being				
% Poor life satisfaction	32.7	35.3	26.7	35.1
% Often feel lonely	47.9	47.7	38.1	51.7
% Often feel useless	57.2	58.3	47.6	60.9
Social media use				
% Use of social media	28.2	25.0	100.0	0.0
Covariates				
% Ages 65–74	64.8	38.0	81.6	58.3
% Ages 75–85	27.1	44.7	17.0	31.0
% Ages 85+	8.1	17.3	1.4	10.7
% Men	47.5	50.5	51.3	49.8
% Han ethnicity	95.5	94.0	95.4	20.7
% Urban residents	52.7	54.9	67.4	49.9
% 0 years of schooling	24.4	23.6	9.7	30.2
% 1–6 years of schooling	39.1	41.2	31.3	42.1
% 7+ years of schooling	36.5	35.2	59.0	27.7
% Economically poor	10.4	11.5	8.7	31.4
% White-collar occupation	10.8	11.7	22.3	6.4
% Blue-collar occupation	27.5	29.9	40.7	22.3
% Agricultural workers	61.7	58.4	37.0	71.3
% Currently Married	78.1	75.3	86.8	43.4
% Having 2+ close family members	80.5	79.7	85.3	41.0
% Having 2+ close friends	71.4	70.6	78.2	46.4
% Frequent engagement in leisure activity	82.1	83.2	89.4	40.6
Positive views on internet impact (0–8)[a]	2.12	2.08	3.33	1.64
Negative views on aging (7–35)[a]	21.32	21.41	20.76	21.54
Negative perceived aging (8–40)[a]	24.09	24.02	23.25	24.42
%Having 1+ diseases	79.6	80.4	76.8	80.8
% IADL disabled	18.7	24.2	9.4	22.3
% ADL disabled	11.3	15.1	7.9	12.7
% Cognitively impaired	24.5	30.4	10.8	29.9
% Good self-rated health	50.3	46.8	62.6	45.5
% East China	38.5	36.1	57.2	31.2
% Central China	27.1	25.7	18.3	30.6
% West China	25.7	24.8	14.7	30.0
% Northeast China	8.6	13.4	9.7	8.2

Note: (1)[a], the mean score of the variable. (2) *ADL* activities of daily living, *IADL* instrumental ADL

Table 20.2 Odds ratios of social media use in predicting poor life satisfaction, 2020, CLASS

	Model I	Model II	Model III	Model IV	Model V	Model VI
Use of social media (no)	0.69***	0.79***	0.71***	0.90+	0.82***	1.09
Ages 75–85 (65–74)	1.15**	1.13**	1.13**	1.10*	0.98	0.95
Ages 85+ (65–74)	1.53***	1.50***	1.42***	1.39***	1.08	1.01
Men (women)	0.92*	0.96	0.96	0.94	1.01	1.06
Han ethnicity (minority)	0.93	0.91	0.93	0.90	0.72***	0.72***
Urban (rural)	0.79***	1.00	0.78***	0.84***	0.81***	0.99
1–6 years of schooling (0)		0.99				1.11+
7+ years of schooling (0)		0.81***				1.01
Economically poor (no)		1.20**				1.04
Blue-collar occupation (white-collar)		1.18*				1.35***
Agricultural workers (white-collar)		1.66***				1.71***
Currently married (no)			0.77***			0.85**
Having 2+ close family members (<2)			0.77***			0.90
Having 2+ close friends (<2)			0.94			0.85**
Freq. leisure and social activity (no)				0.78***		0.74***
Positive views on internet impact (0–8)				0.90***		0.93***
Positive views on aging (7–35)				0.97***		0.98**
Positive perceived aging (8–40)				0.92***		0.93***
Having 1+ diseases (no)					1.13*	1.12+
IADL disabled (no)					1.00	0.94
ADL disabled (no)					1.24**	1.25**
Cognitively impaired (no)					1.19***	1.11*
Good self-rated health (no)					0.18***	0.19***
Central China (East China)	0.94	0.87*	0.93	0.98	0.89+	0.84**
West China (East China)	1.16**	1.06	1.09	1.13*	1.20**	1.02
Northeast China (East China)	1.68***	1.66***	1.65***	1.47***	2.01***	1.69***
- Log likelihood	7145.5	7093.3	7111.1	6913.1	6321.4	6155.3
Degree of freedom	9	14	12	13	14	26
LR Chi square	288.7	393.1	357.5	753.6	1936.8	2269.2
No. of individuals	11,228	11,228	11,288	11,228	11,228	11,228

Note: (1) The results were based on logistic regression models. (2) The category of a variable in the parentheses is the reference. (3) *ADL* activities of daily living, *IADL* instrumental ADL. (4) +$p < 0.1$, *$p < 0.05$, **$p < 0.01$, ***$p < 0.001$

Table 20.3 Odds ratios of social media use in predicting loneliness, 2020, CLASS

	Model I	Model II	Model III	Model IV	Model V	Model VI
Use of social media (no)	0.69***	0.71***	0.73***	0.83***	0.78***	0.91+
Ages 75–85 (65–74)	1.10*	1.09*	1.07	1.07	1.03	1.00
Ages 85+ (65–74)	1.57***	1.54***	1.32***	1.49***	1.31***	1.12+
Men (women)	0.89**	0.90**	0.98	0.89**	0.92*	1.00
Han ethnicity (minority)	0.84*	0.83*	0.85+	0.77**	0.76**	0.74***
Urban (rural)	0.84***	0.87**	0.84***	0.87***	0.85***	0.87**
1–6 years of schooling (0)		0.92				0.99
7+ years of schooling (0)		0.87*				1.01
Economically poor (no)		1.02				0.93
Blue-collar occupation (white-collar)		0.96				0.97
Agricultural workers (white-collar)		0.99				0.97
Currently married (no)			0.51***			0.52***
Having 2+ close family members (<2)			0.82***			0.91
Having 2+ close friends (<2)			1.18**			1.11*
Freq. leisure and social activity (no)				1.08		1.07
Positive views on internet impact (0–8)				0.91***		0.92***
Positive views on aging (7–35)				0.96***		0.97***
Positive perceived aging (8–40)				0.98***		0.99*
Having 1+ diseases (no)					0.84***	0.83***
IADL disabled (no)					1.15**	1.09
ADL disabled (no)					1.22**	1.18*
Cognitively impaired (no)					1.10*	1.04
Good self-rated health (no)					0.55***	0.58***
Central China (East China)	1.22***	1.22***	1.28***	1.28***	1.24***	1.31***
West China (East China)	1.35***	1.32***	1.37***	1.38***	1.39***	1.44***
Northeast China (East China)	0.70***	0.71***	0.71***	0.67***	0.72***	0.70***
- Log likelihood	7563.9	7560.6	7456.3	7457.7	7410.5	7250.9
Degree of freedom	9	14	12	13	14	26
LR Chi square	413.1	419.6	628.3	625.5	719.9	1039.1
No. of individuals	11,228	11,228	11,288	11,228	11,228	11,228

Note: (1) The results were based on logistic regression models. (2) The category of a variable in the parentheses is the reference. (3) *ADL* activities of daily living, *IADL* instrumental ADL. (4) +$p < 0.1$, *$p < 0.05$, **$p < 0.01$, ***$p < 0.001$

Table 20.4 Odds ratios of social media use in predicting uselessness, 2020, CLASS

	Model I	Model II	Model III	Model IV	Model V	Model VI
Use of social media (no)	0.64***	0.68***	0.65***	0.82***	0.74***	0.90+
Ages 75–85 (65–74)	1.26***	1.25***	1.25***	1.21***	1.12*	1.10*
Ages 85+ (65–74)	1.79***	1.77***	1.72***	1.69***	1.27***	1.26***
Men (women)	0.83***	0.85***	0.85***	0.83***	0.88**	0.90**
Han ethnicity (minority)	1.07	1.06	1.07	0.96	0.98	0.89
Urban (rural)	0.86***	0.94	0.86***	0.89**	0.87**	0.95
1–6 years of schooling (0)		0.93				0.99
7+ years of schooling (0)		0.90+				1.04
Economically poor (no)		1.03				0.92
Blue-collar occupation (white-collar)		1.19**				1.27***
Agricultural workers (white-collar)		1.32***				1.32***
Currently married (no)			0.85***			0.92
Having 2+ close family members (<2)			0.91+			1.04
Having 2+ close friends (<2)			1.16**			1.08
Freq. leisure and social activity (no)				1.34***		1.35***
Positive views on internet impact (0–8)				0.88***		0.90***
Positive views on aging (7–35)				0.95***		0.96***
Positive perceived aging (8–40)				0.94***		0.96***
Having 1+ diseases (no)					1.27***	1.31***
IADL disabled (no)					1.39***	1.33***
ADL disabled (no)					1.37***	1.36***
Cognitively impaired (no)					1.25***	1.17**
Good self-rated health (no)					0.54***	0.60***
Central China (East China)	0.91+	0.89*	0.93	0.97	0.96	1.02
West China (East China)	1.16**	1.13*	1.19**	1.19**	1.25***	1.31***
Northeast China (East China)	0.61***	0.61***	0.61***	0.53***	0.67***	0.60***
- Log likelihood	7400.0	7389.2	7390.6	7166.7	7144.4	6974.5
Degree of freedom	9	14	12	13	14	26
LR Chi square	453.1	474.6	471.9	919.7	964,3	1304.2
No. of individuals	11,228	11,228	11,288	11,228	11,228	11,228

Note: (1) The results were based on logistic regression models. (2) The category of a variable in the parentheses is the reference. (3) *ADL* activities of daily living, *IADL* instrumental ADL. (4) +$p < 0.1$, *$p < 0.05$, **$p < 0.01$, ***$p < 0.001$

Table 20.5 Odds ratios of social media use in predicting poor life satisfaction, loneliness, and uselessness among subgroups, 2020, CLASS

	Poor life satisfaction		Loneliness		Uselessness	
Subgroups	Model I	Model VI	Model I	Model VI	Model I	Model VI
Ages 65–74 (*N* = 4,264)	0.71***	1.09	0.63***	0.79**	0.67***	0.89
Ages 75+ (*N* = 6,964)	0.67***	1.04	0.74***	1.01	0.63***	0.91
Women (*N* = 5,554)	0.64***	1.18	0.67***	0.95	0.64***	1.01
Men (*N* = 5,674)	0.73***	1.03	0.71***	0.88^{+}	0.64***	0.83*
Rural (*N* = 5,061)	0.70***	0.95	0.63***	0.80*	0.63***	0.83*
Urban (*N* = 6,167)	0.69***	1.23	0.74***	0.99	0.65***	0.96
Ethnic minorities (*N* = 672)	0.71	1.25	0.88	1.34	0.97	1.53
Han majority (*N* = 10,556)	0.68***	1.07	0.68***	0.88*	0.63***	0.87*
0–6 years of schooling (*N* = 7,271)	0.75***	1.13	0.73***	0.98	0.68***	0.96
7+ years of schooling (*N* = 3,957)	0.71***	1.03	0.66***	0.80**	0.63***	0.83*
Economically not poor (*N* = 9,937)	0.68***	1.07	0.71***	0.92	0.65***	0.92
Economically poor (*N* = 1, 291)	0.82	1.23	0.59***	0.84	0.60***	0.75^{+}
Blue-collar /agriculture job (*N* = 9,919)	0.75***	1.10	0.70***	0.91	0.68***	0.92
White-collar job (*N* = 1,309)	0.49***	1.05	0.69***	0.95	0.54***	0.88
Not married (*N* = 2,778)	0.81^{+}	1.43*	0.86	1.19	0.64***	1.00
Married (*N* = 8,450)	0.68***	1.01	0.71***	0.86*	0.65***	0.89
Having <2 close family members (*N* = 2,279)	0.72***	1.07	0.92	1.10	0.74***	0.96
Having 2+ close family members (*N* = 8,949)	0.69***	1.08	0.64***	0.87*	0.61***	0.88
Having <2 close friends (*N* = 3,300)	0.69***	1.01	0.86	1.18	0.74**	1.09
Having 2+ close friends (*N* = 7,928)	0.69***	1.06	0.63***	0.84*	0.60***	0.84**
Not freq. engage. in leisure activities (*N* = 1,889)	0.55***	0.73	0.73*	1.09	0.86	1.28
Freq. engagement in leisure activities (*N* = 9,339)	0.73***	1.14*	0.70***	0.88^{+}	0.61***	0.85**
Less positive views on internet tech. (*N* = 3,058)	0.53***	0.68**	0.55***	0.56***	0.63***	0.73*
More positive views on internet tech. (*N* = 8,170)	0.75***	1.11	0.76***	0.96	0.72***	0.95
Positive views on aging (7–22)[a] (*N* = 7,752)	0.73***	1.12	0.76***	0.94	0.71***	0.95
Positive views on aging (23–35)[a] (*N* = 3,476)	0.67***	1.00	0.64***	0.88	0.58***	0.82*
Positive perceived aging (8–25)[a] (*N* = 7,939)	0.80***	1.14	0.78***	1.07	0.75***	1.05

(continued)

Table 20.5 (continued)

Subgroups	Poor life satisfaction		Loneliness		Uselessness	
	Model I	Model VI	Model I	Model VI	Model I	Model VI
Positive perceived aging (26–40)[a] (*N* = 3,289)	0.62***	1.05	0.61***	0.93	0.58***	0.80*
Having no disease condition (*N* = 2,200)	0.55***	0.83	0.91	1.19	0.83+	1.17
Having 1+ disease condition (*N* = 9,028)	0.71***	1.17***	0.66***	0.87*	0.58***	0.84**
IADL not disabled (*N* = 8,510)	0.80***	1.18	0.72***	0.91	0.71***	0.92
IADL disabled (*N* = 2,718)	0.66***	0.92	0.77*	0.93	0.66***	0.92
ADL not disabled (*N* = 9,531)	0.75***	1.11	0.74***	0.94	0.70***	0.93
ADL disabled (*N* = 1,697)	0.86	1.18	0.56**	0.66*	0.51***	0.78*
Cognitively unimpaired (*N* = 7,816)	0.77***	1.13	0.70***	0.85*	0.71***	0.90+
Cognitively impaired (*N* = 3,412)	0.85	1.14	0.89	1.21	0.67***	0.91
Not-good self-rated health (*N* = 5,972)	0.89	1.18	0.74***	0.83*	0.72***	0.94
Good self-rated health (*N* = 5,256)	0.66***	0.96	0.74***	0.96	0.65***	0.87+
East China (*N* = 4,055)	0.72***	1.27*	0.65***	0.74***	0.55***	0.83*
Central China (*N* = 2,883)	0.57***	0.98	0.70***	1.08	0.68***	1.05
West China (*N* = 2,783)	0.63***	0.87	0.87	1.03	0.88	1.04
Northeast China (*N* = 1,507)	0.81+	0.851	0.67***	0.72*	0.77*	0.68**

Note: (1)[a], referring to the score range of the variable. A less positive view of the impact of internet technology on society was defined by a score of 0–3, while a more positive view was indicated by a score of 4–8. (2) *ADL* activities of daily living, *IADL* instrumental ADL. (3) Model I controls for demographic factors only, whereas Model VI controls for all study covariates. (4) $+p < 0.1$, $*p < 0.05$, $**p < 0.01$, $***p < 0.001$

variables are controlled (Model I), social media use is associated with 20–51% lower odds of poor life satisfaction in 35 of 42 subgroups. Similarly, 35 subgroups show 23–49% lower odds of loneliness, and 38 subgroups show 23–45% lower odds of feeling useless. These findings suggest a widespread association between social media use and enhanced subjective well-being (SWB).

However, these relationships are substantially attenuated after adjusting for all covariates (Model VI). For poor life satisfaction, only one subgroup retain significantly reduced odds, while three subgroups unexpectedly show increased odds. No significant associations are found in the remaining subgroups, indicating that the link between social media use and life satisfaction is largely confounded by other factors. By contrast, associations with feelings of loneliness and uselessness remain robust in most subgroups even after full adjustment. Social media use is associated with 13–34% lower odds of feeling lonely in 28 subgroups and 13–32% lower odds of feeling useless in 31 subgroups. This suggests that while the strength of these relationships is moderately reduced, they remain statistically significant, highlighting their resilience to confounding variables.

Overall, the association between social media use and reduced feelings of loneliness and uselessness appear stronger and more consistent among the following subgroups: individuals living in rural areas, those with 7 or more years of schooling, those holding less positive views on the internet's impact on society, individuals with one or more chronic conditions, those with ADL disabilities, and residents of East and Northeast China.

Table 20.6 presents the odds ratios of reporting poor life satisfaction, feeling lonely, and feeling useless by the purposes of social media use. When only demographic factors are controlled (Model I in the left panel), social media use is associated with 27–47% lower odds of reporting poor life satisfaction across various purposes. However, when all covariates are included (Model VI), these associations become not statistically significant and even reversed significantly in the cases of communication and shopping.

In the middle panel, the baseline models (Model I) show that social media use is linked to 31–43% lower odds of feeling lonely, except when the primary purpose is shopping, travel, or health management. After adjusting for all covariates (Model VI), only entertainment and information-seeking remain associated with significantly lower odds (20–26%) of feeling loneliness. Notably, using social media for shopping or travel is associated with 41–44% higher odds of feeling lonely. The right panel shows that social media use initially corresponded with 38–65% lower odds of feeling useless (Model I). Even after full adjustment (Model VI), the associations remain significant in most cases, though the reduced odds are down to 14–46%. However, the associations become not significant for shopping and travel purposes.

Table 20.6 Odds ratios of social media use in predicting poor life satisfaction, loneliness, and uselessness by the purposes of use, 2020, CLASS

	Poor life satisfaction		Loneliness		Uselessness	
Purposes of social media use	Model I	Model VI	Model I	Model VI	Model I	Model VI
Any type of social media use (no)	0.70***	1.09	0.69***	0.91+	0.64***	0.90+
For contacting with family members/friends (no)	0.72***	1.15*	0.69***	0.92	0.62***	0.86**
For reading /following-up news (no)	0.60***	0.92	0.68***	0.90+	0.60***	0.85**
For entertainment (no)	0.65***	1.00	0.57***	0.74***	0.56***	0.78***
For seeking information (no)	0.53***	0.95	0.59***	0.80***	0.52***	0.80**
For online shopping (no)	0.73***	1.47***	0.92	1.44***	0.57***	0.99
For travel (no)	0.63***	1.17	0.94	1.41***	0.56***	0.95
For health management (no)	0.56***	0.95	0.81	1.10	0.35***	0.54***

Note: (1) The results were based on binary logistic regression models. (2) Model I controls for demographic factors and region, whereas Model VI controls for all factors in the table. (3) Category in the parentheses of each purpose is its reference group, which includes non-users. (4) $+p < 0.1$, $*p < 0.05$, $**p < 0.01$, $***p < 0.001$

Overall, using social media for health management is associated with the greatest reduction in odds of reporting poor life satisfaction and feeling useless. Entertainment and information-seeking are the most consistent in associating with less feelings of loneliness and uselessness. Compared to loneliness and life satisfaction, social media use shows a more consistent and stronger association with reduced feelings of uselessness across different purposes.

20.4 Discussion

Based on CLASS, a nationally representative survey with 11,228 older adults aged 65 or older, this study examined social media use and SWB. The findings of this study reveal a nuanced relationship between social media use and SWB among older adults in China, with substantial variations across demographic and socioeconomic subgroups. The results demonstrate that while social media use is broadly associated with reduced feelings of loneliness and uselessness, these benefits are not uniformly distributed. Instead, they are particularly pronounced among specific subgroups: rural residents, those with 7 or more years of schooling, individuals holding less positive views on the internet's societal impact, those with chronic conditions or ADL disabilities, and residents of East and Northeast China. Below, we interpret these findings in depth, explore potential mechanisms, acknowledge study limitations, and outline key policy and research implications of this study.

20.4.1 Social Media Use and Reduced Loneliness/Uselessness: Subgroup Variations

The stronger association between social media use and reduced feelings of loneliness and uselessness among rural residents aligns with prior research highlighting the digital divide in China (Lyu et al., 2022). In rural areas, where geographic isolation and limited healthcare infrastructure are prevalent, social media may serve as a critical lifeline for maintaining social connections and accessing health information. For example, telemedicine services via platforms like *WeChat* can bridge gaps in rural healthcare access, directly improving perceptions of usefulness and reducing isolation (Wang et al., 2020).

The finding that individuals with 7 or more years of schooling benefit more from social media use underscores the role of digital literacy in moderating technology's impact. Higher educational attainment likely enables older adults to navigate digital platforms more effectively, engage in meaningful online activities (e.g., health information-seeking), and avoid negative experiences such as scams or misinformation (Hargittai & Dobransky, 2017). This suggests that interventions targeting digital skills training could amplify social media's benefits, particularly for less-educated older adults.

Surprisingly, those with less positive views on the internet's societal impact derived greater well-being benefits from social media use. This may reflect a "compensatory effect," where skeptical users adopt technology out of necessity (e.g., for family communication) and may be easily pleased by its utility (Schehl et al., 2019). Alternatively, individuals with overly optimistic expectations about the internet may instead experience more disappointment when reality fails to match idealized outcomes (Yang et al., 2021).

The robust benefits observed among older adults with chronic conditions or ADL disabilities highlight social media's role in mitigating health-related isolation. For these individuals, online platforms provide avenues for social participation that physical limitations might otherwise restrict (Cotten et al., 2013). Support groups on *WeChat* or health forums, therefore, can offer emotional support and practical advice, reducing feelings of uselessness (Song et al., 2021).

Finally, the stronger effects on SWB in East and Northeast China may reflect economic and infrastructural disparity of China. Eastern China, with its higher internet penetration and denser social networks, may offer more opportunities for meaningful online engagement. In contrast, Northeast China's aging population and economic stagnation could make digital connectivity a particularly valuable resource for maintaining social ties among older adults (Zhang et al., 2024).

20.4.2 Weak Links Between Social Media Use and Life Satisfaction

While social media use consistently predicted reduced feelings of loneliness and uselessness, its association with life satisfaction was weaker and more susceptible to confounding effects. This discrepancy may stem from the different psychological mechanisms underlying these SWB dimensions. Loneliness and uselessness are more directly tied to social connectedness, which social media can address through communication and informational support (Nimrod, 2020). In contrast, life satisfaction reflects a broader evaluation of circumstances in later life, which may be less malleable to digital engagements (Diener et al., 2018).

The attenuation of this relationship after adjusting for covariates like health status and social support (Table 20.2) suggests that social media's impact on life satisfaction is indirect. For example, an older adult with robust offline social networks may derive little additional benefits from online interactions, whereas someone isolated might experience a more pronounced boost in well-being (Dumitrache et al., 2018).

20.4.3 Purpose Matters: Health and Information vs. Shopping/Travel

The analysis of usage purposes presented in Table 20.6 underscores the significance of goal-oriented social media activities in shaping SWB among older adults. Specifically, health management and information-seeking, two usage purposes, are consistently associated with reduced feelings of loneliness and uselessness. These findings support the notion that purposeful, utility-driven online behaviors, such as seeking health-related knowledge or staying informed, can enhance psychological well-being by fostering a sense of autonomy, competence, and control (Nimrod, 2020). Health-related social media use, in particular, may be especially empowering for older adults managing chronic illnesses, as it allows them to access reliable information, monitor symptoms, and engage in preventive care independently, thus reinforcing their self-efficacy (Lyu et al., 2022).

In contrast, when all confounding factors are taken into account, the use of social media platforms for commercial or leisure-related purposes, such as shopping and travel, is positively associated with higher levels of loneliness. This counterintuitive association may be explained by two interrelated mechanisms. First, such activities may expose users to idealized portrayals of consumerism or luxurious lifestyles, leading to upward social comparisons and reinforcing feelings of social or economic inadequacy (Yang et al., 2021). Second, the increasing commercialization of digital spaces, where algorithm-driven advertising dominates user experiences, may reduce the sense of genuine interpersonal connection and transform these platforms into transactional, rather than relational, environments (Castellacci & Tveito, 2018). This contrast highlights the need to promote meaningful and empowering online engagement, away from passive or consumption-driven interactions.

20.4.4 Strengths and Limitations

This study makes a meaningful contribution to the growing body of research on digital engagement and aging by investigating the impact of social media use on SWB by different subgroups and usage purposes. However, several limitations should be acknowledged to contextualize the findings. First, the use of cross-sectional data limits our ability to draw causal conclusions; future research should employ longitudinal designs to examine how changes in social media use over time influence psychological outcomes such as feelings of loneliness and uselessness (Szabo et al., 2019). Second, reliance on self-reported measures may introduce recall or social desirability bias. Integrating behavioral data, such as screen time records or usage patterns, would capture real-time user behavior and thus enhance measurement validity (Schehl et al., 2019). Third, potential confounding effects from regional and cultural factors, such as the strong influence of filial piety in East China, may shape both social media engagement and well-being outcomes;

qualitative approaches are thus needed to offer deeper insights into such contextual dynamics (Song et al., 2021). Finally, the mechanisms between social media use and SWB have not been examined by incorporating mediators and moderators. Studies have shown the important roles of mediators and moderators in modifying the relationship between social media use and SWB (Wu et al., 2023). Future research should design holistic frameworks to comprehensively disentangle the role of ICT in affecting SWB.

20.4.5 Policy Implications and Further Research Directions

The findings of this study offer several important implications for policy and practice to enhance the well-being of older adults in the digital age. First, there is a pressing need to implement targeted digital literacy programs, especially for rural residents and individuals with lower levels of education. These groups are often disadvantaged in terms of digital access and skills, which can exacerbate social isolation and informational inequality (Hargittai & Dobransky, 2017). Digital training initiatives should go beyond basic instructions to emphasize active and meaningful forms of engagement, such as video calls and interactive discussions, rather than passive consumption like scrolling through feeds. Such engagement has been shown to foster greater emotional connection and a sense of purpose (Nimrod, 2020).

Second, health-oriented platform design presents a promising avenue for improving both access to care and SWB. Collaborations between social media platforms, such as *WeChat*, and healthcare providers could result in the integration of telemedicine services, chronic disease management tools, and mental health resources directly into the platforms commonly used by older adults (Wang et al., 2020). These health-related functionalities can promote autonomy, reduce barriers to care, and empower older users in managing their well-being.

Third, there is an urgent need to address algorithmic harms that disproportionately affect older adults. Commercial algorithms can overexpose users to targeted advertising, potentially leading to financial exploitation or misinformation. Regulatory frameworks should be considered to ensure age-appropriate content and protections from predatory commercial practices (Yang et al., 2021).

As the Chinese government continues to champion digital inclusion for older adults through initiatives such as the "Digital Inclusion for Seniors" (2020–2022) program, which aims to improve internet accessibility, usability, and digital literacy among aging populations, our study offers timely and actionable insights into how these goals can be further refined. Our findings suggest that while internet access is a foundational step, it is the quality and the purpose of digital engagement that truly influence well-being outcomes. Rather than treating digital inclusion as a purely technological challenge, interventions should be grounded in a complete understanding of older adults' psychosocial needs, usage patterns, and vulnerability to online risks. Effective strategies should target not only the expansion of infrastructure but also the development of context-sensitive tools, safeguards, and educational efforts that promote meaningful online participation. In doing so, public policy can move beyond bridging the digital divide toward fostering an age-friendly digital environment that actively supports healthy and dignified aging in the rapidly evolving technological landscape.

Academically, our study suggests that future research should delve deeper into the mechanisms through which social media use affects well-being in later life. For instance, studies should investigate whether increased social support or simple distraction mediates the relationship between online engagement and reduced loneliness among older adults (Hawkley & Cacioppo, 2010). Cross-cultural research comparing collectivist societies like China with individualist contexts could help reveal how cultural values shape digital experiences and their emotional consequences (Degli Antoni & Franco, 2022). Moreover, ethical issues such as data privacy, digital autonomy, and inclusive design need to be systematically explored to ensure that digital platforms are responsive to the specific needs and vulnerabilities of older populations (Schulz et al., 2015).

20.4.6 Conclusions

Social media use offers promising avenues for enhancing SWB in late life, particularly by reducing feelings of loneliness and uselessness. However, these benefits are not evenly distributed. Vulnerable subgroups, such as rural residents, individuals with disabilities, and those with lower educational attainment, are less likely to access or meaningfully benefit from digital platforms, highlighting the urgent need for inclusive and targeted digital policies. Moreover, the potential harms of algorithmic manipulation, commercial exploitation, and passive consumption patterns cannot be overlooked. To fully harness the positive potential of social media while minimizing its risks, policymakers must design interventions to be sensitive to the needs of these diverse older populations. Future research should move beyond cross-sectional snapshots and invest in longitudinal, cross-cultural, and mixed-method studies. Such approaches will allow researchers to unpack causal pathways, examine sociocultural mediators, and offer more nuanced guidance for designing age-friendly digital environments that support well-being across demographic groups and geographic contexts.

Acknowledgement The authors would like to thank the Research Center for Population & Development and the Institute of Gerontology, Renmin University for providing access to the China Longitudinal Aging and Social Survey (CLASS) dataset used in this chapter.

Disclaimer Views expressed in the chapter are solely those of the authors and do not necessarily reflect those of the United Nations, the National University of Singapore, Shanghai University, and the University of Alabama at Birmingham.

References

Antonucci, T. C., Ajrouch, K. J., & Manalel, J. A. (2017). Social relations and technology: Continuity, context, and change. *Innovation in Aging, 1*(3), 1–9.

Benvenuti, M., Giovagnoli, S., Mazzoni, E., Cipresso, P., Pedroli, E., & Riva, G. (2020). The relevance of online social relationships among the elderly: How using the web could enhance quality of life? *Frontiers in Psychology, 11*, 1–10.

Carstensen, L. L., Isaacowitz, D. M., & Charles, S. T. (1999). Taking time seriously: A theory of socioemotional selectivity. *American Psychologist, 54*(3), 165.

Castellacci, F., & Tveito, V. (2018). Internet use and well-being: A survey and a theoretical framework. *Research Policy, 47*(1), 308–325.

China Internet Network Information Center [CNNIC]. (2025). *The 55th statistical report on the development of China's Internet*. China Internet Network Information Center. [in Chinese].

Cotten, S. R., Anderson, W. A., & McCullough, B. M. (2013). Impact of internet use on loneliness and contact with others among older adults: Cross-sectional analysis. *Journal of Medical Internet Research, 15*(2), e39.

Degli Antoni, G., & Franco, C. (2022). The effect of technological behaviour and beliefs on subjective well-being: The role of technological infrastructure. *Journal of Evolutionary Economics, 32*(2), 553–590.

Di Martino, S., & Prilleltensky, I. (2020). Happiness as fairness: The relationship between national life satisfaction and social justice in EU countries. *Journal of Community Psychology, 48*(6), 1997–2012.

Diener, E., Lucas, R. E., & Oishi, S. (2018). Advances and open questions in the science of subjective well-being. *Collabra: Psychology, 4*(1), 15.

Dong, X., Meng, S., & Chen, D. (2022). How does the internet enhance the subjective well-being of elderly individuals in China? *Frontiers in Psychology, 13*, 1036169.

Dong, T., Zhu, Z., Guo, M., Du, P., & Wu, B. (2019). Association between dying experience and place of death: Urban–rural differences among older Chinese adults. *Journal of Palliative Medicine, 22*(11), 1386–1393.

Dumitrache, C. G., Rubio, L., & Rubio-Herrera, R. (2018). Extroversion, social support and life satisfaction in old age: A mediation model. *Aging & Mental Health, 22*(8), 1069–1077.

Hargittai, E., & Dobransky, K. (2017). Old dogs, new clicks: Digital inequality in skills and uses among older adults. *Canadian Journal of Communication, 42*(2), 195–212.

Havighurst, R. J. (1961). Successful aging. *The Gerontologist, 1*, 8–13.

Hawkley, L. C., & Cacioppo, J. T. (2010). Loneliness matters: A theoretical and empirical review of consequences and mechanisms. *Annals of Behavioral Medicine, 40*(2), 218–227.

House, J. S., Landis, K. R., & Umberson, D. (1988). Social relationships and health. *Science, 241*(4865), 540–545.

Jin, Y., & Zhao, M. (2019). Internet access and the elderly's active aging in China—A study based on 2016 China Longitudinal Aging Social Survey. *Population Journal, 6*, 44–55. [in Chinese].

Lei, X., Matovic, D., Leung, W.-Y., Viju, A., & Muthrich, V. M. (2024). The relationship between social media use and psychosocial outcomes in older adults: A systematic review. *International Psychogeriatrics, 36*(9), 714–746.

Li, X., Chen, W., & Popiel, P. (2015). What happens on Facebook stays on Facebook? The implications of Facebook interaction for perceived, receiving, and giving social support. *Computers in Human Behavior, 51*, 106–113.

Lifshitz, R., Nimrod, G., & Bachner, Y. G. (2018). Internet use and well-being in later life: A functional approach. *Aging & Mental Health, 22*(1), 85–91.

Lyu, M., Peng, X., & Zhang, Y. (2022). Internet and the health of the elderly in rural China – Micro evidences and impact mechanisms. *China Economic Studies, 333*(4), 156–169.

Nimrod, G. (2020). Aging well in the digital age: Technology in processes of selective optimization with compensation. *Journal of Gerontology Social Sciences, 75*(9), 2008–2017.

Sagong, H., & Yoon, J. Y. (2022). The effects of smartphone use on life satisfaction in older adults: The mediating role of depressive symptoms. *CIN: Computers, Informatics, Nursing, 40*(8), 523–530.

Schehl, B., Leukel, J., & Sugumaran, V. (2019). Understanding differentiated internet use in older adults: A study of informational, social, and instrumental online activities. *Computers in Human Behavior, 97*, 222–230.

Schulz, R., Wahl, H. W., Matthews, J. T., De Vito Dabbs, A., Beach, S. R., & Czaja, S. J. (2015). Advancing the aging and technology agenda in gerontology. *The Gerontologist, 55*(5), 724–734.

Sims, T., Reed, A. E., & Carr, D. C. (2017). Information and communication technology use is related to higher well-being among the oldest-old. *Journals of Gerontology: Social Sciences, 72*(5), 761–770.

Song, L., Ge, Y., & Zhang, X. (2021). The relationship between WeChat use by Chinese urban older adults living alone and their subjective well-being: The mediation role of intergenerational support and social activity. *Psychology Research and Behavior Management, 14*, 1543–1554.

Szabo, A., Allen, J., Stephens, C., & Alpass, F. (2019). Longitudinal analysis of the relationship between purposes of internet use and well-being among older adults. *The Gerontologist, 59*(1), 58–68.

United Nations. (2024). *World population prospects 2024: Summary of results*. United Nations, Department of Economic and Social Affairs, Population Division. https://population.un.org/wpp/

Wang, J., Liang, C., & Li, K. (2020). Impact of internet use on elderly health: Empirical study based on Chinese General Social Survey (CGSS) data. *Healthcare, 8*(4), 482.

Windsor, T. D., Curtis, R. G., & Luszcz, M. A. (2015). Sense of purpose as a psychological resource for aging well. *Developmental Psychology, 51*(7), 975–986.

Wu, B., Liu, T., & Tian, B. (2023). How does social media use impact subjective well-being? Examining the suppressing role of Internet addiction and the moderating effect of digital skills. *Frontiers in Psychology, 14*, 1108692.

Yang, H., Wu, Y., Lin, X., Xie, L., Zhang, S., Zhang, S., & Zheng, X. (2021). Internet use, life satisfaction, and subjective well-being among the elderly: Evidence from 2017 China General Social Survey. *Frontiers in Public Health, 9*, 1–12.

Zhang, C., Zhang, Y., & Wang, Y. (2024). A study on internet use and subjective well-being among Chinese older adults: Based on CGSS (2012–2018) five-wave mixed interface survey data. *Frontiers in Public Health, 11*, 1277789.

Zou, Y., Wang, H., Chen, W., Shen, K., Huang, K., Gui, J. F., Zhang, G., Feng, Q. S., & Liu, H. Y. (2024). Embrace the past and forge ahead: The China report on the 30th anniversary of the International Conference on Population and Development (ICPD). *China Population and Development Studies, 8*, 239–286.

Chapter 21
Social Media Use and Aging Experiences Among Older Adults in China

Danan Gu, Qiushi Feng, and Fang Yang

21.1 Introduction

By the end of 2024, the number of internet users in China aged 60 and above exceeded 150 million (CNNIC, 2025; see Chap. 2). A large majority of these older adults actively engage with social media platforms. Applications such as *WeChat and QQ, Douyin (akin to TikTok), BiliBili or Xiguan Videos (similar to YouTube), and Xiaohongshu (RedNote, akin to Instagram)* have become vital tools for social connection, self-expression, and information access among older Chinese (CNNIC, 2025). As internet penetration deepens alongside China's rapidly aging population, older adults' digital participation is profoundly reshaping how aging is experienced and perceived.

This demographic and technological convergence underscores an urgent research imperative: to understand whether and how social media use influences subjective experiences of aging, both in terms of older adults' self-understanding and the broader cultural narratives surrounding later life. Often underexamined in mainstream discourses, this intersection is essential to comprehending the evolving relationship between aging and digital life in contemporary China.

Research to date presents a complex and sometimes contradictory picture. On the one hand, social media engagement among older adults has been associated with

D. Gu (✉)
Population Division, UN Department of Economic and Social Affairs, New York, NY, USA
e-mail: gudanan@yahoo.com

Q. Feng
Centre for Family and Population Research/Department of Sociology and Anthropology, National University of Singapore, Singapore, Singapore
e-mail: socfq@nus.edu.sg

F. Yang
School of Sociology, Shanghai University, Shanghai, China

K. Wang et al. (eds.), *ICT Use and Healthy Longevity*, Advances in Studies of Aging and Health 5, https://doi.org/10.1007/978-3-031-98964-3_21

improved mental and physical health, increased social support, and enhanced subjective well-being (Cotten et al., 2013; He et al., 2024; Wang & Gu, 2023a, b; Zhang et al., 2024; see also Chap. 15). These benefits are often more psychological than physical, reflecting the emotional and relational dimensions of digital connectivity (Hunsaker & Hargittai, 2018; Juárez et al., 2016). Within the Chinese context, social media use has been shown to reduce social isolation, foster civic participation, and support community-based interactions that may counter age-related stereotypes (Cheng et al., 2024; Li, 2021; Li et al., 2025; Xiang et al., 2025; Zhang et al., 2024).

On the other hand, digital engagement also brings risks. Scholars have documented potential downsides, including increased depressive symptoms, psychological distress triggered by social comparison, and frequent exposure to ageist content (Levy et al., 2014; Köttl et al., 2023; Nimrod, 2022; Wang & Gu, 2023a, b; Wangler & Jansky, 2023). These adverse outcomes are often tied to passive browsing behaviors, idealized portrayals of youth and success, stereotypes of older adults, and the spread of misinformation. Such patterns may deepen negative older adults' experience of aging and contribute to their emotional strain (Köttl et al., 2021; Levy et al., 2014; Nimrod, 2019, 2022).

Some longitudinal studies, particularly those conducted in Western contexts, caution against drawing overly deterministic conclusions, highlighting the moderating and mediating role of factors such as perceived social support (Cotten et al., 2013; Mariano et al., 2021). In this context, cultural values play a crucial role in shaping both the nature and impact of social media use. In China, longstanding norms of filial piety and strong intergenerational ties influence how older adults engage with digital technologies. Platforms like *WeChat*, for instance, enable frequent communication among geographically dispersed family members, thereby reinforcing emotional bonds and intergenerational solidarity (He et al., 2024; McKenna et al., 2025). At the same time, concerns remain regarding the risks of overuse and the psychological burdens associated with increased digital immersion. These dynamics underscore the importance of contextually grounded and culturally sensitive research in understanding the complexities of social media use among older adults.

Several theoretical frameworks offer valuable insights into the multifaceted effects of digital participation in later life. Social capital theory emphasizes the role of social networks and the resources they provide in supporting well-being (He et al., 2024; see Chaps. 3 and 4), framing social media as a potentially powerful means of maintaining and expanding social connections. The Social Comparison Theory underscores how digital exposure to idealized representations of others can shape older adults' self-perceptions of aging (Nimrod, 2019; see Chaps. 3 and 4). Meanwhile, theories of ageism explore how online content may reinforce or challenge age-related stereotypes, influencing the ways in which older adults internalize and interpret their aging identities (Köttl et al., 2023; Levy et al., 2014; Wangler & Jansky, 2023). Together, these frameworks illuminate the complex, and often ambivalent, implications of digital engagement in later life.

Despite increasing scholarly attention, substantial research gaps remain in the study of older adults' digital engagement. Nationally representative studies focusing specifically on the digital behaviors of older Chinese adults are still limited (Li et al., 2025; Zhang et al., 2024). Moreover, many existing investigations fail to account for critical differences between platforms and types of use, even as growing evidence indicates that active content creation and passive consumption are associated with markedly different psychosocial outcomes (Wang & Gu, 2023b; Zhang et al., 2024). Key factors such as educational attainment, health status, and the strength of pre-existing social networks also remain insufficiently examined. In particular, there is an urgent need for more intersectional approaches to better understand the diverse and layered experiences of internet use among older adults (e.g., Wang et al., 2024).

Given these complexities and ongoing gaps in the literature, examining the relationship between social media use and perceptions of aging among older Chinese adults is both timely and essential. First, older adults' self-perceptions of aging have significant implications for their health behaviors, psychological resilience, and levels of social participation (Cotten et al., 2013; Schlomann et al., 2022; Wangler & Jansky, 2023). Second, the impact of digital engagement warrants closer examinations, as it is often associated with enhanced emotional support, expanded social networks, and improved access to health-related information. These factors can contribute to more active and positive aging experiences (Bernardo et al., 2022; Hu et al., 2024; Zhang et al., 2024). Third, persistent digital inequalities, which are shaped by disparities in education, income, gender, and geography, necessitate a critical assessment of who benefits from digital participation and how (Choi et al., 2020; Wang et al., 2024). Finally, China's distinctive sociocultural context, characterized by rapid modernization, enduring familial norms, and state-led digital inclusion efforts, offers a unique vantage point from which to explore how social media shapes aging perceptions (Lee et al., 2025; Zhang et al., 2024).

This chapter examines whether and how social media use is associated with older adults' subjective experiences of aging in China, using nationally representative data. It investigates the individual and sociocultural factors that may influence this relationship, integrates current empirical findings with relevant theoretical perspectives, and highlights key directions for future research. Ultimately, the chapter seeks to deepen our understanding of the digital lives of older adults and to support the development of inclusive approaches that foster positive aging through responsible digital engagement and improved media literacy.

21.2 Data and Method

21.2.1 Data Sources

We used data from the China Longitudinal Aging Social Survey (CLASS), a nationally representative longitudinal study of older adults in China. A detailed overview of CLASS is provided in Chap. 6 and in prior research (Dong et al., 2019; Jin &

Zhao, 2019). In line with the analyses presented in Chaps. 6, 9, 14, 19, and 20, this chapter relied exclusively on data from the 2020 wave of CLASS. To align with the objectives of this chapter, we restricted our analysis to respondents aged 65 and above, resulting in a final analytical sample of 11,228 individuals.

21.2.2 Measures

Aging Experience

We use views on aging (VoA) and self-perceived aging (or simply perceived aging, PA) to measure aging experience. VoA were assessed using seven statements, comprising four negative and three positive items. The negative statements included: "I feel I am already old," "In my view, aging is a process of loss," "Once I get old, it becomes difficult for me to make new friends," and "Because of my age, I feel isolated by others." The positive statements were: "The older one gets, the greater their ability to cope with daily life," "Knowledge increases with age," and "Aging is a pleasant experience." Each item was rated on a five-point Likert scale ranging from "strongly disagree" to "strongly agree." The three positive items were reversely coded so that higher scores consistently reflected more negative views on aging. The internal consistency of these seven items was modest, with a reliability coefficient of approximately 0.50. For analytical convenience, the item scores were summed to create a composite measure of negative VoA, ranging from 7 to 35. Sensitivity analyses showed that modeling the seven items separately did not alter the study's conclusions.

PA is constructed based on eight items. Four statements captured positive aspects of aging and social participation, including: "If given the opportunity, I am willing to participate in Neighborhood Residential Committee/Village Committee work," "I often wish to contribute to society," "I enjoy learning new things," and "I feel I am still a useful member of society." The remaining four items reflected challenges in adapting to social change: "It is difficult for me to adapt to the rapidly changing environment," "Nowadays, it is difficult for me to accept increasingly common viewpoints," "It is becoming harder for me to accept new social policies," and "Recent social changes have not been beneficial for older adults." The first four items were reverse coded, and all responses were summed up to create a total score ranging from 8 to 40, with higher scores indicating a more negative PA. The measure demonstrated high internal consistency, with a reliability coefficient of 0.81.

Use of Social Media

Consistent with the approach in Chaps. 14, 19, and 20, respondents were classified as non-users of social media if they reported never using any of the 12 commonly used apps or platforms designed in the CLASS questionnaire. These included

WeChat, Douyin (Chinese TikTok), Xigua Videos and Bilibili (both similar to YouTube), Taobao (similar to Amazon), and Didi (similar to Uber), among others.

Covariates

Drawing on the STAM framework and other digital divide models discussed in Chap. 3, we included the full set of covariates used to examine internet use in Chap. 6. These variables offer a comprehensive basis for analyzing aging-related issues and consist of five categories: (1) demographic characteristics, (2) socioeconomic status, (3) family and social support networks, (4) frequency of engagement in leisure activities and attitudes toward internet technology, and (5) health status. The region variable was consistently included as a control in all models. Detailed definitions and coding schemes for these variables are provided in Chap. 6.

21.2.3 Analytical Strategies

Our primary analytical approach involved multiple linear regression models, complemented by descriptive analyses. In line with the strategy outlined in Chap. 6, we first estimated a series of partial models to assess how associations between social media use and VoA and PoA changed with the inclusion of different sets of covariates. However, because of space constraints and in order to enhance clarity, we reported only the base model (only including demographic variables) and the fully adjusted models (including all covariates).

To assess the moderating effects of covariates, we conducted subgroup analyses, following the practice in Chaps. 19 and 20. In total, there are 42 subgroups classified by 20 different covariates. As in Chaps. 6, 9, 14, 19, and 20, the sampling weight was applied to descriptive statistics but not to the regression analyses. All statistical analyses were performed using Stata 18.0.

21.3 Results

Table 21.1 presents both the weighted and unweighted distributions of study variables for the overall sample, along with the weighted distributions separately for social media users and non-users. The differences between the weighted and unweighted mean scores for both negative VoA and negative PA are minimal. The table also reveals that social media users tend to report lower mean scores for negative VoA and negative PA compared to non-users.

Figure 21.1 displays the unweighted density distributions of scores for negative VoA and negative PA. As shown in the density plots, both variables exhibit approximately normal distributions.

Table 21.1 Unweighted and weighted percentage distribution of the analytical sample by study variable, 2020, CLASS

	Overall sample		Selected (weighted)	
	Weighted	Unweighted	Media users	Non-media users
N	11,228	11,228	2,806	8,422
Negative VoA (7–35)[a]	21.32	21.41	20.76	21.54
Negative PA (8–40)[a]	24.09	24.02	23.25	24.42
% Use social media	28.2	25.0	100.0	0.0
% Use WeChat	23.5	21.6	83.5	–
% Use Douyin	16.0	13.5	56.8	–
% Use Xigua Videos	4.4	3.3	15.6	–
% Ages 65–74	64.8	38.0	81.6	58.3
% Ages 75–85	27.1	44.7	17.0	31.0
% Ages 85+	8.1	17.3	1.4	10.7
% Men	47.5	50.5	51.3	49.8
% Han ethnicity	95.5	94.0	95.4	20.7
% Urban residents	52.7	54.9	67.4	49.9
% 0 years of schooling	24.4	23.6	9.7	30.2
% 1–6 years of schooling	39.1	41.2	31.3	42.1
% 7+ years of schooling	36.5	35.2	59.0	27.7
% Economically poor	10.4	11.5	8.7	31.4
% White-collar occupation	10.8	11.7	22.3	6.4
% Blue-collar occupation	27.5	29.9	40.7	22.3
% Agricultural workers	61.7	58.4	37.0	71.3
% Currently Married	78.1	75.3	86.8	43.4
% Having 2+ close family members	80.5	79.7	85.3	41.0
% Having 2+ close friends	71.4	70.6	78.2	46.4
% Frequent engagement in leisure activity	82.1	83.2	89.4	40.6
Positive views on internet impact (0–8)[a]	2.12	2.08	3.33	1.64
%Having 1+ diseases	79.6	80.4	76.8	80.8
% IADL disabled	18.7	24.2	9.4	22.3
% ADL disabled	11.3	15.1	7.9	12.7
% Cognitively impaired	24.5	30.4	10.8	29.9
% Good self-rated health	50.3	46.8	62.6	45.5
% East China	38.5	36.1	57.2	31.2
% Central China	27.1	25.7	18.3	30.6
% West China	25.7	24.8	14.7	30.0
% Northeast China	8.6	13.4	9.7	8.2

VoA views on aging, *PA* perceived aging, *ADL* activities of daily living, *IADL* instrumental ADL
[a]The mean score of the variable

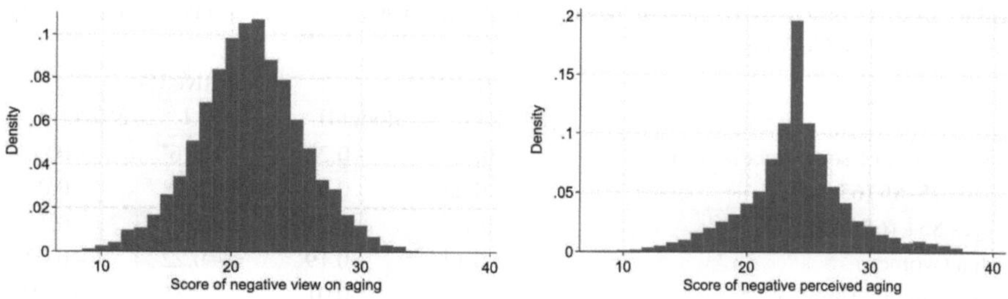

Fig. 21.1 Distribution of density of scores for negative VoA and negative PA, 2020, CLASS

Table 21.2 shows that social media use is associated with a 0.78-point reduction in negative VoA when only demographic variables are controlled for. Although the effect size decreases to 0.22 after adjusting for all covariates, the association remains statistically significant. Regarding negative PA, the corresponding reductions are 1.36 and 0.94, respectively, which is substantially larger than those observed for negative VoA.

Table 21.3 presents the associations between social media use and negative VoA and PA across various subgroups. For negative VoA, when only demographic factors were controlled for (Model I), social media use was significantly associated with reduced scores, ranging from 0.26 to 1.42, across nearly all subgroups. Exceptions included ethnic minorities, individuals with low economic status, those without any diagnosed health conditions, and residents of Western and Northeastern China. These findings suggest that the beneficial effect of social media use in mitigating negative VoA is broadly observed, though not universally.

When all other additional covariates were included in the model (Model II), the strength of the association between social media use and negative VoA diminished in several subgroups, such as those defined by gender, marital status, leisure activity engagement, and cognitive function. This attenuation indicates that the influence of social media use in these groups may be mediated or confounded by other factors.

By contrast, the association between social media use and negative PA appears to be stronger and more consistent across subgroups. In Model I, the coefficients range from 0.56 to 2.56, with the only exceptions for older adults of ethnic minorities and from Northeastern China. The non-significant association among ethnic minorities is likely attributable to a small sample size. After adjusting for all covariates (Model II), the associations remained statistically significant across all subgroups, with a modest reduction in effect sizes to a range of 0.46 to 2.09. Notably, the association became significant among older adults in the Northeast as well. These results suggest that social media use plays a broadly protective role in reducing negative PA, with this effect evident across nearly all demographic and social subgroups.

Table 21.4 examines the role of social media use based on its specific purposes. The results show that, regardless of purpose, social media use is generally associated with lower scores for both negative VoA and negative PA. This association

Table 21.2 Coefficients of having negative VoA and negative PA by social media use and covariates, 2020, CLASS

	Negative VoA		Negative PA	
	Model I	Model II	Model I	Model II
Overall use of social media (no)	−0.78***	−0.22*	−1.36***	−0.94***
Ages 75–85 (65–74)	0.25**	0.06	0.28**	0.07
Ages 85+ (65–74)	0.76***	0.25*	0.61***	0.11
Men (women)	0.11	0.19*	−0.22**	−0.02
Han ethnicity (minority)	0.23	−0.01	−0.15	−0.29+
Urban (rural)	0.00	0.03	−0.23**	0.39***
1–6 years of schooling (0)		0.20*		−0.03
7+ years of schooling (0)		0.02		−0.48***
Economically poor (no)		0.53***		0.01
Blue-collar occupation (white-collar)		0.22+		−0.10
Agricultural workers (white-collar)		−0.06		0.90***
Currently married (no)		0.00		−0.00
Having 2+ close family members (<2)		0.12		0.56***
Having 2+ close friends (<2)		−0.03		0.01
Freq. leisure and social activity (no)		−0.05		0.39***
Positive views on internet impact (0–8)		−0.23***		0.06**
Having 1+ diseases (no)		−0.03		0.36***
IADL disabled (no)		0.40***		0.03
ADL disabled (no)		0.62***		0.53***
Cognitively impaired (no)		0.52***		0.68***
Good self-rated health (no)		−0.47***		−0.89***
Central China (East China)	−1.34***	−1.27***	−0.59***	−0.60***
West China (East China)	−1.29***	−1.22***	0.22*	0.28*
Northeast China (East China)	−1.14***	−1.19***	1.29***	1.51***
Adj *R* square	0.031	0.066	0.044	0.084
Degree of freedom	9	24	9	24
No. of individuals	11,228	11,228	11,228	11,228

Note: (1) The results were based on the ordinary least square linear regression models. The category of a variable in the parentheses is the reference. (2) *VoA* views on aging, *PA* perceived aging, *ADL* activities of daily living, *IADL* instrumental ADL. (3) The score of negative VoA ranges from 7 to 35, whereas the score of negative PA ranges from 8 to 40. (4) The results for *WeChat, Douyin, Xigua Video*, and the number of media use are similar and thus not presented. (5) +$p < 0.1$, *$p < 0.05$, **$p < 0.01$, ***$p < 0.001$

remains significant in all cases except for the use of social media for travel-related purposes, where the effect becomes non-significant after adjusting for all study covariates. Notably, the impact of social media use is consistently stronger in reducing negative PA than in reducing negative VoA.

Table 21.3 Coefficients of having negative VoA and negative PA by social media use among different subgroups, 2020, CLASS

	Negative VoA		Negative PA	
Subgroups	Model I	Model II	Model I	Model II
Ages 65–74 (*N* = 4,264)	−0.77***	−0.36***	−1.22***	−0.97***
Ages 75+ (*N* = 6,964)	−0.61***	−0.03	−1.34***	−0.87***
Women (*N* = 5,554)	−0.84***	−0.17	−1.65***	−1.19***
Men (*N* = 5,674)	−0.72***	−0.26^{+}	−1.09***	−0.74***
Rural (*N* = 5,061)	−0.44**	0.08	−0.72***	−0.38*
Urban (*N* = 6,167)	−0.95***	−0.34*	−1.70***	−1.23***
Ethnic minorities (*N* = 672)	−0.40	0.11	−0.29	−0.17
Han majority (*N* = 10,556)	−0.80***	−0.25*	−1.41***	−0.97***
0–6 years of schooling (*N* = 7,271)	−1.02***	−0.52***	−1.03***	−0.76***
7+ years of schooling (*N* = 3,957)	−0.35*	0.11	−1.24***	−1.05***
Economically not poor (*N* = 9,937)	−0.81***	−0.24*	−1.34***	−0.97***
Economically poor (*N* = 1, 291)	−0.25	−0.04	−1.52***	−0.84*
White-collar job (*N* = 1,309)	−1.48***	−0.56*	−2.41***	−1.68***
Blue-collar /agriculture job (*N* = 9,919)	−0.61***	−0.13	−1.12***	−0.76***
Not married (*N* = 2,778)	−1.10***	−0.32	−1.82***	−1.37***
Married (*N* = 8,450)	−0.68***	−0.21^{+}	−1.24***	−0.87***
Having <2 close family members (*N* = 2,279)	−0.82***	−0.42^{+}	−2.51***	−2.09***
Having 2+ close family members (*N* = 8,949)	−0.76***	−0.14	−1.15***	−0.71***
Having <2 close friends (*N* = 3,300)	−0.79***	−0.43*	−2.56***	−2.18***
Having 2+ close friends (*N* = 7,928)	−0.78***	−0.13	−1.03***	−0.50***
Not freq. engag. in leisure activities (*N* = 1,889)	−0.49^{+}	−0.06	−0.56*	−0.46*
Freq. engagement in leisure activities (*N* = 9,339)	−0.79***	−0.23*	−1.51***	−0.96***
Less positive views on internet tech. (*N* = 3,058)	−0.98***	−0.75**	−2.00***	−1.48***
More positive views on internet tech. (*N* = 8,170)	−0.26*	−0.00	−1.03***	−0.69***
Having no disease condition (*N* = 2,200)	−0.07	−0.17	−1.22***	−0.66**
Having 1+ disease condition (*N* = 9,028)	−0.93***	−0.30***	−1.41***	−1.01***
IADL not disabled (*N* = 8,510)	−0.39***	−0.03	−0.99***	−0.71***
IADL disabled (*N* = 2,718)	−1.42***	−0.97***	−2.33***	−1.79***
ADL not disabled (*N* = 9,531)	−0.45***	−0.11	−1.10***	−0.83***
ADL disabled (*N* = 1,697)	−2.00***	−0.78*	−1.96***	−1.00***
Cognitively unimpaired (*N* = 7,816)	−0.41***	−0.13	−0.96***	−0.84***
Cognitively impaired (*N* = 3,412)	−0.85***	−0.27	−1.63***	−1.11***
Not-good self-rated health (*N* = 5,972)	−0.62***	−0.10	−1.09***	−0.78***
Good self-rated health (*N* = 5,256)	−0.68***	−0.29*	−1.38***	−1.04***
East China (*N* = 4,055)	−1.20***	−0.24	−1.69***	−0.71***
Central China (*N* = 2,883)	−0.86***	−0.49*	−1.24***	−1.02***
West China (*N* = 2,783)	−0.18	0.33	−1.23***	−0.96***
Northeast China (*N*= 1,507)	−0.28	0.31	−0.47	−0.75*

(continued)

Table 21.3 (continued)

Note: (1) The results were based on ordinary least square linear regression models. (2) Model I controls for demographic factors and region, whereas Model II controls for all factors in the table. (3) *VoA* views on aging, *PA* perceived aging. A less positive view of the impact of internet technology on society was defined by a score of 0–3, while a more positive view was indicated by a score of 4–8. (4) The score of negative views on aging ranges from 7 to 35, whereas the score of negative perceptions of aging ranges from 8 to 40. (5) +$p < 0.1$, *$p < 0.05$, **$p < 0.01$, ***$p < 0.001$

Table 21.4 Coefficients of having negative VoA and negative PA by the purposes of social media use, 2020, CLASS

	Negative VoA		Negative PA	
Purposes of social media use	Model I	Model II	Model I	Model II
Any type of social media use (no)	−0.78***	−0.22*	−1.36***	−0.94***
For contacting with family members/friends (no)	−0.90***	−0.34**	−1.20***	−0.75***
For reading /following-up news (no)	−0.47***	−0.34*	−1.23***	−1.03***
For entertainment (no)	−1.08***	−0.20+	−1.37***	−0.76***
For seeking information (no)	−0.95***	−0.31*	−2.47***	−2.10***
For online shopping (no)	−1.20***	−0.56***	−1.50***	−0.95***
For travel (no)	−0.82***	−0.03	−2.09***	−1.64***
For health management (no)	−1.34***	−0.64*	−2.42***	−2.04***

Note: (1) The results were based on ordinary least square linear regression models. (2) Model I controls for demographic factors and region, whereas Model II controls for all factors in the table. (3) Category in the parentheses of each purpose is its reference group, which includes non-users. (4) *VoA* views on aging, *PA* perceived aging. (5) The score of negative views on aging ranges from 7 to 35, whereas the score of negative perceptions of aging ranges from 8 to 40. (6) +$p < 0.1$, *$p < 0.05$, **$p < 0.01$, ***$p < 0.001$

21.4 Discussion

The present study offers empirical evidence on the relationship between social media use and older adults' subjective experiences of aging, with a specific focus on negative VoA and negative PA. Utilizing data from a large-scale, nationally representative survey in China, our analysis reveals that social media use is significantly associated with reductions in both negative VoA and PA, with a stronger effect observed for PA. Notably, these associations remain robust even after adjusting for a comprehensive set of demographic, socioeconomic, health-related, and psychosocial variables. Furthermore, the observed patterns hold consistently across different types of social media platforms. These findings provide valuable insights into the potential mechanisms and pathways through which digital engagement may contribute to more active and positive aging experiences.

21.4.1 Possible Mechanisms Linking Social Media Use to Perceived Aging and Active Aging

Several mechanisms may underlie the observed associations between social media use and reduced negative VoA and PA. First, social media platforms can serve as valuable sources of information, offering older adults' exposure to narratives and images that challenge traditional ageist stereotypes. By participating in online communities, viewing age-diverse content, and witnessing positive experiences of aging, users may internalize more positive self-perceived aging (Leist, 2013; Li, 2021; Wangler & Jansky, 2023).

Second, social media use can facilitate social connectedness, which has been shown to buffer against age-related stigma and decline. Older adults who use social media may benefit from maintaining relationships with family and friends, engaging in intergenerational communication, and expanding their social networks, all of which can enhance their sense of social inclusion and self-worth (Chopik, 2016; Cotten et al., 2013; He et al., 2024). Such relational interactions likely contribute to a more positive self-conception and lower the likelihood of internalizing negative stereotypes about aging.

Third, digital literacy and self-efficacy gained through social media use may foster a greater sense of agency and control, which are key components of active aging. As older adults become proficient in using technology, they may feel more competent and independent, thereby resisting societal narratives that portray aging as a time of inevitable decline (Schlomann et al., 2022; Nimrod, 2019; Wang & Gu, 2023a).

Notably, our findings indicate that the association between social media use negative PA seems stronger than the one between social media use and negative VoA. This may reflect the differing nature of these constructs. While VoA is more reflective of societal-level ageism and cultural scripts, PA encompasses self-directed evaluations about one's own aging process. As such, the personalized and interactive nature of social media may exert a more direct influence on PA, by providing users with positive feedback loops and identity reinforcement within their digital environments (Köttl et al., 2021; Mariano et al., 2021).

21.4.2 Subgroup Analysis: Interpretation of Key Findings

One unique contribution of this study is the subgroup analyses of the relationships between social media use and VoA and PA in 42 subgroups. The analyses reveal important nuances in the relationship between social media use and subjective aging experiences. With regard to negative VoA, the beneficial effect of social media use is broadly observed across demographic subgroups when only demographic variables are controlled for. However, in certain groups, namely, ethnic minorities, individuals with low economic status, those without diagnosed health conditions, and residents of Western and Northeastern China, the association is not statistically significant. These findings may point to differential access, use patterns, or digital inclusion challenges in these populations (Choi et al., 2020; Wang et al., 2024; CNNIC, 2025).

Among ethnic minorities, the non-significant results may reflect limited access to culturally relevant online content or lower levels of digital literacy (Wang & Gu, 2023b). Additionally, the small sample size in this subgroup may have limited statistical power. For individuals with low economic status, limited resources may restrict both the quantity and quality of digital engagement, reducing the potential benefits of social media use (Köttl et al., 2023). Similarly, in regions such as Western and Northeastern China, infrastructural barriers and lower levels of technological penetration may limit social media's influence on subjective experiences of aging (Zhang et al., 2024).

When controlling for all covariates, the strength of the association diminishes in subgroups defined by gender, marital status, leisure activity, and cognitive function. These findings suggest that the effects of social media use may be partially mediated or moderated by psychosocial engagement and cognitive capacity (Leist, 2013; Quinn, 2018). For instance, individuals who are already socially and cognitively active may derive less marginal benefit from social media use, as they possess alternative sources to enhance positive aging experiences (Xiang et al., 2025).

In contrast, the association between social media use and PA remains strong and statistically significant across nearly all subgroups, even after adjusting for all covariates. This consistent pattern underscores the potentially robust and universal impact of social media use on self-directed perceptions of aging. The emergence of significant associations in previously non-significant subgroups (e.g., older adults in the Northeast) after full adjustment may also indicate that once structural disadvantages are accounted for, the psychological benefits of digital engagement become evident (Nimrod, 2022; Li et al., 2025).

21.4.3 Purpose-specific Effects of Social Media Use

Analyses by different purposes of social media use further refine our understanding of how digital engagement influences aging experiences. Regardless of the reason for usage, such as social interaction, information-seeking, or entertainment, social media use is associated with lower scores for both negative VoA and PA. This reinforces the idea that even passive or non-social uses of digital media can contribute to more positive aging experiences (Bernardo et al., 2022; Kebede et al., 2022).

However, travel-related use stands out as an exception. The lack of significance in its association with negative VoA and PA after full adjustment suggests that such engagement may be more aspirational than impactful, particularly for older adults with physical or economic constraints. Unlike social or informational use, which directly fosters connection and competence, browsing travel content may evoke unattainable ideals that do not translate into improved self-perceptions (Chang et al., 2024).

21.4.4 Strengths and Limitations

This study has several strengths. It utilizes a large, representative sample with weighted analyses, enhancing the generalizability of findings to the broader older population. The inclusion of both negative VoA and PA allows for a more nuanced exploration of subjective aging experiences. Moreover, the use of multiple covariates, subgroup analyses, and purpose-specific models contributes to the robustness and specificity of the conclusions (Wang & Ware, 2013).

Nevertheless, several limitations must be acknowledged. First, the cross-sectional design precludes causal inference. While associations are significant, the directionality of the relationship remains uncertain. It is possible that individuals with more positive aging perceptions are more likely to use social media (Wang & Gu, 2023b). Second, self-report bias may affect measures of both social media use and aging experiences (Iverson et al., 2008). Third, despite controlling for a range of covariates, unmeasured confounders, such as personality traits or offline social support, may influence the results (Cheng et al., 2024).

Additionally, the lack of significant findings in certain subgroups highlights potential issues related to digital inequality. Differences in access, content relevance, and digital skills may limit the benefits of social media use for marginalized older adults, warranting further investigation.

21.4.5 Policy Implications and Future Research Directions

The findings of this study have several implications for policy and practice. First, initiatives aimed at enhancing digital inclusion among older adults, particularly those from disadvantaged or underrepresented groups, could serve as a means of promoting active and positive aging. Policies that support affordable internet access, digital literacy training, and age-inclusive content development may help to mitigate disparities in subjective aging experiences (Lee et al., 2025; Leist, 2013).

Second, social media platforms can play a proactive role by curating content that counters ageist stereotypes and showcases diverse aging narratives. Partnerships between government agencies, civil society, and tech companies could foster environments that affirm the dignity and potential of older users through creating and spreading more content against ageism (Levy et al., 2014; Han, 2019).

Third, social prescribing models that integrate digital engagement into health and social care planning deserve to be explored. For example, clinicians and social workers might encourage older adults to join online communities or participate in intergenerational digital programs as a form of psychosocial intervention (McKenna et al., 2025).

Future research should employ longitudinal and experimental designs to better establish causality and explore mechanisms in greater depth. Qualitative studies could provide insight into older adults' subjective experiences of social media use and its influence on self-perception. Furthermore, comparative studies across cultural contexts would help elucidate how societal norms toward aging and digitalization interact.

Lastly, a life course perspective should be integrated into future research, examining how prior exposure to technology and cumulative social experiences shape the trajectory of digital engagement and subjective aging experiences in later life.

21.4.6 Conclusions

Overall, this study adds to a growing body of literature highlighting the potential of digital technologies to promote well-being and resilience in later life. By demonstrating that social media use is significantly associated with reduced negative VoA and PA, particularly the latter, this chapter underscores the importance of fostering digital engagement as part of broader endeavors to enhance active aging. Efforts to ensure equitable access and culturally sensitive digital resources are essential to realizing these benefits across all segments of the aging population.

Acknowledgement The authors would like to thank the Research Center for Population & Development and the Institute of Gerontology, Renmin University for providing access to the China Longitudinal Aging and Social Survey (CLASS) dataset used in this chapter.

Disclaimer Views expressed in the chapter are solely those of the authors and do not necessarily reflect those of the United Nations, the National University of Singapore, and Shanghai University.

References

Bernardo, J., Apóstolo, J., Loureiro, R., Santana, E., Yaylagul, N. K., Dantas, C., et al. (2022). eHealth platforms to promote autonomous life and active aging: A scoping review. *International Journal of Environmental Research and Public Health, 19*(23), 15940.

Chang, F., Wang, G., & Gu, Z. (2024). Navigating challenges and opportunities in community-based interventions for promoting active aging: A systematic review of the roles of technology. *Innovation in Aging, 8*(10), igae077.

Cheng, X., Ge, T., & Cosco, T. D. (2024). Internet use and life satisfaction among Chinese older adults: The mediating effects of social interaction. *Current Psychology, 43*, 717–724.

China Internet Network Information Center (CNNIC). (2025). *The 55th statistical report on China's internet development*. https://www.cnnic.net.cn/n4/2025/0117/c88-11229.html [in Chinese].

Choi, E. Y., Kim, Y., Chipalo, E., & Lee, H. Y. (2020). Does perceived ageism widen the digital divide? And does it vary by gender? *The Gerontologist, 60*(7), 1213–1223.
Chopik, W. J. (2016). The benefits of social technology use among older adults are mediated by reduced loneliness. *Cyberpsychology, Behavior, and Social Networking, 19*(9), 551–556.
Cotten, S. R., Ford, G., Ford, S., & Hale, T. M. (2013). Impact of Internet use on loneliness and contact with others among older adults: Cross-sectional analysis. *Journal of Medical Internet Research, 15*(2), e39.
Dong, T., Zhu, Z., Guo, M., Du, P., & Wu, B. (2019). Association between dying experience and place of death: Urban–rural differences among older Chinese adults. *Journal of Palliative Medicine, 22*(11), 1386–1393.
Han, M. C. (2019). Social media commerce: Next frontier in online shopping focused on Chinese consumers. *Global Business & Finance Review, 24*(1), 80–93.
He, L., Adnan, H. B. M., Fauzi, A., et al. (2024). The effect of social media engagement on social integration of elderly migrants in China: The mechanism of perceived social support and psychological resilience. *Humanities and Social Sciences Communications, 11*, 1100.
Hu, M., Han, S., Ghorbany, S., & Zhang, K. (2024). Healthy aging in place with the aid of smart technologies: A systematic review. *Encyclopedia, 4*(4), 1918–1932.
Hunsaker, A., & Hargittai, E. (2018). A review of Internet use among older adults. *New Media & Society, 20*(10), 3937–3954.
Iverson, S. A., Howard, K. B., & Penney, B. K. (2008). Impact of internet use on health-related behaviors and the patient-physician relationship: A survey-based study and review. *Journal of the American Osteopathic Association, 108*(12), 699–711.
Jin, Y., & Zhao, M. (2019). Internet access and the elderly's active aging in China—A study based on 2016 China Longitudinal Aging Social Survey. *Population Journal, 6*, 44–55. [in Chinese].
Juárez, M. A. R., González, V. M., & Favela, J. (2016). Effect of technology on aging perception. *Health Informatics Journal, 24*(2), 171–181.
Kebede, A. S., Ozolins, L.-L., Holst, H., & Galvin, K. (2022). Digital engagement of older adults: Scoping review. *Journal of Medical Internet Research, 24*(12), e40192.
Köttl, H., Allen, L. D., Mannheim, I., & Ayalon, L. (2023). Associations between everyday ICT usage and (self-)ageism: A systematic literature review. *The Gerontologist, 63*(7), 1172–1187.
Köttl, H., Cohn-Schwartz, E., & Ayalon, L. (2021). Self-perceptions of aging and everyday ICT engagement: A test of reciprocal associations. *Journals of Gerontology Social Sciences, 76*(9), 1913–1922.
Lee, A. R., Liu, D., & Yue, Y. (2025). Empowering China's older adults through online learning: Media literacy and its influence on well-being. *Educational Gerontology*, 1–17.
Leist, A. K. (2013). Social media use of older adults: A mini-review. *Gerontology, 59*(4), 378–384.
Levy, B. R., Chung, P. H., Bedford, T., & Navrazhina, K. (2014). Facebook as a site for negative age stereotypes. *The Gerontologist, 54*(2), 172–176.
Li, K. (2021). The media image of Chinese older people: From stigmatic stereotype to diverse self-representation. *Global Media and China, 6*(3), 281–302.
Li, P.-Q., Sun, G.-Y., Zhao, X.-X., Hu, Z.-X., & Gan, K.-P. (2025). Internet use and self-rated health among Chinese older adults: The role of social engagement and social support. *Frontiers in Public Health, 12*, Article 1504940.
Mariano, J., Marques, S., Ramos, M. R., & de Vries, H. (2021). Cognitive functioning mediates the relationship between self-perceptions of aging and computer use behavior in late adulthood: Evidence from two longitudinal studies. *Computers in Human Behavior, 121*, 106807–106807.
McKenna, B., Cai, W., & Yoon, H. (2025). Chinese older adults' social media use: A study of WeChat from a social practice perspective. *Information Technology & People, 38*(1), 363–379.
Nimrod, G. (2019). Aging well in the digital age: Technology in processes of selective optimization with compensation. *The Journals of Gerontology Series B: Psychological Sciences and Social Sciences, 75*(9), 2008–2017.
Nimrod, G. (2022). Technostress in a hostile world: Older internet users before and during the COVID-19 pandemic. *Aging & Mental Health, 26*(3), 526–533.

Quinn, K. (2018). Cognitive effects of social media use: A case of older adults. *Social Media + Society, 4*(3), 1–9.

Schlomann, A., Memmer, N., & Wahl, H. W. (2022). Awareness of age-related change is associated with attitudes toward technology and technology skills among older adults. *Frontiers in Psychology, 13*, 905043.

Wang, K., Chen, X., Gu, D., Smith, B. D., Dong, Y., & Peet, J. Z. (2024). Examining first and second-level digital divide at the intersection of race/ethnicity, gender, and socioeconomic status: An analysis of the National Health and Aging Trends Study. *The Gerontologist, 64*(gnae079), 1–11.

Wang, K., & Gu, D. (2023a, November 8–12). Does internet use promote older adults' self-perception of aging: Separating within- and between-person effects. In *Paper presented at the 2023 annual meeting of the Gerontological Society of America*.

Wang, K., & Gu, D. (2023b). Reciprocal associations between social media use and self-perception of aging among older adults: Do men and women differ? *Social Science & Medicine, 321*, 115786.

Wang, R., & Ware, J. H. (2013). Detecting moderator effects using subgroup analyses. *Prevention Science, 14*(2), 111–120.

Wangler, J., & Jansky, M. (2023). Media portrayal of old age and its effects on attitudes in older people: Findings from a series of studies. *Humanities and Social Sciences Communications, 10*, 165.

Xiang, S., Deng, Q., & Chen, B. (2025). Relationship between Internet use and offline leisure activities among Chinese older adult people: A moderated mediation model. *Frontiers in Public Health, 12*, 1458413.

Zhang, C., Zhang, Y., & Wang, Y. (2024). A study on Internet use and subjective well-being among Chinese older adults: based on CGSS (2012–2018) five-wave mixed interface survey data. *Frontiers in Public Health, 11*, 1277789.

Section V
Prospects and Conclusions

Chapter 22
Promoting ICT Use and Healthy Aging in the Digital Era

Qiushi Feng, Danan Gu, Kun Wang, and Hee Yun Lee

The rapid advancement of information and communication technologies (ICT) amidst the unfolding Fourth Industrial Revolution presents profound opportunities and challenges for older adults. The digital revolution has transformed modern societies, offering unprecedented opportunities for communication, health management, and social participation. However, despite the potential benefits, many older adults still face challenges in accessing and effectively using ICT due to financial constraints, lack of training, and age-related usability barriers. There has been increasing recognition on the importance of ICT use among older people and the need for inclusiveness to ensure that all older individuals can benefit from digital technology. Such an all-inclusive manner is crucial in the context of the ongoing industrial revolution for older adults to fully participate in the digital transformation of our world. By providing access to digital skills, cutting-edge technologies, and inclusive design, older people can actively participate in the digital economy, contribute to society, and improve their quality of life. This chapter summarizes key insights on promoting ICT use and healthy aging reviewed and discussed in the

Q. Feng (✉)
Centre for Family and Population Research/Department of Sociology and Anthropology, National University of Singapore, Singapore, Singapore

D. Gu
Population Division, UN Department of Economic and Social Affairs, New York, NY, USA
e-mail: gudanan@yahoo.com

K. Wang
Department of Social Work, College of Arts and Sciences, University of Alabama at Birmingham, Birmingham, AL, USA
e-mail: kw2@uab.edu

H. Y. Lee
School of Social Work, University of Georgia, Athens, GA, USA
e-mail: heeyunlee@uga.edu

K. Wang et al. (eds.), *ICT Use and Healthy Longevity*, Advances in Studies of Aging and Health 5, https://doi.org/10.1007/978-3-031-98964-3_22

preceding chapters and outlines prospects for future research. We believe, when promoting ICT use among older people in an all-inclusive manner, the following key aspects should be emphasized: (1) accessibility and affordability; (2) digital literacy, skill development and support, and lifelong learning; (3) user-centered and age-friendly designs; (4) digital divide and social inclusion; (5) adaptability and usability across contexts; (6) innovation and entrepreneurship among older adults; (7) gains in health and well-being; (8) privacy and security; and (9) supportive ecosystems.

22.1 An Overview of the Key Findings of the Book

This book explores the intersection of ICT, particularly use of the internet and social media, and healthy aging, drawing insights from empirical studies conducted across various global contexts. Organized into five thematic sections, it addresses foundational concepts, digital inequalities, links to behavior and health, cognitive and psychosocial outcomes, and the broader implications for aging experiences and policies. The chapters of this book collectively emphasize how digital technologies can promote cognitive, emotional, and social well-being among older adults, highlighting the persistent disparities and structural challenges that confront digital inclusion.

The first section establishes the theoretical base and empirical backdrop for understanding ICT's role in aging. Chapter 1 defines healthy aging as a holistic process encompassing physical, mental, and social well-being, rooted in frameworks like the WHO's *Decade of Healthy Ageing*. It highlights ICT's potential to support the autonomy of older adults and enhance their social inclusion. Chapter 2 maps global trends and patterns of ICT use, showing that older adults remain digitally disadvantaged, particularly in low-income regions, where limited infrastructure and affordability remain barriers. Chapter 3 synthesizes theoretical models such as the Senior Technology Acceptance Model (STAM) to explain digital engagement. These theories emphasize that motivation, self-efficacy, and perceived utility significantly shape older adults' technology adoption. Chapter 4 reviews empirical evidence linking ICT use to healthy aging outcomes. While health benefits are noted in cognitive, emotional, and social domains, it is concluded that disparities in access and methodological limitations persist, especially among the oldest-old and underrepresented populations.

The second section explores structural and demographic disparities in digital access and engagement. Chapter 5 focuses on African American older adults, identifying gender and age-specific patterns, such as depression reducing men in ICT use, whereas physical limitations affecting women. Chapter 6 examines correlates of internet use among older Chinese adults, highlighting the roles of education, urban residence, and health, with socioeconomic status mediating many disparities. Chapter 7 offers a rare cross-cultural comparison of welfare technology use in Korea and the United States, showing that trust, collectivism, and cultural norms shape usage. Chapter 8 expands this view through multinational comparisons (Brazil, China, India, Singapore, Europe, the United States), revealing that education, social network, and urbanization are consistent predictors of digital engagement, though national contexts can mediate outcomes. Chapter 9 categorizes barriers of ICT use in China into access, knowledge, and skill gaps, especially among rural, cognitively impaired, or economically disadvantaged older adults. Chapters 10 and 11 analyze digital divides in the United States, showing that while access has improved among racial minorities, disparities in usage, especially for health and social purposes, remain, and are often shaped by intersecting disadvantages in race, income, and education.

The third section, including Chapters 12 and 13, further assesses how underserved populations use ICT to seek health information. In rural Alabama, as shown by Chapter 12, technology access alone was insufficient; social media use, not device ownership, predicted health information-seeking. Similarly, in rural Vietnam, as discussed in Chapter 13, usage was low and shaped by gender, marital status, and prior healthcare behaviors. Chapter 14 details the various purposes for which older Chinese adults use social media, ranging from chatting to information seeking, demonstrating stratified patterns by gender, region, and education. Chapter 15 finds a reciprocal relationship between self-perceptions of aging and technology use, with gender moderating the strength and direction of effects. These findings underscore that digital inclusion is not just about access of technology but also about context, literacy, and trust of older users.

The fourth section highlights ICT's cognitive and emotional value as well as how ICT shapes subjective experiences of aging. Chapters 16–18 consistently show that ICT access, usage frequency, and diversity are linked to better cognitive outcomes, with depression and perceived control mediating these effects. These findings support the view that ICT is not just a cognitive stimulus but also a psychological resource that fosters autonomy and resilience in later life. Chapters 19 and 20 introduced how social media use is associated with better self-rated health and higher subjective well-being in China, respectively, particularly among rural residents, women, and the less educated. In this regard, using ICT for health seeking or information purposes tends to be more beneficial than for shopping or entertainment purposes. Chapter 21 further shows that social media users report more positive views on aging and lower perceived burden of aging, especially among those with physical or cognitive limitations. These findings highlight ICT's potential to support a more empowered, connected aging experience.

Together, these chapters of this book demonstrate that while social media and broader ICT use hold great potential to support healthy aging, benefits are unevenly distributed. Factors such as socioeconomic status, gender, geographic location, and cultural values all shape how older adults engage with and benefit from digital tools. The book underscores the importance of inclusive digital policies, targeted interventions, and culturally sensitive and age-friendly designs in fostering equitable access to digital health resources and promoting well-being among older populations globally.

22.2 Policy Recommendations: Ways Froward

As societies grapple with the profound demographic shifts of population aging and rapid technological advancement, ensuring the digital inclusion of older adults has become a policy imperative, an issue of social justice. This book has attested that ICTs hold considerable promises for enhancing the health, autonomy, and quality of life of older people across various cultural and socioeconomic contexts. However, realizing this potential requires strategic, inclusive, and context-sensitive policies. Drawing on the insights from across the previous chapters, we outline nine key areas for future action.

22.2.1 Accessibility and Affordability

A foundational step toward inclusive ICT engagement is to ensure that older adults have access to affordable and appropriate digital technology. Multiple chapters, including those focused on global adoption trends (Chapter 2) and digital inequality in China and the United States (Chapters 6, 9, and 10), have highlighted cost as a key barrier, and this is especially true for low-income regions and among marginalized populations, where device costs, internet service fees, and infrastructural deficits remain prohibitive.

Policies must prioritize subsidized access to devices and broadband for older individuals in need, especially those living in rural or underserved communities. Public-private partnerships, such as low-cost tablet distribution or municipal broadband initiatives, have shown promise in narrowing these gaps (UNESCO, 2022). Moreover, universal service frameworks should explicitly recognize older adults as a vulnerable group in digital infrastructure planning.

22.2.2 Digital Literacy, Skill Development, and Lifelong Learning

Digital literacy is a basic condition for older adults to adopt ICT. As shown in Chapters 4 and 9, skill and knowledge deficits often surpass access barriers among older non-users. Even among users, limited digital confidence can inhibit meaningful engagement. More importantly, digital literacy is not a one-time achievement but a continuum of learning, especially as technologies evolve. Thus, the efforts to promote digital literacy must be continuous as a part of lifelong learning (Mo et al., 2025).

Governments and civil societies should develop community-based, intergenerational learning programs that offer hands-on, culturally appropriate training programs for older people to master digital tools. Importantly, these skill development programs must go beyond basic instruction to include teaching on privacy, cybersecurity, and application of digital skills to health, finance, and social participation (Charness & Boot, 2009). Lifelong learning platforms, especially when integrated into libraries, community centers, or aging services, are recommended, which can foster continued digital growth.

22.2.3 User-Centered and Age-Friendly Design

Older adults face physical, cognitive, and sensory changes that make interaction with standard digital interfaces challenging. In this regard, Chapters 3 and 14 underscore the importance of design tailored to aging users, emphasizing the need for accessible font sizes, simplified navigation, voice control, and error-forgiving interfaces.

Policy can support age-inclusive innovation by promoting design guidelines such as the Web Content Accessibility Guidelines and by funding co-design initiatives where older adults collaborate directly with technology developers (Marston et al., 2020). Regulatory standards could mandate usability audits for government and public service apps to ensure their accessibility to older users.

22.2.4 Digital Divide and Social Inclusion

The vulnerability of older adults has been featuring the digital divide in our time. Digital exclusion among older adults exacerbates existing social inequalities and leads to social isolation in later life. Chapters 5, 7, and 11 show that intersectional factors, such as gender, race, ethnicity, and socioeconomic status, compound digital marginalization of older adults.

Policy must target the social dimensions of the digital divide by supporting outreach to the most excluded subpopulations among older adults. This includes translating content into minority languages, fostering culturally tailored support systems, and enabling peer-support networks. Additionally, promoting digital platforms that connect older adults to friends, family, and communities, as evidenced in Chapters 14 and 20 can enhance social inclusion and combat loneliness, and should be considered as a necessary part of the general population health policies.

22.2.5 Adaptability and Usability Across Contexts

A basic principle learnt from previous chapters is that the one-size-fits-all approach is insufficient in addressing the diversity of aging populations in ICT adoption. As shown in Chapters 8 and 13, rural and urban environments require different strategies of promoting ICT use due to varying infrastructure and user needs. Usability also varies based on individual capabilities and purposes, such as whether the user is to manage chronic illness, maintain social connections, or seek employment.

Adaptability issue is thus essential in policy and product design. Cross-national case studies in Chapters 6–8 have provided rich data for benchmarking and adapting successful strategies across borders. Good practices could include promoting modular and scalable technologies that can be customized for different needs, and flexible funding models that support both broadband and mobile-first solutions.

22.2.6 Innovation and Entrepreneurship Among Older Adults

Far from being passive ICT users, older adults can be innovators, entrepreneurs, and contributors in the digital economy. However, few policies nowadays actively foster their participation. Chapter 3 calls attention to activity and self-efficacy theories that frame older adults as capable agents of change. There should be no doubt that older adults could join the young people as active agents in creating the digital era together.

Along this line, public programs should invest in "silver innovation" by funding startups led by or serving older populations and by including older adults in hackathons, technology incubators, and product testing initiatives. Research by the OECD (2020) has highlighted how older entrepreneurship boosts local economies and promotes intergenerational knowledge exchange.

22.2.7 Gains in Health and Well-Being

Chapters 16–20 in this volume demonstrates strong associations between ICT use and improved self-rated health, cognitive performance, and subjective well-being. Purposeful ICT use, particularly for health management, information-seeking, and connectedness, correlates with reduced loneliness in later life and a stronger sense of aging well (see Chapter 21).

Policy frameworks should incentivize the application and integration of digital health tools tailored to older adults, including telehealth, remote monitoring, and medication management platforms. Training caregivers and healthcare providers in digital inclusion strategies can further amplify these tools' effectiveness. Health insurance plans and related government programs might consider reimbursing digital literacy programs as preventive health interventions.

22.2.8 *Privacy and Safety*

As shown in Chapters 2 and 12, older adults are especially vulnerable to online fraud, misinformation, and privacy breaches due to their limited digital literacy and skills, which can erode their trust in technology and thus discourage use. As they become more engaged with digital platforms, robust protection is critical to protect them from possible harms.

Governments must enforce stronger privacy and data protection standards while ensuring these are understandable and transparent to older users. Legal frameworks like the General Data Protection Regulation in the European Union offer a starting point. Additionally, fraud prevention programs and accessible reporting mechanisms should be part of any digital literacy curriculum in the related training.

22.2.9 *Supportive Ecosystems*

Promoting digital inclusion among older adults requires a multisectoral approach. No single actor, government, market, or civil society can address the issue alone. Chapters throughout the book stress the value of partnerships that span medicine, public health, education, urban planning, technology development, and elder services.

National digital strategies aimed to promote inclusiveness should coordinate efforts across ministries, embed digital equity in urban and rural planning, and encourage collaboration with NGOs and tech companies. Community organizations can play a pivotal role in implementation of these initiatives, but they need sustained localized funding and capacity-building support (Gallistl et al., 2020).

22.3 Future Research Directions

While significant progress has been made in understanding the relationship between ICT and aging populations, several critical gaps remain that warrant further investigation. One key area is the long-term effects of ICT use on cognitive decline, social connectivity, and mental health. Although short-term benefits such as improved communication and access to health information have been documented in current literature, there is limited empirical evidence on how sustained ICT engagement influences the progression of cognitive impairments or contributes to emotional well-being over long time among older adults.

Another vital avenue for future research is the cultural variation in technology adoption, particularly in low- and middle-income countries (LMICs). Most existing studies are based on high-income nations, potentially overlooking how socioeconomic, educational, and infrastructural disparities affect the uptake and outcomes of

ICT use among older adults in other settings. Furthermore, the intersectional barriers that influence technology access and usability require closer attention. Factors such as gender, health, literacy, and socioeconomic status often intersect to exacerbating digital exclusion of older adults, which deserve more studies to identify the most vulnerable subgroups within aging populations.

Finally, the development and deployment of ethical artificial intelligence (AI) applications for older adults represent an emerging frontier in this field. Research should explore not only technological feasibility but also ethical concerns, including privacy, autonomy, and potential biases. Inclusive design processes that engage older adults in the creation and evaluation of AI tools will be essential for ensuring technologies serve their intended purpose effectively and respectfully.

22.4 Conclusions

Promoting ICT use among older adults is a complex, multifactorial endeavor that necessitates a holistic, interdisciplinary approach. It requires coordinated attention to diverse yet interconnected domains, including access, affordability, digital literacy, inclusive design, social inclusion, adaptability, health applications, data privacy, and supportive policy frameworks. Despite the multiple aspects of promoting ICT use, one consensus is that as the global population ages, digital equity must become a central pillar of healthy aging initiatives.

To ensure that technology acts as a bridge rather than a barrier, stakeholders, including governments, technology developers, healthcare providers, educators, and community organizations, must collaborate in building inclusive, responsive digital ecosystems. This includes promoting digital access to all older adults, designing technologies that evolve with users' changing needs, offering ongoing digital skills training, protecting older adults from online frauds and privacy breaches, and incorporating older adults in every stage of technology development and deployment.

Future research should prioritize longitudinal studies to understand sustained ICT impacts over time, the scalability of community-based interventions, and the development of ethical, human-centered AI solutions. A life-course approach that recognizes the cumulative effects of social and digital disadvantage is also essential. Ultimately, ensuring older adults are not only passive consumers of digital technology but empowered co-creators of digital futures will determine the success of inclusive innovation in the era of the Fourth Industrial Revolution. The challenge is significant, but so too is the opportunity for transformation towards a better digital world of ours.

Disclaimer Views expressed in the chapter are solely those of the authors and do not necessarily reflect those of the National University of Singapore, the United Nations, the University of Alabama at Birmingham, and the University of Georgia.

References

Charness, N., & Boot, W. R. (2009). Aging and information technology use: Potential and barriers. *Current Directions in Psychological Science, 18*(5), 253–258.

Gallistl, V., Rohner, R., Seifert, A., & Wanka, A. (2020). Configuring the older non-user: Between research, policy and practice of digital exclusion. *Social Inclusion, 8*(2), 233–243.

Marston, H. R., Shore, L., & White, P. J. (2020). How does a (smart) age-friendly ecosystem look in a post-pandemic society? *International Journal of Environmental Research and Public Health, 17*(21), 8276.

Mo, Y., Liu, Y., Yeung, W. J., Koh, W. P., Gu, D., & Feng, Q. (2025). From digital divide to digital equality: The role of learning in older Singaporeans. *Journal of Gerontology: Social Sciences, 80*(7), gbaf090.

Organization for Economic Co-operation and Development (OECD). (2020). *The silver economy as a pathway for growth: Insights from the OECD-GCOA global silver economy forum*. OECD Publishing. https://apo.org.au/sites/default/files/resource-files/2014-06/apo-nid62476.pdf

United Nations Educational, Scientific and Cultural Organization (UNESCO). (2022). *Guidelines for digital inclusion of older persons*. https://unesdoc.unesco.org/ark:/48223/pf0000381629

Chapter 23
Conclusions: Charting Inclusive Digital Futures for Healthy Aging

Kun Wang, Hee Yun Lee, Qiushi Feng, and Danan Gu

The accelerating pace of digital transformation, fueled by the Fourth Industrial Revolution, has coincided with a dramatic global demographic shift: the rapid aging of populations across high-, middle-, and low-income countries. In this context, the intersection between information and communication technologies (ICTs) and aging is not simply a matter of obtaining access and gaining convenience, adoption of ICTs has become a critical determinant of health, equity, and social participation. This book, *ICT Use and Healthy Longevity: Empirical Data and Perspectives*, has brought together an international group of scholars to examine how older adults engage with digital technologies and how such engagement influences their physical, cognitive, emotional, and social well-being. By drawing on evidence from diverse national and cultural contexts, the chapters offer an integrated understanding of both the transformative potential of ICTs for older populations and the persistent inequalities that must be addressed to achieve digital inclusion.

Across the chapters, several major themes have emerged. First, digital technologies are clearly linked to healthy aging outcomes. Older adults who engage with the

K. Wang (✉)
Department of Social Work, College of Arts and Sciences, University of Alabama at Birmingham, Birmingham, AL, USA
e-mail: kw2@uab.edu

H. Y. Lee
School of Social Work, University of Georgia, Athens, GA, USA
e-mail: heeyunlee@uga.edu

Q. Feng
Centre for Family and Population Research/Department of Sociology and Anthropology, National University of Singapore, Singapore, Singapore
e-mail: socfq@nus.edu.sg

D. Gu
Population Division, UN Department of Economic and Social Affairs, New York, NY, USA
e-mail: gudanan@yahoo.com

K. Wang et al. (eds.), *ICT Use and Healthy Longevity*, Advances in Studies of Aging and Health 5, https://doi.org/10.1007/978-3-031-98964-3_23

internet and social media tend to report better cognitive performance, higher levels of subjective well-being, reduced loneliness, and a stronger sense of autonomy and control. These outcomes are well-evidenced, reflecting the role of ICTs as both cognitive and psychosocial resources. For example, engaging in diverse online activities such as information-seeking, managing finances, communicating with family, and learning new skills can support cognitive stimulation and maintain mental sharpness. Similarly, the ability to maintain social ties through digital platforms can mitigate feelings of isolation and enhance life satisfaction.

However, these benefits are not experienced equally by all older adults. A second major theme is the continuing digital divide. While improvements in access are evident in many high income countries, especially among young-old adults, large gaps remain in lower income regions and among groups facing structural disadvantages. The studies in this volume, including those from China, the United States, Vietnam, and Brazil, show that education, income, gender, rural or urban residence, health conditions, and ethnicity all play important roles in shaping access to and engagement with digital technologies. Even when access is available, older adults differ widely in their digital skills, confidence, and ability to use ICTs effectively. Those with higher socioeconomic status are more likely to use ICTs in active and purposeful ways, such as managing their health and accessing information. By contrast, those with fewer resources are more likely to use digital tools for entertainment or passive consumption.

These differences in usage patterns contribute to a third and equally important dimension of inequality: unequal outcomes from ICT engagement. As the evidence in this book shows, older adults who use digital technologies to maintain social relationships or manage their health often experience measurable benefits. By contrast, those whose use is limited to passive entertainment may not enjoy the same advantages and in some cases may even experience increased stress or loneliness. This distinction highlights the need for inclusive policies and programs that go beyond improving access. To ensure that all older adults can benefit from digital transformation, it is essential to strengthen digital literacy, support meaningful forms of engagement, and address the broader social and structural barriers that limit digital participation among disadvantaged groups.

Another central insight is the importance of context. Technology use among older adults cannot be fully understood without reference to the cultural, institutional, and policy environments in which it occurs. Studies from the United States and Korea highlight how socio-cultural values, such as individualism, collectivism, or trust in government, influence not just whether older adults use welfare technologies, but how they evaluate their usefulness and risks. Similarly, research in rural Alabama and Vietnam underscores that digital inclusion involves more than distributing devices, requiring culturally grounded outreach, health literacy, and trusted intermediaries who can bridge gaps in digital trust and competence.

Throughout the volume, digital engagement is also shown to be closely related to how older adults view themselves and their aging process. Older adults who use digital tools often develop more positive self-perceptions of aging and lower levels of perceived aging-related burden. Social media users report feeling less useless and more connected to others, and these perceptions are especially pronounced among those with cognitive or physical limitations. These findings support the notion that digital inclusion not only is about technical skills, but also shapes identity, belonging, and empowerment.

In translating these findings into actionable strategies, the volume highlights several policy directions. Ensuring affordable access to digital tools and broadband is a foundational first step, especially in rural areas and for low-income groups. Subsidized programs, public-private partnerships, and universal service policies must explicitly consider older adults as priority. Yet access alone is not enough. Older adults need ongoing opportunities to build digital literacy and confidence. This requires community-based, culturally tailored education programs that move beyond basic skills to include training of digital safety, the application of technology to daily life, and opportunities for lifelong learning. Intergenerational training models, libraries, and senior centers all play important roles in creating supportive environments for digital learning.

Design also matters. Technologies must be user-centered and age-friendly, accommodating age-related changes in vision, cognition, and dexterity. Inclusive design standards should be mainstreamed into both public and commercial platforms, and older adults should be actively involved in the co-design process. Policymakers should conduct usability audits and provide age-inclusive innovation grants to ensure that older adults are not marginalized in product development.

Broader systems of support are essential. Governments, civil organizations, health providers, and technology companies all have a role to play in building ecosystems that support digital aging. National digital strategies should coordinate across sectors and include measurable goals for digital inclusion among older adults. At the same time, local implementation must be adequately funded and adapted to community needs. Innovations in digital health, including telemedicine and remote monitoring, should be integrated with aging services and supported through health insurance or government subsidies.

Importantly, ethical concerns must be addressed. Older adults are disproportionately targeted by scams and often struggle to navigate complex privacy settings. Ensuring trust in digital systems requires not only strong legal protections but also clear, user-friendly communication of rights and risks. The growing integration of artificial intelligence (AI) into health and social care introduces new ethical challenges around autonomy, bias, and consent. Older adults must not be passive recipients of these tools but be encouraged to active participate in shaping their digital future.

As the global population ages and digital technologies continue to evolve, research must keep pace. Longitudinal studies are needed to assess the long-term impacts of ICT use on cognitive health, emotional well-being, and social integration. More studies are also needed from low- and middle-income countries (LMIC) to understand how different structural and cultural conditions shape older adults' access and engagement with digital technologies. Intersectional research that considers how gender, age, health, race, and income interact is crucial for designing equitable interventions. The field must also explore emerging technologies, such as AI and virtual reality, and assess their potential to support or undermine healthy aging.

Ultimately, the findings in this volume lead to a single, urgent conclusion: healthy longevity in the digital age requires inclusive innovations. Technology must be seen not just as a tool for efficiency, but as a means of advancing equity, dignity, and opportunity for older people. It must be designed and governed in ways that reflect the diverse realities of aging, and older adults themselves must be included in this work not merely as users, but as co-creators of the digital future.

In this rapidly changing world, leaving older adults behind is not an option. Building a future where they are empowered, connected, and thriving in digital societies is not only possible but also essential.

Disclaimer Views expressed in the chapter are solely those of the authors and do not necessarily reflect those of the University of Alabama at Birmingham, the University of Georgia, the National University of Singapore, and the United Nations.

MIX
Papier aus verantwortungsvollen Quellen
Paper from responsible sources
FSC® C105338

If you have any concerns about our products,
you can contact us on
ProductSafety@springernature.com

In case Publisher is established outside the EU,
the EU authorized representative is:
Springer Nature Customer Service Center GmbH
Europaplatz 3, 69115 Heidelberg, Germany

Printed by Libri Plureos GmbH
in Hamburg, Germany

Lecture Notes in Energy

Volume 30

Lecture Notes in Energy (LNE) is a series that reports on new developments in the study of energy: from science and engineering to the analysis of energy policy. The series' scope includes but is not limited to, renewable and green energy, nuclear, fossil fuels and carbon capture, energy systems, energy storage and harvesting, batteries and fuel cells, power systems, energy efficiency, energy in buildings, energy policy, as well as energy-related topics in economics, management and transportation. Books published in LNE are original and timely and bridge between advanced textbooks and the forefront of research. Readers of LNE include postgraduate students and non-specialist researchers wishing to gain an accessible introduction to a field of research as well as professionals and researchers with a need for an up-to-date reference book on a well-defined topic. The series publishes single and multi-authored volumes as well as advanced textbooks.

More information about this series at http://www.springer.com/series/8874

George Giannakidis · Maryse Labriet
Brian Ó Gallachóir · GianCarlo Tosato
Editors

Informing Energy and Climate Policies Using Energy Systems Models

Insights from Scenario Analysis Increasing the Evidence Base

Springer

Editors
George Giannakidis
Laboratory for Energy Systems Analysis
Center for Renewable Energy Sources
Pikermi, Attiki
Greece

Brian Ó Gallachóir
Environmental Research Institute
University College Cork
Cork
Ireland

Maryse Labriet
Eneris Environment Energy Consultants
Madrid
Spain

GianCarlo Tosato
ASATREM
Rome
Italy

ISSN 2195-1284 ISSN 2195-1292 (electronic)
Lecture Notes in Energy
ISBN 978-3-319-16539-4 ISBN 978-3-319-16540-0 (eBook)
DOI 10.1007/978-3-319-16540-0

Library of Congress Control Number: 2015933834

Springer Cham Heidelberg New York Dordrecht London

Printed on acid-free paper

Springer International Publishing AG Switzerland is part of Springer Science+Business Media (www.springer.com)

Foreword

Climate change mitigation and transformation to a global low-carbon economy is a pressing issue in policy discussions and international negotiations. The political debate is supported by the scientific community through a wide range of projections, pathway simulations, and scenario analyses of the global energy system and its development over the next decades. Achieving balance between economic competitiveness and the need to respond to climate change threats and to ensure energy security constitutes a significant challenge policy makers face today.

Efforts to develop energy models began back in the 1960s but it was the first oil crisis in 1973 that highlighted the need for analytical tools to inform strategies and sparkled the development of energy models as instruments aiming to contribute to informed decision-making in energy policy planning. ETSAP[1] was one of the multilateral technology initiatives (formally called Implementing Agreements, or 'IAs') initiated in 1976 under the aegis of the International Energy Agency, IEA, with the aim of carrying out a joint program of energy technology systems analysis. The IEA through its broad range of Implementing Agreements and the Energy Technology Network enables member and nonmember countries, businesses, industries, international organizations, and nongovernmental organizations to share research on technology-related activity that supports energy security, economic growth, environmental protection, and engagement worldwide.

ETSAP evolved from the analysis of existing tools to evaluate R&D strategies in its first year of operation to the combination of the energy flow optimization approach with macroeconomic top-down modeling, technology learning, and stochastic modeling. Today, ETSAP is a unique network of energy modeling teams from approximately 70 countries involving 177 institutions over the world, well beyond the number of its contracting parties, which are the governments of 18 countries and the European Commission.

[1] Energy Technology Systems Analysis Program.

ETSAP's objective was (and still is) to build, maintain, and expand modeling capability in order to assist and support government officials and decision makers in creating the robustness of the evidence base underpinning energy and environmental policy issues by applying these tools for energy technology assessment and analysis. ETSAP developed through cooperation the MARKAL (MARKet ALlocation) and subsequently the TIMES (The Integrated Markal-Efom System) energy systems model generators.

These bottom-up technoeconomic models have been used in Global models like the IEA Energy Technology Perspective model, the global TIMES Integrated Assessment Model and the Global TIMES model of the European Fusion Development Agreement. At national and regional levels, MARKAL-TIMES models for countries in all continents as well as the Pan-European TIMES model were also developed. The latter was used for the evaluation of the RES Directives implementation in EU27 for 2020, an analysis of the future European gas supply, the interplay between the global goal of mitigating climate change and the European goal of reducing dependence and vulnerability of the energy system, the transmission infrastructure development to support sustainable electricity supply, the effect of a White Certificate Trading Scheme in the EU-27 and the analysis of potentials and costs of CO_2 storage in the North Sea. A large number of ETSAP applications also produced Sub-National Models, for example for Western China, Reunion Island (France), Lombardy and Pavia (Italy), Southwest region (Sweden), and Kathmandu (Nepal). Local models for rural areas and cities have been developed, e.g., Madrid (Spain), Beijing, Guangdong and Shanghai (China), and New York City (United States).

The main selling point of the ETSAP modeling frameworks is that they combine a detailed technology rich database with an economically optimizing solver, providing useful guidance into how to achieve policy decisions (e.g., emissions targets) using a least-cost approach.

This book collates together for the first time, in one volume, a range of methodological approaches and case studies of good modeling practice at national and international scale from the IEA-ETSAP energy technology initiative and demonstrates the high degree of flexibility of the ETSAP tools to represent extremely different energy systems from national to global scales. The book captures in a coherent structure the strength and breadth of energy systems modelling undertaken by ETSAP teams. Most chapters provide insights into key methodological features backed up with concrete applications. It demonstrates how energy systems models have been and are being used to answer complex policy questions relating, amongst others, to energy security, climate change mitigation, and the optimal allocation of energy resources.

I trust the readers will find within the book analysis and insights that demonstrate both the complexity and usefulness of energy systems modeling in increasing the robustness of energy and climate policy decisions.

The publication of this book in 2015 coincides with the 40th anniversary of the IEA Implementing Agreement mechanism, in existence for longer than many other international energy technology initiatives, increasingly being recognized as a time-proven, flexible, and effective means of international collaboration on energy technology and science, within and beyond IEA member countries.

January 2015

Alicia Mignone
Chair of the IEA Committee on Energy Research and Technology
Ministry of Foreign Affairs and International Cooperation
Rome, Italy

Preface

This book collates a range of methodological approaches and case study applications of good modeling practice at national and international scales from the IEA Energy Technology Systems Analysis Program (IEA-ETSAP), a collaborative network of energy modeling teams from around 70 countries that has operated for over 40 years. A key objective of IEA-ETSAP is to assist decision makers in robustly developing, implementing, and assessing the impact of energy and climate mitigation policies with the bottom-up technoeconomic models of the MARKAL/TIMES family.

The methodologies and cases studies presented in the book provide a critical understanding of the richness and width of application of energy systems models, demonstrating the underlying methods as well as the policy questions they can address. Energy engineers and technology specialists will find in the book the rationale for innovation in the field of energy technologies and insights into their evolving costs and benefits. Energy economists will gain deep insights into the key future role of energy technologies. Energy and climate policy makers as well as environmental scientists will learn about how energy systems modeling can provide unique perspectives and insights into national energy and environment challenges like climate change. Students and researchers in energy system analysis, sustainable energy, and climate change mitigation will reinforce their knowledge of energy system modeling and may find new ideas of research and applications.

The editors are grateful to the chapter authors and peer reviewers who willingly shared their expertise and contributed their valuable time, without which this book would not have been possible. In addition, the editors acknowledge the English language revision support provided by Seán Collins, Paul Deane, James Glynn, Eamonn Mulholland, Maitiú Ó Ciarain, Fionn Rogan, Clare Watson, and Evelyn Wright.

Athens, Greece — George Giannakidis
Madrid, Spain — Maryse Labriet
Cork, Ireland — Brian Ó Gallachóir
Rome, Italy — GianCarlo Tosato
January 2015

Preface

Contents

Introduction: Energy Systems Modelling for Decision-Making

Alessandro Chiodi, George Giannakidis, Maryse Labriet, Brian Ó Gallachóir and GianCarlo Tosato

Abstract The role that energy modelling plays in improving the evidence base underpinning policy decisions is being increasingly recognized and valued. The Energy Technology Systems Analysis Program is a unique network of energy modelling teams from all around the world, cooperating to establish, maintain and expand a consistent energy/economy/environment/engineering analytical capability mainly based on the MARKAL/TIMES family of models, under the aegis of the International Energy Agency. Energy systems models like MARKAL/TIMES models provide technology rich, least cost future energy systems pathways and have been used extensively to explore least cost options for transitioning to an energy secure system and a low carbon future. This chapter presents an overview of ETSAP's history and objectives, introduces the main principles of energy system modelling and summarizes the different chapters of the book.

Policy makers face significant challenges in balancing on the one hand the drive for economic competitiveness, with the need to respond to the threats posed by climate change and ensuring energy security. Achieving this balance requires a comprehensive and cohesive set of robustly informed long term policies, targets and

A. Chiodi · B. Ó Gallachóir
Energy Policy and Modelling Group, Environmental Research Institute, University College Cork, Cork, Ireland
e-mail: a.chiodi@ucc.ie

B. Ó Gallachóir
e-mail: b.ogallachoir@ucc.ie

G. Giannakidis
Centre for Renewable Energy Sources and Saving (CRES), Athens, Greece
e-mail: ggian@cres.gr

M. Labriet (✉)
Eneris Environment Energy Consultants, Madrid, Spain
e-mail: maryse.labriet@enerisconsultants.com

G. Tosato
ASATREM, Rome, Italy
e-mail: giancarlo.tosato@gmail.com

G. Giannakidis et al. (eds.), *Informing Energy and Climate Policies Using Energy Systems Models*, Lecture Notes in Energy 30,
DOI 10.1007/978-3-319-16540-0_1

strategies, combined with appropriate short and medium term action plans and measures. Increasingly, the important role that energy modelling plays in improving the evidence base underpinning policy decisions is being recognized and valued. There is a wide range (Gargiulo and Ó Gallachóir 2013) of energy modelling tools and typologies available (including simulation, optimisation, partial equilibrium, general equilibrium, sectoral demand, single technology, power system, energy system, etc.). It is important for policy analysts to understand the strengths and weaknesses of the different approaches, in order to determine which type of modelling tool is best suited to the policy question being assessed.

This book focuses on one important branch of energy models, namely energy systems models. Energy systems models provide technology rich, least cost future energy systems pathways and have been used extensively to explore least cost options for transitioning to (initially in the 1970s and 1980s) an energy secure and (more recently, in particular since 2000) a low carbon future.

This chapter introduces energy system analysis and modelling, and summarizes the different applications presented in the book: part I of the book focuses on policy insights obtained from MARKAL/TIMES models at country, regional or global levels; parts II present how to model and assess the sector specificities of the energy system, such as power, oil and end-use sectors; part III proposes model coupling to reinforce the insights obtained with energy models.

1 The IEA Energy Technology Systems Analysis Program

The first energy models developed from the 1960s were focussing on the demand and supply of a single commodity; they were soon succeeded by energy system models. Economic competitiveness and growing environmental awareness added the necessity for improved understanding of the interaction of energy systems with the environment and the economy. Since the beginning of 1970s a plethora of energy models have been developed and used to generate many energy/environment scenarios, and to undertake scientific and technical policy impact evaluations at the global, multi-regional, national and local level. These energy models are formulated using different approaches that vary in terms of model starting point and the type of questions they are designed to answer (Gargiulo and Ó Gallachóir 2013); and they are generally able to provide insights on the energy systems, which, in the absence of a modelling framework, would revert to educated guesswork. Energy models adopt theoretical and analytical methods from several disciplines including engineering, economics, operations research and management science, and apply different techniques, including mathematical programming (especially linear programming), econometrics and related methods of statistical analysis and network analysis (Hoffman and Wood 1976).

The development of energy models is not an end in its self but it is a tools aiming to provide an important contribution to the solution of the energy and environmental issues. Energy policy and planning is getting more and more complex and uncertain as questions related to the availability of primary energy sources are coupled with environmental protection issues, security of supply and related risk. The vision of a low carbon (or even a carbon-free) energy system that has emerged over the last decade needs detailed studies of roadmaps. The technical constraints of the new technologies, their efficiencies, costs and the timing of the commercial introduction contain high uncertainties. Therefore the main policy questions asked today are related to what an energy policy should look like in order to be robust and flexible enough to deal with the uncertainties of the future. Energy models are necessary in order to help in decision making and in the context described above it does not make sense to be used for forecasting (since forecasts are by definition uncertain and wrong). The models should demonstrate the robust steps that have to be taken in the immediate future and at the same time make sure that the chosen path will not be regretted later in time. Of course no single model can give answers to all the possible questions due to the complexity of energy policy issues. Therefore it is always a suit of models that are used in order to support energy planning effectively.

The use of energy models in order to analyze alternative scenarios on a global scale, is an important component of the work of the International Energy Agency (IEA). The IEA started publishing medium to long term energy projections in 1993, using the World Energy Model (WEM) which is a large scale simulation model, trying to replicate the operation of energy markets. The scenarios analyzed in the World Energy Outlook publication are based on the results of the WEM.

The IEA also publishes the Energy Technology Perspectives since 2006, which presents a core analysis of energy technologies and policies. It focuses on the long-term analysis of trends in the energy sector and the technologies that are necessary to reach a secure, low-carbon energy system. The ETP model used in this analysis is made out of four soft linked models: the energy conversion model, the industrial model, the transport model and the buildings model. The energy conversion model, covering energy supply from primary energy to transformation and final energy, is based on the TIMES model generator and is called the ETP-TIMES model.

The ETSAP[1] Implementing Agreement, a multilateral technology initiative, was initiated in 1976, under the aegis of the International Energy Agency (IEA), with the aim of carrying out a joint program of energy technology systems analysis.

In the first year of its operation, ETSAP focussed on the analysis of existing tools for evaluating R&D strategies. Then for the period 1978–1980 the MARKAL model generator development was its only activity. In 1981 the first Annex of the Implementing Agreement was initiated, with a duration of three years and this was the first time that the Energy Technology Systems Analysis Project was used as a title. After this the ETSAP community continued to coordinate for common projects and tools improvement. Environmental issues were always taken into consideration. During the 1980s, SO_2 and NO_x emissions were the main concern. The focus changed towards greenhouse gases since about 1990. The tools development moved towards

[1] Energy Technology Systems Analysis Programme.

the combination of the energy flow optimisation approach with macroeconomic top-down modelling, technology learning, and stochastic modelling.

Today ETSAP is a unique network of energy modelling teams from approximately seventy countries over the world. The contracting parties of ETSAP are the governments of eighteen countries and the European Commission. The key focus of ETSAP was (and still is) to cooperate to establish, maintain and expand a consistent multi-country energy/economy/environment/engineering analytical capability mainly based on the MARKAL/TIMES family of models. The objective was to build modelling capability in order to assist and support government officials and decision-makers in increasing the robustness of the evidence base underpinning energy and environmental policy issues by applying these tools for energy technology assessment and analysis (IEA-ETSAP 2008a). ETSAP developed through co-operation the MARKAL (MARKet ALlocation) and—subsequently—the TIMES (The Integrated Markal-Efom System) energy systems model generators, both based on a multi-regional, multi-period, bottom-up, linear programming, optimization paradigm (Loulou et al. 2004, 2005). These bottom-up techno-economic models have been used to build long term energy scenarios and to provide in-depth national, multi-country, and global energy and environmental analyses.

ETSAP's energy systems models have underpinned a significant body of research studies, as evidenced by the most recent achievements summarised in the ETSAP Annex X and XI reports (IEA-ETSAP 2008b, 2011). This research and analysis contributes to building a rich knowledge base in energy systems, impacts of policy decisions, climate change mitigation and energy security. Experiences have been mixed with respect to effectiveness in directly influencing the policy-making process.

The work of ETSAP members using the MARKAL/TIMES tools includes a wide range of models, from global to city models, used to support decision-making in the energy, environment and economy fields. This book presents applications of several of these models.

2 Energy Systems Modelling

Energy systems models approach energy as a system rather than as a set of elements. This has the advantage of providing insights into the most important substitution options that are linked to the system as a whole and that cannot be understood when analysing a single technology, or commodity, or sector. A focus on the electricity sector, for example, risks excluding possible unforeseen step changes in electricity demand, due to say, the electrification of transport or of heating. Current energy systems are the result of complex country dependent, multi-sector developments. By considering energy supply and demand across all sectors simultaneously, systems analysis applies systems principles to aid decision-makers in problems of identifying, quantifying, and controlling a system.

Building an energy systems model requires a number of key components, namely a model generator, a solver, interfaces for handling data and results and a detailed database. Energy systems models also require key exogenous inputs, comprising the demand component (energy service demands), the supply component (resource potential and costs) and the policy component (scenarios).

Two model generators have been developed and made available via the ETSAP collaboration, namely MARKAL (MARKet ALlocation) in the 1980s and subsequently during the early 2000's TIMES (The Integrated Markal-Efom System). Both MARKAL and TIMES are written in GAMS (General Algebraic Modelling Software) code and CPLEX and XPRESS are typically the solvers used. A key characteristic of these model generators is that the code is transparent and well documented (Loulou et al. 2004, 2005; IEA-ETSAP), distributed free of charge, and maintained, improved and updated through a collaborative research initiative co-ordinated by ETSAP.

ETSAP has also been instrumental in generating two interfaces for data and results, namely ANSWER (developed by Noble-Soft Systems) and VEDA (VErsatile Data Analyst, developed by KanORS). The database required includes both energy supply side and demand side technologies and contains technical data (e.g. thermal efficiency, capacity), environmental data (e.g. emission coefficients) and economic data (e.g. capital costs) that vary over the entire time horizon.

MARKAL and TIMES model generators are currently in use in 177 institutions across 70 countries. They are have been and are being used to generate MARKAL and TIMES energy systems models for local, national or multi-regional energy systems, providing a technology-rich basis for estimating energy dynamics over a long-term, multi-period time horizon. They are usually applied to the analysis of the entire energy sector, but may also be applied to study individual sectors in detail. They compute a dynamic inter-temporal partial equilibrium on integrated energy markets with the objective (objective function) of producing least-cost energy systems while respecting environmental and many technical constraints. The energy system cost includes investment costs, operation and maintenance costs, plus the costs of imported fuels, minus the incomes of exported fuels, minus the residual value of technologies at the end of the horizon. The main *selling point* of the ETSAP modelling frameworks is that they combine a detailed technology rich database with an economically optimizing solver. They are able to generate robust energy policy scenarios over medium to long time horizons and are able to offer strategic insight into long-term policy formation. This is especially important for the energy sector, which has such large capital investments with long project lifetimes. The modelling perspective of these tools is that of a benevolent central planner: as if there was a single decision-maker (mono-objective) taking rational choices surrounding all energy-related issues on technologies and fuels at the lowest cost to the economy and to society. This clearly does not reflect reality, where there are many decision makers and not all decisions are rational, but it does provide very useful guidance into how to achieve policy decisions (e.g. emissions targets) using a least-cost approach. The complex dynamics (incorporating technologies, fuel prices, infrastructures and capacity constraints) of the entire energy system can be analysed through this modelling approach to better inform policy choices.

Like all energy models, MARKAL and TIMES models also have a number of limitations which should be considered when interpreting the results and scenario analyses. In some instances, these are simply limitations born of the structure of the model; they are inevitable based on the way the model is built. In other instances, they could be considered weaknesses and in these cases, research should be carried out to generate improvements. The following list presents the main limitations: (i) *Time resolution*: Long term energy systems model are generally inadequate to capture daily supply and demand curves. Even though there are no limitations on the number of time-slices in MARKAL/TIMES models; it would become computationally unwieldy if the model had to make decade long decision as well as hourly decisions. (ii) *Macro-economic assumptions*: The results of the scenarios are tied to the assumption and results of the macro-economic model, which by themselves are inherently uncertain. While scenario analysis, by its nature, tries to counteract this uncertainty by producing a range of results, this uncertainty is nevertheless present. (iii) *Limited macro-economic feedback*: MARKAL and TIMES models are generally not able to take account feedbacks between the output of the energy system analysis and the macro-economy. (iv) *Behaviour*: ETSAP models have the limited capacity to simulate behavioural aspects. This is a limitation of most energy (and indeed macro-economic) models, in that consumer behaviour is generally limited to simple price response and non-price related behaviour is generally very poorly treated. (v) *Power system operational characteristics*: Technical characteristics, such as minimum stable generation, ramps rates and minimum up and down times play an important role in actual power system operation and planning, in particular systems with high levels of variable

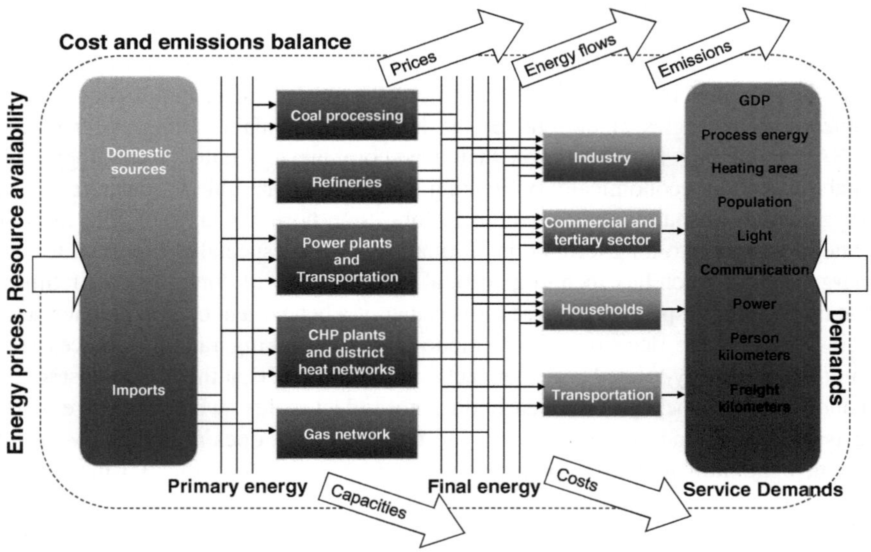

Fig. 1 TIMES model schematic (Remme et al. 2001)

renewables and these are generally not adequately incorporated into energy system models.

ETSAP energy systems models are able to generate a vast number of outputs, assessing implications for (i) the economy (including energy prices, investments in the energy system, marginal CO_2 abatement costs, etc.), for (ii) the energy mix (fuels and technologies) and energy dependence, and for (iii) the environment (in particular greenhouse gas emissions). Figure 1 shows in schematic form how a MARKAL and TIMES models operate. The exogenous model inputs are shown entering from the left hand side (energy supply) and right hand side (energy service demands) of the model. The model outputs are shown on the top and bottom.

3 Overview of the Book

This book collates together for the first time in one volume a range of methodological approaches and case studies of good modelling practice at national and international scale from the IEA-ETSAP energy technology initiative. Most chapters provide insight into key methodological features backed up with concrete applications. The book demonstrates the high degree of flexibility of the modelling tools which haves been used to represent extremely different energy systems, from national to global levels. It demonstrates how energy systems models have been and are being used to answer complex policy questions relating to energy security, climate change mitigation, the optimal allocation of energy resources, amongst others.

The book is carefully structured into three parts which focus on policy decisions that have been underpinned by energy systems models (Part I), specific aspects of supply and end-use sector modelling, including technology learning and behaviour (Part II) and how additional insights can be gained from linking different models (Part III).

3.1 Part I—From Policy Insights to Policy Decisions

Chapter by **Chiodi et al**. presents four case studies, in which there is clear evidence of a direct link between the use of MARKAL/TIMES scenario modelling activities and policy decisions. The lessons learned, along with the role of policy makers and stakeholders in the modelling process are discussed. The case studies assess how the (i) UK MARKAL model informed the development of energy and climate mitigation policy in the UK (Energy White Papers of 2003 and 2007, Climate Change Act in 2008); (ii) Irish TIMES model informed the development of climate mitigation legislation in Ireland in 2014 and Ireland's negotiating position regarding the EU 2030 Climate Energy Package in 2014; (iii) TIMES_PT model informed climate policy in Portugal in the last 10 years and has supported the design of climate mitigation policies; (iv) IEA ETP Model informed the G8 in responding to the 2005 Gleneagles Plan of Action and has supported the work of the Major Economies Forum and Clean Energy Ministerial.

Chapter by **Kumpener et al.** compares the global renewable energy roadmap to double the share of renewables in the global energy mix by 2030 compared to 2010, called REmap 2030 and published by the International Renewable Energy Agency (IRENA) in 2014, with the methods and results obtained with the IEA-ETSAP models. It discusses the advantages that ETSAP models have, by accounting for trade-offs between renewable energy and energy efficiency activities, system planning issues like grid infrastructure, competition for scarce resources in the commodity prices, or dynamic cost developments as technologies get deployed over time. Authors conclude how the REmap tool and the ETSAP models have complementary roles to play in engaging policy makers and national energy planners to advance renewables.

One key question facing policy makers is that of defining *one* course of action in a context of uncertainties, what is proposed by stochastic programming. Chapter by **Labriet et al.** explains how stochastic programming, combined with a parametric analysis of the probability of the future outlooks, and robust optimization are useful to analyze climate and energy decisions in uncertain context, and applies the methods using respectively TIAM-WORLD at the global level and MIRET in the case of France. "Super-hedging" actions can even be identified, which penetrate more in the hedging strategy than in *any* of the perfect forecast strategies (gas is a good candidate). One of the drawbacks of stochastic programming is the computational requirements. Robust optimization is an alternative since it offers parsimonious ways of dealing with problems of high dimensionality, requiring minimal information about the true probability distributions of uncertain parameters.

Pursuing the study of climate issues, chapters by **Kypreos and Lehtilä**, and by **Kober et al.** explore the allocation of greenhouse gas emission quotas to different countries under a 2 °C long-term climate policy framework using respectively the Integrated TIMES and MERGE Model (ITMM), which integrates hybrid top-down and bottom-up models, and the TIAM-ECN model, which assesses a per-capita-based scheme, and an economic capability-based scheme. Appropriate certificate trading mechanisms of course need to be in place, and depending on the certificate allocation scheme the future trade of carbon certificates might become as important as energy trade.

The next four chapters present applications of energy modelling at regional and national levels. **Fais and Blesl** evaluate how bottom-up energy system models may be utilised to evaluate the long-term effects of energy and climate policy instruments; more particularly, emissions trading systems and different support systems for renewable electricity are outlined and applied to the German energy system. **Kerimray et al.** explore the energy efficiency potential of Kazakhstan in a TIMES-based model. The model suggests significant and economically viable energy efficiency improvements. **Cabal et al.** estimate socioeconomic and environmental impacts associated to energy technologies in the current and future Spanish Energy System using the national energy optimization model TIMES-Spain. **Koljonen and Lehtilä** analyze the implications of low carbon policies with a special focus on the

Finnish energy system. They use the global ETSAP-TIAM model as well as an applied general equilibrium model and a forest sector partial equilibrium model for estimating the impacts on the overall economy as well as land-use change and forestry.

3.2 *Part II—Focussing on Specific Aspects of Supply and End-Use*

The power sector is a key element of the energy system, in terms of energy services, infrastructure and environmental impacts. Chapter by **Kannan et al**. provides a broad overview of temporal features in the MARKAL/TIMES energy modelling framework directly related to the modelling of electricity dispatch. This includes the trade-offs between model time horizon and intra-annual time resolution, the solver algorithm capabilities, data availability and methodological limitations. The trade-offs and benefits of an integrated system approach are discussed with a set of scenarios from the Swiss TIMES electricity and energy system models.

Nijs et al. describe a methodology to integrate DC power flow modelling and N-1 security into the JRC-EU-TIMES model, a multiregional TIMES energy system model developed by the European Joint Research Centre—Institute for Energy and Transport. The methodology improves the accuracy of modelling cross-border transmission expansion especially for energy systems with higher penetration of renewable energy sources. One of the grid representations proposed in the chapter uses the newly developed Integrated TIMES–NEPLAN Software that couples JRC-EU-TIMES energy system modelling with NEPLAN-based electricity grid modelling.

Wright and Kanudia extend the modelling of power sector of the USA to the representation of unit-level emissions of all existing coal-fired plants within the FACETS TIMES model of USA, reflecting the soon-to-be-implemented Mercury and Air Toxics (MATS) regulation. Covered emissions and retrofit costs depend in a detailed way on unit configuration and coal quality, forcing development of new techniques to handle the enormous expansion in model size and detail.

The oil industry currently plays a major role in the Canadian economy. In the future, further developments of the oil sector will be affected by the ability to transport crude oil (mainly from Western Canada) to consuming regions in Canada and abroad. Based on the use of a multi-regional TIMES energy model for Canada, chapter by **Vaillancourt et al**. analyzes different crude oil exportation scenarios based on existing pipeline expansions and the development of new pipelines.

The costs of technologies often fall over time due to a range of processes including learning-by-doing. This is a well-characterized concept in the economics of innovation, in which learning about a particular technology, and hence cost reduction, is related to cumulative investments in that technology. **Anandarajah and McDowall** explore the modelling challenges of applying technology learning endogenously in a TIMES model in a case study based on a multi-cluster learning approach in the transportation sector, where key technologies (fuel cells, automotive batteries, and electric drive trains) are shared across a set of transport modes and technologies. The multi-region TIAM-UCL Global energy system model has been used to model the multi-cluster approach. The analysis is used to explore the competitive and/or complementary relationship between hydrogen and electricity as low-carbon transport fuels.

Chapter by **Daly et al.** also focuses on the transportation sector, and more particularly the representation of travel behavioural change in MARKALT/TIMES models in addition to increased vehicle efficiency and low-carbon fuels as climate mitigation options. Modal choice within passenger transport, which to date has been exogenously modelled (with no competition allowed between alternative modes) is integrated here into a TIMES model, allowing competition between modes, while also imposing a constraint in the system on overall travel time.

The appropriate representation of energy service demands is a crucial factor of MARKAL/TIMES models, which are driven by energy service demands. In China, the growth trend in energy service demand will be a critical factor in the level of energy consumption and carbon emissions in future. Within this context, **Chen et al.** propose various approaches, including stock-based method, saturation model, discrete choices model, to project energy service demands in different sectors of the Chinese economy. The projection of energy service demand are then used as inputs in the China TIMES-ED model to generate a reference scenario.

3.3 Part III—Gaining Additional Insights Through Model Coupling

Linking MARKAL/TIMES models with carefully selected complementary models can provide useful additional insights into the results from standalone models when the multi-model approach succeeds in taking advantage of the individual strengths of different modelling approaches. Chapter by **Deane et al.** collates methodologies and results from a number of soft-linking exercises with TIMES. Two specific examples are given. Firstly the soft-linking of TIMES to a power system model to investigate the TIMES results and provide additional insights into power system flexibility, reliability and market issues. Secondly, the soft-linking of a TIMES model to a power system and a housing stock model to explore the impacts of increased electrification of residential heating on the power system and associated emissions from the residential sector. These examples show how a multi-model approach and soft-linking can provide a strong complementary analysis to TIMES modelling exercises and generate insights into results that otherwise would be difficult to achieve with a single model approach.

Key questions for policy makers surround the economic implications of future changes in the energy system, for example what will be the implications for economic growth of moving to a low carbon energy system? which sectors of the economy will thrive and which sectors will suffer? what are the implications for jobs?, etc. In a climate constrained future, hybrid energy-economy model coupling can provide rich additional insight into interregional competition, trade, industrial delocalisation and overall macroeconomic consequences of decarbonising the energy system. The two chapters by **Glynn et al.** summarize modelling methodologies developed in the ETSAP community to assess economic impacts of decarbonising energy systems at national and global levels. For example: combining MARKAL and TIMES models with the MACRO model, a simplified single-sector general equilibrium model, which maximizes an inter-temporal utility; coupling MARKAL/TIMES models with computational general equilibrium models, in which energy results (costs) from the energy systems models are fed into the CGE model which in turn generates revised energy service demands as inputs into the energy systems models; linking energy systems models with other types of economic models (e.g. econometric models) to understand the interactions between energy systems and the economy.

Chapter by **Labriet et al**. explores another field of model linkages: the coupling of the World TIMES Integrated Assessment Model (TIAM-WORLD) with an emulated version of the climate model PLASIM-ENTS to assess the impacts of future temperature and precipitation changes on the heating and cooling subsector and available hydropower. Such a coupling is important to assess regional temperature increases and therefore the possible impacts of climate change on the energy system at a regional level. The climate module of TIAM-WORLD does not compute the regional or seasonal temperature changes required for a relevant representation of the possible heating and cooling adjustments due to climate change. The coupling of TIAM-WORLD with an emulator of the climate model PLASIM-ENTS provides this additional information.

Coupling may also occur between different MARKAL/TIMES models. **Gerboni et al**. present an application of the coupling of the global TIMES Integrated Assessment Model and the Pan European TIMES model through a series of trade links characterised into a corridor model. The application focuses on the analysis of security of supply to Europe via energy corridors. A new methodology for the assessment of energy security, addressing the risk associated to each supply, is presented together with a scenario analysis related to the European Union (EU) as a whole and to some of the most populated EU's Member States.

4 Conclusion

This book captures in a coherent structure the strength and breadth of energy systems modelling undertaken by ETSAP teams. It focuses on recent analysis that builds on a unique, collaborative, international research effort over the past 40 years. It demonstrates both the complexity and usefulness of energy systems modelling and acts as a bridge between the many energy systems modelling teams and the wider analytical, research and policy community interested in increasing the robustness of energy and climate policy decisions.

References

Gargiulo M, Ó Gallachóir B (2013) Long-term energy models: Principles, characteristics, focus, and limitations. Wiley Interdiscip Rev Energy Environ 2(2):158–177. doi:10.1002/wene.62

Hoffman KC, Wood DO (1976) Energy system modeling and forecasting. Annu Rev Energy 1 (1):423–453. doi:10.1146/annurev.eg.01.110176.002231

IEA-ETSAP (2008a) ETSAP Strategic Plan (2009–2013). Annex XI: joint studies for new and mitigated energy systems. Energy Technology Systems Analysis Programme

IEA-ETSAP (2008b) Global energy systems and common analyses. Final Report of Annex X (2005–2008). Energy Technology Systems Analysis Programme

IEA-ETSAP (2011) Joint studies for new and mitigated energy systems. Final Report of Annex XI (2008–2010). Energy Technology Systems Analysis Programme

Loulou R, Goldstein G, Noble K (2004) Documentation for the MARKAL family of models. Available from http://www.iea-etsap.org/web/MrklDoc-I_StdMARKAL.pdf. Energy Technology Systems Analysis Programme (IEA-ETSAP)

Loulou R, Remme U, Kanudia A, Lehtila A, Goldstein G (2005) Documentation for the TIMES model. Available from http://www.etsap.org/documentation.asp. Energy Technology Systems Analysis Programme (IEA-ETSAP)

Remme U, Goldstein GA, Schellmann U, Schlenzig C (2001) MESAP/TIMES—advanced decision support for energy and environmental planning. In Chamoni P, Leisten R, Martin A, Minnemann J, Stadtler H (eds) Operations research proceedings 2001. Selected papers of the international conference on operations research (OR 2001), 3–5 September, Springer, Duisburg, Germany, pp 59–66

Part I
From Policy Insights to Policy Decisions

Energy Policies Influenced by Energy Systems Modelling—Case Studies in UK, Ireland, Portugal and G8

Alessandro Chiodi, Peter G. Taylor, Júlia Seixas, Sofia Simões, Patrícia Fortes, João P. Gouveia, Luís Dias and Brian Ó Gallachóir

Abstract A key objective of IEA-ETSAP is to assist decision makers in robustly developing, implementing and assessing the impact of energy and climate mitigation policies. This chapter focuses on four case studies, in which there is clear evidence of a direct link between the use of MARKAL and TIMES scenario modelling activities and the resulting policy decisions. The case studies selected assess how the (i) UK MARKAL model informed the development of energy and climate mitigation policy in the UK, focusing on the Energy White Paper in 2003, the Energy White Paper in 2007 and the Climate Change Act in 2008; (ii) Irish TIMES model informed the development of climate mitigation legislation in Ireland

A. Chiodi (✉) · B. Ó Gallachóir
Energy Policy and Modelling Group, Environmental Research Institute,
University College Cork, Cork, Ireland
e-mail: a.chiodi@ucc.ie

B. Ó Gallachóir
e-mail: b.ogallachoir@ucc.ie

Peter G. Taylor
Centre for Integrated Energy Research, University of Leeds,
Leeds, UK
e-mail: p.g.taylor@leeds.ac.uk

J. Seixas · S. Simões · P. Fortes · J.P. Gouveia · L. Dias
CENSE, Faculdade Ciências e Tecnologia, Universidade Nova de Lisboa,
Lisboa, Portugal
e-mail: mjs@fct.unl.pt

S. Simões
e-mail: sgcs@fct.unl.pt

P. Fortes
e-mail: p.fs@fct.unl.pt

J.P. Gouveia
e-mail: jplg@fct.unl.pt

L. Dias
e-mail: luisdias@fct.unl.pt

G. Giannakidis et al. (eds.), *Informing Energy and Climate Policies Using Energy Systems Models*, Lecture Notes in Energy 30,
DOI 10.1007/978-3-319-16540-0_2

in 2014 and Ireland's negotiating position regarding the EU 2030 Climate Energy Package in 2014; (iii) TIMES_PT model informed climate policy in Portugal in the last 10 years and has supported the design of climate mitigation policies; (iv) IEA ETP Model informed the G8 in responding to the 2005 Gleneagles Plan of Action and has supported the work of the Major Economies Forum and Clean Energy Ministerial. This chapter collates methodologies and results from these different case studies and summarizes some key findings regarding (i) policy frameworks and goals; (ii) how policy makers have been intertwined with the modelling tool during the modelling process; (iii) the role of the economic stakeholders dialogue; (iv) main insights from the modelling exercises; (v) lessons learnt: from effective contributions to real limitations and (vi) recommendations.

1 Introduction

This chapter presents a collection of four case studies where this direct linkage between ETSAP modelling tools and the policy-making process took place at national (United Kingdom, Ireland and Portugal) and supra-national level (G8 countries). The purpose is to show how ETSAP energy systems models have informed the environmental and energy policy choices, but also discussing the main lessons learnt, the current limitations, and recommendations both for modellers and policy makers.

The chapter structure is as follows. Section 2 presents the experience of UK MARKAL which informed energy and environmental policy in Great Britain. Section 3 focuses on Irish TIMES model which informed the Irish Government. Section 4 discusses details of TIMES_PT being used to inform climate policy in Portugal in the last decade. Section 5 presents the case of IEA ETP Model, which informed the G8 in responding to the 2005 Gleneagles Plan of Action and supported the work of the Major Economies Forum and Clean Energy Ministerial. Section 6 concludes with some discussions regarding common issues, lessons learned and some recommendations for model developers.

2 The Experience of UK MARKAL

The MARKAL energy systems model has a long history of use in the UK dating back to early versions of the model developed in the late 1970s (Finnis 1980). Yet, for most of the next two decades its impact on the energy policy process was minimal (Taylor et al. 2014). However, around the year 2000 climate change emerged as a key political issue in the UK and, since then, results from MARKAL have been used extensively to inform energy policy as the question of how to reduce greenhouse gas (GHG) emissions has become the defining challenge.

2.1 The 2003 Energy White Paper

In 2000, the Royal Commission on Environmental Pollution (RCEP)[1] recommended that by 2050 the UK should plan to reduce its energy-related carbon dioxide emissions by 60 % (Royal Commission on Environmental Pollution 2000). This conclusion had a significant impact on the Government who set up a review of energy policy in 2001, eventually leading to the publication of an Energy White Paper (EWP) in 2003 (DTI 2003a). As part of this review, the Department of Trade and Industry (DTI) commissioned AEA Technology plc to develop a new UK MARKAL model and to use it to explore future trends in carbon dioxide emissions from the UK energy sector up to 2050 and identify the technical possibilities and costs for the abatement of these emissions. The work considered three levels of abatement by 2050: 45, 60 and 70 % reductions relative to emissions in 2000, combined with three scenarios (Baseline, World Markets and Global Sustainability) for the possible future development of the UK economy and the associated demands for energy related services (DTI 2003b).

The new model database contained a wide variety of low carbon technologies including many types of renewable energy, fossil fuels with carbon capture and storage, nuclear power, efficient demand-side technologies and fuel cells and hydrogen. Two workshops with industry and academic experts were held to review the cost and performance data for low carbon power generation and infrastructure for transmission and distribution of hydrogen.

By running each of the three scenarios without any CO_2 emissions constraints and then with the three level of abatement levels described above, 12 "core" runs of the model were generated. However, these were then supplemented by 70 other "sensitivity" runs to test how the results changed with alternate assumptions on a range of issues including the availability of technologies and fuels, fuel prices and taxes, discount rates and alternative emission paths. While the model results contained a huge amount of information about future technology and fuel mixes, including at the sectoral level, the key use of the modelling in the 2003 EWP was to calculate the costs to the economy of the different abatement levels (DTI n.d.).[2] The results led the 2003 EWP to conclude that "*the cost impact of effectively tackling climate change would be very small—equivalent in 2050 to just a small fraction (0.5–2 %) of the nation's wealth, as measured by GDP*".

The results on costs proved quite controversial, with some experts arguing that they were too low (Great Britain House of Lords 2005). Despite these

[1] The Royal Commission on Environmental Pollution was an independent standing body established in 1970 to advise the Queen, the Government, Parliament and the public on environmental issues.

[2] Ironically, this calculation had to be done off model using output from MARKAL because the choice at the start had been to use the standard MARKAL model (and not MARKAL-MACRO).

controversies, a report by the Institute for European Environmental Policy, an independent institute, concluded that the results from MARKAL "*overcame a key barrier to acceptance of the 60 % target, and appears greatly to have helped develop a positive attitude to carbon reductions in government*" (IEEP 2005).

2.2 The 2007 Energy White Paper

While the 2003 EWP established the principle that emissions reduction was the key policy challenge, it left much of the detail unresolved. In addition, rapid rises in gas and oil prices from mid-2004 led to the issue of energy security joining carbon mitigation as a priority for energy policy (Pearson and Watson 2012). Therefore within a couple of years the government was planning another EWP and once again turned to MARKAL to help inform its decisions.

The UK Energy Research Centre (UKERC), a grouping of UK universities, and AEA Technology worked together on a project commissioned by the DTI using both the standard version of MARKAL and the newly developed MARKAL-MACRO (M-M). The final report focused on a set of 11 M-M model scenarios (Strachan et al. 2007) that were used as the main inputs to the 2007 EWP. The scenarios may be classified as:

1. Base-case, CO_2 emissions in 2050 constrained to 60 % of 2000 levels and alternate CO_2 emission trajectory implemented linearly from 2010;
2. Resource import (high and low) price scenarios, from DTI projections;
3. Technology scenarios: restricted innovation (limited to either 2010 or 2020 levels of improvement), no-nuclear, no-CCS or no-nuclear/CCS scenarios.

Key outputs included primary and final energy mixes, sectoral contributions to CO_2 reductions, detailed technology selection in the electricity and transport sectors, the role of demand side reductions, CO_2 prices, energy system costs and GDP impacts. In total, over 50 scenarios sets were run (including standard model runs) with results from additional scenarios being used to explore key trade-offs between mitigation pathways.

In contrast to the rather narrow use of MARKAL in the 2003 EWP, the 2007 EWP explains its use of M-M in the following terms: "*for the period to 2050, we have used a model of the entire UK energy system (UK MARKAL-Macro model) to explore the changes to the amount and use of energy required if we are to deliver our goal of reducing carbon emissions by 60 % by 2050 at least cost*" (DTI 2007a). This central role given to MARKAL by the 2007 EWP is reflected in over fourteen direct references to various insights from the modelling work, complemented by numerous graphical figures (Fig. 1) in the supplementary material supporting the White Paper (DTI 2007b).

Of particular note, is the fact that the MARKAL results were used to support a significant change in the view of nuclear power compared to the 2003 EWP, with the 2007 EWP noting "*Our modelling indicates that excluding nuclear is a more*

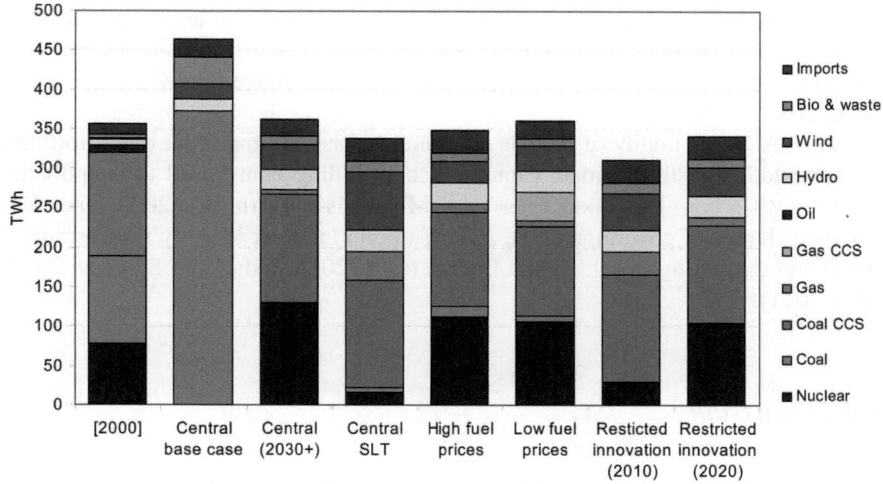

Fig. 1 Example of M-M results for the 2007 EWP: Generation mix in 2050, central and sensitivity scenarios (DTI 2007b)

expensive route to achieving our carbon goal even though in our modelling, the costs of alternative technologies are assumed to fall over time as they mature" (DTI 2007a).[3]

2.3 The 2008 Climate Change Act

Following the 2007 EWP, the Government published a draft Climate Change Bill, which became an Act of Parliament in 2008 (Great Britain 2008). This put in place a new legislative framework of five-year carbon budgets and established an independent Committee on Climate Change (CCC) to advise government on the level of these budgets. A long-term emissions target was written into the Act, but strengthened from the original 60 % recommended by the RCEP to become an 80 % emissions reduction target by 2050.

The impact assessment for the Bill (compulsory for most UK policy proposals) draws on MARKAL-MACRO analysis by AEA Technology looking at the additional impacts (economic and technological) of moving to an increasingly carbon constrained energy system, with reductions in CO_2 of 70 and 80 % by 2050 and the implications of including international aviation within the targets (DECC 2009). In a parallel exercise MARKAL-ED (a variant of MARKAL in which the level of

[3] Interestingly the modelling work for the 2003 EWP had also shown a similar result, but this appears to have been ignored as at the time the Government focus was on delivering carbon reductions through energy efficiency and renewables.

demand for energy services varies according to the costs of meeting them) was used by the CCC to examine the economic and technological implications for reducing carbon emissions by 80 or 90 % by 2050 to inform its advice to government (CCC 2008; AEA 2008a, b).

The MARKAL family of models continues to play an important role informing implementation of the Climate Change Act, including being used to support the 2009 Low Carbon Transition Plan (Her Majesty's Government 2009) and, following a change of government, the 2011 Carbon Plan (Her Majesty's Government 2011) and the setting of 4th carbon budget (CCC 2010; Usher and Strachan 2010; AEA 2011).

2.4 Discussion

Since 2000, the MARKAL family of models have become embedded as key tools used to inform UK climate and energy policy. Three attributes of MARKAL would appear to have been particularly important in facilitating its role to support ambitious climate targets. First, MARKAL is not bound by historical relationships of the kind that underpin econometric and macro-economic modelling and is therefore able to postulate radically different energy system configurations that will be needed for deep reductions in GHG emissions. Second, MARKAL is able to make the necessary changes tangible through its detailed technological representation, which has suited a prevailing techno-centric view of the mitigation challenge. Third, MARKAL's objective function is cost and this accord with the dominance of cost-benefit analysis as a tool for policy appraisal and selection in the UK. Finally, while MARKAL is far from readily comprehensible to all and sometimes criticised for being a "black-box", substantial efforts have been made by the modelling community to increase the transparency and completeness of the model structure and assumptions, including through a range of stakeholder events, expert peer review and publication of the model documentation.

3 The Experience of Irish TIMES

Irish TIMES is a mono-regional model of the entire Irish energy system that was originally extracted from the Pan European TIMES (PET) model (Ó Gallachóir et al. 2012). It has been updated and expanded since 2009 by the Energy Policy and Modelling Group in University College Cork and has been used to build a range of energy and emissions policy scenarios to explore the dynamics behind the transition to low carbon energy systems (Chiodi et al. 2013a, b), to analyse energy security (Glynn et al. 2014), to assess impacts of limited bioenergy resources (Chiodi et al. 2015a) and to explore new modelling approaches (Deane et al. 2012; Chiodi et al. 2015b). However its impact on the policy making process has been limited till 2013, when, over the period June 2013–September 2014, the Irish TIMES model has been extensively used to inform two key policy developments, namely the development of (i) national legislation on climate change and (ii) Ireland's negotiation position regarding the proposed EU 2030 Carbon and Energy Policy Framework.

3.1 Low Carbon Energy Roadmap to 2050

The Irish Government is planning to legislate for Climate Action and Low Carbon Development and published a Heads of Bill (*General Scheme of a Climate Action and Low Carbon Development Bill (CA&LCD Bill))* in 2013 (DECLG 2013). This raises key questions regarding the evolution of Ireland's future energy system to enable the transition to a low carbon future. According to Head 4 of the CA&LCD Heads of Bill, "*the Government shall arrange for the adoption and implementation of plans [...] to enable the State to pursue and achieve transition to a low carbon, climate resilient and environmentally sustainable economy in the period up to and including the year 2050. Article 5 stipulates that a key objective of a National Low Carbon Roadmap is to articulate a national vision for the transition to a low carbon, climate resilient and environmentally sustainable economy over the period to 2050*".

In the period June–December 2013, the Department of the Environment, Community and Local Government commissioned UCC to produce a *Low Carbon Energy Roadmap for Ireland to 2050* using the Irish TIMES model (Deane et al. 2013). The focus of this analysis was on technological changes in the energy system and the associated implications. A key policy question underpinning the analysis focused on the dynamics of the energy system moving towards a low carbon economy for two key time horizons, i.e. to 2050 and to 2030. The process involved modelling analysis and regular meetings and discussions with a number of Government Departments providing technical advice and guidance on the development of a long term strategy for Ireland.

The purpose of the roadmap is to explore possible routes towards decarbonisation of the energy system, with a focus on achieving this at least cost to the economy and to society. The key issue is making well informed policy choices. Hence this roadmap does not stipulate which policies are necessary to achieve the transition; it rather focuses on the key drivers and its implications for the energy system of moving to a low carbon economy. The roadmap presents three distinct scenarios to explore transitions to a near zero CO_2 future.

1. A business as usual (*BaU*) scenario which does not impose emissions targets and efficiency improvements and is used as a base case (counterfactual) against which to compare the two distinct near-zero CO_2 scenarios.
2. An 80 % CO_2 reduction (*CO_2-80)* scenario in which CO_2 emissions are constrained across the entire time horizon to be no greater than 80 % below 1990 levels in 2050.

Table 1 Ireland's low carbon roadmap to 2050

Sector	2030 relative to 1990		2050 relative to 1990	
	BaU (%)	Low carbon (%)	BAU (%)	Low carbon (%)
Electricity	45	−56 to −58	31	−84 to −94
Buildings	−11	−53	−11	−75 to −99
Services	*5*	*−33*	*−6*	*−70 to −99*
Residential	*−16*	*−59*	*−13*	*−77 to −98*
Transport	226	104 to 122	285	−72 to −92
Total	50	−29 to −31	55	−80 to −95

Services and Residential are sub-groups of 'Buildings' chategory

3. A 95 % CO_2 reduction (*CO_2-95*) scenario in which CO_2 emissions are constrained across the entire time horizon to be no greater than 95 % below 1990 levels in 2050.

The roadmap provides insights into when changes in the fuel mix are likely to occur (e.g. transitioning from oil to biogas and biomass), the timing of new technologies (e.g. when and to what extent will electric vehicles penetrate the transport fleet) and the future role of electricity and gas infrastructure. It also emphasizes the scale of the challenge ahead, assessing macro-economic implications of decarbonisation,[4] and points to a number of areas of opportunity for Ireland as it transitions for a low carbon future. Moreover it provides guidance to possible sectoral targets, with the allocation of CO_2 emissions reductions (Table 1), between the key energy sectors in the *BAU* scenario and the range of results arising from the two low carbon scenarios considered (*CO_2-80* and *CO_2-95*).

The analysis also provides useful indications of the impact of different policy metrics to the whole energy systems, resulting with different allocations of fuels, sectors, efficiencies, but also energy dependency, as testified by the energy systems snapshots of alternative future energy systems provided by the Sankey diagrams shown in Fig. 2.

3.2 *Assessment and Implications of EU 2030 Climate and Energy Policy Framework for Energy Policy in Ireland*

In the period January–September 2014, the Irish TIMES model was used to inform Ireland's negotiating position with respect to the European Commission's proposal of a Climate and Energy Policy Framework for 2030 (EC 2014a). Here it was used

[4] The economic impacts were assessed by the Economic and Social Research Institute using outputs from the Irish TIMES model as inputs to the HERMES macro-economic model (Deane et al. 2013).

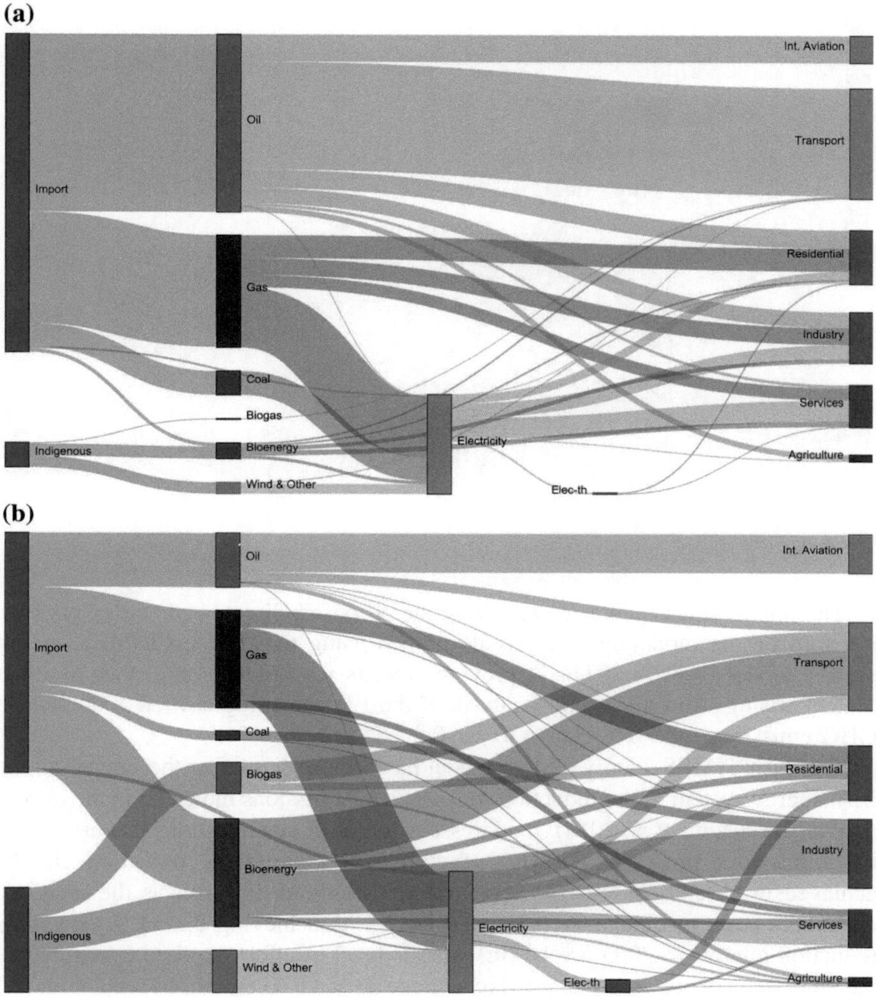

Fig. 2 2050 Sankey Diagrams for Ireland's energy system under BaU, CO_2-80 and CO_2-95 scenarios. **a** BaU scenario. **b** CO_2-80 scenario. **c** CO_2-95 scenario

to examine and provide answers to key questions arising from the proposed targets and in particular to scrutinise the findings of the modelling exercise accompanying the proposal (EC 2014b).

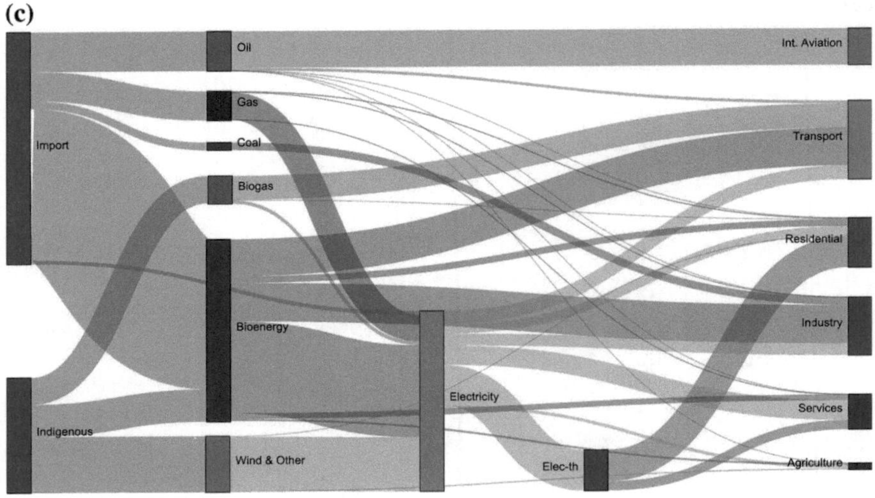

Fig. 2 (continued)

The impact assessment accompanying the proposed climate and energy package is based on the modelling analysis developed using mostly the PRIMES energy system model (NTUA 2011). It provides results for Ireland (and other Member States) arising from a scenario analysis of the EU achieving a 40 % reduction in GHG emissions by 2030 relative to 1990.[5]

The Irish TIMES energy system model has been to scrutinize the impact on the Irish energy system of the reduction in Irish GHG emissions indicated in the impact assessment (Cahill et al. 2014). It addresses a series of key questions that arise from the framework proposal: (i) what level of GHG emissions reduction can be achieved in Ireland up to 2030 at a cost of €40/tonne; (ii) what is the marginal abatement costs in Ireland in 2030 associated with achieving the 33 % emissions reduction relative to 2005 levels; (iii) what is level of effort required (measured as the increase in energy systems cost) to achieve 33 % GHG emissions reduction; (iv) what is the role of renewables in achieving the 33 % emissions reduction; (v) what is the cost optimal effort distribution between ETS and non-ETS sectors of the economy. The analysis addressed these five questions through scenario analysis

[5] The results for Ireland suggest that GHG emissions can be reduced by 33 % below 2005 levels (or 14.8 % below 1990 levels) by the year 2030 at a marginal abatement cost of €40/t CO_2eq. The impact assessment shows that the contribution from non-ETS sectors of the economy is a 21 % reduction in 2030 relative to 2005 levels. This implies that total non-ETS emissions in 2030 would be 36.4 $MtCO_2$ and ETS emissions would account for the remaining 11.5 $MtCO_2$.

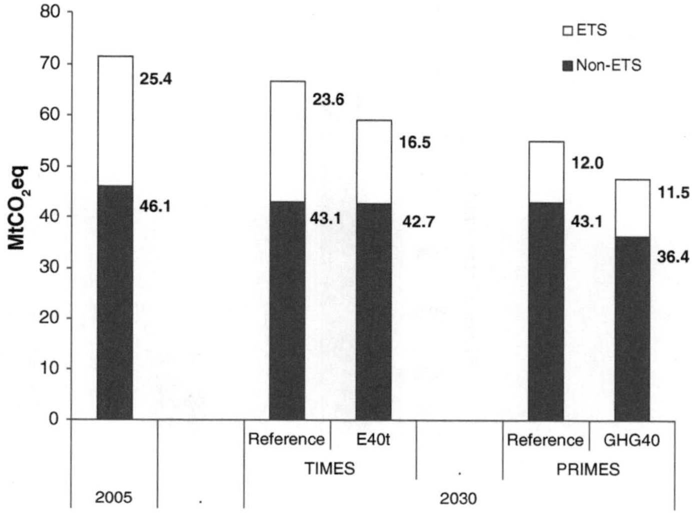

Fig. 3 GHG Emissions Scenario in Ireland in 2030—PRIMES versus Irish TIMES

and a number of sensitivity runs to test impacts of alternative emissions pathways, renewable targets and taxation levels. Additional analysis was undertaken using the outputs of the Irish TIMES scenario analyses as inputs to a macroeconomic model (Bergin et al. 2013) to investigate the macroeconomic impacts of achieving a specific level of emissions reduction by 2030.

Key outputs from Irish TIMES suggest that a 33 % GHG emissions reduction can be achieved at marginal abatement cost of €151/t, significantly higher than the €40/t resulting from the PRIMES scenario analysis, while only 21 % GHG emissions reduction can be delivered at a marginal abatement cost of €40/t (Fig. 3).

Another key difference is also shown in the modal distribution of renewable energy (Fig. 4). Although both analyses indicate renewable energy increases from 7 % currently to 25 % in 2030 as a share of gross final energy consumption, the PRIMES results point to a higher share of electricity from renewables (60 % RES-E compared with 51 % RES-E from Irish TIMES). By contrast, the Irish TIMES scenario analysis points to share of thermal energy from renewables (38 % compared with 17 % in the PRIMES analysis).

The feedback on the analysis undertaken with Irish TIMES was very positive from the Irish delegation negotiating the Climate and Energy Policy Framework for 2030 in the weeks before the European Council meeting in October 2014. It was clear that the modelling analysis was received as being robust and very useful and that is strengthened Ireland's position.

Fig. 4 Modal shares of renewables in gross final consumption in 2030—PRIMES versus Irish TIMES

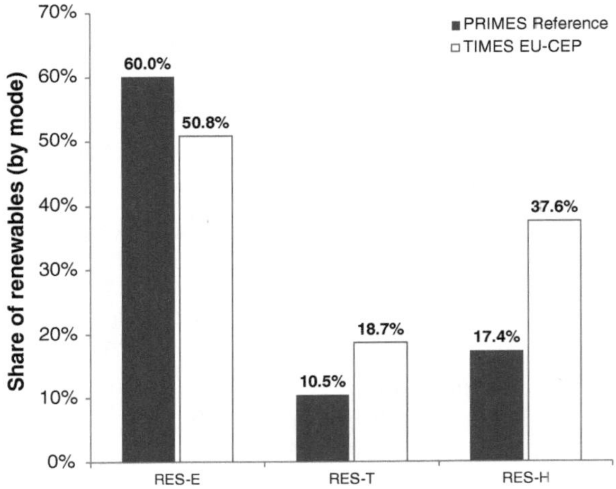

3.3 Discussion

The use of TIMES modelling tools to inform policy decision is quite recent in Ireland. Before 2009, when Irish TIMES project commenced, no similar modelling tools were in fact available in Ireland. This limited Ireland's negotiating strength in EU deliberations regarding 2020 targets for emissions reduction (Chiodi et al. 2013a). The absence of a *whole energy systems approach* has also contributed to a dominant policy renewable energy focus on wind-generated electricity (Ó Gallachóir et al. 2014). The Irish TIMES model has demonstrated the capacity of the energy system to respond directly to a number of key policy issues, facilitating the comprehension of the key challenges towards a low carbon economy and providing direct evidences on Irish negotiating position regarding new policy developments. However the major challenges have been increasing the trust on the analysis via substantial efforts made in respect of the transparency, the completeness of the model structure and assumptions, through stakeholder events, peer-reviewed publications and the online publication of model documentation and main input assumptions.[6] Moreover stakeholder input contributed directly to the development of the model, proving information and data inputs which have been used to update the model databases, i.e. the techno-economic assumptions of the electricity generation portfolio and bioenergy resource potentials and costs. Including stakeholder engagement and input into model development is challenging; however it does contribute enormous added value in terms of transparency and consistency.

[6] Available online at http://www.ucc.ie/en/energypolicy/irishtimes/.

4 The Experience of TIMES_PT

4.1 Use of TIMES_PT in Policy Support

The development of the TIMES_PT (Simões et al. 2008) model started within the EU research project NEEDS and the national research project E^2POL during 2004. Although its implementation was motivated by research goals, during the past decade the model has become a major tool supporting national climate mitigation policies (Gouveia et al. 2012a), and to a lesser extent, air pollution policies (Fig. 5). The Low Carbon Roadmap 2050 (Seixas et al. 2012) is a flagship policy document currently used as the Portuguese long term view on mitigation goals, while the PNAC—National Plan on Climate Change (Seixas et al. 2014) includes the visions up to 2030 from stakeholders from other policy areas, as transportation and industry. The negotiations for the revisions of the National Emission Ceilings Directive for 2020 and 2030 (Seixas et al. 2009; Ferreira et al. 2014) were supported by projections generated by TIMES_PT. More recently, TIMES_PT was linked with a national CGE model (Fortes et al. 2014), which has motivated its use in the Green Tax Reform (Seixas and Fortes 2014).

4.2 Portugal CLIMA2020

The CLIMA2020 project was the first policy support study using the TIMES_PT model as a reference tool for national climate and energy analysis. The project's main objective was the development of 2020 GHG national emission scenarios and assessment of technical and economic implications for different targets on emissions (ETS and non-ETS) and renewable energy shares. The results were provided to advise the Executive Committee of the Portuguese Climate Change Commission (CECAC)—Ministry of Environment on the EU Climate and Energy Policy Package negotiation.

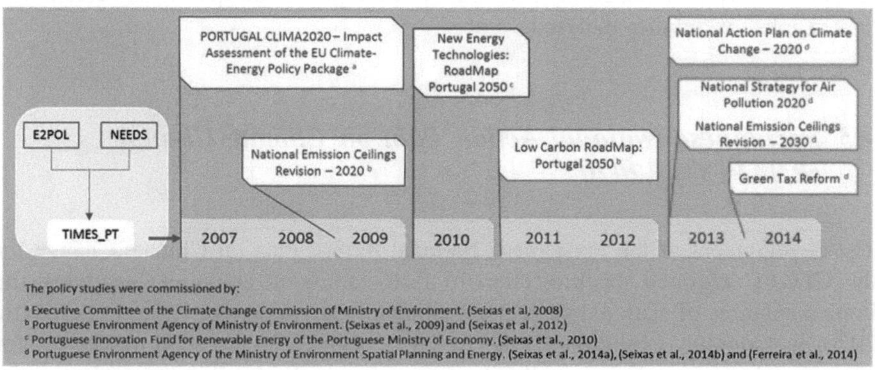

Fig. 5 Overview of the policy support studies using TIMES_PT

4.3 New Energy Technologies: Roadmap Portugal 2050 (NETRP)

The NETRP project assessed the role of new energy technologies, renewable mostly electricity generation, on the national energy system through the development of different national scenarios and focusing on endogenous resources. The work was commissioned by the Portuguese Innovation Fund of the Ministry of Economy. It emphasized the main economic and technical conditions for the competitiveness of the different renewable technologies (solar—PV, CPV and CSP—wind—onshore and offshore—geothermal) in Portugal in the long term. For this, the TIMES_PT model database was upgraded by integrating new technologies or more individual technologies like different photovoltaic and wind offshore technologies. A range of consultations with national industry and experts was held concerning the review and validation of the technical and economic parameters of the TIMES_PT technology database. The scenarios developed included different levels of CO_2 emissions constraints, and progressive reductions on the cost (investment and O&M) of mentioned renewable electricity technologies and electric vehicles.

4.4 Low Carbon Roadmap: Portugal (LCRP) 2050

The ambition to transition to a future low carbon economy in Portugal requires significant effort in achieving the necessary reduction of GHG emissions without compromising the economic and social development. The LCRP—2050 was commissioned by CECAC and established the vision for this by providing an analysis of the technical and economic feasibility of emission reduction trajectories of GHG in Portugal, focusing on modifications in the national energy system and evaluating their economic impact. The scenarios constructed with TIMES_PT covered very different economic growth trajectories and strict GHG emission targets, −60 and −70 % GHG facing 1990 values, in line with the EU low carbon roadmap. The additional co-benefits in terms of improved air quality and creation of "green jobs" were also analysed.

4.5 Portuguese National Action Plan on Climate Change (PNAPCC)—2020

The development of the Portuguese National Action Plan on Climate Change for the CECAC required the projection of GHG emission activities, assuming the implementation of national targets for climate mitigation policy and energy by 2020, and adopting exploratory goals by 2030, inspired by the 2030 framework for climate and energy policies and the positions taken by Portugal in the context of the

EU debate. The GHG national emissions trajectories evaluated by 2030 using TIMES_PT, considered two contrasting socio-economic scenarios, technological evolution scenarios, varied primary energy prices, and the national policy framework. Beyond that, it also analysed the impact of a more conservative view of the national stakeholders on the coal power plants utilization (5 more years than the expected decommissioning), and also a higher availability of the identified cost effective technologies, like solar PV technical and economic potential. Additional runs were made in order to identify potential alternatives on the significant penetration of electric vehicles, the effect of applying a CO_2 tax in sectors not covered by the EU ETS and the potential for renewable production for export, having been based on the assumption of increased interconnections with Europe for the transport of electricity.

4.6 Common Key Findings and Results

A wide number of scenarios were modelled in the policy studies above, depending of the policy requests (Table 2 provides selected examples). Typically two distinct macro-economic scenarios were considered for the long term, encompassing uncertainty. These were combined with different levels of implementation of policies and measures (P&M) according to established policy goals (e.g. National Plan for Energy Efficiency), from deployment of RES power plants to biofuels in transport. The scenarios used common assumptions on primary energy prices (imports of coal, oil and natural gas), on electricity trade with Spain and on hydrological availability, which were then varied in sensitivity analyses. Addition to the reported scenarios, the modellers typically developed more scenarios (often at the request of policy makers) to test how each assumption affects the results. Most of these “extra” scenarios are not directly used in policy support and are instead relevant for research work and model improvements.

The TIMES_PT model, by providing scenarios, has been acting as a central piece for Portuguese policy formulation. The model has been directly used in 7 major national policy development initiatives in climate mitigation, air pollution strategies and green tax reform. The model outputs have supported national communications to the European Commission, the CLRTAP[7] and the UNFCCC and led directly to a number of legislative documents.[8] The transparent approach followed by the modellers and the ongoing engagement with policy makers, has built confidence and trust in model results and contributed for the acceptance of policy proposals.

[7] United Nations Convention on Long-Range Trans boundary Air Pollution.

[8] Such as the Council Minister Resolution (RCM) 119/2004 of July 31st, RCM 104/2006 of August 23rd, or the RCM ° 1/2008 of January 4th.

Table 2 Overview of selected studies using TIMES_PT for policy support

Project name (time horizon)	Project goals	Main TIMES_PT assumptions
Portugal Clima 2020 (2000–2020)	Assess impact of EU 20-20-20 policy package (Seixas et al. 2008)	Two macro-economic scenarios (2–3 % GDP growth), 84 USD_{2010}/bbl in 2020. No GHG caps
New energy technologies: roadmap Portugal 2050 (NETRP) (2005–2050)	Assess competitiveness of renewable technologies within the Portuguese energy system, identifying the critical drivers for their deployment (Seixas et al. 2010)	Two macro-economic scenarios (1–3 % GDP growth), 101 USD_{2010}/bbl in 2020. −20 % GHG cap from 1990 in 2020. Cost reduction in specific renewable technologies
Low carbon roadmap: Portugal (LCRP) 2050 (2005–2050)	Assess the feasibility of achieving a low carbon scenario for Portugal in the long term. Identification of the energy drivers/technologies for achieving a reduction of −60 % and −70 % of energy related and process GHG emissions in 2050 (Seixas et al. 2012)	Two macro-economic scenarios (0.7–3 % GDP growth), 118 USD_{2010}/bbl in 2020. +1 % GHG cap from 1990 in non-ETS in 2020
Portuguese national action plan on climate change (PNAPCC)—2020 (2005–2030)	Develop cost-effective GHG mitigation policies and measures for 2020 (Seixas et al. 2014)	Two macro-economic scenarios (0.39–3 % GDP growth), 115 USD_{2010}/bbl in 2020. +1 % GHG cap from 1990 in non-ETS in 2020. Explicit EU-ETS prices

We believe this has been fundamental to success, since during the past decade several changes have been influencing the model leading to different results for the same modelled year (Fig. 6). For example, there has been a successive downwards adjustment on the GHG projections and upwards on the RES electricity share. These differences are driven by a number of factors, e.g. differences in scenario formulation, expectations on macro-economic growth; primary energy prices, discount rates, etc. Energy systems are intrinsically dynamic and are affected by a myriad of stakeholders and factors. Therefore, any valuable energy system model has to be continually updated and improved. This is only possible if there are enough resources allocated to this time/consuming task and if there is a dedicated modelling team ensuring continuity. In our experience, such has been possible because of the continued model usage for policy making.

On a different note, common key-findings of all the policy support scenario modelling work are the cost-effectiveness of hydro and wind electricity generation technologies from 2020 onwards, and of the PV electricity plants only with the

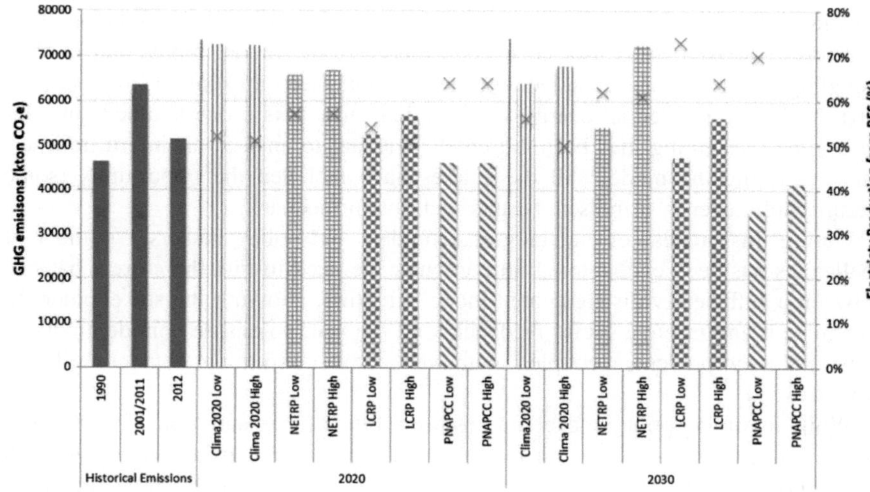

Fig. 6 Projections of GHG emissions (*left axis*) and share of electricity production from RES (*right axis*) for 2020 and 2030 from TIMES_PT within different policy support studies

more recent lower cost data. On the end-use sectors the deployment of electric vehicles is selected, subject to variations in investment costs of around 30 %. On the other hand, the deployment of heat pumps is cost-effective regardless of the several cost updates.

4.7 Discussions and Lessons Learnt

The development of policy studies relies in close cooperation between the modellers and the policy makers that commission them, complemented with frequent meetings with other policy makers and private agents. This process has proven extremely effective for strengthening the role of modelling for policy making, since it enabled the establishment of trust and a common language.

Most of the model inputs have been defined in cooperation with the policy makers that commissioned the studies, particularly the macro-economic assumptions, primary energy import prices, availability of hydrological resources and defining which P&M are in each scenario. The assumptions on energy technologies have been validated with other stakeholders, through a consolidated process (Fortes et al. 2015) including workshops, bilateral meetings and extensive information exchange with the following: Bank of Portugal, Ministry of Economy, Ministry of Transport, associations for production of pulp and paper, chemicals, ceramic, glass and cement; refining companies; electricity utilities; consumer organizations; local and national energy agencies; academia; renewable technologies manufacturers and suppliers and architects. As part of the stakeholder validation process, the files that constitute the model inputs are provided to the stakeholders for validation. Furthermore, extensive work has been done reporting the model inputs and outputs including how the data is generated when applicable (see for example Gouveia et al. (2012b) for the residential energy services demand). This process, albeit substantially time consuming, has been extremely relevant to ensure maximum transparency regarding the model. All the studies have included the opportunity, some within public events, to present results and obtain feedback.

During this process of engaging stakeholders and policy makers a number of challenges has been encountered, in particular the need to find the correct balance between a sufficiently disaggregated model structure, allowing the stakeholders to recognize it and provide useful feedback, and the need to ensure confidentiality in some industry processes coupled with very time consuming data compilation processes.

While involving policy makers, it has been difficult to ensure that TIMES_PT is used as much as possible as an optimization model when it is constrained with assumptions and parameters imposed by policy makers, usually reflecting their expectation of near-term developments, their knowledge on policies that are not fully included in the model or even concerns with eventually politically unacceptable model outcomes. Examples of such assumptions are for example renewable technologies availability factors and minimum activity for certain fossil fuel power plants (Simões et al. 2013). Additionally, policy makers are very demanding on testing new scenarios, perceived as relevant by the policy makers, and are not aware on how time-consuming this task can be. Some of these scenarios do not translate in substantial differences in model outcomes (Simões et al. 2014), particularly CO_2 emissions, which sometimes is very disappointing for policy makers. Finally, a difficulty that should be underlined refers to the need to educate policy makers on the fact that model results provide insights much more than deterministic answers to questions. Although a range of scenarios and results are generated in each policy support process, in several occasions, policy makers have stated: "*Yes, I see all these results, but I just want a number!*"

In conclusion, after ten years of supporting policy makers we have learned the following lessons: (i) opening the model to the stakeholders, public and private, involved in the policy framework is essential to ensure trust and understanding on the model outcomes; (ii) the knowledge on the continuous updates of the model data bases creates a sense of confidence on its outcomes, although they can be different from one modelling exercise to another. This is especially important if the same policy body commissions similar works along the years; (iii) the generation of disruptive scenarios totally different from possible future pathways as perceived by policy makers, usually proposed by the modellers, is very important to give the sense of true alternatives for policy goals and to assess how conservative are the "new" P&M being proposed by policy-makers; (iv) a continuous work with a policy body allows for a high-level cooperation and the recognition that a modelling tool as TIMES_PT, although with limitations, is crucial for policy design, which is directly related with policy evidence.

5 The Experience of IEA ETP Model

5.1 Model Development, Scenarios and Key Findings

In 2001, the Secretariat of the International Energy Agency in Paris launched the Energy Technology Perspectives (ETP) project, with the support of the Energy Technology Systems Analysis Programme (ETSAP) to develop a 15 region global MARKAL model that would be at the heart of the ETP modelling framework.[9] The purpose was to analyse how the deployment of new energy technologies could affect fuel markets, greenhouse gas emissions and energy security (IEA-ETSAP 2001). Over the following four years the model was progressively developed and used to help inform a number of IEA technology studies (IEA 2004, 2005). The ETP project was given significant impetus by the G8 meeting held in Gleneagles, Scotland in July 2005. This meeting launched the G8 Gleneagles Plan of Action on climate change, clean energy and sustainable development and asked the IEA to "*advise on alternative energy scenarios and strategies aimed at a clean clever and competitive energy future*" (G8 2005). As part of its response the IEA began working on a new publication: *Energy Technology Perspectives: Scenarios and Strategies to 2050* (IEA 2006a), which was published in June 2006. This used the ETP MARKAL model to create a "*series of scenarios to demonstrate the role energy technologies that are already available or under development can play in future energy markets*".

The main scenarios were:

1. *Baseline* scenario: includes the effects of technology developments and improvements in energy efficiency that can be expected on the basis of government policies already enacted.
2. *ACT Map* scenario: investigates the potential of energy technologies and best practices aimed at reducing energy demand and emissions, and diversifying energy sources. Focuses on technologies which either exist today or will become commercially available in the next two decades and assumes the successful implementation of a wide range of policies and measures aimed at overcoming barriers to their adoption. Four variants of the ACT scenario were also developed that explore more limited progress in each of four technology areas: renewables, nuclear, carbon capture and storage (CCS) and energy efficiency.
3. *TECH Plus* scenario: makes more optimistic assumptions about the progress for promising energy technologies. Specifically, the scenario assumes greater cost reductions for fuel cells, renewable electricity generation technologies, biofuels and nuclear technologies compared with the ACT Map scenario.

[9] The ETP modelling framework has evolved over time, with the ETP MARKAL (later TIMES) model being supplemented with detailed demand-side models for all major end-uses in the industry, buildings and transport sectors and MARKAL/TIMES models for individual countries and regions.

Based on the results of these scenarios, ETP 2006 concluded that the world was not on course for a sustainable energy future, but that this outlook could be changed. Specifically it proposed a way forward based on strong energy efficiency gains in the transport, industry and buildings sectors, significantly decarbonising the power-generation mix through shifts towards nuclear power, renewables, natural gas and coal with CCS and increased use of biofuels for road transport. The publication highlighted that this would require strong policy action including making energy efficiency the top priority, increasing the budgets for well-focused R&D programmes, creating stable policy environments that promote low carbon options and bridge the *valley of death* between R&D and deployment and increasing international co-operation including between developed and developing countries (Fig. 7).

The key findings from ETP2006 were reported to the St Petersburg G8 summit held in July 2006 and welcomed in a statement from world leaders on Global Energy Security (IEA 2006b). Over the following two years, work continued to develop the ETP model in preparation for a second edition of the ETP publication, including responding to a request from IEA countries for an even more ambitious scenario to address climate change. The next edition of the ETP publication released in June 2008 therefore replaced the *TECH Plus* scenario with a scenario known as *BLUE Map* (plus variants) which envisages a very rapid change in direction of the energy sector leading to a halving of global CO_2 emissions by 2050—consistent with a long term temperature rise of 2–3 degrees (IEA 2008). The ETP2008 modelling showed that halving CO_2 emissions would not be possible with the technologies currently available. Using relatively optimistic assumptions about progress in technology performance and costs, the *BLUE Map* scenario had a marginal cost in 2050 of USD

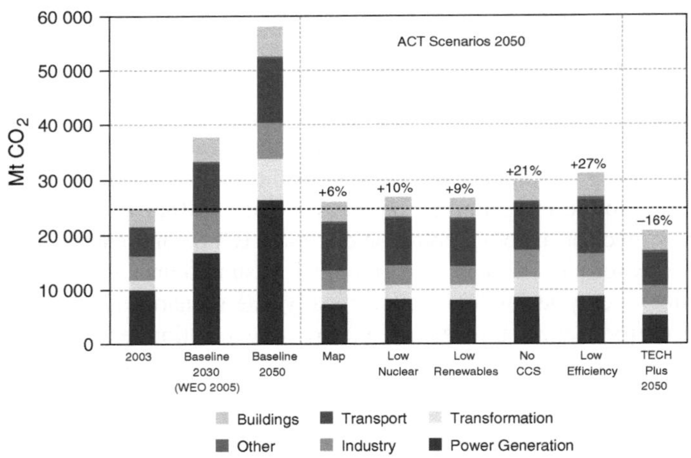

Fig. 7 Global CO_2 emissions in the Baseline Scenario, ACT scenarios and TECH Plus scenario of ETP2006. Based on IEA data from Energy Technology Perspectives © OECD/IEA 2006, IEA Publishing, Fig. 2.1 page 46, License: www.iea.org/t&c/termsandconditions

200 per tCO_2 saved and the technology mix included wide deployment of CCS in the fuel transformation and industry sectors and hydrogen fuel cell vehicles in transport.

By the time the next ETP was released in July 2010 there was a growing realisation that historically high oil prices were starting to impact the world economy. The issues of energy security and economic growth were therefore of significant interest to IEA member countries and this edition used the detailed technological and fuel cost information in the MARKAL model to demonstrate that tackling climate change and improving energy security through lower dependence on fossil fuels were not incompatible with economic priorities. The analysis showed that while realizing the *BLUE Map* scenario would require investments of USD 46 trillion more than the *Baseline* scenario over the period to 2050, over the same period, fuel savings of USD 112 trillion would result. Even if both the investments and fuel savings over the period to 2050 are discounted back to their present values using a 10 % discount rate, the net savings amounted to USD 8 trillion (IEA 2010).

ETP2010 also broke new ground by working with MARKAL analysts and experts in key countries and regions to further develop the regional representation in MARKAL and so present detailed results for OECD Europe, United States, China and India. In the *BLUE Map* scenario, all countries show considerable reductions from the *Baseline* scenario: emissions in 2050 (compared to 2007) were 81 % lower for the United States, 74 % lower for OECD Europe and 30 % lower in China, while India's emissions rose by 10 %.

The 2012 edition of ETP renamed the scenarios according to the long-term temperature rise that was likely to result from each emissions pathway. The baseline scenario therefore became the *6DS* (6° scenario), while the *BLUE Map* scenario became *2DS* and a *4DS* was introduced (somewhat analogous to the previous *Act MAP* scenario). The heart of the modelling framework covering the conversion sector (i.e. transformation of power and fuel) in ETP 2012 was transferred from MARKAL to The Integrated MARKAL-EFOM System (TIMES) model generator, which covered 28 regions and a more detailed depiction of load curves for electricity and heat. The new model was used by ETP2012 to explore the development of three important sub-systems within the energy sector: electricity, heating and cooling and hydrogen. Expanded regional coverage also allowed results to be presented for the first time for Brazil, Russia, South Africa and the ASEAN[10] region (IEA 2012).

The latest edition of ETP published in 2014 focused on the role of electricity in a decarbonized energy system, examining the actions needed to support deployment of sustainable options for generation, distribution and end-use consumption (IEA 2014). All the ETP2014 scenarios showed that electricity's role in the energy system grows faster than any other source and in ETP2014 refined chronological load curves in the TIMES model were used to explore the challenge of balancing supply and demand in greater detail than had previously been possible.

[10] Association of South East Asian Nations.

5.2 Impact of ETP on Global Energy Policy

Over five editions, Energy Technology Perspectives has established itself as the IEA's most important technology publication and a leading source of information for the global energy community. The technology scenarios have been used extensively by a wide range of stakeholders including national governments, international organisations and initiatives, the IEA itself and by academics and other researchers. This success has been due to (i) a flexible framework provided by ETSAP's MARKAL/TIMES model that combines the ability to analyse the technology characteristics of energy systems incorporating both economic and environmental performance data and (ii) access to technology expertise and up-to-date data through the IEA's technology network, consisting of more than 40 multilateral technology initiatives (Implementing Agreements) and more than 6000 specialists covering almost every conceivable energy technology.

A number of national governments have made significant use of the ETP scenarios to support policy-making. For instance, the 2010 and 2011 versions of the US Department of Energy Critical Materials Strategy used the ETP2010 scenarios to develop low and high estimates for materials consumption over the short and medium terms (USDOE 2010, 2011). The report find that many clean energy technologies in the ETP scenarios rely on raw materials with potential supply risks and identifies strategies for addressing these risks. The UK Department of Energy and Climate Change has used the results from ETP2010 to help frame its 2012 science and innovation strategy, highlighting, in particular, the likely large market for clean energy technologies based on the global investment figures from the *BLUE Map* scenario (DECC 2012).

The ETP scenarios are also a key input to many IEA publications including the technology roadmap series, which themselves have proved highly influential in informing the international debate about how best to accelerate the development and deployment of a range of clean energy technologies.[11] Over 20 roadmaps have been published for key low carbon and enabling technologies, describing the potential for transformation across various technology areas, and outlining actions and milestones for the levels of deployment seen in the *BLUE Map/2DS* scenario.

Progress with technology deployment is also monitored in a regular IEA publication *Tracking Clean Energy Progress* that has become an annual input to the Clean Energy Ministerial (CEM).[12] This report tracks each technology and sector against the progress needed to achieve in the IEA BLUE/2DS scenarios. A number of the CEM initiatives have also drawn heavily on ETP scenarios to inform their activities and work programmes including the Bioenergy Working Group, the Carbon Capture, Use and Storage (CCUS) Action Group and the Electric Vehicle Initiative.[13]

---

[11] See http://www.iea.org/roadmaps/.

[12] See http://www.iea.org/etp/tracking/.

[13] See http://www.cleanenergyministerial.org/Our-Work/Initiatives.

The ETP publications have also been referred to extensively in the peer reviewed literature, with over 1500 citations in the peer reviewed literature since 2006, including internationally leading journals such as *Nature* and *Science*.

6 Conclusions

This chapter has presented a selection of case studies which recognize the value of ETSAP modelling tools in providing guidance to decision makers on developing energy and climate mitigation policies. The four case studies showed not only the value of providing quantitative assessments of the key challenges and decisions facing governments in the energy and climate policy space. They also provide insights which helped on overcoming the key barriers to acceptance of the transition to a low carbon future.

6.1 Key Lessons for Modellers

The development of powerful, detailed and robust energy systems model expands the capability for developing and analysing technology roadmaps and assessing the impacts of key climate and energy policies. However this is generally not sufficient in itself to establish trust with policy makers and to underpin policy decisions. Energy systems models are by nature complex, very detailed and not easily accessible, and ensuring transparency and understanding of the model outcomes is not simple. However, the experiences presented in this chapter recognize engagement and dialogue to achieve confidence as a key element for a successful outcome. An open and ongoing engagement between modellers, policy makers and stakeholders; frequent meetings and extensive information exchange via peer-reviewed and online publications have proven to be extremely effective for strengthening the role of modelling for policy making, even though this is very time and resource consuming. Sensitivity analysis and runs are also time consuming, but as was demonstrated they generally contribute to increase the robustness perception of the modelling analysis.

Recent analysis also points to need for expanding the range of outputs from energy systems analysis, from a technology-oriented analysis to a more comprehensive approach, assessing the macro-economic impacts (e.g. impacts on GDP, employment, etc.), impacts on land-use patterns, on non-CO_2 emissions, and the impacts of specific sets of technologies (e.g. storage, wind energy, …), etc. of low carbon economies. Additional insights are needed beyond the direct results that are generated by ETSAP models. Further work is required to investigate new methods for gaining additional insights about these new areas.

6.2 Indications for Policy

This chapter demonstrates how IEA-ETSAP energy systems models can provide unique insight to policy makers. They provide a mean of testing the impacts of single (or groups) of policy targets and assessing the implications of alternative future energy system pathways. They also expand the capability of understanding dynamics behind the interactions between the economy (technology choices, prices, output, etc.), the energy mix and the environment. Energy systems models can contribute to move from a *silos-based* approach (focused on single sets of technologies or specific sectors), to a *whole system* approach, where wide sets of technologies, sectors, and regions are analysed together in a robust and integrated manner. The case studies showed how energy systems model can support policy, how they can point to the feasibility of undertaking challenging climate and energy targets and can also help to change the perception of these challenges to governments, stakeholder and public opinion.

However the development of these modelling tools is extremely complex and time consuming; in which the production of scenarios and the analysis represents only a minimal part of the process. To allow models to continue to expand and increase in capability and robustness, sustained resources need to be allocated to establish and maintain a dedicated modelling team, ensuring continuity. The costs associated with energy systems modelling are dwarfed by the economic benefits of robust, well informed policy decisions.

References

AEA (2008a) MARKAL-MED model runs of long term carbon reduction targets in the UK: Phase 1. AEA Technology

AEA (2008b) MARKAL-MED model runs of long term carbon reduction targets in the UK: Phase 2. AEA Technology

AEA (2011) Pathways to 2050—detailed analyses. MARKAL model review and scenarios for DECC's 4th carbon budget evidence base. AEA Technology

Bergin A, Conefrey T, Fitz-Gerald JD, Kearney I, Žnuderl N (2013) The HERMES-13 macroeconomic model of the Irish economy. Working Paper No. 460, July 2013. Econ Soc Res Inst, Dublin, Ireland

Cahill C, Deane P, Curtis J, Chiodi A, Fitzgerald J, Gargiulo M, Ó Gallachóir BP (2014) EU 2030 climate and energy policy framework. Preliminary assessment and implications for climate policy in Ireland. Report prepared by UCC, ESRI and E4SMA for the Department of Environment, Community and Local Government

CCC (2008) Building a low-carbon economy—the UK's contribution to tackling climate change. The Stationery Office, London

CCC (2010) The fourth carbon budget. Reducing emissions through the 2020s

Chiodi A, Gargiulo M, Deane JP, Lavigne D, Rout UK, Ó Gallachóir BP (2013a) Modelling the impacts of challenging 2020 non-ETS GHG emissions reduction targets on Ireland's energy system. Energy Policy 62(0):1438–1452. doi:http://dx.doi.org/10.1016/j.enpol.2013.07.129

Chiodi A, Gargiulo M, Rogan F, Deane JP, Lavigne D, Rout UK, Ó Gallachóir BP (2013b) Modelling the impacts of challenging 2050 European climate mitigation targets on Ireland's energy system. Energy Policy 53(0):169–189. doi:http://dx.doi.org/10.1016/j.enpol.2012.10.045

Chiodi A, Deane P, Gargiulo M, Ó Gallachóir BP (2015a) The role of bioenergy in Ireland's low carbon future is it sustainable. J Sustain Dev Energy, Water and Environment Systems 3(2):196–216

Chiodi A, Donnellan T, Breen J, Deane JP, Hanrahan K, Gargiulo M, Ó Gallachoir B (2015b) Integrating agriculture and energy to assess GHG emissions reduction—a methodological approach. Clim Policy. doi:10.1080/14693062.2014.993579

Deane JP, Chiodi A, Gargiulo M, Gallachóir BPÓ (2012) Soft-linking of a power systems model to an energy systems model. Energy 42(1):303–312. doi:10.1016/j.energy.2012.03.052

Deane P, Curtis J, Chiodi A, Gargiulo M, Rogan F, Dineen D, Glynn J, Fitzgerald J, Ó Gallachóir BP (2013) Low Carbon Energy Roadmap for Ireland. Technical support on developing low carbon sector roadmaps for Ireland. Report prepared by UCC, ESRI and E4SMA for the Department of Environment, Community and Local Government

DECC (2009) Climate Change Act 2008 impact assessment

DECC (2012) DECC science and innovation strategy 2012. London

DECLG (2013) General scheme of a climate action and low carbon development bill (CA&LCD Bill) 2013

DTI (2003a) Energy white paper. Our energy future—creating a low carbon economy. Department of Trade and Industry, London

DTI (2003b) Options for a low carbon future. Economics Paper No. 4. Department of Trade and Industry, London

DTI (2007a) Meeting the energy challenge. Department of Trade and Industry, London

DTI (2007b) The UK MARKAL energy model in the 2007 energy white paper. Department of Trade and Industry, London

DTI (n.d.) White paper modelling—use of the MARKAL energy model. Available from www.gov.uk/government/uploads/system/uploads/attachment_data/file/48122/file21348.pdf. Department of Trade and Industry, London

EC (2014a) COM (2014) 15 final. A policy framework for climate and energy in the period from 2020 to 2030. Communication from the Commission to the European Parliament, the Council, the European Economic and Social Committee and the Committee of the Regions. Available from http://ec.europa.eu/clima/policies/2030/docs/com_2014_15_en.pdf

EC (2014b) SWD (2014) 15 Commission Staff Working Document. Impact assessment. A policy framework for climate and energy in the period from 2020 up to 2030

Ferreira F, Seixas J, Barroso J, Tente H, Monjardino J, Dias L, Gomes P, Miranda A, Monteiro A, Ferreira J, Martins H, Ribeiro I, Fernandes P (2014) National Strategy for air pollution 2020—projections and scenarios for 2020. [Estratégia Nacional para o Ar 2014–2020—Cenários e Projeções para 2020] Study for the portuguese environmental agency. Lasting values, Lda, CENSE—FCT of the New University of Lisbon and CESAM & Department of Environment and Planning, University of Aveiro, Lisbon (in Portuguese)

Finnis W (1980) Phase II—final report of MARKAL Studies for the United Kingdom: report of the IEA energy systems analysis project

Fortes P, Pereira R, Pereira A, Seixas J (2014) Integrated technological-economic modeling platform for energy and climate policy analysis. Energy 73(0):716–730. doi:http://dx.doi.org/10.1016/j.energy.2014.06.075

Fortes P, Alvarenga A, Seixas S, Rodrigues S (2015) Long term energy scenarios: bridging the gap between socio-economic storylines and energy Modeling. Technol Forecast Soc Chang 91:161–178. doi:j.techfore.2014.02.006

G8 (2005) Gleneagles communiqué. G8 Gleneagles

Glynn J, Chiodi A, Gargiulo M, Deane JP, Bazilian M, Gallachóir BÓ (2014) Energy security analysis: the case of constrained oil supply for Ireland. Energy Policy 66(0):312–325. doi: http://dx.doi.org/10.1016/j.enpol.2013.11.043

Gouveia JP, Dias L, Fortes P, Seixas J (2012a) TIMES_PT: integrated energy system modeling. In: Proceedings of the 1st Int'l workshop on information technology for energy applications (IT4ENERGY'2012)—CEUR workshop proceedings, Lisbon, Portugal, 6–7 September 2012
Gouveia JP, Fortes P, Seixas J (2012b) Projections of energy services demand for residential buildings: Insights from a bottom-up methodology. Energy 47(1):430–442. doi:http://dx.doi.org/10.1016/j.energy.2012.09.042
Great Britain (2008) Climate change act 2008: Elizabeth II. The Stationery Office, London
Great Britain House of Lords (2005) The economics of climate change, vol II: evidence. HL (2005–06, 12-II)
Her Majesty's Government (2009) The low carbon transition plan: national strategy for climate and energy. Analytical Annex
Her Majesty's Government (2011) The carbon plan: delivering our low carbon future
IEA-ETSAP (2001) ETSAP to have key role in IEA energy technology perspectives. ETSAP News, vol 7
IEA (2004) Prospects for CO_2 capture and storage. International Energy Agency, OECD Energy, Paris
IEA (2005) Prospects for hydrogen and fuel cells. International Energy Agency, OECD Energy, Paris
IEA (2006a) Energy technology perspectives 2006. Scenarios and strategies to 2050. International Energy Agency, OECD Energy, Paris
IEA (2006b) Toward a clean, clever and competitive energy future. IEA Report to G8 Summit in St. Petersburg. International Energy Agency, OECD Energy, Paris
IEA (2008) Energy technology perspectives 2008. Scenarios and strategies to 2050. International Energy Agency, OECD Energy, Paris
IEA (2010) Energy Technology perspectives. Scenarios and strategies to 2050. International Energy Agency, OECD Energy, Paris
IEA (2012) Energy technology perspectives. Pathways to a Clean Energy System. International Energy Agency, OECD Energy, Paris
IEA (2014) Energy technology perspectives. Harnessing electricity's potential. International Energy Agency, OECD Energy, Paris
IEEP (2005) Evaluation of the 22nd report of the royal commission on environmental pollution, energy: the changing climate. Final report. Institute for European Environmental Policy
NTUA (2011) The PRIMES energy system model. Summary description. European Commission Joule-III Programme. Athens. Available from http://www.e3mlab.ntua.gr/manuals/PRIMsd.pdf. Accessed March 2014
Ó Gallachóir BP, Chiodi A, Deane P (2014) Renewable electricity is not enough: Increasing renewable heat and transport. In: Proceedings of energy Ireland 2014 Croke Park, 18th–19th June, Dublin
Ó Gallachóir BP, Chiodi A, Gargiulo M, Deane P, Lavigne D, Rout UK (2012) Irish TIMES energy systems model. EPA climate change research programme 2007–2013. Report Series No. 24. UCC, Johnstown Castle, Co.Wexford. http://erc.epa.ie/safer/reports
Pearson P, Watson J (2012) UK Energy Policy 1980–2010: a history and lessons to be learnt
Royal Commission on Environmental Pollution (2000) Energy—the changing climate: Twenty-second report. The Stationery Office, London
Seixas J, Fortes P (2014) Evaluation of the impact of CO_2 taxes in the Portuguese energy system using TIMES_PT model, Annex III [Avaliação do impacto da tributação do CO_2 no sistema energético em Portugal, usando o modelo TIMES_PT (Anexo III)]. Study for the Green Tax Reform Commission. CENSE, FCT of New University of Lisbon, Lisbon, p 39
Seixas J, Simões S, Cleto J, Fortes P, Barroso J, Alves B, Dinis R, Pisco P, Faria P, Finote S (2008) Relatório Final: Portugal Clima 2020—Avaliação do Impacto da Proposta Energia-Clima da Comissão Europeia para Portugal [Final report: Portugal climate 2020—impact evaluation of the EU energy-climate policy package for Portugal]. Study for the Executive Committe of the Climate Change Commission and for the Portuguese Environment Agency. E-value, SA and FCT of New University of Lisbon, Lisbon (in Portuguese)

Seixas J, Barroso J, Dias L, Dinis R, Alves B, Pisco F (2009) PTEN2020—Emissões de Gases Acidificantes e Partículas em 2020—Revisão do protocolo de Gotemburgo da CPATLD e da Diretiva Tetos de Emissão Nacionais [National Emission Celings Program 2020- Emissions of acidifying gaases and particles in 2020—Review of the CLRTAP Gothenburg protocol and national emission ceilings directive]. Study for the Portuguese Environment Agency. E-value, SA and FCT of New University of Lisbon (in Portuguese)

Seixas J, Simões S, Fortes P, Dias L, Gouveia J, Alves B, Mauricio B (2010) New Energy Technologies: RoadMap Portugal 2050—analysis of new national energy technologies & impact scenarios on the national energy system—D3: Competitiveness Assessment of New Energy Technologies, Portuguese Innovation Fund for Renewable Energy of the Ministry of Economy, Lisbon, pp 1–88. (in Portuguese)

Seixas J, Fortes P, Dias L, Dinis R, Alves B, Gouveia J, Simões S (2012) Low Carbon RoadMap—Portugal 2050—Energy and Waste Greenhouse emissions, [Roteiro Nacional de Baixo Carbono—Portugal 2050—Modelação de gases com efeito estufa, Energia e Resíduos. Study for the Executive Committee of the Climate Change Commission. E-value, SA and FCT-UNL of New University of Lisbon, Lisbon (in Portuguese)

Seixas J, Fortes P, Dias L, Barroso J, MArtinho S, Gouveia J, Ferreira F, Gomes P, Tente H, Baptista P (2014) GHG Emission scenarios and technological options for decarbonization in Portugal in 2020 and 2030 [Cenários de emissões de GEE e opções tecnológicas de descarbonização para Portugal em 2020 e 2030]. Study for the Portuguese Environmental Agency. Lasting values, Lda and CENSE, FCT of New University of Lisbon. Lisbon, pp 1–53 (in Portuguese)

Simões S, Cleto J, Fortes P, Seixas J, Huppes G (2008) Cost of energy and environmental policy in Portuguese CO_2 abatement—scenario analysis to 2020. Energy Policy 36(9):3598–3611. doi:http://dx.doi.org/10.1016/j.enpol.2008.06.004

Simões S, Seixas J, Fortes P, Huppes G (2013) The savings of energy saving: interactions between energy supply and demand-side options—quantification for Portugal. Energy Eff 7(2): 179–201. doi:10.1007/s12053-013-9217-7

Simões S, Fortes P, Seixas J, Huppes G (2014) Effects of exogenous assumptions in GHG emissions models—A 2020 scenario study for Portugal using the Times model. Technol Forecast and Soc. In Press October 2014. doi:10.1016/j.techfore.2014.09.016

Strachan N, Kannan R, Pye S (2007) Final report on DTI-DEFRA scenarios and sensitivities, using the UK MARKAL and MARKAL-MACRO energy system models. Policy Studies Institute and UK Energy Research Centre, London

Taylor PG, Upham P, McDowall W, Christopherson D (2014) Energy model, boundary object and societal lens: 35 years of the MARKAL model in the UK. Energy Res Soc Sci 4(0):32–41. doi:http://dx.doi.org/10.1016/j.erss.2014.08.007

USDOE (2010) Critical materials strategy, Office of Policy and International Affairs

USDOE (2011) Critical materials strategy, Office of Policy and International Affairs

Usher W, Strachan N (2010) UK MARKAL modelling—examining decarbonisation pathways in the 2020s on the way to meeting the 2050 emissions target. Final report for the committee on climate change

A Global Renewable Energy Roadmap: Comparing Energy Systems Models with IRENA's REmap 2030 Project

Ruud Kempener, Edi Assoumou, Alessandro Chiodi, Umberto Ciorba, Maria Gaeta, Dolf Gielen, Hiroshi Hamasaki, Amit Kanudia, Tom Kober, Maryse Labriet, Nadia Maïzi, Brian Ó Gallachóir, Deger Saygin, Júlia Seixas, Nicholas Wagner and Evelyn Wright

Abstract In 2014, the International Renewable Energy Agency (IRENA) published a global renewable energy roadmap—called REmap 2030—to double the share of renewables in the global energy mix by 2030 compared to 2010 (IRENA, A Renewable Energy Roadmap, 2014a). A REmap tool was developed to facilitate a transparent and open framework to aggregate the national renewable energy plans and/or scenarios of 26 countries. Unlike the energy systems models by IEA-ETSAP teams, however, the REmap tool does not account for trade-offs between renewable

R. Kempener (✉) · D. Gielen · D. Saygin · N. Wagner
International Renewable Energy Agency, IRENA Innovation and Technology Centre, Bonn, Germany
e-mail: rkempener@irena.org

D. Gielen
e-mail: dgielen@irena.org

D. Saygin
e-mail: dsaygin@irena.org

N. Wagner
e-mail: nwagner@irena.org

E. Assoumou · N. Maïzi
Centre for Applied Mathematics, MINES ParisTech, PSL Research University, Paris, France
e-mail: edi.assoumou@mines-paristech.fr

N. Maïzi
e-mail: nadia.maizi@mines-paristech.fr

A. Chiodi · B. Ó Gallachóir
Energy Policy and Modelling Group, Environmental Research Institute, University College Cork, Cork, Ireland
e-mail: a.chiodi@ucc.ie

B. Ó Gallachóir
e-mail: b.ogallachoir@ucc.ie

G. Giannakidis et al. (eds.), *Informing Energy and Climate Policies Using Energy Systems Models*, Lecture Notes in Energy 30,
DOI 10.1007/978-3-319-16540-0_3

energy and energy efficiency activities, system planning issues like path dependency and investments in the grid infrastructure, competition for scarce resources—e.g. biomass—in the commodity prices, or dynamic cost developments as technologies get deployed over time. This chapter compares the REmap tool with the IEA-ETSAP models at two levels: the results and the insights. Based on the results comparison, it can be concluded that the REmap tool can be used as a way to explicitly engage national experts, to scope renewable energy options, and to compare results across countries. However, the ETSAP models provide detailed insights into the infrastructure requirements, competition between technologies and resources, and the role of energy efficiency needed for planning purposes. These insights are particularly relevant for countries with infrastructure constraints and/or ambitious renewable energy targets. As more and more countries are turning to renewables to secure their energy future, the REmap tool and the ETSAP models have complementary roles to play in engaging policy makers and national energy planners to advance renewables.

U. Ciorba · M. Gaeta
ENEA—Italian National Agency for New Technologies, Energy and Sustainable Economic Development, Central Unit Studies and Scenarios, Rome, Italy
e-mail: umberto.ciorba@enea.it

M. Gaeta
e-mail: maria.gaeta@enea.it

H. Hamasaki
Japan and Centre for International Public Policy Studies, Fujitsu Research Institute, Tokyo, Japan
e-mail: hiroshi.hamasak@jp.fujitsu.com

A. Kanudia
KanORS-EMR, Noida, India
e-mail: amit@KanORS.com

T. Kober
Policy Studies Department, Energy research Centre of the Netherlands (ECN), Petten, The Netherlands
e-mail: kober@ecn.nl

M. Labriet
Eneris Environment Energy Consultants, Madrid, Spain
e-mail: maryse.labriet@enerisconsultants.com

J. Seixas
CENSE, Departamento de Ciências e Engenharia do Ambiente, Faculdade de Ciências e Tecnologia, Universidade Nova de Lisboa, Lisbon, Portugal
e-mail: mjs@fct.unl.pt

E. Wright
Sustainable Energy Economics, Rosendale, NY, USA
e-mail: evelyn.l.wright@gmail.com

1 Introduction

In 2012, the UN Secretary General initiated the Sustainable Energy for All (SE4ALL) initiative with a political call to double of the share of renewable energy in the global energy mix by 2030 compared to 2010. The International Renewable Energy Agency (IRENA) joined the SE4ALL initiative as the hub for renewable energy in the same year. With the United Nations General Assembly declaring 2014–2024 the decade of Sustainable Energy for All, the SE4ALL initiative is now formalized and supported by a global facilitation team.

As an intergovernmental organisation, IRENA was asked by its Members to explore potential pathways to achieve this aspirational target of doubling the share of renewable energy in the global energy mix. This request resulted in the development of a global renewable energy roadmap—REmap 2030—launched in January 2014 (IRENA 2014a).

The main challenge in developing a global roadmap is that the starting point and the potentials to accelerate the deployment of renewables are different per country and per region. For example, the USA and Tonga are two of the REmap countries, but their energy systems are very different from each other. Furthermore, the level of expertise and studies available to explore renewable energy options differs substantially among the IRENA Member countries. Third, the methods used to define renewable energy, renewable energy targets and renewable energy plans differ across countries.

To ensure an accurate representation of country-specific challenges, IRENA developed an analytical framework based on a bottom-up analysis of renewable energy potential in individual country members. In each country, existing renewable energy plans and additional renewable energy options in the 2010–2030 timeframe are identified, and then aggregated at a global level. The 26 countries selected account for around 75 % of global energy consumption, and are representative of different continents.

The tool developed to support this exercise is a relative simple accounting framework. The tool allows national experts to identify additional renewable energy options on top of existing renewable energy expansion plans up to 2030. The advantage of this tool is that it can be applied to all countries and that it provides a transparent way to communicate results with the national experts. However, it does not take into consideration any system constraints, path dependencies or competition for resources that affect both the potential and costs of additional renewable energy (RE) deployment.

There are, however, other tools available to provide a far more detailed analysis of the evolution of energy systems. Among the most widely applied tools are those developed by the Energy Technology Systems Analysis Programme (ETSAP), an implementing agency of the International Energy Agency (IEA). Established in 1976, the programme functions as a consortium of member country teams, mainly using MARKAL and TIMES models to compile long-term energy scenarios. These ETSAP models are bottom-up system engineering tools using least-cost optimisation to satisfy certain system constraints and/or policy objectives. The models can investigate scenarios for the evolution of the energy system, and can also be used to explore which pathway of renewable energy technologies achieves a national renewable energy target with the lowest overall system costs. 20 out of the 26 countries analysed under REmap actually have institutions within their country that are using ETSAP tools.

The ETSAP models are technically far more sophisticated than the REmap tool, but there are a number of specific commonalities and differences between the REmap tool and the ETSAP models that make this comparison of interest. First, both methods are based on technology-specific data, but the REmap tool is limited to energy-supply technologies and electricity-consuming heat and transportation options in the end-use sectors. In contrast, the MARKAL and TIMES models also include the whole range of energy-consuming technologies as well as energy system technologies, like transmission and distribution lines, storage options, etc. Furthermore, in TIMES models, technology deployment in one sector (and region in the case of mult-regional models) will have impacts on deployment levels in the other sectors, while in the REmap tool deployment options are chosen independently. Second, the REmap tool only examines three time instances: 2010, 2020 and 2030. The ETSAP models create time series and the TIMES models even allow for user-defined and flexible length time periods. Third, the TIMES models allow the user to model the construction phase and dismantling of facilities that have reached their end of life internally. The REmap tool assumes that considerations of life time and construction lead times are conducted prior to the selection of additional renewable energy options. Fourth, the ETSAP models allow for multiple regions to be coupled to construct geographically integrated instances, whilst the REmap tool can only be applied to individual countries. Fifth, in the REmap tool energy demand and commodity prices are set exogenously, whilst ETSAP models may include elastic energy demand in the end-use sectors as well as endogenous price setting of commodity prices and energy costs.

The aim of this study is twofold. The first aim is to understand whether the simplified REmap tool creates comparable results with the more sophisticated ETSAP models. The second aim is to understand the appropriateness and complementarity of the usage of both the REmap tool and ETSAP models.

2 Methodology

This methodology section discusses the REmap tool as well as the methodology used to compare the results of ETSAP models with the REmap results.

2.1 REmap Methodology

REmap is based on a bottom-up analysis of existing renewable energy plans and additional renewable energy options between 2010 and 2030 in 26 countries located

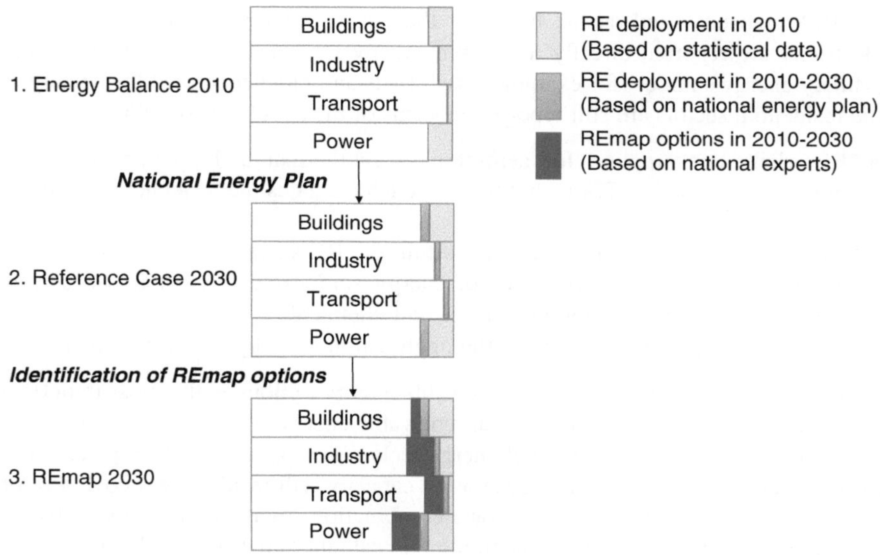

Fig. 1 The analytical steps to develop the REmap analysis

on five different continents (Saygin et al. 2015). For each country analysis, IRENA works together with a REmap expert nominated by the country. Figure 1 shows the three steps in the REmap process. First, data on the national energy balance in 2010 is collected by IRENA and verified by the country expert. Second, the REmap expert provides information on existing renewable energy plans between 2010 and 2030. Based on this information, a national energy balance for 2030 is derived. This is called the **Reference Case**. If no national energy plans are available, IRENA works with national REmap experts to make a business-as-usual projection based on data collected from literature and other sources. Third, together with the national REmap experts and based on existing reports and studies, additional renewable energy options are identified. These are called the **REmap Options**. The technical feasibility of each additional REmap Option is assessed based on resource availability, constraints in the local supply chain, and policies in place promoting or inhibiting further growth of renewables.

At each step, the renewable energy share for both the national energy system and the different subsectors of buildings, industry, power and transport is calculated. The renewable energy share is measured as a percentage of total final energy consumption (TFEC) within a given country or region or sector.[1] Within TFEC—in particular in

[1] The approach is in line with the Global Tracking Framework (GTF) of the SE4ALL initiative, but differs from the EU Directive on Renewable Energy (Article 5, 2009/28/EC) which calculates the RE share based on **gross** final consumption, which includes any RE based electricity and/or heat transmission and distribution losses, including in-house load in power plants.

the IEA statistics used as the basis for the national energy balances—heat and electricity are reported directly in the form ready for consumption although other primary energy sources (for example, fossil fuels and bioenergy used for heating in the residential sector) are still reported in terms of their fuel content. Furthermore:

- Electricity consumption for aerothermal, geothermal and hydrothermal heat pumps is included in TFEC, but the approach excludes the heat energy captured by these pumps.
- RE that is exported is not included within the RE share.
- TFEC excludes non-energy uses of energy sources such as their use as raw material for the production of plastics and chemicals.
- TFEC is computed according to the aggregation used by the IEA statistics.

The identification of additional renewable energy options is the most important step of the process. For each additional renewable energy option, the REmap expert has to determine what conventional energy technology option will be replaced. For example, additional wind power generation capacity will result in less coal, gas, or nuclear power generation capacity (or a combination) built in the period between 2010 and 2030. For each replacement, the tool calculates the so-called 'substitution costs', which is based on the difference in costs of the conventional energy technology—assumed to be in place in 2030—and the renewable energy option that has replaced the conventional energy technology.

Based on this approach, each country analysis results in the creation of a cost supply curve (Fig. 2). The x-axis represents the share of RE in final energy consumption in 2030. The y-axis represents the cost difference per unit of energy consumed [in real 2010 US Dollars per gigajoule (USD_{2010}/GJ)] between renewable and conventional energy technologies. This so-called "annualized incremental cost of substitution"[2] is calculated for each RE technology based on the costs to substitute one unit of final energy generated by non-RE technologies with the costs of one unit of final energy generated by the RE technology. The costs are based on national projections for the capital and operational and maintenance (O&M) costs, and the technical performance of conventional and RE technologies.

To allow for comparison and aggregation of results across multiple countries, standardized energy commodity prices for oil, gas and coal (without any subsidies, taxes, or levies),[3] a standardized cost calculation for electricity prices (based on the maximum RE penetration in 2030), and a fixed 10 % discount rate based on IRENA's costing studies (IRENA 2013) are used to calculate the annualized costs of both RE and conventional technologies. The fixed discount rate (for all countries and technologies) is chosen to allow for comparable results, whereby 10 % is

[2] Referred as "substitution cost" throughout this report.

[3] For coal, natural gas, biomass and electricity, exceptions were made as it is not possible to assign global values that are representative for all countries. Coal and natural gas prices are distinguished between exporting and importing countries. Biomass prices are determined at a regional level with a breakdown by energy crops, residues and waste. Electricity prices are determined for each country.

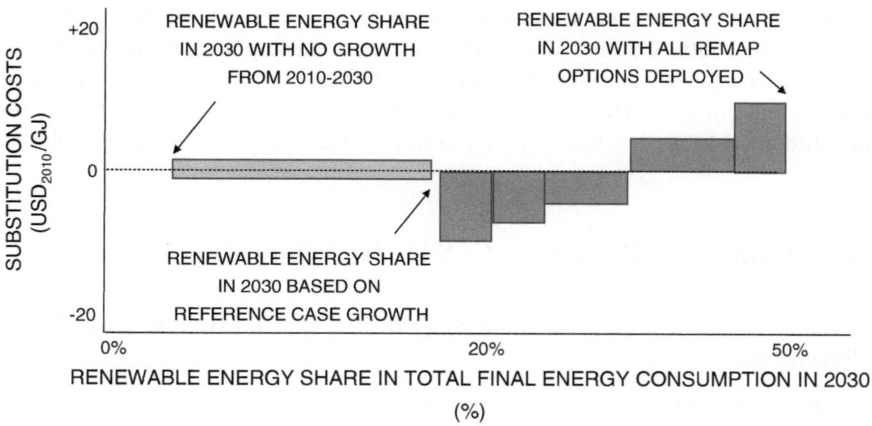

Fig. 2 The REmap cost supply curve

chosen as a middle ground between the costs of capital for energy projects in developing countries (indicative range of 15–20 %) and OECD countries (indicative range of 6–12 %). The costs are expressed in USD_{2010}/GJ.

In the electricity and heat sector, one unit of final energy generated by an RE technology substitutes the same amount of energy produced by a non-RE technology. In other words, one MWh of coal-based electricity production would be replaced by one megawatt-hour (MWh) of solar-based electricity production. For the end-use sectors, one unit of final energy used by an RE technology substitutes the units of final energy which would have been otherwise used by a non-RE technology to deliver the same amount of useful energy. Electricity consumption of heat pumps to generate heat (e.g. for space heating) from various sources including air, geothermal, hydrothermal, is included in the TFEC of the respective end-use sectors (e.g. residential sector). However, heat consumed by the end-use sectors is not reported separately in the TFEC. Substitution costs of heat pumps are expressed in USD per GJ of heat produced. To estimate heat production, the co-efficient of performance (COP) is used. The costs are calculated as follows:

Substitution cost of an RE technology for the energy transformation sector is estimated as "*(annualized costs of RE technology to generate 1 petajoule (PJ) of electricity or heat—annualized costs of non-RE technology to generate 1 PJ of electricity or heat)/total RE electricity or heat generated*".

Substitution cost of an RE technology for the end-use sectors is estimated as "*(annualized costs of RE technology to generate 1 PJ of useful energy—annualized costs of non-RE technology to generate 1 PJ of useful energy) /total RE final energy used to generate 1 PJ of useful energy*".

The cost supply curve contains two separate sets of data (Fig. 2). The first part of the curve represents the increase in the renewable energy share between 2010 and 2030 based on the Reference Case. Since the existing national energy plans are assumed to be the baseline, no costs are associated with the renewable energy expansion in the Reference Case. The second part of the curve shows the REmap Options. The width of each REmap Option is determined by the absolute amount of renewable energy consumption entering the system, and is represented on the x-axis as an increase in the renewable energy share in 2030. For each REmap options, the substitution costs are determined by the conventional energy option being replaced.

2.2 Comparing REmap and ETSAP Modelling Results

For the comparison of the results, IRENA provided the ETSAP modellers with the following data:

- Data sources for Reference Case and REmap Options;
- Total energy consumption and RE deployment in the Reference Case per sector, expressed in PJ or GWh;
- The assumed commodity prices and discount factors for 2030. These assumptions impact the cost calculations;
- List of REmap Options, expressed in PJ and with associated substitution costs;
- RE shares in the end-use sectors in 2030 in the Reference Case as well as after the REmap Options.

Based on this information, the ETSAP modellers performed clusters of multiple model runs for the year 2030 for the specific purpose of this chapter. The first model run targets the RE share in 2030 as suggested by the Reference Case. Each subsequent model run increases the RE share by a certain percentage up to the RE share achieved by the REmap Options. The RE share are only applied at a national level, and not to individual subsectors.

The approach is illustrated with the Irish TIMES model (Ó Gallachóir et al. 2012). The x-axis shows the total share of RE in TFEC by 2030, while the y-axis shows the system cost difference of each REmap scenario from the *Reference Case*. For each target scenario pathway, a scenario file has been created (e.g. in the case of Ireland, as shown in Fig. 3 we have the *Reference Case* with 16 % by 2020, and 16 % by 2030; the *REmap-18* case with 16 % by 2020, 18 % by 2030, etc.). The supply curve was built comparing differences in total system costs between scenario runs. The costs of additional RE options are only positive (incremental), because, unlike in the REmap analysis, the negative costs (savings) are already embedded in the *Reference Case* (objective minimization of total system cost).

Given the nature of MARKAL-TIMES models (vertical and horizontal competition), multiple substitution technologies and/or efficiency measures are selected as the model optimizes for an increasing share of renewables in the system. The contributions of individual renewable energy technologies (and the conventional technologies that have been substituted) are identified afterwards from results analysis, as shown in Fig. 3.

Furthermore, each scenario is run individually, which means that the system changes (i.e. electrification of the transport sector) under a 16 % scenario target

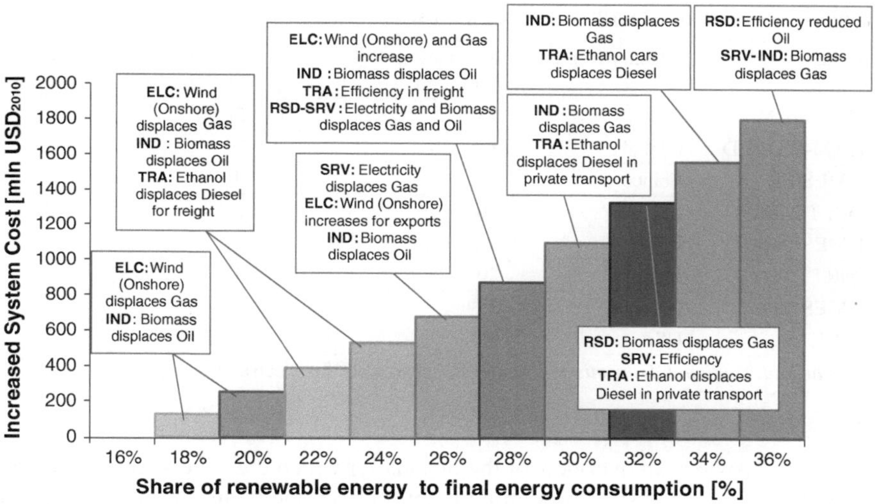

Fig. 3 Illustrative cost supply curve for Ireland. Information on the x-axis and y-axis show the share of RE in TFFC and the increased system costs, respectively

might not apply to the 18 % scenario target. Furthermore, some system changes might be reversed at a later stage. Any discontinuities are highlighted in the results analysis.

Implementation of REmap scenarios in the Irish TIMES model

The implementation in single MARKAL-TIMES models strongly depends on the model structure. In Irish TIMES the cost supply curve has been built performing a cluster of 11 model runs with the Reference Case as a starting point, in which Ireland's energy system must deliver at least 16 % renewable energy penetration by 2020 (the EU RE Directive target for Ireland for the year 2020), and is then assumed to maintain this share in the period 2020–2030. Each individual *REmap* scenario run then increases the RE share by 2 percentage points resulting in a final scenario of 36 % RE share by 2030 (Fig. 3).

Furthermore, the amount of RE consumed (measured as a share of total final energy consumption, or TFEC) was simply evaluated as the sum of green certificates produced by renewable technologies in the electricity generation sector and the end use sectors. In Irish TIMES green certificates are automatically generated by the model when renewable fuels are consumed in electricity, heat and transport sectors. The EU Directive sectoral specific target of 10 % renewables in the transport sector (with different weightings for different biofuels) was excluded in the Irish TIMES *REmap scenarios*.

Table 1 Overview of ETSAP models and the assessed range of RE share in TFEC in 2030

Model	Country/Region	RE share in Reference Case (%)	RE share with REmap Options (%)
TIAM-ECN	Global	18	36
TIAM-WORLD	Global	18	37
TIMES-FR	France	27	42
Irish TIMES	Ireland	16	36
TIMES-Italy	Italy	9.5	19
JMRT[a]	Japan	20	44
TIMES-PT	Portugal	33	62
FACETS	USA	8.3	16.7

[a] *Japan Multi-regional Transmission Model* RE shares are for electricity sector only

Table1 provides an overview of the models for which the results were compared with the REmap analysis. The starting point for each model has been the RE share in the Reference Case. For the case of Ireland and Portugal, the Reference Case was based on the EU RE Directive target for 2020 and extended towards 2030. For the case of Italy, the government's new energy strategy (*Strategia Energetica Nazionale*, SEN) was used as the *Reference Case* and the ETSAP model was used to identify and quantify the REmap Options.

In the following two subsections, the results of these comparative analyses are used to explore the aims and main questions outlined at the outset of this chapter:

1. How do the REmap Options identified by national experts compare to the renewable energy deployment identified in ETSAP models (Sect. 3)?
2. How can the different insights derived from the ETSAP models and the REmap tools be used to support policy makers (Sect. 4)?

3 Comparing Results

This section answers the question of whether the results of the simplified REmap tool are in line with the results of the more sophisticated ETSAP models. The results of the REmap tool and the ETSAP models are compared on three levels:

- Deployment of renewable energy technologies (in PJ or GWh) in 2030 (Sect. 3.1);
- The sequence with which renewable energy technologies are deployed to increase the share of RE (Sect. 3.2);
- The additional overall system costs compared to the Reference Case (Sect. 3.3).

3.1 Comparing Results: Deployment Levels in 2030

Table 2 presents some comparative deployment numbers in the ETSAP models and REmap results for France, Japan and the world (Ireland and Portugal were not part of the initial set of 26 REmap countries).

These results show that considering the differences in the overall RE share in 2030 (ranging between 0 and 5 %) in each country, the deployment levels of individual renewable energy technologies between the ETSAP models and the REmap results are comparable. In the case of France and Japan, the national REmap experts have assumed higher deployment levels of hydropower but lower levels of solar photovoltaics than the ETSAP models. This might be due to the fact that in the ETSAP models the deployment levels are a function of their techno-economic characteristics in 2030, whilst the deployment levels in the REmap tool is a deliberate choice of the national experts. For technologies like solar photovoltaics that are currently at a relative low deployment level, it might be difficult for these national experts to envision their rapid growth of deployment. Similarly, the biggest difference can be found in solar photovoltaics deployment at a global level, but this might also be explained by the fact that the TIAM-WORLD model targets 37 % RE share, whilst the REmap analysis only achieves 28 %.

3.2 Comparing Results: Substitution Choices

The comparison of absolute deployment levels in Sect. 3.1 provides a static picture of the deployment levels in 2030. The REmap model, through its cost supply curve, and the ETSAP models also allow for a comparison of the relative costs of different RE options. In the case of the REmap cost supply curve, individual RE options

Table 2 Comparison of deployment levels of renewable power generation in ETSAP models and the REmap tools in 2030

	TFEC (EJ)	RE share (%)	Hydro (TWh)	Wind (TWh)	Solar PV (TWh)
TIMES-FR	5.1	42	67	89	33
REmap France	5	40	83	89	30
TIMES-IT[a]	115.8	40	48	29.3	28.7
REmap Italy[a]	115	40	50	29.4	29
JMRT[b]	4	43.7	93	188	146
REmap Japan[b]	4	40	127	113	121
FACETS	68	16.7	251	650	361
REmap USA	66	27	430	994	235
TIAM-WORLD	491	37	5673	4043	3150
REmap World	448	28	5907	5279	1807

[a] TIMES-IT was used to populate the REmap tool for Italy

[b] Power sector only

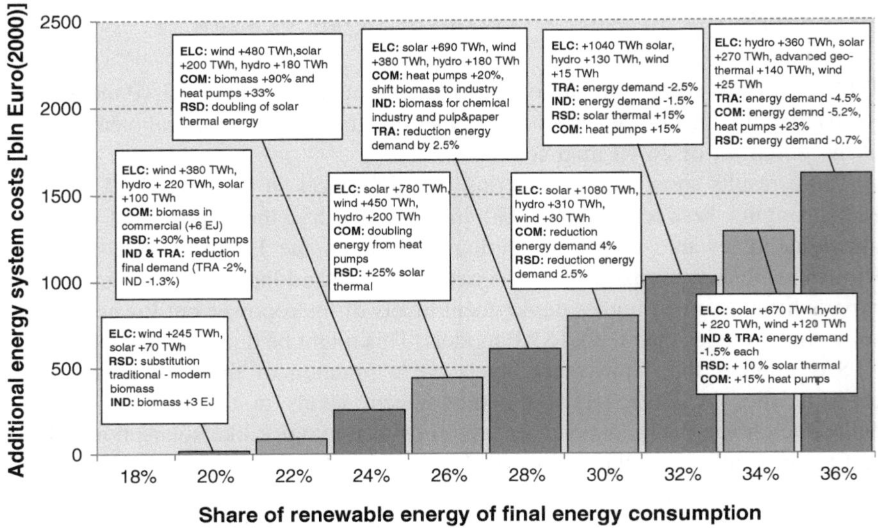

Fig. 4 Global marginal cost curve for the renewable energy share of gross final energy consumption in 2030 based on TIAM-ECN. *N.B.* (1) additional system costs refer to the Reference Case with a renewable energy share in 2030 at today's level of 18 %. (2) Descriptions in the boxes refer to effects of the incremental increase. (3) Abbreviations for sectors *ELC* elcectricity, *IND* industry, *COM* commercial and agriculture, *RSD* residential, *TRA* transport

contributing to the RE share in 2030 are displayed in order of increasing costs. The ETSAP models, by virtue of their economic cost optimization, choose the most economic options contributing to an increasing RE share. This means that the REmap Options on the left side of the curve (the cheaper options) would also be the first options that would be chosen by the ETSAP models to increase the RE share. A key difference between the REmap tool and the ETSAP models is that the latter also may choose energy efficiency options or structural changes to the energy system to increase the RE share.

Figures 4 and 5 show the sequences of RE options identified by the TIAM-World and TIAM-ECN models as the RE share increases from 18 to 36 %. These results can be compared to the global REmap cost supply curve.

The TIAM-ECN [for model description see Rösler et al. (2011), Keppo and van der Zwaan (2012), Kober (2014)] model shows that early opportunities to increase the RE share arise from the shift of biomass from traditional use to modern biomass use in the residential sector, but also an increased biomass use in the commercial sector and in industry.[4] Additional least cost opportunities to accelerate RE growth in the residential and commercial sectors include heat pumps and solar thermal appliances for room

[4] Traditional uses of biomass is not included in the renewable energy share, hence a shift to modern uses of biomass increases the share of RE.

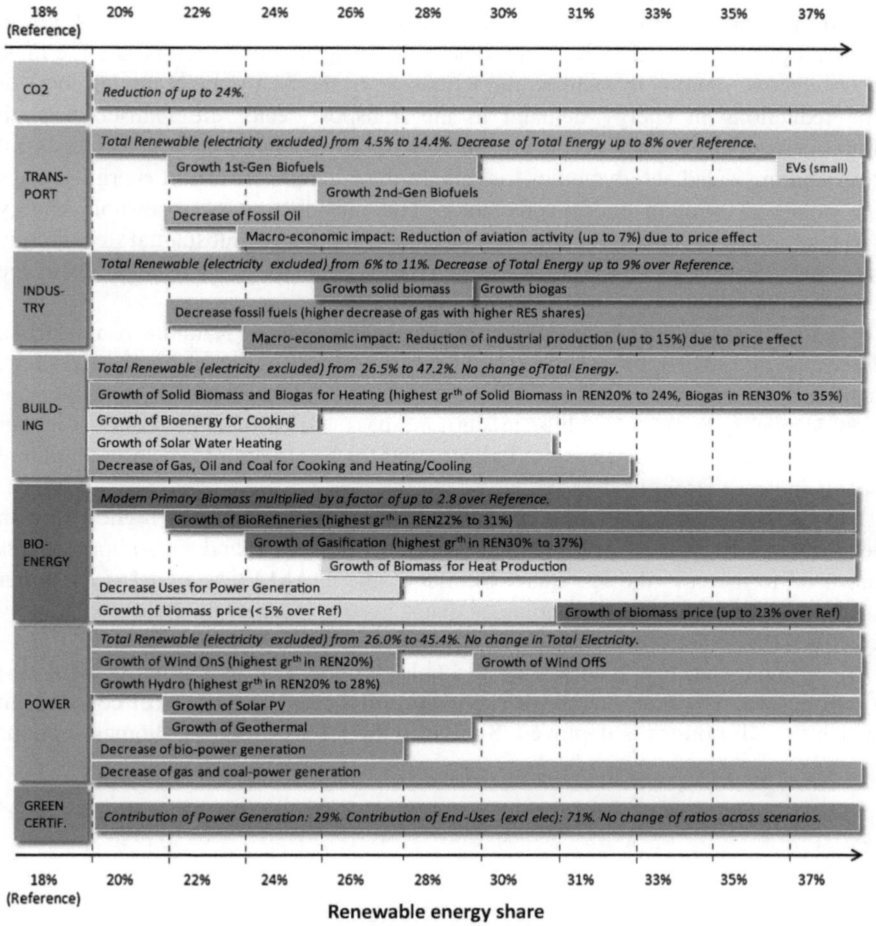

Fig. 5 Technology options with increasing RE share in the TIAM-WORLD model

heat and warm water production. For electricity generation from RE, wind offshore technology represents the least cost option, and contributes with additional 1000 TWh to increase the RE share of gross final energy consumption from 18 to 26 %.

The more costly options for increasing the RE share, which are deployed at shares higher than 26 %, include measures and technologies to diminish the total final energy demand, such as more efficient engines for road transport, and also more expensive options for the production of RE-based electricity. For RE-targets above 28 %, electricity generation from wind (onshore and offshore) is almost fully deployed (in total about 1300 GW), and additional capacity from RE technology is commissioned based on solar (mainly CSP and PV at sites with lower full load hours), small hydro power plants and advanced geothermal power plants.

At high levels of RE shares, strong reductions in energy demand use (−4.5 % in the transport sector, −5 % in the commercial and agricultural sectors) are the most cost-effective options to increase the RE share. In the TIAM-ECN model, most of the reductions in energy demand in the transport sector are realised through improvements of energy efficiency, such as more efficient engines, low resistant tires and improved aerodynamics for cars. In the commercial sector, energy savings are achieved through energy efficiency. The introduction of renewable energy targets failed to provide sufficient incentive for more substantial technology switches, such as electric cars, hydrogen vehicles or fuel cell technology in the commercial sector.

In the TIAM-WORLD model [see recent applications in Kanudia et al. (2014); Labriet et al. (2012)], bioenergy also plays a crucial role in increasing the RE share, especially in the end-use sectors. More specifically, biomass-based power generation decreases up to 26 % whilst modern biomass and biofuels increase. At higher RE shares (>30 %), biogas use in industry and for heating purposes in the building sector increase strongly (Fig. 5).

In the power sector, hydropower and onshore wind exhibit the highest growth levels at low RE shares. At higher RE shares, offshore wind and solar photovoltaics are used to increase the RE share. Similar to the TIAM-ECN model, solar water heating is one of the early technologies that is used to increase the RE share. Battery electric vehicle are only deployed at RE shares above 35 %.

In comparison, Fig. 6 shows the technology options of the REmap global cost supply curve. The brackets above each option indicate the number of countries in which the RE options is deployed. Similar to the ETSAP models, biomass options

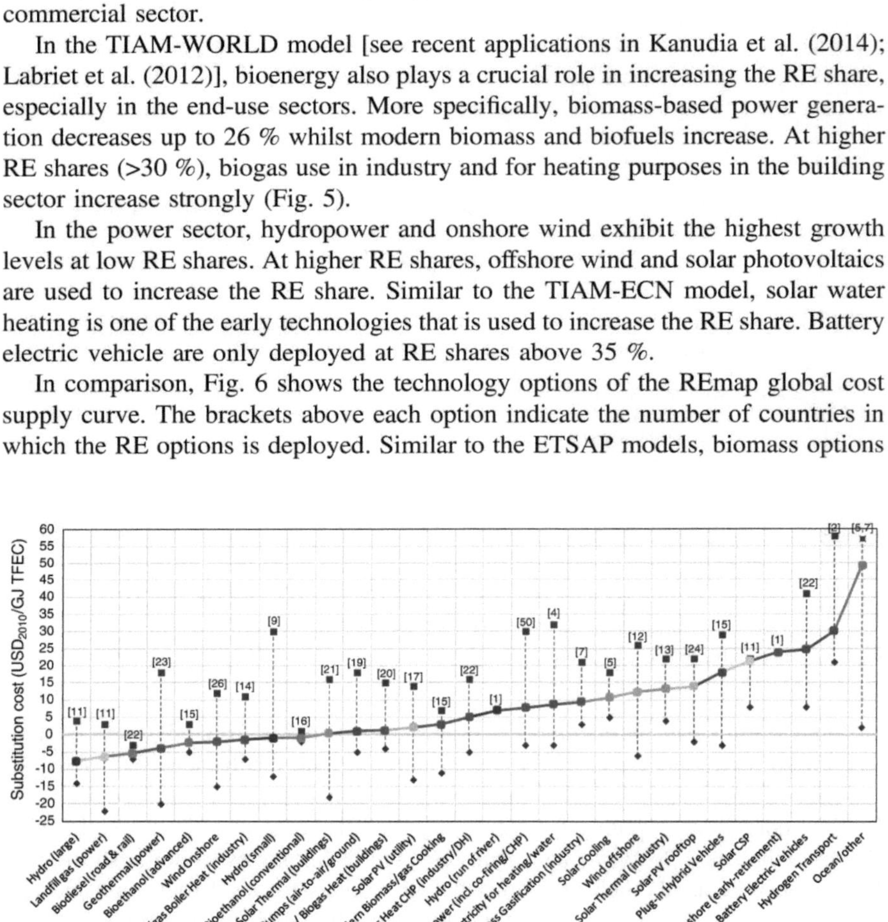

Fig. 6 Ranges of substitution costs of REmap Options in the 26 REmap countries based on the perspective of governments in 2030

are among the least-cost options to increase the RE share of modern energy use, except for biomass gasification. Solar thermal and heat pumps are cost-effective options in the buildings sector. In the power sector, hydro, wind and geothermal are the least cost options followed by solar photovoltaics. The more expensive options are solar photovoltaics on rooftops, solar concentrated solar power, and the upgrading/repowering of existing wind parks [indicated as "wind onshore (early retirement)"]. Similar to the TIAM-WORLD model, battery electric vehicles are one of the most expensive options to increase the RE share.

A similar analysis is possible at a country level. Figure 7 shows the REmap cost supply curve of the USA (IRENA 2014b). Figure 8 shows the RE options contributing to an increasing RE share in the FACETS model (for model description see Wright and Kanudia (2014) and http://facets-model.com).

The results from the FACETS model and the REmap tool show that the main contributors (wind, solar PV, biomass heat and electricity production, and biofuels) to an increasing renewable energy share are the same, but they differ in terms of the sequence with which they are deployed. These differences are partly due to the different RE targets for 2030. Wind power (nr. 4 in Fig. 7) is one of the cheaper options in the REmap tool, but is only chosen at a later stage in the FACETS model. Similarly, biofuels seem to be a technology option that is relatively cheap in the REmap tool (nr. 7 in Fig. 7), deployed at later stages in the FACETS model.

One explanation for the differences is the explicit choice for substitution technologies that is offered by the REmap tool. In the USA analysis, national REmap analysts determine that the additional renewable power generation would mainly

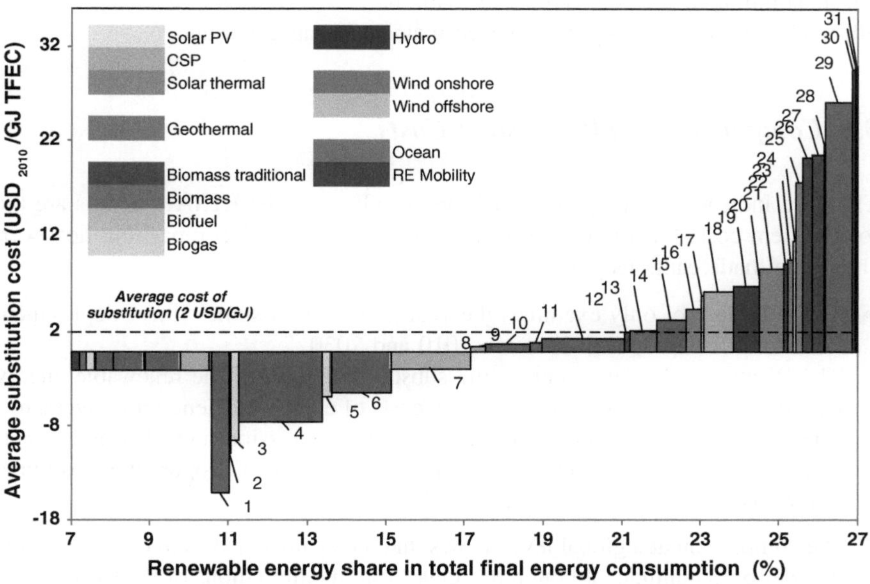

Fig. 7 REmap Options cost supply curve, government perspective, by resource

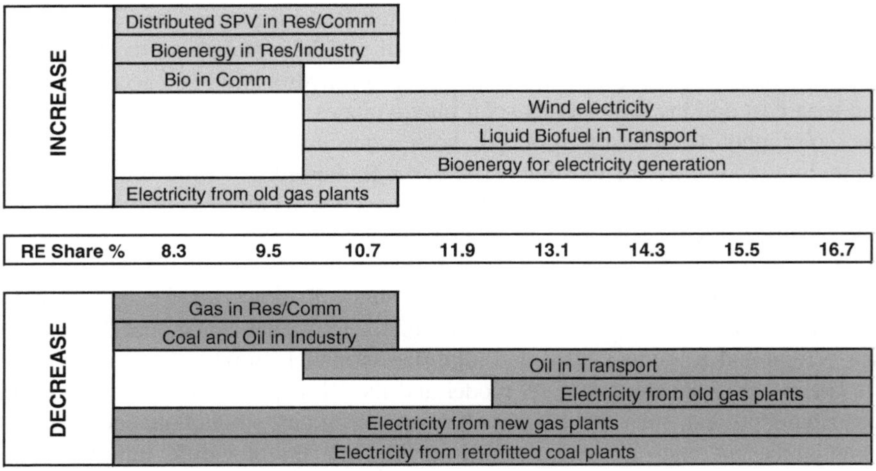

Fig. 8 RE technology options in the FACETS model

replace United States Environmental Protection Agency (EPA) compliant conventional coal (89 %), new nuclear (6 %) and advanced coal carbon capture and storage (CCS) (5 %). In contrast, the FACETS model chooses to rely on electricity production from old inefficient gas plants to support the variable renewable power generation production from distributed solar photovoltaics, and replace both new and old gas plants as the renewable energy share is increased. In the industry sector, the substitution choice is also different with the FACETS model replacing coal and oil, whilst the national experts replaced mainly natural gas usage.

3.3 Comparing Results: System Costs

The third indicator to compare the REmap results with the ETSAP models are the total system costs for a transition towards renewables. This comparison, however, should be made cautiously as:

- The REmap tool only examines the year 2030, and assumes linear deployment rates for RE deployment between 2010 and 2030;
- The REmap tool only examines the substitution costs of the renewable energy technologies, and does not consider the costs of energy efficiency improvements;
- The REmap tool does not consider costs in transmission and distribution networks, or other infrastructural investments, required to support the additional renewable energy deployment (Table 3).

The comparison at a global level shows that the estimated system costs are in the same order of magnitude, although it is clear from the limitations of the REmap tool that ETSAP models are better suited for an assessment of system costs. For the year

Table 3 Comparison of incremental systems costs over the Reference Case for the ETSAP models and the global REmap results

Model	Incremental system costs (USD_{2010})[a] (billion)	Discount rate (%)
Global REmap	1450	10
TIAM-ECN	1980	10
TIAM-WORLD	5582	5
TIMES-FR	58	10
Irish TIMES	1.8	6
TIMES-PT[b]	5.6	10
FACETS	865	5

[a] The costs are converted into USD_{2010} using the official exchange rates and consumer price indexes provided by the World Bank (http://data.worldbank.org/indicator/PA.NUS.FCRF and http://data.worldbank.org/indicator/FP.CPI.TOTL)

[b] For decentralized solar PV on residential rooftops, a discount rate of 17.5 % was used to reflect family decisions

2030, the REmap tool estimates total additional system costs of USD_{2010} 145 billion. An approximate level of additional system costs over the 2010–2030 period would be USD_{2010} 1450 billion assuming linear increasing deployment levels of renewables.[5] In comparison, the total additional energy system costs estimated by the TIAM-ECN model are around USD_{2010} 1980 billion, and for the TIAM-WORLD model USD_{2010} 5580 billion (discount rate of 5 %). The higher system costs observed in TIAM-WORLD are explained by the lower discount rate (system costs obtained with a 10 % discount rate are in the range of USD_{2010} 1340 billion.

The incremental system costs for the national models highly depends on the system size, national cost assumptions, absolute deployment levels as well as the different financial indicators used. More detailed information would be required to make a one by one comparison across the national results.

4 Comparing Insights

The second question is how the different insights derived from the ETSAP models and the REmap tools can be used to support policy makers, and when and where the REmap tool and ETSAP models are appropriate to use. One clear advantage of the ETSAP models is their ability to examine changes at each time step, whilst the REmap tool only provides results for a single year (essentially assuming that all

[5] For a proper comparison, additional assumptions would be required in terms of the energy commodity prices (oil, coal, gas, biomass, electricity, etc.), and capital and operational cost development for both renewable and conventional energy technologies over the 2010–2030 period.

system changes occur instantaneously). However, there are also a number of other features that are included in the ETSAP models but excluded from the REmap tool:

- The inclusion of infrastructural systems to examine the transition towards renewables (Sect. 4.1);
- The dynamic interaction and competition between different renewable energy technologies and resources (Sect. 4.2);
- The inclusion of both energy efficiency and renewable energy options (Sect. 4.3).

Furthermore, we explore the use of ETSAP models as input into the REmap tool.

4.1 Comparing Insights: Infrastructural Features

The REmap tool assumes that any costs associated with infrastructural investments that will take place in the Reference Case will also support the deployment of renewable energy options. In the ETSAP models, these infrastructural requirements can be explicitly modelled and taken into consideration. The results of the JMRT model show this most clearly (Hamasaki and Kanudia 2013). The model comprises 10 grids with weak inter-grid connections, using geographically specific resource data and GIS data to calculate distances to and from roads and grids, as well as seabed depth. In Japan, the greatest potential for onshore wind lies in the Northern regions, while the Southern region has great demand but limited potential, resulting in geographical supply-demand mismatch. Given the current state of Japan's power grids, the full potential of onshore wind in the north cannot be tapped without new interconnecting facilities.

Grid expansion changes the portfolio of renewable energy technologies selected under a 44 % renewable energy target. Onshore wind deployment levels increase and geothermal and offshore wind decrease (±10 % on deployment levels). The model also shows that despite the increased costs for the interconnecting facilities, the overall system costs will be marginally lower with grid expansion.

The impacts of infrastructure on the deployment levels of renewable energy technologies is an important insight for policy makers, especially since in the case of Japan they substantially alter perspectives for onshore versus offshore wind deployment. However, the JMRT model also shows that substantial model enhancements are needed to address these issues, including the introduction of sub-regions, increased data requirements and higher computing power.

In general, it seems that the inclusion of infrastructural constraints increases the insights provided by the ETSAP models, but the demand for model development and data requirements are also substantially higher than the REmap tools. As the renewable energy shares, especially those of wind power and solar photovoltaics, increase, the insights from the ETSAP models on infrastructural requirements and investments will become more important for policy makers.

4.2 Comparing Insights: Competition of Technologies and Resources

The REmap tool allows the national policy makers to identify additional individual renewable energy options to be deployed above and beyond the Reference Case. The deployment levels for these additional RE options should be based on an assessment of the available resources, energy demand, supply chain constraints and political barriers for each of the individual RE options. However, the REmap tool does not force the analyst to consider competition between different REmap Options, except for the fact the overall deployment levels are limited to the energy demand within a given sector.

In the ETSAP models, there is endogenous competition between the different RE technologies to satisfy the RE share that is set for the year 2030 most cost effectively. Figure 9 shows this competition for the case of TIMES-FR (Assoumou and Maïzi 2011). The results show the difference in deployment levels between the *Reference Case* to achieve a 27 % RE share, and higher RE shares. The results show increasing levels of solar heating deployed to satisfy the increasing shares of RE. However, beyond 36 % it becomes more cost-effective to deploy solar photovoltaics systems rather than solar water heaters. Due to space limitations associated with rooftops, this leads to a decrease in the deployment of solar water heaters. Similarly, the results show that to achieve higher shares of RE the deployment levels of biofuels in the transport sector drop in favour of biomass usage for heat and power. Furthermore, additional biogas production based on energy crops is used to increase biomass usage at higher renewable energy shares.

Fig. 9 Increase of renewables per source (vs. 27 % case) in TIMES-FR

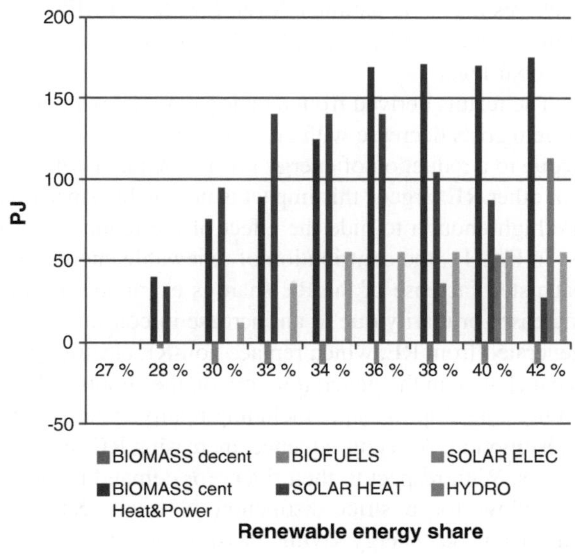

Similar dynamics can be observed in the Irish TIMES model (Fig. 3). In that particular case, the deployment levels of biomass in the commercial sector decreases in favour of increased levels of biofuel usage in the transport sector as the renewable energy share increases from 30 to 32 %.

The competition between renewable energy resources and technologies is an important insight that can be gained from the ETSAP models, and that can inform the deployment levels of renewable energy technologies considered in the REmap tool. These insights seem to be particularly relevant for biomass, which is a renewable energy technology that can be used in the power sector as well as all of the end-use sectors. Consequently, countries that have high levels of biomass use should complement any REmap analysis with more detailed ETSAP models to understand how competition between the different end-use sectors may affect both the prices of biomass commodities as well as the deployment levels.

4.3 Comparing Insights: Energy Efficiency and Rational Use of Energy

Energy efficiency can substantially contribute to higher shares of renewables by reducing overall energy consumption. The REmap tool only considers energy efficiency measures that have been considered in the Reference Case, and as such determine the national energy balance in 2030. In contrast, the ETSAP models explicitly consider additional energy efficiency measures to increase the share of renewables.

All of the ETSAP models show that energy efficiency measures and the reduction of energy service demand are very important tools to increase the RE share, especially when RE shares are reaching levels above 30 %. Figure 10 shows such results at a national level for the TIMES-PT model created for Portugal (Simoes et al. 2008), whilst Fig. 11 shows the impact of energy efficiency options at a global level.

The results derived from a national model with elastic demand show that the total system costs decrease with an increasing share of renewables from 40 to 41 %. This is due to a reduction of energy service demand with impact in the total system costs. For other RE targets, this impact is not visible since other costs like investment costs are high enough to hide the effect of the reduction of services demand.

In Fig. 11, the contribution of renewable energy and energy efficiency options in each step increase of the RE share is examined. From 26 to 34 %, the share of RE increases primarily due to an increase in consumption of electricity and district heat generated from RE, which replace non-RE electricity. In this range of RE targets, we see a change in the generation mix on the supply side rather than substantial changes on the consumption side, including relatively small changes in the total final energy consumption. As a consequence, increasing RE supply outweighs demand-reduction-effects. With respect to the drivers for demand reductions, the model approach does not allow for a strict distinction between technology-related energy efficiency improvements, energy saving measures and demand reductions due to changes in the

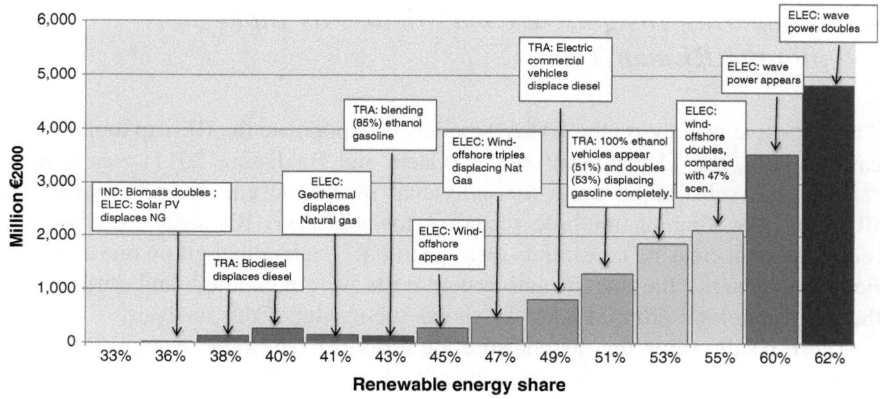

Fig. 10 National cost supply curve for Portugal from the TIMES-PT model

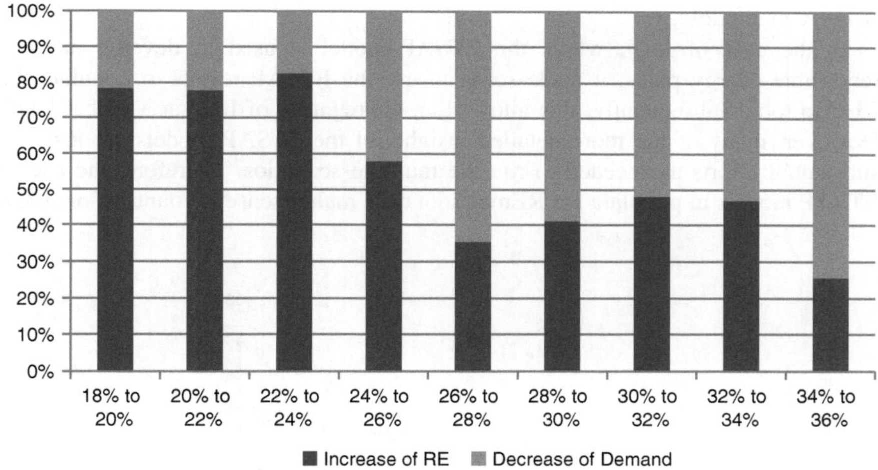

Fig. 11 Decomposition of RE and demand (TFEC) effects for each step to increase the RE share in the TIAM-ECN model

demand pattern. However, in general two thirds can be allocated to reductions in energy services demand, which also include energy saving measures, and one third to technology-based energy efficiency uptake.

In conclusion, the REmap tool seems to be sufficient to examine and explore deployment levels of renewable energy options up to around 30 % of TFEC. However, as countries are moving towards higher shares of renewables they simultaneously need to consider additional energy efficiency options available to decrease overall energy consumption and therefore increase the renewable energy share.

4.4 Comparing Insights: ETSAP Models as Input into the REmap Tool

An alternative way to use the ETSAP models is to populate the REmap tool. For the case of Italy, the TIMES-Italy model (Gaeta and Baldissara 2011) was used to estimate the substitution costs for individual renewable energy technologies (in EURO/GJ) by running multiple scenarios towards a set RE share in 2030, and removing or decreasing constraints on a specific RE technology group one at a time. For each scenario, the incremental system costs were computed, and attributed to the RE technology group. Figure 12 shows the results of this analysis.

These results show that the substitution costs per renewable energy option are comparable to the substitution costs identified in other REmap countries and at a global level. For example, Fig. 12 shows that the range of substitution costs between −10 and +50 USD/GJ in the case of Italy falls within the range of substitution costs from −20 to +60 USD/GJ identified in the REmap tool (Fig. 6). The renewables share at the x-axis does not include traditional biomass, as in the IRENA methodology.

In the case of Italy, where the ETSAP model is used to develop national renewable energy plans, it made sense to use the ETSAP results to populate the REmap tool. Subsequently, this allowed an aggregation of Italy at a global level. However, many of the more detailed insights of the ETSAP models are lost and substantial efforts are needed to run the multiple scenarios. Therefore, the use of ETSAP models to populate the REmap tool only makes sense if countries' national

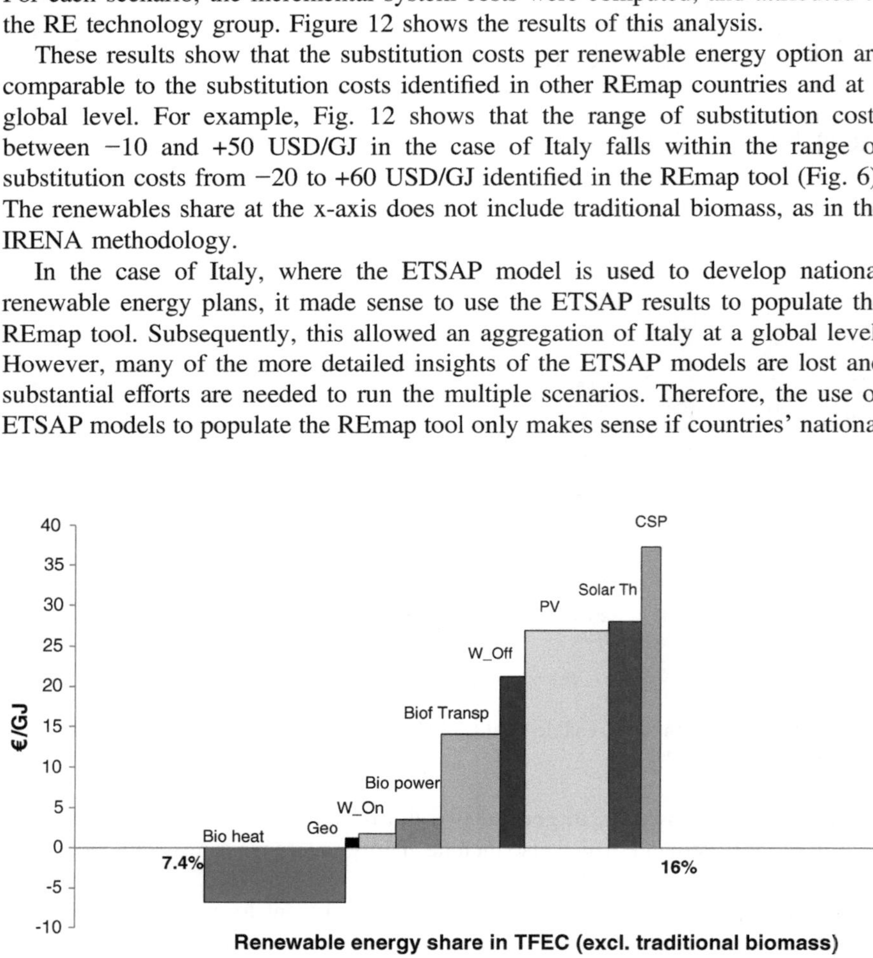

Fig. 12 Substitution costs of REmap Options by TIMES-Italy

renewable energy plans are based on ETSAP models and these plans need to be simplified to compare and aggregate at a global level.

5 Conclusions

In this chapter, we have examined a number of indicators to determine whether the simplified REmap tool creates comparable results with the more sophisticated ETSAP models, and to understand the appropriateness and complementarity of the usage of both the REmap tool and ETSAP models.

For the comparison of the results, we have examined the deployment levels, the substitution choices, and the system costs. The comparison of deployment levels of renewable energy options in 2030 shows that the results are similar. The major difference is in the deployment levels of solar photovoltaics, which could be explained by the reluctance by national REmap experts to envision radical changes in deployment levels. The comparison of substitution choices and the REmap cost supply curve shows that the REmap results correspond with the sequence in which the ETSAP models choose renewable energy options to satisfy an increasing RE share. The difference in results is mainly due to the political choices made by REmap experts. For example, in the case of the USA the national REmap experts choose to only substitute coal-fired power stations, whilst the ETSAP model chooses a mixture of conventional technologies depending on their economics. The results on system costs are far more robust for the ETSAP models than for the REmap tool, mainly because of the single time step (2030) used in the REmap tool. However, the difference in system costs between the two global ETSAP models also shows that system costs are highly affected by parameter choices, such as the discount factors.

From the comparison of results, it can be concluded that the REmap tool is a useful and appropriate tool to engage national experts and policy makers in the assessment and comparison of renewable energy options and renewable energy targets within and across countries. However, the REmap tool is not an appropriate tool for detailed national renewable energy planning. The results of the ETSAP tools show that they can provide far more detailed analyses, including the assessment of uncertainty, required to determine national renewable energy targets and associated policies. Furthermore, the comparison has demonstrated the value of multiple ETSAP model runs to examine progressively higher renewable energy shares as it demonstrates how a specific target may lock-in certain renewable technology options and infrastructures that are less economic for higher shares of variable renewables.

Considering the additional features of the ETSAP models, it is clear that they can provide more detailed insights than the REmap tool. In this chapter, the comparison considered three of these features: the infrastructure requirements for higher shares of renewables in the energy system, the role of competition between renewable energy technologies and resources, and the role of energy efficiency. For the specific case of Japan, the results show that infrastructural changes can have an important impact (±10 %) on the deployment levels of individual RE technologies considered. However, detailed analysis of grid infrastructure impacts requires the ability for inter-regional modelling, is data-intensive and is especially relevant for those countries with grid issues or with high shares of variable renewables.

The comparison also shows that the ability to provide insights on the role of competition between different renewable energy technology options and resource use among sectors is an important feature that is lacking in the REmap tool. In the REmap cost supply curve, the renewable energy options are presented as independent options to increase the renewable energy share within a country. Only through a qualitative discussion of the results can policy makers be informed about the possible interactions between these options. In the ETSAP models, the interaction and competition is made explicit, and this provides a valuable and important mechanism to support policy makers in their energy planning. The results show that this issue is particularly relevant for countries where there is competition for biomass in the different end-use sectors, and for examining different renewable energy options in the residential sector (rooftop photovoltaics versus solar thermal systems versus heat pumps).

The same applies for the insights that the ETSAP models provide on the competition and complementarity between energy efficiency options and renewable energy options to increase the overall RE share with an energy system.[6] Especially at higher levels of RE shares, the ETSAP models show that energy efficiency options become the dominant option to increase RE shares cost effectively.

The overall conclusion of this comparative analysis is that tools need to be geared towards the specific purpose of the exercise, but that it is important to collaborate between the different institutions that are supporting policy makers in their decision making process. The purpose of the REmap process is to explicitly engage national experts in the process of comparing and aggregating national renewable energy plans across a diverse set of countries. However, such an exercise should not be seen in isolation. For detailed national renewable energy planning, any use of the REmap tool should be complemented with ETSAP models as they provide a more flexible and robust tool to examine renewable energy options. In particular, the ETSAP tools can provide insights on system interactions, more detailed insights on the overall system costs, including possible investments in infrastructural changes, and provide insights on the competition of renewable energy options, renewable resources, and energy efficiency options once renewable energy targets have been set. The latter features become particularly relevant as countries continue to move to higher renewable energy targets.

[6] Please note that this competition is driven to achieve a certain renewable energy target, which is different from competition to satisfy greenhouse gas emission reductions.

References

Assoumou E, Maïzi N (2011) Carbon value dynamics for France: a key driver to support mitigation pledges at country scale. Energy Policy 39(7):4325–4336

Gaeta M, Baldissara B (2011) Il modello energetico TIMES-ITALIA. Struttura e dati. ENEA report ENEA-RT-2011-09, Rome, Italy

Hamasaki H, Kanudia A (2013) System analysis of Japanese renewable energy. Fujitsu, no. 404. http://jp.fujitsu.com/group/fri/downloads/report/research/2013/no404.pdf. April 2013

IRENA (2013) Renewable power generation costs in 2012: an overview. IRENA. www.irena.org/costing. January 2014

IRENA (2014a) REmap 2030: a renewable energy roadmap. IRENA.www.irena.org/remap. June 2014

IRENA (2014b) Renewable energy prospects: United States of America, REmap 2030 analysis. IRENA. www.irena.org/remap. November 2014

Kanudia A, Labriet M, Loulou R (2014) Effectiveness and efficiency of climate change mitigation in a technologically uncertain World. Special Issue on "The EMF27 Study on Global Technology and Climate Policy", Clim Change 123(3–4):543–558

Keppo I, van der Zwaan BCC (2012) The impact of uncertainty in climate targets and co_2 storage availability on long-term emissions abatement. Env Model Assess 17:177–191

Kober T (2014) Impact of energy efficiency measures on greenhouse gas emission reduction. Energy research Centre of the Netherlands (ECN report ECN-E- 14 -038), Petten, Netherlands

Labriet M, Kanudia A, Loulou R (2012) Climate mitigation under an uncertain technology future: a TIAM-WORLD analysis. Energy Econ 34(Supplement 3):366–377

Ó Gallachóir BP, Chiodi A, Gargiulo M, Deane P, Lavigne D, Rout UK (2012) Irish TIMES energy systems model. EPA climate change research programme 2007–2013. Report Series No. 24. UCC, Johnstown Castle, Co.Wexford, Ireland http://erc.epa.ie/safer/reports

Rösler H, Bruggink JCC, Keppo IJ (2011) Design of a European sustainable hydrogen model—model structure and data sources. Energy research Centre of the Netherlands (ECN) report ECN-E-11-041, Petten, Netherlands

Saygin D, Kempener R, Wagner N, Ayuso M, Gielen D (2015) A renewable energy roadmap for doubling the share of renewables in the global energy mix between 2010 and 2030. Manuscript under review

Simoes S, Cleto J, Fortes P, Seixas J, Huppes G (2008) Cost of energy and environmental policy in Portuguese CO_2 abatement-scenario analysis to 2020. Energy Policy 36(9):3598–3611

Wright E, Kanudia A (2014) Low carbon standard and transmission investment analysis in the new multi-region US power sector model FACETS. Energy Econ 46:136–150

Energy Decisions in an Uncertain Climate and Technology Outlook: How Stochastic and Robust Methodologies Can Assist Policy-Makers

Maryse Labriet, Claire Nicolas, Stéphane Tchung-Ming, Amit Kanudia and Richard Loulou

Abstract Uncertain conditions may deeply affect the relevance of deterministic solutions proposed by optimization or equilibrium models as well as leave the decision maker in a quandary at the moment of defining policy. This chapter presents two applications of stochastic programming and robust optimization to climate and energy decisions using respectively TIAM-WORLD at the global level and MIRET in the case of France. At the global level, stochastic analysis demonstrates that the hedging strategy usually presents a smoother technology transition and is not equivalent to an average of deterministic solutions. Combined with a parametric analysis of the probability of the future outlooks, the approach produces a hedging strategy where the energy system prepares early for high mitigation even in the case of a low probability for such an outcome. Moreover, some technologies appear to be particularly appealing since they penetrate more in the hedging than in deterministic strategies; the penetration of gas power without carbon capture and sequestration in China, coal power plants with carbon capture in India, renewable electricity in Central and South America are examples of these "super-hedging"

M. Labriet (✉)
Eneris Environment Energy Consultants, Madrid, Spain
e-mail: maryse.labriet@enerisconsultants.com

C. Nicolas
UPOND and IFPEN, Rueil-Malmaison, France
e-mail: claire.nicolas@ifpen.fr

S. Tchung-Ming
IFPEN, Rueil-Malmaison, France
e-mail: stephane.tchung-ming@ifpen.fr

A. Kanudia
KanORS-EMR, Noida, India
e-mail: amit@KanORS.com

R. Loulou
McGill University, Montréal, Canada
e-mail: richardloulou@gmail.com

G. Giannakidis et al. (eds.), *Informing Energy and Climate Policies Using Energy Systems Models*, Lecture Notes in Energy 30,
DOI 10.1007/978-3-319-16540-0_4

choices. In the case of the French transportation sector, robust optimization illustrates the crucial role of biofuels as a robust mitigation strategy in both moderate and severe emission reduction cases.

1 Introduction

Uncertainty in the long-term energy, economy and climate outlook may deeply affect the relevance of the proposed solutions as well as leave the decision maker in a quandary at the moment of defining policy. The cause of uncertainty may be prediction error, affecting parameters of the model, as well as the absence of precise knowledge on the operation of certain processes or mechanisms, which forces modelers to use simplified representations of physical processes (Ben-Tal and Nemirovski 2002).

Many aspects of climate change and of energy systems are uncertain. First, the nature and extent of future climate change is not precisely known, as shown for instance by the uncertain parameters in the carbon cycle and the sensitivity of the climate to concentration of greenhouse gases (GHGs). Both the inherent variability of the climate system, that is, the natural fluctuations that arise in the absence of any radiative forcing of the planet, and the response of the climate system to changes in radiative forcing, are uncertain, and the level of uncertainty increases at the local or regional level (Hawkins and Sutton 2009). Moreover, greenhouse gas emission scenarios are uncertain, depending on techno-economic, development and policy choices, which depend themselves on climate changes, amongst other factors. Secondly, the actions to mitigate GHG emissions depend on the technical-economic characteristics of key technologies (efficiencies, investment and operation costs, which depend on research and development, economies of scale, spillover effects, etc.), the type of socio-economic development, the social willingness to modify behaviors as well as the dynamics of international negotiations and the time-horizon considered in the decision framework.

The most recent assessment report of the Intergovernmental Panel on Climate Change (IPCC) insists on the importance of considering uncertainties surrounding climate, technology, and social and political characteristics in supporting transitional adaptation and mitigation strategies, and recognizes the lack of consistent tools to deal with these uncertainties (IPCC 2013, 2014; Clarke and Jiang 2014; Kunreuther and Gupta 2014).

Optimal solutions elaborated with optimization or equilibrium models like TIMES are based on a complex, high cardinality set of exogenous assumptions (except to some extent in the case of endogenous learning) on the data populating the models. In short, optimization will sort technologies by decreasing economic merit order to meet various policy objectives in a cost efficient manner. Consequently, different sets of assumptions could yield different relative costs, and in turn to a different optimal technological portfolio. It could lead to an underestimation of the cost of the chosen strategies or to induce the policy maker into implementing a suboptimal policy.

To tackle these questions, *deterministic multi-scenario analysis* is a useful attempt to scope the range of impacts of key parameters on the possible climate adaptation and mitigation responses (Kunreuther and Gupta 2014). It constitutes a usual approach where alternative scenarios of plausible future developments are formulated. In such an approach, unknown parameters can be given extreme values, one at a time, with the intention of circumscribing the space of possibilities. The scenarios thus defined form *ensembles* of scenarios. Systematic ways of choosing parameter values to cover the space of possibilities efficiently are based on design of experiments. Amongst the different possible scenarios, "representative sets" may be identified and play a crucial role as guides for scenario analysis by the research community. In the climate change arena, multi-scenario analysis is frequent, as proposed by the scenarios of the IPCC or the modelling exercises of the Energy Modelling Forum (Weyant and Kriegler 2014), among others. Scenario/ensemble analyses can be performed without quantifying the uncertainty of the underlying unknown parameters. However, this also implies an unavoidable ambiguity in interpreting ensemble results since they tend to be used in a deterministic fashion without recognizing that they may have a low probability of occurrence and are only one of many possible outcomes (Clarke and Jiang 2014; Kunreuther and Gupta 2014). Moreover, such scenarios leave the policy adviser in a quandary as to *what policy to initiate now, given the often widely diverging courses of action solutions proposed by each of the alternative scenarios, even in the short term.*

Stochastic programming and *robust optimization* provide other rigorous frameworks applied on decision making models (Wets 1989). One of the main advantages of the stochastic programming approach is to obtain an explicit single hedging strategy while uncertainty prevails, contrary to classical multi-scenario analysis. Its main drawback is computational: it quickly leads to large-scale instances of the original model. Moreover, probability distribution have to be defined over the entire tree of events. Robust optimization offers parsimonious, computationally efficient ways of dealing with problems of high dimensionality requiring minimal information about the true probability distributions (Ben-Tal and Nemirovski 2002).

This chapter presents two different applications of stochastic programming (Sect. 2) and robust optimization (Sect. 3) to climate and energy decisions using TIMES models: TIAM-WORLD at the global level and MIRET in the case of France. Each section introduces the main principles of the methodology and describes results obtained in different cases.

2 Climate and Energy Decisions Under Stochastic Programming

2.1 Methodological Principles of Stochastic Programming

One key question facing policy makers is that of defining *one* course of action for example for the next 20 years, a time horizon relevant to energy investment, in a context of long-term uncertainties. From the viewpoint of a policy adviser, it is highly desirable to obtain a recommendation for a single *hedging strategy*, which strikes a good compromise between the costs of the many ways of "guessing wrong" (Kanudia and Loulou 1998; Loulou et al. 2009). The main objective is that there be no ambiguity as to *how to act now*, *before uncertainty is resolved*, thus alleviating the main defect of traditional deterministic scenario analysis which computes multiple strategies even prior to the resolution date, leaving the decision maker in a quandary.

This is the essence of decision under risk, and in particular of stochastic programming (Wets 1989). Stochastic programming produces an optimal single strategy, the hedging strategy, until the first date of resolution of the uncertain event (s). After that, the hedging strategy has as many *contingent* strategies as there are possible outcomes of the random event(s), each such strategy being a recourse against the corresponding outcome. Robust actions are those actions chosen in the hedging strategy. In fact, hedging is deemed relevant if decisions prior the resolution of uncertainty are different from those in the base case (i.e. the no-action scenario). Otherwise, "*wait and see*" is a good policy. But one of the most striking advantages of stochastic programming is that the hedging strategy is not necessarily an average of deterministic strategies and could represent solutions that could not easily be found otherwise.

Moreover, "super-hedging" actions can be identified, which are actions that penetrate more in the hedging strategy than in *any* of the perfect forecast strategies (i.e. strategies obtained from the traditional multi-scenario analyses). The existence of such actions seems counter-intuitive, since they lie outside the limits defined by the perfect forecast strategies, but their existence confirms that stochastic analysis of future climate and energy strategies may propose decisions that are beyond any combination or interpolation of the deterministic strategies (Kanudia and Loulou 1998).

Another very desirable property of the hedging strategy is that it greatly attenuates the well-known "razor edge" effect of Linear Programming (i.e. abrupt switches between two actions), as it tends to identify a robust portfolio of technologies instead of merely choosing the least-cost technology (Loulou and Kanudia 1999). It thus proposes a more diversified mix of technologies to attain the desired climate target, and that mix evolves more smoothly over time.

One of the computational drawbacks of stochastic programming is that it quickly leads to large-scale instance of the original model, whenever the number of random events and/or the number of outcomes of each event, become too large. Moreover, the probabilities associated with the different events are themselves not always easily available (Baker et al. 2007).

Our proposal to overcome this limit is to conduct a systematic exploration of the hedging strategies, while varying the probabilities of the expected outcomes. Such a parametric exploration constitutes a useful and original complement to the computation of hedging strategies and contributes to identify those technologies that are robust under a wide set of probabilities, and those that are not.

2.2 Mathematical Formulation of Stochastic Programming in TIMES Models

The detailed mathematical formulation is described in Loulou and Lehtila (2012). A typical stochastic linear program is written as in Eqs. 1 and 2, in the simpler two-stage case where all uncertainties are resolved at a single date θ, and where the optimization is done on the expected value of the total system cost (equivalent to maximizing total expected surplus).

$$\text{Minimize} \sum_{t} \beta(t) \sum_{s=1 \text{ to } S} C(t,s) \cdot X(t,s) \cdot p(s) \tag{1}$$

$$\text{Subject to: } A(t,s) \times X(t,s) \geq b(t,s) \tag{2}$$

and $X(t, 1) = X(t, 2) = \cdots = X(t,S)$, if $t <$ resolution date θ
where

- s represent the possible *states of the world* (sow), s = 1, 2, …, S
- $p(s)$ is the probability that sow s realizes
- C and b are respectively the cost and the right hand side (RHS) vectors of the Linear Program (LP). Their elements may also depend on s and t
- A is the matrix of LP coefficients under sow s at time t
- $X(t, s)$ is the vector of decision variables at time t, under state-of-the-world s.
- $\beta(t)$ is the discount factor.

Very many parameters of TIMES models that may be stochastic, such as: demand projections, bounds on total installed capacities, cumulative bounds on commodity production (net or not), seasonal distribution of a commodity, cumulative bound on an energy flow or on a process activity, process efficiency, process investment cost, seasonal availability factor, right hand side constant of user constraint, damage cost of net production of commodity, bound on maximum level of climate variable, climate module constants (climate sensitivity and thermal capacity of the atmosphere).

The current version of the TIMES implementation for stochastic programming is based on directly solving the above deterministic problem. This is the most straightforward approach, which may be applied to all problem instances. As this may lead to very large problem instances, stochastic TIMES models are in practice limited to a relatively small number of sow's.

In order to avoid the simplifying assumption of risk neutrality, two alternative candidates for the objective function have been proposed and used on TIMES models. In each, the objective function is replaced by a version that introduces varying degrees of risk aversion: expected utility criterion with linearized risk aversion and Minimax Regret (Savage) criterion (Loulou and Kanudia 1999). The first alternative has been fully implemented in the stochastic version of TIMES, providing a feature for taking into account that a decision maker may be risk averse, by defining a new utility function to replace the expected cost. The approach is based on a modified version of the classical E-V model (an abbreviation for Expected Value-Variance). In the E-V approach, it is assumed that the variance of the cost is an acceptable measure of the risk attached to a strategy in the presence of uncertainty (Loulou and Lehtila 2012). The second approach is also possible with TIMES, but requires a three step implementation of TIMES using the sensitivity analysis and the stochastic programming features of TIMES (Loulou and Lehtila 2012). Doing so requires substantial manual operations by the user.[1]

2.3 Applications in TIAM-WORLD

2.3.1 Overview of TIAM-WORLD

The TIMES Integrated Assessment Model (TIAM-WORLD) is a technology-rich model of the entire energy/emission system of the World split into 16 regions,[2] providing a detailed representation of the procurement, transformation, trade, and consumption of a large number of energy forms (Loulou 2008; Loulou and Labriet 2008).

It is an incarnation of the TIMES (The Integrated MARKAL-EFOM System) economic paradigm and computes an inter-temporal dynamic partial equilibrium on energy and emission markets based on the maximization of total surplus, defined as the sum of suppliers and consumers surpluses. In other words, the model finds optimal (cost-efficient) energy and technology mixes to satisfy demands for energy services like lighting, cooking, heating, cooling of houses, kilometers driven by cars, trucks, tons of aluminum, cement to be produced, etc. Each demand may vary endogenously in alternate scenarios, in response to endogenous price changes.

The model contains explicit detailed descriptions of more than 1500 technologies and several hundreds of energy, emission and demand flows in each region. Such technological detail provides a precise description of technology and fuel competition in the entire energy system, where changes in one sector may have direct and indirect impacts on other sectors. The model is set-up to explore the development of the World energy system until 2100. It is calibrated to 2005 energy statistics of the International Energy Agency (IEA 2013a, b).

TIAM-WORLD integrates a climate module for the modeling of global changes related to greenhouse gas concentrations, radiative forcing, and temperature increase. The module includes separate cycles for CO_2, CH_4, and N_2O, and also

---

[1] Interested readers may want to consult the online forum of this topic at http://www.iea-etsap.org/forum/forum_posts.asp?TID=95.

[2] Africa, Australia, New Zealand, Canada, United States, Mexico, Central and South America, China, India, Japan, South Korea, Other Developing Asia, Middle-East, Europe of 27 + Switzerland, Norway and Iceland, Other East Europe, Russia, Central Asia and Caucasia + OPEC and Non-OPEC disaggregation when relevant.

accounts for the additional forcings introduced by other causes, natural and anthropic. The total atmospheric forcing is then introduced into equations that simulate the changes in mean temperatures of two layers: surface, and deep ocean. The climate module provides a very useful means of simulating scenarios with specific climate targets, be they on concentration, forcing, or temperature.

2.3.2 Uncertain Climate Context

Climate variability is one of the many elements of uncertainty involved in energy planning and decision-making. Assessing the vulnerabilities of energy systems and incorporating them into long-term energy planning and operation is becoming imperative for the development of policies that aim to cope with climate change but also to better understand the possible impacts of climate change on the energy system in terms of timing and sequencing of decisions. This section focuses on cases where the future mitigation level is considered as a random event.

First, in order to explore the uncertainties associated with the climate sensitivity (*Cs*) of the climate module of the model, defined as the equilibrium response of global surface temperature to a doubling of the equivalent CO_2 concentration, Labriet et al. (2009) considered four possible values of *Cs* with respective probabilities (between brackets) as follows, and according to Yohe et al. (2004): 1.5 °C (25 %), 3.0 °C (45 %), 5.0 °C (15 %) and 8.0 °C (15 %). It is assumed that the uncertainty on *Cs* will be fully resolved in 2040. The research focuses on climate strategies to keep long-term temperature increase below the 2.5 °C target. One of the findings of the study is that when *Cs* = 1.5 °C, the base case as modeled with this version of the model satisfies the climate target at all times. In other words, the Perfect Foresight scenario with *Cs* = 1.5 °C and a climate target of 2.5 °C is identical to the Base Case. Moreover, additional hydroelectricity, sequestration by forestry and the shutdown of coal power plants without carbon capture are identified as hedging decisions. While carbon capture penetrates early in the most pessimistic PF with *Cs* = 8.0 °C, it penetrates much later in the hedging strategy. In the end-use sectors, fuel switches in industry (to biomass and gas), biomass in residential buildings, and methane abatement actions are identified as super-hedging actions: they penetrate more in the hedging than in any PF strategy.

Second, Loulou et al. (2009) is part of a multi-model study sponsored by the Energy Modeling Forum, which suggests three scenarios, each with a specific alternative value for total forcing (2.6, 3.7 and 4.5 W/m^2). The study proposed a probabilistic interpretation of these three PF scenarios by converting the problem into a stochastic problem with a *single target* on long-term global temperature change (2.45 °C), while assuming that three possible values of the climate sensitivity were possible, each with a specific probability: 2.0 °C (50 %), 2.9 °C (35 %), 5.0 °C (15 %). Greenhouse gas emissions in the hedging are close to those in the PF scenario with a 2.6 forcing target, showing the strong influence of this severe target on the hedging strategy. The composition of the electricity supply shows that the amount of electricity produced with carbon capture and sequestration (CCS) in the hedging strategy is higher than in any deterministic strategy in year 2040, but not so in preceding periods. Overall, the hedging strategy presents a smoother transition from the initial electricity mix to a radically different one in 2040, than the PF strategies with 3.7 or 2.6 forcing targets. This "smoothing" property was also observed in Labriet et al. (2009), as described above. Usually observed in hedging strategies, such a smooth transition is one great advantage of hedging strategies and is easier to implement in practice.

Finally, another manner to explore climate uncertainties is to define uncertain climate targets to be respected in the long term. Based on this approach, TIAM-WORLD was used to analyze the impact of two contrasted climate outlooks with a severe (450 ppm CO_2 equivalent) and a loose (650 ppm CO_2 equivalent) climate target imposed on the energy system. Due to the expected impacts of climate change, heating and cooling needs as well as the price of bioenergy are also considered uncertain, and were defined based on the coupling of TIAM-WORLD and respectively a climate model, PLASIM-ENTs (see chapter by Labriet et al. at the end of this book), and a land-use model, MAgPIE (Leimbach et al. 2013). All the other parameters of the models remain unchanged. Since the probability of each of the two proposed climate target remains fully unknown, a systematic exploration of the hedging solution is proposed with probabilities of the second state of the World varying from 0 to 1, in 0.1 increments. The two runs where the probability is equal to 0 or to 1, correspond to perfect forecasts of the future climate outlook (Fig. 1).

The scenario naming convention is as follows: The first 3 digits represent the probability of the High Mitigation scenario, the next 3 digits represent the probability of the Low Mitigation scenario, * represents the High Mitigation branch after bifurcation.

As already discussed, the main value of stochastic analysis is to assess the decisions made in the hedging, prior to the definition of the uncertain parameters. Total net CO_2 emissions help understand how the hedging varies between the two perfect foresight scenarios when the probability of scenarios varies (Fig. 2): the

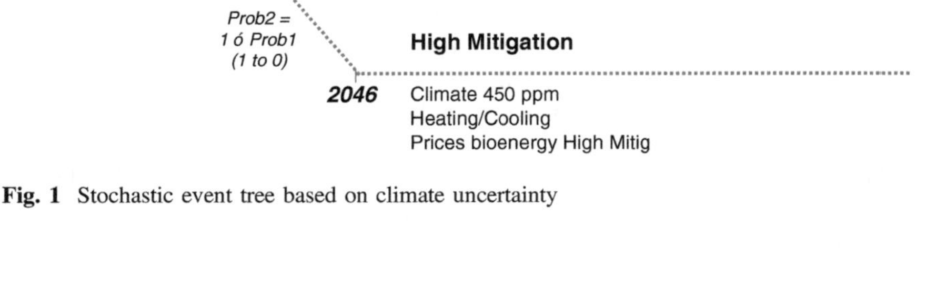

Fig. 1 Stochastic event tree based on climate uncertainty

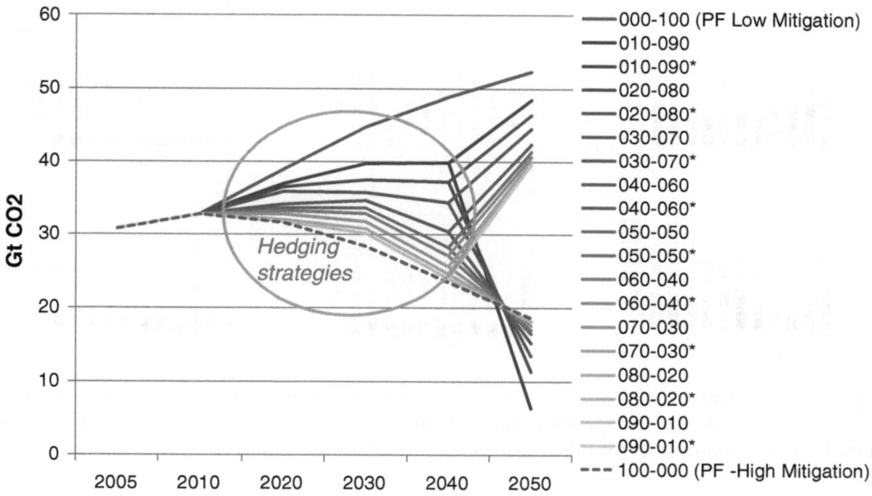

Fig. 2 Net CO_2 emissions under each of the 11 cases

hedging does not vary uniformly within the range defined by the two perfect foresight cases; a small probability of high mitigation (10 %—scenario 010–090) forces the energy system to adopt decisions quite different from the "PF Low Mitigation". In other words, some energy decisions deserve an early implementation "in any case".

The analysis of the capacity mix of power plants in 2030 shows that significant changes occur in most regions as soon as the probability of the High Mitigation case reaches 10 % (Fig. 3): coal and gas are substituted by wind, hydro and nuclear. This implies that the 2030 electricity system fully prepares for the high mitigation scenario even if the latter has low (but non zero) probability. Other changes, specific to some regions, are observed around 30–40 % of probability of High Mitigation, such as the penetration of CCS in China and India, or the increase of the share of renewables in Central and South America. In 2040, just before the state of the world is revealed, significant changes also occur when the probability of High Mitigation goes from 0 to 10 %, but some "clusters" also appear in several regions (Fig. 4). Amongst them, three levels of electrification of the economy are observed in China (with changes observed for a probability of the High Mitigation of 40 and 70 %), the role of coal power plants with CCS only for intermediate probabilities in India, while gas power plants with CCS, which is cleaner but more expensive, starts gaining share with 70 % probability and is preferred to coal + CCS at the end. This peaking of coal power plants with CCS at intermediate probabilities in some regions reveals a unique value that the stochastic approach adds over deterministic scenario analysis: coal CCS penetration in India, as well as in Japan and Russia (not shown here) is higher around 40–50 % probability of high mitigation compared to either perfect foresight cases; such a mitigation option is a "super-hedging".

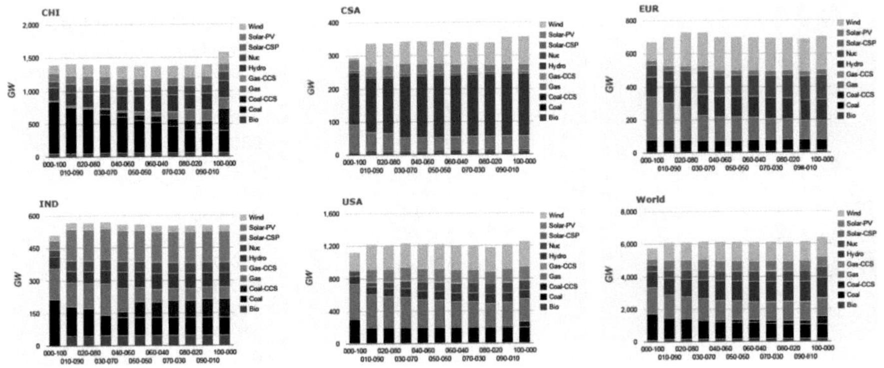

Fig. 3 Power plant capacity in 2030. The first 3 digits of scenario names on the x-axis represent the probability of the high mitigation scenario, the next 3 digits represent the probability of the low mitigation scenario (results for other regions are available upon request)

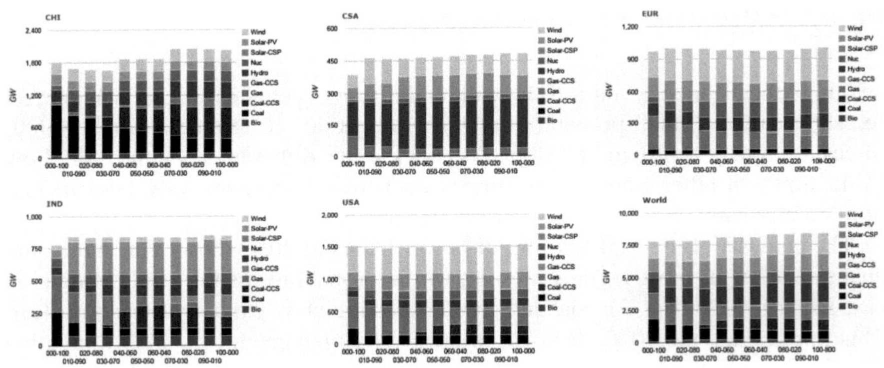

Fig. 4 Power plant capacity in 2040. The first 3 digits of scenario names on the x-axis represent the probability of the high mitigation scenario, the next 3 digits represent the probability of the low mitigation scenario (results for other regions are available upon request)

2.3.3 Uncertain Technology Outlooks

The impacts of the long-term technology context on the optimal evolution of the World energy system are now explored in a stochastic framework where the availability and characteristics of future technologies are uncertain, and the level of mitigation is no longer modelled as a random event, but rather as a discrete parameter on which sensitivity analysis is performed (targets of 2.6 and 3.7 W/m^2).

Two contrasted sets of assumptions are made on the future energy system of the World are considered after 2040: one (the Renewable Outlook) is focused on renewable energy and improvement of the energy intensity of the economy, while CCS and nuclear power are assumed not to play an important role; the other one

(Conventional Outlook) is centered on fossil (with or without CCS) and nuclear energy, where renewable energy is expected to be more expensive, biomass potentials and improvements of the energy intensity lower (Labriet et al. 2012). This dichotomy is of course a simplified view of the various technological futures since it is not at all clear that the technologies included in each state of the World are so well correlated that they can be lumped together in a single state of the World. Probabilities of each branch varied from 0 to 1 in 0.05 increments.

Analysis of the hedging strategies in the case of a stringent climate target (2.6 W/m^2) shows that mitigation actions are quite stable when probabilities vary from the Conventional Outlook to the Renewable Outlook (Fig. 5 top). In other words, for stringent targets, the need for rapid de-carbonization severely restricts the set of effective options, and the most effective mitigation actions are used in the mid-term almost irrespective of the values of future probabilities of technology outlooks.

For the moderate climate target (3.7 W/m^2), the degree of uncertainty of the technology outlook has a larger impact on mid-term hedging energy decisions (Fig. 5 bottom). Indeed, mitigation scenarios are much milder but more volatile, reflecting a lower robustness of actions across the range of probabilities associated to the technology outlook. Without the pressure of a rapid decarbonization required by a severe climate target, mitigation remains moderate and quite flexible, and the nature of the mitigation options is highly dependent on the nature of the technology outlook.

Regional results show that natural gas appears as an appealing options in several countries, such as in China, in an uncertain technology context. Its use in power plants without CCS is even considered as a "super-hedging" mitigation option, penetrating more in the hedging solution than in any of the deterministic scenarios (Fig. 6). In other words, when the future availability and characteristics of key energy technologies is uncertain and long term emissions must be reduced in a moderate manner (3.7 W/m^2), power plants without CCS is a good "install-now" strategy and allows "wait-and-see" for other options given its relatively low emissions and the low capital cost of associated technologies. By implementing such a technology option, the policy maker keeps a middle-of-the-road position that does not emit too much GHG and that can be modified without too much "regret" in terms of economic losses, when uncertainty is resolved on the more effective options.

3 Robust Optimization

3.1 Methodological Principles of Robust Optimization

One drawback of stochastic programming is that probability distributions, possibly parameterized, have to be defined over the entire tree. When whole probability distributions are defined for the uncertain events, Monte-Carlo type of analysis may ensue: in such a case, sets of values are randomly sampled from the distributions, and series of deterministic runs are performed (MIT 2011). However, both

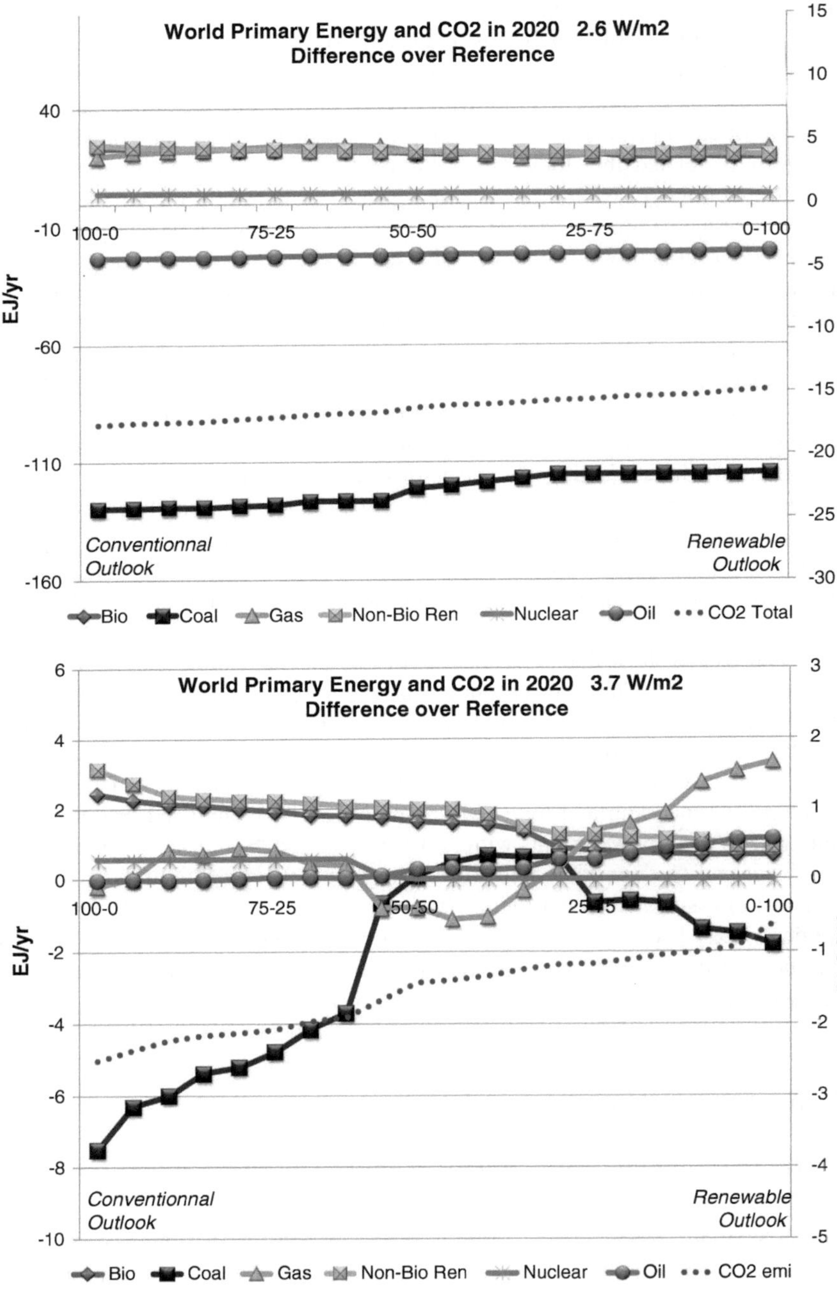

Fig. 5 Mitigation options in the power sector in 2030 at the world level in two climate cases (*top* 2.6 W/m²; *bottom* 3.7 W/m²), measured as the difference over the reference case. The first 3 digits of scenario names on the x-axis represent the probability of the conventional outlook, the next 3 digits represent the probability of the renewable outlook

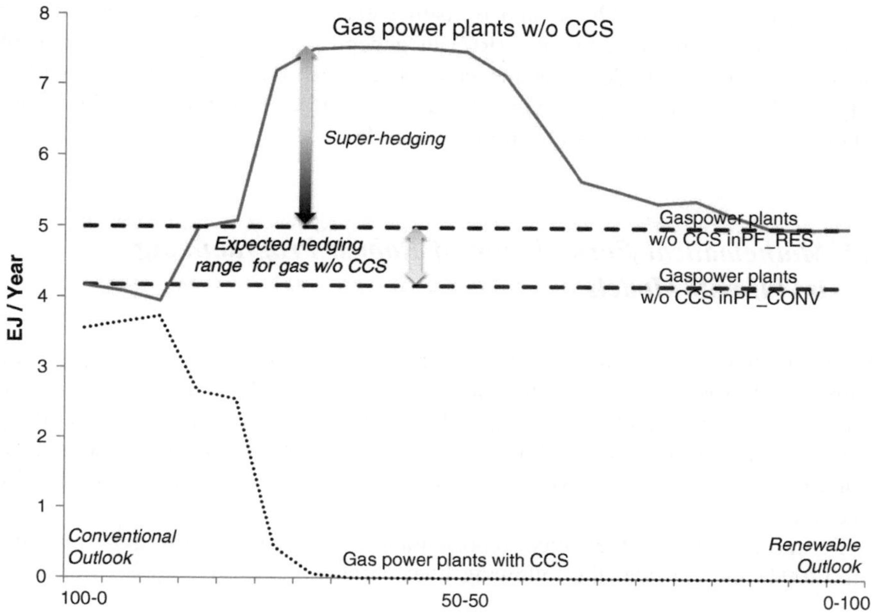

Fig. 6 The role of gas power plants without CCS as a super-hedging strategy in China, 2030, 3.7 W/m^2. The first 3 digits of scenario names on the x-axis represent the probability of the conventional outlook, the next 3 digits represent the probability of the renewable outlook

techniques are rapidly confronted with the intractability issue in numerical computations as problem size grows. Robust optimization (RO) is an alternative approach for coping with uncertainty. RO formulations offer parsimonious ways of dealing with problems of high dimensionality, requiring minimal information about the true probability distributions.

Early developments of RO date back to Soyster (1973) who initiated an approach for obtaining relevant (i.e. feasible) LP solutions when matrix coefficients are inexact. RO has known many developments in the last 15 year by generalizing Soyster approach (Bertsimas and Sim 2004) or using different formalisms (Ben-Tal and Nemirovski 2002; El Ghaoui et al. 1998). Its applications to energy and environment problems are currently emerging as a promising technique for practitioners. For example, Babonneau et al. (2011) applied it to the TIAM-WORLD model to study the security of supply to the European energy system.

The general principle of RO consists in immunizing a solution against adverse realizations of uncertain parameters within a given *uncertainty set*. The basic requirement for a robust solution is that constraints of the problem are not violated whatever the values of the parameters in that set. The main modelling issue then consists in identifying, depending on the model class and the nature of the uncertainty region, computable robust counterparts for the initial optimization program. Ben-Tal et al. (2014) and Bertsimas et al. (2010) review techniques for building such robust counterparts (RC) in general cases. One particular case of interest for TIMES modelers is the case of a linear program combined with a polyhedral uncertainty set, for which the RC is itself a linear program. The application presented below is based on this principle.

3.2 Mathematical Formulation of Robust Programming in TIMES Models

As mentioned above, while stochastic or Monte-Carlo frameworks require the definition of probability density functions, the principle of RO consists in set-based descriptions of uncertainties. As such, only the *extent* to which parameters are likely to vary needs to be known (although this information may be itself difficult to acquire), but not its likelihood. This corresponds to the support of the density functions.

To introduce the mathematical representation of RO, we follow Bertsimas and Sim (2004) and consider the following linear problem (Eq. 3):

$$(\mathrm{P})\begin{cases}\min\ c^T x\\ \text{s.t. } Ax \leq b\\ x \in \mathbb{R}^+\end{cases} \tag{3}$$

We assume that the uncertainty only affects the coefficients $a_{i,j} (i \in I, j \in J)$ of the matrix A. The coefficients can vary in a symmetric range: $a_{i,j} \in \left[\overline{a_{i,j}} - \widehat{a_{i,j}}, \overline{a_{i,j}} + \widehat{a_{i,j}}\right]$ where $\overline{a_{i,j}}$ is the nominal value of the parameter and $\widehat{a_{i,j}}$ the uncertainty set half-length. No specific probability distribution is needed.

We can now introduce the parameter $\Gamma \in [0, |I| + |J|]$ named the budget of uncertainty whose role is to adjust the robustness of the methodology against the level of conservatism of the solution.

By writing $a_{i,j} = \overline{a_{i,j}} + z_{ij}\widehat{a_{i,j}}$, $z_{ij} \in [-1, 1]$ we can reformulate the problem (P) and write its robust counterpart ($\mathrm{P_{rob}}$) as shown in Eq. 4:

$$(\mathrm{P_{rob}})\begin{cases}\min\quad c^T x\\ \text{s.t.}\quad \sum\limits_j \overline{a_{i,j}} x_j + \max_{z_{ij}} \sum\limits_j z_{ij}\widehat{a_{i,j}} x_j \leq b_i \quad \forall i \in I, j \in J\\ z_{ij} \in [-1, 1] \quad \forall i \in I, j \in J\\ \sum\limits_{i,j} |z_{ij}| \leq \Gamma \quad \forall i \in I, j \in J\\ x \in \mathbb{R}^+\end{cases} \tag{4}$$

More generally, by limiting the number of parameters allowed to deviate, Γ represents the degree of pessimism on the problem parameters. When $\Gamma = 0$, the robust problem is identical to the nominal one and when $\Gamma = |I| + |J|$, it is equal to the "worst case" problem. The concept of the uncertainty budget is based on the fact that it is highly unlikely that all the parameters take their worst case value at the same time.

Using strong duality, the maximization problem in the constraint becomes a minimization problem which can be reinjected into the original problem. Hence, the robust counterpart of the problem is still a linear programming problem (a little bit bigger) and conserves the good properties of this class of model in terms of tractability and computational time (Bertsimas and Thiele 2006).

The robust counterpart of the initial problem includes variables that traduce the deviations of the worst-case parameters with respect to their nominal values (the number of potentially deviating coefficients being controlled by the uncertainty budget).As an outcome, the solution of the problem is immune to variations of the uncertain parameters within their set. Moreover, it has nice connections with attitudes of the decision maker towards risks (Bertsimas et al. 2010), and provides probabilistic guarantees of constraints violation.

3.3 Application in MIRET

3.3.1 Overview of MIRET

As a TIMES instance, the MIRET model (Lorne and Tchung-Ming 2012) is a technology-explicit, sectoral model of the French energy-transport sector. It describes in detail the supply of primary energy (fossils, agricultural and woody biomass), energy conversion through detailed refinery modeling, first and second generation biofuel production units, biogas, and a simple model of the electricity sector. Transport end-uses are detailed through a hundred of vehicle technologies for passenger and freight road transport, rail transport, air transport and navigation. Its scope is continental France, and the time horizon is 2050, with 2007 as a calibration year; it works as a long-term, dynamic inter-temporal partial equilibrium model. The version used here was built as a partial equilibrium model, including demand-side reactions to the endogenously formed energy services prices.

3.3.2 Scenarios: Meeting Transportation Abatement Objectives Under Cost Uncertainty

One major issue arising from the many possible uncertainties of the techno-economic parameters of the model is the following: *how robust is an optimal technological trajectory to* (*which*) *techno-economic assumptions*? In other words, decision makers may wish to analyze solutions that are immune to adverse realizations of these parameters.

To illustrate the methodology, we built two alternate sets of normative scenarios: reductions of 50 % (Cap1) and 66 % (Cap2) of GHG emissions are imposed in the

Table 1 Parameters affected by uncertainty

Scenario component	Sector	Uncertainty source
Primary energy supply	Fossils (oil, coal, gas)	Price (maximum: +10 % above nominal value)
	Biomass (agricultural, wood)	
Energy conversion	Oil refining	None
	Biofuels	Investment cost (maximum: +10 % above nominal value)
	Electricity generation	
End-use	Road transport (passenger cars, buses, trucks)	
	Rail transport (all trains)	

French transport sector in 2050 compared to 2007. For each of these emission caps, we conduct a sensitivity analysis on the uncertainty budget. This application is particularly helpful to better understand the impact of cost uncertainties in the definition of mitigation policies in the French transportation sector.

The uncertainty set is as follows. We assume that the investment cost of new technologies available from 2020 and beyond is not known with certainty. For each of these technologies, the uncertainty model consists in assuming that the investment cost can rise by 10 % above its nominal value. On top of that, it is assumed that the unit costs of primary energy are also subject to uncertainty. This concerns fossil primary energy (crude, natural gas and coal), biomass (agricultural crops, imported vegetable oils, dedicated energy crops and agricultural and forest residues). These assumptions are summarized in Table 1. Because of the number of costs involved in this exercise, we do not distinguish between the fuels and processes and we use the same value (10 %) to create the uncertainty set of costs. We are aware that the investment cost for mature technologies is much less uncertain than the one of new technologies. In that sense, the threshold is to be understood as a sensitivity experiment, rather than an attempt to calibrate uncertainty bounds for all affected technologies.

The overall uncertainty set comprises around 120 parameters, including technology investment costs and energy prices. Under the uncertainty model chosen, this makes a total of around 900 constraints to be added to the original model. The original TIMES modeling framework does not include such equations; consequently, they were added manually. In the sequel, the uncertainty budgets at each period are varied proportionally: if $\Gamma = (\Gamma_t)_{t \geq t_0}$ is the vector of uncertainty budgets over time, then we vary $h \in [0, 1]$ such that $\Gamma_h = h\Gamma$.

3.3.3 Results

Results are presented for the two carbon caps imposed in the transport sector. The uncertainty budget Γ corresponds to the number of coefficients allowed to vary; it is between 0 (no coefficient deviates from the nominal value: this is the deterministic case) and the maximal value of around 120 (all coefficients can deviate from the nominal value). Results are presented as percentages of this maximal uncertainty budget. For example, the scenario Cap 1–10 % corresponds to the −50 % carbon cap (Cap1), and allowing 10 % of the cost and price coefficients to drift from their nominal value.

What is the cost of robustness? Figure 7 presents the evolution of the objective function for the two emission cap scenarios and for different ratios of the uncertainty budget. We observe the usual increasing concave shape of the objective function. Total cost increases by up to 11 % over the case without uncertainty in both Cap1 and Cap2 (absolute total cost is of course higher in the case of Cap2 given the more severe emission reduction imposed in this scenario). The main part of the additional cost is the *additional cost of using uncertain technologies/energy sources*; it is due to limitations in substitution options: even if the price of oil is 110\$/bbl rather than 100 \$/bbl, some fossil fuels will still be used in the transportation sector and the price increase will directly impact the objective function. Another part of the cost corresponds to the *additional costs of technical substitution*, due to changes in the relative costs of technology which induce different technology investment paths. For example, if the apparent price of oil is 110\$/bbl instead of 100\$/bbl, some diesel or gasoline vehicles may be replaced by gas vehicles or fossil fuels may be substituted with biofuels. When the uncertainty budget reaches 30 %, the objective function is almost stable. Indeed, the costs and prices impacting a lot the objective function have already deviated and the technical substitutions have been done or even undone (when lots of costs can vary, the relative cost of technologies does not vary hence the investment trajectories are not necessarily impacted).

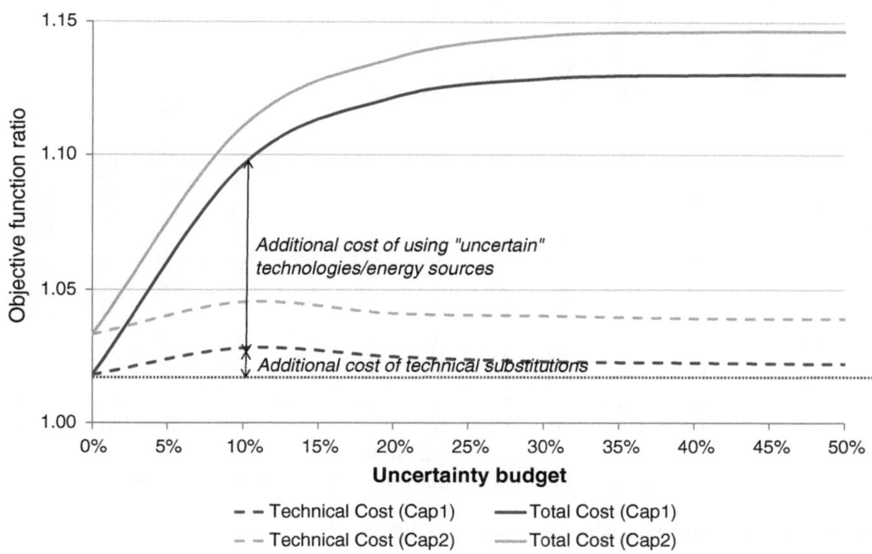

Fig. 7 Objective function value ratio (change over reference case)

What are the main technological hedges in the transportation sector? Figures 8 and 9 highlight some of the hedging strategies for the two caps and uncertainty budgets until 50 % (no major changes occur after this threshold). In Cap1 and for low uncertainty budgets, hedging consists in raising the share of gasoline and diesel in transport to replace natural gas (Fig. 8). The share of gas increases again for higher uncertainty budget. The underlying biofuels incorporation consists in adding more ethanol into gasoline and in blending more hydrotreated vegetable oil in diesel (Fig. 9). The 10 % uncertainty budget corresponds to the highest integration of biofuels in the energy mix of transport in absolute terms; this is consistent with the peak observed in the trajectory of cost of technical substitutions (Fig. 7). In Cap2 scenarios, gasoline substitutes diesel in all cases (Fig. 8). This substitution is motivated by a higher blending rate with ethanol, as observed in Cap1 scenarios. In Cap2 scenarios, this strategy is accompanied by a strong substitution of hydrotreated vegetable oil by biomass-to-liquids biodiesel in the low uncertainty budget. In Cap2–10 %, the decreasing market share of diesel vehicles in the fleet impacts the consumption of biofuels for diesel car, leading to a small decrease of biofuel consumption compared to Cap2. In both emission cases, using more biofuels appears to be a robust strategy to hedge against uncertain costs. Results also show that the fuel diversity increases under uncertainty, more particularly when the uncertainty budget constraint is more stringent. This confirms the common conclusion among model users working with uncertainty: diversification is a good hedging strategy.

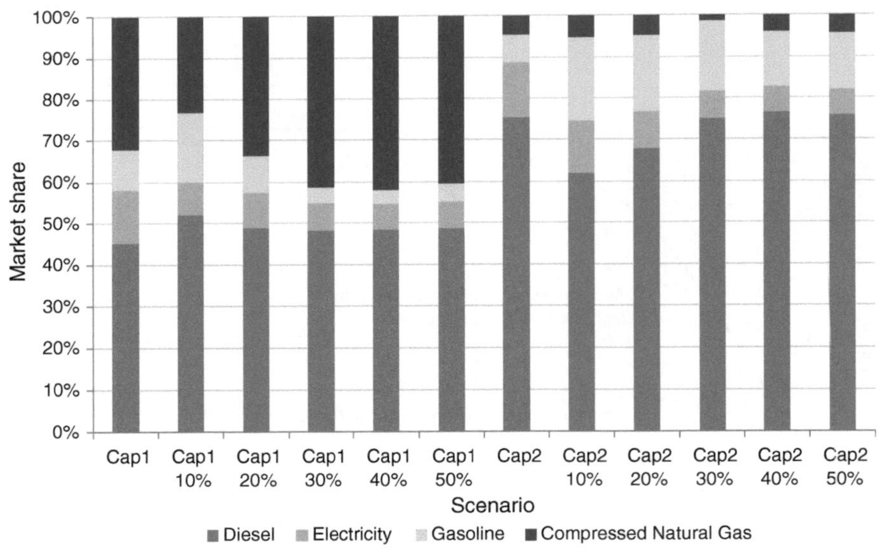

Fig. 8 Fuel mix in the French transport sector in 2050

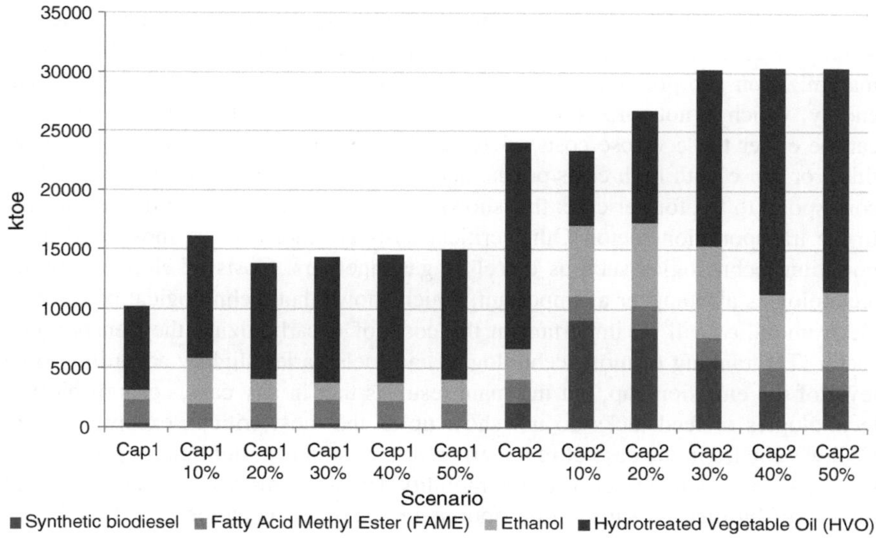

Fig. 9 Biofuels mix in the French transport sector in 2050

Finally, and consistently with the evolution of the objective function, the integration of pathways which are sensitive to the level of uncertainty does not vary monotonically: the use of substitution is higher for low uncertainty budgets—where relative costs are perturbated most.

Which costs are the most critical? Table 2 illustrates the most critical costs, for a 10 % uncertainty budget and the two emission caps. The 10 % uncertainty budget is particularly interesting since it corresponds to the most important technological hedging (Fig. 7). The technologies and fuels in Table 2 are those whose cost variation impacts most the objective function. They were sorted by decreasing

Table 2 Most critical costs in the two scenarios

	Cap1 10 %	Cap2 10 %
1	Crude oil import	Crude oil import
2	Natural gas import	Medium diesel car
3	Medium diesel car	Natural gas import
4	Diesel light utility vehicle	Biodiesel light utility vehicle
5	Small gasoline car	Diesel light utility vehicle
6	Jet fuel import	Small gasoline car
7	Small diesel vehicle	Small diesel vehicle
8	Medium electric vehicle	Medium electric vehicle
9	Naphtha import	Jet fuel import
10	Small CNG vehicle	Electric car battery

shadow value of the robust counterpart of the energy problem: the higher the shadow value, the higher the impact on the optimum objective function of the maximization sub-problem is. The most impacting costs are related with primary energy, which is not surprising. Indeed, the most sensitive technologies and fuels can be either those whose costs/prices are low and which are used in large quantities, or those with high costs/prices, and used in small quantities. Oil-based fuels correspond to the former case; this shows the difficulty of reducing oil dependency in the transportation sector. Other critical costs are those of the most used transportation technologies such as diesel or gasoline cars. Costs of electric mobility technologies also appear as important, which shows that technological progress on electromobility will be important in the costs of decarbonizing the transportation sector. The ranking of most technologies and fuels varies slightly according to the level of the emission cap, but the main result is that in any case, costs of biofuels technologies or feedstocks do not show up as the most critical, except for Light Utility Vehicles in the case of more stringent emission cap, but light utility vehicles represent only a small fraction of the mobility demand. This result is consistent with the use of biofuels as substitution options in uncertain scenarios.

4 Relevance for Policy-Making

Stochastic programming and robust optimization are crucial to support decision-making in an uncertainty context.

Stochastic programming produces an optimal single strategy, the hedging strategy, providing outcomes about how to act now, before uncertainty is resolved, thus alleviating the main defect of traditional deterministic scenario analysis which leaves the decision maker in a quandary. The hedging strategy is not necessarily an average of deterministic strategies and could represent solutions that could not easily be found otherwise; "super-hedging" actions can even be identified, i.e. actions that penetrate more in the hedging strategy than in *any* of the perfect forecast strategies. For example, natural gas in power and industrial sectors appears as an appealing robust option in several countries, being even considered as a "super-hedging" mitigation option; in other words, gas is a good "install-now" strategy given its relatively low emissions and the low capital cost of associated technologies; it allows policy makers to keep a middle-of-the-road position that does not emit too much GHG and can be modified without too much "regret" in terms of economic losses, when uncertainty is resolved on the more effective options.

Since probabilities of future outlooks are usually unknown, a parametric exploration of the hedging strategies with varying probabilities constitutes a useful complement to identify those technologies that are robust under a wide set of probabilities, and those that are not. For example, results show that the electricity system should fully prepare for the high mitigation scenario even with a less than even chance of the latter. The need for rapid de-carbonization severely restricts the set of effective options, and the most effective mitigation actions are used almost irrespective of the values of future probabilities. At the opposite, for moderate climate targets, mitigation scenarios are much milder but more volatile, reflecting a lower robustness of actions across the range of probabilities associated to the technology outlook.

Implementing RO principles in full-scale energy models also offers useful insights for policy-makers. From a normative systems analysis standpoint, it may not be obvious to identify the most influential technological parameters to reach a given policy objective (emission reduction targets, financing constraints, etc.). RO offers a parsimonious way to do so. Conversely, some parameters may have a far smaller role than could be anticipated. Hence, (i) key technologies to specific policy objectives are easily identified (ii) optimal technology mixes for these policies are made robust to random realizations in the techno-economics of the key technologies. In short, potential risks and hedging potentials of future technologies can be assessed all at once, within a technology mix that remains compliant with modeled objectives. In the case presented in this chapter, insights for policy makers include the interest in relying on a more diversified use of biofuels when future costs are uncertain. Finally, the policies and targets may themselves be subject to uncertainty. Making solutions robust to these uncertainties is particularly relevant, and should be part of future research agendas.

5 Conclusion

Understanding the sensitivity of short-term mitigation decisions to the long-term technology and climate outlook is of particular interest for the decision-makers in order to define relevant climate and energy policies in the context of uncertainty. Stochastic programming combined with a systematic exploration of the hedging strategies while varying the probabilities of the possible futures is particularly interesting to identify preferred energy and climate strategies in an uncertain context, which may even penetrate more in uncertain scenarios than in deterministic ones, as well as clusters of decisions valid for a large range of probabilities.

Robust optimization is illustrated with an example where uncertainty weighs on costs. From the theoretical viewpoint, it allows to manage large uncertainty sets while preserving linearity and tractability. The application in energy system models can prove useful in elaborating robust long-term strategies, and help identify what combinations of parameters are the most critical, or conversely do not really impact solutions. The technique may be relevant to study other sources of uncertainty in models. An on-going research consists in applying it to climate model parameters of the TIAM model. In this context, robust optimization will contribute to better know the most sensitive parameters, whether and how the uncertainty affects the mitigation strategies as well as the mitigation cost increment induced by uncertainty.

References

Babonneau F, Kanudia A, Labriet M, Loulou R, Vial JP (2011) Energy security: a robust optimization approach to design a robust European energy supply via TIAM-WORLD. Environ Model Assess 17(1–2):19–37

Baker E, Clarke L, Keisler J, Shittu E (2007) Uncertainty, technical change, and policy models. College of Management Working Papers and Reports. Paper 10. 30 p

Ben-Tal A, Nemirovski A (2002) Robust optimization—methodology and applications. Math Program 92(3):453–480

Ben-Tal A, Hertog D, Vial JP (2014) Deriving robust counterparts of nonlinear uncertain inequalities. Math Program, Series A, Available online

Bertsimas D, Brown DB, Caramanis C (2010) Theory and applications of robust optimization. SIAM Rev 53(3):464–501

Bertsimas D, Sim M (2004) The Price of Robustness. Oper Res 52(1):35–53

Bertsimas D, Thiele A (2006) A robust optimization approach to inventory theory. Oper Res 54 (1):150–168

Clarke L, Jiang K (2014) Chapter 6. Assessing transformation pathways. In: Climate change 2014, Mitigation of climate change. Contribution of Working Group III to the Fifth Assessment Report of the Intergovernmental Panel on Climate Change. Cambridge University Press, Cambridge, United Kingdom and New York, USA

El Ghaoui L, Oustry F, Lebret H (1998) Robust solutions to uncertain semidefinite programs. Society Indus Appl Math 9(1):33–52

Hawkins E, Sutton R (2009) The potential to narrow uncertainty in regional climate predictions. Bull Am Meteorol Soc 90(8):1095–1107

IEA (2013a) Energy statistics of non-OECD countries. International Energy Agency, Paris

IEA (2013b) Energy statistics of OECD countries. International Energy Agency, Paris

IPCC (2013) Summary for policymakers. In: Climate change 2013: The physical science basis. In: Stocker TF, Qin D, Plattner G-K, Tignor M, Allen SK, Boschung J, Nauels A, Xia Y, Bex V, Midgley PM (eds) Contribution of working group I to the fifth assessment report of the intergovernmental panel on climate change. Cambridge University Press, Cambridge, United Kingdom and New York, USA

IPCC (2014) Summary for policymakers. In: Field CB Barros VR, Dokken DJ, Mach KJ, Mastrandrea MD, Bilir TE, Chatterjee M, Ebi KL, Estrada YO, Genova RC, Girma B, Kissel ES, Levy AN, MacCracken S, Mastrandrea PR, and L.L. White (eds) Climate change 2014: impacts, adaptation, and vulnerability. Contribution of Working Group II to the Fifth Assessment Report of the Intergovernmental Panel on Climate Change. Cambridge University Press, Cambridge, United Kingdom and New York, NY, USA

Kanudia A, Loulou R (1998) Robust responses to climate change via StochasticMARKAL: the case of Quebec. Eur J Oper Res 106(1):15–30

Kunreuther H, Gupta S (2014) Chapter 12. Integrated risk and uncertainty assessment of climate change response policies. In: Climate change 2014, Mitigation of climate change. Contribution of working group III to the fifth assessment report of the intergovernmental panel on climate change. Cambridge University Press, Cambridge, United Kingdom and New York, USA

Labriet M, Loulou R, Kanudia A (2009) Modeling Uncertainty in a Large scale integrated Energy-Climate Model. In: Filar JA, Haurie AB (eds) Environmental Decision Making under Uncertainty, 51–77

Labriet M, Kanudia A, Loulou R (2012) Climate mitigation under an uncertain technology future: a TIAM-WORLD analysis. Energy Economics 34(3):S366–S377

Leimbach M, Dietrich J, Popp A, Klein A, Labriet M, Kanudia A, Slavin P, Bauer N, Biewald A, Bodirsky B, Humpenöder F, Lenz T, Schultes A (2013) Deliverable 7.1. Macro-economy agriculture link. EU-FP7 ERMITAGE project

Lorne D, Tchung-Ming S (2012) The French biofuels mandates under cost uncertainty—an assessment based on robust optimization Les Cahiers de l'économie, No. 87

Loulou R (2008) ETSAP-TIAM: the TIMES integrated assessment model part II: mathematical formulation. CMS 5:7–40

Loulou R, Kanudia A (1999) Minimax regret strategies for greenhouse gas abatement: methodology and application. Oper Res Lett 25:219–230

Loulou R, Labriet M (2008) ETSAP-TIAM: the TIMES integrated assessment model part I: model structure. CMS 5:41–66

Loulou R, Lehtila A (2012) Stochastic Programming and Tradeoff Analysis in TIMES. TIMES version 3.3 User Note, Energy technology systems analysis programme. http://www.iea-etsap.org/web/Docs/TIMES-Stochastic.pdf

Loulou R, Labriet M, Kanudia A (2009) Deterministic and stochastic analysis of alternative climate targets under differentiated cooperation regimes. Energy Econ 31(Suppl 2—International, US and EU Climate Change Control Scenarios: Results from EMF22: S131–143

MIT (2011) The future of natural gas—an interdisciplinary MIT Study. Massachusetts Institute of Technology. Available at https://mitei.mit.edu/system/files/NaturalGas_Report.pdf

Soyster LA (1973) Convex programming with set-inclusive constraints and applications to inexact linear programming. Oper Res 21(5):1154–1157

Wets RJB (1989) Stochastic programming. In: Nemhauser G, Kan R, Todd M (eds) Handbooks in operations research and management science, vol 1. Elsevier Science Publishers, Amsterdam

Weyant J, Kriegler E (2014) Preface and introduction to EMF 27. Clim Change 123:345–352

Yohe G, Andronova N, Schlesinger M (2004) To hedge or not against an uncertain climate future? Science 306:416–417

Schemes for the Regional Allocation of Emission Allowances under Stringent Global Climate Policy

Tom Kober, Bob van der Zwaan and Hilke Rösler

Abstract In this chapter we investigate burden-sharing regimes for the allocation of greenhouse gas emission reduction obligations under a 2 °C long-term climate policy framework, and present our findings derived from an integrated energy-economy-climate assessment. In our analysis we focus on two different allocation schemes: a per-capita-based scheme, and a scheme aiming at equalising the climate policy costs among the world regions with respect to their economic capability. We find that, under a per capita based burden-sharing scheme, the amount of carbon certificates traded on the carbon market yields a cumulative capital transfer of 20 trillion US$ between 2020 and 2050, which is on average 680 billion US$/year. The main certificate selling regions are Africa and India and the main buyers South America and the Middle East. Conversely to the per capita based scheme, a burden-sharing regime that aims at equalising regional climate policy costs leads to a cumulative carbon market capita flow until 2050 of about one quarter with average annual certificate transactions worth 180 billion US$/year, with China and Other Developing Asia being the major certificate sellers and Western Europe the main buyer. Comparing both burden-sharing schemes with regard to the compensation of non-OECD countries' climate change mitigation efforts via revenues from the global carbon certificate market reveals an advantage of the scheme based on climate policy costs over the per capita scheme, because the policy cost related

T. Kober (✉) · B. van der Zwaan · H. Rösler
Policy Studies Department, Energy research Centre of the Netherlands (ECN), Petten/Amsterdam, The Netherlands
e-mail: Kober@ecn.nl

B. van der Zwaan
e-mail: vanderzwaan@ecn.nl

H. Rösler
e-mail: rosler@ecn.nl

B. van der Zwaan
School of Advanced International Studies, Johns Hopkins University, Bologna, Italy

B. van der Zwaan
Faculty of Science, University of Amsterdam, Amsterdam, The Netherlands

G. Giannakidis et al. (eds.), *Informing Energy and Climate Policies Using Energy Systems Models*, Lecture Notes in Energy 30,
DOI 10.1007/978-3-319-16540-0_5

scheme covers 12 % of the non-OECD's climate policy costs of the first half of this century, whereas 4 % under the per capita scheme only.

1 Introduction

At the 19th Conference of the Parties (COP-19) of the United Nations Framework Convention on Climate Change (UNFCCC) in 2013 in Warsaw governments decided on further important steps towards a new binding climate change agreement as successor to the Kyoto Protocol. To reach such an agreement policy makers from developed and developing countries will have to negotiate their countries' contribution to the world's climate change efforts taking an equitable allocation of emission reduction obligations into account.

In this chapter we present our work on the cost and carbon certificate trade impacts of two different regimes of inter-regional burden-sharing for the allocation of GHG emission reduction obligations needed to reach stringent global climate change stabilisation. This work, among other research topics, was conducted in the context of the LIMITS project which focussed on the main world regions.[1] Project results regarding burden-sharing schemes are described as a cross-model comparison study in Tavoni et al. (2013) and for one model in particular in Kober et al. (2014). Compared to the latter publication, this chapter reports more regionally detailed results and provides additional insights for selected countries as to the implications of the different burden-sharing schemes.

We focus our investigation on the distribution of emission allowances and carbon certificate trade effects, as well as carbon market capital flows emanating from the introduction of equitable burden-sharing between regions that undertake collective effort in mitigating global climate change. In Sect. 2 we provide a brief characterisation of the model that we apply, as well the approach and main assumptions used. In Sect. 3 we highlight our main results regarding the main dynamics of the two emission allocation schemes analysed here, including their main differences in terms of certificate trade and carbon market capital flow. In Sect. 4 we report our overall conclusions and reflect upon these in the light of implications for policy makers.

---

[1] The LIMITS project was funded by the European Union Seventh Framework Programme FP7/ 2007–2013 under grant agreement no. 282846. Further information on the project is available under www.feem-project.net/limits.

2 Approach and Socio-economic Assumptions

The analysis of regional burden-sharing schemes under stringent climate policy control is conducted through a scenario analysis using a global energy system model.

2.1 TIAM-ECN Energy System Model

TIAM-ECN is the global TIMES Integrated Assessment Model (TIAM) of the Energy research Centre of the Netherlands (ECN). Its general structure is similar to the ETSAP-TIAM model, as well as the linear optimisation algorithm, in which the total discounted energy system costs are minimised over whole time horizon until 2100. For its 15 regions it contains the abstracted structure of the entire energy economy from resource extraction to energy end use. It features many region-specific details associated to energy resource availability, conversion and demand. As a technology-rich bottom-up model, it contains many possible fuel transformation and energy supply pathways, and encompasses technologies based on fossil, nuclear and renewable energy resources. According to the technologies' economic and energy system constraints the models determines the most cost-efficient energy transformation pathways in order to satisfy energy demand. Regarding the representation of GHG emission reductions, the model covers abatements options for carbon dioxide (CO_2), methane (CH_4) and nitrous oxide (N_2O) related to energy conversion, industrial processes and other GHG emission sources, such as agricultural activities. More detailed model descriptions and examples of the application of TIAM-ECN can be found in Rösler et al. (2011, 2014), Keppo and van der Zwaan (2012), van der Zwaan et al. (2013a) and Kober et al. (2014), as well as several references therein. Although the model has been applied to the time horizon to 2100 in order to reflect the very long-term dynamics of selected GHG emissions, we focus our investigation around burden-sharing schemes on the first half of this century as this period better corresponds to the scope of the current climate policy debate.

The demand of useful energy in TIAM-ECN is derived based on socio-economic parameters. For the global development of the gross domestic product (GDP)[2] we assume more than a tripling of over four decades, from 68 trillion US$ in 2010 to 247 trillion US$ in 2050 while the world population grows to 9 billion persons in 2050. This population development is based on the medium fertility projections of the United Nations (UN 2011), with a particular strong growth in Africa, India and Other Developing Asia with a population in 2050 of 2.1, 1.7 and 1.4 billion respectively. China's population is expected to peak at 1.4 billion people around

[2] GDP is expressed in terms of purchasing power parity (PPP) and monetary values in US$ (2005), if not indicated otherwise.

2025, and to decline thereafter to 1.3 billion people in 2050. For most of the countries of the Organisation for Economic Cooperation and Development (OECD) the population remains comparably stable, with a total average increase of 0.1 %/year for the period 2010–2100. The number of households, which has an impact on the demand for space heating for instance, is assumed to increase more rapidly than the population due to changes of the living patterns towards smaller household sizes. The total number of households doubles from 2 billion to 4 billion households between 2010 and 2050. Further model assumptions and a description of model input data, including the availability of future energy technology, can be found in Kriegler et al. (2013), van der Zwaan et al. (2013b) and Kober et al. (2014).

2.2 Burden-Sharing Regimes

An energy system that allows the provision of energy services while attaining deep GHG emission reductions in order to mitigate climate change is more costly compared to a system not subjected to GHG emission reductions if one neglects damages to the energy system due to climate change. To achieve stringent climate policy targets as cost-effective as possible, substantial expenditures are required in all regions worldwide, independent of their economic development status. These additional cost vary across regions due to various reasons, and in some regions there may exist more low-cost GHG abatement options than in others. To unlock the world's least-cost GHG mitigation options, some regions may need to disproportionally contribute to global climate change mitigation efforts, for which they would need to be compensated. Regional compensation mechanisms, also named burden-sharing schemes, aim to establish a more equitable distribution of the financial burdens associated with climate change mitigation by shifting costs attributed to GHG emission reduction across regions. Examples of burden-sharing mechanisms are the emission reduction targets of the member states of the European Union (EU), which are subjected to emissions not covered by the European Emissions Trading Scheme (EU 2013), and the intra-EU burden sharing of the 2010 EU target under the Kyoto Protocol based on the "Triptych approach" (Phylipsen and Blok 2013). Burden-sharing schemes that have different indicators in common, which can be based on socio-economic variables, energy- and emission's parameters and/or cost factors, are used to formulate the equity principle underlying each scheme and to determine a region-specific allocation of emission allowances. Through exchange of these allowances on a carbon certificate market, both cost-efficient allocation of GHG emission reductions and financial compensation of regions can be realised. The literature provides studies of many different burden-sharing schemes which have been analysed over the past. An overview is compiled in Tavoni et al. (2013). This publication also explains the methodological background of two burden-sharing schemes that we use for our study. Tavoni et al. (2013) also provide the outcomes of the LIMITS cross-model comparison study on the two burden-sharing schemes. Further comparative assessments of different burden-sharing principles can be found, for instance, in den Elzen et al. (2008), Hof et al. (2008), Jacoby et al. (2008) and Ciscar et al. (2013).

Our study concerns two different burden-sharing schemes. The first scheme, which we refer to as "resource-sharing" scheme uses a population based indicator, and the second scheme, the so-called "effort-sharing" scheme, considers climate policy costs and economic development. The resource-sharing scheme describes an allocation mechanism for emission permits according to the level of GHG emissions allowed per capita. For this scheme we assume a transition phase for the period 2020–2050 in which the regional per capita emissions converge from status-quo towards the global average while the global average converges according to the GHG reduction obligation in order to achieve stringent climate targets. For an explanation of the terminology 'contraction and convergence' see Meyer (2000). The goal of the effort-sharing scheme is to equalise the mitigation costs across regions with the paradigm that all regions should incur the same climate change control costs in percentage terms of their GDP after emissions trading. Hence, revenues or expenses from carbon certificate trade are included in climate change control costs. Starting in 2020, the regions' shares of total climate change mitigation costs should be equal to the world average. This implies that regions with higher relative mitigation costs compared to the global average receive additional carbon certificates. Each region gains revenue from the carbon market through the sale of excess carbon certificates, which provides compensation (at least partly) for their mitigation costs. This effect leads to an equalisation of climate change mitigation efforts across regions. Conversely to contraction and convergence under the resource-sharing scheme, we assume no transition phase under the effort-sharing scheme.

The two burden-sharing schemes are investigated under a framework of stringent climate policy goals achieving a long-term stabilisation of the global mean temperature increase at 2 °C with respect to the pre-industrial level. For the calculation of the regional allowance allocation we apply a 2 °C climate stabilisation scenario in which the regional allocation of GHG emission certificates corresponds to the regional emissions under a global least-cost GHG reduction pathway. This scenario is referred to as the 'reference' scenario. In both burden-sharing schemes the amount of worldwide available emission allowances equals the reference scenario in each period. The duration of one trading period is 10 years while banking or borrowing between trading periods is not allowed.

The model implementation of the burden-sharing schemes, which is described in more detail in Kober et al. (2014), is realised through pre-optimisation procedures for the calculation each region's overall allocations of permits. The calculated certificate quantities are introduced as user constraints to the optimisation problem. Key input parameters for the calculation of the allocation of emission allowances under the resource-sharing scheme are the population development assumptions, the regional GHG emissions per capita in 2020 and the future evolution of the global average of per capita GHG emissions. For the calculation of the regional per capita emissions in 2020 and the global average specific emissions from 2020 onwards, we used those derived from the reference scenario. Each regions' per capita emissions contract beyond their respective starting points in 2020 and converge in subsequent decades by 2050. Under the effort-sharing scheme target policy costs are calculated for every region and period. These regional costs are the product of the world total climate change control costs as percentage of global GDP and the GDP of the respective region. The difference between all regions' effort-sharing target policy costs and their policy costs under global least-cost climate change mitigation is divided by the global carbon certificate price for each period. The resulting quantity per period is added to the regions' emission levels calculated under least-cost mitigation criteria, which then equals the regional effort-sharing certificate allocation.

3 Results

We focus the presentation of our results on the time period to 2050. Nevertheless, long-term energy system effects past 2050 are considered in our study due to our model approach with perfect foresight for the time horizon until 2100.

3.1 GHG Emissions Development and Associated Costs in the Reference Scenario

The reference scenario is characterised through a GHG emissions reduction pathway with fragmented weak national climate policies in the near-term that reflect the unconditional Copenhagen pledges. For the period after 2020 we anticipate a global coordinated action to achieve climate stabilisation at 2 °C average atmospheric temperature increase, which is implemented through a maximum radiative forcing level of 2.8 W/m^2 in 2100.[3] A detailed description of the policy framework and assumptions of this scenario can be found in Kriegler et al. (2013).

The GHG emissions of the reference scenario are displayed for the 15 model regions disaggregated by emission source in Fig. 1. The development of the regional emissions in 2020 mimic the countries' Copenhagen pledges as described in Kriegler et al. (2013). Global level GHG emissions reach their maximum in 2020 with 51 GtCO_2e and decrease afterwards to 21 GtCO_2e in 2050. Undoubtedly, industrialised countries and emerging economies have to reduce their GHG emissions drastically in order achieve the global 2 °C climate change control target at

[3] This forcing target refers to all anthropogenic radiative agents with the exception of three agents: nitrate aerosols, mineral dust aerosols, and land use albedo changes. According to our model approach we adjusted the forcing target to be applied to the three GHG emissions represented in the TIAM-ECN.

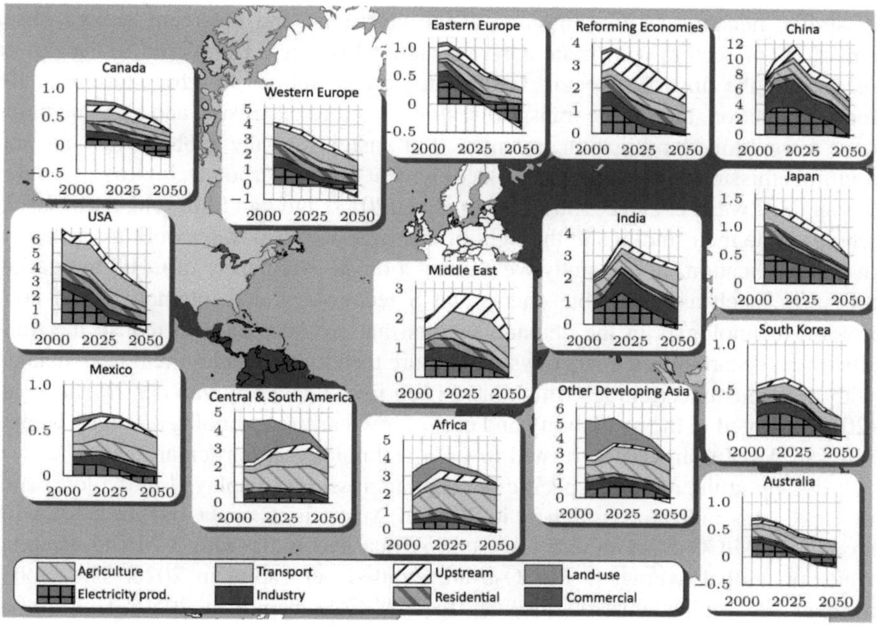

Fig. 1 GHG emissions by sector in the reference 2 °C climate change control scenario with least-cost long-term GHG mitigation (units in $GtCO_2e$)

least costs. For most of the industrialised regions GHG emissions never exceed 2010 emission levels. Deepest emission reductions in relative terms are realised in Eastern and Western Europe, Canada and Australia where 2050 emission levels are at least 80 % below 2010 emissions. In most of the non-OECD regions, which are characterised by either a strong economic growth and/or a significant increase of population, GHG emissions continue to increase until 2020 and decline rapidly afterwards. A modest increase of emissions in the two regions Central and South America and Other Developing Asia towards 2020 can be observed as a result of compensation of increasing emissions from fossil fuel combustion and agricultural activities by decreasing emissions from land-use and land-use change and forestry (LULUCF). The emissions from LULUCF follow a declining trend which can partly be attributed to policy measures due to the benefits related to conservation of natural area and biodiversity. There are only four out of the 15 regions with emission reductions in 2050 compared to 2010 of less than 40 %, which are Africa, Central and South America, India and the Middle East.

In general, we observe most of the GHG emission reductions being realised through abatement of CO_2, in particular in the upstream sector and in the power sector which in some regions even allow for negative net emissions. Negative emissions occur when biomass is converted in technologies with carbon dioxide capture and storage (CCS), e.g. for the production of electricity, biofuels or hydrogen. For instance, in Eastern and Western Europe, the USA, Canada and

Australia, negative GHG emissions of the electricity and upstream sectors offset emissions of sectors with more costly abatement options. Compared to the power sector and the upstream sector, GHG emission reductions in agriculture, e.g. for food production, and in the transport sector, are more expensive and in some cases have very limited mitigation potential. For insights in the global, regional and sectoral emission reductions and the deployment of low-carbon technology we refer to van der Zwaan et al. (2013b), Calvin et al. (2013) and van Sluisveld et al. (2013) who provide their findings in the light of the same scenario framework as presented in this publication. In our study we assume a broad availability of GHG mitigation measures, such as renewable energy, CCS technology and alternative fuel conversion technologies in the demand sectors that are necessary to realise the transition to a decarbonised energy system. Future technology deployment is associated with a various uncertainties which have been investigated by van der Zwaan et al. (2013b) related to the availability and cost of low-carbon technology, and by Keppo and van der Zwaan (2012) related to CCS technology in particular.

Looking at the regions' specific per capita emissions, displayed in the left panel in Fig. 2, this indicator is highest in 2020 in Australia, Canada and the USA with around 20 $MtCO_2e$/capita and lowest in Africa and India with 3 $MtCO_2e$/capita, while on global average 7 $MtCO_2e$ are emitted per capita in 2020. The global average per capita emission declines to 2 $MtCO_2e$/capita in 2050. This global average in 2050 represents the convergence target for the emission allocation under the resource-sharing scheme. The regional per capita emissions in 2050 range from 6 $MtCO_2e$ per capita for Reforming Economies to less than zero for Eastern Europe.

The carbon certificate price that corresponds to the emission trajectory in order to attain the 2 °C climate target increases from 70 US$/$tCO_2e$ in 2020 to

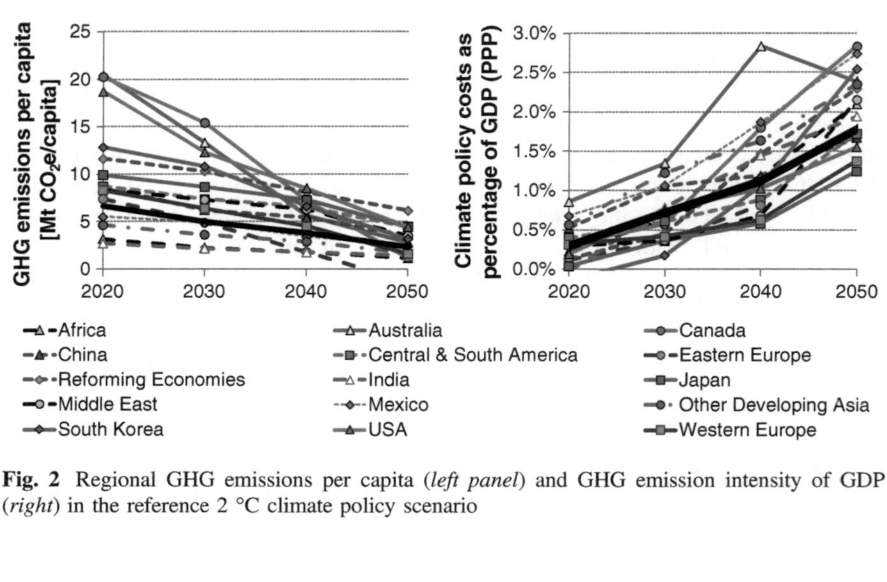

Fig. 2 Regional GHG emissions per capita (*left panel*) and GHG emission intensity of GDP (*right*) in the reference 2 °C climate policy scenario

130 US$/t$CO_2$e in 2030, and to 390 US$/tCO_2e in 2050. According to our model approach, this price path represents the marginal overall GHG emission abatement cost, and it applies to all regions and sectors of the global energy system. In 2020 the certificate prices are strongly influenced by the stringent Copenhagen/Cancun pledges we imposed, and prices in the long-run are determined by the availability and cost of the GHG mitigation measures. These abatement prices are in line with the prices stated by other models which span a range between 200 and 900 US$/t$CO_2$e in 2050 with a median at 200 US$/t$CO_2$e (see Kriegler et al. 2013). The Global Energy Assessment reports a CO_2 price above 110 US$/t$CO_2$e that is associated with a global GHG emission reduction down to about 25 GtCO_2e by 2040 (GEA 2012). The worldwide aggregated energy system costs (including costs to avoid non-energy related GHG emissions), to which we refer as 'climate policy costs',[4] accumulate to 77 trillion US$ for the entire first half of the century with 0.3 trillion US$ in 2020, and around 4 trillion US$ in 2050. In 2020, the highest costs occur in China (90 billion US$), followed by Western Europe (50 billion US $). For India in 2020 we observe a slightly positive cost effect due to reduced fossil energy imports under climate policy. In absolute terms, China faces highest climate policy costs throughout the whole first half of the century, with about one fifth of the global costs in 2050, and India's costs grow substantially in this timeframe that India becomes the country second highest climate policy costs by 2050 (16 % of the global costs).

For the effort-sharing scheme of particular importance, we provide the climate policy costs in relative terms to GDP in the right panel in Fig. 2, which shows that these costs on global level correspond to 0.3 % in 2020 and 1.7 % in 2050. Australia faces comparably high costs until 2040 due to the fact that the country undergoes a substantial change of its domestic energy supply structure and its revenues from coal export decline drastically as a result of reduced coal demand under climate change policy. After 2030/2040 this effect applies also to the Middle East, Reforming Economies and Canada, which experience extensive net fossil fuel exports under absence of climate policy and possess few local GHG reduction potential. Under stringent climate policy their fossil fuel exports reduce significantly in the long-run associated with a decline of their revenues from the oil and gas markets, which consequently leads to an increase of their climate policy costs. In China until 2030 and in Mexico and Other Developing Asia over the whole period, relative policy costs are higher than the world average, which results from the large expected increases in their respective energy demands and thus massive investment requirements in renewable energy for power production and energy efficiency improvements on the demand side. Western Europe and Japan are

---

[4] Policy costs in the context of our bottom–up modelling approach refer to undiscounted costs for the entire energy system, including expenditures for technology investments, operation and maintenance, other variable costs as well as costs associated with changing demand patterns. Policy implementation and transaction costs are excluded. Climate policy costs are calculated as the difference between the total costs under certain policy conditions and the costs in the reference case.

regions with relative climate policy costs below the global average for most of the time until 2050, which is driven by their low energy intensity of GDP, their reduction of energy imports under climate change policy and their good potentials to deploy low-carbon technology. This includes for both regions the continuation of electricity production from nuclear power until 2050 with an installed power plant capacity at around 2005 level.

3.2 Allocation of Emission Allowances

Based on the development of GHG emissions in the reference scenario and the burden-sharing schemes' calculation methods, regional allowance endowments are determined as displayed in Fig. 3. Independent of the burden-sharing scheme China is the region which receives most of certificates equivalent to cumulative emissions for the period 2020–2050 of about 250 $GtCO_2e$. The figure also illustrates that for the majority of the regions the allocation according to the effort-sharing deviates less from the regions' cost-optimal GHG emission trajectories than the distribution under the resource-sharing scheme.

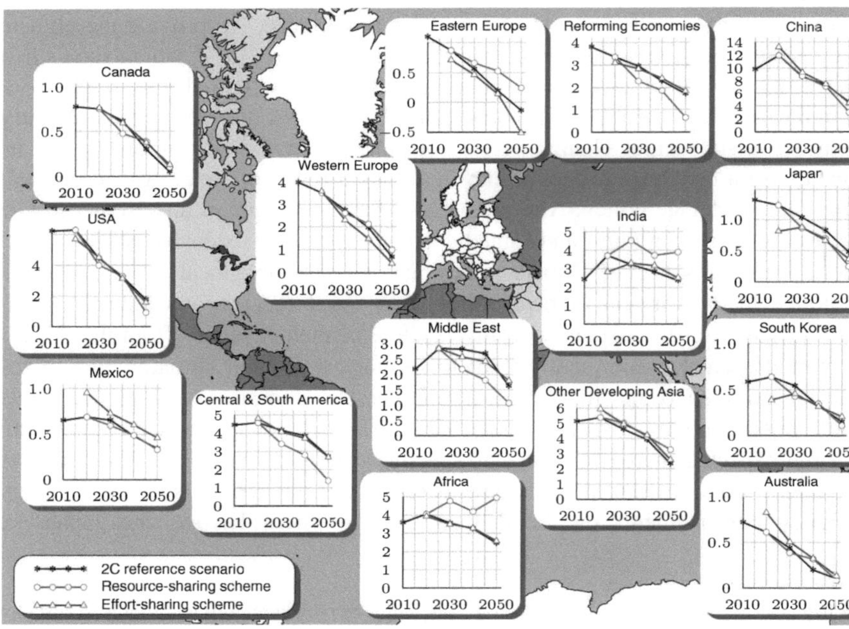

Fig. 3 GHG emissions in the reference scenario and emission allowances allocation under the two burden-sharing regimes (units in $GtCO_2e$)

The resource-sharing method favours regions with a high population growth, such as Africa and India. For both regions the amount of emission permits increases from 2020 to 2030, and for Africa also from 2040 to 2050. All other regions receive less certificates in the periods past 2020. The endowment of certificates to Other Developing Asia is higher than the emission reductions of the reference pathway as a result of the initially low per capita emissions in 2020 and the high population growth in this region. In regions with low or even negative population growth rates, the number of emission rights of regions declines drastically in particular when the initial number of GHG emissions allowances is high, such as for China, Japan, the USA, Central and South America and Reforming Economies.

The effort-sharing scheme favours regions which are characterised by comparably high costs for GHG emission reduction with respect to their overall economic capability. China receives emission permits between 2020 and 2050 of cumulatively 256 $GtCO_2e$, which exceeds the reference GHG emissions by 14 $GtCO_2e$ (6 %). Also Other Developing Asia, Mexico and Australia can profit from additionally available certificates worth about 18 $GtCO_2e$ until 2050. In contrast, Western Europe and Japan as a region with a high expected GDP and moderate climate policy costs get 16 $GtCO_2e$ less allocated in the same timeframe compared to its reference emission pathway.

When comparing the certificate allocation under the two burden-sharing schemes, significant differences can be observed for Africa, India, Latin America, the Middle East and Reforming Economies. Africa, for example, receives under the resource-sharing allocation in total 34 $GtCO_2e$ more emission permits until 2050 than under the effort-sharing scheme. The different endowments affect the carbon certificate trade and hence the extent to which the regions are compensated for their climate change mitigation efforts.

3.3 *Carbon Certificate Trade*

Emission certificate trade allows a return from an initial certificate allocation to the overall cost-optimal mitigation pathway, if one assumes the existence of a perfect carbon certificate market (as we here do). The traded quantities are determined by the allocation of GHG emission rights and the region's technological potentials to reduce GHG emissions. The trade of certificates in the resource-sharing scheme starts after the year of grandfathering in 2020. A cumulative amount of certificates equivalent to 83 $GtCO_2e$ is traded until 2050 under the resource sharing scheme. 60 % (50 $GtCO_2e$) less certificates are traded under the effort-sharing scheme in the same period due to the fact, that the allocation under the effort-sharing regime comes closer to each regional cost-optimal GHG emissions reduction pathways than under the resource sharing scheme.

Under the resource-sharing regime the total annually traded quantity of emission rights reaches its maximum with 6 $GtCO_2e$ in 2050, which represents about a quarter of the global GHG emissions and half of the global CO_2 emissions in that year. Most of the emission certificates are sold by Africa and India (Table 1). These two regions combined sell emission rights equivalent to a cumulative amount of 63 $GtCO_2e$ until 2050, which corresponds to about 80 % of all certificates sold in this period. Around 80 % of the tradable permits in this time frame are bought by Central and South America, China, the Middle East and the Reforming Economies due to their rapidly increasing GHG emissions and modest or even negative population growth rates.

Table 1 Emission certificate trade and carbon market capital flow cumulative between 2020 and 2050 for the two burden-sharing schemes

Resource-sharing scheme			Effort-sharing scheme		
	Certificates sold ($MtCO_2e$)	Revenues from the carbon market (billion US$)		Certificates sold ($MtCO_2e$)	Revenues from the carbon market (billion US$)
Certificate selling regions					
Africa	33984	8473	China	13873	1327
India	29375	6574	Other Dev. Asia	10620	1831
Other Dev. Asia	10937	2809	Mexico	3883	693
Eastern Europe	6233	1614	Australia	3171	505
Western Europe	1870	797	Canada	951	290
Australia	586	165	India	366	788
	82984	20432		32865	5435
Certificate buying regions					
South America	−24549	−5854	Western Europe	−10272	−2151
Middle East	−17850	−3823	Japan	−5899	−936
Ref. Economies	−16432	−3905	USA	−4461	−760
China	−9632	−3605	Middle East	−4207	−553
USA	−8403	−2150	Eastern Europe	−4139	−1022
Japan	−4146	−953	South Korea	−1902	−106
South Korea	−1119	−174	South America	−1087	−366
Mexico	−569	−79	Ref. Economies	−627	272
Canada	−283	112	Africa	−273	186
	−82983	−20432		−32866	−5435

Associated to the trade of emission allowances is the capital transfer on the global carbon market, which is determined by the amount of certificates traded and the corresponding price of emission certificates. As a result of the exponential increase of the carbon certificate price, the carbon market capital flow is increasingly determined by the certificate price, rather than by the traded quantities. Under the resource-sharing scheme the total carbon market capital flow accumulates to 20 trillion US$ until mid of this century with annual capital transfers of 400 billion US$ in 2030 to 620 billion US$ in 2040 and to 2200 billion US$ in 2050 (Table 1). Over the entire timeframe Africa and India receive together 70 % of the worldwide generated revenues from sales of certificates. Conversely, Central and South America's spends about 30 % of the total global expenditures for certificate purchases, and the Middle East, Reforming Economies and China about 20 % each.

Comparing the global capital flows of the carbon certificate market under the resource-sharing scheme with the climate policy costs associated with the 2 °C climate stabilisation target, reveals, that the cumulative carbon market capital flows represent 30 % of the global policy costs during the first half of the 21st century (Fig. 4). Of course, this indicator deviates regionally. For the group of non-OECD countries, in total 4 % of the policy costs can be compensated by revenues from the carbon market until 2050. Looking at single regions, we can observe for Africa on the one hand total cumulative revenues from the carbon market of 8.5 trillion US$ which is almost 2.5 times the cumulative climate policy costs (3 trillion US$) in the

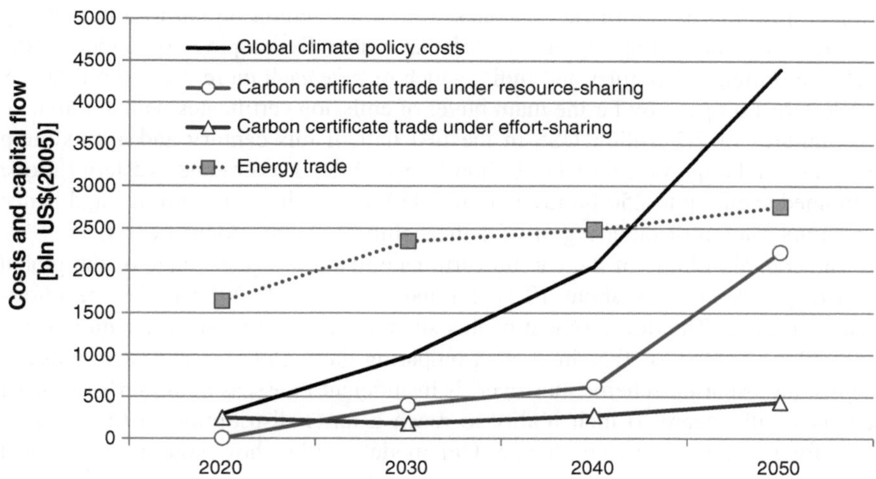

Fig. 4 Climate policy costs and capital flows for trade of carbon certificates, energy and captured CO_2 under the resource-sharing scheme (based on Kober et al. 2014) *N.B.* Capital flows refer to trade among the 15 regions represented in the model. Market capital volumes would increase if results are shown based on a higher geographical resolution

period to 2050. On the other hand, Reforming Economies' expenses for certificate purchases are about 50 % higher than their climate policy costs in the reference scenario for the period 2020 to 2050. These two cases indicate that the resource-sharing regime analysed in this study is unsuitable to compensate all developing and transition countries at once. This underpins the drawback of the resource-sharing scheme, which refers to the allocation regardless of each region's capabilities to reduce GHG emissions. Especially, if a regions' population growth is rather moderate, or even negative, and emission abatement measures are costly, the region is hardly compensated for their cost to mitigate climate change. The case of Africa also shows that the resource-sharing scheme might also over-compensate the financial efforts of GHG emission reduction measures of selected emerging regions. This finding has also been observed by Jacoby et al. (2008).

Under the effort-sharing scheme certificate trade reaches its maximum with almost 3 $GtCO_2e$ in 2020 and declines in the subsequent periods until 2050 to about 1 $GtCO_2e$ annually. The resulting annual carbon market volume ranges between 170 and 270 billion US$ in the period 2020 until 2040 and peaks at 430 billion US$ in 2050. The corresponding cumulative capital flow until 2050 (5 trillion US$) represents one quarter of the volume under the resource-sharing scheme. China and Other Developing Asia are prime certificate selling regions under the effort-sharing regime, and receive 30 and 40 % respectively of the total global carbon market revenues until 2050. China is particular important in the near-term with a share of global certificate sales values of 50 % in 2020 (95 billion US$). In the decades beyond 2020, China's carbon market revenues decline, and towards mid-century China's position on the market changes from a net selling region to a net buying region. The main selling regions in 2050 are Other Developing Asia, the Middle East, Reforming Economies and India, which receive each more than 50 billion US $. Western Europe is by far the main buyer of emission certificates with cumulative expenditures of 2.2 trillion US$ in the first half of this century and a maximum annual capital requirement of 110 billion US$ in 2050. Eastern and Western Europe combined spent up to 250 billion US$ in 2050 for purchases of permits, and hence for compensation of other regions for their climate change control costs.

The capital volume of the carbon certificate market as percentage of the global climate policy costs is about 10 % for the period 2020–2050 under the effort-sharing regime. The development of this share over time reveals a declining trend from 70 % in 2020 to 10 % in 2050. Comparing these global shares, with those of the resource-sharing scheme, however, is insufficient to assess both burden-sharing schemes with regard to their ability to reach a fairer distribution of the region's costs for mitigating climate change. Our model results show significant regional differences between the two burden-sharing schemes with respect to the regions revenues or expenditures on the carbon market versus their climate policy costs. In 2020, China and Central and South America are able to recover almost all their climate policy costs through revenues from the carbon market, and Other Developing Asia at least 30 %. Overcompensation, as observed for Africa under the resource-sharing scheme, is less significant under the effort-sharing regime. The effort-sharing regime allows all non-OECD countries combined, to cover 12 % of their climate policy costs using revenues from the carbon certificate market during the first half of the century, with a maximum of 27 % in 2020 and a minimum of 9 % in 2040. Comparing the two burden-sharing schemes we conclude, that the effort-sharing regime is better capable to compensate less developed economies for their costs under a global 2 °C climate policy framework. The effect of burden-sharing—generating generally higher policy costs for the cluster of OECD countries and lower ones for non-OECD countries—is larger for the effort-sharing scheme than the resource-sharing scheme.

The certificate exchanges and associated capital volumes to realise either of the two burden-sharing schemes indicate the importance of the existence of an appropriate carbon certificate market to cost-efficiently reach climate change mitigation goals. In particular under the resource-sharing scheme, the capital transfer of the carbon market would almost reach the level of energy market capital flows around the middle of the century (Fig. 4). For the assessment presented here we assumed perfectly functioning markets for both carbon certificates and energy commodities. It might be difficult, to establish perfect carbon market conditions, and market distortions of many different types could arise. For an analysis of the impacts of an imperfect carbon certificate trade we refer to Kober et al. (2014), who investigate in particular effects related to timing issues, regional trade implications, certificate price effects, and global climate policy costs.

4 Conclusions

In this study we analysed the two different regional burden-sharing schemes for the allocation of GHG emission allowances, the resulting carbon certificate trade, and carbon market capital flows under a 2 °C climate policy regime. To achieve this climate target at least-cost, global GHG emissions must reduce by half between 2010 and 2050, which is in line with recent publications (see Kriegler et al. 2013; IPCC 2014; IEA 2014). Thereby sectors in which abatement is costly, such as agriculture, industry and transportation, would be compensated by extensive emissions reductions in other sectors which even become negative net emitters in selected regions around the middle of the century.

We investigated a population-based certificate allocation regime (resource-sharing) versus a scheme which aims at equal distribution of the economic burden across regions (effort-sharing). We find that under the resource-sharing regime the regional allocation of emission certificates deviates more from the region's emission trajectories under a global least-cost reference mitigation pathway than observed under the effort-sharing scheme. Consequently, significant differences between the two burden-sharing schemes occur regarding the amount of certificates traded on a global certificate market, and the resulting carbon market capital flow. Between 2020 and 2050 under the resource-sharing scheme almost three times more certificates are traded than under the effort-sharing scheme. Establishing a proper functioning of a global carbon certificate market is essential when implementing burden-sharing schemes, as it allows the unlocking of a regions' least cost GHG mitigation potential. If carbon certificate trade possibilities are limited global costs to attain the 2 °C climate target might even increase by 20 % (Kober et al. 2014).

The resource-sharing method favours regions with a high population growth, such as Africa and India. Both regions are net seller of certificates on the certificate market with cumulative sales of permits equivalent to 63 $GtCO_2e$ until 2050 which corresponds to an aggregated capital flow of 15 trillion US$. With these revenues from the carbon market, both regions combined can cover their climate policy costs until 2050. The most important certificate-buying regions until 2050 are Central and South America, the Middle East, Reforming Economies and China due to their low or even negative population growth.

The effort-sharing scheme favours regions which are characterised by comparably high costs for GHG emission reduction with respect to their overall economic capability. China and Other Developing Asia face comparable high climate policy costs in the near-term and receive excess emission permits which they sell on the carbon market and gain combined revenues worth 140 US$ in 2020. These revenues offset the regions' climate policy costs in that year. Towards 2050 China becomes a net buying region as a result of its strong economic growth and comparable advantage in terms of its GHG emissions reduction potential. An important determinant of climate policy costs in the long-run are changes in fossil fuel trade, which occur as consequence of global fuel shifts towards low-carbon energy and demand reductions to meet the stringent climate targets. This increases climate policy costs of traditional fossil fuel exporting regions (Middle East, Reforming Economies and Australia) because of substantial reductions of their import revenues from fossil fuel trade. Western Europe, which has relatively low climate policy costs as percentage of its GDP, is the main buyer of emission certificates with cumulative expenditures of 2.2 trillion US$ in the first half of this century and a maximum annual capital requirement of 110 billion US$ in 2050.

Comparing both burden-sharing schemes, with regard to the compensation of non-OECD countries' climate change mitigation efforts via revenues from the global carbon certificate market, reveals an advantage of the effort-sharing scheme over the resource-sharing scheme. Under the effort-sharing regime, for all non-OECD countries combined, about 12 % of their climate policy costs can be covered by revenues from the carbon certificate market during the first half of the century, with a maximum of 27 % in 2020. The average annual capital needed to realise this compensation until 2050 amounts to about 140 billion US$. Comparing these means, with the 100 billion $US\$_{2020}$ targeted to be mobilized by the Green Climate Fund under the Copenhagen accord by 2020, (UNFCCC 2014) advocates for continuation of this financial instrument in future and to increase its budget, if a higher compensation of less developed economies is aimed for.

References

Calvin K, Wise M, Klein D, McCollum D, Tavoni M, van der Zwaan B, van Vuuren D (2013) A multi-model analysis of the regional and sectoral roles of bioenergy in near-term and long-term carbon mitigation. Clim Change Econ 4(4):1–31

Ciscar J, Saveyn B, Soria A, Szabo L, van Regemorter D, van Ireland T (2013) A comparability analysis of global burden sharing GHG reduction scenarios. Energy Policy 55:73–81

den Elzen M, Höhne N, van Vliet J, Ellerman C (2008) Exploring comparable post-2012 reduction efforts for AnnexI countries. MNP report 500102019/2008, Netherlands Environmental Assessment Agency (MNP), Bilthoven

European Union (2013) Decision of the European parliament and of the council on the effort of Member States to reduce their greenhouse gas emissions to meet the Community's greenhouse gas emission reduction commitments up to 2020. 406/2009/EC

GEA (2012) Global energy assessment—towards a sustainable future. Cambridge University Press, Cambridge

Hof A, den Elzen M, van Vuuren D (2008) Environmental effectiveness and economic consequences of fragmented versus universal regimes: what can we learn from model studies? Int Env Agreements: Politics, Law Econ 9(1):39–62

IEA (2014) Energy technology perspectives. International Energy Agency, Paris

IPCC (2014) Climate change 2014: mitigation of climate change. In: Edenhofer O, Pichs-Madruga R, Sokona Y, Farahani E, Kadner S, Seyboth K, Adler A, Baum I, Brunner S, Eickemeier P, Kriemann B, Savolainen J, Schlömer S, von Stechow C, Zwickel T and Minx JC (eds) Contribution of working group III to the fifth assessment report of the intergovernmental panel on climate change. Cambridge University Press, Cambridge, United Kingdom and New York, NY, USA

Jacoby H, Babiker M, Paltsev S, Reilly J (2008) Sharing the burden of GHG reductions. Report No. 167, MIT joint program on the science and policy of global change, Cambridge, MA, USA

Keppo I, van der Zwaan B (2012) The impact of uncertainty in climate targets and CO_2 storage availability on long-term emissions abatement. Environ Model Assess 17:177–191

Kober T, van der Zwaan B, Rösler H (2014) Regional burden sharing regimes for reaching a global long-term 2 °C climate change control target. Clim Change Econ 5(1):0–32

Kriegler E, Tavoni M, Aboumahboub T, Luderer G, Calvin K, De Maere G, Krey V, Riahi K, Rösler H, Schaeffer M, van Vuuren D (2013) What does the 2 °C target imply for a global climate change agreement in 2020? The LIMITS study on implications of Durban platform action scenarios. Clim Change Econ 4(4):1–30

Meyer A (2000) Contraction and convergence—the global solution to climate change. Schumacher Briefings 5, Green books for the Schumacher society, Bristol, USA

Phylipsen, D, Blok C (2013) European experiences with burden sharing in climate change—lessons learned for the post-2020 negotiations. Report published under the MAPS programme

Rösler, H, Bruggink J, Keppo I (2011) Design of a European sustainable hydrogen model—model structure and data sources. Energy research Centre of the Netherlands (ECN) report ECN-E-11-041, Petten

Rösler H, van der Zwaan B, Keppo I, Bruggink J (2014) Electricity versus hydrogen under stringent climate change control. Sustain Energy Technol Assess 5:106–118

Tavoni M, Kriegler E, Aboumahboub T, Calvin K, De Maere G, Jewell J, Kober T, Lucas P, Luderer G, McCollum D, Marangoni G, Riahi K, van Vuuren D (2013) The distribution of the major economies' effort in the Durban platform scenarios. Clim Change Econ 4(4):0–25

United Nations (UN) (2011) World population prospects: the 2010 revision. http://www.un.org/en/development/desa/population/. Accessed 31 Mar 2012

UNFCCC (2014) Financial, technology and capacity-building support. http://cancun.unfccc.int/financial-technology-and-capacity-building-support/new-long-term-funding-arrangements/. Accessed 31 July 2014 van der Zwaan B, Keppo I, Johnsson F (2013a) How to decarbonize the transport sector? Energy Policy 61:562–573

van der Zwaan B, Rösler H, Kober T, Aboumahboub T, Calvin K, Gernaat D, Marangoni G, McCollum D (2013b) A cross-model comparison of global long-term technology diffusion under a 2 °C climate change control target. Clim Change Econ 4(4):1–24

van Sluisveld M, Gernaat D, Otto A, Isaak M, van Vuuren D, Mouratiadou I, Ashina S, Garg A, Shukla P, Calvin K, Rao S, Lucas P, van Vliet J (2013) A multi-model analysis of post-2020 mitigation efforts of five major economies. Clim Change Econ 4(4):1–24

Assessment of Carbon Emissions Quotas with the Integrated TIMES and MERGE Model

Socrates Kypreos and Antti Lehtila

Abstract The success of climate change mitigation depends on the modalities for the extension of the Kyoto protocol after 2020. This refers to the appropriate level of GHG reduction imposed as emissions quotas in line with the 2 °C commitment. We perform a parametric analysis where increasingly stringent cumulative and global emission quota bounds are applied using the integrated TIMES and MERGE model (ITMM). The model integrates in one set of equations two hybrid top-down and bottom-up models both able to analyze technological change. The study assumes efficient policies and measures where all world regions accept a binding protocol in 2020 while mitigation policies will start already in 2015. However, this early introduction of efficient policies needs capital transfers for a fair burden sharing in favor of countries with low income and in that sense the model assumptions are critical. Marginal cost of carbon control of these optimistic policies are high (600–1000 \$/t of carbon by 2050) but global GDP losses remain moderate and below 1.5 % per year.

1 Introduction

The Copenhagen Conference of Parties (COP15), as endorsed by the COP16 in Cancun, reached an agreement described in the so-called Copenhagen Accord (CA) (UN-FCCC/CP/2009). The accord aims to combat global warming with differentiated reduction targets of greenhouse gas emissions and by mobilizing resources supporting adaptation and carbon-free technology in developing countries. Unfortunately, both conferences and the subsequent ones failed to negotiate a binding

S. Kypreos (✉)
Paul Scherrer Institute, Villigen, Switzerland
e-mail: socrateskypreos@gmail.com

A. Lehtila
VTT Technical Research Centre of Finland, Espoo, Finland
e-mail: antti.lehtila@vtt.fi

G. Giannakidis et al. (eds.), *Informing Energy and Climate Policies Using Energy Systems Models*, Lecture Notes in Energy 30,
DOI 10.1007/978-3-319-16540-0_6

agreement to combat global warming. The COPs approved to negotiate and to arrange by 2015 the initiation of such legal binding commitment from 2020 onwards. Nevertheless, the final outcome on mitigation depends on the modalities for the extension of the protocol. Therefore, the legitimate question is which levels of GHG reduction would be sufficient to serve as a Post-Kyoto policy framework aiming to stabilize GHGs concentration at levels that would prevent dangerous anthropogenic interference with the climate system (UNFCCC Art. 2).

Also, as such an agreement will start with global commitments in 2020, while the Kyoto protocol is not supported by significant countries like USA, Canada and eventually Japan and Russia, it is justified to question if it is not already too late to sustain global warming below 2 °C. This is especially the case, in a period following the economic recession of 2008, where governments and markets become increasingly hesitant to mitigate global warming supporting a globally binding agreement. On the other hand, the CO_2 concentration and the mean temperature in the earth atmosphere and the oceans are increasing. These are the overarching questions of the present study. The analysis is based on MERGE (Manne et al. 1995) integrated with the TIMES-MACRO model of USA (Remme and Blesl 2006) both being able to analyze technological change. Emphasis is given to model US, a key player for mitigation policy, as we need to analyze details of technological change including among others the end-use markets not available in MERGE.

A significant study that helps to quantify the probability to sustain global warming below 2 °C as function of cumulative GHGs reduction bounds has been published in Nature (Meinshausen et al. 2009). This study, based on comprehensive probabilistic analysis, claims that cumulative emissions up to 2050 are robust indicators of the probability that twenty-first century warming will not exceed 2 °C relative to pre-industrial temperatures. Limiting cumulative CO_2 emissions over 2000–2050 to 273 GtC yields a 25 % probability of warming exceeding 2 °C—and a limit of 392 GtC yields a 50 % probability—given a representative estimate of the distribution of climate system properties. Similarly, an intermediate probability level is obtained by limiting emissions to 316 GtC (33 % probability) while a limit of 242 GtC yields a 20 % probability. Therefore the results of Meinshausen et al. (2009) may serve as an acceptable benchmark to define cumulative targets for our analysis. Finally, for comparison we refer to the Synthesis Report of the Fifth Assessment Report of the Intergovernmental Panel on Climate Change (IPCC). This report estimates a similar value of 273 GtC as the remaining amount of carbon emissions quotas from 2011 onwards for a global warming below 2 °C with a probability of 66 % and 355 GtC for a 50 % probability.

As part of the Copenhagen Accord, Annex I Parties (industrialized countries) and non-Annex I Parties (developing countries) have submitted reduction proposals (pledges) and mitigation actions to the UNFCCC secretariat. Based on these pledges and some extra assumptions compiled by Labriet (2010), emissions for 2020 are estimated to be around 39 $GtCO_2$ (10.64 GtC) and have been adopted in our analysis. This level is lower than the ranges discussed in Den Elzen et al. (2011). Then, for the subsequent periods between 2020 and 2060, we run scenarios postulating different levels of carbon emissions quotas, aiming to assess the feasibility and the implications of the Durban COP17 outcome. Simultaneously the global target of CO_2 emissions in the period 2015–2020 remains free but below the level of 39 $GtCO_2$.

2 The Baseline

The baseline development considered in MERGE is based on the assumptions made in the EU project ADAM, Edenhofer et al. (2010), fine-tuned with the baseline scenario development generated by the TIMER model (Van Vuuren and van Ruijven et al. 2006; Magné et al. 2010) for that project. The baseline excludes any consideration of climate policies or damages due to climate change. The MERGE regions refer to the WEUR (European Union), EEFSU (Eastern Europe and former Soviet Union), CANZ (Canada, Australia and New Zealand), MOPEC (Mexico and OPEC), China, India, Japan and ROW (rest of world). USA which is the ninth world region, is analyzed based on the assumptions and database of the IEA-ETSAP TIAM project (Loulou and Labriet 2008a, b).

ITMM is a large scale NLP model that maximizes the Negishi weighted regional utilities of all world regions. It is solvable directly with only one TIMES region represented explicitly, in our case this is USA. Similar analysis can be done with the global TIMES model but concentrating on the energy system policies without considering the macro-economic feed-backs and implications of such policies. Studies with a model like ITMM can put emphasis either on the global dimension of the issue or could focus on the national consequences of global policies or both, as in this study.

In the baseline, electricity production increases (as a consequence of population and economic growth with a moderate improvement in energy intensity), from 19.2 PWh in 2010 to 62 PWh in 2050, while the annual primary energy use increases from 455 EJ in 2010 to 976 EJ in 2050. Existing fossil fuel-based thermal plants are progressively phased out and replaced initially by a combination of pulverized coal and natural gas combined cycle (NGCC), followed then by integrated gasification combined cycle coal (IGCC) plants due to their outstanding high efficiency and low fuel cost. Next to IGCC, wind turbines followed by nuclear reactors are the most competitive power generation systems. Wind power complements the power supply up to 27 % of overall electricity generation. Primary energy is mainly provided by coal followed by renewable energy forms and biomass, complemented with gas and oil. As a consequence, energy and industry related carbon emissions reach a level of 15 GtC while the atmospheric concentration of CO_2 becomes 545 ppmv in 2050 (642 ppmv, if all Kyoto gases are included). This moderate increase of CO_2 in the atmosphere is the consequence of learning by doing (LbD) and learning by research (LbS) options available in the model. These options refer to wind, solar PV, nuclear, advanced coal and gas with carbon capture and sequestration, biofuels, hydrogen and synthetic fuels. See also Barreto and Kypreos (2004) and Kypreos (2007). These options reduce the specific investment cost (eventually to the level of their floor cost) as function of experience and research spending, making for example wind energy a competitive baseline option.

Next we perform a parametric analysis with different cumulative CO_2 emission reduction targets aiming to restrict temperature change below 2 °C for different probabilities. This policy goal was initially accepted by the European Parliament (European Commission 2007) and has been confirmed in Cancun. The MERGE model describes the emissions of all other Kyoto GHGs based on a baseline development and their marginal abatement supply curves while TIMES defines an explicit treatment of mitigation technologies for CH_4 and N_2O. We have concentrated on the CO_2 cumulative emissions as this was the most demanding part in the cumulative integral of GHGs in the study of Meinshausen et al. (2009).

3 Global Emissions Quotas, Concentrations and Marginal Costs

In this section we present different results obtained, in particular: the level of emission reduction and the associated probabilities to exceed the 2 °C of post-industrial warming; the implied global carbon taxes; and finally the economic implications for USA and other world regions in respect to the baseline developments. The description of the induced changes in the primary energy use and power production and the related technology implications follow afterwards. All scenarios are estimated with a descriptive utility discount rate of 3 %.

3.1 Global Remaining Emissions Quotas

Figure 1 illustrates the emission levels estimated when different cumulative budgets are imposed for the period 2020–2060 guided by the four emission budgets of Meinshausen et al. (2009) between 242 GtC (20 % probability) and 392 GtC (50 % probability). Simultaneously another constraint ensures that at least the global annual emissions of CO_2 emissions by 2020 remains below the level of 39 $GtCO_2$ (10.64 GtC). Otherwise, the model was free to select optimal emission levels for the period of 2010. As consequence of this flexibility, when stringent cumulative CO_2 bounds are imposed the global emission level for 2020 becomes less than the total level of the Copenhagen pledges of 39 $GtCO_2$. This implies an optimistic view assuming that the signatory countries of the extended Kyoto protocol will opt for policies consistent with the stringency of this constraint already by 2015. Another possibility would have been to simulate the COP17 decisions and force the Copenhagen pledges for 2020 in all scenarios. But this would give high levels of emissions for 2020 making it more difficult and expensive to satisfy the sustainability targets afterwards.

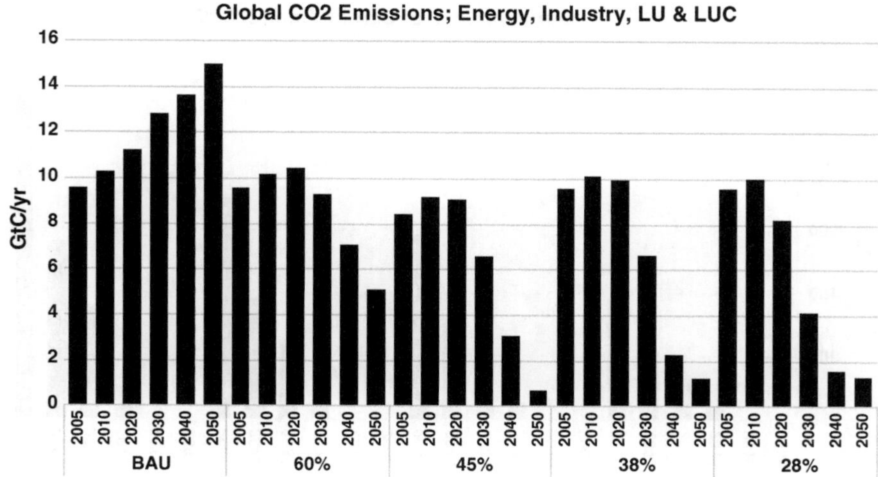

Fig. 1 Annual carbon emissions for the baseline and under different cumulative emissions quotas with 60, 45, 38 and 28 % probability of exceeding 2 °C

Examining the column of cumulative emissions 2000–2050 of Table 1 estimated by multiplying the annual emission levels with 10 (years per period), we confirm that cumulative emissions are above the levels proposed by Meinshausen et al. (2009). Also the probability to exceed 2 °C associated with the cumulative emissions is between 60 % and 28 %. This is a consequence of the optimization freedom given for the years 2010–2020 and the bounds from 2020 to 2060. Results given in Fig. 2 indicate that: (a) the associated shadow prices in our parametric analysis are becoming quite high when approaching low probability levels. For example the marginal costs for 2050 increase above $1000/tC for the 28 % probability case starting from $400/tC in the 60 % case (b) emission in 2020 follow the stringency of the cumulative constraint while there are doubts that the potential signatory countries of the Kyoto protocol and the less developed countries will reduce emissions to the levels estimated in the model for the period 2010–2020. See for example the conclusions of the FEEM report of Bosetti et al. (2011).

Table 1 Model estimates of global CO_2 emissions from energy, industry, land use and land use change in GtC/year; cumulative emissions quotas 2000–2050 for the scenarios analyzed and their corresponding probability for not exceeding 2 °C

2010 (GtC/a)	2020 (GtC/a)	2030 (GtC/a)	2040 (GtC/a)	2050 (GtC/a)	2000–50 (GtC/a)	Probability obtained (%)
10.28	11.23	12.8	13.62	14.99	593	
10.20	10.47	9.32	7.10	5.14	436	60
10.13	10.13	7.74	4.15	1.58	369	45
10.12	10.0	6.65	2.27	1.25	336	38
10.02	8.23	4.13	1.58	1.28	286	28

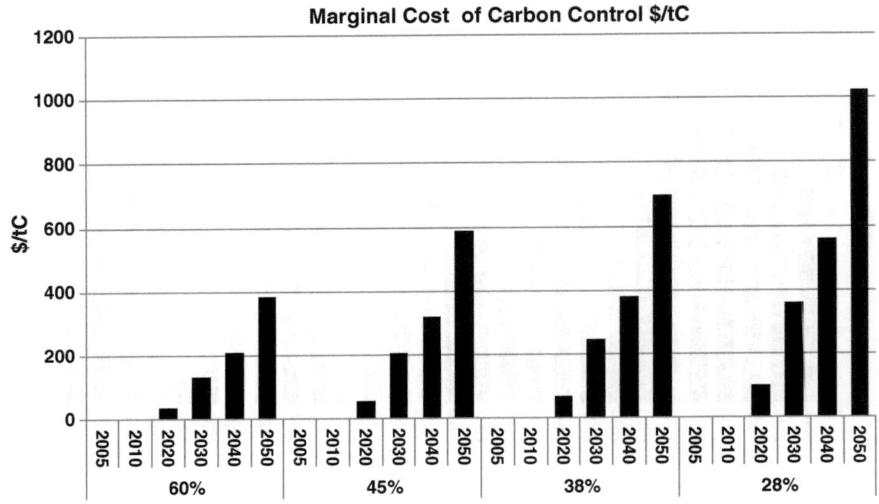

Fig. 2 Marginal cost of carbon control estimated with ITMM under cumulative and global emission for different probabilities of exceeding 2 °C

Finally, as the results demonstrate the benefits of early mitigation policies (e.g., the feasibility to meet the policy target at low economic cost), we have decided not to repeat the estimations lowering the cumulative bounds until to reach the exact probabilities of Meinshausen et al. (2009). Notice that our probability level for three scenarios is below 50 %.

3.2 Emissions and Concentrations

Figure 2 presents the marginal costs that correspond to the imposed cumulative constraints. The emission profiles for the low probability cases indicate significant reductions for the year 2020 already which needs the initiation of effective policies by the year 2015. The CO_2 concentration for the 28 % probability case is 410 ppmv while the other unconstrained GHGs add another 100 ppmv of CO_2eq. It is expected that imposing global constraints in form of CO_2 equivalent emissions could move the global GHGs concentrations to 450 ppmv by 2050 at similar marginal emission reduction cost, as given for example by Den Elzen in his default case (2010).

3.3 GDP Development and Economic Burden by Region

Most of the economic growth in the future will take place in the less developed countries. These countries will also consume more energy having higher shares of carbon emissions than the industrialized countries.

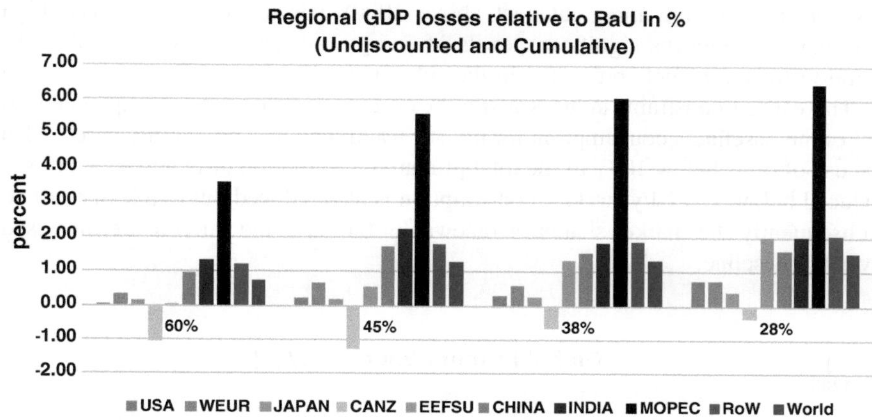

Fig. 3 Regional cumulative and undiscounted GDP losses relative to BAU

Figure 3 defines the undiscounted GDP losses for the period of 2010–2050. The cumulative constraint on CO_2 emissions defines efficient solutions across time and regions but is not considering any compensation transfers as in the case of Cap and Trade policies or in the case of technology protocols to counter balance these losses.

The estimated global GDP losses relative to baseline development for the different scenarios are low. However the impacts are significant for some developing world regions (e.g., the oil exporting countries), as shown in Fig. 3. The losses for the OPEC regions have a maximum of 6.5 % as not only oil and gas exports are reduced but also their prices. The cost for the industrialized world is a fraction of the cost for the other world regions with CANZ having a net benefit mainly due to the use/export of domestic resources. This explains why the now less developed countries are reluctant to join a globally binding protocol without compensation measures. On the other hand a full compensation of economic losses will conclude to very high capital transfers from the industrialized countries (Jacoby et al. 2009). Notice that the undiscounted GDP losses of the global and cumulative economic output for the period of analysis are low (1.2–1.5 %). The net losses are even lower as secondary benefits from reduced local pollutions (due to lower fossil fuel use) and the reduced damages due to lower temperature increase are not assessed in the analysis.

3.4 Primary Energy and Power Generation

This section presents the primary energy consumption (PEC) and power generation for the baseline and the carbon constrained cases. We have already realized (Figs. 1 and 2) that the strong emission reduction obtained for the 28 % probability case is associated with high marginal cost above 1000$ per ton of carbon. The high marginal cost induces significant levels of energy conservation (Fig. 4) and substitution for fossil fuels presented in the subsequent Figs. 4 and 5.

The carbon constraint induces a significant change in energy use equivalent to 1/3 of the baseline's consumption for the 38 % and the 28 % probability cases. Also the use of oil is below 10 % of the total primary consumption or in absolute terms is reduced below 100 EJ/year. Gas consumption is also reduced but to a lesser extent. Consequently the market shares of renewable, biomass and nuclear are increased over the baseline.

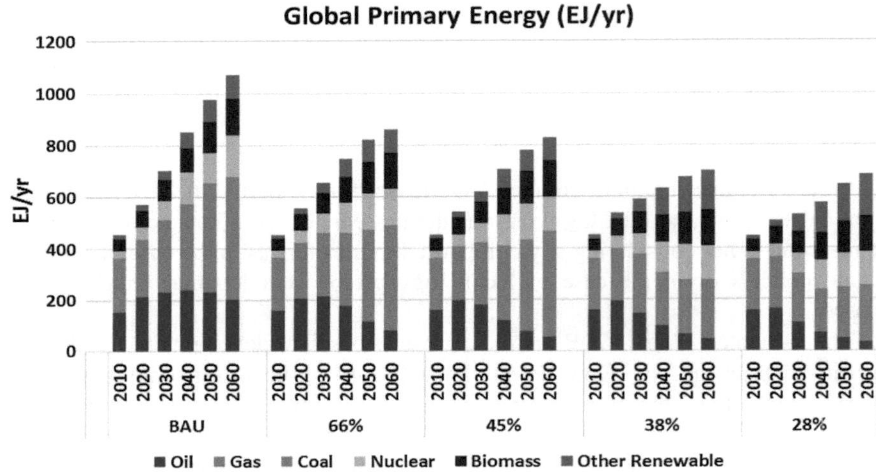

Fig. 4 Global primary energy consumptions for all cases and the BAU

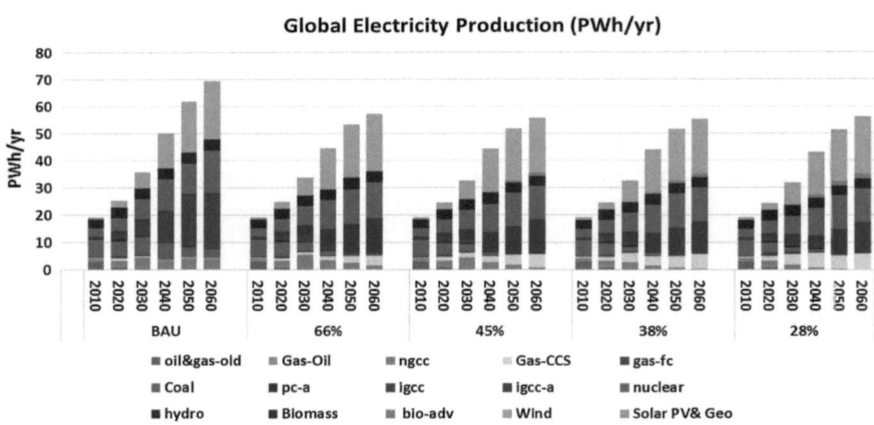

Fig. 5 Global electricity production for all cases analyzed

The level of electricity production is reduced by about 7 PWh/year or by 10 % relative to baseline for the three most stringent constrained cases. The production changes in power generation are drastic as carbon free options are becoming mature dominating the market while the level of production is reduced following the stringency of the carbon constraint. Winners are wind energy, nuclear energy and coal based on IGCC and gas combined cycle (GCC) with carbon capture and sequestration (CCS) options. Advanced biomass systems with CCS options having negative carbon emissions begin to penetrate in 2040.

4 Specific Results for USA

The previous sections explained the consequence of global and binding carbon constraints to the energy system necessary to restrict temperature change below 2 °C. The bounds and the induced carbon prices act as driving forces for technological change needed to establish a carbon free world. The last part of this report (Figs. 6, 7, 8 and 9) presents and discusses the implications of the global constraint to the national USA energy system and carbon emissions.

The reduction of carbon emissions in USA follows the general pattern that appears on the global level where the industry and transport sectors are less efficient to reduce emissions than the power generation industry and the households where

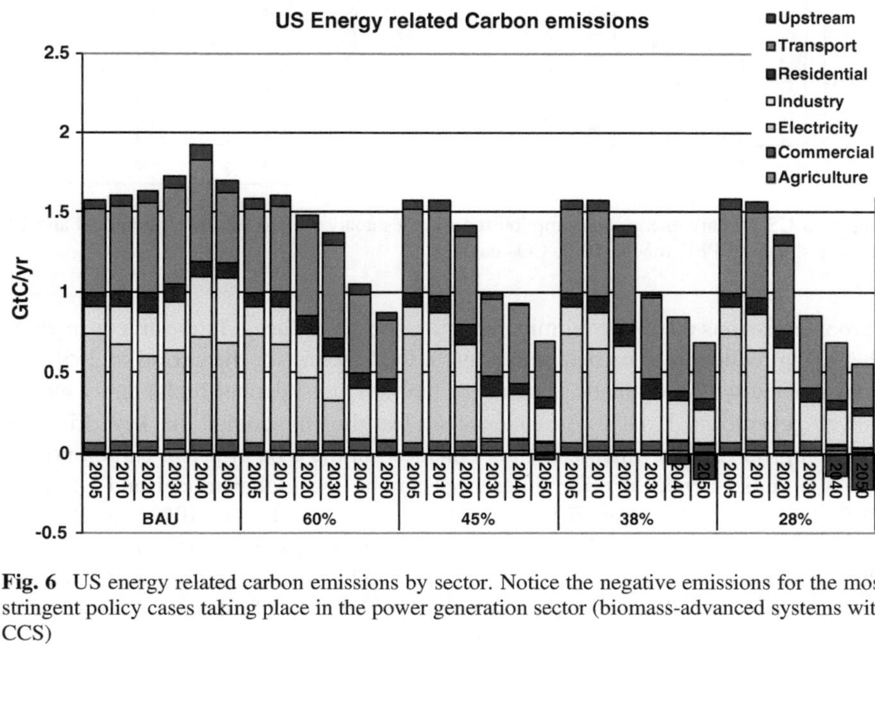

Fig. 6 US energy related carbon emissions by sector. Notice the negative emissions for the most stringent policy cases taking place in the power generation sector (biomass-advanced systems with CCS)

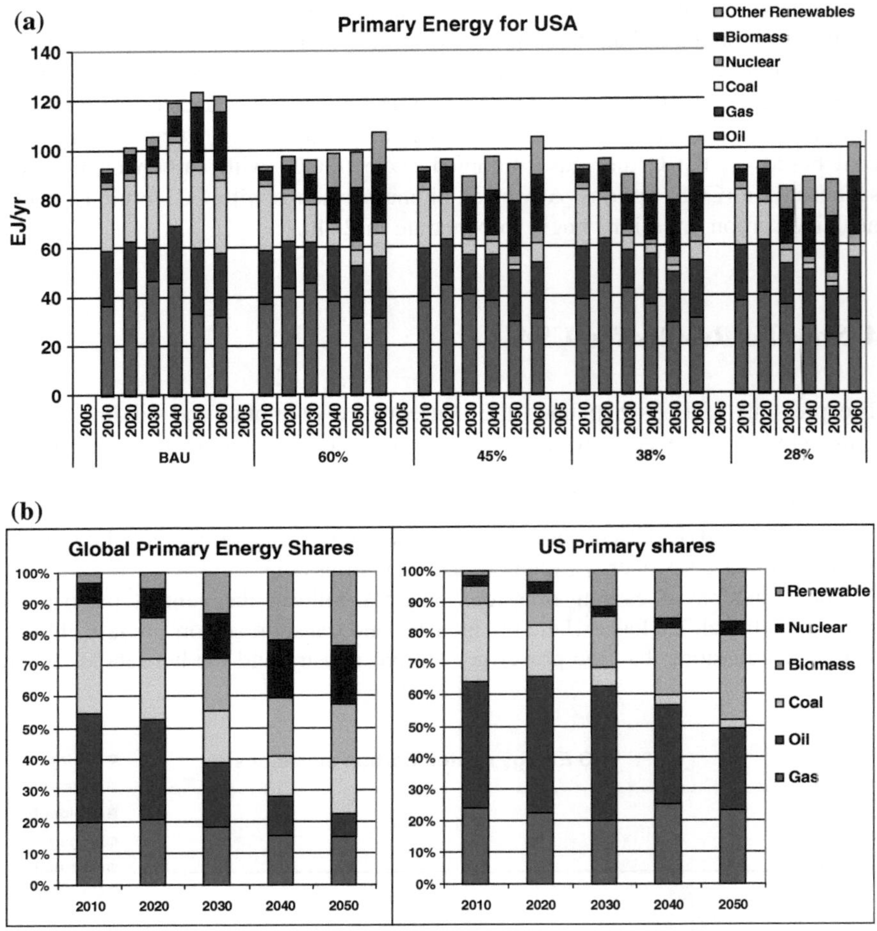

Fig. 7 **a** US primary energy consumption for all cases analyzed and the BAU. **b** Global and US relative shares of PEC for the 28 % CO_2 case

carbon emissions are totally eliminated or drastically reduced. Interesting is anyhow the strong reduction of carbon emissions in the baseline for the period of 2050 that is associated with a dramatic increase of biomass use (alcohol fuels) and wind for power generation. It is a consequence of learning by doing, the key driver of technological change which is further enhanced in the case of active carbon policy.

As a consequence of price differences among the global model and USA the PEC shares in the US (Fig. 7b) and for the most stringent cases, differ significantly from the corresponding global shares. For the US, oil and gas share covers 50 % of PEC followed by biomass (27 %) and renewable (16 %) while coal (3 %) and nuclear (4 %) are almost insignificant. At the global level oil and gas cover only 22 % while IGCC, coal with CCS and nuclear attain significant market shares

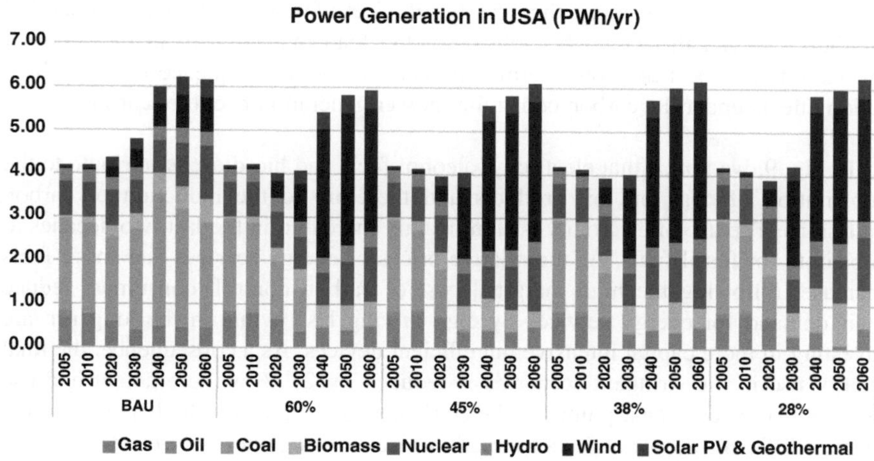

Fig. 8 US electricity generation for the constrained cases and the BAU

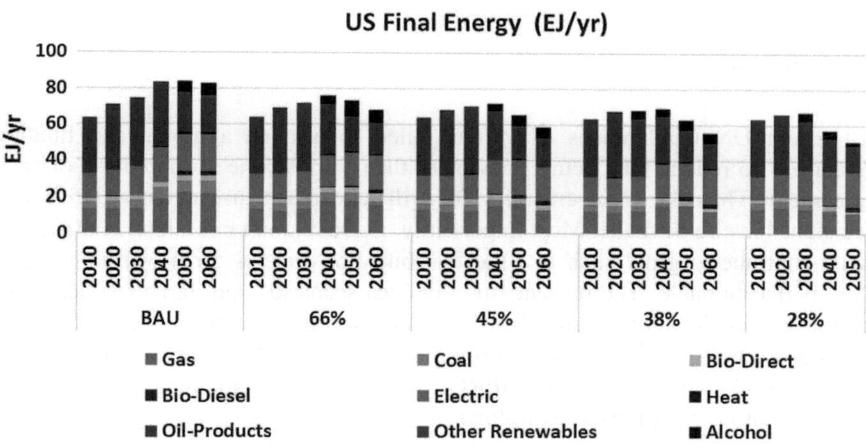

Fig. 9 US final energy use by fuel for all cases and the BAU

complemented with biomass and other renewables. PEC in USA is increased over time by 1/3rd in the baseline case (Fig. 7a) following the economic growth but remains almost stable in the carbon constrained cases. Thus coal substitution by renewable is significant, oil and gas defend their market position while nuclear energy is not free to recover market shares.

Again in the power generation sector (Fig. 8) coal is substituted by wind followed by biomass and nuclear energy under the carbon constraint. Most of the cases show a stabilization in production for the first decades followed by strong penetration of renewable electricity in the last decades as electricity substitutes for fossil use. Geothermal options and solar PV are also introduced in the last periods of analysis. Wind covers more than 53 % of electricity generation and solar PV another 2 % and this could be critical for the load management in the future if production will be based on intermittent systems. As consequence of the substitution effects under the carbon constraint, power generation becomes carbon-free in the US.

In Fig. 9, we notice that electricity, alcohol fuels and bio-diesel contribute to the substitution of coal and oil products and therefore to the reduction of carbon emissions. The use of electricity is significantly increased in the last two decades to substitute for fossil fuels. As the relative prices of energy services and fossil fuels increase, following the high marginal cost of carbon control, consumers reduce their demand for energy services by e.g., driving less, while in the long run are investing in more capital intensive but efficient devices. As a consequence, the final energy use in the stringent scenarios is reduced by 27 % while efficient end-use devices like electric heat pumps and electric cars as well as bio-fuels penetrate the market. Efficient devices and conservation measures together with electricity substitution for oil, contribute to the de-carbonization of the US economy for the stringent scenarios in the last decades.

5 Conclusions

All recent UN Conferences of Parties failed to arrange a global and binding agreement to reduce GHG emissions other than to postpone the initiation of such agreement. Thus the most critical COP will take place in Paris in 2015 where decisions have to be made. Most importantly, global carbon emissions in the recent years continue to grow such that the feasibility of policies for a warming below 2 °C is questionable. The present study defines scenarios and derives conclusions on the economic impacts and this feasibility question, with the help of a new integrated assessment approach merging TIMES-MACRO (a hybrid model) for critical world regions, with the MERGE model for the remaining regions. Conclusions can be summarized as follows:

- The study assumes efficient policies and measures where all world regions accept a binding protocol in 2020 while policies could be initiated already in 2015. However, this needs compensation transfers for countries with low income and in that sense the model assumptions for the early periods are critical. Further delays beyond 2015–2020 or low participation to the protocol will make the goal of 2 °C warming a difficult, but not impossible task, as efforts are postponed towards the second half of the century. This leads to higher marginal prices and costs (see also Den Elzen et al. 2010). These extra costs are related to the inertia of the infrastructures in the energy system that locks-in conventional production technologies and the foregone learning by doing cost reductions. Obviously moderate targets can be satisfied at lower cost but at higher risks of damages.

- Some carbon-free technologies like wind and advanced nuclear reactors together with more efficient end-use devices like conventional but advanced vehicles are contributing to the reduction of carbon emissions already in the baseline. Other systems like solar PV and advanced carbon capture and sequestration options for power generation and transportation fuels need the introduction of high carbon taxes or other instruments to become better competitive.
- Bio-fuel production and advanced power generation based on biomass with CCS options with negative carbon emissions appear already in the 2040s and have the potential to become one of the key future technological options to mitigate carbon emissions and reach the 2 °C constraint.
- Conservation options in buildings and the transportation sector together with efficiency improvement are key end-use policy options contributing to the reduction of carbon emissions as shown implicitly in Fig. 9 in the case of USA. We notice also the importance of electricity, alcohol fuels and bio-diesel for the substitution for coal and oil products in the end-use markets.
- Although the net undiscounted GDP reduction on the global level and for the most stringent carbon constraint remains below 1.5 %, the impact of the carbon constraint in the oil exporting regions and non-OECD regions is significant, asking for counterbalancing actions and measures and a fair burden sharing.

There is work remaining for the scientific community as almost 22 years after the Earth Summit in Rio de Janeiro in 1992 or after 20 years with the Framework Convention on Climate Change into force in 1994, we are neither successful in reducing global emissions nor able to emphasize enough the uncertainties and risks in the physics and economics of climate change convincing the public and politicians to take serious actions. Better scenario analyses with differentiated emission reductions focusing on the historical responsibility of the industrialized world must be balanced with the expected projections of future emissions of developing countries to prepare better UN Conferences and negotiations. Scientists should quantify better not only the mitigation strategies but also the expected damages and the cost of adaptation options in order to improve the allocation of capital and technology transfer between word regions and among mitigation and adaptation options.

References

Barreto L, Kypreos S (2004) Emissions trading and technology deployment in an energy-systems "bottom-up" model with technology learning. Eur J Oper Res 158(1):243–261. doi:10.1016/S0377-2217(03)00350-3

Bosseti V, Paltzev S, Reilly J, Carraro P (2011) Emissions pricing to stabilize global climate. FEEM Nota di Lavoro 80:2011

Den Elzen M, van Vuuren D, van Vliet J (2010) Postponing emission reductions from 2020 to 2030 increases climate risks and long-term costs. Clim Change 99:313–320. doi:10.1007/s10584-010-9798-5

Den Elzen M et al (2011) The emissions gap between the Copenhagen pledges and the 2 °C climate goal: options for closing and risks that could widen the gap. Glob Environ Change 21 (2):733–743

Edenhofer O et al (2010) The economics of low stabilisation: exploring its implications for mitigation costs and strategies. Energy Journal 31(1):11–48 ISSN: 0195-6574

European Commission (2007) Communication from the commission to the council, the european parliament, the european economic and social committee and the committee of the regions—limiting global climate change to 2 degrees Celsius—the way ahead for 2020 and beyond COM (2007) 2

Jacoby et al (2009) Sharing the burden of GHG reductions in post-Kyoto international climate policy. In: University Cambridge (ed) Aldy J, Stavins R. Press, Cambridge, pp 753–785

Kypreos S (2007) A MERGE model with endogenous technological change and the cost of carbon stabilization. Energy Policy 35(11):5327–5336

Labriet M (2010) Private communication

Loulou R, Labriet M (2008a) ETSAP-TIAM: the TIMES integrated assessment model. Part I: model structure. CMS 5(1):7–40

Loulou R, Labriet M (2008b) ETSAP-TIAM: the TIMES integrated assessment model. Part II: mathematical formulation. CMS 5(1):41–66

Magné B, Kypreos S, Turton H (2010) Technology options for low stabilization pathways with MERGE. In: Edenhofer K, Leimbach B (eds) 31(Special Issue):83–107, ISSN: 0195-6574

Manne A, Mendelsohn R, Richels R (1995) MERGE: a model for evaluating regional and global effects of GHG reduction policies. Energy Policy 23(1):17–34

Meinshausen M et al (2009) Greenhouse-gas emission targets for limiting global warming to 2 °C. Nature 458:1158–1162. doi:10.1038/nature08017

Remme U, Blesl M (2006) Documentation of the TIMES-MACRO model. http://www.etsap.org

UN-FCCC/CP/2009/L.7, Copenhagen Accord, 18 Dec 2009

Van Vuuren DPB, van Ruijven B et al (2006) TIMER 2: model description and application. Integrated modelling of global environmental change. In: An overview of IMAGE 2.4, Netherlands Environmental Assessment Agency (MNP), Bilthoven, The Netherlands, pp 39–59

Integrating Policy Instruments into Energy System Models—From Theory to Application to Germany

Birgit Fais and Markus Blesl

Abstract This chapter provides an overview of the use of bottom-up energy system models to evaluate the long-term effects of energy and climate policy instruments. The major benefits of this type of model for policy evaluation are the inclusion of all interactions within the energy system as well as the high level of technological detail. Progress, on the other hand, needs to be made in terms of the representation of the decision-making behavior of different economic agents and the inclusion of macroeconomic feedbacks. Flexible, endogenous modelling approaches for two important instrument categories are then outlined and applied to a case study on the German energy system: emissions trading systems and different support systems for renewable electricity. This scenario analysis shows how the explicit modelling of policy instruments in energy system models can provide quantitative policy insights, e.g. to analyze the interaction between different types of instruments or to compare alternative policy mechanisms which can be applied for the same political target.

1 Introduction

Over the last two decades energy policy has grown more and more complex. Ambitious and, in some cases, conflicting targets have been established regarding climate change, energy security, the affordability of energy and the deregulation of energy markets. Especially in the area of climate policy, the introduction of a large variety of new policy instruments on different regional levels could be observed in recent years. In this process, policy makers need to have the possibility to back up

B. Fais (✉)
UCL Energy Institute, London, UK
e-mail: b.fais@ucl.ac.uk

M. Blesl
Institute of Energy Economics and the Rational Use of Energy, Stuttgart, Germany
e-mail: Markus.Blesl@ier.uni-stuttgart.de

G. Giannakidis et al. (eds.), *Informing Energy and Climate Policies Using Energy Systems Models*, Lecture Notes in Energy 30,
DOI 10.1007/978-3-319-16540-0_7

their decisions with comprehensive and scientifically sound research on ex-ante and ex-post evaluation of policy instruments in order to arrive at a consistent and efficient policy framework.

Technology-rich, bottom-up energy system models have been used for a long time to represent and analyze complex systems in an understandable form as well as to determine cost-efficient technological pathways to reach energy savings or emission reduction targets. The aim of this chapter is firstly to assess the usefulness of such models for the quantitative evaluation of the long-term impact of climate policy instruments on the energy system and the interaction between various policy tools. In addition, modelling approaches for the explicit representation of two central types of policy instruments are outlined briefly: emissions trading systems and different support mechanisms for renewable electricity. Using the German energy and climate policy as a case study, a comparative scenario analysis is then conducted to explore the interaction between these two instruments and to contrast the long-term effects of alternative renewable support systems.

2 Current State of Research: The Use of Energy System Models for Policy Evaluation

Energy system analyses have for a long time played a crucial role in supporting the political decision-making process by identifying sustainable technology pathways and contrasting the impacts of alternative energy futures. In order to assess the suitability of energy system models for the evaluation of specific policy instruments, the approach initiated by Jaccard et al. (2003) provides a valuable starting point. It identifies three attributes that an ideal model should comprise when used for the assessment of different types of policy instruments: (1) technological explicitness; (2) microeconomic realism (i.e. representation of consumer behaviour); and (3) macroeconomic completeness.

The main advantage of bottom-up engineering models is easily identified in their high level of technological detail. Hence, it is the only approach that can be applied to evaluate the effect of technology-specific measures and, even more importantly, to incorporate the impact of new technologies and technological breakthroughs for which no historical data is yet available (Hoffman and Jorgenson 1977). Bottom-up energy system models also provide the possibility to model technology competition and learning.

However, conventional bottom-up energy system models have often been criticized for their representation of the decision-making behaviour of different economic agents, since strong emphasis is put on financial costs as the key decision variable for technology choice assuming that technologies that provide the same energy service can be regarded as perfect substitutes (Jaccard 2009). However, in reality investment decisions by households or firms depend on a large variety of parameters which can explain why the most cost efficient option is not always chosen.

In recent years, various attempts have been made to improve the representation of consumer behaviour in energy system models. A basic approach to model investment barriers has consisted for a long time in using high implicit discount rates, also referred to as hurdle rates (Mundaca et al. 2010). A more sophisticated method has been developed for the hybrid model CIMS. To account for behavioural aspects, the calculation of the market shares of competing technologies is not only based on financial costs but also on additional parameters: the weighted average time preference rate, a cost term representing intangible costs, and a market heterogeneity parameter (Jaccard 2009). Within the scope of the optimising energy system model SOCIO-MARKAL, the effect of awareness campaigns is modelled by introducing "virtual technologies" which include the cost of the awareness campaign and, if used, directly have an effect on the investment decision (Nguene et al. 2011). Another example is the TIMES-Household model where a variety of household types are differentiated to account for household behavior and heterogeneity (Cayla and Maïzi 2015).

Apart from the shortcomings in terms of behavioural realism, the limited consideration of macroeconomic feedbacks is often highlighted as the second shortcoming of energy systems models when used for policy evaluation. A first comparatively simple step to increase the economic flexibility consists in assigning own-price elasticities to the different demand categories in the model such that the economic agents can react more flexibly to changes in the scenario assumptions (Loulou et al. 2005). However, it has to be pointed out that in order to account for all macroeconomic feedbacks, some sort of coupling with a macroeconomic model is necessary (Böhringer and Rutherford 2005): either through a soft-link with an existing large-scale macro-model (e.g. Schäfer and Jacoby 2006), or by hard-linking an energy system model with a reduced from representation of a computable general equilibrium (CGE) model (cf. for example Loulou et al. 2004).

A more detailed discussion on the theoretical background of modelling policy instruments in energy system models can be found in Götz et al. (2012a).

3 Modelling Approaches to Represent Policy Instruments in Energy System Models

In the following chapter specific modelling approaches are briefly outlined for two important instrument categories: emissions trading systems and support schemes for renewable electricity generation.

3.1 Emissions Trading Systems

In general, the modelling of a cap and trade system in an energy system model is straightforward by putting a constraint on total emissions in the participating sectors. The optimization approach of the model then ensures that, as in a trading system, the most cost efficient way of fulfilling the cap is realized. The dual variable of the user constraint representing the cap equals the marginal costs of the last (most expensive) unit of emission abated to fulfil the constraint. It can be therefore interpreted as the certificate price that would arise in the trading system under the modelled conditions (Remme et al. 2009).

However, due to computational and data constraints in most cases, models with limited regional scope are applied for policy evaluation. The challenge therefore often consists in the fact that the modelled region does not cover the entire trading region (31 countries in the case of the EU emissions trading system (EU ETS)). So far this issue has usually been addressed in two manners: either by setting a fixed emission reduction path for the respective country (e.g. Anandarajah and Strachan 2010), or by integrating fixed certificate prices into the model (e.g. Unger 2010). In the first case the drawback consists in the fact that the emission trade with the remaining trading region is neglected, while in the second case the influence of changing national framework conditions on the certificate price is ignored.

To overcome these shortcomings, a modelling approach has been developed that makes it possible to determine both the emission reduction in the national (in this case German) ETS sector and the ETS certificate price endogenously within the model. With this procedure, the cap can be put on total EU ETS emissions instead of on Germany alone. While the emission mitigation in the German ETS sector is still determined endogenously within TIMES-D based on the explicit modelling of technologies within the reference energy system, the reduction options in the rest of the countries participating in the EU ETS are added to the model with the help of a CO_2 abatement cost curve, modelled as a step function containing the CO_2 reduction potentials in the ETS sectors outside of Germany at different certificate price levels. Through the optimization approach, marginal abatement costs for Germany and the rest of the ETS sectors are equalized and a uniform certificate price for the whole system will be determined as the shadow price of the upper bound on total ETS emissions.

To implement this modelling approach, comprehensive data on the emission reduction potentials at different certificate price levels in the ETS sectors outside of Germany are required. This information can be either obtained by an extensive literature research, by conducting a quantitative model analysis at European scale or by aggregating the results from several national model analyses. For the case at hand, a version of the Pan-European TIMES model—TIMES PanEU (Blesl et al. 2009, 2010)—which comprises of 30 regions (EU-27 plus Switzerland, Norway and Iceland) with a less detailed time resolution (12 time slices) and less sectoral detail than TIMES-D, is applied. The basic model assumptions, i.e. on energy prices or technology parameters, are harmonized between the two models. In order to determine the various steps of the abatement cost curve, several model runs with different ETS certificate price levels are executed in the Pan-European model. The difference in emission abatement between one model run and the next represents the reduction efforts that would occur in the entire ETS sector at the corresponding allowance price level. When using an abatement cost curve for the remaining trading region, one has to keep in mind that one specific cost curve represents the reduction potentials under a specific set of assumptions. If it is assumed that the framework conditions in the remaining trading region change, the cost curve needs to be adjusted.

Further information on the technical details of modelling supranational emission trading system in national energy system models is provided in Götz et al. (2012b).

3.2 Support Systems for Renewable Electricity

Specific support schemes for the deployment of renewable electricity technologies form an integral part of the climate policy of many countries. However, in energy systems modelling so far the effects of such instruments have in most cases only been taken into account in an indirect and inflexible way by exogenously setting the expected minimum amounts of electricity produced from different types of renewable energies without making reference to the characteristics of a specific support system (e.g. Capros et al. 2010; Blesl et al. 2010). This, however, clearly reduces the flexibility of the model as generally no changes in the electricity generation from renewable sources will occur when the scenario assumptions are altered and the effects on electricity prices are often not accounted for. Some first attempts have been made in recent years to incorporate renewable electricity generation in the optimisation approach and to explicitly represent specific support instruments (cf. the Green-X model (Ragwitz et al. 2007), the PERSEUS-RES-E model (Möst and Fichtner 2010), and the simulation model in Frontier Economics (2012)). However, renewable electricity generation is in most cases analysed in an isolated manner, i.e. electricity prices are set exogenously such that no interactions with conventional power generation are considered and the effects on the demand side are neglected. Apart from that the support systems for renewable electricity are generally modelled in a very simplified and abstract manner without keeping in mind the often complex structure of the real-world application of such instruments.

In the following, methodological approaches for the explicit representation of the most important support mechanisms for renewable electricity, fixed feed-in tariffs (FIT), tradable green certificate (TGC) systems as well as tendering procedures, in energy system models are presented. Further information on the modelling of instruments to promote renewable electricity is provided in Götz et al. (2012c).

3.2.1 Feed-in Tariff Systems

To illustrate the modelling approach for a FIT scheme, the example of the German system is used which since the year 2000 offers fixed, technology-specific tariffs and has been highly successful in promoting renewable electricity generation raising its share in gross final electricity consumption from 6 % in 2000 to 23 % in 2012. The methodology is divided into the modelling of the payment side (e.g. the tariffs) and the cost side (e.g. the FIT surcharge, a levy on retail electricity prices).

From the point of view of the renewable plant operator, the tariffs can be understood as a subsidy on the renewable electricity generation. They are therefore integrated into the model by using the TIMES parameters developed to display subsidies such that for each unit of electricity generated a subsidy (equal to the real-world tariff, expressed as a negative cost factor in the model) is assigned to the renewable generation process. Moreover, the modelling approach takes into account a number of distinctive features of the German FIT system, as these have a substantial impact on the competitiveness of renewable electricity generation: the payment period is limited to 20 years, tariffs decrease as a function of the vintage year and tariffs remain constant in nominal terms which results in a reduction in real terms over the years.

After integrating the tariffs into the model, one has to bear in mind that this only constitutes one part of the FIT system. The tariffs are not a subsidy by the state, but are financed through a levy on retail electricity prices (the FIT surcharge). The level of this surcharge depends on the actual expansion of renewable electricity, i.e. on the model results for the generation side. Therefore, subsequent to the first model run, where only the tariffs are implemented, the FIT surcharge is calculated and integrated into the model framework (as additional costs on final electricity demand). Afterwards, as the integration of the FIT surcharge and the associated increase in end-use electricity prices causes modifications in the electricity consumption and consequently also in electricity generation, an iterative process of several model runs is needed to adjust FIT payments and the FIT surcharge to one another.

The main advantage of this methodology lies in the fact that both the amount of renewable electricity generation and the effects on the demand side are determined endogenously within the model.

3.2.2 Quantity-Based Support Schemes for Renewable Electricity

In comparison, modelling tradable green certificate schemes and tendering procedures in an energy system model is much more straightforward, as this type of instrument establishes the quantity of renewable electricity to be produced rather than its price. Target values for relative shares of renewable energies in electricity generation (either technology-specific or -unspecific) can be easily integrated in the model with the help of user-defined constraints. As it would be the case in the trading system for green certificates or the tendering process, in the optimization process the cheapest generation options to fulfil the quota are chosen. The shadow price of such a user constraint is equivalent to the difference between the generation costs of the most expensive generation technology required to fulfil the quota and the electricity price (given in the model as the dual variable of the electricity commodity balance) and can therefore be interpreted as the certificate price in the trading system or bidding process. Furthermore, it directly impacts electricity generation costs and electricity prices in the model. Generation costs of conventional plants (outside of the quota) increase by the costs that arise from the purchase of green certificates, while generation costs of renewable plants decrease through the selling of certificates (cf. Remme et al. (2009) for further information on the interpretation of dual solutions in a TIMES model).

4 Scenario Analysis on the German Energy and Climate Policy

In order to illustrate how the explicit modelling of policy instruments can benefit the long-term evaluation of policy impacts on the energy system, the results of a scenario analysis focusing on Germany will be briefly outlined in the following section. This analysis uses the national energy system model TIMES-D which depicts the entire German energy system with high technological detail from primary energy supply to energy services demand (for further information see Götz et al. 2013).

The scenario analysis focuses on two important issues of the German energy and climate policy based on the scenario shown in Table 1. Firstly, in order to explore the interactions between the EU ETS and the German FIT system for renewable electricity, three scenarios with varying assumption on these two policy instruments are contrasted. The reference case (REF) combines the currently implemented EU ETS target of −21 % until 2020 compared to 2005 with the present version (as of 2012) of the German FIT system, while the other two scenarios only consider one of the two instruments (ETS_Only and FIT_Only).

Secondly, to compare the current German FIT scheme with different types of alternative support schemes for renewable electricity, the scenario REF is contrasted against three additional scenarios which represent different renewable support instruments and are set up such that one specific effect relevant in the

Table 1 Scenario overview

Scenario	Renewable support	ETS target
REF	Current German FITs (2012 version)	−21 % until 2020 compared to 2005; −1.74 % p.a. afterwards
ETS_Only	–	
FIT_Only	Current German FITs (2012 version)	–
FIT_Neut	Technology-neutral feed-in tariff system reaching the same absolute amount of renewable electricity as in the reference case	−21 % until 2020 compared to 2005; −1.74 % p.a. afterwards
TGC_Neut	Technology-neutral quota system reaching the targets for the renewable share in gross electricity consumption of the German Energy Concept	
TGC_Spec	Technology-specific quota system reaching the same shares for each renewable source in gross electricity consumption as in Qu_Neut	

comparison of these instruments can be quantified with each of them. First of all, a technology-neutral FIT system (scenario FIT_Neut) it used to explore the impacts of promoting only the most cost efficient technologies as opposed to the current technology-specific variations in the support level without changing the absolute amount of renewable electricity generated (technology effect). In the next step, the FIT systems are contrasted with quantity-based tradable green certificate schemes which have the advantage that compliance with the previously set political targets can be guaranteed (quantity effect). In the scenario TGC_Neut, a technology-neutral quota is put on the entire renewable generation reflecting the official government target values of the German Energy Concept (BMWi and BMU 2011). In contrast, in the scenario TGC_Spec a technology-specific TGC system is implemented (using the cost efficient shares from the scenario TGC_Neut) which allows to evaluate the advantages of a technology-specific scheme in terms of limiting the profits of renewable generators (windfall effect). It needs to be pointed out that all scenarios account for the historical development of the FIT system, i.e. it is assumed that all plants installed until the end of 2012 remain in this system and continue to receive the fixed tariffs.

4.1 Interaction Between European Emission Trading and the German Support Scheme for Renewable Electricity

The impacts of introducing a support instrument for renewable electricity on a national level while having a supranational emissions trading system in place become clearly visible when looking at the emission reduction in Germany under the different scenario assumptions (Fig. 1). Due to the strong expansion of renewable sources in electricity generation, overall emission mitigation efforts in the German ETS sectors are higher for the reference case in which the FIT system is in place. Hence, the implementation of a national support instrument affects the burden sharing within the EU trading system with German contribution to the 21 %-target in 2020 varying between 26 % (REF) and 13 % (ETS_Only). On the EU level, however, the national scheme does not stimulate any additional emission abatement, but results in a system-wide decrease of the ETS certificate price. Given that Germany is responsible for almost a quarter of total ETS emissions, the model results indicate quite substantial price differences of up to 6 €/t CO_2 until 2030 between the scenarios REF and ETS_Only.

Additional insights on the interaction effect can be gained by looking at the development of the German electricity sector (Fig. 2). With the FIT system in place renewable generation is further increased to almost 46 % in 2020 and 54 % in 2030 to gross electricity consumption such that the targets of the German energy concept of 35 and 50 % are clearly exceeded. In the scenario without the FIT system, the extension of renewable electricity generation remains rather limited (shares of 25 % in 2030), underlining the fact that supporting renewable electricity generation does

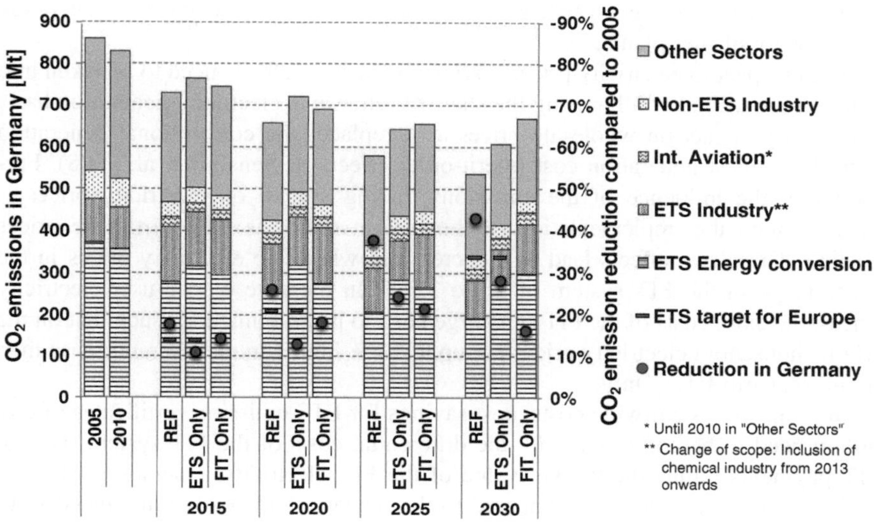

Fig. 1 CO_2 emissions in Germany and emission burden sharing under different assumptions regarding the FIT scheme and the EU ETS (based on Fais et al. 2014a, cf. www.tandfonline.com)

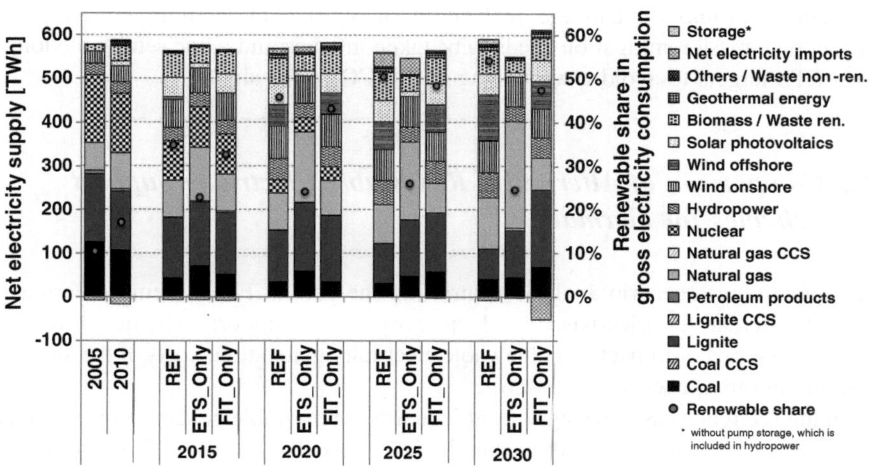

Fig. 2 Net electricity supply in Germany under different assumptions regarding the FIT scheme and the EU ETS

not constitute a cost efficient emission abatement strategy for Germany. Under the premises that only the FIT system but not the EU ETS is implemented (FIT_Only), renewable electricity generation in Germany still rises considerably until 2020. After that, however, growth rates slow down significantly when compared to the reference case indicating that in the long term the EU ETS has a supporting effect on the expansion of renewable electricity in Germany by raising the generation costs for fossil fuel plants.

With respect to electricity prices, various interaction effects need to be taken into consideration. First of all, raising the share of renewable electricity generation has a dampening impact on wholesale prices as it replaces the conventional generation with the highest generation cost (merit-order effect, cf. Sensfuß et al. 2008). Furthermore, the influence of the emissions trading system on electricity prices is lowered with the implementation of the feed-in tariffs as ETS certificate prices decline. These two effects lead to a decrease in wholesale electricity prices in the scenarios with the FIT system of up to 22 %. In the case of end-user electricity prices, the extra costs of the FIT surcharge need to be accounted for such that on the whole, household electricity prices are up to 23 % higher in the reference case than in the scenario ETS_Only.

In terms of system-wide costs, cost savings for ETS emission certificates of €57 billion need to be contrasted with the differential costs of the FIT system (i.e. the FIT payments minus the market value of the FIT electricity generation) of €320 billion in the reference case compared to the scenario ETS_Only (cumulated from 2013 to 2030). Thus, the scenario analysis shows that the additional support mechanism for renewable electricity deteriorates the cost efficiency of emission mitigation in Germany and affects the EU-wide carbon price. Hence, even though these measures might be justified by additional policy targets, most importantly technology promotion and the realization of substantial learning effects, their impact on emission mitigation needs to be taken into account when setting the long-term ETS targets to avoid a weakening of the CO_2 price signal.

4.2 *Comparison of Alternative Renewable Electricity Support Schemes for Germany*

The quantitative scenario analysis contrasting the current FIT system in Germany against alternative price-based and quantity-based support schemes provides insights in terms of impacts on renewable electricity generation, costs of the support system, and total energy system cost.

In the reference case, the significant increase in renewable generation is strongly based on comparatively costly technologies, (especially solar PV and offshore wind) for which the tariff level is comparatively high. Switching to a technology-neutral support system (scenario FIT_Neut) leads to significant shifts in the structure of renewable generation, as heavier reliance is put on comparatively low-cost technologies (especially onshore wind in less favourable locations and large-scale biomass plants) (Fig. 3). With the quantity-based support systems, the targets of the German energy concept are precisely complied with, such that renewable electricity generation drops by a quarter (66 TWh) in 2020 and by 11 % (36 TWh) in 2030 compared to the reference case. With respect to the composition of renewable electricity generation, some similarities with the scenario FIT_Neut are

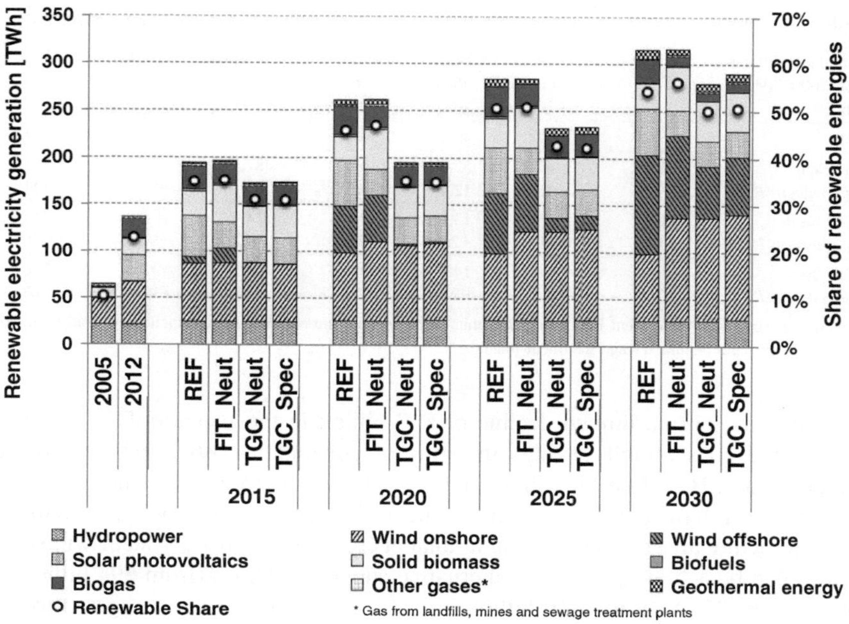

Fig. 3 Comparison of renewable electricity generation in the scenarios with different support schemes for renewable electricity

discernible. The lower overall generation level affects in particular the development of offshore wind energy. However, even when reducing renewable generation to the policy target levels, an exploitation of relatively costly technologies like offshore wind energy is still required under the chosen scenario assumptions.

The stronger emphasis on cost efficiency under the technology-neutral support system is reflected in a reduction of cumulated generation costs for all renewable generation units installed between 2013 and 2030 of €117 billion in the scenario FIT_Neut in relation to the reference case. If, in addition, the amount of renewable generation is lowered to the policy targets (scenarios TGC_Neut and TGC_Spec), this cost difference sums up to €208 billion.

The additional costs that arise under the different support systems are best represented by their differential costs. Here, a general difference in the remuneration level caused by technology-neutral and -specific systems needs to be kept in mind: uniform remuneration tends to lead to an over-subsidisation of less costly technologies resulting in high profit margins for producers, while technology-specific tariffs that reflect disparities in generation costs of renewable technologies can limit the producer surplus and the additional costs for consumers (Ragwitz et al. 2007).

Accordingly, considerable increases in differential costs for renewable technologies with relatively low investment costs can be observed in the scenarios with technology-neutral support systems (Table 2). This leads to a rise in cumulated differential costs of almost €33 billion between 2000 and 2032 in the scenario

Table 2 Cumulated differential cost under different support schemes for renewable electricity

Cumulated differential cost, 2000–2032 (Bn €)[a]	Hydro-power	Wind onshore	Wind offshore	Solar photovoltaics	Biomass[b]	Geothermal energy	Total
REF	5.5	47.2	40.5	126.6	86.9	13.1	319.7
FIT_Neut	13.5	84.1	52.9	110.1	87.3	4.7	352.5
Difference to REF	7.9	36.9	12.4	−16.5	0.4	−8.4	32.8
TGC_Neut	11.3	76.5	13.9	109.3	74.9	3.8	289.7
Difference to REF	5.8	29.3	−26.6	−17.3	−12.0	−9.3	−30.0
TGC_Spec	3.4	51.7	14.7	109.3	69.3	3.4	251.8
Difference to REF	−2.2	4.5	−25.8	−17.3	−17.6	−9.7	−68.0

[a] The costs arising from the current FIT system for units installed until the end of 2012 are included for all scenarios
[b] Incl. gas from landfills and sewage treatment plants

FIT_Neut and only a limited decline of €30 billion in the scenario TGC_Neut in spite of the considerable savings in terms of generation costs compared to the reference case. Based on the differentiation in the tariff structure, higher cost savings of €68 billion are realized under the technology-specific quota system. A different picture arises when looking at total energy system costs. System-wide cost savings can be achieved under all alternative support schemes (from €94 billion in the scenario FIT_Neut to €416 billion in the scenario TGC_Spec compared to the reference case, cumulated from 2013 to 2030). It needs to be pointed out, however, that energy system costs do not contain any information on the distribution of these costs across the system.

Thus, the scenario comparison at hand indicates that when strictly adhering to the principle of cost efficiency the long-term development of renewable electricity in Germany would change considerably and generation costs could be lowered significantly. However, it is also shown that it is not guaranteed that consumers benefit from a technology-neutral support system that promotes the most cost efficient renewable technologies.

5 Conclusion

This chapter has given an overview on the use of bottom-up energy system models to assess the long-term impacts of energy and climate policy instruments by explicitly including such instruments in the modelling framework. For further information on the two applications for the German energy system see Fais et al. (2014a, b).

Using flexible, endogenous modelling approaches for policy instruments in bottom-up energy system models provides several contributions to policy evaluation, most importantly: (1) explore how changing scenario assumptions, for example on fossil fuel prices, affect the outcomes of a certain policy instrument; (2) evaluate the interactions between different policy instruments and (3) compare alternative policy instruments which can be applied for the same political target.

Some general lessons can be drawn from this modelling exercise:

- The real-world application of climate and energy policy instruments often differs substantially from the abstract, theoretical representation in textbooks. This additional complexity has to be accounted for in the modelling approach to arrive at a realistic depiction of the policy impact. This means that generally a highly detailed model, comprising a large variety of technologies, is required.
- Quantity-based measures, like emissions trading systems or tradable green certificate schemes, are generally much more straightforward to model than price-based instruments like FITs as in the latter case additional cost terms have to be introduced.
- When using a comprehensive energy system model for policy evaluation, one has to make sure that all effects that a policy instrument causes are included in the modelling approach. For example, when modelling a FIT system for renewable electricity, the impacts on electricity demand as well as on the electricity grid and the required storage capacity need to be taken into consideration.
- Finally, it has to be noted that when using energy system models for policy evaluation entails a change in perspective. Traditionally, such models assume the perspective of a social planner simultaneously minimizing total discounted costs of the entire system using a social discount rate (Keppo and Strubegger 2010). For policy evaluation, however, the individual perspectives and decision-making behaviour of the various economic agents need to be taken into consideration.

If the aim consists in integrating all effects of a certain measure into the model in an endogenous manner, the modelling approach can prove to become relatively complex. So, it needs to be highlighted that the choice of the modelling tool and the sophistication of the methodology should always depend on the specific research question that is analysed.

References

Anandarajah G, Strachan N (2010) Interactions and implications of renewable and climate change policy on UK energy scenarios. Energy Policy 38:6724–6735. doi:10.1016/j.enpol.2010.06.042

Blesl M, Cosmi C, Cuomo, V et al (2009) Final report on the integrated Pan-European Model (Technical Report no T5.20—RS 2a). NEEDS new energy externalities developments for sustainability integrated project. http://www.needs-project.org/. Accessed 15 Nov 2014

Blesl M, Kober T, Bruchof D et al (2010) Effects of climate and energy policy related measures and targets on the future structure of the European energy system in 2020 and beyond. Energy Policy 38:6278–6292. doi:10.1016/j.enpol.2010.06.018

Böhringer Ch, Rutherford T (2005) Integrating bottom-up into top-down: a mixed complementarity approach. ZEW Discussion Paper No. 05–28, Zentrum für Europäische Wirtschaftsforschung (ZEW). ftp://zew.de/pub/zew-docs/dp/dp0528.pdf. Accessed 13 Aug 2014

Capros P, Mantzos L, Tasios N et al (2010) European energy and transport—trends to 2030, update 2009. European Commission (EC). http://ec.europa.eu/energy/observatory/trends_2030/doc/trends_to_2030_update_2009.pdf. Accessed 13 Aug 2014

Cayla JM, Maïzi N (2015) Integrating household behavior and heterogeneity into the TIMES-households model. Appl Energy 139:56–67. doi:10.1016/j.apenergy.2014.11.015

Fais B, Blesl M, Fahl U et al (2014a) Analysing the interaction between emission trading and renewable electricity support in TIMES. Climate Policy. doi:10.1080/14693062.2014.927749

Fais B, Blesl M, Fahl U et al (2014b) Comparing different support schemes for renewable electricity in the scope of an energy systems analysis. Appl Energy 131:479–489. doi:10.1016/j.apenergy.2014.06.046

Federal Ministry of Economy and Technology (BMWi), Federal Ministry for the Environment, Nature Conservation and Nuclear Safety (BMU) (2011). The Federal Government's energy concept of 2010 and the transformation of the energy system of 2011. http://www.bmubbund.de/en/service/publications/downloads/details/artikel/the-german-governments-energy-concept-long-term-strategy-for-future-energy-supply/. Accessed 01 Dec 2014

Frontier Economics (2012) Die Zukunft des EEG - Handlungsoptionen und Reformansätze. Bericht für die EnBW Energie Baden-Württemberg AG, London. http://www.frontier-economics.com/documents/2014/05/die-zukunft-des-eeg-handlungsoptionen-und-reformansatze.pdf. Accessed 15 Nov 2014

Götz B, Blesl M, Fahl U et al (2012a) Theoretical background on the modelling of policy instruments in energy system models. Report on Work Package A of the ETSAP Project "Integrating policy instruments into the TIMES Model", Institute for Energy Economics and the Rational Use of Energy (IER), University of Stuttgart. Available via ETSAP. http://www.iea-etsap.org/web/Projects/ETSAP_PI_WPA_IER.pdf. Accessed 13 Aug 2014

Götz B, Blesl M, Fahl U et al (2012b) The representation of emission trading schemes in national energy system models. Report on Work Package B-2 of the ETSAP Project "Integrating policy instruments into the TIMES Model", Institute for Energy Economics and the Rational Use of Energy (IER), University of Stuttgart. Available via ETSAP. http://www.iea-etsap.org/web/Projects/ETSAP_PI_WPB2-IER.pdf. Accessed 13 Aug 2014

Götz B, Blesl M, Fahl U et al (2012c) The explicit modelling of support systems for renewable electricity in TIMES. Report on Work Package B-1 of the ETSAP Project "Integrating policy instruments into the TIMES Model", Institute for Energy Economics and the Rational Use of Energy (IER), University of Stuttgart. Available via ETSAP. http://www.iea-etsap.org/web/Projects/ETSAP_PI_WPB1.pdf. Accessed 13 Aug 2014

Götz B, Blesl M, Fahl U et al (2013) Application: scenario analysis with the TIMES-D model. Report on Work Package C of the ETSAP Project "Integrating policy instruments into the TIMES Model", Institute for Energy Economics and the Rational Use of Energy (IER), University of Stuttgart. Available via ETSAP. http://www.iea-etsap.org/web/Projects/ETSAP_PI_WPC.pdf. Accessed 13 Aug 2014

Hoffman K, Jorgenson D (1977) Economic and technological models for evaluation of energy policy. Bell J Econ 8(2):444–466. doi:10.2307/3003296

Jaccard M (2009) Combining top down and bottom up in energy economy models. In: Evans J, Hunt L (eds) International handbook on the economics of energy. Edward Elgar, Cheltenham, pp 311–331

Jaccard M, Nyboer N, Bataille C et al (2003) Modeling the cost of climate policy: distinguishing between alternative cost definitions and long-run cost dynamics. Energy J 24(1):49–73. doi:10.5547/ISSN0195-6574-EJ-Vol24-No1-3

Keppo I, Strubegger M (2010) Short term decisions for long term problems—the effect of foresight on model based energy systems analysis. Energy 35(5):2033–2042. doi:10.1016/j.energy.2010.01.019

Loulou R, Goldstein G, Noble K (2004) Documentation for the MARKAL family of models, part II: MARKAL-MACRO. Energy technology systems analysis programme (ETSAP), international energy agency (IEA). http://www.iea-etsap.org/web/MrklDoc-II_MARKALMACRO.pdf. Accessed 13 Aug 2014

Loulou R, Remme U, Kanudia A et al (2005) Documentation for the TIMES Model, part I. Energy technology systems analysis programme (ETSAP), international energy agency (IEA). http://www.iea-etsap.org/web/Docs/TIMESDoc-Intro.pdf. Accessed 13 Aug 2014

Möst D, Fichtner W (2010) Renewable energy sources in European energy supply and interactions with emission trading. Energy Policy 38(6):2898–2910. doi:10.1016/j.enpol.2010.01.023

Mundaca L, Neij L, Worrell E et al (2010) Evaluating energy efficiency policies with energy-economy models. Annu Rev Environ Resour 35:305–344. doi:10.1146/annurev-environ-052810-164840

Nguene G, Fragnière E, Kanala R et al (2011) SOCIO-MARKAL: integrating energy consumption behavioral changes in the technological optimization framework. Energy Sustain Dev 15 (1):73–83. doi:10.1016/j.esd.2011.01.006

Ragwitz M, Held A, Resch G et al (2007) OPTRES—assessment and optimisation of renewable support schemes in the European electricity market. Final report, European Commission Directorate-General for Energy and Transport. http://ec.europa.eu/energy/renewables/studies/doc/renewables/2007_02_optres.pdf. Accessed 15 Nov 2014

Remme U, Blesl M, Kober T (2009) The dual solution of a TIMES model: its interpretation and price formation equations—Draft. Energy technology systems analysis programme (ETSAP), international energy agency (IEA). http://www.iea-etsap.org/web/Docs/times_interpetation_dual.pdf. Accessed 13 Aug 2014

Schäfer A, Jacoby HD (2006) Experiments with a hybrid CGE-MARKAL Model. Energy J Spec Issue #2: 171–177. doi:10.5547/ISSN0195-6574-EJ-VolSI2006-NoSI2-9

Sensfuß F, Ragwitz M, Genoese M (2008) The merit-order effect: a detailed analysis of the price effect of renewable electricity generation on spot market prices in Germany. Energy Policy 36:3086–3094. doi:10.1016/j.enpol.2008.03.035

Unger T (ed) (2010) Coordinated use of energy system models in energy and climate policy analysis—lessons learned from the Nordic Energy Perspectives project. Nordic Energy Perspectives. http://www.nordicenergyperspectives.org/modellrapport.pdf. Accessed 13 Aug 2014

Improving Efficiency in Kazakhstan's Energy System

Aiymgul Kerimray, Kanat Baigarin, Aidyn Bakdolotov, Rocco De Miglio and GianCarlo Tosato

Abstract Kazakhstan is one of the most energy-intensive countries in the world, almost 4 times higher than the world average and 7 times higher than the OECD average. There are various reasons for inefficiencies in Kazakhstan's energy system: administrative and economic (statistical double counting of energy flows, above normative losses and low profitability), geographic (the extremely continental climate and low population density) and technical considerations (high share of coal in generation mix, high wear on main and auxiliary equipment in energy intensive sectors, high wear on electric lines, dilapidation of housing stock, and an absence of control systems for energy savings) all contribute to the high energy intensity. This study explores energy efficiency potential by analyzing the evolution of the Kazakh energy system. All the technical inefficiencies have been taken into consideration through the explicit representation of existing inefficient technologies/chains in a TIMES-based model. Under the assumptions of a market-oriented development of the economic system, even without specific policies (Business as Usual), the model suggests significant energy efficiency improvement: 22 Mtoe (million tons of oil equivalent) by 2030 and a 40 % reduction in energy intensity of GDP by 2030. The more ambitious policy target of reducing energy intensity of GDP by 40 % by 2020 also appears easily achievable via economically viable solutions.

A. Kerimray (✉) · K. Baigarin · A. Bakdolotov
NURIS—Nazarbayev University Research and Innovation System, Nazarbayev University, Astana, Kazakhstan
e-mail: aiymgul.kerimray@nu.edu.kz

K. Baigarin
e-mail: kbaigarin@nu.edu.kz

A. Bakdolotov
e-mail: aidyn.bakdolotov@nu.edu.kz

R. De Miglio
E4SMA, Turin, Italy
e-mail: rocco.demiglio@gmail.com

G. Tosato
ASATREM, Rome, Italy
e-mail: giancarlo.tosato@gmail.com

G. Giannakidis et al. (eds.), *Informing Energy and Climate Policies Using Energy Systems Models*, Lecture Notes in Energy 30,
DOI 10.1007/978-3-319-16540-0_8

1 Introduction

The high energy intensity of the Republic of Kazakhstan can be explained better by deconstructing the fuel-energy balance—as published by the Committee on Statistics of the Republic of Kazakhstan (2013) and the International Energy Agency (2013). For the present analysis, the fuel-energy balances of the Committee on Statistics were reclassified according to the IEA format, cross-checked with available information on technology and infrastructure and compiled with other local sources of information.

The total primary energy supply of Kazakhstan was 64.5 Mtoe in 2011 (million tons of oil equivalent): almost half of which was consumed by the energy sector (including losses). The International Energy Agency reported an energy intensity of GDP of 0.93 toe/thousand USD (at 2005 prices) in 2011, 3.7 times higher than the world average and 6.6 times higher than the OECD average.

As represented in Fig. 1, the ratio of total final consumption over total primary energy supply (TFC/TPES) is significantly higher in other countries, 55 % in Kazakhstan. The world average is 69 %, while the share is 64 % in the Russian Federation and 79 % in Canada (IEA 2013).

Power plants' transformation losses account for 15 Mtoe: 23 % of the country's total primary energy supply (TPES). This is explained by the fact that most power plants were inherited from Soviet Union days, and that 41 % of generating capacity have been operating for more than 30 years (ME RK 2010). Efficiency at the largest coal fired electric power plants is no more than 40 % while that at heating plants does not exceed 65–70 %. The introduction of new heating plants may increase efficiency by up to 85–90 %. Coal is the most commonly used fuel at power plants, accounting for 67 % of total generating capacity.

Another 8 % of TPES (4.8 Mtoe) is attributed to losses, most of which are heat losses (1.9 Mtoe). According to the Ministry of Energy of the Republic of Kazakhstan (ME RK 2010), between 2010 and 2011, 37 % of generated heat was lost. The country's severe climatic conditions require high consumption of heat since the average winter temperatures are −19 °C in the North and −5 °C in the South.

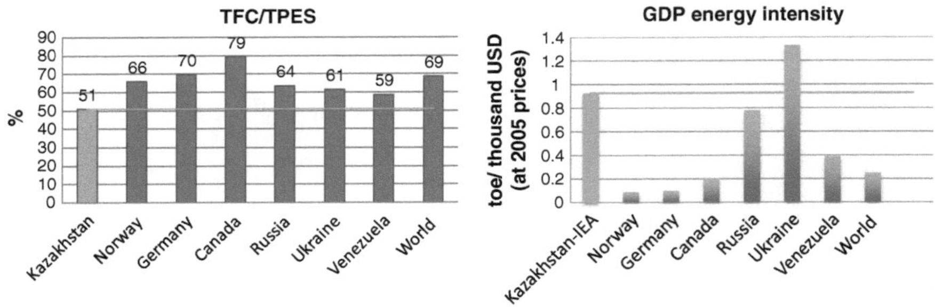

Fig. 1 Benchmarking analysis of TFC/TPES and TPES/GDP

Heating networks have deteriorated, with more than 60 % of components in use for over 20 years. Electricity losses are also high, at 9.3 % of total generation, due to long distance transmission and severe climatic conditions, and wear and tear is significant, at 50–60 %.

There are significantly high rates of self-consumption in the oil and gas sector—4.6 Mtoe (7 % of TPES). Kazakhstan is a net exporter of crude oil and natural liquids: 71.3 Mtoe in 2011 (110 % of domestic TPES). Gas is also exported, at lower volumes—most recently, 10.1 Mtoe. Power plants's self-consumption account for another 2 Mtoe: 11 % of the electricity generated.

On a demand side, industry is the biggest consumer in Kazakhstan—12 Mtoe (19 % of TPES). The energy efficiency of industry in Kazakhstan is low, at 45–60 %, as equipment is old and worn out. Until recently, there were no energy efficiency policies or programmes. Also, the prices of energy commodities were too low to result in reduction of energy consumption. Industry in Kazakhstan is mainly represented by energy intensive and heavy industries.

The residential sector is the second largest consumer of energy in Kazakhstan—9.7 Mtoe. Climatic conditions force households to use 2.3 Mtoe of heat, 2 Mtoe of coal, 2 Mtoe of gas and another 1.6 Mtoe of oil products, mainly for heating purposes. The Ministry of Energy of the Republic of Kazakhstan reports that, on average, buildings consumed 270 kwh/m^2 of heat in 2010: 1.5–2 times higher than in other countries with a similar climate (ME RK 2010).

Kazakhstan has significant potential for improving its energy efficiency and reducing its GHG emissions across most sectors of its economy. The Government of Kazakhstan has already taken steps to reduce its energy consumption through the direct and indirect policies discussed in the next section. The main aim of this chapter is to investigate the energy efficiency potential of Kazakhstan, using techno-economic modeling instruments.

2 Policies and Measures in Energy Efficiency in Kazakhstan

On 12th January 2012, the Law on Energy Saving and Improving Energy Efficiency (2012) was adopted. It covers the creation of the State Energy Register, and mandatory energy audits on major industrial sites and public services. In 2014, the Government planned to establish voluntary agreements on energy saving with industrial companies. The residential sector is affected by a law promoting metering, with differentiated pricing of district heating depending on the availability of metering devices. Provision of heat, electricity and gas is prohibited to new sites unless meters are fitted, and sales and production of electricity consuming devices are prohibited unless class of efficiency is indicated. Sales and production of incandescent lamps are also now prohibited.

In 2013, the Concept of the Republic of Kazakhstan for Transition to a Green Economy (2013) was approved. It sets concrete targets for six key sectors: water resources, agriculture, energy efficiency, the power sector, air pollution and waste utilization. It aims to ensure that renewable energy and nuclear power account for half of all electricity generation by 2050. The plan is also for gas fired power plants to account for 30 % of total electricity generation by 2050. This requires investment into gas infrastructure across the Northern, Eastern and Southern regions of the country.

To realize these ambitious targets, the Energy Saving—2020 programme was adopted in 2013 (ME RK). This defines strategies to improve energy efficiency across the industry, transport and residential sectors, and electricity and heat distribution systems. The final target is to reduce energy intensity of GDP use by 40 % by 2020 (compared to 2008 levels).

3 Approaches to Modelling of Improving Energy Efficiency

3.1 Energy Efficiency Chains

The model of the Kazakh energy sector (TIMES-KZK), calibrated to the reclassified national energy balances of 2009–2012 and further broken-down by end-uses in each demand sector, makes explicit the stocks and technical characteristics of existing technologies, as well as the energy flow through the system, resulting emissions, and associated costs, thereby reproducing the present inefficiencies in Kazakhstan.

The TIMES-Kazakhstan single region model represents all steps in the energy chain: from extraction of primary resources to their supply to primary energy markets; from transformation of primary energy carriers to their transmission and distribution to the final energy sectors (residential, commercial, industry, transport, agriculture); and from the use of final energy commodities to the satisfaction of end users demand for energy services (space heating and cooling, water heating, lighting, private and public mobility, iron and steel production, etc.). This process-oriented model provides a consistent framework with which to explore various paths towards energy efficiency within the coming 15–20 years.

Energy efficiency improvements (EEI) are virtual commodities of the model, representing energy not consumed whenever an existing technology is substituted with something better, at extra cost (Sarbassov et al. 2013). Equations 1 and 2 make explicit the efficiency gaps (EG) between an existing reference technology (ET) and the new ones (NT) available for the same energy sector/service (j), as well as the virtual savings due to the use of more efficient technologies (Q(NT)). Alternative options (NT) are included in a technology repository and characterized by an additional attribute representing the efficiency gap. Per each unit of output of the new technology (i), $EG_{i,j}$ units of improvements (units of losses avoided) are generated.

$$EG_{i,j} = \left(EFF(NT_i)_j - EFF(ET)_j\right) \quad (1)$$

$$EEI_{i,j} = EG_{i,j} * Q(NT_i)_j \quad (2)$$

EG efficiency gap
NT new technology
ET reference technology
EFF energy efficiency of the technology, which can be expressed as a ratio between energy output of the technology to its input
EEI energy efficiency improvement
Q savings
i indicator for a generic new technology
j energy service

EEI index must be intended as an approximate measure of efficiency improvement due to the chain of commodities and technologies before and after the system point where each measure applies. In terms of primary energy supply equivalent, the amount of avoided losses is greater; in terms of final energy consumption it is slightly lower.

In particular, new-generation electricity consumption meters are explicitly described through investment costs (US$2 at prices of 2000 per GJ per activity) and savings potential (up to 4 % of the unnecessary electricity consumption, based on authors estimation), while the installation of heat meters (with automatic regulation of the radiator temperature) could reduce the consumption by about 35 % (Sarbassov et al. 2013) with reference to the present situation, at a cost of about US$25 at prices of 2000 per GJ per activity.

The main technical causes for inefficiencies have been taken into consideration in current analysis, through the explicit representation of existing inefficient technologies and chains, as well as of some more efficient alternatives for the future development of the Kazakh system. To reduce tampering, which causes the above normative losses, the possible installation of meters has been considered. Thus, the model is able to track improvements in electricity, heat and natural gas transmission/transport and distribution, as well as in the oil, coal and gas transformation and uses.

The development of demand toward 2030 is driven by assumed population, and GDP (a medium variant projection by the Committee on Statistics of the Republic of Kazakhstan). From 2009 to 2030, the population is predicted to grow by 30 % (at 1.25 % pa), while GDP is assumed to rise at an annual rate of 6 % pa until 2020, followed by 5 % pa later on (300 % growth by 2030).

3.2 *Internalising Energy Policy Instruments*

Energy efficiency improvements result from investments into upgrading, affecting primary energy supply and resulting emissions. Through tracking technologies and energy flow, analysts can determine improvements in efficiency across the system, checking where specific measures bring cost-effective changes.

Standards and carbon taxes are often considered in order to reduce consumption across energy systems, and such regulatory-based and market approaches are usually combined in a multi-policy instrument, aiming to enhance additive energy and carbon reducing effects. Moreover, the explicit modelling of existing and new technological options allows for the use of subsidies (directly stimulating energy efficiency improvements), by applying an incentive per unit of loss avoided. Such a new instrument, generally called energy efficiency feed in tariffs—EEFiTs, has not been used for the scenarios presented in this paper, but it is fully embedded in the last version of the Kazakhstan model.

The present study aims to test two alternative approaches across the entire system: targeting energy intensity of GDP (a regulatory-based approach), and testing a CO_2 tax (a market-based approach).

4 Scenarios and Results

Two scenarios were run for this study, to quantify the potential for energy efficiency improvements in the Kazakhstan's system, subject to two types of energy measures. The first envisages reducing energy intensity of GDP by 40 % by 2020 (compared to the 2008 level) as set in the Energy Saving-2020 programme (ME RK 2013). The second offers an incentive of US$20 (at 2000 prices) per ton of CO_2 equivalent reduced starting from 2020 (CO_2TAX). The results, presented in Fig. 2, show the strong impact of energy intensity on reducing TPES (which is the denominator of the indicator, the reduction is due largely to improved efficiency in the coal chain), and the relevant impact of CO_2 taxation on emissions and the penetration of natural gas.

The Business as Usual (BaU) scenario doubles TPES by 2030, with coal remaining the dominant fuel (57 % of TPES). Assuming rigid GDP growth[1] (inelastic energy service demand), the target for GDP energy intensity would lower TPES by more than 22 Mtoe both in 2020 as well as in 2030, almost halving the coal supply compared to BaU. The overall efficiency of the system (the amount of energy consumed per unit of energy supplied) will reach 72 %: comparable to the levels in

[1]Domestic GDP is strongly tied to oil and gas export volumes. In the present analysis, all the scenarios share the same assumptions about export increases, which are consistent with the assumed GDP growth rate.

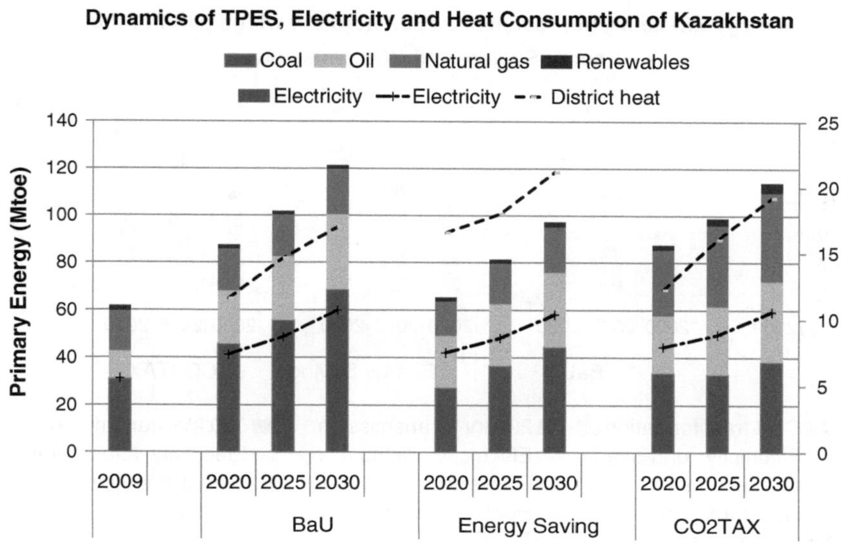

Fig. 2 Dynamics of TPES, electricity and heat consumption

Norway and Germany. The impact of CO_2 taxation[2] on TPES is less evident. The total supply in 2020 would be almost the same as in the BaU case, with reduction by 2030 to around 7 Mtoe.

In terms of reducing emissions, regulatory-based measures are much less effective than taxation-based measures. The dynamic of CO_2 in the former case is very similar to the BaU dynamic, while the latter produces an evident reduction in emissions (more than 25 %). Such a reduction is mainly due to the strong penetration of natural gas (from 19.5 Mtoe to 37.5 Mtoe in TPES) in the generation and final consumption sectors, and to the significant improvement of the efficiency of natural gas-fired stations, as shown in Figs. 3 and 4. Reducing the growth of CO_2 emissions in Kazakhstan—from the average annual 12–8 %—would require significant change in the configuration of the energy system and the involvement of gas. Currently, most of the gas extracted is reinjected; therefore, issues on gas production, processing and transportation should be resolved, to provide additional gas to the domestic market.

Figure 3 shows that even in the BaU case, energy savings may reach 10 Mtoe by 2020 and 22 Mtoe by 2030—mainly through more efficient coal transformation and electricity end-use sectors. This scenario reduces energy intensity of GDP by 18 % by 2020 and by 40 % by 2030 (compared to current levels). Meanwhile, the

[2]Such an approach simulates policies and measures already announced, for instance in the Concept of the Republic of Kazakhstan for Transition to a Green Economy (2013), and (more in general) aims to stimulate a market-based renovation and improvement of those technologies which become competitive at a low CO_2 price.

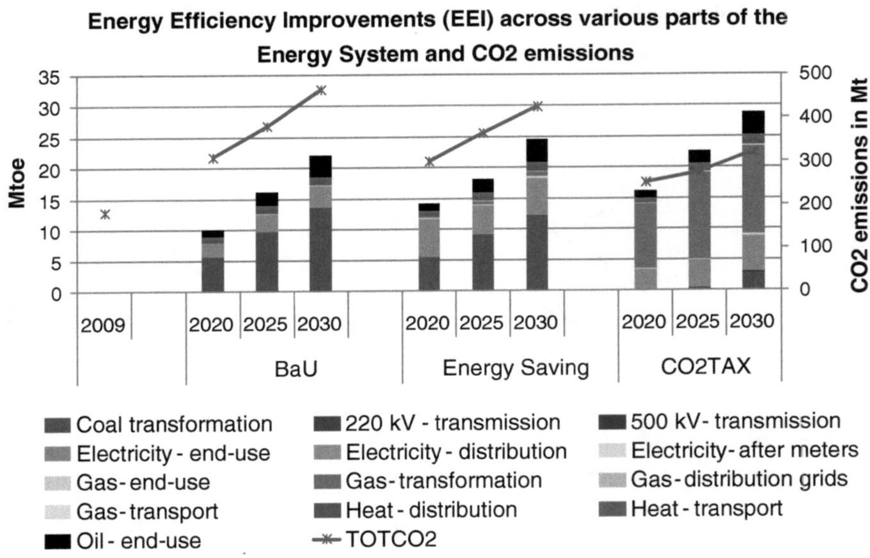

Fig. 3 Energy efficiency improvements across various parts of the energy system and CO_2 emissions

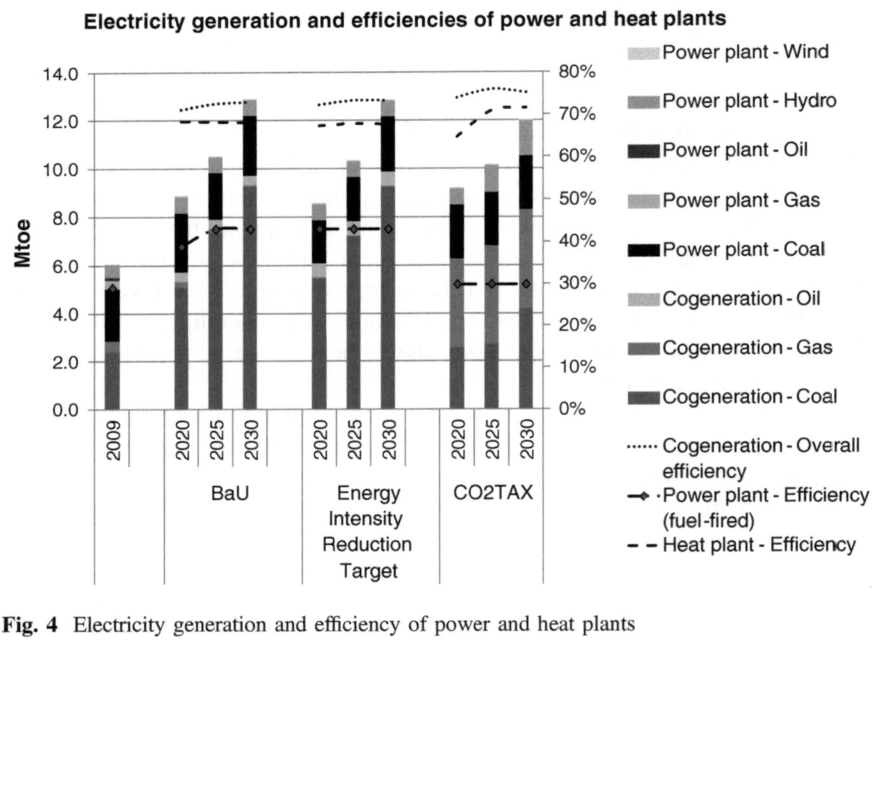

Fig. 4 Electricity generation and efficiency of power and heat plants

TFC/TPES indicator rises to 62 % by 2030. This means that most energy efficiency improvements are economically feasible and can be easily achieved once administrative and regulatory barriers are eliminated.

For all considered scenarios, most improvements are due to higher efficiency of generation (mainly coal-based in the BaU and in the Energy Intensity Reduction Target scenario, and mainly gas-based in the CO_2TAX case). Also, improvements are evident in the substitution of old electrical appliances with more efficient options, and new vehicles for the transport sector.

By 2030, the efficiency of CHP plants will rise by 9 % (maximum) while that of heat plants rise by 7 %. Figure 4 also demonstrates that CHP plants prevail in the new capacity-mix, rather than fuel fired pure electricity plants—mainly because climatic conditions force high demand for heating (as well as increasing levels of housing stock per capita). This is consistent with the recent Energy Saving Law, which aims to increase the use of cogeneration plants.

In absolute terms, the effects of the two efficiency-oriented alternative measures are hardly distinguishable in the demand side, as the total final consumption is almost the same over the three scenarios (slight reductions of 5 and 6 Mtoe compared to the BaU case for 2030), although the share of resources shifts, with natural gas partially replacing coal for heating.

5 Conclusions

The BaU case suggests significant energy efficiency improvement, meaning some significant cost-effective improvement (in particular regarding generation) can be gained, even without a specific energy policy to reduce (eliminate) market barriers (low priority of energy issues, incomplete markets for energy efficiency, distortionary fiscal and regulatory policies, and insufficient, or inaccurate information).

More than 50 % of energy efficiency improvement in the BaU case can be obtained by replacing old, coal-fired stations with modern coal plants. The efficiency of the energy system (TFC/TPES) increases from the current level of 55–62 % in the BaU scenario and to 72 % in the Energy Intensity Reduction Target scenario, by 2030, reaching the current level of Norway and Germany.

The reduction of energy intensity of GDP by 40 % by 2020 (compared to the 2008 level) can be achieved with economically viable options and without significant structural changes to the energy system: using timely technology updates and no market barriers. On the contrary, reduction of CO_2 would require significant efforts to increase the share of gas in the fuel mix.

References

Committee on Statistics of the Republic of Kazakhstan (2013) Fuel-energy balance of the Republic of Kazakhstan, statistical publication. http://www.stat.gov.kz/faces/wcnav_externalId/publicationsCompilations?_afrLoop=2066156156088395#%40%3F_afrLoop%3D2066156156088395%26_adf.ctrl-state%3Dd4l68r1uu_168. Accessed 24 Sep 2014

International Energy Agency (2013) Key World Energy Statistics. Kazakhstan: balances for 2011. http://www.iea.org/. Accessed 24 Sep 2014

ME RK (2010) Programme on the development of the power system of the Republic of Kazakhstan for 2010–2014. Ministry of Energy of the Republic of Kazakhstan (in Russian)

ME RK (2013) Energy saving—2020 programme. Ministry of Energy of the Republic of Kazakhstan. http://www.gosexpertiza.kz/sites/gosexpertiza/files/pp_rk_no904_ot_29.08.2013g._programma_energosberezhenie-2020.pdf. Accessed 24 Sep 2014 (in Russian)

The Concept of the Republic of Kazakhstan for Transition to a Green Economy (2013) http://www.led-ca.net/assets/files/Concept_Rus-GreenEcon-Kaz.pdf. Accessed 24 Sep 2014, in Russian

Sarbassov Y., Kerimray A., Tokmurzin D., Tosato G., De Miglio R. (2013) Electricity and heating systems in Kazakhstan exploring energy efficiency improvement paths. Energy Policy 60: 431–44

Ex Post and Prospective Analyses of Renewable Policies in Spain

Helena Cabal, Yolanda Lechón, Natalia Caldés, Cristina de la Rúa, Diego García-Gusano, Elena López-Bernabé, Inés López-Dóriga and Marta Santamaría

Abstract In this work, socioeconomic and environmental impacts associated to energy technologies in the current and future Spanish Energy System have been estimated. This information has provided the base from which to conduct two kinds of analyses. First, an Ex post analysis of renewable policies in Spain, where the net impact on social welfare associated to the progressive introduction of those energies in the energy system has been assessed using a partial cost-benefit analysis. Then, a prospective analysis of the Spanish energy system where the optimum energy mix, which leads to the largest social welfare under different energy scenarios, taking into account a medium-long term time horizon (2035), has been estimated using the national energy optimization model TIMES-Spain. The results of the Ex post analysis of the period 2005–2012 show an increase on social welfare due to the introduction of renewable energies. Nevertheless, when assessing the total expenditure of renewables support policies, the results show this support exceeds the

H. Cabal (✉) · Y. Lechón · N. Caldés · C. de la Rúa · D. García-Gusano · I. López-Dóriga · M. Santamaría
Center for Energy, Technology and Environmental Research (CIEMAT), Madrid, Spain
e-mail: helena.cabal@ciemat.es

Y. Lechón
e-mail: yolanda.lechon@ciemat.es

N. Caldés
e-mail: natalia.caldes@ciemat.es

C. de la Rúa
e-mail: cristina.delarua@ciemat.es

D. García-Gusano
e-mail: diego.garcia@ife.no

I. López-Dóriga
e-mail: inesldoriga@gmail.com

M. Santamaría
e-mail: marta.santamaria@ciemat.es

E. López-Bernabé
Universidad de Castilla-La Mancha, Albacete, Spain
e-mail: Elena.Lopez12@alu.uclm.es

G. Giannakidis et al. (eds.), *Informing Energy and Climate Policies Using Energy Systems Models*, Lecture Notes in Energy 30,
DOI 10.1007/978-3-319-16540-0_9

economic value of the socioeconomic and environmental externalities calculated in this work. The prospective analysis results for the period 2010–2035 definitely recommend a support for renewable electricity generation technologies and the redesigning of renewables support policies to better reflect their external benefits with respect to the fossil alternatives.

1 Introduction

This work has been carried out within the framework of the INER project, funded by the Spanish R+D Plan. INER stands for Study of the Net Social, Economic and Environmental Impacts of the Promotion of Renewable Energies in the Spanish Energy System. The aim of INER was to estimate the socioeconomic and environmental impacts associated to the introduction of the renewable energy technologies in the current and future Spanish Energy System.

The first Plan of Promotion of Renewable Energy in Spain, PPER 2000–2010 (IDAE 1999), started in 2000 to strengthen the energy policy objectives of security and quality of electricity supply and environment protection in order to meet Spanish international commitments. Afterwards, a reviewed plan was published, Plan of Renewable Energy, PER 2005–2010 (IDAE 2005), whose main indicative targets were to reach 12.1 % of total energy consumption with renewables and to contribute 30.3 % to the total gross electricity production by 2010. This objective was fully met with a share of 35.4 % of renewable electricity (REE 2011). Biofuels would account for 5.83 % of the gasoline and diesel consumption in transport. The total investment needed by the plan was estimated in 23,598,641 Million Euro. After PER 2005–2010, a new plan, PER 2011–2020 (IDAE 2011), was elaborated with new objectives by 2020.

Besides fiscal support of investments and tax exemptions, the successful deployment of renewable technologies in the electricity system has been mainly due to a feed-in tariff scheme (FIT) which has been working in Spain from 1998. This scheme, regulated by Royal Decrees 2818/1998, 436/2004, 661/2007, 1578/2008 and 1565/2010, has facilitated the penetration of renewables in the electricity market and their technological development until 2012 when the Government, in an attempt to reduce the growing high electric tariff deficit, approved Royal Decree-Law 1/2012 suspending the remuneration pre-assignment procedure and removing incentives for new electricity installations.

Despite this growth experienced by renewables, there is still a high foreign energy dependence which strongly affects the sustainability of our energy system (SEE 2013). Among others, in addition to not meeting the greenhouse gas emissions reductions committed in the Kyoto Protocol (SEMA 2014), the country, with high external energy dependence, is very vulnerable to fossil fuel price fluctuations and faces serious risks in energy supply security. In the current energy market, where only private generation costs are taken into account, fossil energies are more cost competitive than renewable energies and thus, keep their dominant role in the energy system. However, renewable energies have other advantages that should be taken into account. They contribute to the diversification and continuity of energy supply and the reduction of environmental impacts, and represent a good alternative way of generating prosperity and employment and facilitating the access to energy in isolated rural areas. Therefore, the competitiveness of renewables improves substantially when, besides the private costs of the technologies, their externalities are also considered. For that and to also guarantee a sustainable energy system which maximizes the society welfare, policy makers should make use of economic instruments to internalize externalities and to design energy policies which take into consideration social welfare.

In this context, this work performs a cost assessment of the most recent energy policies in Spain, not only considering the private cost of electricity production but also the environmental and socioeconomic costs. First, external costs have been quantified and monetized so that the total cost of electricity has been estimated for all the technologies in the Spanish electricity system. Two main results have been obtained from this analysis: the net impact on the social welfare associated to the progressive substitution of fossil technologies by renewable technologies up to 2010, and the optimal electricity system in the medium and long term under different scenarios.

2 Total Costs of Current and Future Electricity Technologies

First of all, a comprehensive literature review was carried out to identify relevant publications on socioeconomic impacts of energy technologies. Then, a data gathering task was performed regarding the different components of the total cost of energy technologies, such as private costs, environmental burdens and damages, direct employment, etc. For this purpose, national and international data sources were consulted.

2.1 Levelised Electricity Costs

Levelised electricity costs (LEC) and their projections were calculated from investment and operation and maintenance costs data (IDAE 2011; IEA 2010; BCG 2011) for the different technologies in the Spanish electricity system, according to the IEA methodology (IEA 2010). Results showed that, in 2010, most of the renewable technologies were not cost competitive compared with conventional ones. Only LEC for hydropower was close to LEC for nuclear and fossil technologies (Fig. 1).

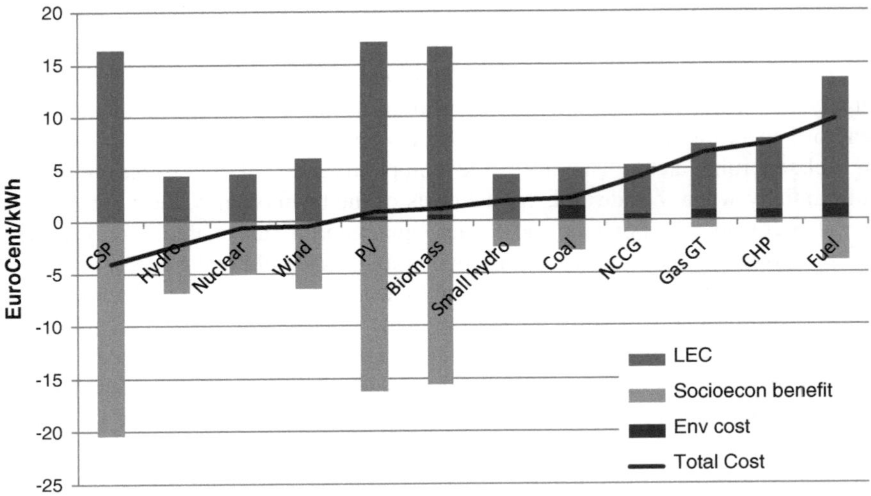

Fig. 1 Disaggregated total cost by technology in 2010 (Caldés et al. 2014)

Nevertheless, over the next periods, LEC for fossil and nuclear technologies is expected to increase. In the case of fossil technologies, this is due to increasing prices for CO_2 and emission allowances as well as fuel prices (Kost et al. 2013). In the case of nuclear technologies, such a trend is due to the longer construction times and changes in regulatory requirements in nuclear (IAEA 2013). On the other side, LEC for renewables is expected to reduce, except for hydropower. It should be noted that there is a relevant change in the LEC for solar technologies which will drop by up to 40 % by 2030 mainly due to the effects of increased learning.

2.2 Environmental Externalities

Data from the CASES project (Cost Assessment for Sustainable Energy Systems, 6th FP), where ExternE methodology (EC 2005) was applied, has been used to estimate the environmental external costs of the technologies. Environmental damages have been estimated from the inventory of emissions of the different technologies during their whole life cycle and using damage factors for the main global and local atmospheric pollutants adapted to the Spanish conditions. The environmental costs for renewable technologies, as can be seen in Fig. 1, are lower than those from conventional fossil ones, with the highest costs attributed to coal and oil technologies. Among renewables, the lowest environmental costs correspond to hydro and wind technologies while the highest costs correspond to biomass technologies.

2.3 Socioeconomic Externalities

The domestic impact on economic activity of the main electricity technologies in Spain has been estimated using the Input-Output table for 2009 from the WIOD project (Timmer 2012) and real data on investment and operation and maintenance costs for each technology. The domestic direct and indirect economic activity generated by each technology has been calculated, as a way to estimate the impact on Value Added. As with the environmental externalities, renewable technologies present the largest socioeconomic external benefits. This result is especially positive taking into account that renewable energy projects are usually located in rural areas with a lower socioeconomic development than cities. It has been considered that all the goods and services have been produced in Spain. If this assumption is relaxed, for instance due to an increase in solar panels imports from China, the socioeconomic positive impacts of renewables would be substantially reduced. To account for such effects, a sensitivity analysis on this subject will be carried out in future studies.

3 Impact of the Renewable Penetration on the Social Welfare

All the previous results have been integrated into a partial Cost-Benefit Analysis (CBA) to evaluate the total costs of electricity generation during the period 2005–2010, when the first PER was in force. Factors considered in the analysis are shown in Table 1.

For this purpose, three scenarios have been considered: (i) BASE scenario, which considers the actual RES deployment, (ii) PER scenario, where the Spanish energy mix matches the PER objectives for RES, and (iii) NoRES scenario. In this last scenario, it has been assumed that the renewable capacity installed in 2004 remained constant over the whole period and that the demand not met with renewables would have been met with natural gas combined cycle plants.

The total electricity system cost has been estimated for the three scenarios adding the external costs and benefits to the private costs.

The scenario without renewable growth (NoRES) presents the highest total costs. It is followed by the BASE scenario where the difference in the generation costs of renewables is compensated by higher external benefits. Finally, the scenario where PER is met presents the lowest total costs. Comparing BASE and PER scenarios, the higher cost in the first is mainly due to a huge installation of solar technologies, which in 2008 surpassed in 2500 MW the installed capacity foreseen in the PER.

Once the total cost of the electricity system was calculated for each scenario, the difference between BASE and NoRES scenarios was estimated. This comparison provided the net impact associated with renewable technologies penetration in terms of private costs, and environmental and socioeconomic externalities.

Table 1 Factors considered in the partial CBA (Caldés et al. 2014)

Relevant factor	Cost or benefit for society	Measurement indicators	Monetized (monetization method)	Considered in this CBA?
Electricity generation costs	Private cost	Levelised electricity cost	Yes	Yes
Economic activity	Socio-economic externality	Value added	Yes	Yes
Local environmental effects	Environmental externality	Various environmental impact indicators/kWh	Yes (Extern-E and Cases)	Yes
Global environmental effects	Environmental externality	CO_{2equiv}/kWh	Yes (Extern-E and Cases)	Yes
Renewable support expenditures	Public cost	Feed in tariffs expenses	Yes	Yes
Employment	Socio-economic externality	Jobs created	Yes	Estimated but not included
Tax revenues	Public benefit	Tax revenues from energy related activities	Yes	No
Fossil fuel imports	Public benefit	Oil and gas imports	Yes	No
Other renewable support polices	Public cost	Tax exemption, investment subsidies, etc.	Yes	No
Transaction costs	Public costs	Not measured	Not measured	No
Merit order effects	Public and private benefit	Not measured	Not measured	No
Increase in RES exports	Private benefit	Not measured	Not measured	No
Rural development	Public benefit	Not measured	Not measured	No

The differences in total external cost between renewable and non-renewable technologies have been compared with the cost of the renewable support policies in the power generation sector (feed-in tariffs) for the years between 2005 and 2010. The results (Fig. 2) show that the cost of the feed-in tariff system exceeds the net environmental and socioeconomic externalities. From this result it can be concluded that the feed-in tariff scheme should have been designed in such a way that private costs and social benefits of renewable were better balanced and therefore result in lower policy costs.

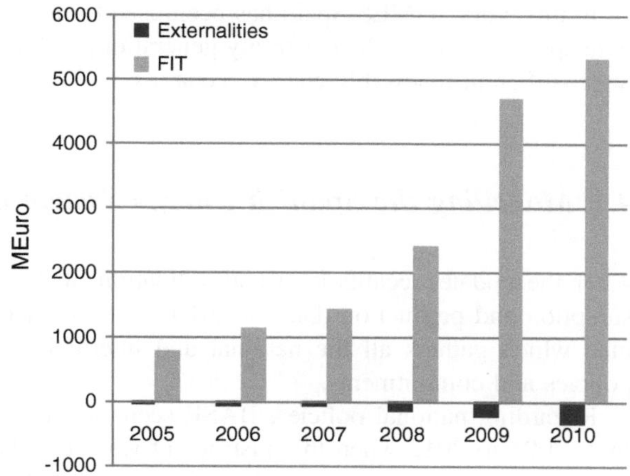

Fig. 2 Costs for feed-in tariff and total externalities for renewable technologies

Other benefits that could be incorporated in future analysis include the savings in fossil fuel imports, tax revenues, merit order effects and job creation, which could be monetized. Additionally, there are also other benefits derived from the support for renewable energies in this period worthy of mention such as the increase in technology exports resulting from the market leadership of some Spanish companies.

An alternative scenario to NoRES scenario was considered for sensitivity analysis purposes. Under this alternative scenario, the demand not met with renewables would have been met with coal instead of gas. Results show that the total cost for the scenario with gas is higher than that for the scenario with coal. Looking at the total cost components, although the coal has higher environmental costs it also presents higher socioeconomic benefits mainly because coal consumed is an indigenous resource while gas is imported and most of its associated economic activity stimulation takes place outside of Spain's borders and has not been evaluated. In addition, coal also has lower private generation costs.

4 Optimum Energy System in the Medium and Long Term

TIMES-Spain is a national energy model part of the Pan European Times model (PET) developed within the NEEDS project (New Energy Externalities Development for Sustainability, 6th FP) in 2004. From then, TIMES-Spain has continuously been updated and improved within the framework of several European Commission and national projects such as RES2020 (Monitoring and Evaluation of the RES directives implementation in EU27 and policy recommendations for 2020, IEE) (Labriet et al. 2010), REACCESS (Risk of Energy Availability: Common Corridors for Europe Supply Security, 7th FP), COMET (Towards an infrastructure for CO_2 transport in the Western Mediterranean, 7th FP) and INER.

In this work, TIMES-Spain has been used to model the Spanish energy system, with special focus on the electricity generation, within the 2010–2035 time horizon under different renewable energy scenarios.

4.1 Modelling the Spanish Energy System in 2020–2035

After the update, recalibration and validation of the model with the energy consumption and production data for 2010, a first scenario has been built, the BASE one, which gathers all the national and international energy and environmental policies and commitments.

Regarding national policies, BASE scenario includes the feed-in tariff scheme from 2005 to 2012 when this instrument was abolished for new renewable, CHP and residues facilities (Decree-Law 1/2012). The BASE scenario also considers subsidies to investments on renewable technologies in the commercial and residential sectors.

As far as international commitments are concerned, BASE scenario includes the commitments in force related to Directive 28/2009/EC on the promotion of the use of energy from renewable sources, Directive 29/2009/EC to improve and extend the greenhouse gas emission allowance trading scheme of the Community, and Directive 2001/81/EC on national emission ceilings for certain atmospheric pollutants. Those commitments set by 2020 have been kept at the same level until the end of the time horizon. Such Directives are included as a constraint in the model setting a series of objectives such as 20 % renewable energy from final energy consumption and a maximum emission of 258.4 Mt of CO_2 by 2020, and SO_2 and NOX emission ceilings up to 746 and 847 kt respectively from 2015 to 2035.

The inclusion of those policies leads to renewable technologies reaching 44 % share of electricity generated by 2020 (39 % when electricity from industry is considered), and 100 % in 2035 (97 % including electricity from industry). The robustness of this result should be further analysed. The model includes average availability factors for each seasonal time slice. A higher level of disaggregation should be considered to properly assess this point. The highest contribution among renewables in 2020 corresponds to wind power. Later on, particularly by 2030, there is a considerable penetration of solar technologies which, by 2035, generate 38 % of the total electricity. For simplicity reasons, in this exercise, impacts on the electricity grid, storage requirements and Demand Side Management (DSM) have not been taken into account.

Comparing the objectives of PER 2011–2020 (IDAE 2011) with the results of the optimization, some discrepancies have been found (Fig. 3). It should be noted that PER 2011–2020 estimations were done under an optimistic demand projection. According to the results of the modelling exercise, electricity with biomass does not enter the Spanish electricity system, in fact the objective for this technology in PER is quite modest. Additionally, there is a delay in wind offshore which participates in the system with a negligible share of 0.08 % by 2020 and reaches 0.4 % in 2035.

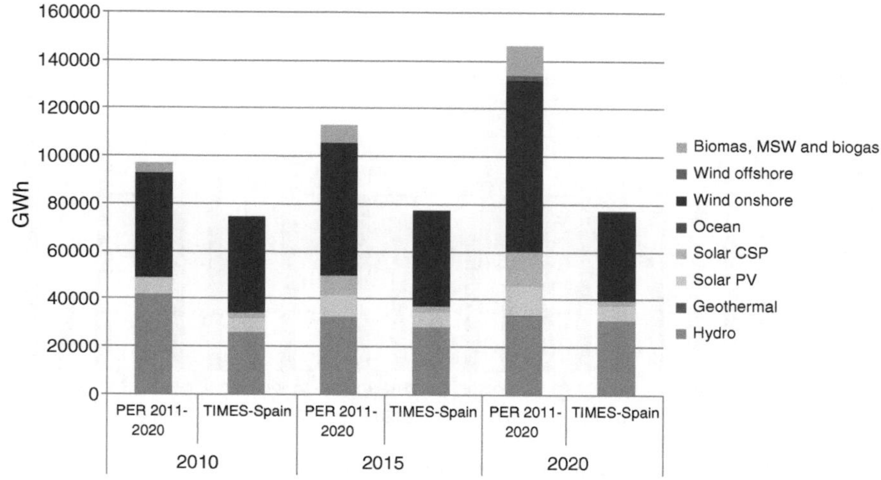

Fig. 3 RES forecasted penetration in BASE scenario versus PER 2011–2020 objectives

4.2 Energy, Environmental and Socioeconomic Scenarios

In addition to the BASE scenario, two alternative scenarios have been built:

- ZERO scenario, which considers the evolution of the energy system when there are no restrictions or targets to emissions and renewable technologies penetration set by the policies in force.
- INTER scenario, which considers the internalization of the environmental and socioeconomic external costs for all the electricity technologies estimated in the previous sections. Socioeconomic externalities have been calculated as an increase in economic value added into the Spanish economy associated to technology investment and operation. They resulted only in benefits (Fig. 1). They have been introduced in the objective function by reducing the investment and operation and maintenance costs of each technology from the amount of the socioeconomic externalities. Environmental externalities have been introduced in the model as an additional variable operation and maintenance cost. As in ZERO scenario, INTER scenario does not include any restriction or target either.

Results of the ZERO scenario show a mix with a huge participation of fossil technologies, a high share of coal (also via CHP) and a lower but still relevant share of renewables in 2020 (33 %) and 2035 (25 %), mainly hydro and wind technologies.

Penetration of renewable technologies in the final energy consumption in the INTER scenario is higher than in the BASE scenario (62 % in 2020 and 68 % in 2035). The electricity production with natural gas disappears from the system in 2015 and is replaced by renewable electricity, mainly wind and solar power. This

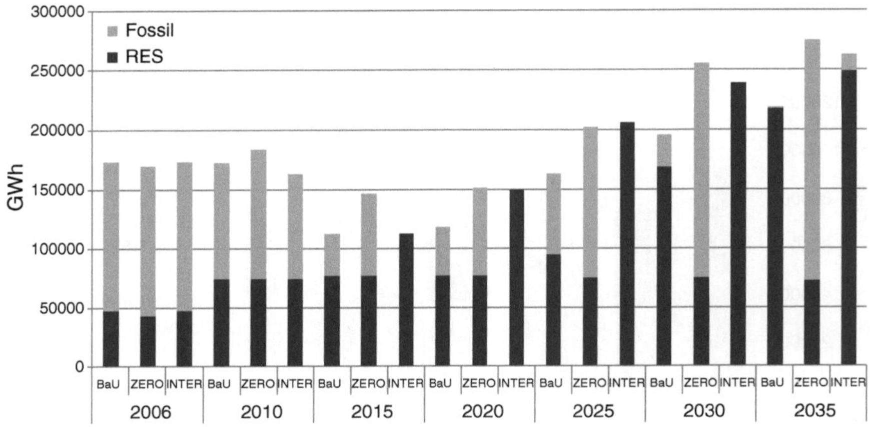

Fig. 4 Fossil and renewable technologies production in the three scenarios

result might appear unrealistic because of the large investments in natural gas combined cycle (NGCC) plants made in Spain over recent last years. However this is what is actually happening as many NGCC plants are producing at 10 % of their capacity or even in standby because of the high penetration of renewable electricity into the system. At the end of the time horizon, both scenarios present an electricity mix almost completely renewable with the rest being produced with gas through CHP in the BASE scenario, and CHP and NGCC in the INTER.

Figure 4 shows the production of electricity with fossil technologies (except for CHP) and renewables.

5 Conclusions and Recommendations

Based on the results from the partial Cost-Benefit Analysis some conclusions have been drawn. The positive impact on social welfare associated to the renewable energies is higher than the impact associated to fossil energies. Thus, the Government should restart the promotion of the penetration of renewable technologies in the national electricity mix by means of support policies, as in the past. Nevertheless, this support has to be well designed and diversified in order to avoid past imbalances. Various policies such as public support to R+D in less mature but promising renewable technologies and a well-designed investment incentive system (e.g. feed-in tariffs and tenders) should be put in place. Also, the expansion of technologies in the system should not overpass the target assigned to them, which could be estimated as the amount of capacity that maximizes the welfare of the society. Besides, the magnitude of socioeconomic benefits associated to renewable energies is very sensitive to the origin of the components and services. Consequently, industrial policies should be designed to strengthen the domestic production of those goods and services. Finally, there was a huge growth of renewable technology installation from 2005 to 2010 which resulted in a capacity expansion for some technologies well above the objectives set by the PER 2005–2010. This led to an unexpected increase in the support policy costs which over-passed the associated environmental and socioeconomic benefits. A more accurate design of the level of feed-in tariffs and a limit to the new capacity installed according to the PER estimates could have reduced the costs of those support policies.

Regarding the modelling exercise, the main conclusion is that it is possible to meet the objectives of renewable technologies penetration and emission reductions set by the European Directives internalizing the external costs and benefits of electricity technologies. Thus, renewable support policies through financial instruments which reflect the external benefits with respect to fossil technologies should be reestablished.

Acknowledgments This work has been carried out within the framework of the INER project, co-funded by the Spanish R+D Plan.

References

BCG (2011) Evolución tecnológica y prospectiva de costes de las energías renovables. Estudio técnico PER 2011–2020. Boston Consulting Group, Madrid

Caldés N et al (2014) What are the costs and benefits associated to RES deployment in Spain?—Evidence for the period 2005–2010. Paper presented at the 14th IAEE European energy conference, Rome, 28–31 Oct 2014

EC (2005) ExternE. Externalities of Energy. Methodology 2005 update. Report EUR 21951. In: Bickel P, Friedrich R (eds) European commission, directorate-general for research, sustainable energy systems, Luxembourg (ISBN 92-79-00423-9)

IAEA (2013) Energy, electricity and nuclear power estimates for the period up to 2050. Reference data series No. 1. International Atomic Energy Agency, Vienna (ISBN 978–92–0–111910–0)

IDAE (1999) Plan de Fomento de las Energías Renovables en España 2000–2010. Instituto para la Diversificación y Ahorro de la Energía, Ministerio de Industria, Energía y Turismo, Madrid

IDAE (2005) Plan de Energías Renovables para España 2005–2010. Instituto para la Diversificación y Ahorro de la Energía, Ministerio de Industria, Energía y Turismo, Madrid

IDAE (2011) Plan de Energías Renovables 2011–2020. Instituto para la Diversificación y Ahorro de la Energía, Ministerio de Industria, Energía y Turismo, Madrid

IEA (2010) Projected costs of generating electricity, 2010th edn. OECD, International Energy Agency, Paris

Kost C et al (2013) Levelised cost of electricity renewable energy technologies study. Fraunhofer Institute for Solar Energy Systems ISE, Freiburg

Labriet M, Cabal H, Lechón Y, Giannakidis G, Kanudia A (2010) The implementation of the EU renewable directive in Spain. Strat Challenges Energy Policy 38(5):2272–2281

REE (2011) El sistema eléctrico español 2010. Red Eléctrica de España, Madrid

SEE (2013) La energía en España 2012. Secretaría de Estado de la Energía, Ministerio de Industria, Energía y Turismo, Madrid

SEMA (2014) Inventarios nacionales de emisiones a la atmósfera 1990–2012. Documento resumen. Secretaría de Estado de Medio Ambiente, Ministerio de Agriculturas, Alimentación y Medio Ambiente, Madrid
Timmer MP (ed) (2012) The world input-output database (WIOD): contents, sources and methods, WIOD working paper number 10

Modelling Pathways to a Low Carbon Economy for Finland

Tiina Koljonen and Antti Lehtilä

Abstract Concretizing the roadmaps outlined for moving to a low carbon economy by 2050 into detailed policies is a challenging task. Using ETSAP-TIAM as the central modeling tool, we have analyzed the implications of low carbon policies within Europe, with a special focus on the Finnish energy system. The main objective of the work was to identify cost-effective pathways for moving into a low carbon economy by 2050, by creating a set of different storylines for the future society and economy. The analysis involved also linking the energy system model to an applied general equilibrium model and a forest sector partial equilibrium model for estimating the impacts on the overall economy as well as land-use change and forestry. The scenario results indicate that Finland has good opportunities for achieving its low carbon targets by 2050 due to its large natural resources. The major uncertainties are related to the application of carbon capture and storage (CCS) and possible sustainability criteria for biomass.

1 Introduction

The Government of Finland adopted the Foresight Report on Long-term Climate and Energy Policy in 2009 setting a target to reduce Finland's greenhouse gas (GHG) emissions by at least 80 % from the 1990 level by 2050 as part of an international effort (PMO 2009). Finland's long term climate target is in line with the strategies and emission targets set by the European Commission for achieving the low carbon economy by 2050 (EC 2011a, b). The government of Finland established a Parliamentary Committee on Energy and Climate Issues on summer 2013 with the task of preparing an energy and climate roadmap for Finland up to

T. Koljonen (✉) · A. Lehtilä
VTT Technical Research Centre of Finland, Espoo, Finland
e-mail: tiina.koljonen@vtt.fi

A. Lehtilä
e-mail: antti.lehtila@vtt.fi

G. Giannakidis et al. (eds.), *Informing Energy and Climate Policies Using Energy Systems Models*, Lecture Notes in Energy 30,
DOI 10.1007/978-3-319-16540-0_10

2050. The Energy and Climate Roadmap 2050 report was published on October 2014 (MEE 2014) which builds up strategic guidelines for Finland in order to achieve a low carbon society.

The central supporting research and analysis work for the Energy and Climate Roadmap preparation was a scenario building and modelling of alternative low carbon pathways for Finland, which was assessed by the multidisciplinary research project Low Carbon Finland 2050 platform (LCFinPlat) in collaboration with VTT Technical Research Centre of Finland, the Government Institute for Economic Research (VATT), the Geological Survey of Finland (GTK), and the Finnish Forest Research Institute (Metla). The analyses presented in this paper are based on the results of the LCFinPlat project (Koljonen et al. 2014), which included integrated assessments with energy system, general equilibrium, and sectoral models for mining industry, building sector, and forest sector. The scenario building and analysis included large and multidisciplinary consultation between industries, non-governmental organizations (NGOs), scientists, and policy makers. Also, interview of 1000 private energy consumers were carried out to analyze the motivation and potential barriers for GHG mitigation.

The primary focus of this paper is on energy system modelling of alternative low carbon scenarios for Finland with TIMES-VTT model. The impacts of low carbon emission targets on national economies and the use of natural resources are also shortly reviewed. The modelling and analysis of low carbon targets on Finland's, Nordic, and EU's energy systems with TIMES-VTT model were partly based on earlier work (Koljonen et al. 2012; IEA 2013; Knopf et al. 2013) but in the LCFinPlat project a new setup of scenarios and more detailed modelling of forest and mining industries were included. The paper is structured as follows: Sect. 2 describes the alternative low carbon pathways and Sect. 3 the modelling methodology. In Sects. 4 and 5 the modelling results of alternative low carbon scenarios and selected sensitivity analysis are presented, including a summary of the impacts on national economy and the use of natural resources of Finland. Section 6 concludes the analysis presented and gives some recommendations for future work.

2 Senario Definition

Five low carbon scenarios were created: Continued growth, Stagnation, Save, Change, and Base-80 %. The scenario matrix for the first four scenarios was formulated according to Jim Dator, who has compressed the range of futures into four archetypes—continued growth, collapse/decline, conserver/disciplined society, and high tech transformation. The Base-80 % scenario was built around the Baseline scenario defined in the National Energy and Climate Strategy (MEE 2013). The low carbon societal scenarios are based on both narrative storylines (Table 1) and systematic modelling (Sect. 2 and Table 2).

The development and analysis of scenarios aimed at broad-based utilization of viewpoints of different interest groups and consumers, and, on the other hand,

Table 1 Characteristics of the low carbon scenario storylines

Scenario	Main characteristics from Finland's perspective
Baseline	"Business as usual", including existing national and EU's energy and climate policies, like EU's and Finland's 2020 targets. No major changes to industrial or community structures. Conservative development of technologies
Base-80 %	Similar assumptions as in the Baseline, despite the minimum 80 % emission reduction target by 2050 for Finland and the rest of the EU region
Continued growth "smart society"	Global agreement on 2 °C climate target, economic prosperity, internationalizing, open society, rapid development of technology, structural change in industry, increasing density of urban and regional structures
Stagnation "climate crisis"	Rise of global mean temperature of over 4 °C ⇒ economic crisis, closed society, slow development of technology, current industrial structure, current urban and regional structures
Save "modern oil crisis"	Delayed global agreement on 2 °C climate target ⇒ forward-leaning climate policy of the EU, conservative development of technology, emphasis on energy and material efficiency, current industrial structure, current urban and regional structures
Change "smart consumer"	Global agreement on 2 °C climate target, radical innovations emphasized, developments in economic structure ⇒ role of services emphasized, intertwining work and leisure time, internationalizing, open society, slight dispersal in urban and regional structures, major changes in industrial structure

utilizing the assessments of sustainable use of natural resources. The interactive platform was implemented by a series of seminars, workshops, consultations between different interest groups and between experts, as well as a broad questionnaire targeted at private consumers, contributing as a whole to the target of interactivity. As a result of these viewpoints, a set of quantitative inputs were formulated by the broad group of experts, including VTT's experts on technologies, foresight and energy systems, VATT's and Metla's economists, Metla's experts on forestry, and GTK's geologists.

The central assumption for the scenarios is set by a globally binding climate agreement reflecting the 2 °C climate change mitigation target. In the Save scenario, it is assumed that the global climate agreement is delayed and the EU takes a lead in climate policies by setting the 80 % mitigation target by 2040. In the Stagnation scenario, global climate policies fail and the global mean temperature rises of over 4 °C.

The development of new low carbon technologies and changes in industrial as well as urban and regional structures vary between the scenarios as central drivers of future development. In the Continued growth and Change scenarios optimistic development and implementation of new technologies were assumed while in the other scenarios base (i.e. more conservative) assumptions were used. In the Continued growth and Change scenarios the urban and industrial structures were also

Table 2 Main assumptions of the low carbon scenarios modeled (in the TIMES-VTT model, EU is approximated by the group of six European regions included)

Scenario characteristic	Base-80 %	Growth	Save	Stagnation	Change
Climate policy	EU—80 % by 2050 global 2 °C	EU—80 % by 2050 global 2 °C	EU—80 % by 2040 global 2 °C	EU—80 % by 2050 regional, ~4 °C	EU—80 % by 2050 global 2 °C
GDP growth	Good	High	Moderate	Slump	High
Industrial structure	As in official Baseline[a]	Focus on value added	Conventional	Focus on traditional strengths	Focus on value added and services
Technology development	Normal	Rapid for all sectors	Focus on end-uses[b]	Slow	Very rapid
Nuclear power in Finland	2 new plants + refurbishments	≤5 GW in 2050	≤7.2 GW in 2050	≤3.4 GW in 2050	Moratorium
CCS availability	EOR/EGR	Full potential	Full potential	EOR/EGR + depleted fields	EOR/EGR + depleted fields
Buildings	Conventional	Low energy concepts	Focus on renovation	Slow improvements	Low energy concepts
Transport	Slow technological changes	Rapid technological change	Modal shifts, new infra, savings	Mostly conventional	Rapid technological change

[a] Refers to the Baseline of the 2013 updated national energy and climate strategy of Finland (MEE 2013)
[b] High investments and deployment of energy efficiency measures assumed

assumed to change from the current development path. In the Change scenario urbanisation is high, which provide industrial innovations in information and communication technologies (ICT) and related industry. In the Change scenario more local, small scale industries are assumed to emerge, and regional structure moves in a more decentralized direction enabling distributed energy solutions to emerge.

In addition to the four low carbon scenarios, a Baseline scenario corresponding to the main characteristics of an updated national energy and climate strategy (MEE 2013) until 2025 was analyzed. Furthermore, the Base-80 % scenario, including similar assumptions as the Baseline, despite the 80 % emission reduction target by 2050, was analyzed. The scenario assessments also include sensitivity analyses with respect to the most essential uncertainties. Table 1 summarizes the main characteristics of the alternative low carbon scenarios for Finland while the main assumptions of the low carbon scenarios modeled in the TIMES-VTT are described below in Sect. 3.2 and Table 2.

3 Modeling Methodology

3.1 Models Used

In the low carbon scenario analysis we employed five different models, of which the TIMES-VTT energy system model was the core tool. The four other models were soft-linked with the TIMES model, as illustrated in Fig. 1.

The energy system model TIMES-VTT is a global multi-region model originally developed from the global ETSAP-TIAM model (Loulou 2008; Loulou and Labriet 2008). It is based on the IEA TIMES modeling framework (Loulou et al. 2005), and is characterized as a technology-rich, bottom-up type partial equilibrium model. TIMES-VTT model consists of 17 regions, which include four regions for the Nordic countries (Denmark, Finland, Norway, Sweden), Western Europe, Eastern

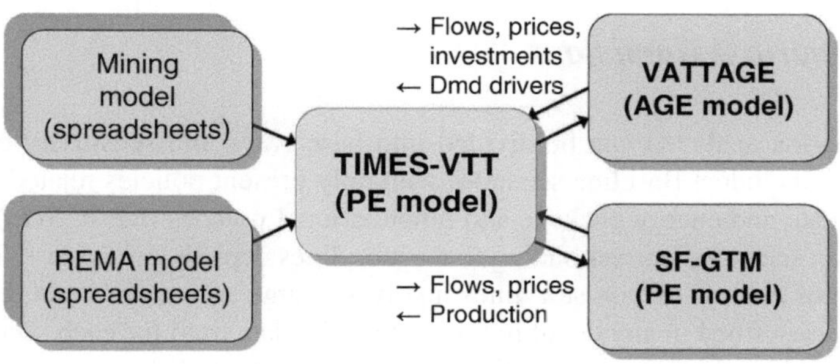

Fig. 1 The linked models used for analyzing the scenarios. *PE* Partial equilibrium, *AGE* applied general equilibrium

Europe, CIS (Former Soviet Union excluding the Baltic countries), Africa, the Middle East, India, China, Japan and South Korea, Other Developing Asia, Canada, the USA, Latin America, and Australia and New Zealand. For the Nordic regions, the district heat production and demand is divided into four sub-regional areas for better modeling of the heat networks in these countries (Koljonen et al. 2012; Lehtilä et al. 2014).

The time horizon of the model is flexible, and can be extended to 2100 or even beyond. For the low carbon scenarios, we used a horizon extending to 2065, divided into successive periods of 5–10 years duration, each representing an average year of the period. To reflect seasonal and diurnal variations in supply and demand, each year is divided into five seasons and two daily time segments.

For gaining further insights into the macroeconomic impacts of the low carbon pathways, the VATTAGE applied general equilibrium model, developed at the Government Institute for Economic Research (VATT), was soft-linked with the TIMES model (Honkatukia 2009). A detailed spatial partial equilibrium model of the Finnish forest sector, SF-GTM, was linked for obtaining more detailed results concerning the LULUCF (i.e. Land Use, Land Use Change and Forestry) effects and the use of regional biomass resources (Kallio et al. 2013). Furthermore, spreadsheet models are used to provide input data for the modeling of various sectors. Two such models were specifically used for the low carbon scenarios, namely, a long-term mining sector model developed by the Geological Survey of Finland (GTK) for modeling the developments in the mining industries (Tuusjärvi et al. 2014), and the bottom-up REMA model for estimating the energy use in various segments of the building stock (Tuominen et al. 2014).

The TIMES model incorporates also an integrated climate module, with a three-reservoir carbon cycle for carbon dioxide (CO_2) concentrations and single-box decay models for the atmospheric methane (CH_4) and nitrous oxide (N_2O) concentrations, and the corresponding functions for radiative forcing. Additional forcing induced by other natural and anthropogenic causes is taken into account by means of exogenous projections. Finally, the changes in mean temperature are simulated for two layers, surface, and deep ocean (Loulou et al. 2010).

3.2 Scenario Assumptions

The scenarios analyzed can be divided into base cases and sensitivity cases. The base cases include a Baseline scenario, with only present policies related to the EU 2020 climate and energy package and other national policies (MEE 2013), and five low carbon scenarios corresponding to the storylines depicted in Table 1. The actual modeling of the low carbon storylines involves a large amount of input data, which cannot be described in any detail in this paper. The data used for each scenario have been tailored to the storylines with respect to the demand drivers for all sectors, assumptions on technological development, constraints on the deployment of certain technologies (e.g. nuclear power, carbon capture and storage, bio-refineries), and development of building standards. The main assumptions in the low carbon scenarios are summarized in Table 2.

As in bottom-up models in general, by far the largest amount of input data is required for the various existing and new technologies available in the energy system. The technology data have been collected from numerous sources, and have been classified into base estimates and optimistic ones. In the scenarios with rapid technological change, optimistic estimates have been used for the technical and economic development of many key technologies for achieving a low carbon society, such as wind and solar power technologies, new bioenergy technologies and end-use technologies in different sectors (Koljonen et al. 2012; MEE 2014).

A second important category of input data is related to energy resources and potentials, which are also based on numerous literature sources as well as the ETSAP-TIAM database (Loulou 2008; Koljonen and Lehtilä 2012; IEA 2013). For these data, assumptions are not varied across scenarios but base estimates are used for all scenarios. However, due to differing projections for the forest industries and agricultural production, biomass potentials implicitly vary across scenarios.

The sensitivity cases are variants of the base case scenarios, where the assumptions concerning certain key assumptions have been changed in order to see how much they affect the solution. Within our project, we have mainly considered the assumptions regarding nuclear power, biomass sustainability criteria and the commercial availability of carbon capture and storage (CCS) for the sensitivity cases, which were assumed to be the most critical uncertainties for Finland based on the stakeholder interviews. These cases are described in more detail later in this section.

The global climate policies of at most 2 °C global temperature increase, as shown in Table 2, have been modeled by limiting the total radiative forcing to at most 3 W/m^2 until 2100, in line with the median estimates by Meinshausen et al. (2009). The Stagnation scenario has been modeled assuming no new global agreements on climate change policies, but only regional climate policies according to the pledges presented by various countries, leading roughly to about 4 °C increase in the global temperature (De Cian et al. 2013).

In the scenario analysis, we assumed only the EU-wide targets binding, and that they must be reached solely by reductions within the EU. The so-called flexible mechanisms, where measures outside the EU could also be credited, were thus excluded from consideration. Moreover, changes in emissions related to land use, land use change and forestry (LULUCF) were also excluded from the EU-wide emission targets in the energy system model runs, and were only assessed separately with the SF-GTM forestry sector model (Kallio et al. 2013, 2014). However, we did take into account BECCS (i.e. CCS integrated to biomass fired energy production, pulp and paper industries, and 2nd generation liquid biofuel production) as an option for reducing emissions, as it has already been accepted in the inventories submitted to the UNFCCC (IEA 2011).

4 Results from the Basic Scenario Variants

4.1 Energy and Emission Scenarios of the Alternative Low Carbon Pathways

Like most European countries, Finland has also a national GHG reduction target for 2050, which is the same as the EU-wide target, i.e. 80 % compared to the 1990 level, and it concerns all greenhouse gas emissions of the Kyoto protocol. The results from the basic scenario variants indicate that the EU-wide emission target for 2050 would lead to closely comparable emission reductions in Finland, as illustrated in Fig. 2. In the Baseline scenario (current policies, the proposed EU's 2030 climate and energy targets not included), total emissions would be reduced only by about 30 % by 2050. On the other hand, in the low carbon scenarios the EU-wide targets would entail reductions in Finland amounting to 67–85 % of the 1990 emission levels by 2050. The Stagnation scenario is the only one clearly left behind the national targets, while in the Growth, Save and Change scenarios the national targets related to a low carbon society appear to become well achieved also in Finland.

In Finland, the total primary energy consumption was about 1500 PJ in 2010, of which 52 % consisted of fossil fuels, including peat. The use of renewable energy is already at a high level, close to 30 %, and the role of nuclear energy is also considerable, about 18 %. In the low carbon pathways the contribution of fossil fuels decreases steeply, dropping to around 20 % in 2050, while the share of renewable energy increases to 44–60 % of total primary energy (Fig. 3a). In all

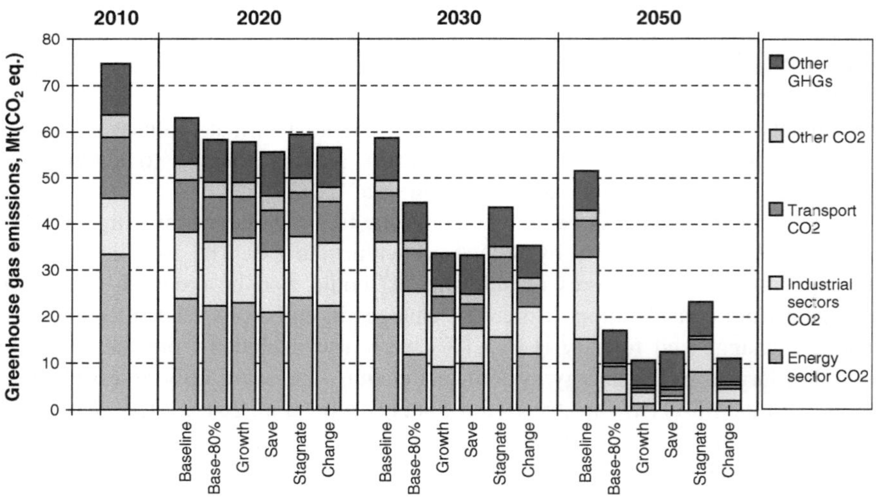

Fig. 2 Development of GHG emissions in Finland in the base scenario variants (other CO_2 includes CO_2 emissions in all other sectors)

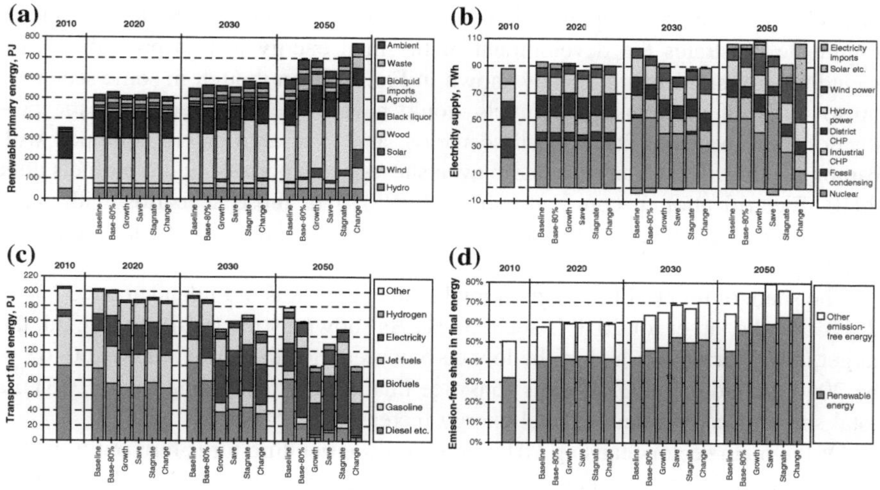

Fig. 3 Development of electricity supply (**b**), renewable primary energy (**a**), final energy in transport (incl. aviation) (**c**), and emissions-free final energy (**d**) in the base variants of the low carbon scenarios considered

scenarios bioenergy remains the most important renewable energy source in Finland.

The development of electricity supply is illustrated in Fig. 3b. The results clearly illustrate that in the low carbon economy electricity generation should become practically free of GHG emissions. That appears to shrink the economic potential for combined heat and power (CHP) and district heating, which may seem somewhat unexpected in view of the high efficiency of CHP generation. However, because basically all thermal generation should be based either on biofuels, carbon-free synthetic fuels, or fossil fuels with CCS, it tends to become both logistically difficult and uneconomical to maintain a very high share of CHP generation. According to the results CCS may indeed become competitive also in CHP plants producing district heat for large urban areas, especially combined with oxyfuel combustion technology, as it enables maintaining high total energy efficiency in CHP generation. The Change scenario depicts a high penetration of solar power, which may be realistic only under the optimistic assumptions concerning energy storage technologies in this scenario.

In final energy consumption the impacts of continued electrification, which are pronounced in the low carbon pathways, are clearly seen in the results. Along with high efficiency improvements e.g. in the building and transport energy use, the share of industry in final energy consumption tends to increase in the case of Finland. As an example, the average specific energy consumption for heating and hot water decreases by up to 60 % in the scenarios, compared to the present levels.

Concerning the transport sector, our scenario results indicate that along with second generation liquid biofuels and electrification in the longer term, the obstacles to achieving deep emission cuts also in this sector will be much reduced. Figure 3c illustrates the development of the final energy in transport, the corresponding emissions being already shown in Fig. 2. Even though in some scenarios up to 40 % of the transport biofuels would have to be imported, domestic production becomes significant in all scenarios, and to a large extent equipped with carbon capture. The Change scenario even shows net exports of liquid biofuels after 2030. Electrification becomes dominant by 2050 in those scenarios with rapid technological change, turning the market share of liquid biofuels eventually downwards.

The share of renewable energy in total final energy was in Finland about 32 % in 2010, and the target for 2020 is set at 38 %. As shown by the results in Fig. 3d, the target is well achieved, and in the low carbon scenarios the share reaches 60–65 % by 2050. Including all GHG emissions-free final energy (excluding fossil CCS) the total share of carbon-neutral final energy increases to 75–80 %.

Of the main sectors causing GHG emissions, agriculture turns turn out to be the one where achieving substantial reductions is the most difficult. In our scenarios, the decrease in agricultural emissions were at the highest 44 % in the Change scenario, but that was to a large extent due to the assumed decrease in agricultural production in that storyline, and only to a lesser degree through advanced technical abatement measures or changes in fertilizer use and cultivation practices. The decrease in domestic production was based on the assumed favorable development of global trade.

As the emission targets were EU-wide, the GHG emission prices were the same for all European countries. According to the results, the marginal prices would rise to 100–125 €(2010)/tonne (CO_2 eq.) in 2050, depending on scenario. The prices are within the range of carbon values (85–264 €(2010)/tonne) reported in the assessment of the EU 2030 climate and energy policy framework (EC 2014).

As practically no suitable geological CO_2 storage capacity has been identified within the territory of Finland, the transportation and storage related to CCS applications in Finland have been estimated by assuming that the storage site is located either in the North Sea or the Barents Sea (Teir et al. 2010). Despite the considerable costs for CO_2 transportation, the results indicate that CCS could still have a notable role in Finland, if the storage technology will be commercialized on a wide scale. That was assumed to take place in the Base-80 %, Growth and Save scenarios, which also show the highest proportions of emission reductions occurring within the emission trading sectors. The scale of the emission abatement by CCS is illustrated in Fig. 4 for the basic scenario variants.

One of the characteristics of the Finnish energy system is the use of biomass for large-scale energy conversion, currently mainly within the pulp and paper industry and in public power and heat generation, but in the future also in bio-refinery plants producing liquid biofuels. Due to the substantial forest resources, this opens up the possibilities for negative emissions via BECCS, thereby facilitating deeper cuts in overall emissions. According to the results, BECCS accounts for the majority of the

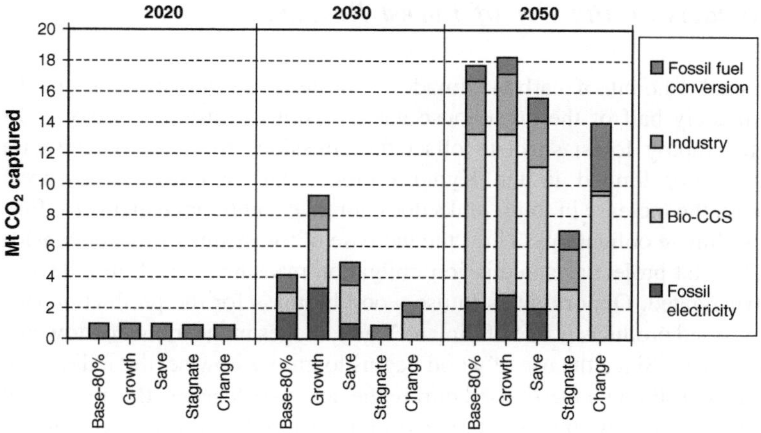

Fig. 4 Emission abatement by CCS

CCS potential in Finland, and appears to be a particularly attractive option in bio-refinery plants, where carbon can be captured from an almost pure CO_2 stream. The potential for fossil-based CCS appears to be limited, and is mostly related to large multi-fuel CHP plants using also biomass, as well as hydrogen production. Within industry, the most promising CCS option appears to be enhanced blast furnace process with top gas recycling and oxygen injection.

4.2 Impacts on the National Economy

The build-up of the LCFinPlat scenarios on the national economy did not directly aim at comparability. The Base, Base-80 %, Save, and Stagnation scenarios show similarities from an economic viewpoint. Compared to Baseline, the 80 % emission reduction does not imply a major decrease in gross domestic product (GDP), partly due to the moderate reduction of emissions already in the Baseline, partly due to the fact that majority of the reductions can be implemented by new technology, which was assumed to be commercially available, when needed. On the basis of the Baseline and Base-80 % scenarios, the macroeconomic effect of 80 % emission reduction is mild: the growth of GDP is lower by less than 1 % in comparison to the Baseline in 2050. Assuming slow technological development and thereby the need for increased supports for new technology implementation the GDP losses will increase. Climate policy has also an impact on the structure of the economy by slightly diminishing the external balance—that is, the share of exporting sectors decreases compared to the Baseline (Honkatukia et al. 2014).

4.3 Impacts on the Use of Forest Resources

The annual amount of carbon dioxide sequestered by forests in Finland equals approximately half of the greenhouse gas emissions from other sectors. Opportunities to employ forest sinks to offset the emissions from the other sectors are, however, very limited in the Kyoto Protocol and in consecutive agreements. Therefore, the increase in forest sinks does not give additional benefits for Finland to meet its climate obligations. Thus, the increase of forest sinks was not considered in the LCFinPlat project as an emission mitigation measure even if their development was investigated. Opportunities to use wood biomass for the production of energy and processed products is one of Finland's advantages in the transition towards a low carbon society. Since the use of wood begins to grow stepwise, the felling potential[1] of forests will still be underutilised during the next two decades. Because the planned use of wood is below the growth, the volume of Finnish forests keeps on growing. This also contributes to a growth of carbon sinks. That is, forests store carbon from the atmosphere more than it is emitted back due to felling and the decaying process of natural mortality. By 2050 the carbon sinks could be more than doubled compared to current levels (70–90 Tg CO_2/a in 2050), indicating the net carbon sinks might be much larger than Finland's GHG emissions (Kallio et al. 2014).

5 Results from the Sensitivity Cases

The low carbon pathways depicted by the scenarios contain many inherent uncertainties that require further sensitivity analysis with respect to the key factors influencing the results. In addition, as the scenario storylines were also quite different from each other, sensitivity analysis can also help identifying the main similarities and differences between scenarios to arrive at robust conclusions regarding the low carbon pathways. As mentioned above, we analyzed sensitivities to three significant uncertainties the stakeholders identified important for the Finnish energy system: (1) new nuclear power (N), (2) biomass sustainability (B), and (3) the commercial availability of CCS (C). Lastly, we also looked into the case where these three uncertainties are applied simultaneously (R). Selected results from the sensitivity analyses are shown in Fig. 5 for the Save and Growth scenarios.

In the first sensitivity analysis case (N), we assumed that no new nuclear power plants would be installed in Europe after those currently under construction. As there have been plans for several new plants in the relatively small energy system of Finland, the uncertainties related to nuclear power have a particularly high impact on the low carbon pathways in Finland.

[1] The felling potential corresponds to the sustainable harvesting potential of roundwood, which is estimated from harvesting suggestions obtained from the national forest inventory.

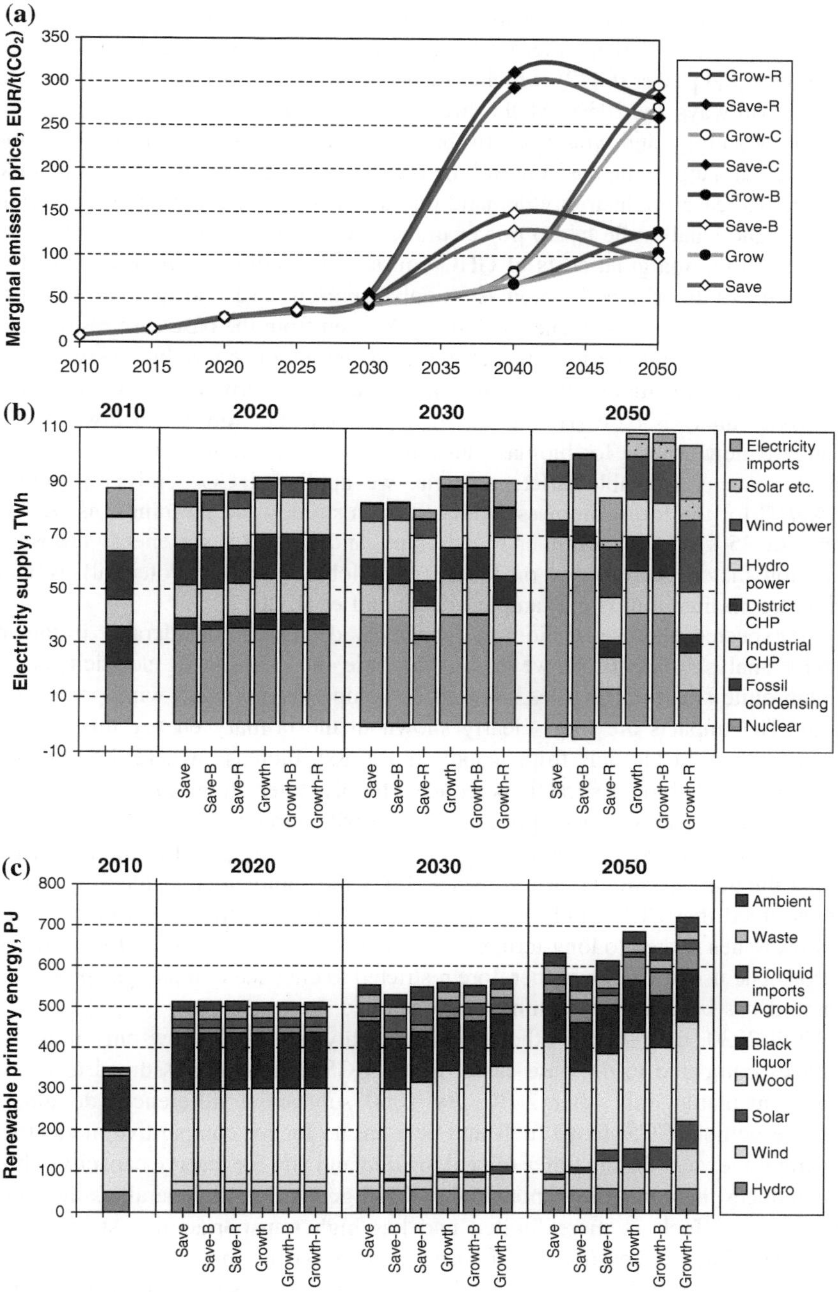

Fig. 5 Marginal GHG emission prices (**a**), electricity supply (**b**) and renewable primary energy (**c**) in Finland in the Save and Growth scenarios, with sensitivity variants B and R

As expected, the nuclear power case (N) shows its strongest impacts on the electricity system. Perhaps the most significant impact is seen in the role of combined heat and power (CHP), which now becomes much more prominent in the low carbon pathways by 2050. At the highest, CHP would cover 40 % of the total electricity supply, and would mostly be based on biomass but also on fossil fuels with CCS in large scale pass-out turbine plants. Other substantial changes include a notable decrease in electricity demand due to higher prices, and larger penetration of wind and small scale hydro power in the N case. However, it turns out that the impacts on the marginal costs of GHG emission reduction remain quite small.

Sustainability criteria for biomass supply represent a second important factor of uncertainty for the Finnish energy system. As seen from the base case results, in all of our scenarios, bioenergy remains the most important renewable energy source, and plays a very important role in attaining the low carbon targets. The second sensitivity analysis case (B) thus attempts to find out, how the pathways might change if new criteria for biomass sustainability would be implemented in future. To simulate conceivable stricter criteria, we applied a CO_2 emission factor of 65 kg/GJ for the forest biomass produced from stumps and thinnings, as well as a factor of 25 kg/GJ for all other forest chips, and 20 kg/GJ for energy crops. The emission factors were based on GWP (i.e. Global Warming Potential) estimates presented in literature (for example in Pingoud et al. 2012).

As expected, the use of biomass for energy decreases considerably in the sensitivity analysis case B. However, in this case the changes in electricity supply remain quite small. CHP loses some of its competitiveness and wind power gains some. The impacts are most clearly shown in the primary energy mix and production of liquid biofuels from woody and grassy biomass, where the use of the least sustainable biomass fractions reduces sharply. Interestingly, there is also some increase in electricity consumption due to electrification in this case. The marginal GHG emission prices rise about 25 % in 2040–2050 compared to the base cases.

For the third sensitivity case considered (C), the commercial availability of CCS, we assumed that CCS would not become a commercial option in Europe, due to various issues related to long-term storage, like public acceptance, or for some other reason. The use of CCS was therefore restricted to enhanced oil and gas production, where it has been already commercially applied.

Until 2030, the results in the sensitivity analysis case C show only minor differences compared to the base cases, as the CCS option was assumed to become widely available only after 2030. By 2050 substantial differences do emerge, because without CCS, fossil fuels and peat are no longer competitive in electricity generation, except during times of peaking demand and for reserve capacity. This in turn reduces the competitive potential of CHP generation in general, as the supply of non-fossil fuels is more limited and has high transportation costs over long distances. The decreasing fossil-based generation is mostly compensated by increases in electricity imports and larger wind and solar power production. However, the demand for electricity is not reducing, because the opportunity costs related to electrification remain favorable. The strength behind these impacts can be understood by looking at the marginal GHG emission prices, which are in this case more than doubled, rising over 250 €/tonne. The impacts on bioenergy use are two-fold: higher marginal costs increase it, while the unavailability of CCS reduces it. Yet steeper increases in marginal costs of GHG reduction have been reported earlier by Remme and Blesl (2008).

Finally, to see the combined effect of the three factors described above, we also ran the scenarios assuming that all the three main uncertainties described above are simultaneously applied. The results from this case (R) indicate the availability of CCS being indeed the most significant uncertainty for the low carbon pathways. The results are in many respects similar to the sensitivity case (C), and the marginal abatement costs are only 10 % higher. However, in the (R) case the demand for electricity is now in many scenarios notably lower than in the base cases, as the incentives for demand reduction are finally exceeding those of electrification. Note that in case (R) investment in nuclear power was prohibited in Finland only and not in the rest of the EU. In the case (N) new nuclear power was prohibited in Europe as well.

It may also be of interest to look at the impacts of the sensitivity cases on the projected European-wide electricity supply due to EU-wide cap of GHG emissions and, on the other hand, due to the increasingly integrated electricity markets within the EU. The results for some of the cases are illustrated in Fig. 6, where the base case results are shown for the Save and Growth scenarios, and the sensitivity cases B, C and R for the Growth scenario. From the results one can clearly see the high importance of wind and solar power for reaching the low carbon targets on the European level, as well as the influence of CCS availability on the results. Without CCS, fossil fuel based generation should become practically negligible also on the

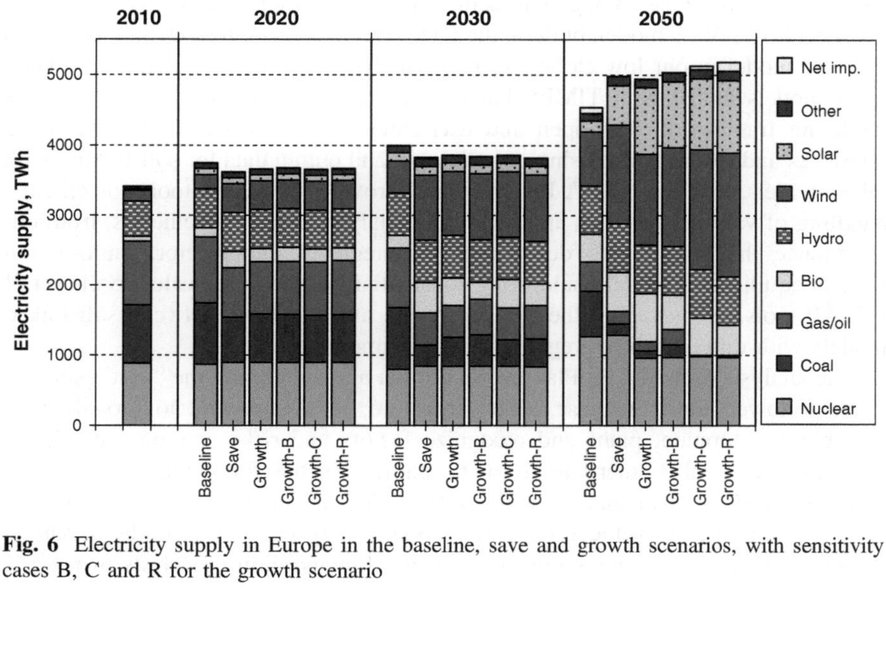

Fig. 6 Electricity supply in Europe in the baseline, save and growth scenarios, with sensitivity cases B, C and R for the growth scenario

European level, leading to yet higher and more costly dependence on variable renewable generation. But with CCS, one can see BECCS having potential also on the wider European scale.

6 Conclusions

The recently published Energy and Climate Roadmap 2050 for Finland (MEE 2014) builds up strategic guidelines in order to achieve a low carbon society. The modelling and analysis work by the LCFinPlat project formed the basis of the low carbon strategies for the government. An important part of the LCFinPlat project was also the established interactive platform, which was implemented by a series of seminars and workshops held during the project, consultations between different interest groups and experts, as well as a broad questionnaire targeted at private consumers, contributing as a whole to the target of interactivity. The platform served policy makers through the whole period of formulation of the Energy and Climate Roadmap 2050 for Finland and also policy makers gave feedback on preliminary results of the impact assessments. The platform proved to be an essential part of the whole scenario building and modelling framework because of large uncertainties related to long term scenarios. The consultations, seminars and workshops through the project period also increased the transparency and common understanding of the challenges and opportunities of the transition to a low carbon society. On the other hand, it was also shown that multidisciplinary and systematic modelling of alternative low carbon pathways is needed to identify the major uncertainties, risks, opportunities, and strengths of alternative low carbon pathways and to build up robust strategies in achieving the assessed climate targets.

The TIMES-VTT model, built on the ETSAP energy system modeling tools, was the core model in our low carbon scenario analysis. The combined use of several other models linked with TIMES has demonstrated the flexibility of the TIMES modeling framework. The open and user-extensible GAMS code facilitates the interfaces and tailored processing of both input and output data for soft-linking with other models, and the VEDA-FE user shell provides powerful tools for efficient handling of various scenarios and sensitivity analysis cases. Nonetheless, from our experience there seems no doubt that an integrated multi-sector, multi-region general equilibrium model could bring substantial further added value to the set of ETSAP tools, as managing the data exchange and iterations between soft-linked models with different disaggregations can be time-consuming.

The analysis of the LCFinPlat project did not aim at defining the "best" pathway to be followed until the year 2050. Therefore, it is important to broadly map possible development paths and recognize factors and risks common for all the pathways potentially emerging from the choices in the following decades. The modelling and scenario analysis with TIMES-VTT model showed that Finland has good opportunities to achieve the low carbon society because of its large natural resources. However, in the Stagnation scenario Finland didn't reach its own 80 %

GHG reduction target expect by buying emission allowances indicating, that at least EU level and preferably global level climate target should be agreed before implementing national low carbon targets and policies. In all the low carbon scenarios bioenergy remains the most important renewable energy source, and plays a very important role in attaining the low carbon targets. Therefore the impacts of possible future sustainability criteria for biomass was analyzed with sensitivity analysis, which showed that the marginal GHG emission prices rose about 25 % in 2040–2050 compared to the base cases. However, both the stakeholder consultancy and sensitivity analysis showed that commercialization of CCS represents the major uncertainty: the marginal GHG emission prices more than doubled, rising over 250 €/tonne if we assumed that CCS would not be available as a mitigation option. Without CCS, fossil fuel based generation should become practically negligible also on the European level, leading to yet higher and more costly dependence on variable renewable generation. But with CCS, one can see BECCS having large potential in Finland but also on the wider European scale.

In many impact analyses of low carbon policies, alternative technology portfolios and technology learning rates have been considered (EC 2011b; Knopf et al. 2013). On the other hand, alternative scenarios for the changes in the community structures, industrial structures, or economy structures are usually not considered at all, expect in the more detailed sectoral analysis. In the LCFinPlat project it was shown that there is a clear advantage of analyzing these to create robust scenarios and to better identify risks and opportunities in the transition to the low carbon society. It also important to integrate multidisciplinary expertise in formulating and analyzing alternative low carbon pathways even though more resources and time would be needed to create common low carbon visions and strategies.

Acknowledgments The work presented in this paper was based on research work of above twenty researchers from VTT, VATT, Metla and GTK. The impacts of low carbon policies on national economics was analysed by Juha Honkatukia from VATT and the impacts on the use of forest resources was analysed by Maarit Kallio and Olli Salminen from Metla. The authors greatly acknowledge collaboration between the whole research group and the financial support from Tekes—the Finnish Funding Agency for Technology and Innovation, VTT, VATT, GTK, and Metla.

References

De Cian E, Keppo I, Bollen J, Carrara S, Förster H, Hübler M, Kanudia A, Paltsev S, Sands RD, Schumacher K (2013) European-led climate policy versus global mitigation action: implications on trade, technology, and energy. Clim Change Econ 4(1):28

EC (2011a) European Commission. Communication form the Commission to the European Parliament, the Council, the European Economic and Social Committee and the Committee of the Regions. A Roadmap for moving to a competitive low carbon economy in 2050, Brussels, 8.3.2011, COM (2011) 112 final

EC (2011b) European Commission. Communication form the Commission to the to the European Parliament, the Council, the European Economic and Social Committee and the Committee of the Regions. Energy Roadmap 2050, Brussels, 15.12.2011 COM (2011) 885 final

EC (2014) A policy framework for climate and energy in the period from 2020 up to 2030. Impact assessment. European Commission, SWD (2014) 15 final, Bussels

Honkatukia J (2009) VATTAGE—a dynamic, applied general equilibrium model of the Finnish economy. VATT Research Reports 150. http://www.vatt.fi/file/vatt_publication_pdf/t150.pdf

Honkatukia J, Tamminen S, Niemi J (2014) Development of economy in low carbon scenarios: Finland report of the low carbon Finland 2050 platform project [Kansantalouden kehitys vähähiiliskenaarioissa: low carbon Finland 2050—platform—hankkeen loppuraportti]. VATT Tutkimukset 178/2014 (in Finnish, English abstract)

IEA (2011) Combining bioenergy with CCS. Reporting and accounting for negative emissions under UNFCCC and the Kyoto protocol. International Energy Agency, Paris

IEA (2013) Nordic energy technology perspectives. Pathways to a carbon neutral energy future. International Energy Agency, Paris. http://www.iea.org/media/etp/nordic/NETP.pdf

Kallio AMI, Salminen O, Sievänen R (2013) Sequester or substitute—consequences of increased production of wood based energy on the carbon balance in Finland. J Forest Econ 19 (4):402–415

Kallio M, Salminen O, Sievänen R (2014) Low carbon Finland 2050 platform: scenarios for the forest sector [low carbon Finland 2050 platform: skenaariot metsäsektorille]. Metlan työraportteja 308 (in finnish). http://www.metla.fi/julkaisut/workingpapers/2014/mwp308.htm

Knopf B, Chen Y-HH, De Cian E, Förster H, Kanudia A, Karkatsouli I, Keppo I, Koljonen T, Schumacher K, van Vuuren DP (2013) Beyond 2020—strategies and costs for transforming the European energy system. Clim Change Econ 4(1):38

Koljonen T, Lehtilä A (2012) The impact of residential, commercial, and transport energy demand uncertainties in Asia on climate change mitigation. Energy Econ 34(3):410–420

Koljonen T, Similä L, Sipilä K, Helynen S, Airaksinen M, Laurikko J, Manninen J, Mäkinen T, Lehtilä A, Honkatukia J, Tuominen P, Vainio T, Järvi T, Mäkelä K, Vuori S, Kiviluoma J, Sipilä K, Kohl J, Nieminen M (2012) Low carbon Finland 2050. VTT clean energy technology strategies for society. VTT visions: 2. VTT, Espoo, 75 p. http://www.vtt.fi/inf/pdf/visions/2012/V2.pdf

Koljonen T, Similä L, Lehtilä A, Grandell L, Airaksinen A, Tuominen P, Järvi T, Laurikko J, Sipilä K, Helynen S, Honkatukia J, Kallio M, Salminen O, Kivinen M, Vuori S, Kihlman S, Lauri L (2014) Low carbon Finland 2050 platform: summary report [low carbon Finland 2050—platform: vähähiilipolkujen kiintopisteet ja virstanpylväät. Yhteenveto hankkeen tuloksista ja johtopäätöksistä]. VTT, VTT Technology 167, Espoo (in finnish, extended abstract in English)

Lehtilä A, Koljonen T, Airaksinen M, Tuominen P, Järvi T, Laurikko J, Similä L, Grandell L (2014) Low carbon Finland 2050—platform. Energy system pathways towards a low carbon society. [Energiajärjestelmien kehityspolut kohti vähähiilistä yhteiskuntaa]. VTT, VTT Technology 165, Espoo (in finnish, English abstract)

Loulou R (2008) ETSAP-TIAM: the TIMES integrated assessment model. Part II: mathematical formulation. CMS 5(1–2):41–66

Loulou R, Labriet M (2008) ETSAP-TIAM: the TIMES integrated assessment model. Part I: model structure. CMS 5(1–2):7–40

Loulou R, Remme U, Kanudia A, Lehtilä, A and Goldstein G (2005) Documentation for the TIMES model. Energy technology systems analysis programme (ETSAP). http://www.iea-etsap.org/web/Docs/TIMESDoc-Intro.pdf

Loulou R, Lehtila A, Labriet M (2010) TIMES climate module (Nov. 2010). TIMES version 2.0 user note, energy technology systems analysis programme. http://www.iea-etsap.org/web/Docs/TIMES-Climate-Module2010.pdf

MEE (2013) Ministry of economy and the employment. National energy and climate strategy. Government Report to Parliament on 20 Mar 2013. http://www.tem.fi/files/36292/Energia-_ja_ilmastostrategia_nettijulkaisu_ENGLANNINKIELINEN.pdf

MEE (2014) Ministry of economy and the employment. Energy and climate roadmap 2050. Report of the Parliamentary Committee on 16 Oct 2014. Publications of the ministry of employment and the economy. Energy and the climate 50/2014. http://www.tem.fi/files/41483/Energy_and_Climate_Roadmap_2050.pdf

Meinshausen M et al (2009) Greenhouse-gas emission targets for limiting global warming to 2 °C. Nature 458:1158–1162

Pingoud K, Ekholm T, Savolainen I (2012) Global warming potential factors and warming payback time as climate indicators of forest biomass use. Mitig Adapt Strat Glob Change 17:369–386

PMO (2009) Prime Minister's office Finland. Government foresight report on long-term climate and energy policy: towards a low-carbon Finland. Prime Minister's Office Publications 30/2009. Helsinki University Print, Helsinki. http://vnk.fi/julkaisukansio/2009/j28-ilmasto-selonteko-j29-klimat-framtidsredogoerelse-j30-climate_/pdf/en.pdf

Remme U, Blesl M (2008) A global perspective to achieve a low-carbon society (LCS): scenario analysis with the ETSAP-TIAM model. Clim Policy 8:60–75

Teir S et al (2010) Potential for carbon capture and storage (CCS) in the Nordic region. VTT Technical Research Centre of Finland, Espoo, VTT Research Notes 2556

Tuominen P, Holopainen R, Eskola L, Jokisalo J, Airaksinen M (2014) Calculation method and tool for assessing energy consumption in the building stock. Build Environ 75:153–160

Tuusjärvi M, Mäenpää I, Vuori S, Eilu P, Kihlman S, Koskela S (2014) Metal mining industry in Finland—development scenarios to 2030. J Cleaner Prod (in press)

Part II
Focussing on Specific Aspects of Supply and End-Use

Methodological Significance of Temporal Granularity in Energy-Economic Models—Insights from the MARKAL/TIMES Framework

Ramachandran Kannan, Hal Turton and Evangelos Panos

Abstract One of the key attributes that distinguishes bottom-up energy modelling frameworks is the temporal depiction. In any given bottom-up model, the depiction across two dimensions—viz. model time horizon and intra-annual time resolution—has an implicit meaning for the framework and research questions to be answered. There are also tradeoffs between these two temporal dimensions in model design driven by computational resources, solver algorithm capabilities, data availability and methodological limitations. In the TIMES framework, the option to apply a higher intra-annual time resolution offers the potential to generate additional powerful insights into the electricity sector where fluctuations in supply and demand are significant, even though this feature alone is still less suitable for analyzing fully the dynamics of the sector. Nonetheless, the TIMES integrated system approaches offer additional capabilities which are not available in single-sector modeling approaches. This chapter provides a broad overview of temporal features in the MARKAL/TIMES energy modelling framework. The significance in terms of higher time resolution, along with trade-offs and benefits of an integrated system approach are discussed with a set of scenarios from the Swiss TIMES electricity and energy system models.

R. Kannan (✉) · H. Turton · E. Panos
Energy Economics Group, Laboratory for Energy Systems Analysis, Paul Scherrer Institute, 5232 Villigen, Switzerland
e-mail: kannan.ramachandran@psi.ch

H. Turton
e-mail: hal.turton@psi.ch

E. Panos
e-mail: evangelos.panos@psi.ch

G. Giannakidis et al. (eds.), *Informing Energy and Climate Policies Using Energy Systems Models*, Lecture Notes in Energy 30,
DOI 10.1007/978-3-319-16540-0_11

1 Background

Energy models have emerged as a useful methodology for energy research aimed at evaluating future energy supply options and generating insights for policy design. Energy models covering a wide range of analytical approaches have been developed for specific objectives with a predefined methodological scope and limited applications (Kannan and Turton 2013; Foley et al. 2010; Pfenninger et al. 2014). One of the key attributes that distinguishes bottom-up energy modelling frameworks is temporal representation, among others. It has two dimensions viz. time horizon and intra-annual time resolution. The time horizon is often important to explore the evolution of the energy system over multiple years/decades while the intra-annual granularity can accommodate variability in demand and supply. Both of these temporal dimensions have an implicit meaning for the framework and research questions to be answered. In addressing long-term policy goals, e.g. climate change mitigation and increasing integration of renewable energy sources, requires analytical approaches that combine a sufficiently long time horizon and an appropriate level of intra-temporal resolution. In practical terms, the tradeoffs between these two temporal dimensions are driven by a range of factors such as: computational resources; solver algorithm capabilities; data availability; and methodological limitations. Nevertheless, advances in computational power and solver algorithms have facilitated the emergence of modelling frameworks with the potential to combine a long time horizon and detailed intra-annual time resolution for representing electricity load curves. For instance, the TIMES framework has the capacity to represent any number of intra-annual timeslices and time periods. To some extent, combining these features enables analysis of the long-term evolution of energy system along with energy balancing mechanisms in a single model. We describe the application of the Swiss TIMES electricity and energy systems models, denoted as STEM-E and STEM respectively, with an hourly timeslice resolution and a century-long time horizon.

Section 2 provides a broad overview of the temporal significance in energy modelling frameworks with their strengths and shortcomings. Insights from two scenarios analysed using the STEM-E and STEM models are presented as a case study to support the discussions in Sect. 3. A summary of approaches for improving model development in MARKAL/TIMES frameworks are highlighted in Sect. 4 with conclusion in Sect. 5.

2 Temporal Dimensions in Energy Models

The following subsections describe the two temporal dimensions of bottom-up energy modelling framework.

2.1 Time Horizon

The time horizon in energy models is defined according to the number of periods represented and the number of years in each period. Frameworks have either a pre-defined period definition, a choice of fixed (equal) period lengths, or options for unequal period length. The choice of model time horizon depends on the research and policy questions to be answered. The long time horizon is critical when the research is concerned with long-term energy challenges such as resource depletion, technology spillover effects, climate change mitigation, investment cycles and evolution of long-lived infrastructure (e.g. power plants, gas pipelines, electric grid) and so on. Given that integrated energy system models are often applied to explore these issues, almost all employ a long time horizon of multiple years and decades. Clearly, uncertainties affecting the energy system increase over longer time horizons, as underlying driving factors like economic growth and technology development become less certain. In some modelling frameworks like TIMES, the long-term uncertainties can be represented while maintaining a greater focus on near- to mid-term developments, through the definition of unequal time periods in the model, describing the near term in a higher level of temporal detail.

2.2 Intra-Annual Time Split

The inter-annual time split is the number of daily, weekly and seasonal time splits within a year. A high level of intra-annual time resolution is very important when the balancing of demand and supply of time-dependent energy commodities is likely to have a large impact on energy system technology options development. For example, electricity is a highly time-dependent energy commodity because both energy (e.g. kWh) and capacity requirements (e.g. MW) must be met at every instant. In sectoral electricity modelling approaches, the intra-annual resolution is often high and covers intervals ranging from seasons to a few minutes. These approaches have been used for scheduling electricity dispatch and planning and operation of power system (e.g. Deane et al. 2014; IAEA 2001; Energy Exemplar 2014).

2.3 Trade Offs

Figure 1 illustrates two key temporal dimensions in energy model applications. Energy system models conventionally adopt a long time horizon because their primary application is to assess long-term issues (e.g. climate change mitigation, resource depletion, etc.). In most of these models (as well as in integrated assessment models), the intra-annual resolution is simplified and electricity demand is

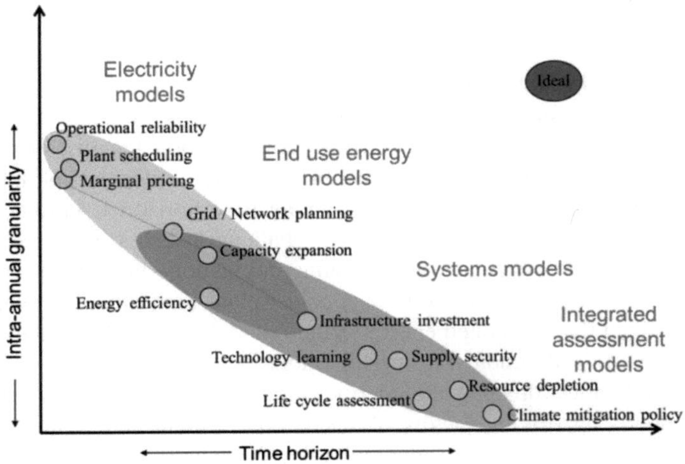

Fig. 1 Temporal representation in bottom-up energy models

often tracked by annual flows, and therefore dynamic electric peaks are not fully accounted. This intra-annual simplification is often due to the already-high level of computational complexity required in these models to represent the entire energy system and multi-year and decadal time horizons. In some energy system models like LEAP, MARKAL, TIMES, POLES and NEMS a simplified algorithm is included to represent some of the basic intra-annual features (e.g., approximate capacity demands), but they are not comparable to power sector specific models [e.g. WASP (IAEA 2001), PLEXOS (Energy Exemplar 2014)]. In comparison, sectoral energy models and electricity dispatch models often have high levels of intra-annual time resolution because they aim to represent balancing mechanisms and/or assess inter-temporal variations. However, even in sectoral (i.e., single sector) modelling approaches, intra-annual details may also need to be simplified with longer modelling time horizons because of computational and data issues (Kannan and Turton 2013).

Ideally, models of energy system development should combine a sufficiently long time horizon and an appropriate level of intra-temporal resolution for the given analysis—all in one model. In practical terms, the tradeoffs between these two temporal dimensions are driven by a range of factors, including computational resources and data availability. Importantly, these modelling tradeoffs could also affect model solutions, and thus it is important to find the right balance given the practical constraints and the specific analytical policy application. Some approaches combine two or more modelling frameworks to integrate the two temporal aspects (Chaudry et al. 2009; Johnsson 2011; Welsch et al. 2014).

2.4 MARKAL/TIMES Framework

MARKAL and TIMES have a long track record of policy and academic research. In the early application of MARKAL models, the year is divided into six timeslices using two indices: three seasonal (Winter, Summer and Intermediate) and two diurnal (Day and Night). Only electricity and heat are tracked via these six intra-annual timeslices whereas all other energy-commodities are tracked via annual flows. A "flexible timeslicing" feature was introduced in the MARKAL framework, enabling more detailed representation of variations in energy demand and supply, including operating characteristics of specific technologies. This flexible timeslicing was first implemented in the UK MARKAL model (Kannan 2011).

The TIMES framework—the successor to MARKAL—has the capacity to represent any number of intra-annual timeslices and unequal time periods, which enables a wide range of additional applications of energy system modelling. A Swiss TIMES electricity systems model (STEM-E) was developed with an hourly timeslice resolution and a century-long time horizon with unequal time periods (Kannan and Turton 2012a). The primary objective of developing STEM-E was to understand the long-term evolution of the Swiss electricity system. At the same time, it is intended to provide insights into electricity generation scheduling.

2.4.1 Swiss TIMES Electricity Model

STEM-E is a single-region model, covering the entire Swiss electricity system from resource supply to end use electricity demands. It has a time horizon of 110 years (2000–2110) in 14 unequal time periods. The time periods are specified to a length of 2 years in the short term and between five and 20 years in length in the medium and long term. The intra-annual resolution depicts four seasonal, three daily and 24 hourly timeslices. Thus the model has 288 timeslices for each year (or, technically for the milestone year in each period). Electricity demands are given exogenously and the model then selects (via the optimization process) across a range of existing and new electricity generation technologies to satisfy demands. Temporal factors affecting the generation from each of these technologies is represented across the 288 timeslices (e.g., hydro availability, solar irradiance, wind). Given the importance of electricity trade in Switzerland (including the import of cheap off-peak electricity, pumped storage, and export during other periods), electricity import and export interconnectors with neighboring markets are also modeled in STEM-E. We analysed an extensive number of electricity supply scenarios using STEM-E (Kannan and Turton 2012b). To showcase the incremental insights provided by the high intra-annual resolution, we compared the basic version of STEM-E with a second version of the model in which the 288 timeslices are aggregated[1] to a level

[1] The 288 hourly timeslices of STEM-E are aggregated into eight timeslices (two diurnal timeslices viz. Day and Night in four seasons and the representation of different days of the week is removed).

similar to most TIMES/MARKAL models (Kannan and Turton 2013). All other inputs, e.g. technology characterization, demands and cost data remain the same in both models. The objective of this aggregated model was to illustrate the differences between the solutions of the two models, and thus the potential influence of temporal factors on optimal energy technology deployment.

This comparative analysis identified the risk that models with an aggregated intra-annual time resolution may overestimate the potential contribution of large base-load power plants (Box 1), and underestimate the need for supply-demand management and storage (because the aggregation is liable to smooth peaks and troughs in supply and demand). Thus, it appears to be a significant value added by the higher intra-temporal resolution available in the TIMES framework, in providing an enhanced representation of load-balancing in the electricity system.

Box 1: Aggregated and disaggregated intra-annual time splits in STEM-E

The STEM-E model was applied to analyze the potential strengths and shortcomings of a disaggregated hourly model compared to an aggregated model. Although STEM-E is a model of the Swiss electricity sector, for this illustration we analyzed a hypothetical electricity system excluding some of the unique features in Switzerland in order to derive insights into the wider applicability of a TIMES model for dispatch modelling. We analyzed two scenarios with this hypothetical system—the *Hyp* scenario using STEM-E with the disaggregated 288 timeslices, and an otherwise identical *Hyp-A* scenario using an aggregated version of STEM-E.

The figure below shows the electricity schedule in 2048 (mid-year of period 2041–2055) on a winter day for the *Hyp* scenario (with the 288 disaggregated timeslices) compared to the aggregated *Hyp-A* scenario. The figure shows that the hourly model deploys a large capacity of flexible gas plant, whereas the aggregated model chooses a large deployment of base-load gas generation. For example, the total capacity of base-load plants in 2048 is 10.8 GW in the hourly model compared to 14 GW in the aggregated model. This occurs because the dynamic load curve in the hourly model is most cost-effectively managed with new investments in flexible (i.e. dispatchable) gas plant, whereas in the aggregated model the smaller variation in demand is more readily supplied with (cheaper) base-load gas plants and existing dam hydro plants. The flexible gas plants are scheduled only during winter weekdays and therefore have a low capacity factor. Resource cost is significantly higher in the hourly model compared to the aggregated model because of the flexible gas plant with relatively low efficiency. Electricity system cost differs ($\sim$8 % in 2048) between the two models. The higher system cost in the hourly model is also attributable to the need for additional installed capacity to manage the higher peak compared to the aggregated model. Some additional scenarios analysed with both models are discussed in Kannan and Turton (2013).

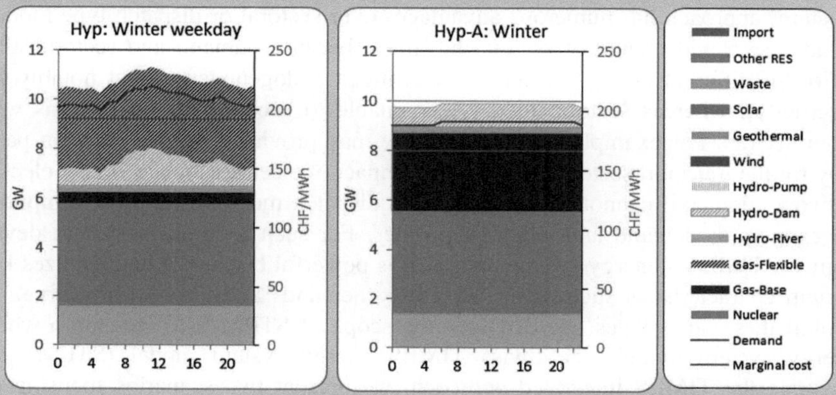

Electricity generation schedules on a winter day from both models in 2048

3 TIMES Versus Other Modelling Approaches

3.1 TIMES Versus Traditional Dispatch Models

It is evident that a higher time resolution can provide powerful insights into the generation schedule and choice of technology. However, the current TIMES framework cannot account for reliability and stochastic characteristics of the electricity system, or probable unserved energy or loads, which are typically represented in electricity dispatch models (e.g. WASP, PLEXOS). For example, in the TIMES framework, technology is assumed to be available on average throughout the year up to its availability factor. However, in real-world operation some generation capacity may be completely unavailable during planned and unplanned outages. Similarly, time required for start-up, shut-down, unit commitment, are inadequately represented.

3.2 TIMES Integrated System Approach

Although the TIMES framework does not account for some features available in typical electricity dispatch type models, its integrated system approach is complementary. For example, dispatch models represent only the electricity sector and are generally static in terms of generation stock. Thus, they are not intended for analysing dynamics and emerging energy system developments in other sectors that affect the electricity sector. TIMES's integrated system approach is suitable for analysing dynamics in other sectors that affect the electricity sector. This energy 'system' approach has numerous advantages over sectoral or dispatch type models to address a wide range of policy objectives, because demand and sectoral allocation of different energy carriers is determined endogenously (most notably for electricity), whereas sectoral models are unable to account for interactions with other sectors. For example, electric mobility may provide a decarbonisation pathway for the transport sector. However, the impact of electric vehicles on the electric network (demand) cannot be analysed with dispatch models without assumptions on exogenous demand and charging profiles. For such a complex system development, TIMES's energy system approach is powerful because it endogenizes key system characteristics such as the electricity demands and load profile/curve. To exploit these advantages, we extended the scope of STEM-E to develop a whole energy system model—the Swiss TIMES energy system model (STEM). To illustrate the TIMES integrated approach, we present two scenarios focusing on interaction between e-mobility and the electricity sector.

3.2.1 Swiss TIMES Energy System Model

The Swiss TIMES energy system model (STEM) is the full energy system—an extension to STEM-E to include all end-use energy service demands (ESDs), and calibrated to the Swiss national energy statistics (Kannan and Turton 2014). However, due to computational complexity of representing the entire energy system, the number of timeslices was aggregated to 144 (weekdays and weekends in three seasons) from the 288 timeslices in STEM-E. Figure 2 shows the temporal structure of STEM.

A selection of scenarios have been analysed using STEM and the input assumptions and results are described in Kannan and Turton (2014). In this chapter we highlight insights from two scenarios to illustrate the significance of combining the TIMES system approach with a high intra-annual time resolution. Figure 3 shows car fleet technology mix from two low-carbon scenarios, which achieve a 60 % reduction in CO_2 emissions by 2050 with and without options to invest in centralised natural gas combined cycle power plants—denoted as *LC60* and *LC60-NoCent* respectively. In the *LC60* scenario, plug-in hybrid electric vehicles (PHEVs) and full battery electric vehicles (BEVs) penetrate from 2035 and 2050 respectively. The car fleet is nearly decarbonized on a tank-to-wheel basis in 2050.

Figure 4 shows the electricity supply mix in the two scenarios. The existing nuclear power plants are gradually replaced by natural gas turbine combined cycle (GTCC) power plants (reflecting government policy precluding new investment in nuclear). By 2035, one third of the electricity supply is from GTCC plants. Renewable electricity generation contributes 22 % of the total supply by 2050, with

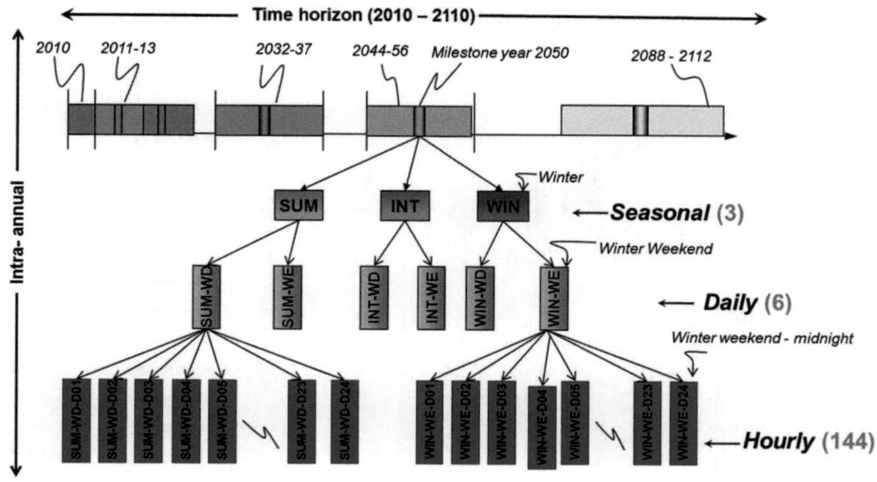

Fig. 2 Temporal depiction in STEM. *SUM* summer, *INT* intermediate, *WIN* winter, *WD* weekday, *WE* weekends

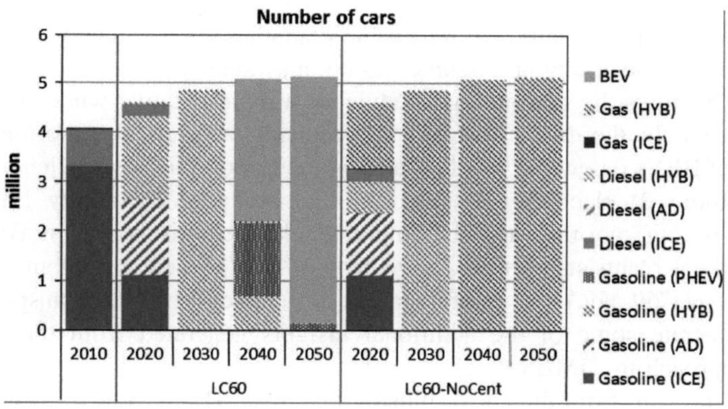

Fig. 3 Car fleet in *LC60* and *LC60-NoCent* scenarios. *BEV* Full battery electric vehicle, *HYB* hybrid vehicle, *PHEV* plug-in hybrid electric vehicles, *ICE* internal combustion engine, *AD* advanced ICE

almost all of the domestic renewable potential exploited. Despite the carbon cap in the *LC60* scenario, centralised gas power plants are deployed to facilitate increased electrification to enable decarbonisation of the car fleet (and other end-use applications, e.g. space heating through heat pumps). However, in the absences of centralized gas electricity supply (*LC60-NoCent* scenario) the car fleet switches to natural gas hybrid vehicles (Fig. 3) due to the absence of additional alternative low-

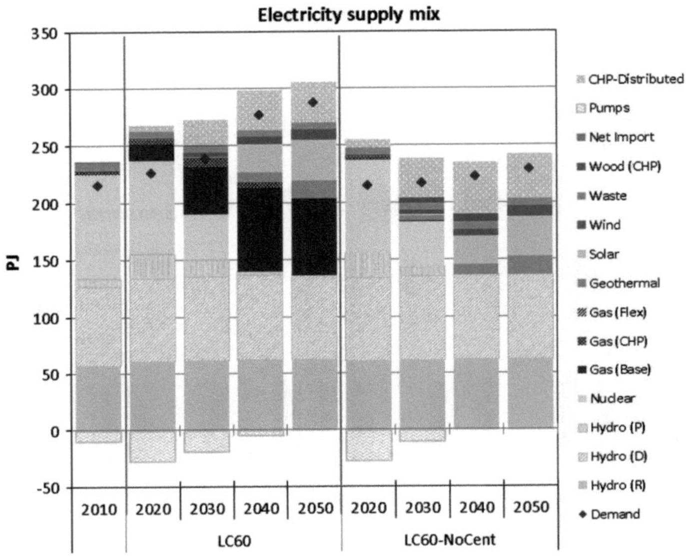

Fig. 4 Electricity supply mix in *LC60* and *LC60-NoCent* scenarios

carbon sources of electricity, i.e. renewable potentials are assumed to be finite and net imports[2] of electricity are assumed to be unavailable.

Figure 5 shows the generation schedule on a representative winter weekday in the scenarios. In the *LC60* scenario the demand peaks in the morning due to charging of BEVs (shown in purple shades in the Export plot) using cheap imported (See Footnote 2) electricity assumed in this scenario. Electricity imports are attractive during morning and the imported electricity is stored in BEVs. The centralized gas plants support the deployment of BEVs whereas without centralized gas plants (*LC60-NoCent*), natural gas is cost effective in car transport. These results illustrate some of the additional insights generated from the integrated system approach in TIMES.

As can be seen from the above illustrations from STEM, a novel feature of the integrated model with higher intra-annual time resolution is that it has the potential to provide insights into electricity demand and supply balancing mechanisms across sectors. Unlike electricity models, for which the electricity demand and profile are exogenously given, the integrated system framework, like MARKAL and TIMES, determines both the demand and its profile endogenously based on end-use technology choice, even though the demand (or user) pattern of ESDs is itself exogenously given (Kannan 2011). This feature enables the exploration of different electricity demand trajectories through demand reduction or peak shaving

[2] A self-sufficiency constraint is introduced requiring that net electricity trade is roughly in balance over the year, but the timing of electricity trade is left unconstrained.

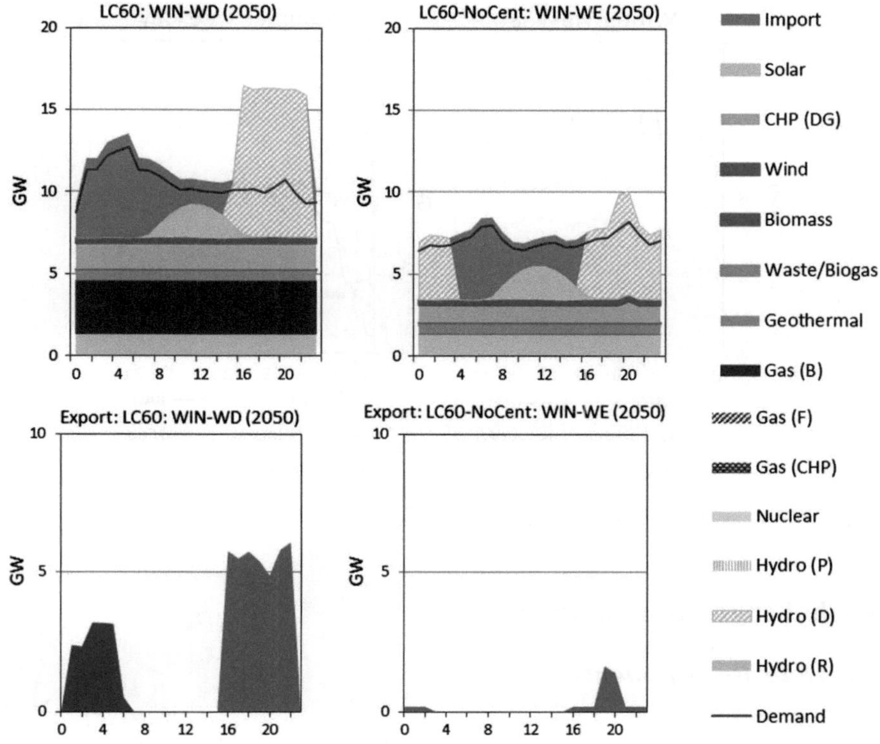

Fig. 5 Electricity generation schedule on winter weekdays

measures. To illustrate this feature, Fig. 6 shows the electricity demand profile for a set of scenarios from STEM. Depending up on technology and/or carbon constraints, the electricity demand diverges across scenarios (Kannan and Turton 2014 for more detail). Compared to a daytime peak in 2010, demands peak during early morning hours in the *LC60* and *BAU* scenarios because of charging of BEV using cheap electricity.[3] On the other hand, without centralised gas power plants (*BAU-NoCent* and *LC60-NoCent*), demand is lower because there is less electrification (neither heat pump or BEV) of end uses. This demonstrates the strength of the integrated modelling framework with flexibility to adjust electricity demands endogenously.

[3] It should be noted that the availability of cheap electricity during the early morning is an assumption applied in the analysis (based on historical electricity import prices), which may change if the demand profiles in electricity trading partners were to vary substantially (for example, as a result of charging of BEVs).

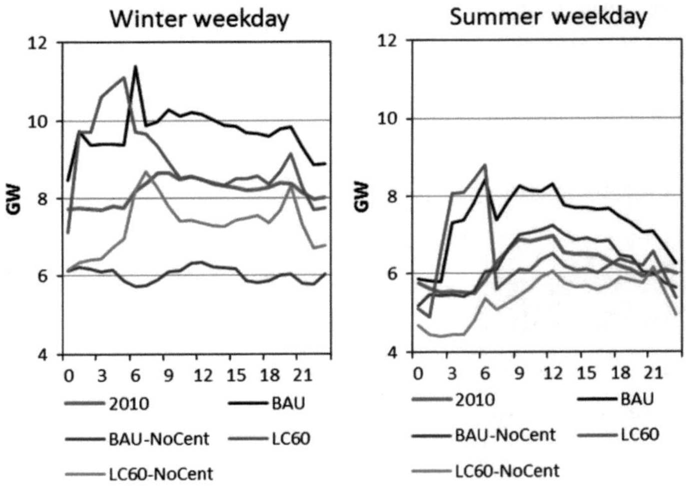

Fig. 6 Electricity demand profiles of 2050

4 Challenges and Solutions

4.1 Data Requirements

Clearly, the high intra-annual resolution in STEM is demanding in terms of data requirements—e.g. performance of demand technologies, load profile of ESDs, resource availability, etc. at the same resolution as that of the intra-annual timeslices. Such data are not commonly available in many countries, meaning that a large number of assumptions and approximations may be needed, which risks undermining the reliability of the detailed intertemporal model. Therefore, the availability of input data is one of the key determinants in choosing an appropriate intra-annual resolution. If the data availability is poor or subject to high uncertainty, an aggregated model could be a more suitable choice. Again, the choice of timeslices also depends on the energy system in question, and the policy and research applications of interest. For some applications, an aggregated model can still provide some robust insights (Kannan and Turton 2013).

4.2 Computational Complexity

The large number of timeslices considerably increases computational resource requirements. Therefore, introducing a high time resolution in a model with an already large number of equations and variables requires careful choice of timeslices and use of an appropriate solver; and involves trade-offs in terms of

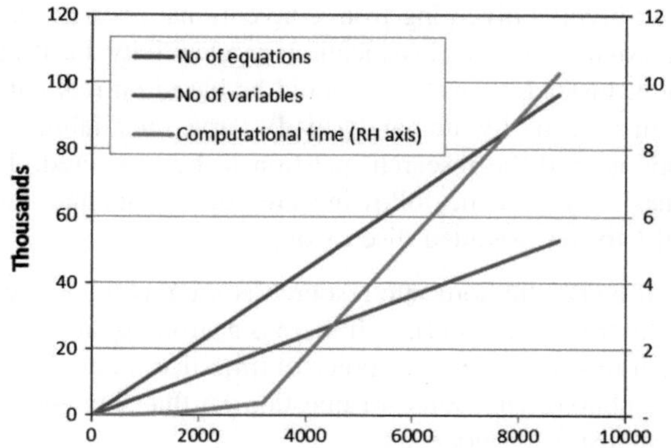

Fig. 7 Timeslice versus matrix size and computational time in TIMES framework

representing other features such as lumpy investment or endogenous technology learning. Figure 7 shows some simple correlations between the number of timeslices and the number of variables and equations in a TIMES framework. It is based on a highly simplified reference energy system with one typical process and two commodities fully characterised for one period; variables and equations relevant for storage, inter-regional exchange, user constraints and vintage are not generated and have been excluded. The model matrix size grows approximately linearly with number of timeslices, but computational time[4] is increasing nearly exponential.

The computational complexity is not only limited to the solution time, but memory and numerical problems may also arise. To reduce computational time in linear programming (LP) formulations, interior point algorithms such as CPLEX/Barrier can be used (Wright 2004; Dantzig and Thapa 2003) at the expense of memory.[5]

4.3 Alternative Approaches

To address the computational and data availability issues, a number of alternatives are possible to approximate some elements of a more detailed load curve in a conventional energy system model to improve electricity sector depiction. Most of

[4] The computational time includes both model generation and solution time using CPLEX solver in 8-cores Intel processor with 24 GB RAM.

[5] For example, some specific CPLEX/Barrier options for improving the performance of the algorithm includes *BarColz*, *BarEpComp*, *BarOrder*, *BarStartAlg*, etc. However, the use of CPLEX/Barrier requires large memory, which can be addressed with solver options like *MemoryEmphasis*, *Names*, *WorkMem* to conserve memory (GAMS 2014). Numerical difficulties can occur during the optimisation if large LP problems are ill-defined due to large differences in the magnitude of coefficients in an equation. In such a case, the solver reports the problem as unscaled infeasibility. This can be diagnosed by *GAMSCHK* option described in Bruce (2013) and accordingly input data has to be adjusted to avoid large numerical differences in coefficients.

these involve diverging from conventional approaches of defining timeslices based on usual seasonal classification or electricity tariff-based definitions of day and night. Instead, timeslicing should be based on real data on intertemporal variations in the electricity demand (load) curve; availability of energy resource supply options; and the research question to be answered. There is no rule of thumb in timeslicing, but the following are some guidelines (also see Kannan and Turton 2013 for an extended discussion).

- If a specific domestic resource is seen as the key electricity supply option (e.g. hydro, solar, wind), or if there is a strong policy interest on a specific technology or resource, then the choice of timeslices could be based on characteristics of the technology/resource in question so that their operational characteristic can be realistically modelled.
- When the number of intra-annual timeslice is small, this leads to an averaging of capacity demands and thus underestimates the real demand peak. This can be partly addressed by defining the timeslices in a way that ensures a better representation of the peak, such as with:
  - An uneven seasonal time split to capture some of the seasonal variations in demand and/or resource supply.
  - A non-uniform diurnal time split. For example, a time split that defines 'day' according to the peaking hours in each season could be chosen, or according to daylight hours if solar PV has a significant potential.
- An alternative to ensure the impact of large variations in demand is represented in the choice of base-load and dispatchable generation technology, is to introduce a share constraint for base-load and dispatchable technologies. This could be determined from the highest and lowest electricity demand hours in each season. However, any such constraint could have negative implications for future years.
- Similarly, a non-conventional electricity reserve margin (Kannan 2011) could be applied based on the differences between the average capacity demand and hourly peak demand. This reserve margin would need to be larger than prevailing rule-of-thumb values used by electric utilities to cover the instantaneous peak and spinning reserves. However, while this approach may ensure a more appropriate representation of total capacity requirements, it does not represent generation and dispatch at the peak.
- In some countries, weekly (weekdays vs. weekends) demand variations are more significant than seasonal variation (e.g., in tropical countries) which imply additional limitations on the operation of large base-load plants (operational control in case of nuclear plants and part load efficiency penalty for fossil fuel plants). In such cases, a time split can be applied at the weekly level.
- Insofar as an hourly TIMES model can represent some features of electricity dispatch model, it cannot fully replace an electricity dispatch model. Therefore approaches have been explored to soft-link integrated energy system model with

aggregated timeslices and detail electricity model to generate issues specific to the electricity system such as reliability and stochastic characteristic of technologies (Chaudry et al. 2009; Deane et al. 2014; Welsch et al. 2014).

5 Conclusions

We used the TIMES framework to develop models of the Swiss electricity and energy systems combining detailed technology pathways, an hourly load curve and a long model horizon. The long time horizon facilitates the analysis of long-term goals and challenges, and accounts for the long lifetimes of energy-related capital infrastructure. The high level of intra annual detail in this model provides richer insights into the operational schedule of power plants. Despite the computational and data intensity of this model, the higher time resolution leads to solutions that appear to be more realistic from a technical and 'real-world' standpoint compared to an equivalent aggregated intra-annual model. Therefore, there are considerable benefits in investing in data collection and exploiting developments in computational and solver power. Nonetheless, there is no one-size-fits-all approach for intra-annual timeslicing. The ideal number of timeslices to represent in a model depends on energy system characteristics, the research question to be answered and, most importantly, the availability of data at the timeslice level. TIMES models can represent some of the features of electricity dispatch, but cannot fully replace such models, and instead can be viewed as providing complementary insights and inputs. However, the TIMES framework's integrated system approach and flexible temporal depictions are equally important for the application of this framework in supporting policy and other decision makers; and exploring different strategies for the long-term development of the energy and electricity systems.

References

Bruce AM (2013) McCarl expanded GAMS user guide. http://www.gams.com/mccarl/mccarlhtml/gams_user_guide_2005.htm

Chaudry M, Dougamas A, Ekins P, Kannan R, Shakoor A, Skea J, Strbac G, Wang X (2009) A resilient UK energy system: building in resilience, UKERC Research Report. http://www.ukerc.ac.uk/support/tiki-download_file.php?fileId=618

Dantzig GB, Thapa MN (2003) Linear programming 2: theory and extensions. Springer, New York

Deane JP, Drayton G, Ó Gallachóir BP (2014) The impact of sub-hourly modelling in power systems with significant levels of renewable generation. Appl Energy 113:152–158

Energy Exemplar (2014) PLEXOS for power systems. http://www.energyexemplar.com

Foley AM, Ó Gallachóir BP, Hur J, Baldick R, McKeogh EJ (2010) A strategic review of electricity systems models. Energy 35(12):4522–4530

GAMS (2014) CPLEX solver manual

IAEA (2001) Wien automatic system planning (WASP) package—a computer code for power generating system expansion planning. International Atomic Energy Agency, Vienna

Johnsson F (2011) Methods and models used in the project used in the project pathways to sustainable European energy systems, alliance for global sustainability. http://www.energy-pathways.org/pdf/Metod_reportJan2011.pdf

Kannan R (2011) The development and application of a temporal MARKAL energy system model using flexible time slicing. Appl Energy 88(6):2261–2272

Kannan R, Turton H (2012a) Documentation on the development of the swiss TIMES electricity model (STEM-E), PSI Bericht 11-03. Paul Scherrer Institute, Switzerland. http://www.psi.ch/eem/PublicationsTabelle/2011_Kannan_STEME.pdf

Kannan R, Turton H (2012b) Cost of ad-hoc nuclear policy uncertainties in the evolution of the Swiss electricity system. Energy Policy 50:391–406

Kannan R, Turton H (2013) A long-term electricity dispatch model with the TIMES framework. Environ Model Assess 18(3):325–343

Kannan R, Turton H (2014) Switzerland energy transition scenarios—development and application of the swiss TIMES energy system model (STEM). Final Report to the Swiss Federal Office of Energy, Bern. http://www.psi.ch/eem/PublicationsTabelle/2014-STEM-PSI-Bericht-14-06.pdf

Pfenninger S, Hawkes A, Keirstead J (2014) Energy system modeling for twenty-first century energy challenges. Renew Sustain Energy Rev 33:74–86

Welsch M, Deane P, Howells M, Ó Gallachóir B, Rogan F, Bazilian M (2014) Incorporating flexibility requirements into long-term energy system models—a case study on high levels of renewable electricity penetration in Ireland. Appl Energy 135:600–615

Wright MH (2004) The interior-point revolution in optimization: history, recent developments, and lasting consequences. Bull Am Math Soc 42(1):39–56

Improved Representation of the European Power Grid in Long Term Energy System Models: Case Study of JRC-EU-TIMES

Wouter Nijs, Sofia Simoes, Alessandra Sgobbi, Pablo Ruiz-Castello, Christian Thiel, George Giannakidis, John Mantzaris, Kostas Tigas, Dionisios Dimitroulas, Pavlos Georgilakis and Costas Vournas

Abstract This chapter describes a methodology to integrate DC power flow modeling and N − 1 security into JRC-EU-TIMES, a multiregional TIMES energy system model. It improves the accuracy of modeling cross-border transmission expansion especially for energy systems with higher penetration of renewable energy sources (RES). We describe three grid representations with increasing accuracy of modeling power flow constraints: (1) basic trade flow without DC power flow, (2) DC power flow with fixed line characteristics and (3) DC power flow with a discretization algorithm, endogenous grid characteristics and N − 1 contingency analysis. The last approach uses the newly developed Integrated

The views expressed are purely those of the authors and may not in any circumstances be regarded as stating an official position of the European Commission.

W. Nijs (✉) · S. Simoes · A. Sgobbi · P. Ruiz-Castello · C. Thiel
European Commission—Joint Research Centre—Institute for Energy and Transport, Petten, The Netherlands
e-mail: wouter.nijs@ec.europa.eu

S. Simoes
e-mail: sofia.simoes@ec.europa.eu

A. Sgobbi
e-mail: alessandra.sgobbi@ec.europa.eu

P. Ruiz-Castello
e-mail: pablo.ruiz-castello@ec.europa.eu

C. Thiel
e-mail: christian.thiel@ec.europa.eu

G. Giannakidis · J. Mantzaris · K. Tigas
Centre for Renewable Energy Sources and Saving (CRES), Athens, Greece
e-mail: ggian@cres.gr

J. Mantzaris
e-mail: jmantzaris@cres.gr

K. Tigas
e-mail: ktigas@cres.gr

G. Giannakidis et al. (eds.), *Informing Energy and Climate Policies Using Energy Systems Models*, Lecture Notes in Energy 30,
DOI 10.1007/978-3-319-16540-0_12

TIMES–NEPLAN Software (ITNS) that couples JRC-EU-TIMES energy system modeling with NEPLAN-based electricity grid modeling. To evaluate the improvement of the JRC-EU-TIMES modeling mechanisms, the three grid representations are compared. We conclude that cross border transmission expansion is cost efficient regardless of the grid representation. The impact of power flow constraints is limited for the analyzed case study under the assumption of perfect markets. However, integrating these constraints is leading to slightly higher cross-border capacities for most countries mainly in periods with limited availability of variable renewable electricity. This occurs when grid extensions and peaking power in some strategic countries are more competitive than local peaking power for each country. This is possible without a substantial increase in model running time.

1 Introduction

The combined generation and transmission expansion planning (CGTEP), also called composite or coordinated, or integrated resource planning, is a very complex non-linear and non-convex optimization problem (El-Debeiky and Hasanien 2000; Alvarez Lopez et al. 2007; Roh et al. 2007; Tor et al. 2008; Sepasian et al. 2009; Bent et al. 2011; Hemmati et al. 2013b). The large integration of renewable energy sources (RES) into modern power systems has made the CGTEP problem even more challenging, because the greatly increased uncertainties introduced often require new transmission lines in order to maintain a satisfactory level of power system security and adequacy (Contaxi et al. 2012; Orfanos et al. 2013). CGTEP is typically split into generation expansion planning (GEP) (Kabouris and Contaxis 1991; Zhu and Chow 1997; International Atomic Energy Agency 2001; Chuang et al. 2001) and transmission expansion planning (TEP) (Romero et al. 2002; Georgilakis 2010; Hemmati et al. 2013a) to improve computational tractability. Comprehensive reviews on CGTEP, GEP, and TEP can be found in Zhu and Chow (1997), Hemmati et al. (2013a, b), respectively. However, in planning for RES, the complete decoupling of the two problems is not necessarily the best approach. The potential to generate energy is highly dependent on where the generators are built and the distances to connect RES to existing systems bring the relative costs of transmission and generation closer in scale.

D. Dimitroulas · P. Georgilakis · C. Vournas
National Technical University of Athens (NTUA), Athens, Greece
e-mail: ddimitr@power.ece.ntua.gr

P. Georgilakis
e-mail: pgeorg@power.ece.ntua.gr

C. Vournas
e-mail: vournas@power.ece.ntua.gr

Examples of a coupling between energy model and electrical network model can be found in UKERC (2009), REALISEGRID (2010), Sakellaridis et al. (2011), Deane et al. (2012), Hamasaki (2014). More specifically, the MARKAL-MED energy model is combined with the WASP GEP (International Atomic Energy Agency 2001) model and a combined gas and electricity network model in UKERC (2009) in order to assess how the UK system can move to a secure and low-carbon energy system over the period to 2050. The combined use of MARKAL, WASP and Cost (Stochastic modeling tool) for the analysis of the electricity system under high RES penetration is presented in Sakellaridis et al. (2011). The use of TIMES and Stochastic Analysis for the analysis of the electricity system under high RES penetration is also presented in Sakellaridis et al. (2011). TIMES is used to model the energy system and a tool is developed for planning cross-border transmission capacity expansion in REALISEGRID (2010). Geographical information system (GIS) gathered renewable energy potential data are coupled with a multiregional TIMES energy system model to study the effect of feed-in tariff (FIT) in the development of wind turbines for the Japanese electricity system (Hamasaki 2014). A soft-linking methodology that employs detailed simulation outputs from a dedicated power systems model to gain insights and understanding of the generation electricity plant portfolio results for the electricity sector from a separate energy systems model is presented in Deane et al. (2012).

The previous analysis has shown that there is an open challenge to establish a link between an energy system model and an electricity network model. This challenge is even bigger, if the objective is to create a link between a well-established energy model and a widely used network analysis model. The work presented in this chapter is designed so as to fill the above mentioned gap, because the objective is to provide interfaces for the integration of TIMES-based energy system modeling with NEPLAN electricity grid modeling.

The TIMES energy system model is a long-term energy planning model that finds the least-cost solution of the evolution of a specific energy system in terms of time resolution and of a Reference Energy System simulating the real energy system (Loulou et al. 2005). TIMES is a bottom-up, partial equilibrium energy model based on maximizing total societal surplus. Main inputs in TIMES are the evolution of the economy resulting in scenarios of useful energy demand, a forecast of international fuel prices and technology roadmaps including specific costs and efficiencies for a time period of several decades.

The TIMES model does not consider in detail the analysis of the electrical power system. It includes a rather elementary approach for dispatching generation, use of transmission and integration of non-dispatchable renewable generation. As a result, the optimal technology mix computed by TIMES may not be optimal when considering the geographically specific transmission grid investments resulting from that technology mix. In addition, renewable investments economic analysis should normally include costs related to transmission grid expansions necessary for penetration in geographical areas with a high potential of renewables, and costs related to balancing measures required due to variations of renewable generation, such as pumped storage plants, gas turbines.

NEPLAN is a well-established software tool to analyze, plan, optimize and simulate electrical, water, gas and district heating networks (BCP Busarello+Cott +Partner Inc. 2014). The NEPLAN Programming Library (NPL) allows to access NEPLAN data and calculation algorithms through a C/C++ written program (BCP Busarello+Cott+Partner Inc. 2014). NPL allows developing user defined algorithms.

This chapter proposes a methodology for the integration of DC power flow modeling into a multiregional TIMES energy model. More specifically, the chapter proposes an Integrated TIMES–NEPLAN Software (ITNS) that provides interfaces for the integration of TIMES-based energy system modeling with NEPLAN-based electricity grid modeling. Among others, the ITNS allows more accurate estimation of maximum permissible penetration of RES in a system.

The ITNS incorporates economical and technical parameters of transmission grid expansion planning to the solution of TIMES and modifies its solution in order to include transmission line investment costs. These parameters are either incorporated in the TIMES solver directly or are incorporated through available loading coefficients of the transmission lines. In this sense, constraints and costs imposed by transmission system operators when determining an expansion plan of the transmission grid are taken into account and affect the generation expansion planning proposed by TIMES. Thus, the solution calculated through ITNS is more realistic than the basic TIMES solution as it incorporates costs of transmission investments, which cannot be evaluated otherwise, since network reinforcements depend on the generation expansion plan. Reversely, cost of these reinforcements should be weighed against a more expensive dispatching that demands fewer investments in transmission network. This interaction may be modeled only with an integrated approach.

The ITNS software incorporates the N − 1 security criterion[1] to the expansion planning determined by TIMES. Although the optimality of the solution is not guaranteed, the solution exported by ITNS can be considered at least near-optimal, thanks to an iterative optimization algorithm, which is the core innovation of ITNS. Major constraints are incorporated in the objective function, while other constraints can be accounted for by a fine tuning and do not affect significantly the TIMES solution. The ITNS and its optimization algorithm have been fully adopted by EU-JRC within the JRC-EU-TIMES model. Application results of JRC-EU-TIMES indicate the value and the usefulness of the proposed approach.

To evaluate the improvement of the JRC-EU-TIMES modeling mechanisms, three grid representations are compared in scenarios with free and fixed transmission expansion.

[1] The N − 1 criterion for system operation requires that the system is able to tolerate the outage of any one component (line, generator, transformer) without disruption of the operation of the electrical system.

2 Methodology

2.1 General Description of the JRC-EU-TIMES Model

The JRC-EU-TIMES model represents the EU28 energy system plus Switzerland, Iceland and Norway (hereafter EU28+) from 2005 to 2050, where each country is modeled as a single region. Each year is divided into twelve (12) time-slices that represent an average of day, night and peak demand for every one of the four seasons of the year.

The materials and energy demand projections used in JRC-EU-TIMES for each country are differentiated by economic sector and end-use energy service, using as a starting point historical data of 2005 and macroeconomic projections from the GEM-E3 model and in line with the values considered in the EU Energy Roadmap 2050 reference scenario. From 2005 till 2050 the exogenous useful energy services demand grows by 32 % in agriculture, 56 % in commercial buildings, 28 % in other industry, 24 % in passenger mobility and almost doubles (97 %) in freight mobility. On the other hand, the exogenous useful energy services demand for residential buildings is 12 % lower in 2050 than in 2005 due to the assumptions on energy efficiency improvements in buildings.

Energy consumption data from Eurostat is used to derive country and sector-specific energy balances, which determine the characterization of energy technology profiles for supply and demand technologies in the base year. Beyond the base year, new energy supply and demand technologies are compiled in an extensive database with detailed technical and economic characteristics. The model considers power plants in operation and under construction as well as plants to be decommissioned and built, allocating a specific vintage to each electricity generation technology. Cumulative CO_2 storage capacity is derived from the GEOCAPACITY research project,[2] and does not include national policy decisions restricting storage possibilities, such as only storing in offshore sites, or no storage. We consider country-specific wind and solar annual availability profiles for an average year for the 12 modeled time-slices.

Regarding electricity grids, in its basic configuration, JRC-EU-TIMES considers both import/export processes regarding the existing infrastructures (capacity and flows) and possible new investments both within EU28+ and with the rest of the world. In the basic JRC-EU-TIMES configuration there are three levels of electricity voltage and conversion between levels, while no DC power flow is considered. Transmission grids have an associated cost of in euros/kW based on the electricity transport tariff for 2011 for each country from Eurostat.

In this section as well as in Sect. 2.2 certain procedures of the methodology will be presented. The overall methodology will be presented in Sect. 2.3.

[2] http://www.geology.cz/geocapacity.

2.2 *Incorporating DC Power Flow Equations and Power Flow Scenarios Formulation*

2.2.1 DC Power Flow Equations into TIMES and Regional Interconnection Costs

A special version of the TIMES model generator developed by CRES, VTT, NTUA and JRC incorporates Power Flow Analysis into the calculations of TIMES. This version is applicable to all TIMES models and was also implemented in JRC-EU-TIMES. In particular, a linear (DC) power flow algorithm, which is a linearized approach of the Power Flow problem and calculates power flows of a rather aggregated transmission grid of the studied system, was incorporated into TIMES. The grid used for the power flow analysis is not necessarily identical to the region split used in a multiregional TIMES model. For example, Fig. 1 presents a simplified network where R1–R4 represent the regions in which the energy system is split in the TIMES model. As it can be seen, each region of TIMES may include several network nodes.

Trade (transactions between regions) and internal flows within a region should comply with the restrictions imposed by network capacity. The equations to calculate the power flow in each power line of the network are Eqs. 1 and 2 (Seifi and Sepasian 2011).

For every bus (node) i:

$$P_{G,i} - P_{L,i} = P_{T,i} \quad i = 1, \ldots, N \tag{1}$$

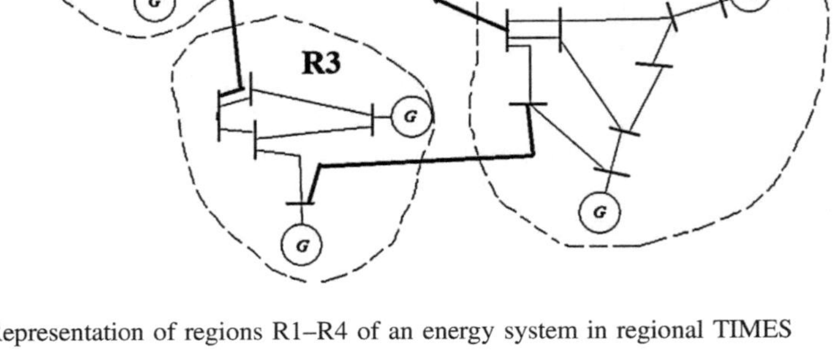

Fig. 1 Representation of regions R1–R4 of an energy system in regional TIMES

and

$$P_{T,i} = \sum_{j=1}^{M} P_{flow,ij} = \sum_{j=1}^{M} B_{ij} \cdot \left(\delta_i - \delta_j\right) \quad i = 1, \ldots, N \tag{2}$$

where

N	the total number of nodes
M	the number of branches that are connected with node i,
$P_{G,i}$	active power injected into node i by generators
$P_{L,i}$	active power withdrawn in node i by loads
$P_{T,i}$	total active power injected into node i
P_{flowij}	branch active power flow between nodes i and j
B_{ij}	susceptance of the branch connecting nodes i and j
δ_i	voltage phase angle of node i with respect to a reference angle

Rewriting the nodal active power balance equations, in matrix notation:

$$[B_r] \cdot [\delta] = [P_T] \tag{3}$$

where

B_r is the reduced admittance matrix by the line and column corresponding to the slack bus—(N − 1) × (N − 1),

δ is the nodal voltage angle vector (except for slack bus)—1 × (N − 1)

In addition, the branch power flow equation is

$$\left[\tilde{B}\right] \cdot [\delta] = [P_{flow}] \tag{4}$$

where

P_{flow} is the matrix of power flows in every power line,

$\tilde{B}$ being the flow admittance matrix—M × N

$$[P_{flow}] = \left[\tilde{B}\right] \cdot [B_r]^{-1} [P_T] \tag{5}$$

where

P_{flow} is the power flow in every power line,

P_T is the power injection in every bus except for the slack bus—(N − 1) × 1.

Regional interconnection costs are given as exogenous input by the user, in terms of cost per unit of power transmission capacity (euros/MW). It should be noted that investments calculated by TIMES are indicative as they do not correspond to actual line types, as it will be explained in detail in the next sections.

2.2.2 Allocation of Additional Capacity, Generation and Demand

The solution of TIMES results in the total quantity (in terms of energy) of generation and demand of electricity for each type of generation technology (CCNG, wind, PV, etc.) or demand category (industry, households, etc.) for each time slice modelled. In addition TIMES results define the capacity of electricity production plants in every region for every generation technology. Based on these information, power flow scenarios are formed for each time slice.

First of all energy quantities (generation and demand) are translated into power, based on the duration of each time slice. The following step is the allocation of these quantities to the grid nodes. As it is referred in Sect. 2.2.1 multiple nodes may be included in a single region. Thus, the aggregated quantities (generation, demand and capacity of power plants) should be allocated to the existing nodes for every region. The allocation of generation and demand can be performed based on a set of criteria:

- The first is to use a predefined distribution scheme based on statistical data, for the nodes of each region. For example, if the solution of TIMES show industrial load to increase in a region, there should be a predefined distribution of industrial load among the region's nodes. Therefore, certain nodes near industrial areas will undertake the additional loads, while others in urban or mountainous areas will not. This approach is used in order to allocate electricity demand.
  The same criterion is also used in allocating the capacity of distributed generation plants. This procedure is also based on statistical data derived from suitable sites for expansion of distributed plants ensuring that development of new distributed power plants (e.g. wind, solar or CHP) will take place in sites with high RES or CHP potential.
- The second criterion is applied for (non-distributed) generation expansion allocation and is to mark predetermined sites for new plants. This applies mostly to conventional plants, for which sites for a new power plant of a certain type (e.g. coal, nuclear) inside a region can easily be determined in advance.

2.2.3 Synchronous and Asynchronous Connections

Before analyzing synchronous and asynchronous connections, it is necessary to define the notion of a corridor. In a transmission network, multiple circuits may link the same network nodes. In the current analysis, every group of such circuits is merged and substituted by one equivalent line, which is called "a corridor". In case that the circuits of a corridor operate at different voltage levels, transformers at both ends of the circuit together with the circuit are substituted with an equivalent admittance.

Depending on the type, a connection may be synchronous (AC connections) or asynchronous (DC connections). Asynchronous connections are capable of controlling power flow due to the converter stations that exist at both ends of the line. DC connections are usually used in interconnections between countries or isolated areas. Since power flow is controlled, the flows in asynchronous connections are considered in TIMES as normal trade processes. In the power flow problem, asynchronous lines are omitted from the network and substituted with a positive power injection in one end and an equal negative power injection in the other end of the line.

Power injection at synchronous connections is not controlled. Power flow in these lines is calculated through DC power flow equations, based on the network admittance matrix. However, in the realization of the algorithm a third category of lines arises, which are radial connections. Radial connection is a connection between two nodes, that if it is opened, one node becomes isolated from the rest of the power grid. In such connections, the flow depends only on positive or negative injections of power from generation and load demand. Thus, the excess of production or load of a radially connected node equals the power flow in the connection line. These circuits are considered as DC connections (predefined power flow).

In Fig. 2, a simplified network of Western Europe is shown as an example of the method that has been used with the JRC-EU-TIMES model. United Kingdom (UK) and Ireland (IR) are connected through DC lines, while Spain (ES) and Portugal (PT) are radially connected through AC lines.

The corridor PT-ES is radial and therefore flow in this corridor is determined by the excess or the shortage of power generation comparing to the demand in nodes of PT and ES. Asynchronous and radial connections have been modeled with the traditional trade approach and synchronous with the flow based methodology developed.

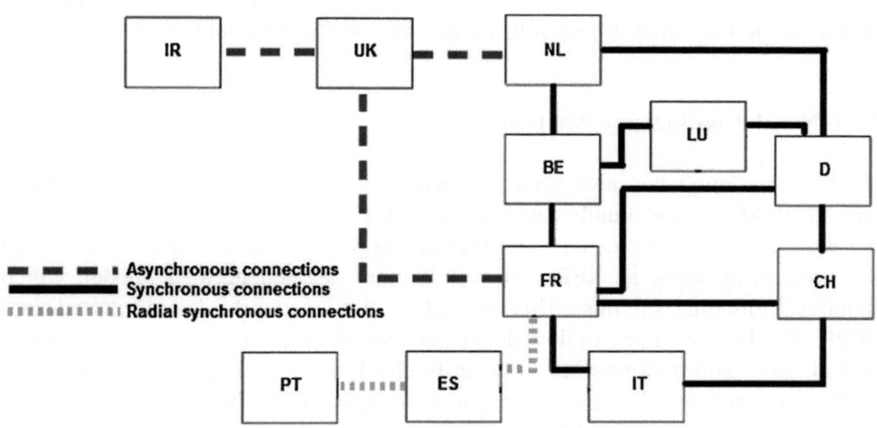

Fig. 2 Simplified network

2.3 Incorporating N − 1 Security Constraints Integrating TIMES with NEPLAN

Incorporating N − 1 security constraints in TIMES directly is not possible as this would make the problem non-linear. Therefore, N − 1 security analysis is performed indirectly using a usability coefficient (ε) which determines the acceptable loading of a corridor. The basic concept is that through this coefficient it is possible to limit the loading of a corridor in N (normal) state—which is modeled in TIMES through DC power flow—so as to avoid overloading in N − 1 (emergency) conditions. In particular, incorporation of the N − 1 security constraint is being performed using an iterative method through which the value of the usability coefficient (ε) is determined. This coefficient expresses the percentage of acceptable loading for a certain corridor in N state in order to fulfill N − 1 criterion. This acceptable loading depends on the characteristics of the corridor, as well as on the surrounding network. The initial value of the usability coefficient is determined by Eq. 6:

$$\varepsilon_{ij} = \begin{cases} \dfrac{\min\left\{\sum_{n_{ij}-1} \mathrm{P}_{\mathrm{k}}^{\mathrm{max}}\right\}}{\sum_{n_{ij}} \mathrm{P}_{\mathrm{k}}^{\mathrm{max}}}, & \text{if} \quad n_{ij} > 1 \\ 0.9, & \text{if} \quad n_{ij} = 1 \end{cases} \tag{6}$$

where $\mathrm{P}_{\mathrm{k}}^{\mathrm{max}}$ is the transfer capacity of circuit k of corridor ij and n_{ij} is the number of circuits constituting corridor ij.

Equation 6 expresses the acceptable loading of a corridor so that after a trip of the circuit with the maximum transfer capacity, the corridor will not be overloaded. In other words, by applying this criterion we assure that if power flows do not change after a circuit trip, the loading of corridor ij will be within predefined limits. As it is well known, a modification of a network, such as a circuit trip, modifies all power flows in the network. Yet, this is an approximate way of determining the initial value of the usability coefficient ε. For corridors that consist of only one circuit, the initial value of usability coefficient ε is taken equal to 0.9.

2.3.1 N − 1 Contingency Analysis

The N − 1 contingency analysis is performed through an iterative procedure that uses NEPLAN and eventually calculates usability coefficients (ε). As it is described in Sect. 2.2 for every time slice a corresponding power flow scenario is formulated and used as an input in NEPLAN with a more detailed network model, which includes individual circuits. This procedure uses network data imported into NEPLAN, along with power flow data calculated through the procedures described in Sect. 2.2.2 and performs N − 1 security check using NEPLAN functions.

The overloading of a circuit computed through NEPLAN has to be translated into a restriction for the loading of the corresponding corridor, in order to be used by TIMES (usability coefficient). Through this procedure a correction factor of the initial value of usability coefficient is calculated.

Suppose that for the m contingency (i.e., the contingency of circuit m), circuit k gets overloaded. The overload indicator L_{km} is then computed as follows (Eq. 7):

$$L_{km} = \begin{cases} \frac{P_{km}}{P_k^{\max}}, & \text{if} \quad P_{km} \geq P_k^{\max} \\ 0, & \text{if} \quad P_{km} < P_{km}^{\max} \end{cases} \quad (7)$$

where

L_{km} overloading indicator of circuit k under the contingency of circuit m
P_{km} loading of circuit k under the contingency of circuit m
P_k^{max} upper limit of loading (capacity) of circuit k

For each overloaded circuit and for each contingency, we compute the indicators I_m and J_k as follows (Eqs. 8 and 9):

$$I_m = \sum_{k=1}^{n_{lines}} L_{km} \quad (8)$$

$$J_k = \sum_{m=1}^{n_{cont}} L_{km} \quad (9)$$

where

n_{lines}, n_{cont} total number of circuits and total number of contingencies, respectively.

In practice, indicator I_m is the total overloading that appears in all circuits under contingency m. Similarly, indicator J_k is the total overloading of circuit k under all contingencies.

The overloading of circuit j is computed by selecting the maximum value of J and the value of the maximum J as follows (Eq. 10):

$$J_j = \max_k \{J_k\} \quad (10)$$

We compute the contingency i with the maximum I and the value of the maximum I as follows (Eq. 11):

$$I_i = \max_m \{I_m\} \quad (11)$$

Using these two parameters, we calculate the value of the correction factor K_c for each corridor. The correction factor K_c for each corridor indicates the required reduction of the value of usability coefficient ε according to the N − 1 security analysis results. In other words, the correction factor K_c reduces the acceptable loading of a corridor in case it is overloaded when a contingency occurs.

There are two cases of correction requirements:

Case 1: $J_j \geq I_i$, which means that circuit j (belonging to corridor c) has to be reinforced. In this case, the value of K_c for the corridor c is computed as follows (Eq. 12):

$$\mathrm{K_c} = \frac{1}{\mathrm{L_{ji}}} = \frac{1}{\max\limits_{\mathrm{m}} \{\mathrm{L_{jm}}\}} \tag{12}$$

$$L_{ji} = \max_{m}\{L_{jm}\} = \max\{L_{j1}, L_{j2}, \ldots, L_{ji}, \ldots, L_{jn_{cont}}\} \tag{13}$$

where L_{ji} denotes the overloading of circuit j during the contingency i.

Case 2: $J_j < I_i$, which means that in this case we have to avoid contingency i, i.e., we have to reinforce the corridor c in which the circuit i belongs, the outage of which results in the contingency i. In this case, in order to force TIMES to add a new circuit in the corridor c, the value of K for corridor c is defined as (Eq. 14):

$$\mathrm{K_c} = 0.5 \tag{14}$$

The new value of the usability coefficient is calculated through Eq. 15:

$$\varepsilon_{ij}^{new} = K_{ij}\varepsilon_{ij}^{old} \tag{15}$$

2.3.2 Discretization of Line Investments

Corridor reinforcements indicated by the TIMES model solution is a continuous variable (since TIMES gives a linear programming solution). A mixed integer programming solution with discrete investments can be calculated, however this will considerably increase the computational time. Since investment costs depend on the types of circuits constructed or upgraded, there is a need for a discretization algorithm, which rationalizes the reinforcements and associated investments indicated by the TIMES solution.

As mentioned in Sect. 2.2.3, every corridor consists of several circuits of different capacities. In the methodology used it is assumed that each corridor may be reinforced by a predefined type of circuit, based on certain criteria (e.g. topological features of transmission grid). In other words, the characteristics of each corridor indicate acceptable reinforcements and investments. If the additional capacity requirement calculated from the TIMES solution exceeds a predefined percentage of the capacity of the predefined reinforcement, the investment is approved by the algorithm. Otherwise the investment is not approved, and the network is not reinforced.

2.4 Iterative Process Coupling JRC-EU-TIMES with Neplan (ITNS)

The individual procedures analysed in Sects. 2.2 and 2.3 are assembled in a process that constitutes ITNS, the overall methodology of coupling between JRC-EU-TIMES and NEPLAN and is analysed in the current section. This coupling is performed through an iterative process, which allows both models to approach a minimum cost solution, taking into account the transmission expansion costs. A simplified flow chart of the algorithm is shown in Fig. 3 and the steps that should be followed are:

First step: This step includes three elements. First of all it includes an external procedure that imports the initial values of all parameters and variables into the JRC-EU-TIMES model (e.g. circuit admittance, cost, network parameters). The second element is the execution of JRC-EU-TIMES and the third is an external function that extracts the results of JRC-EU-TIMES into ASCII files. The extracted results are the generation and demand of electricity for every region, the generation and load type as well as the generation capacity expansion.

Second step: This is performed in an external function that formulates power flow scenarios. Demand, generation and generation expansion are allocated at the nodes of each region of JRC-EU-TIMES for every time slice. Thus, for every year, a load flow scenario is formulated, for each time slice (instances of grid operation). In addition, new circuit investments are calculated in JRC-EU-TIMES and then they are discretized according to method presented in Sect. 2.3.2.

Third step: This step is similar to the first step. Updated data from the second step are imported into JRC-EU-TIMES through an external procedure. These data are the adjusted allocation factors for generation and demand and the line investments calculated through the discretization process presented in Sect. 2.3.2. These grid reinforcements are imported as fixed line investments.

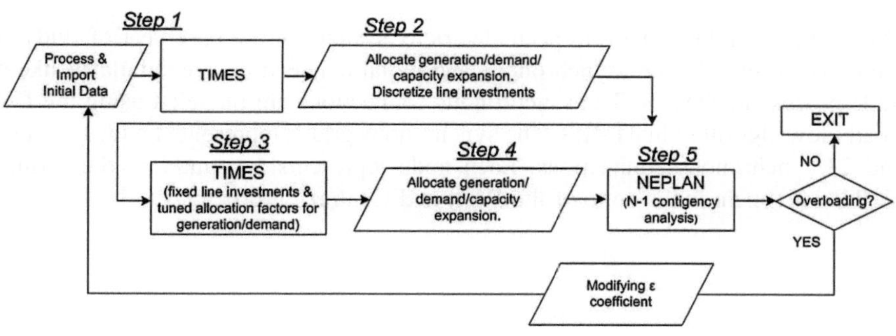

Fig. 3 Flow chart of the coupling between JRC-EU-TIMES and NEPLAN software (ITNS)

JRC-EU-TIMES is re-executed with the updated values calculated in the second step and the new results are extracted in ASCII files.

Fourth step: This step is similar to the second step. It is an external procedure that uses the JRC-EU-TIMES results produced in step three and reallocates demand, generation and generation expansion to the nodes of every region of TIMES for every time slice and for every year studied.

Fifth step: This step consists of three procedures. The first procedure imports data into the NEPLAN software (circuit investments which is the discretization output, injections of generation and demand). The second procedure is the N − 1 security analysis, which is performed using NEPLAN, and the calculation of the overloading of circuits under all contingencies. The third procedure is the calculation of the correction factor of usability coefficients (K_c) through an external procedure (see Sect. 2.3.1).

Sixth step: This is an external procedure that is a logic check for the termination of the iteration. If the solution of NEPLAN does not indicate overloading calculated through the N − 1 contingency analysis, the iterations are terminated. In the opposite case, the iteration starts again from step 1. The execution of JRC-EU-TIMES is performed with new epsilon coefficients calculated by multiplication of the initial ε with the K_c coefficients using Eq. 15.

In Fig. 3, the flow chart of the overall methodology is presented. Every iteration presupposes that NEPLAN detects overloading of circuits under N − 1 conditions. Usability coefficients are then reduced (through K coefficient). Thus, in every iteration the JRC-EU-TIMES solution reduces the loading of corridors. This may be accomplished by modifying the dispatch of electricity (allocation of generation to the different nodes), or by reinforcing the electricity network. The reduction of circuit/corridor loading after each iteration, leads to the convergence of the algorithm.

2.5 Power flow representation in JRC-EU-TIMES

The simplified grid of the European electricity system for the base year of study is presented in Fig. 4. The asynchronous and radial connections are simulated like a trade process in TIMES. The synchronous connections are modeled using the DC Load Flow algorithm in TIMES. The synchronous grid is represented with 13 nodes and 23 synchronous connections. Each node represents a country of the former UCTE 1st synchronous zone of the West and Central Europe.

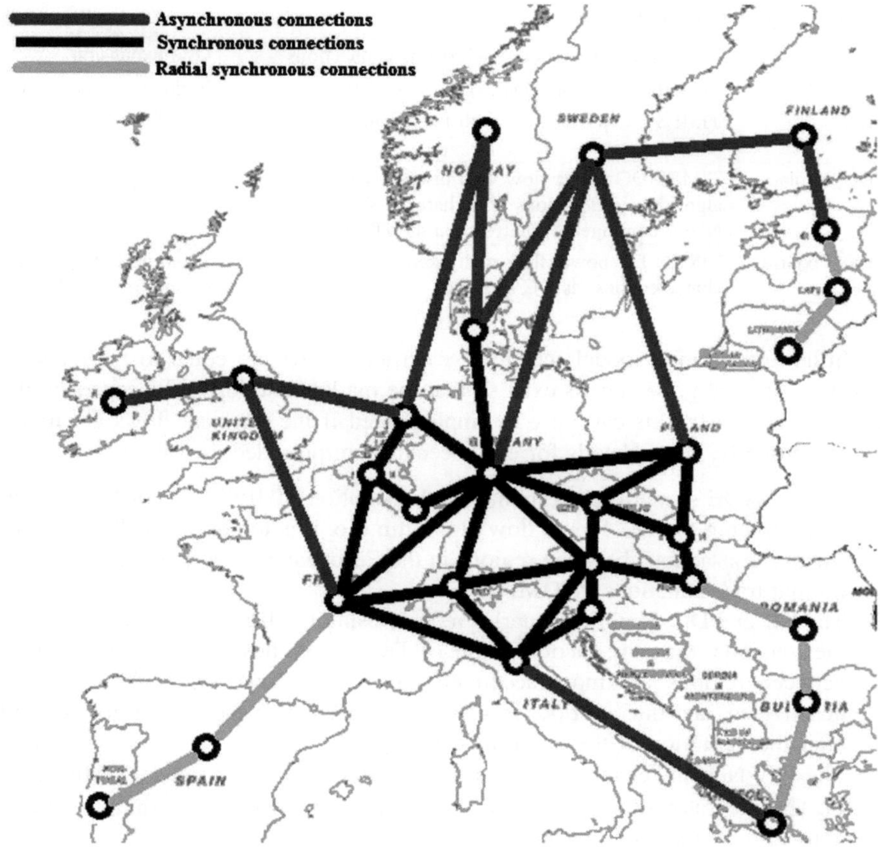

Fig. 4 Simplified model of European grid at the base year of study

3 Scenarios to Assess Integrating Grid Constraints in JRC-EU-TIMES

To assess both the impact of DC Power flow modeling and ITNS in JRC-EU-TIMES results, we developed four scenarios as shown in Table 1. To determine the effect of the different grid representations we compare the optimal solutions of the basic TIMES code with the more advanced approaches. Asynchronous and radial connections are always modeled with the traditional trade approach. However, synchronous connections have been modeled with both the traditional trade approach as well as with the new flow based methodologies. The three grid representations are compared in the scenarios TRADE, DC and DC_Neplan where the transmission expansion is free after 2025. The last scenario, DC_FixGrid, has a fixed transmission expansion up to 2050.

Table 1 Scenario description

Scenario	Grid representation of synchronous connections	Grid expansion
TRADE	Trade based (basic TIMES)	Endogenous grid expansion (after 2025)
DC	TIMES DC power flow with fixed grid characteristics	
DC_Neplan	TIMES DC power flow with discretization algorithm, endogenous grid characteristics and N − 1 contingency analysis via the ITNS	
DC_FixGrid	TIMES DC power flow with fixed grid characteristics (as DC scenario)	Fixed grid expansion (fixed up to 2050)

In an optimization model scheduled electricity flows are equal to the physical flows as optimal price signals exist so that the market solutions fully represent the physics. However, this can only be implemented if the physical flows are represented properly. More details for each scenario are provided as follows:

- The TRADE scenario corresponds to the solution of JRC-EU-TIMES without incorporating the DC Power flow algorithm (i.e. it is the basic TIMES model). Energy transactions between regions in the European system are calculated like normal trade functions in TIMES.
- The DC and DC_FixGrid scenarios refer to using the JRC-EU-TIMES model in the versions with the incorporation of DC power flow, where power flows between regions are more accurately estimated. However, ITNS loops are deactivated, and thus corridor reactances and allocation factors are not updated after the definition of the initial investment plan.
- The DC_Neplan scenario refers to the execution of the complete TIMES-NEPLAN integrator software (ITNS), including discretization algorithm, endogenous grid characteristics and N − 1 contingency analysis.

In all scenarios an 80 % CO_2 emission cap was considered compared to 1990 values. Moreover, all scenarios have in common the following assumptions: (i) No consideration of specific policy incentives to RES (e.g. feed-in tariffs, green certificates); (ii) three additional constraints to ensure: (1) sufficient reserve capacity, (2) realistic representation of variable RES generation and (3) sufficient storage charging capacity. Variable RES (wind, solar, PV and ocean) cannot operate during the winter peak time slice to account for reserve capacity considerations; and (iii) countries without nuclear power plants (NPPs) will not have these in the future (Austria, Portugal, Greece, Cyprus, Malta, Italy, Denmark and Croatia). NPPs in Germany are not operating after 2020 and Belgium NPPs are not operating after 2025.

The main objective of the case study is to evaluate the improvement of the JRC-EU-TIMES modeling mechanisms by including grid related constraints. Note that when looking into the results of our case study regarding the impact on the power system there are several limitations, such as that the insights that are gained from the current configuration are most useful when the consumption and production of electricity are similar to the assumed averages of the 12 time slices. Ideally, one would include a higher number of time slices, regions as well as the national grids to represent different conditions for power plant availability, weather conditions and volatility of fuel prices. This allows including in JRC-EU-TIMES representative day patterns with much more combinations of normal and more extreme events as well as regional differences in renewable availability. Moreover, more differences will be visible when more disruptive situations are modeled based on less perfect circumstances.

4 Results

In the JRC-EU-TIMES model, cross border transmission expansion is cost efficient regardless of the grid representation. The most important factors determining cross border electricity flows as well as the cost efficiency of transmission expansion are (1) the electricity price difference between the countries strongly driven by technology specificity, (2) the transfer capacity limits active in the model and (3) storage possibilities in JRC-EU-TIMES. The results show that a more accurate representation of the grid is possible and worthwhile in a large energy system model. However, we observe that the impact of DC Power Flow is limited for the analyzed case study. Figure 5 shows the net electricity export in 2035 for the four scenarios. The large export from Norway is notable as well as the export from France in the scenario with limited grid expansion (DC_FixGrid). At this level of detail, there are very limited differences between the three grid representations TRADE, DC and DC_Neplan.

Remarkably, unscheduled flows do not appear in the DC scenario because the physical grid limitations are fully internalized in JRC-EU-TIMES. The TRADE scenario does not have grid constraints so unscheduled flows, deviations between scheduled flows and physical flows, take place. Including DC Power Flow triggers

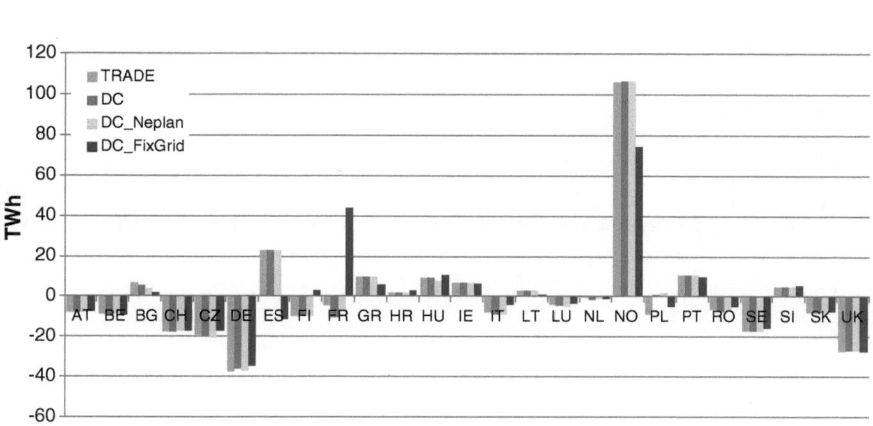

Fig. 5 Net electricity export in 2035

grid extensions but also a shift in generation and consumption to make the physical flows stay in the limits of the grid network. As we compare a market that does not have physical limitations (copper plate) except net transfer capacity with a market that has physical limitations (grid with power flow constraints) one could consider the changes of generation and consumption as some kind of redispatch, however based only on limitations of interconnectors.

In the JRC-EU-TIMES model the Summer Day and Summer Peak represent times with vast amounts of available solar energy. In fact, because of the limited number of time slices, the Summer Day and Summer Peak show a homogenous high level of solar energy across the regions. The Winter Peak represents times without any contribution from variable renewables. Under these somewhat disruptive circumstances we observe increased investments in interconnection capacity.

First, we look at the impact of summer solar electricity production. In the TRADE scenario, the DC scenario as well as the DC_Neplan scenario, more than 10 GWe cross-border capacity is built between Spain and France. This allows transferring electricity from Spain and Portugal in the summer to Northern Europe. As a consequence, we observe a reduced use and capacity of nuclear power plants in France when compared to the DC_Fixgrid scenario that has limited grid expansion possibilities. Interestingly, when the grid expansion is limited, there is an increased deployment of electric cars in Spain. The reason is that in the year 2035, there is a trade-off between storing part of the solar electricity into the batteries of electric cars and using the grid to export. We conclude that the impact of DC Power Flow and NEPLAN is low although the summer solar production induces grid expansions.

In the Winter Peak no variable renewable electricity is available. This a somewhat extreme assumption—not all countries will be without wind, solar and ocean activity at the same time—which leads us however to an interesting finding. As Fig. 6 shows, in the Winter peak time slice important flows occur making Poland, Belgium, Italy and UK exporting electricity to mainly Switzerland, Sweden and

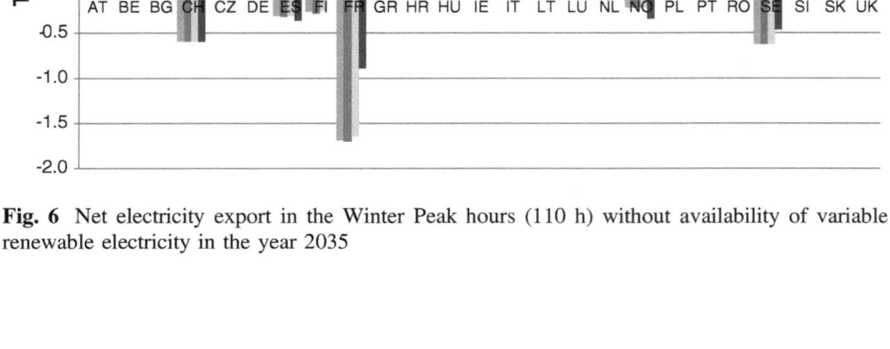

Fig. 6 Net electricity export in the Winter Peak hours (110 h) without availability of variable renewable electricity in the year 2035

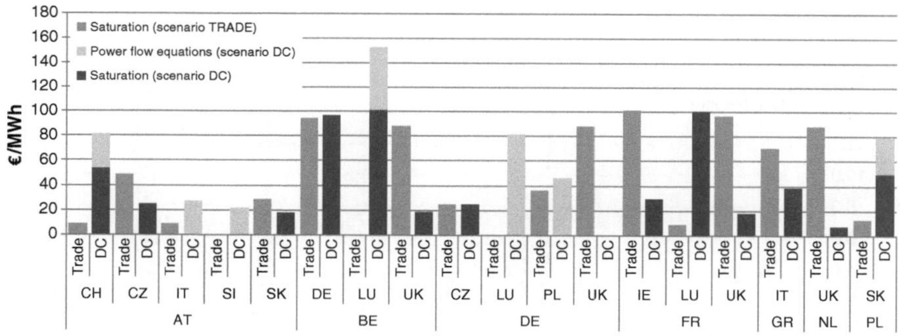

Fig. 7 Electricity price difference between countries in the scenarios TRADE and DC and decomposition for the Winter Peak in 2035

France. Also, the representation of the grid has an impact on some countries such as Germany and Poland.

The electricity market in JRC-EU-TIMES is optimal in this way that it does not have external costs when DC Power Flow is included and it implements nodal pricing in each of the 13 nodes of the synchronous central European grid. The market value of the transmission connection is with nodal pricing equal to the price difference between the areas arising from differences in marginal production cost as well as from congestion costs. Figure 7 shows for the situation in 2035 without available variable renewables the electricity price differences between countries. In the TRADE scenario, electricity price differences are only based on marginal production costs. In contrast, the DC grid representation has another component arising from the power flow constraints. In some connections like Austria-Italy or Germany-Poland it only has the component of power flow constraints.

The traditional representation of the grid, the TRADE approach, uses the network as optimal as possible with the only limitation that the sum of the inflows and outflows in a node is zero. With such a representation, many possible combinations of trade are possible for a given consumption and production in each node. However, the DC power flow approach represents also the physical electricity flows, directed by the grid characteristics. With a given consumption and production in each node (country in our case) and with given trade in radial and asynchronous connections, only one solution of the electricity flow exists in the synchronous grid and investments in new lines are triggered by a combination of regional cost of electricity production and physical limitations. The added value of DC power flow is that it models the physical flow of electricity. This usually leads to higher investments in grid lines than in the TRADE approach.

When the price difference is large enough for a sufficient long period, this can cause a grid expansion at least when this grid expansion is not too costly. Figure 8 shows most of the grid expansions for the three scenarios where investments are free. Most of the connections have higher cross-border capacities when power flow constraints are included such as Austria and Slovakia with all its neighboring

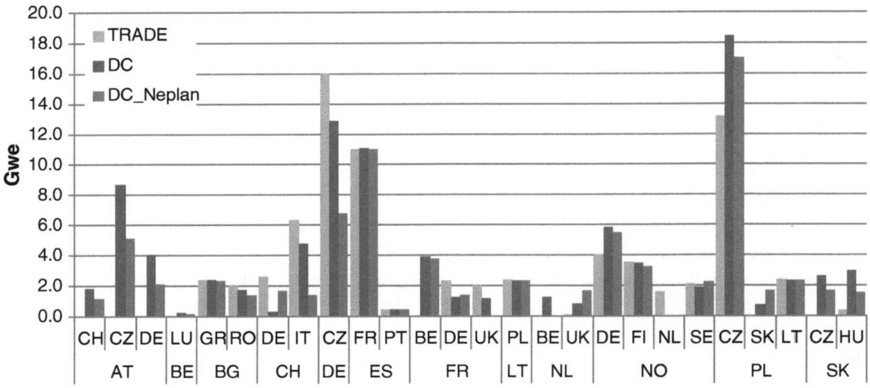

Fig. 8 Electricity grid expansions between countries in the scenarios TRADE, DC and DC_Neplan

countries but also the connection Germany-Norway and Poland-Czech Republic. The main driver for the optimal electricity path is the cost of the combined grid expansions. Typically this cost of the grid expansion is a factor 10–100 lower than the value of the traded commodities. However, the impact of the price component of the power flow constraints is often even smaller than the cost differences between possible grid expansions. Because of this reason the model will typically not drastically change the grid expansion as there are preferred routes based on the cost of these interconnections. We conclude that power flow constraints have an impact on optimal grid expansion and that the accuracy of the grid expansion costs is crucial for proper grid flow analysis.

We evaluated the improvement of the JRC-EU-TIMES modeling mechanisms by including grid related constraints. No substantial increase in modeling time was observed when static DC power flow equations are added to the JRC-EU-TIMES model. However, mainly the discretization loop of the ITNS is time consuming. Depending on the number of new investments, the total ITNS cycle needs 10 up to 100 iterations.

5 Conclusions

To evaluate the improvement of the JRC-EU-TIMES modeling mechanisms, three grid representations are compared in scenarios with free and fixed transmission expansion. We conclude that the impact of power flow constraints is limited for the analyzed case study. However, integrating these constraints has a relevant impact on the value of future possible grid expansions mainly in periods with limited availability of variable renewable electricity, without a substantial increase in model running time and leading to slightly higher cross-border capacities for most countries.

Future research can define restrictions based on the output of the total ITNS cycle so to prevent the iterative procedure of the soft coupling of TIMES with NEPLAN. Further work can also include increasing the number of regional differences such as renewable availability as well as stochastic generation or consumption. This would trigger more disruptive situations that are necessary to understand the true value of grid extensions. We conclude that the perfect foresight assumption of JRC-EU-TIMES requires special attention of the modeler. Indeed, some of the robustness of the JRC-EU-TIMES should be removed in order to get a possibly less optimal distribution of power plants and consumption patterns, as we observe today in many members states. We expect to see more differences between the three grid representations for situations that are more disruptive and less perfect.

Under these conditions, we conclude that the decision making process on transmission expansion can strongly be affected by tools like JRC-EU-TIMES as there is a strong competition between grid extension, storage options, local peak power as well as demand side management.

References

Alvarez Lopez J, Ponnambalam K, Quintana VH (2007) Generation and transmission expansion under risk using stochastic programming. IEEE Trans Power Syst 22:1369–1378

BCP Busarello+Cott+Partner Inc. (2014) NEPLAN software. http://www.neplan.ch. Accessed 14 Sep 2014

Bent R, Berscheid A, Loren Toole G (2011) Generation and transmission expansion planning for renewable energy integration. Paper presented at the 17th power systems computation conference, Stockholm, Sweden, 22–26 Aug 2011

Chuang AS, Wu F, Varaiya P (2001) A game-theoretic model for generation expansion planning: problem formulation and numerical comparisons. IEEE Trans Power Syst 16:885–891

Contaxi E, Vournas CD, Kabouris J (2012) A probabilistic methodology for transmission planning under severe uncertainties. Paper presented at the 12th international conference on probabilistic methods applied to power systems, Istanbul, Turkey, 10–14 June 2012

Deane JP, Chiodi A, Gargiulo M, Gallachoir BPO (2012) Soft-linking of a power systems model to an energy systems model. 8th World Energy System Conference, WESC 2010, vol 42, pp 303–312

El-Debeiky SM, Hasanien NE (2000) Rule-based system for determining unit locations of a developed generation expansion plan for transmission planning. IEE Proc Gener Transm Distrib 147:62–68

Georgilakis PS (2010) Market-based transmission expansion planning by improved differential evolution. Int J Electr Power Energy Syst 32:450–456

Hamasaki H (2014) Analysis on the design of Japan FIT after Fukushima disaster using GIS and TIMES integrated model. J Energy Power Eng 8:217–225

Hemmati R, Hooshmand RA, Khodabakhshian A (2013a) State-of-the-art of transmission expansion planning: comprehensive review. Renew Sustain Energy Rev 23:312–319

Hemmati R, Hooshmand RA, Khodabakhshian A (2013b) Comprehensive review of generation and transmission expansion planning. IET Gener Transm Distrib 7:955–964

International Atomic Energy Agency (2001) Wien automatic system planning (WASP) package: a computer code for power generation system expansion planning, Version WASP-IV User's manual. http://www-pub.iaea.org/MTCD/Publications/PDF/CMS-16.pdf. Accessed 14 Sept 2014

Kabouris J, Contaxis GC (1991) Optimum expansion planning of an unconventional generation system operating in parallel with a large scale network. IEEE Trans Energy Conv 6:394–400
Loulou R, Remme U, Kanudia A, Lehtila A, Goldstein G (2005) Documentation for the TIMES model. http://www.iea-etsap.org/web/Docs/TIMESDoc-Intro.pdf. Accessed 14 Sep 2014
Orfanos GA, Georgilakis PS, Hatziargyriou ND (2013) Transmission expansion planning of systems with increasing wind power integration. IEEE Trans Power Syst 28:1355–1362
REALISEGRID (2010) Research, methodologies and technologies for the effective development of pan-European key grid infrastructures to support the achievement of a reliable, competitive and sustainable electricity supply. http://realisegrid.rse-web.it/content/files/File/Publications%20and%20results/Interim%20report.pdf. Accessed 14 Sept 2014
Roh J, Shahidehpour M, Fu Y (2007) Market-based coordination of transmission and generation capacity planning. IEEE Trans Power Syst 22:1406–1419
Romero R, Monticelli A, Garcia A, Haffner S (2002) Test systems and mathematical models for transmission network expansion planning. IEE Proc Gener Transm Distrib 149:27–36
Sakellaridis N, Mantzaris J, Nakos C, Giannakidis G, Tigas K (2011) Hellenic power generation system: towards meeting the national targets up to 2020. Paper presented at the 10th international conference on environment and electrical engineering, Rome, Italy, 8–11 May 2011
Seifi H, Sepasian MS (2011) Electric power system planning—issues, algorithms and solutions. Springer, Berlin
Sepasian MS, Seifi H, Foroud AA, Hatami AR (2009) A multiyear security constrained hybrid generation-transmission expansion planning algorithm including fuel supply costs. IEEE Trans Power Syst 24:1609–1618
Tor OB, Guven AN, Shahidehpour M (2008) Congestion-driven transmission planning considering the impact of generator expansion. IEEE Trans Power Syst 23:781–789
UKERC (2009) Making the transition to a secure and low-carbon energy system. http://www.ukerc.ac.uk/Downloads/PDF/U/UKERCEnergy2050/0906UKERC2050.pdf. Accessed 14 Sept 2014
Zhu J, Chow M (1997) A review of emerging techniques on generation expansion planning. IEEE Trans Power Syst 12:1722–1728

Highly Detailed TIMES Modeling to Analyze Interactions Between Air Quality and Climate Regulations in the United States

Evelyn Wright and Amit Kanudia

Abstract This chapter describes highly detailed modeling of existing coal-fired units in the US power sector within the FACETS TIMES model. Such detailed modeling is necessary wherever the existing stock plays a key role in determining policy cost. The soon-to-be-implemented Mercury and Air Toxics (MATS) regulation imposes unit-level emissions rate constraints on nearly 1100 coal-fired units, forcing retrofit or retire decisions at a large portion of the existing fleet. Covered emissions and retrofit costs depend in a detailed way on unit configuration and coal quality, forcing development of new techniques to handle the enormous expansion in model size and detail. These retrofit/retire decisions are being made under uncertainty about future carbon policies for the sector. FACETS was used to compare "foresight" scenarios in which the model could "see" both the MATS requirements and a power sector clean energy standard (CES) to "myopic" scenarios in which the MATS decisions made in the Reference scenario are fixed in the model solution up through the MATS compliance window in model year 2018, after which the model is free to begin responding to the CES. The overall national costs of myopia were found to be small, except when the carbon policy ramps up very quickly after air quality compliance decisions are made, but significant regional heterogeneity exists. Stranded asset costs from retrofitted units that must be underutilized or abandoned later range from $2 to 8 billion in the myopic cases. Substantially fewer retrofits are undertaken in the foresight cases, reducing stranded asset costs in some regions by up to 100 %.

E. Wright (✉)
Sustainable Energy Economics, Rosendale, NY, USA
e-mail: Evelyn.L.Wright@gmail.com

A. Kanudia
KanORS-EMR, Noida, India
e-mail: amit@kanors.com

G. Giannakidis et al. (eds.), *Informing Energy and Climate Policies Using Energy Systems Models*, Lecture Notes in Energy 30,
DOI 10.1007/978-3-319-16540-0_13

1 Introduction

Carbon policy is slowly becoming a reality in many parts of the world. As this happens, analysis needs are evolving from abstract consideration of goals, timing, and high-level strategies to rigorous evaluation of the costs, incidence, and risks of specific policy designs. In the United States power sector, a key determinant of the economic impacts of carbon policy is the fate of the substantial existing stock of coal-fired units.

Over the next few years, these units are subject to implementation of historic new air emissions regulations, including a tightening of standards for sulfur dioxide (SO_2) and nitrogen oxides (NO_x), as well as new standards under the Mercury and Air Toxics (MATS) rule for air toxins including acid gases, mercury, and other heavy metals (US EPA 2014a). The MATS standards differ from most major regulations recently implemented (and modeled) in an important way. These pollutants are subject to toxic hot spots, and thus the standards impose unit-level emissions rate constraints, not regional cap and trade budgets. Each of the country's nearly 1100 coal-fired units above 25 megawatts (MW) capacity faces the requirement to individually comply with these standards or retire.

At the same time, the stringency and timing of future carbon regulations for the sector remain uncertain. Although the Obama administration has recently proposed standards under the Clean Air Act (US EPA 2014b) prohibiting new coal plants without carbon capture and storage (CCS) and imposing moderate medium-term emissions rate reductions on existing plants, it remains unclear whether these proposed rules will survive legal challenge, and in any case they are expected to serve as only a prelude to eventual new, dedicated climate legislation.

The MATS compliance deadline is 2015, with possible extensions through 2017, so owners of non-compliant units will need to make costly decisions to retrofit or retire these units without certainty about how much longer these units will remain economic to operate under future carbon policy. The cost of carbon policy, in turn, depends on the decisions made regarding MATS compliance: how large is the existing stock of vulnerable units, and how significant are recent stranded investments in air compliance equipment when carbon policy becomes stringent enough to start forcing these units to retire.

Of equal importance is the *regional distribution* of carbon policy cost impacts. Previously analyses (Pizer et al. 2009; Rausch et al. 2011; Wright and Kanudia 2014) have shown that cost impacts may vary several-fold across the US, and it appears that these differences have played at least some role in the difficulty reaching consensus on a federal carbon policy (Wheeler 2008). The stock of coal-fired units, and their age, size, and existing emissions control equipment, are distributed unequally around the country, so the interactions between air quality and carbon policy can be expected to impact different regions more significantly than others.

Because air toxin emissions depend in quite a detailed way on unit configuration, coal quality, and existing emissions control equipment, it has been necessary to model the stock of existing units and their many retrofit options in a highly detailed, unit-level manner. These challenges are described in the next section. In addition to presenting this analysis, this chapter is designed as an illustration of how the TIMES platform can be used to analyze problem spaces that are much more highly detailed than has been common previously. Thus the modeling discussion in Sect. 3 assumes some familiarity with VEDA-FrontEnd[1] and interest in the details of the technique. Some new features have been developed to deal with the volume of data required, but much of the work has been done by using existing features in new ways. We hope this discussion will be useful to other modelers who are also wrestling with the need for incorporating more detail into their analyses. Other readers can feel free to scan or skip this section, as the remainder of the discussion does not depend on it.

To investigate the interaction between air quality compliance demands and carbon policy uncertainty, and demonstrate the application of these modeling techniques, the FACETS US TIMES model (Wright and Kanudia 2014) was used to compare "foresight" scenarios in which the model could "see" both the MATS requirements and a power sector clean energy standard (CES) that imposes a national cap and trade program forcing a reduction of the carbon intensity of generation over time to "myopic" scenarios in which the MATS decisions made in the Reference scenario are fixed in the model solution up through the MATS compliance window in model year 2018, after which the model is free to begin responding to the CES. Three versions of the CES policies with different stringency ramping rates were tried.

Section 4 presents this analysis, including the scenarios assessed, and the resulting system configurations, costs, and emissions results at national and regional levels. The chapter concludes with a discussion of the implications of the results, and considers the recently proposed Clean Power Plan carbon regulations for existing units in light of our findings.

2 Challenge of Modeling MATS Emissions and Compliance

MATS requires each unit to meet standards for several toxins. Three of the most significant were modeled here: an acid gas standard, using emissions of hydrochloric acid (HCl) as the measurement proxy; a mercury standard; and a standard for non-mercury metal toxins using filterable particulate matter (PM) as a surrogate for compliance measurement. Emissions of HCl and mercury depend on boiler type, coal quality, and emissions control equipment, and several compliance routes may be available to each unit. This section describes the rule's requirements and the emissions control retrofit options made available in the modeling.

[1] http://www.kanors-emr.org/VedaSupport/.

The acid gas standard requires emissions below approximately 0.002 pounds per million British Thermal Unit (lb/MM BTU) of coal consumed.[2] HCl emissions are a function of the chlorine content of coal and emissions control equipment for SO_2. The higher ash content of subbituminous and lignite coals neutralizes much HCl before emission, leading to an effective range of uncontrolled emissions among US coals ranging from 0.281 pounds per million BTU (lb/MM BTU) to 0.0015 lb/MMBTU, or more than two orders of magnitude, implying that between zero and more than 99 % reduction is necessary to comply, depending on the coal type used.

Plants can retrofit to reduce HCl emissions with either flue gas desulphurization (FGD) or direct sorbent injection (DSI). Capital and operating costs depend on unit size and existing emissions control configuration, as DSI requires a fabric filter (FF) in place, but in general, FGD is a high capital cost, low operating cost technology, whereas DSI requires a lower upfront capital cost, but three-fold higher variable operating and maintenance (O&M) cost. FGD removes a much higher percentage of the HCl (99 vs. 90 %), providing more coal type flexibility. As discussed below, FGD also makes a contribution to mercury removal, and may provide an important compliance route for the mercury standard, depending on a unit's other characteristics. Table 1 summarizes retrofit device cost and performance assumptions for all devices made available in the modeling.[3]

Mercury emissions depend on the mercury content of the coal burned along with boiler type and emissions control equipment for SO_2, NO_x, PM, and an optional dedicated activated carbon injection (ACI) for mercury removal. The latter also requires the unit to have either an electrostatic precipitator (ESP) or FF. The mercury standard requires emissions below approximately 1.2 pounds per trillion BTU of coal consumed.[4] As coal mercury contents range from 1.8 to 34.7 lb/TBTU, removal of 33–97 % of the mercury content is required.

Many different unit configurations will lead to compliant mercury control for units burning bituminous coals. For example, most boiler types will achieve 90 % reductions when equipped with FGD and selective catalytic reduction (SCR) and burning bituminous coal, and a fluidized bed unit with FF achieves a 95 % reduction. Non-ACI controls are less effective at removing mercury from subbituminous and lignite coals, but ACI will remove 90 % of incoming mercury content from any coal type. Overall, 510 units, or nearly half, achieve 90 % or greater mercury reductions under their existing configurations when burning bituminous

[2]The standards for HCl and mercury are given in mass per electricity generated for units below a heat rate threshold of 10,000 BTU per kilowatt-hour (kWh) and mass per unit of coal combusted for units above, in order to provide some flexibility for high heat rate units. Thus the precise standard is dependent on the characteristics of each unit. The threshold values are used here to provide an approximate sense of the requirements of compliance. The unit-specific standards were used in the modeling described below.

[3]Characteristics derived from US EIA (2011a) and US EPA (2010, 2011a, b).

[4]For plants burning bituminous or subbituminous coals. Plants burning lignite are subject to a different standard, which was implemented in the modeling but neglected here for simplicity of discussion.

Table 1 Emissions control retrofit options and characteristics

Equipment	Capital cost ($/kW)[a]	Addition to fixed O&M ($/kW years)	Addition to variable O&M (mills/kWh)	Removes	Removal rate
FGD	378–662	5.9–18.0	1.9	SO_2	95 %
				HCl	99 %
				Hg	Depends on configuration
DSI alone	30–110	0.4–2.0	5.9	SO_2	70 %
				HCl	90 %
DSI plus FF	154–291	0.4–2.0	5.9	SO_2	70 %
				HCl	90 %
SCR	154–219	0.5–2.3	1.1	NO_x	90 %
				Hg	Depends on configuration
ACI alone	5–27	0.0	2.4	Hg	90 %
ACI plus FF	144–228	0.5–0.9	0.5	Hg	90 %

[a]All costs presented in 2004$

coal, enough for compliance burning most bituminous coals, while just over 100 achieve 90 % when burning subbituminous coal, largely through existing ACI.

The remaining plants must install some combination of retrofits, or in some cases, switch to a lower mercury coal type, in order to continue operation. Depending on their existing configuration, their HCl compliance needs, and the value of SO_2 and NO_x reductions in their region, this may be as simple and inexpensive as adding ACI, at a relatively low capital cost, or it may be necessary or optimal to upgrade their SO_2, NO_x, or PM control equipment as well or instead, at costs up to nearly two orders of magnitude higher.

Finally, enhanced filterable PM controls are required at many units to control emissions of other toxins under MATS. US EPA (2011b) evaluated existing coal units and found that 393 units would be required to upgrade their existing ESP or install a new FF. These upgrades were exogenously imposed on each unit in the modeling described below, with capital costs imposed as an increment to annual fixed O&M charges of $5.5–20.4 $/KW, depending on the upgrade required.

Because of this great diversity in compliance costs and the unit-level nature of the MATS requirements, analysis of the regulation's impact based on average or typical plant characteristics, as would be required in a model with coarse geography, would fail to represent the very detailed supply curve for the survival of existing plants. And importantly, it would also fail to capture the regional diversity of retrofit costs and the need to build replacement capacity for those plants that retire. This geographic information is essential for the analysis of carbon regulations because the costs of implementing low carbon technologies depend on geographical relationships between low carbon resources, electricity generation and transmission infrastructure, and loads. The distribution of low carbon resources, including wind, solar, geothermal, and access to CO_2 sequestration sites, is highly heterogeneous, leading to significant regional differences in the costs of emission reduction (Wright and Kanudia 2014).

3 Modeling the Power Sector in FACETS

The Framework for Analysis of Climate-Energy-Technology Systems (FACETS) multi-region US TIMES model has been designed to enable such geographically rich analysis of the US energy system. Specifically, FACETS has been designed with unit-level detail in the power sector, including a rich set of emissions control retrofit options for coal-fired units, and a regional structure that emphasizes existing infrastructure and key geographical relationships. This section describes the FACETS power sector and associated fuel supplies, with a focus on the techniques used to handle the challenges described in the previous section. The rule-based VEDA-TIMES system was essential to handle the enormous level of detail required, and was enhanced on both the input and output sides. In particular, we describe three things: the use of VEDA rules to describe the existing control equipment at each unit and its retrofit options and resulting emissions; the use of a topology insert table to create coal input options specific to each unit, and the VedaViz system to support analyzing the correspondingly large volume of results data.

The data source for the power sector is the US EPA National Electric Energy Data System database (US EPA 2010), which provides capacity, cost, efficiency, availability, emissions, and emissions control equipment data for just over 15,000 units in the lower 48 states. Plants are grouped into 32 regions that represent regional transmission organizations (RTOs), independent system operators (ISOs) and key transmission bottlenecks. A matrix of transmission capacities and costs describes the potential flows between these regions, and data from the US Department of Energy (DOE) National Energy Modeling System (NEMS, US EIA 2009) provides capital costs for additions to this capacity.

In order to preserve this infrastructure information, the 32 power sector regions were implemented as regions within FACETS, with the transmission capacities serving as a trade matrix. Electricity demand[5] takes place in a different set of regions: the nine Census divisions that US DOE uses to track sectoral consumption data. A matrix of user constraints prescribes the share of each consumption region's electricity that must be provided by each of its corresponding electricity regions.

[5]Although FACETS contains a full representation of end use sectors, for this study, which focuses on power sector policies, only the power sector and its fuel supplies were used. The demand for electricity consumption was driven by Annual Energy Outlook projections (US DOE 2011a).

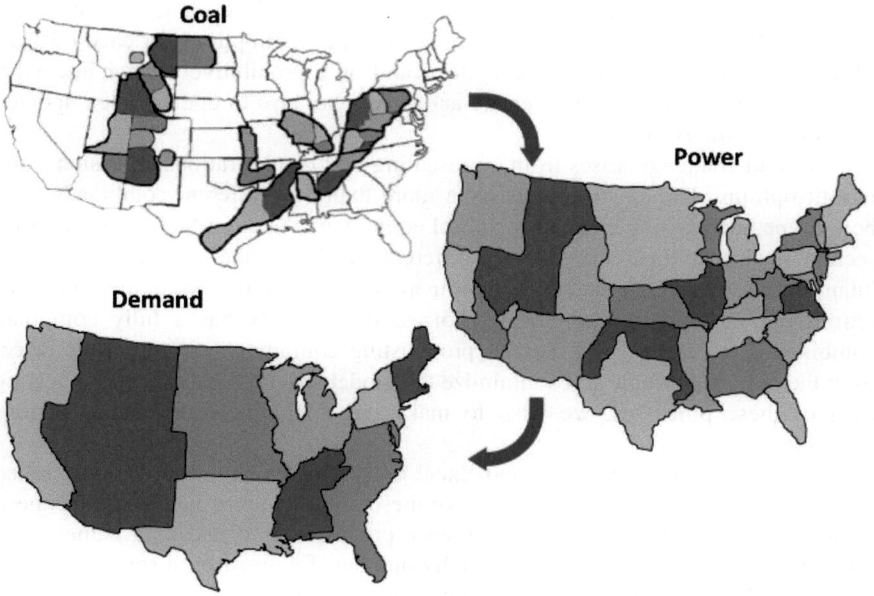

Fig. 1 FACETS coal, power, and demand regions

This matrix is based on historical data and represents the physical location of homes, businesses, and facilities within each power region's territory.

On the input side, coal and biomass are sourced from their own sets of regions and traded to the power sector regions using trade matrices, as illustrated in Fig. 1. (Because of high cost of transport, biomass may only be traded to geographically overlapping regions.) Finally, when the model implements carbon capture and storage, the CO_2 flows are traded to a set of sequestration regions, each with their own "supply" cost curves for accepting CO_2, and again governed by a trade cost matrix from the power regions.

Within the power sector, the nearly 3800 hydroelectric units, whose production is governed by seasonal capacity factors, are aggregated by power region and state. The remaining 11,200 units are modeled individually. While much of the data for these units can be read in a single Excel table built directly around the source data, a major data handling challenge is presented by the need to describe the input fuel choice, emissions, and emissions retrofit options for the 1100 coal units.

A TIMES model is based on network topology. The inputs and output of each process must be specified in order to provide the links that "hook" the network together. FACETS includes 85 bituminous, subbituminous, and lignite coals, distinguished by rank, source region (and hence transportation cost to each unit) and sulfur level, each with its own sulfur, mercury, and chlorine content. Each unit may burn some subset of these fuels, depending on its configuration, location, equipment, and permitted sulfur emissions level. Some units are restricted to only one rank, while others are flexible. And beginning in 2017, each is subject to its individual MATS constraints. Enumerating the input fuel options for each of these 1100 units line by line in an Excel file would be a prohibitively labor intensive, error-prone process, not only to create and check, but also to update when updated data sources are available.

A second challenge arises from representing unit configurations, emissions, and retrofit options. The existing units have more than 100 different combinations of boiler type and existing emissions control equipment. As described in the previous section, each combination removes a different fraction of the content of each pollutant in the source coal, and each combination is also eligible for a different set of retrofit options, ranging from zero choices, if it already has a fully compliant combination, to eleven, if it has no pre-existing equipment, and can fully select from the options in Table 1. To minimize the model size implications of duplicating each of these processes, we wish to make only potentially improving options available.

VEDA's rule-based approach and Excel lookup tables have been heavily relied upon to build the specifications. To drive these specifications, heavy use has been made of information embedded within each process's short and long names. Unit short names consist of the federal unit ID number, followed by a seven character code that describers its boiler configuration and NO_x, acid, PM, and mercury emissions control equipment specifications and indicates whether it is the original (mother) unit or one of its retrofitted replacements. Unit descriptions are packed with information as follows:

> EPLT -<Plant name>.<Fuels>.<Coal transport cost category>.<County>-<State>.<Plant type>.<Plant size category>.<Optional code for retrofit equipment>

For example, *EPLT—E C Gaston.CoaB.ALR3.Shelby-Alabama.CST.SC3.EmRf C* describes a coal steam (CST) unit at E C Gaston plant in Shelby County, Alabama, that burns bituminous coal only, is approximately 300 MW in size, has been retrofitted with SCR, and receives coal according to transport cost category ALR3. The unit size categories are used to specify costs for emissions control retrofits. This information allows emissions, retrofit, and fuel choice data to be input by rules based on process name and description, rather than manual data entry.

The code in each unit's short name is used in the input template to look up from a source data table of emission modification factors the amount of each pollutant "scrubbed" from the input coal. All emissions constraints are then written in terms of the net of raw minus scrubbed emissions. Another lookup table specifies which retrofits are available to plants with each code. For example, plants with existing wet scrubbers but no post-combustion NO_x or mercury controls are eligible for retrofits with SCR, ACI, or SCR + ACI. A set of process declaration tables references this table using each unit's code to declare or not declare each possible option. A set of simple update tables then references the codes in the process description to add the corresponding capital cost and modify the unit's operating costs and efficiency.

Table 2 Topology insert table for coals to coal-fired units

~TFM_TOPINS			
PSET_SET	PSET_PD	CSET_CN	All regions
ELE	*.CoaB.*	ECoal-__-B*	IN
ELE	*.CoaB/CoaS.*	ECoal-__-B*,ECoal-__-S*	IN
ELE	*.CoaL.*	ECoal-__-L*	IN
ELE	*.CoaL/CoaS.*	ECoal-__-L*,ECoal-__-S*	IN
ELE	*.CoaS.*	ECoal-__-S*	IN

User constraints limit the total capacity of each group of mother plus retrofit units to the capacity of the original unit. In principle, lumpy investment in each retrofit choice would be a more precise way to model the retrofit choice, as the current approach could lead to partial retrofits. However, with this many units, lumpy investment would be prohibitive in terms of solve time, and because of the unit-level nature of the constraints, in practice this behavior has been minor.

To manage the fuel inputs, all units that take a single input energy carrier—for example, dedicated natural gas units, and renewable units with dummy inputs—have that specification directly entered in the base year (2012) input template, reading from the source data. All other inputs have been created by means of a Topology Insert table using rules based on the process description. Table 2 shows the portion of the table for coal-fired units. The first row assigns *all* bituminous coal types as inputs to every bituminous unit. Two restrictions are then applied to limit the coals actually available to the unit. First, the coal transport cost matrix specifies the actual list of some 1200 allowable links and their costs, which range from very small costs and single links for mine-mouth plants, to high costs for cross-country rail transport. One single-line table bounds out all possible transport links, and another reads the transport matrix, releases the bounds on allowed links, and assigns them the correct cost. Finally each unit has a permitted sulfur emissions rate, which in conjunction with its scrubber efficiency (if any) will further restrict its allowable fuels. This limit is imposed via user constraint on each unit restricting the net sulfur emissions per electricity generated.

The rich detail of the model creates data handling challenges on the output side as well. In particular, the regional information and trade flows between regions are crucial to understanding the model behavior and extracting meaning from the results. But trade flows in particular are difficult to interpret in a table of numbers. The regions themselves are many and do not correspond to political, social, or cultural boundaries. Because regions are of different geographic size, viewing, for example, capacities of retrofits or retirements by model region may not give and accurate sense of how these changes are distributed in the country.

To help interpret these results, a geographic information systems (GIS) results mapping system has been developed within the VedaViz[6] online results processing

[6]http://vedaviz.com.

and visualization tool. VedaViz was developed to facilitate collaborative interpretation of model results by analysts who are not themselves TIMES modelers or VEDA users. Originally developed as part of the Energy Modeling Forum EMF-27 study (Weyant and Kriegler 2014), it begins with a set of standard high-level summary variables, including primary energy, electricity generation and capacity, final energy consumption, emissions, and cost data, which are then made available online for quickly generating summary graphs and tables using a set of flexible forms based on Google Chart tools[7] and the D3 JavaScript visualization library.[8] Dimensions including scenarios, regions, variables, years, and (for multi-model comparisons) models may be pivoted, and small multiples may be created for side-by-side comparisons.

This system makes high-level results available online to any domain-aware analyst without them needing to be experts in the model Reference Energy System (RES). The tool is designed facilitate collaborative analysis and results dissemination. One can create and save views for others to view, post and respond to comments on views, and generate links from any view to publish online. We now use VedaViz as a primary tool for a first, high-level graphical view of the patterns in the results, combined with VEDA-BE for drilling down into RES details as needed.

The GIS system is based on Google Maps components. Each region in the model is represented by a map coordinate, allowing values to be "graphed" on the map using pie or bar charts. Trade flows may be visualized using arrows, whose width corresponds to the size of the flow (example in Fig. 5). In the FACETS power sector, each unit is coded in the input data with its latitude and longitude, so that unit-level data may also be visualized to see how retirements, retrofits, and emissions "clump" geographically (Fig. 6).

To create a VedaViz online project for a set of results, the VD files[9] are read into an SQL server database, which creates the variable names, processes the raw VD results into the variable values. It can then can do further operations on them, including scenario differences, period averages, shares, capacity utilization, and so on. These variables and calculations are data driven, and customized for each application. In addition to standard charts and maps, a host of other graphical features are available, including animated bubble charts, and Sankey diagrams.

4 Analysis

This section describes the scenarios modeled and the national, regional, and unit level results.

[7]https://developers.google.com/chart/.

[8]http://d3js.org/.

[9]Standard results files from TIMES runs.

4.1 Scenarios Modeled

In addition to the MATS regulations described above, which are assumed to be fully in effect in 2017, the Reference scenario includes regional cap and trade standards for SO_2 and NO_x under the Clean Air Interstate Rule (CAIR), and the proposed New Source Performance Standard (NSPS) for CO_2. The NSPS is implemented as a ban on new coal units without CCS.

The new CO_2 policy analyzed here is a power sector clean energy standard (CES), similar to that analyzed by US EIA (2011b). Like a renewable portfolio standard (RPS), a CES requires a minimum fraction of generation to be obtained from specified sources, in this case a range of zero and low carbon technologies. One full CES credit is awarded to generators per MWh of zero-carbon generation, and partial credit is awarded for some other types in rough proportion to their degree of carbon emissions reduction from coal steam generation (Table 3).

The percentage of CES credits as a share of total national generation ramps up from 2010 levels of roughly 42.5–90 % in 2050, the last model year, with the constraint first binding in model year 2023, after MATS compliance decisions are final. Three different CES trajectories were tested, representing a range of aggressive to delayed action, as illustrated in Fig. 2. The scenarios are named 85, 65, and

Table 3 CES credits by generation type

Generation type	CES credits per MWh
Biomass, geothermal, hydro, nuclear, solar, wind	1.0
Gas combined cycle	0.5
Coal or gas with CCS	0.9

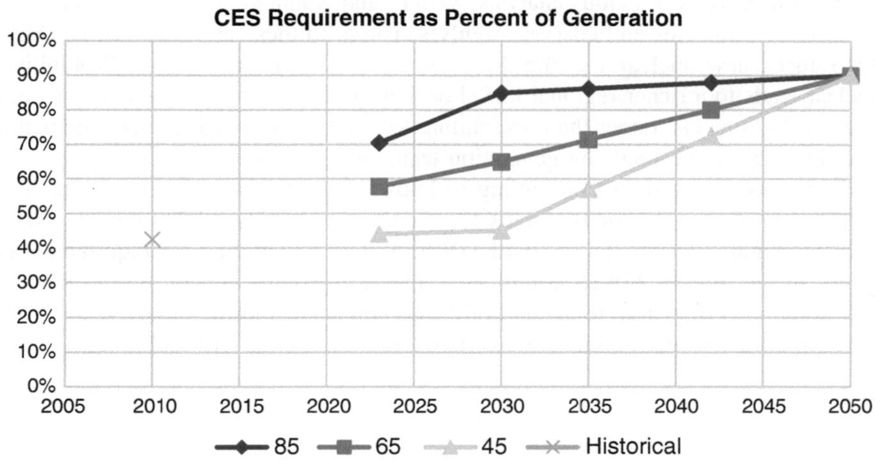

Fig. 2 CES trajectories

Table 4 Build rate constraints

Plant type	Annual build limit before cost penalty incurred (GW/year)			
	2010	2020	2035	2050
Coal/Gas with CCS	1.3	2.6	3.9	5
Photovoltaic	5	15	45	450
Offshore wind	0.5	1.5	10	100
Onshore wind	10	30	90	900

45, for the share required in 2030. The 65 trajectory increases linearly to 2050, while the 85 trajectory ramps up much more aggressively, reaching nearly the full level by 2030, and the 45 trajectory postpones most action until after 2030. Banking and borrowing are not permitted.

New power plant cost and performance characteristics are derived from AEO 2013 (US EIA 2013). All plant options face the same cost of capital. However, plants also face capital cost supply step adders that vary by plant type, representing short-term increases in costs for labor and materials when the model seeks to build new capacity faster than the rates shown in Table 4. These steps are based on a review of similar build rate adders in IPM (US EPA 2010) and NEMS (US EIA 2011c), as well as recent historical maximum annual builds (US EIA 2012) for these capacity types. Plant types with complex engineering requirements and limited recent builds (coal/gas with CCS and offshore wind) have more stringent limits that increase more slowly over time than types with simpler engineering and more rapid recent capacity additions. All supply steps relax over time to represent the potential for development of increased national construction capacity for in-demand plants.

New nuclear builds are prohibited. The cost and social acceptance of new nuclear builds in the US is highly uncertain, as no new plants have been completed for several decades. Previous analysis (Wright and Kanudia 2014) found that CES compliance strategies and cost are highly sensitive to these assumptions. At AEO 2013 costs, new nuclear was the dominant strategy in many regions. Prohibiting nuclear leads to a richer regional mix. For these runs, electricity demand was kept fixed at AEO levels, rather than responding to price changes using elastic demand, in order to keep the focus on generation technology changes.

To assess the impact of the timing of knowledge about the CES when making MATS compliance decisions, each CES scenario was analyzed in two variations. The "foresight" version is a standard TIMES run, in which the CES requirement is "seen" at the time of MATS compliance. In the "myopic" version, the Reference case solution is frozen up to the end of the compliance window (model year 2018), after which the model is free to make new decisions about CES compliance.

5 Results

5.1 National Results

As shown in Table 5, the cost of the CES policy is very sensitive to policy ramping speed. The slow-ramping 45 scenario increases total system cost—which can be interpreted in this instance as the total net present value cost of delivering electricity to all US end users—by about eight percent. The 65 scenario roughly doubles this impact to around 15–16 %, and the fast-ramping 85 scenario increases it further. The cost impacts of myopia depend even more dramatically on CES stringency. In the 45 scenario, lack of foreknowledge about the carbon policy increases the policy's cost by only one percent, or approximately 4 billion dollars. In the 65 and 85 scenarios, these increases are far more significant, at 9 and 23 %.

Figure 3 shows how the CES compliance strategies vary with policy ramping speed and foresight versus myopia. The difference between the foresight and myopic cases derive from two factors: the relative build rates of different low carbon generation types, and the extra retrofitted coal stock in the myopic cases.

In 2018, the 65 and 85 foresight scenarios have begun to deviate significantly from the Reference case. They undertake significantly less coal retrofitting, and make up the difference with new gas combined cycle builds and, in the 85 case, small amounts of gas and coal with CCS. By scenario design, the three myopic scenarios are frozen to the reference case in this period, and the 45 foresight case requires CES compliance so far down the road that it deviates from Reference hardly at all.

By 2023, the 85 foresight scenario is generating more than 10 % of its electricity from CCS plants, and the lead over the myopic scenario in building these plants persists over the model horizon. The myopic scenario relies on quicker-to-build wind and combined cycle to meet the suddenly tightening CES. In the two 65 cases, total generation from existing coal units is similar, at around 19 % of total generation, but the myopic case is more heavily relying on the retrofits it has invested in, whereas the foresight case is splitting generation roughly evenly between retrofits and retained original equipment. The early compliance strategy for both of these scenarios is an investment in new combined cycle capacity.

Table 5 Scenario system cost impacts

Scenario	Increase over reference (%)	Increase due to Myopia (%)
85-MY	35.6	23
65-MY	16.5	9
45-MY	8.1	1
85-FS	28.9	
65-FS	15.1	
45-FS	8.0	

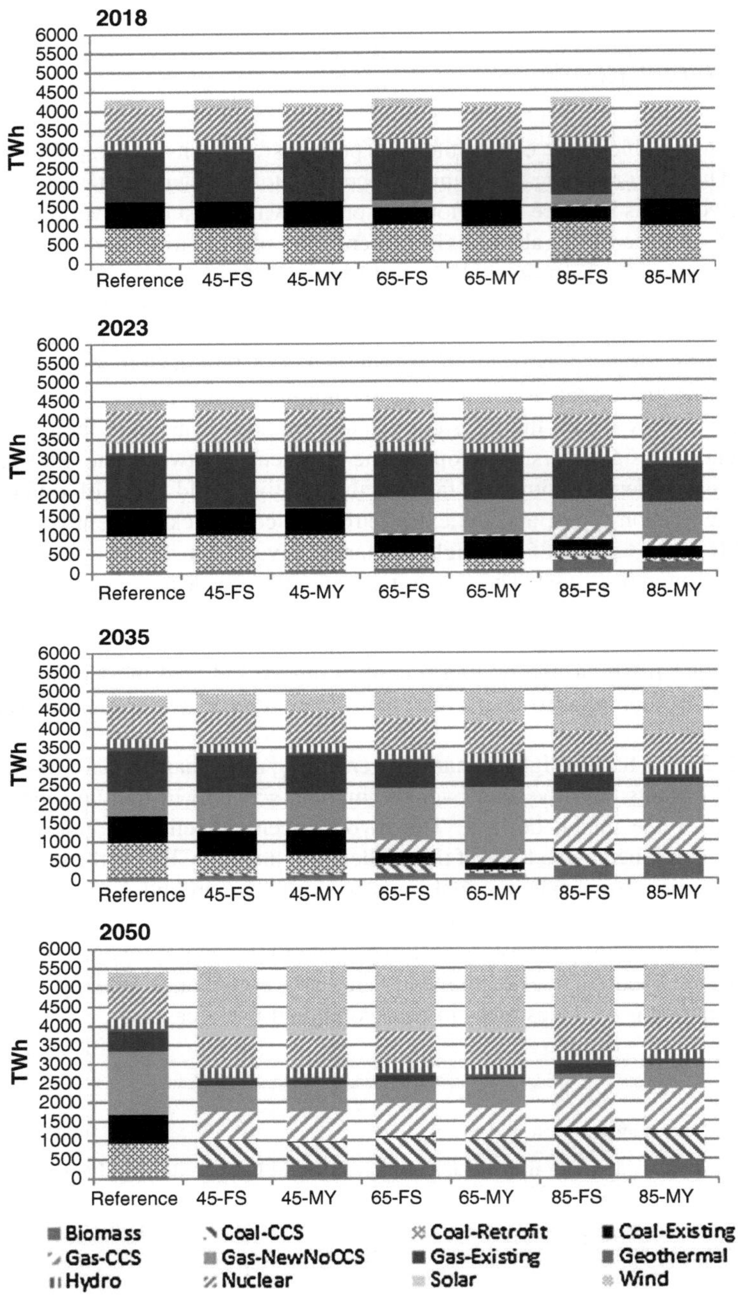

Fig. 3 National generation mix across scenarios

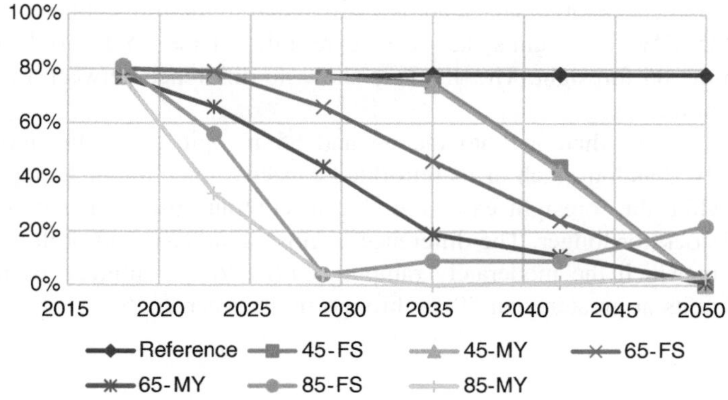

Fig. 4 Utilization of retrofitted coal units

By 2035, the 65 foresight case is still operating nearly half of the coal capacity it retrofitted, covering this non-compliant generation with more CCS than the myopic case, which has abandoned most of its retrofits (Fig. 4). The 45 cases have begun investing in wind and combined cycle, but are still operating most of their retrofit capacity. The differences between the foresight and myopic cases are minimal.

2050 brings a convergence of all the CES policies to the same 90 % requirement, but the compliance strategies differ significantly depending on the route taken over the previous periods. The 85 foresight case relies most heavily on the CCS it has been building steadily over the entire horizon, followed closely by the 85 myopic case. The foresight case is still operating around a quarter of its retrofit capacity. The other cases include more wind and solar, whose cost has come down, and the differences between the myopic and foresight cases have largely evaporated.

Table 6 summarizes retrofits and retirements by scenario. 76 GW of capacity retires rather than retrofit in the Reference and myopic cases, with an additional 30 GW in the 65 foresight case and a further 9 GW in the 85 foresight. Most of the foregone retrofits are additions of ACI to control mercury, along with some decrease in SCR and FGD. Perhaps surprisingly, DSI retrofits, which have lower

Table 6 Coal unit retirements and retrofits by scenario (GW)

	85-MY	65-MY	45-MY	85-FS	65-FS	45-FS	Reference
Retirements	76	76	76	115	106	76	76
Retrofits—ACI	71	71	71	44	49	71	71
Retrofits—SCR	4	4	4	0	0	4	4
Retrofits—DSI	11	11	11	13	4	11	11
Retrofits—FGD	41	41	41	8	23	41	41
Retrofits—All[1]	100	100	100	55	65	100	100

[1]Retrofits do not sum to totals because some units receive more than one retrofit

capital but higher operating costs, are not stimulated in the foresight cases. Overall, there are 35 GW fewer units that receive retrofits in the 65 foresight case and 45 GW in the 85 foresight. The 45 cases show no difference between myopic and foresight choices.

Figure 4 shows that, in both the 65 and 85 myopic cases, the model must precipitously abandon much of its retrofitted capacity, once the unanticipated CES kicks in, while the foresight cases are able to continue using their more modest retrofitted stock for longer. The difference is most significant and prolonged in the 65 cases, in which the moderately ramping CES allows continued utilization of retrofitted units at greater than 50 % through model year 2035.

5.2 Regional and Unit-Level Results

Figure 5 shows the generation mix and inter-regional trade flows in 2035 for the 85 foresight and myopic scenarios. (Pie and wedge sizes in the figure are proportional to generation, and arrow widths are proportional to interregional flows.) A mix of compliance strategies are visible, with heavy investment in wind and biomass in the resource-rich Plains and Upper Midwest. Coal and gas with CCS are concentrated in Southeast and Gulf Coast regions with good access to sequestration sites, and other regions rely on new gas combined cycle and existing nuclear and hydro.

Table 7 shows the net present value change of the costs to each region of supplying its own consumers' electricity demand, including capital, operating, and fuel costs, along with net costs/earnings for inter-regional electricity and CES permit trades. The values are then scaled by 2012 generation in order to allow impacts on regions of different sizes to be compared.

The CES hits the small, gas-dependent regions of New York City and Long Island hardest, with both higher gas prices and the need to import CES credits. Other high cost regions are those that have fewer (Kentucky) and/or more expensive (Southwest Power Pool—South) compliance options, or that have significant existing coal fleets that must be abandoned and replaced (PJM). Those regions that already have (Upstate and Downstate New York, Commonwealth Edison, and Pacific Northwest) or can relatively cheaply build (Northwest Power Pool—East, and Midwest Regional Organization) significant supplies of compliant generation experience a net benefit from the CES.

Myopia imposes costs on most regions, especially under the high-cost 85 CES. But some regions benefit under myopia from being able to export higher cost credits to regions with more constrained options. For example, regions in the Upper Midwest (Midwest Regional Organization) and Plains (Southwest Power Pool—North) with strong wind and biomass resources are able to become large exporters of power and CES credits in the myopic scenarios, and experience a net cost gain from myopia as a result (Fig. 5).

Those who are impacted most by not knowing about the CES before retrofit decisions must be made are, of course, the owners of the coal plants affected.

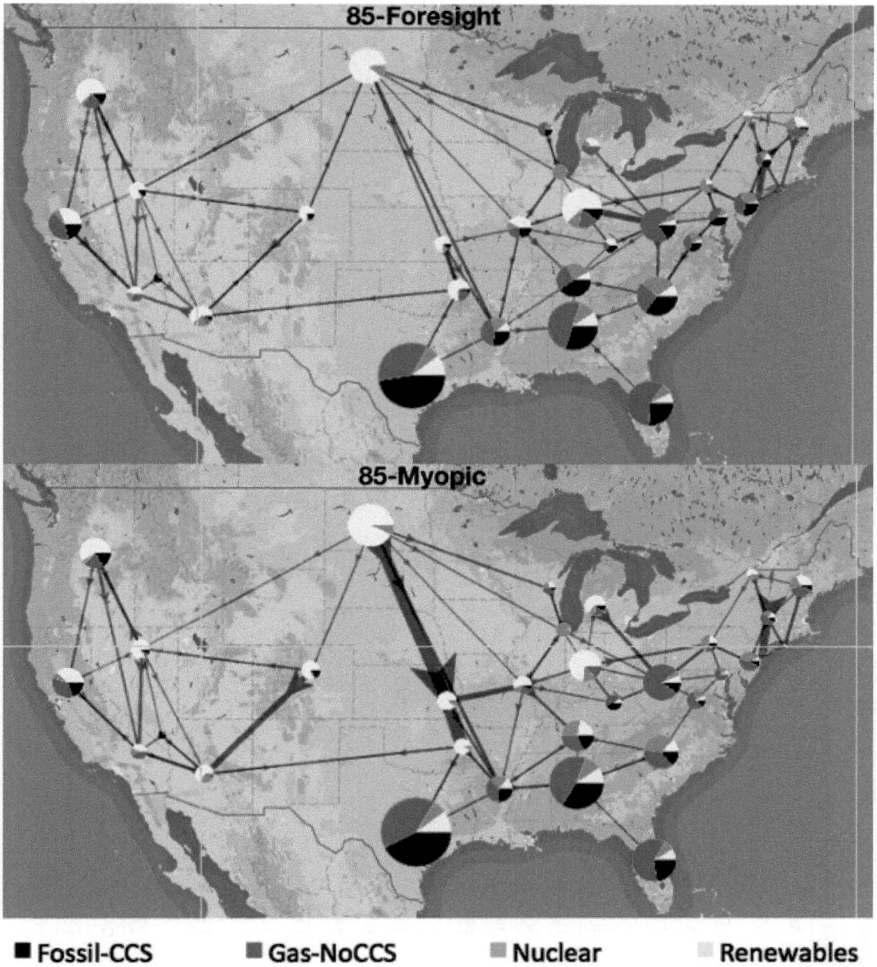

Fig. 5 2035 generation mix and inter-regional trade in the 85 foresight and myopic scenarios

Table 8 shows the cost of stranded retrofitted capacity, measured by regional annualized investments in retrofits multiplied by the difference in utilization between the Reference case (taken to be normal utilization rates) and each scenario's regional utilization. These costs range several orders of magnitude across regions, up to more than $1 billion in some regions. Regions with the lowest costs have little or no retrofitted capacity even in the Reference scenario, whereas the highest cost regions tend to be those with the largest retrofit capacities (Southwest Power Pool—South, Texas Regional Entity, and Midwest Regional Organization), along with those that must abandon retrofit capacity most precipitously (Southern Company and MISO).

Table 7 Net present value regional cost of electricity supply (M2004$/MMBTU)

Region	Cost increase over reference (scaled)						Cost of Myopia		
	85-MY	65-MY	45-MY	85-FS	65-FS	45-FS	85	65	45
Arizona—New Mexico	72	6	42	58	25	36	13	−19	6
California North	60	6	20	121	12	13	−61	−6	7
California South	351	100	37	308	126	41	43	−26	−4
Commonwealth Edison	−242	−177	−34	−143	−209	−21	−98	32	−13
Downstate New York	−1190	−681	−200	−948	−645	−190	−241	−35	−9
Kentucky	403	202	147	240	203	104	162	−1	43
MISO	105	65	−9	63	91	−5	41	−26	−4
PJM	501	254	89	313	242	89	187	13	0
Entergy	263	87	32	123	59	41	140	28	−9
Texas Regional Entity	183	89	35	114	108	34	68	−19	1
Florida Reliability Coordinating Council	321	134	45	227	125	45	94	9	0
Long Island Lighting Company	959	433	149	711	456	152	248	−24	−3
Mid-Atlantic Area Council—East	102	25	16	84	32	20	18	−7	−4
Mid-Atlantic Area Council—South	351	124	44	95	174	42	256	−50	2
Mid-Atlantic Area Council—West	178	39	17	151	26	21	28	12	−4
Gateway (Illinois-Missouri)	327	178	43	170	198	43	156	−20	0
Michigan Electric Coordination System	110	78	18	116	29	26	−5	49	−8
Midwest Regional Organization	−116	34	0	−40	61	−6	−77	−27	6
New England Power Pool	76	−59	−12	24	−56	−12	52	−3	0
Northwest Power Pool East	−271	−58	−35	−190	−48	−50	−81	−11	15
New York City	960	440	132	719	463	128	241	−23	4
Pacific Northwest	−180	−140	−29	−92	−149	−19	−87	9	−10
Rocky Mountain Power Area	−67	89	10	26	99	11	−92	−9	−2

(continued)

Table 7 (continued)

Region	Cost increase over reference (scaled)						Cost of Myopia		
	85-MY	65-MY	45-MY	85-FS	65-FS	45-FS	85	65	45
Southern Nevada	95	−25	−158	−81	−59	−141	176	34	−17
Southern Company	210	129	46	144	97	44	66	32	2
Southwest Power Pool—North	−445	−13	−28	−123	−14	−39	−321	1	11
Southwest Power Pool—South	571	221	68	283	229	68	289	−8	0
Tennessee Valley Authority	192	66	27	82	67	28	109	−1	−2
Upstate New York	−447	−282	−66	−283	−304	−66	−163	22	0
Virginia-Carolinas	151	46	29	43	47	31	108	−1	−2
Dominion Virginia Power	219	65	39	177	24	29	42	41	10
Wisconsin-Upper Michigan	265	101	39	312	103	42	−47	−2	−3

Table 8 Net present value cost of abandoned retrofit capacity (M2004$)

Region	Cost of lost retrofit utilization						Cost of Myopia		
	85-MY	65-MY	45-MY	85-FS	65-FS	45-FS	85	65	45
Arizona—New Mexico	209	99	42	107	53	40	102	46	2
California North	0	0	0	0	0	0	0	0	0
California South	3	2	1	3	1	1	0	1	0
Commonwealth Edison	1	1	0	1	0	0	0	0	0
Downstate New York	0	0	0	0	0	0	0	0	0
Kentucky	85	40	17	0	0	16	84	40	0
MISO	878	563	174	330	152	156	548	411	18
PJM	756	469	170	37	92	163	719	376	7
Entergy	459	314	100	0	40	97	459	275	3
Texas Regional Entity	470	359	109	227	215	116	243	144	−7
Florida Reliability Coordinating Council	254	165	57	3	38	57	251	127	0
Long Island Lighting Company	0	0	0	0	0	0	0	0	0
Mid-Atlantic Area Council—East	0	0	0	0	0	0	0	0	0
Mid-Atlantic Area Council—South	0	0	0	0	0	0	0	0	0
Mid-Atlantic Area Council—West	224	57	52	60	31	53	164	26	−1
Gateway (Illinois-Missouri)	265	176	51	145	72	51	120	105	−1
Michigan Electric Coordination System	95	68	23	15	25	21	80	44	2
Midwest Regional Organization	770	531	250	338	215	239	432	316	11
New England Power Pool	2	1	1	0	1	0	2	0	0
Northwest Power Pool East	205	128	57	146	53	59	58	74	−1
New York City	0	0	0	0	0	0	0	0	0
Pacific Northwest	1	1	0	0	0	0	1	1	0
Rocky Mountain Power Area	145	77	39	48	38	38	97	39	1

(continued)

Table 8 (continued)

Region	Cost of lost retrofit utilization						Cost of Myopia		
	85-MY	65-MY	45-MY	85-FS	65-FS	45-FS	85	65	45
Southern Nevada	0	0	0	0	0	0	0	0	0
Southern Company	1053	675	231	22	11	217	1031	664	14
Southwest Power Pool—North	372	217	104	122	101	102	249	115	2
Southwest Power Pool—South	1311	768	331	395	371	310	916	396	21
Tennessee Valley Authority	724	479	165	240	139	148	484	340	17
Upstate New York	0	0	0	0	0	0	0	0	0
Virginia-Carolinas	158	82	32	12	6	30	146	76	2
Dominion Virginia Power	128	65	23	0	0	23	128	65	0
Wisconsin-Upper Michigan	106	93	30	0	0	32	106	93	−3
Total	8673	5430	2057	2254	1656	1971	6335	3709	41

The additional costs imposed by myopia also vary greatly, even among the high cost regions, with some regions able to eliminate most or all of these costs with foresight, even in the 85 case, through reduced retrofit investments and longer utilization of the retrofitted stock. For example, the PJM region foregoes more than 5 GW of capital-intensive FGD retrofits, retaining only 0.3 GW of FGD and 1.4 GW of ACI, substantially reducing its lost investments when these units must be shut down under the increasing CES. Overall, foresight saves more than $6 billion in stranded asset costs in the 85 case and nearly $4 billion in the 65 case.

Figure 6 compares the distribution of the retrofitted units in the 85 foresight and myopic scenarios. The concentration of additional myopic retrofits—and hence the costs of myopia—in the Ohio Valley and Southeast is clearly visible.

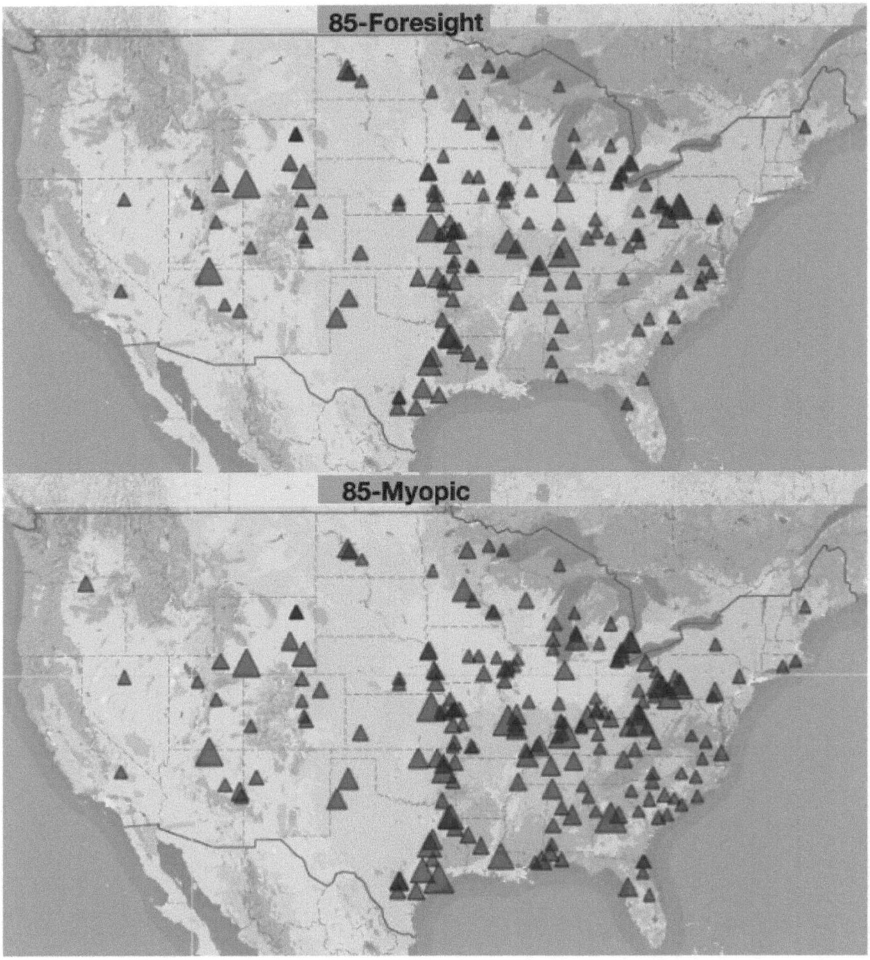

Fig. 6 Retrofitted units in 85 foresight and myopic scenarios

6 Conclusions

This chapter has described and illustrated the techniques used to conduct highly detailed modeling of existing coal-fired units in the US power sector. Such detailed modeling is called for in situations where the existing stock plays a key role in determining policy cost and incidence, and will be increasingly necessary for analyzing real climate policies. It also permits the application of TIMES modeling to policies that are far nearer-term than has been commonly practiced.

In the analysis presented here, the FACETS model was used to analyze the interactions between air quality and carbon policies, when the timing and stringency of the carbon policy is uncertain. The overall national costs of myopia were found to be small (1–10 % of overall carbon policy cost), except when the carbon policy ramps up very quickly after air quality compliance decisions are made. However, these national results obscure significant regional heterogeneity. Some regions experience substantial cost increases from myopia, while others that can export valuable credits actually experience a net benefit. The cost of retrofitted units that must be underutilized or abandoned later range from $2 billion in the slow-ramping 45 cases to more than $8 billion in the 85 myopic case. Substantially fewer retrofits are undertaken in the foresight cases, reducing stranded asset costs in some regions by up to 100 %. Because elastic demand was not used for these runs, we would expect the real world cost and generation mix impacts to be somewhat muted as electricity demand responded to price changes.

Recently US EPA (2014) has released draft regulations for carbon emissions from existing power plants under section 111d of the Clean Air Act, known as the Clean Power Plan (CPP). The CPP is similar to the CES modeled here, imposing a maximum carbon emissions rate for covered generation in each state, where covered units include existing fossil plus non-hydro renewables. Existing hydro and most existing nuclear are excluded, reducing or eliminating the windfall gains found herein for regions with substantial shares of hydro and nuclear capacity in their existing mix. The CPP requirements ramp in over the period 2020–2030, reaching approximately midway in stringency between our 45 and 65 cases, and require no further reductions beyond 2030.

The analysis conducted here suggests that the overall costs of the CPP are likely to be modest, although some regions may experience substantially greater cost impacts than others. Assuming any new, additional carbon policy would not take effect until after the CPP's compliance period ends in 2030, additional costs from having taken MATS decisions more than a decade earlier without foreknowledge of the future carbon policy will be small. If, however, the need for additional carbon emissions reductions from the power sector comes to be seen as more urgent, the potential for significant costs from stranded assets rises.

Because the CPP will be implemented at the state level, each state will need to conduct its own analysis of compliance strategies, based on its own existing stock and resource base. An analysis of the CPP using FACETS is underway.

References

Pizer W, Sanchirico JN, Batz M (2009) Regional patterns of U.S. household carbon emissions. Clim Change 99:47–63

Rausch S, Metcalf GE, Reilly JM (2011) Distributional impacts of carbon pricing: a general equilibrium approach with micro-data for households. Energy Econ 33:S20–S33

US Energy Information Administration (2009) The national energy modeling system: an overview, Washington, DC. DOE/EIA-0581(2009)

US Energy Information Administration (2011a) Assumptions to the annual energy outlook 2011, Washington, DC. DOE/EIA-0554(2011)

US Energy Information Administration (2011b) Analysis of impacts of a clean energy standard as requested by Chairman Hall, Washington, DC

US Energy Information Administration (2011c) Electricity market module of the national energy modeling system, Washington, DC. DOE/EIA-M068(2011)

US Energy Information Administration (2012) Annual energy review 2011, Washington, DC DOE/EIA-0384(2011)

US Energy Information Administration (2013) Annual energy outlook 2013, Washington, DC DOE/EIA-0383(2013)

US Environmental Protection Agency (2010) Documentation for EPA base case v.4.10 using the integrated planning model, Washington, DC. EPA #430R10010

US Environmental Protection Agency (2011a) Documentation supplement for EPA base case v4.10_PTox—updates for proposed toxics rule, Washington, DC. EPA #430-R-11-006

US Environmental Protection Agency (2011b) Documentation supplement for EPA base case v.4.10_MATS—updates for final Mercury and Air Toxics Standards (MATS) rule, Washington, DC. EPA #430-F-11-066

US Environmental Protection Agency (2014) Carbon pollution emission guidelines for existing stationary sources: electric utility generating units—proposed rule, Washington, DC. EPA-HQ-OAR-2013-0602

US Environmental Protection Agency (2014a) Mercury and Air Toxics Standard. http://www.epa.gov/mats/. Accessed 25 Nov 2014

US Environmental Protection Agency (2014b) Air pollution and the clean air act. http://www.epa.gov/air/caa/. Accessed 25 Nov 2014

Weyant J, Kriegler E (2014) Preface and introduction to EMF 27. Clim Change 123:345–352. doi:10.1007/s10584-014-1102-7

Wheeler D (2008) Why Warner-Lieberman failed and how to get America's working families behind the next cap-and-trade bill. Center for Global Development, Working Paper 149, Washington, DC

Wright E, Kanudia A (2014) Low carbon standard and transmission investment analysis in the new multi-region US power sector model FACETS. Energy Econ 46:136–150. http://dx.doi.org/10.1016/j.eneco.2014.09.013

An Analysis of the Impacts of New Oil Pipeline Projects on the Canadian Energy Sector with a TIMES Model for Canada

Kathleen Vaillancourt, Yuri Alcocer and Olivier Bahn

Abstract The oil industry currently plays a major role in the Canadian economy. In the future, further developments of the oil sector will be affected by the ability to transport crude oil (mainly from Western Canada) to consuming regions in Canada and abroad. This chapter analyzes different crude oil exportation scenarios based on existing pipeline expansions and the development of new pipelines. We use for this a multi-regional TIMES energy model for Canada. Our results indicate that: (i) the exporting capacity will be an important driver for oil production levels in Canada, and (ii) impacts on the other Canadian energy sectors are rather limited.

1 Introduction

It is an understatement to allege that the oil industry plays a major role in Canada's economy and development. Considering crude oil alone, with over $69 billion of private investment in 2013, it represents nearly a fifth of Toronto's Stock Exchange value and pays over $18 billion to the provincial and federal governments in taxes and revenues each year (CAPP 2014a). Providing over 550,000 direct and indirect jobs in the country, the oil industry is the backbone of Canada's actual economy and financial stability.

K. Vaillancourt (✉)
ESMIA Consultants, Montréal, QC, Canada
e-mail: kathleen@esmia.ca

Y. Alcocer
HEC Montréal and North Atlantic Refining, St-John's, NL, Canada
e-mail: yuri-ernesto.alcocer-morales@hec.ca

O. Bahn
GERAD and Department of Decision Sciences, HEC Montréal, Montréal, QC, Canada
e-mail: olivier.bahn@hec.ca

G. Giannakidis et al. (eds.), *Informing Energy and Climate Policies Using Energy Systems Models*, Lecture Notes in Energy 30,
DOI 10.1007/978-3-319-16540-0_14

In 2013, Canada's crude oil production reached an approximate total of 3.5 million barrel/day (bbl/d), of which 1.9 were produced from oil sands. It is expected that by 2030, Canada will produce a total of 6.4 million bbl/d, with crude oil from bitumen representing over 90 % of this augmentation (CAPP 2014b). Even if new techniques and technologies improve the actual life expectancy of conventional oil reserves, oil sands, with a fast expending capital investment and the recent confirmation of new reserves, is where the growth is expected. Of the 339 billion barrels of crude oil that represent Canada's estimated resources by the end of 2012, oil sands bitumen and conventional crude are in a respective proportion of 90 and 10 % (NEB 2013). All of Canada's bitumen resources can be found in Alberta and Saskatchewan. Canada owns the third largest reserves of oil in the world, just after Saudi Arabia and Venezuela.

However, every actor in the industry agrees that in order to achieve such a progression in production, Western Canada's oil must find a demand for its offer. As Alberta and Saskatchewan are inland provinces, without access to tidewater ports, they are in need to develop their capacity to export this expected production. It is now becoming a political, economic and national security matter that this oil finds access to tidewater and export opportunities (McKenna 2013). As for their actual markets, maintenance on existing pipelines and the necessity of upgrading refineries receiving the crude oil from Western Canada, create bottleneck in the distribution system that furthermore puts pressure on expected growth. Already, the impact of this surplus in crude, and the inability to reach external markets, produces negative effects for the industry. Furthermost, is the price discount that Canadian oil producers must pay for their inability to reach markets, putting negative pressure on their profits. From 2011 and 2012, the Western Canadian Select (WCS), the price reference for Canadian heavy crude, traded up to US$19/bbl below West Texas Intermediate (WTI). This price reflects also the difference in quality of the two products (CAPP 2014b).

Seeing how, in the short term, production is straining pipeline capacity and will soon exceed transportation capacity, implementing only long term solutions may jeopardize this intended growth. On the order hand, short term solutions may prove useful in the interim, as such, the transport by rail cars may prove an interesting temporary solution. Rail cars shipping is expected to increase in Canada from about 200,000 bbl/d in late 2013 to 700,000 bbl/d by the end of 2016 (CAPP 2014c), about the transport capacity of a major pipeline. Even with this rapid development, Western Canada must increase dramatically its capacity to export.

The objective of this chapter is to analyze different crude oil exportation scenarios based on existing capacity expansion and new pipeline projects taking off from the *Western Canadian Sedimentary Basin* (WCSB) to reach North American, Asian or domestic markets. For the maximum levels of oil exports corresponding to the available pipeline capacity in each scenario, we compare both the impacts on the final energy demand and on the crude oil production profiles.

This chapter is organized as follows. Section 2 gives an overview of the different markets opportunities for supplying Canadian oil while Sect. 3 presents the database structure for the oil sector. Section 4 details our scenario definition. Section 5 provides contains the analysis of all scenarios, namely the impacts on the Canadian oil sector in particular and on the energy system in general. In Sect. 6, we compare some of our results with results from existing outlooks before concluding in Sect. 7.

2 Canadian Oil Exportation Options

It falls to the industry and governments to find and open new markets in order to achieve a significant increase in oil production. Three markets are therefore considered: (1) Central and South USA markets, (2) Canadian and USA West coasts and Asia, and finally (3) East Canada and Eastern USA.

2.1 Central and South USA Markets

The Midwest or PADD II district (Petroleum Administration for Defense District), is currently the largest market for Canada's oil, for an approximate amount of 1.7 million bbl/d. These markets are connected to Canada by two major pipelines, Enbridge Mainline and TransCanada Keystone. Both of these networks are suffering from overload capacity and are in need of major improvements. Secondly, PADD II's refineries are already receiving most of their foreign oil (98 % in Eastern district) from Canada, allowing less space for new market shares. Finally, recent years have seen an increase in tight and crude oil, as well as in natural gas in the USA. This new production is mainly directed in this district, competing directly with Canada's oil (EIA 2014). With these constraints, demand is anticipated to reach only 2.2 million bbl/d in 2020.

The main hope for future exportation resides in PADD III, Gulf district. It is home to half the refining capacity of the USA, with over 9.4 million bbl/d (EIA 2014). From this amount, 3.7 million bbl/d of crude were imported, mainly from Saudi Arabia, Mexico and Venezuela. But this share is diminishing rapidly with the surge in local oil, 17 % in 2012 alone. Mexico is producing slightly less each year and Venezuela is constantly threatening to diminish its offer to USA markets as a political lever. These trends, and the fact that the refineries in the Gulf are the most sophisticated in North America, already able to receive and transform Canada heavy crude, makes it an excellent option for exportation. Since this is a remote region from Western Canada, to reach this market, the authorities have been pushing its project of TransCanada Keystone XL for over 5 years now. If completed, it would provide an additional 830,000 bbl/d of capacity.

2.2 Canadian and USA West Coasts and Asia

By improving the pipeline network of Kinder Morgan Trans-Mountain (+590,000 bbl/d) and by developing the Enbridge Northern Gateway (525,000 bbl/d) between Edmonton and Kitimat, Western producers wish to accede to tidewater and therefore to Asian and Western USA markets. However, most of the extra capacity of the Kinder Morgan Trans-Mountain is already locked by firm 15–20 years' contract to Washington's refineries. It is primarily the Northern Gateway project, with its tidewater port at Kitimat, that could open the new and avid markets of India and China for Canada's crude oil. Singapore and Japan could also become interesting markets for light crude since they already have an extended refining industry for this product. Furthermore, the cost of transportation by tankers is also on par with the pipeline tariffs to USA refining markets (Wood-Mackenzie 2011). A tidewater access could also mean reaching PADD III and its attractive refining industry.

2.3 Eastern Canada and Eastern USA

Moreover, Western producers are also considering new markets on the other side of the country. Refineries in Québec and Atlantic Provinces import more than 80 % of their crude oil (642,000 bbl/d) from international markets, which makes them perfect targets for the expanding production. It is an argument in favor of the country's energy security. These regions' four refineries can handle heavier crude without much modification to their installation and their products could therefore be exported to Eastern USA. There is also the advantage of an existing, but incomplete network of pipelines that could be used to transport large amount of crude to these regions. In Ontario, in 2013, the refineries processed 380,300 bbl/d of crude oil from Canadian producers (94 % of capacity) with the first phase of the re-reversal of Enbridge line 9 of the same facilitating transportation. PADD I district is also a potential market that, if reached, may want to change its international imports to a more local and secure supply. Two pipeline projects are key to open these new markets, the re-reversal of Enbridge line 9 A and B, and the TransCanada Energy East Pipeline. If they were to be accepted in their actual form, they would add respectively 300,000 bbl/d and 1 million bbl/d to Québec's and Atlantic refineries.

3 Modeling the Canadian Oil Sector

The multi-regional energy model used for this study is an application of the TIMES model generator (Loulou et al. 2005) supported by the Energy Technology Systems Analysis Program (ETSAP 2014) of the International Energy Agency. More precisely, this TIMES model for Canada is part of a larger modeling framework: The North American TIMES energy model (ESMIA 2014).

The model covers the energy system of the 13 Canadian provinces and territories. The model spans 90 years (2011–2100) and this study will cover 2011–2050 through nine time periods and 16 annual time slices: four seasons (spring, summer, fall and winter) and four intraday periods (day, night, morning peak, evening peak). All costs are in 2011 Canadian dollars (CAD$). The global annual discount rate has been set to 5 % for this study. The model is driven by a set of 70 end-use demands for energy services and the database includes more than 4500 technologies and 800 commodities in each jurisdiction, logically interrelated in a reference energy system. As a result of our calibration process, the TIMES model for Canada yields for 2011 energy balances and greenhouse (GHG) emissions consistent with official statistics (Statistics Canada 2011, 2012; OEE 2011; NEB 2013; Environment Canada 2013) for the different province and territories.

In particular, Fig. 1 gives a simplified representation of the oil sector in the model. Supply curves have been built from the latest data available from NEB (2013) and CAPP (2013) for the different types of oil (conventional and non-conventional), reserves (located reserves, enhanced recoveries and new discoveries) and extraction techniques (mined and in situ). Most of the Canadian oil reserves (93 %) are located in the WCSB spread in four main provinces (Alberta, Saskatchewan, British Columbia, Manitoba). Extraction technologies are modeled for each type of oil and reserves, including several new methods for in situ extraction. Most of the mined bitumen (95 %) is currently upgraded into synthetic oil, while

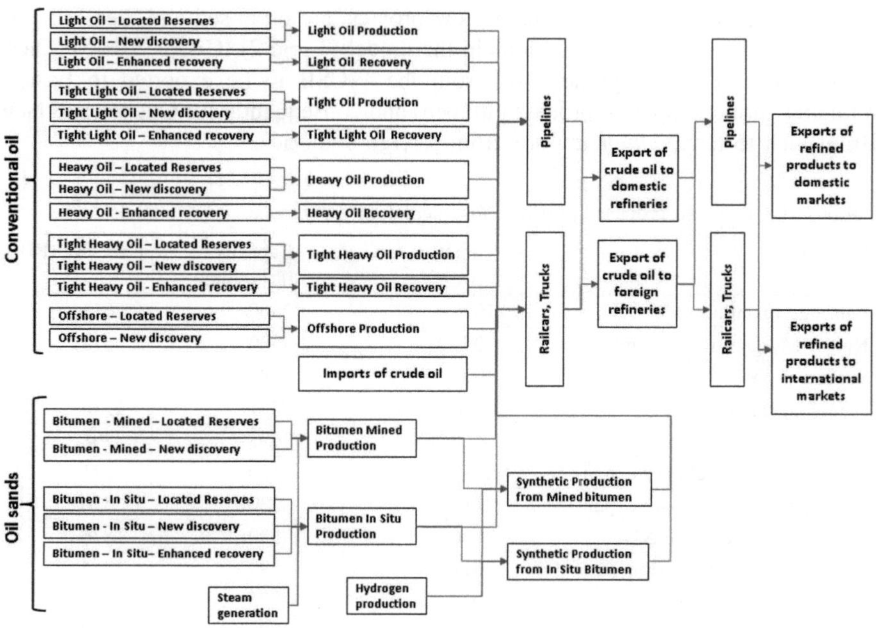

Fig. 1 Simplified representation of the oil supply sector

the in situ bitumen is mixed with condensates to produce a diluted bitumen appropriate for transport by pipeline.

Downstream activities includes six upgraders with a total capacity of 1.2 million barrels per day and 19 refineries with a total capacity of 2.06 million barrels per day and producing a full range of refined products (CAPP 2014b). Only a small number of refineries in Ontario and Alberta are currently configured to upgrade bitumen directly. All technologies are characterized by different costs and energy requirements. An important quantity of natural gas is use for steam generation (bitumen recovery) and hydrogen production (bitumen upgrading). Corresponding GHG emissions from fuel combustion and fugitive emissions are accounted at each step of the supply chain as well as flaring and venting emissions.

The model database includes the current existing transportation capacity as well as already planned projects for existing capacity expansion or new infrastructure. Due to the location of the main production centers in the WCSB and of the major markets in the USA Midwest and Gulf Coast regions, the pipeline network in North America has a strong North-South linkage. There are actually four main pipelines exiting the WCSB with a total capacity of 3.67 million barrels per day. The existing pipelines as well as planned projects are listed in Table 1 for exports from the WCSB to international destinations; they can all be visualized on maps in CAPP (2014b). In addition, rail transportation capacity has evolved quickly from 46 thousand barrels per day in 2012 to 300 thousand barrels per day in 2014 (CAPP 2014b). The growth in available rail capacity is expected to slow down and reach a maximum of 945 thousand barrels per day in 2050.

As for domestic trade, two major new projects are proposed and they are considered as future investment options in the model (Table 2) (CAPP 2014b). These projects would allow synthetic oil from the WCSB to be exported to Eastern refineries (not equipped to process bitumen) and consequently for Quebec and New Brunswick to reduce their imports from foreign countries.

Table 1 Existing and proposed pipelines for international exports

Pipeline	Target in-service	Capacity (k bbl/day)	Capacity (PJ)
Enbridge mainline	1950	2500	5651
Kinder Morgan trans mountain	1953	300	678
Spectra express	1997	280	633
TransCanada keystone	2010	591	1336
Total existing capacity		3671	8298
Enbridge Alberta clipper expansion	2014	120	271
Enbridge Alberta clipper expansion	2016	230	520
TransCanada keystone XL	2020	830	1876
Trans mountain expansion	2017	590	1334
Enbridge northern gateway	2017	525	1187
Total proposed capacity		2295	5188
Total capacity		5966	13,486

Table 2 New pipelines for domestic exports

Pipeline	Target in-service	Capacity (k bbl/day)	Capacity (PJ)
Enbridge line 9 reverse	2015	300	678
TransCanada energy east	2018	850	1921
Total proposed capacity		1150	2599

The model captures six types of oil commodities that can be transported by pipelines and/or other means (trucks, trains and tankers) from primary production wells to different types of destinations: domestic refineries, USA refineries and export terminals (e.g. Kitimat in BC) reaching two aggregated international regions (Rest of the World—East and Rest of the World—West). While international trade movements are modeled using fix prices and limits on quantities by origins and destinations, domestic trade movements within Canada are determined endogenously.

4 Description of Scenarios

For this study, end-use demand have been projected using a coherent sets of socio-economic drivers (NEB 2013), together with coefficients capturing demand sensitivity to these drivers. This approach builds on Vaillancourt et al. (2014) where five different baselines were developed and characterized by different assumptions on oil prices or economic growth covering a large range of uncertainties related to possible future trends. We have used here the central baseline scenario consistent with an oil price reaching US$123/barrel in 2050.

4.1 Pipeline Capacities in the Baseline Scenario

Baseline (BAU): This scenario illustrates the situation where all new projects would take place. The following assumptions are used to define the real availability of pipelines for exportation from the WCSB (CAPP 2014b):

- Enbridge Mainline: The pipeline is used at 70 % of its existing capacity for international exports (USA) and at 5 % for domestic exports (Ontario), while the remaining portion (25 %) is not available due to the competition with the oil entering the pipeline on the other side of the USA border.
- Enbridge Alberta Clipper Expansion: About 90 % of the total capacity will be used for international exports and 10 % for domestic exports (Ontario).
- Kinder Morgan Trans Mountain and Expansion: Most of the capacity is currently used to export oil to the USA (70 %), and to the rest of the world through

terminals in British Columbia (26 %). A small portion (4 %) is already used for carrying oil to domestic refineries in British Columbia.
- Spectra Express and TransCanada Keystone: These pipelines are available at 100 % to export oil to USA.
- TransCanada Keystone XL: This pipeline would be available at 100 % to export oil to USA.
- Enbridge Northern Gateway: This pipeline would be available at 100 % to export oil to ROW.
- Enbridge Line 9 reverse & TransCanada Energy East: These pipelines would be available at 100 % to export oil to Central and Eastern Canada.

Given these assumptions, the remaining available capacity is 4858 PJ and is expected to be doubled by 2020 with an additional 4986 PJ of capacity (Table 3).

A breakdown by type of destinations gives a better illustration of the saturation levels and potential for increases. Most of the existing capacity is used to export oil to Southern markets (capacity used at 97 %), while only a marginal portion is sent to Western markets (used only at 15 %). The addition of new capacity will allow increasing current exportation levels to the Southern markets by 1.79 times and to the Western markets by 65 times.

4.2 Pipeline Capacities in Three Alternate Scenarios

We have defined three alternate scenarios which differ in terms of the pipeline capacity available to supply the WCSB oil on various markets.

- **Southern markets (No South)**: This scenario represents a situation where there would be less additional options for WCSB oil to reach South and Central USA markets. The following project would never occur: TransCanada Keystone XL (1876 PJ of additional capacity for international trade).

Table 3 Available pipeline capacity for oil exports by destination

	Existing capacity (PJ)	New capacity (PJ)	Total capacity (PJ)	Exports in 2011 (PJ)	% of capacity in 2011
Southern markets	4679	3448	8127	4546	97
Western markets	179	1538	1717	27	15
Total international	4858	4987	9844	4573	90
Eastern: up to Quebec		678	678		
Eastern: up to new Brunswick		1921	1921		
Total domestic		2600	2600		

- **Western markets (No West)**: This scenario builds on the previous one and represents a situation where there would be also less additional options for WCSB oil to reach Canadian and USA West Coast and consequently Asian markets. The following projects would never occur: TransCanada Keystone XL (1876 PJ of additional capacity for international trade) as well as the Enbridge Northern Gateway (1187 PJ of additional capacity for international trade).
- **Eastern markets (No East)**: This scenario represents a situation where there would be no additional options allowing WCSB oil to reach refineries in Central and Eastern Canada (more precisely Quebec and New Brunswick). The following projects would never occur: Enbridge Line 9 reverse and TransCanada Energy East (2600 PJ of additional capacity for domestic trade).

5 Analysis of Scenarios

In this section, we present the impacts on the Canadian oil production levels and trade movements both within and outside Canada in all four scenarios: on the oil sector specifically (Sect. 5.1) and on the overall energy system in general (Sect. 5.2).

5.1 Impacts on the Canadian Oil Sector

These results show the evolution of the total oil production to 2050 to meet both the domestic demands and international exports. Figure 2 illustrates the breakdown of crude oil production by type in all scenarios. In the BAU scenario, oil production increases by 1.72 times between 2011 and 2030 level and peaks at 12,045 PJ in

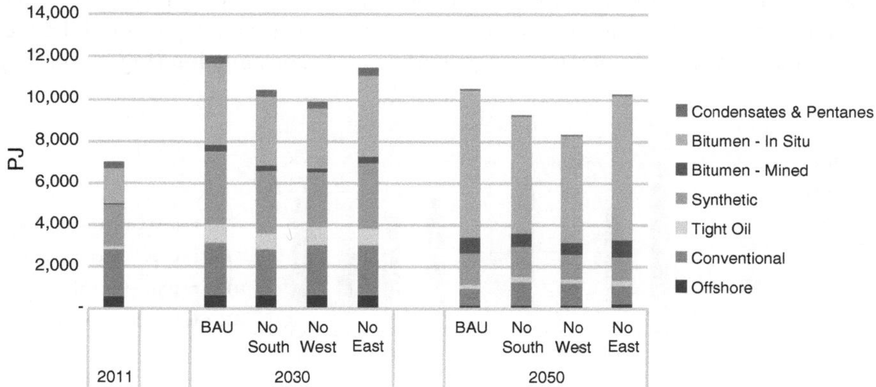

Fig. 2 Oil production by type in all scenarios

2030 before starting its decline to reach 10,492 PJ in 2050. The highest growth occurs between 2020 and 2030 after all pipeline projects have been built and the available capacity for exports has reached its maximum. The stability in the share of conventional oil between 2011 and 2030 is due to the availability of enhanced oil recovery options extending the life of some wells and the extraction of tight oil. However, conventional and tight oil *production* declines by significant faster rates between 2030 and 2050, representing only 10 % of the total oil production in 2050. While oil sands represented already half of the total oil production in 2011, it is expected to represent 88 % of the production in 2050. The proportion of oil sands extracted via in situ techniques alone is expected to represent 67 % of the overall production in 2050. A significant portion of this oil sands production via mined or in situ techniques is converted to synthetic oil.

Oil production levels in the three alternate scenarios show the significant impacts of available pipeline capacity for international exports: total oil production is 18 % lower in the No West scenario than in the BAU scenario in 2030 and 21 % lower in 2050. Conversely, the impacts of available pipeline capacity for domestic exports are non-significant, with only a 2 % decrease in 2050. As most of the production is exported, the international demand for Canadian crude is the main driver of oil production levels. A very large proportion of all the oil produced in the WCSB is exported to international destinations: 64 % in 2011 to 82 % in 2050 (Fig. 3). Consequently, the availability of the pipeline capacity for international exports has direct impacts on oil production levels while the effect of domestic exports is minor. In terms of international destinations, oil exports are almost exclusively oriented to USA markets by pipeline in 2011 but diversify on the long term both in terms of transportation means and other destinations due to (the assumed) higher oil prices.

5.2 Impacts on the Canadian Energy System

The availability of pipeline capacities do not significantly affect final energy consumption in Canada, even if fossil fuels continue to represent a large part of the fuel mix in the long term. Looking at the primary energy consumption (Fig. 4), energy

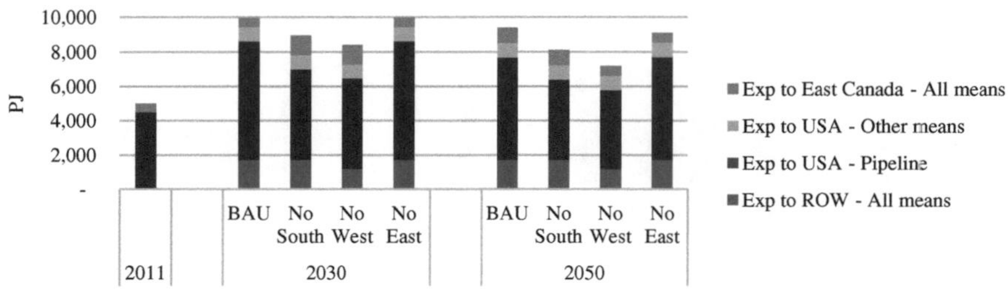

Fig. 3 Oil exports by destination in all scenarios

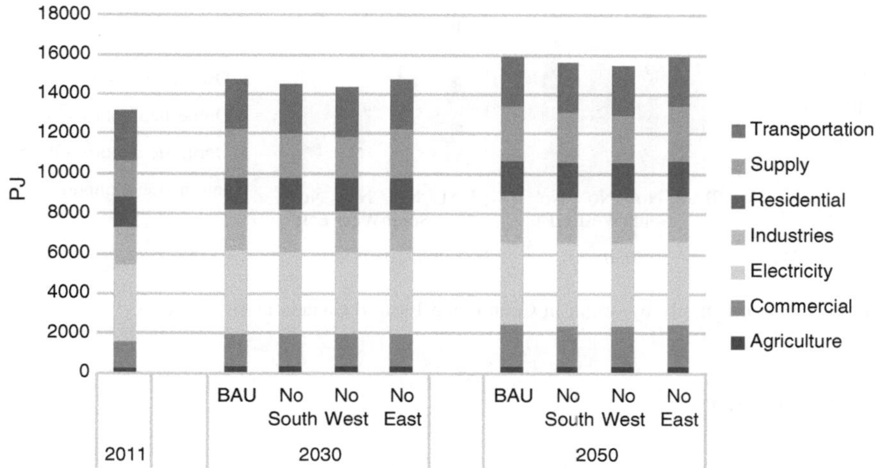

Fig. 4 Primary energy consumption by sector in all scenarios

uses in the supply sector is reduced along with the decline in oil production and exports: energy uses in the supply sector reach 2729 PJ in the BAU scenario, but only 2302 PJ in the No West scenario. However, the impacts on the primary energy consumption are minor. Less energy is required for oil extraction, upgrading and transportation of crude oil, but a portion of this decline is offset by an increase of energy uses for natural gas production, another resource largely available in Canada especially with the tight and shale gas.

The origin of crude oil used in the Central and Eastern regions of Canada (Fig. 5) indicates a strong trend toward the replacement of international light crude oil with domestic synthetic crude through the reversed Enbridge Line 9 and the TransCanada Energy East pipeline. The No East scenario shows that the high dependence Central and Eastern provinces would have to maintain imports from global markets, a situation with many energy security concerns. Only domestic supply is limited to the imports of WCSB bitumen and synthetic crude in Ontario through the existing pipeline network. In all scenarios, the need for crude oil is decreasing significantly toward 2050 due to two main factors: (1) a larger diversification of fuel used in transportation as well as important energy efficiency improvements for the various types of vehicles, and (2) an important decline in the exports of offshore oil from Newfoundland & Labrador to the USA.

In the BAU scenario, the level of GHG emissions reaches 704 Mt CO_2-eq in 2050. Due to changes in the primary energy consumption patterns, GHG emissions are lower in the scenarios where the exporting capacity is limited: 686 Mt CO_2-eq in the No South scenario (a 2.5 % reduction from the BAU level) and 673 Mt CO_2-eq in the No West (a 4.4 % reduction from BAU). The variations in GHG emissions are more significant than the variations in primary energy due to the fact that oil sands production is more energy intensive than natural gas production.

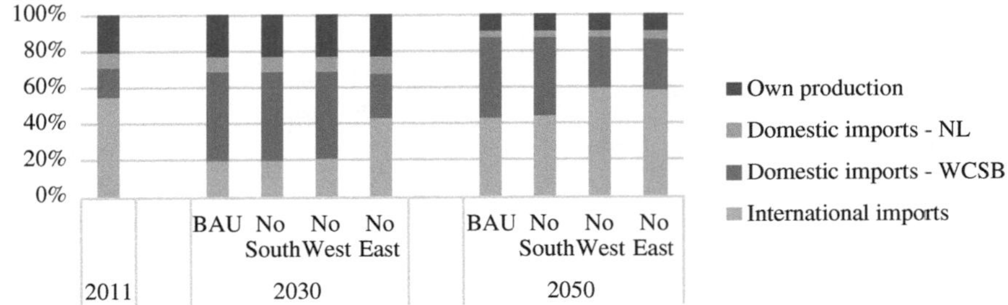

Fig. 5 Crude oil supply by origin in Central and Eastern Canada in all scenarios

6 Discussion

It is interesting to see how these oil projections compare with official Canadian outlooks. Figure 6 displays the oil production in all scenarios until 2035: oil production stabilizes at 9691 PJ in 2035 in the most conservative scenario (No West) and to 12,014 PJ in the most optimistic scenario with all pipeline projects (BAU). In all cases, these production levels are conservative compared with the central and high scenarios of the NEB (2013), where oil production reaches up to 13,201 PJ (NEB–Med) and 14,806 PJ (NEB-High) in 2035 respectively and with the scenario of the Canadian Association of Petroleum Producers (CAPP) (CAPP 2014b). These outlooks build on an optimistic view about the global demand for Canadian unconventional oil and the corresponding infrastructure capacity necessary to supply global markets: not only the available options (pipelines and/or other means) should include all projects already proposed but additional ones equivalent to the Enbridge Northern Gateway project for the NEB-Med scenario and to both Enbridge Northern Gateway and TransCanada Keystone XL projects in the NEB-High scenario.

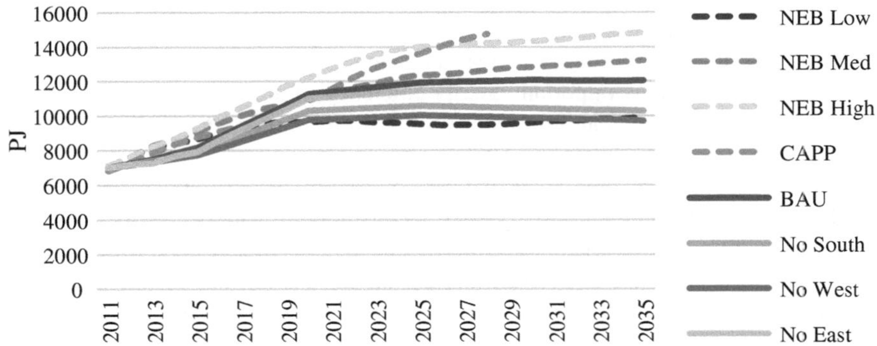

Fig. 6 Oil production levels compared with Canadian outlooks

These projections could appear as rather optimistic in the face of the many uncertainties surrounding the development of some pipeline projects that have the highest potential for increasing the exporting capacity. For instance, the TransCanada Keystone XL is currently facing vivid political opposition in the USA, augmenting the project's uncertainty.

7 Conclusion

We have presented the oil sector of a multi-regional TIMES energy model for Canada, a bottom-up optimization model that represents, in details, the whole integrated energy system from primary to useful energy in all provinces. We have also defined different exportation scenarios based on existing pipeline capacity expansion proposals and new projects taking off from the WCSB to reach North American and Asian markets. For corresponding maximum levels of conventional and unconventional oil exports, we have compared both the impacts on the crude oil production profiles and on final energy consumption mix. Results show that the exporting capacity will be an important driver for oil production level in Canada. Outside the oil sector, impacts on the energy system are limited. In particular, final energy consumption patterns are similar across scenarios since fossil fuels remain the basis for the economy whatever the origin of crude oil.

If Western oil producers are experiencing uncertainty as per which market they will be able to occupy, and by when, what is certain is that, default by them and the interested governments to find new avenue to a fast growing production will result in lower price for Canadian oil and postpone major investments and expected financial development. Variation of oil prices on international markets have indeed major impacts on the Canadian oil sectors in addition to pipeline capacities. Future works will study the impacts of different oil price forecasts on the Canadian energy system.

Acknowledgments The authors wish to acknowledge financial support from the Natural Sciences and Engineering Research Council of Canada (individual grant of Olivier Bahn) as well as research assistance from Cedric Gagnon-Ducharme.

References

CAPP (2013) Statistical handbook for Canada's upstream petroleum industry. Canadian Association of Petroleum Producers. Technical report

CAPP (2014a) Basic statistics. Canadian Association of Petroleum Producers. http://www.capp.ca/library/statistics/basic/Pages/default.aspx

CAPP (2014b) 2014 Crude oil forecast, markets and transportation. Canadian Association of Petroleum Producers

CAPP (2014c) Transporting crude oil by rail in Canada. 240914-v9. Canadian Association of Petroleum Producers

EIA (2014) Annual energy outlook 2014. Energy Information Agency. http://www.eia.gov/forecasts/aeo/pdf/0383(2014).pdf

Environment Canada (2013) National inventory report 1990–2011: greenhouse gas sources and sinks in Canada. http://www.ec.gc.ca/ges-ghg/default.asp?lang=En&n=1357A041-1

ESMIA (2014) The North American TIMES energy model (NATEM). Information available online. http://www.esmia.ca/

ETSAP—Energy Technology Systems Analysis Program (2014) Information available online. http://www.iea-etsap.org/web/index.asp

Loulou R, Remme U, Kanudia A, Lehtila A, Goldstein G (2005) Documentation for the TIMES model, energy technology systems analysis program. http://www.iea-etsap.org/web/Documentation.asp

McKenna B (2013) Oil export markets crisis has been years in the making. The globe and mail, p B3. 25 Feb 2013

NEB (2013) Canada's energy future 2013—energy supply and demand projections to 2035—an energy market assessment. National Energy Board

OEE (2011) Comprehensive energy use database. Office of Energy Efficiency Online. http://oee.nrcan.gc.ca/corporate/statistics/neud/dpa/home.cfm

Statistics Canada (2011) Report on energy supply-demand in Canada. Catalogue N. 57-003-XIE

Statistics Canada (2012) The supply and disposition of refined petroleum products in Canada. Data for 2011. Catalogue no. 45-004-X

Vaillancourt K, Alcocer Y, Bahn O, Fertel C, Frenette E, Garbouj H, Kanudia A, Labriet M, Loulou R, Marcy M, Neji Y, Waaub J-P (2014) A Canadian 2050 energy outlook: Analysis with the multi-regional model TIMES-Canada. Appl Energ 132:56–65

Wood-Mackenzie (2011) West coast export capacity netback impact analysis. Wood-Mackenzie for Alberta Department of energy, 16 Dec 2011

Multi-cluster Technology Learning in TIMES: A Transport Sector Case Study with TIAM-UCL

Gabrial Anandarajah and Will McDowall

Abstract The costs of technologies often fall over time due to a range of processes including learning-by-doing. This is a well-characterized concept in the economics of innovation, in which learning about a particular technology, and hence cost reduction, is related to cumulative investments in that technology. This chapter provides a case study applying technology learning endogenously in a TIMES model. It describes many of the key challenges in modelling technology learning endogenously, both in terms of the interpretation and policy relevance of the results, and in terms of methodological challenges. The chapter then presents a case study, exploring a multi-cluster learning approach where many key technologies (fuel cells, automotive batteries, and electric drivetrains) are shared across a set of transport modes (cars, buses and LGVs) and technologies (hybrid and plug-in hybrid fuel cell vehicles, battery electric vehicles, hybrid and plug-in hybrid petrol and diesel vehicles). The multi-region TIAM-UCL Global energy system model has been used to model the multi-cluster approach. The analysis is used to explore the competitive and/or complementary relationship between hydrogen and electricity as low-carbon transport fuels.

1 Introduction

Energy system models inform policymakers about the potential importance of particular technologies by examining whether their presence or absence (at a given cost/performance) influences the overall costs of decarbonisation. In examining the potential of new technologies, technology-rich models like TIMES and MARKAL

G. Anandarajah (✉)
UCL Energy Institute, University College London, London, UK
e-mail: g.anandarajah@ucl.ac.uk

W. McDowall
UCL Institute for Sustainable Resources, University College London, London, UK
e-mail: w.mcdowall@ucl.ac.uk

G. Giannakidis et al. (eds.), *Informing Energy and Climate Policies Using Energy Systems Models*, Lecture Notes in Energy 30,
DOI 10.1007/978-3-319-16540-0_15

take one of three approaches, which can be varied with different model runs or scenarios, for the capital cost of a technology:

1. Assume no technological change to examine whether, with stock turnovers, current technologies are sufficient to meet energy system goals.
2. Use exogenous forecasts of technological development, drawn from a range of sources. This is the approach that is typically taken with MARKAL and TIMES model.
3. Endogenise technological change into the model structure (by implementing "Endogenous Technology Learning" or ETL).

Most bottom-up energy system models adopt the second approach, using exogenous forecasts of technological development to represent technology improvements. These forecasts come from diverse sources, for which underlying assumptions are not always clear. Typically, it is recognized that while significant cost reduction is possible as a result of research and development (R&D) before a technology enters markets, there is further cost reduction after market introduction, as a result of learning-by-doing, economies of scale, continued R&D and other factors such as maturing supply chains. Some technological forecasts are produced on the basis of learning curve studies that posit a particular level of deployment of the technology. This can lead to several problems:

- First, the models' technology choice is resting on inputs that already assume the success of particular technologies. If the analyst is interested in optimal technology portfolios, this is clearly problematic: the input data already incorporates assumptions about which technologies will be most widely deployed.
- Second, exogenous technology learning allows the energy system to get the benefits of learning for free. There is no need to deploy expensive first-of-a-kind technologies, because in later years the costs will have fallen. It is possible that this appears to implicitly advocate a wait-and-see mode of technology deployment (it is not cost effective yet, so it should not be deployed yet); and it understates the total investment requirements and costs of decarbonisation, since learning costs are ignored. This has been described as 'learning without doing' (Seebregts et al. 1999).

Endogenous technology learning thus improves the internal consistency of the models (Grubb et al. 2002), and can be more appropriate for analysis attempting to gauge the relative importance of different technologies. Multi-cluster ETL-enabled models also allow insights into technology dynamics, which may suggest that technologies are worth supporting even if they are not in themselves the least-cost option, because they support learning that enables other lower cost solutions.[1]

[1]For example, fuel cell buses may not themselves be the least-cost bus technology in a carbon constrained future; but they may 'earn' their position in a least-cost solution if their deployment results in learning that can be applied to cars.

This chapter provides a case study applying technology learning endogenously in TIMES model. It applies a multi-cluster approach where many key technologies (fuel cells, automotive batteries, and electric drivetrains) are shared across a set of transport modes (cars, buses and LGVs) and technologies (hybrid and plug-in hybrid fuel cell vehicles, battery electric vehicles, hybrid and plug-in hybrid petrol and diesel vehicles). The analysis is used to explore the synergies and interactions between key component technologies, and the competitive and/or complementary relationship between hydrogen and electricity as low-carbon transport fuels.

2 Background: Modelling Technology Learning and the Experience Curve

The relationship between cumulative deployment and capital cost—described as the "learning curve"—is a well-characterized concept in the economics of innovation. Learning curves have been determined empirically for a wide range of energy technologies (McDonald and Schrattenholzer 2001). The most common formulation of the learning curve is described by Eq. 1 below:

$$C_t = C_0 * (Q_t/Q_0)^{-b} \tag{1}$$

where C_0 and Q_0 are the initial capital cost and initial installed capacity respectively, while C_t and Q_t are the capital cost and cumulative installed capacity respectively at time t. The parameter b is not intuitively easy to grasp, so is usually expressed as the progress ratio ($PR = 2^{-b}$) or the learning rate ($LR = 1 - PR$). The learning rate is the cost reduction achieved for a doubling of cumulative capacity, and is typically around 15–20 % for new energy technologies (Gritsevskyi and Nakićenovic 2000; Seebregts et al. 1998).

The learning curve equation, based on cumulative capacity, is an intuitive and analytically tractable account of how deployment relates to technological change. As a result, it has become the most widespread approach to implementing technology learning endogenously within energy-economy models. However, a growing literature—from both quantitative analysts and more qualitative 'innovation studies' scholars (Winskel et al. 2013) highlights the complexities that such a basic formulation overlooks. Perhaps unsurprisingly, representing technology dynamics effectively in energy systems and integrated assessment models is recognised as one of the great challenges for the field (Grubb et al. 2002). Here, we highlight three key methodological challenges and issues in modelling ETL, and the ways in which previous analysis has addressed them.

First, empirically derived learning curves capture changes that are both time dependent (typically thought to reflect learning 'by research'), and scale dependent (including returns to scale, and maturation of supply chains). For this reason, some scholars prefer the term 'experience curve'. Disentangling those different factors is not always straightforward, and the estimation of true 'learning by doing' can thus be challenging. Other factors come into play too—commodity costs, supply-chain bottlenecks, and the processes of 'forgetting' (described by economists as depreciation of knowledge stocks) that can occur when an industry experiences pauses or set-backs, as has occurred with the nuclear industry in many countries. The wider innovation literature highlights the existence of regulatory and wider socio-technical processes (such as socially conferred 'legitimacy' and the establishment of political lobbying power) that also go hand in hand with successful deployment, and help to reinforce allocation of R&D budgets and reduction in regulatory and transaction costs (Bergek et al. 2008). Some authors have suggested that the specification of future learning rates in models should therefore be dependent on the policy scenario (Winskel et al. 2014).

Some authors have attempted to disaggregate these diverse learning and other effects. For example, the separate processes of learning-by-doing and learning-by-research have been modelled by adopting a 'two-factor' learning curve, in which both cumulative capacity, and some measure of the R&D knowledge stock, influence rates of learning (e.g. Totschnig and Keppo 2007; Criqui et al. 2014). Others have developed three-factor or multi-factor models (Yeh and Rubin 2012). However, such approaches add analytic complexity, and may not be appropriate for a large, technology rich model. In any case, an innovation system perspective suggests that it is rare that technologies are fostered solely through R&D or solely through deployment with no accompanying R&D. It seems possible that a single learning curve, though undoubtedly a simplification, may be well placed to represent aggregate capacity-cost relationships that emerge from a wide range of processes, including both true 'learning' and other correlated processes. A similar point is made by Watanabe et al. (2000) and Kahouli-Brahmi (2008), and a good discussion of the issues is provided by Yeh and Rubin (2012). An alternative to two-factor or multi-factor learning is to model exogenous learning as a function of time in addition to learning-by-doing.

Second, technologies are often closely related, and cost reductions in one application often leads to cost reductions for a related technology in a different application, even where slightly different characteristics are required. In modelling ETL, it is possible to create 'clusters' of closely-related technologies, which share learning, to account for this effect. Examples of cluster-based learning include Totschnig and Keppo (2007), who assessed clusters around several key technologies for cars (fuel cells, hydrogen tanks, hybrid systems, and onboard fuel reformers); and Gritsevskyi and Nakićenovic (2000), who modelled ETL for fuel cells, with full spill-overs between different types of fuel cell for cars (e.g. running on hydrogen vs. on methanol), and partial spill-overs between automotive and stationary fuel cells. Krzyzanowski et al. (2004) explored clusters in which learning in hybrid drive trains is shared between light trucks and cars, and it appears that Krzyzanowski et al. (2008) explored cluster learning in which fuel cell learning was shared between buses and cars, but this is not made explicitly clear in the paper. Gül et al. (2009) applied learning to clusters of hydrogen and electricity production technologies, but the representation of transport technologies does not use a cluster approach, and so does not enable spill-overs between e.g. fuel cell cars and battery electric light goods vehicles.

The degree of spill-over between particular technologies is an important assumption in such analysis, but it is not clear that such relationships can be forecasted with any accuracy. Past practice has tended to make assumptions about the degree of relatedness and spill-over, largely on the basis of modeller judgement rather than empirical evidence. Furthermore, it is not necessarily straightforward to define the level of aggregation at which to study (and model) the experience curve. Components (such as wind turbine blades or nacelles) may develop at different rates from the aggregate wind turbine.

A third methodological challenge relates to the perfect foresight nature of bottom-up energy system models such as MARKAL/TIMES. Many earlier studies applying ETL in MARKAL/TIMES or other bottom-up optimization models (e.g. Mattsson and Wene 1997; Seebregts et al. 1998; de Feber et al. 2003) found that the model tends to deploy the 'learning technology' very rapidly and to the greatest extent possible—or not at all. In terms of interpretation, this raises questions about the feasibility of very rapid transitions from one technology to another, as well as questions about the relationship between deployment speed and learning rate. An observation from the rapid roll-out of flue-gas desulphurisation in Germany during the 1980s was that simultaneous deployment across a large number of power stations inhibited effective learning because the same mistakes were being made at the same time (Eames 2000). There was no time to learn from one installation and apply those lessons to the next, since they were not occurring sequentially. The implications of this observation for system models is that the relationship between learning rates and deployment rates (and rate constraints) should be considered, at least in the interpretation of results if not endogenously within the model.

The immediately-or-never pattern of deployment of a learning technology within an ETL model has led some authors to advocate caution in modelling ETL: if the resulting model dynamics are simply the result of exogenous rate constraints and upper bounds, then there may be few additional insights derived from the considerable effort required to endogenise learning in the model (Loulou et al. 2005). However, the approach presented in the case study in this chapter appears to reduce the problem of immediately-or-never deployment in an ETL model. This case study applies multiple clusters in which key vehicle components (automotive batteries, fuel cells, and electric drivetrains) undergo learning that is then combined within and shared across vehicle modes (buses, HGVs, cars). As the analysis shows, the model does not show the immediately-or-never behavior typical to previous work with ETL in energy system models.

3 Endogenous Technology Learning in TIMES

To represent learning-by-doing in TIMES, the investment cost (INVCOST) of the learning technology will decrease with the cumulative investment of the learning technology. The investment cost of the learning technology becomes a variable investment cost. This is represented by Eq. 2.

$$INVCOST = aC_t^{-b} \tag{2}$$

where, a is initial investment cost, C is cumulative investment and b represents learning. Since the relationship between the investment cost and learning rate is non-linear (Eq. 1), the TIMES model's objective function will yield a non-linear expression, which as a linear programming model it is unable to solve. To avoid a non-linear relationship, the investment cost in the objective function will be represented by piecewise linear approximation of total investment cost (*TCt*) as shown in Fig. 1. The cumulative learning curve is approximated by linear segments and binary variables are used—leading to mixed integer programming, which increases computing time.

Learning in one technology often enables cost reductions in closely related technologies. To account for this effect, a cluster approach can be used in TIMES, in which a group of technologies sharing a common component—the 'key technology'—learn together. The technologies constituting a cluster are related by multiple links that contribute to magnify their economic, social and environmental impacts (Grübler et al. 1999). These multiple relations ensure that progress in one technology contributes, directly or indirectly, to progress for other members of the cluster, as it helps to reinforce their own position in the marketplace.

In TIMES, it is possible to apply learning for a single technology at a regional level or global level. When learning is global, deployment yields cost reductions for users of the technology worldwide regardless of which region has deployed the technology—learning is said to spill over globally.

For each learning technology, the user provides:

The progress ratio pr [$pr = 2^{-b}$; $1 - pr$ (learning rate) is the cost reduction incurred when cumulative investment is doubled];
One initial point on the learning curve, denoted (C_0, TC_0) and floor cost;
The maximum allowed cumulative investment $C_{\max}$ (from which the maximum total investment cost $TC_{\max}$ may be inferred);

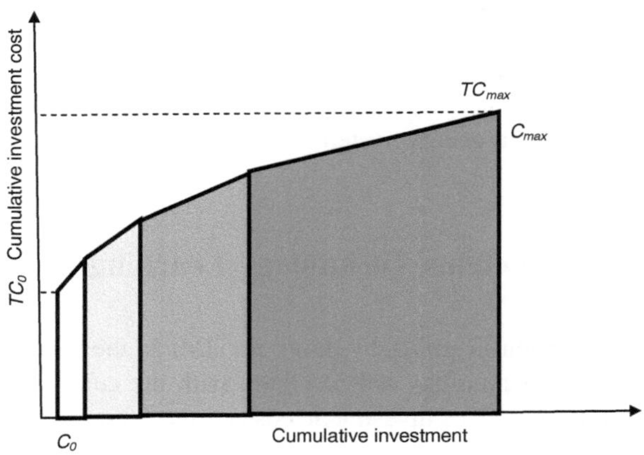

Fig. 1 Segment approximation of the cumulative cost curve

The number N of segments for approximating the cumulative learning curve over the (C_0, C_{max}) interval (note that N may be different for different technologies).

As noted above, many previous applications of ETL within MARKAL/TIMES models have observed that the model tends to select learning technologies, and invest massively in early periods in these technologies in order to lower future cost. The resulting unrealistically rapid deployment can be prevented by additional constraints (build rate). Results are then conditioned by the exogenous upper bound. The discount rate provides an incentive for postponing investments. Investing early allows the unit investment cost to drop immediately, and thus allows much cheaper investments in the learning technologies in the current and all future periods. The resulting dynamics depend on the learning rate and the discount rate.

4 Case Study

4.1 Introduction

Both hydrogen and electricity have been widely discussed as possible fuels for decarbonising road transport, as long as hydrogen and/or electricity is produced in a sustainable manner. Yet deployment of such vehicles is currently limited, as battery electric and fuel cell technologies are too expensive to compete techno-economically with internal combustion vehicles using fossil fuels. This case study, which draws on Anandarajah et al. (2013), analyses the long-term role of hydrogen and electricity in facilitating decarbonisation of the global transport sector by implementing global learning endogenously in the TIAM-UCL multi-regional global energy system model. The 16-region TIAM-UCL model has been developed at UCL through the UK Energy Research Centre (UKERC) by breaking out the UK from the Western Europe Region in the 15-Region ETSAP-TIAM model, which is the global multiregional incarnation of the TIMES model generator (Loulou et al. 2005; Loulou and Labriet 2008).

4.2 Technology Learning

The cluster approach adopted in this paper uses single factor learning, where a group of technologies sharing a common component—the 'key technology'—learn together. For example, fuel cells are an example of a key component technology, and members of the corresponding cluster of 'shell' technologies in which the component is used are hybrid- and plug-in hybrid-fuel cell vehicles both in cars and light goods vehicles (LGVs) as well as in buses. Three key component technologies undergo learning in the model, and are thus explicitly represented in the model as technologies in their own right, in addition to the vehicle 'shell' systems in which they are deployed (Fig. 2):

Fuel cell systems ($/kW)
Electric drivetrains ($/kW)
Automotive battery systems ($/kWh)

Only investment costs undergo learning. As a result, the component technologies in the model only carry investment costs. Efficiency and O&M costs are attributes of the vehicles (shell) themselves. Each of these component technologies is embedded in vehicles that use them. For example, a hybrid hydrogen fuel cell vehicle uses electric drivetrain, battery, and a fuel cell system. A plug-in hybrid petrol car, in contrast, uses an electric drivetrain and battery but no fuel cell. Table 1 shows the vehicle types, the acronyms used to describe them in this paper, the fuels they use, and which of the component 'key technologies' they use. Data are not shown in the table, for brevity, since the capacity of each key technology differs depending on whether the vehicle type is deployed as a car, bus or LGV. Data can be found in McDowall (2012).

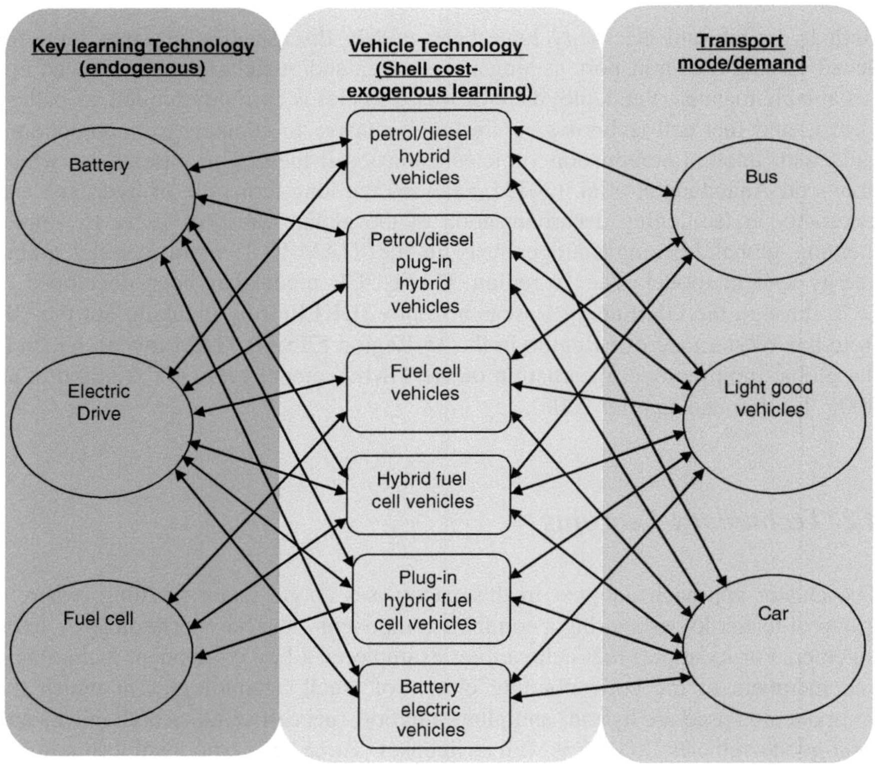

Fig. 2 Multi-cluster learning approach modelled in TIAM-UCL

Table 1 Vehicle types in the model. All vehicle types are available as cars and light goods vehicles (LGVs), only those marked with an asterisk are available as buses

Vehicle type	Acronym	Fuels used	Key technologies		
			Battery	Electric drive	Fuel cell
Petrol vehicle	Petrol ICE	Petrol or ethanol	✗	✗	✗
Diesel vehicle*	Diesel ICE	Diesel or biodiesel	✗	✗	✗
Petrol hybrid vehicle	Petrol HEV	Petrol or ethanol	✓	✓	✗
Diesel hybrid vehicle*	Diesel HEV	Diesel or biodiesel	✓	✓	✗
Petrol plug-in hybrid vehicle	Petrol PHEV	Petrol or ethanol and electricity	✓	✓	✗
Diesel plug-in hybrid vehicle	Diesel PHEV	Diesel or biodiesel and electricity	✓	✓	✗
Fuel cell vehicle	FCV	Hydrogen	✗	✓	✓
Fuel cell hybrid vehicle*	FCHV	Hydrogen	✓	✓	✓
Fuel cell plug-in hybrid vehicle	FCPHEV	Hydrogen and electricity	✓	✓	✓
Battery electric vehicle	BEV	Electricity	✓	✓	✗
Natural gas vehicle*	CNG	Natural gas	✗	✗	✗
LPG vehicle	LPG	Liquefied petroleum gas	✗	✗	✗

Learning for a component takes place regardless of the vehicle type in which it is deployed. i.e. cost reductions that arise from deployment of fuel cells in buses also apply to fuel cells for use in cars. Shared learning of this kind is thought realistic by the automotive industry, which sees opportunities for hybrid vehicles to provide a stepping stone into electric vehicles, whether battery powered or fuel cell powered (Lipman and Hwang 2003). Similarly, Zaetta and Madden (2011) suggest that a plausible route for bus fuel cell system development is through shared learning with car fuel cells.

4.3 Data

Documentation for TIAM-UCL is available in the website of the UK Energy Research Centre, and data and assumptions for vehicle characteristics and learning technologies are fully documented in McDowall (2012) and McDowall and Dodds (2012). For brevity, only the key technology learning parameters (learning rate, initial cost, initial capacity and floor cost) are presented in Table 2. It is assumed that learning can start from 2015. All costs are in year 2005 US$.

Table 2 Data on key learning technologies. Detailed assumptions found in McDowall (2012)

	Fuel cell system	Electric powertrain	Automotive batteries
	$/kW	$/kW	$/kWh
Initial cost	883	244	756
Floor cost	27	24	151
Learning rate	18 %	10 %	7 %
	GW	GW	GWh
Initial installed capacity	1.1	250	6.5
Number of doublings of capacity to reach floor cost	18	23	23

5 Scenarios

Five groups of scenarios have been run in order to examine the role of learning in determining the optimality of electricity and hydrogen in the global road transport sector. All scenarios are greenhouse gas (GHG) reduction scenarios, in which cumulative carbon-equivalent (CO_2e) emissions are constrained to a total of 1980 $GtCO_2e$ during 2010–2100 (consistent with a 50 % likelihood of global mean temperatures rising no more than 2 °C above pre-industrial levels). This scenario does not force the model to meet commitments made by particular countries to reduce emissions. Instead, the model is free to determine the least-cost global abatement.

1. ***Static technological development***. Transport technologies undergo no learning; transport technology costs are constant across the model time horizon.
2. ***ETL base case scenario***. Transport technologies undergo ETL; roll-out of hydrogen and electric vehicles occurs only when they become cost effective.
3. ***ETL Early hydrogen deployment scenarios***. Cases in which countries deploy hydrogen vehicles before they are part of a cost-optimal carbon abatement solution. There are several scenario variants:

Three scenarios examine differing levels of non-optimal early deployment of fuel cell cars, representing efforts made by countries to launch fuel cell vehicles domestically in order to capture first-mover advantages in this technology. The first of these scenarios envisages Germany and Japan each deploying 15,000 vehicles in 2020. The importance of early deployment is further tested by running scenarios with twice and four times this early deployment level.

An additional early deployment scenario examines early deployment of fuel cell buses. This scenario supposes that some cities force uptake of fuel cell buses for air quality reasons.

4. ***ETL No CCS scenario***. Deployment of carbon capture and storage (CCS) technologies is prevented; otherwise same as ETL base case scenario
5. ***ETL Late action scenario***. Global mitigation is delayed; no emissions reductions against the base case are possible before 2020 in this scenario; otherwise same as ETL base case scenario.

The global availability of bioenergy is uncertain, and it may have an important effect on the cost-effectiveness of low-carbon vehicle technologies, since biofuels derived from biomass might be expected to compete with hydrogen and electricity in a low carbon scenario. The base case scenarios assume that global availability of biomass is broadly in line with the more optimistic scenarios of Erb et al. (2009). However, Slade et al. (2011) note that the literature encompasses estimates of significantly greater global biomass availability. Each of the above scenarios has therefore also been tested under more optimistic assumptions about the global availability of biomass, in which the availability of biomass is twice that in the base case.

6 Results

6.1 Roles for Hydrogen and Electricity in the Transport Sector

Static Technology Scenario: Without significant learning, hydrogen and electric vehicles remain too expensive, and hence play a minimal role, appearing only in 2095, in the transport sector even under a stringent carbon constraint.

Endogenous Technology Learning base scenario (*ETL*): When the model is allowed to benefit from learning-by-doing, hydrogen and electricity both play a substantial role. Learning brings down the cost of fuel cells and electric vehicle components, enabling hydrogen and electricity to become cost-effective transport fuels.

Early Hydrogen Deployment Scenarios: The forced early deployment in these scenarios does not change long-term transport sector hydrogen or electricity consumption patterns as compared to the ETL scenario. While early deployment reduces vehicle costs, these technologies and their associated infrastructure remain too expensive to justify deployment until marginal abatement costs have risen further.

Later Action Scenario: Combined consumption of electricity and hydrogen in the transport sector substantially exceeds that in the ETL base case scenario. This is because the model is unable to reduce emissions before 2020, and must therefore 'work harder' to reduce emissions after this date to remain within the cumulative carbon emissions budget.

No CCS scenario: This scenario shows a similar pattern to the late action scenario. In the absence of CCS technologies, the model must reduce emissions more quickly in end-use sectors including transport, and so deploys both battery electric vehicles and fuel cells more rapidly than in the ETL base case.

Sensitivity scenarios on Biomass Availability: In the base case runs, the model deploys bioenergy in the power sector and in industry, often in combination with CCS, rather than in the transport sector. One might imagine that in scenarios with greater availability of bionenergy, the model might select biofuels rather than electricity or hydrogen.

However, the results of the biomass resource sensitivity scenarios do not support this view. Instead, increasing biomass resource availability increases the ability of the model to deploy bio-CCS (which is assumed to be net carbon negative). As a result, the model delays the entry of hydrogen and electricity into the transport sector, with little early deployment of either, as end-use sectors need less decarbonisation thanks to the greater contribution from bio-CCS to emissions reductions.

6.2 Transport Technology Deployment Pathways

Within each of the vehicle classes, the results suggest a sequence of vehicle technology transitions. In all vehicle types, the sequence begins with hybridisation of the vehicle fleet, reducing the fuel consumption and deploying a significant number of electric drive-trains and automotive battery systems. Later, these hybrids are replaced, sometimes followed by plug-in hybrid technology as an intermediate stage, and ultimately followed by hydrogen fuel cell technologies, and for cars some battery electric vehicles. An example of this pattern is shown in Fig. 3.

Many studies applying endogenous technology learning find that the model seeks to deploy in early periods a very large amount of the ultimate technology (in this case usually fuel cell vehicles), since early deployment drives down costs and

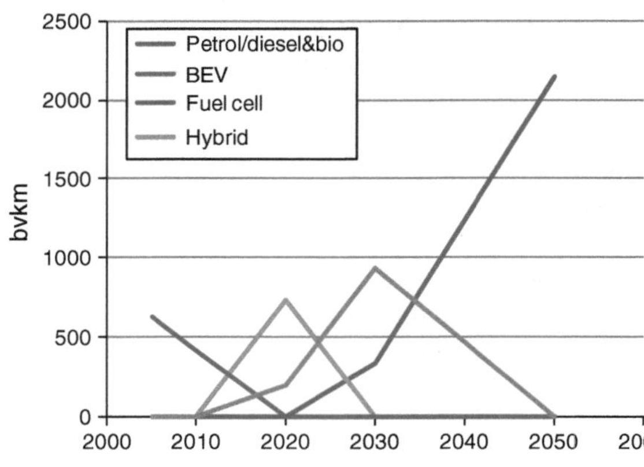

Fig. 3 Sequential deployment of different vehicle technologies (2005–2050) in light goods vehicles (ETL-base case scenario)

those lower costs can be enjoyed for the rest of the modelling period. However, with components sharing learning, and recombined across different vehicle modes and platforms (and across different global markets in the 16 regions of the model), the model can reduce the costs associated with moving down the learning curve by sequential deployment of technologies that contribute to learning without incurring the high costs associated with an early massive deployment of not-yet cost-effective technologies.

There is also a sequence in terms of the timing of deployment of low-carbon technologies across vehicle types. Fuel cells are deployed first in buses and LGVs, which have higher average annual mileage than cars, and which therefore prioritise lower running costs (and hence higher efficiency) more highly than cars. In LGVs, the model first deploys hydrogen, and ultimately transitions to electric vehicles after 2075 in many scenarios. This is likely to be because the efficiency of electric vehicles is higher than that of hydrogen, but so is the capital cost. It is only later in the period, when carbon abatement costs have become very high, that the model prefers the greater efficiency of battery electric vehicles.

The deployment of vehicles results in the deployment of the key technologies that undergo learning. Fuel cell technology becomes cost effective first in buses and LGVs, and then in cars following the cost reductions associated with deployment. Electric drive trains and batteries are cost effective starting in hybrid vehicles, and are subsequently deployed in all other low-carbon vehicle types.

6.3 Implications of ETL for Vehicle Cost

Cumulative investment brings down the costs of key technologies (fuel cell, electric battery and electric drive) in all scenarios in which ETL is applied (ETL base case scenario is shown in Fig. 4). Since the learning rate for fuel cells (18 %) is relatively high compared to that of batteries (7 %) and electric drive-trains (10 %), the cost of fuel cells decreases more rapidly. Battery costs fall quickly to just over $300/kWh,

Fig. 4 Unit cost of key technologies in the base case ETL scenario

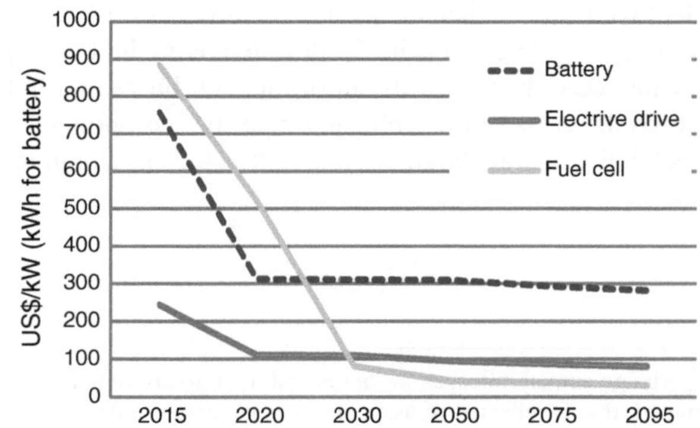

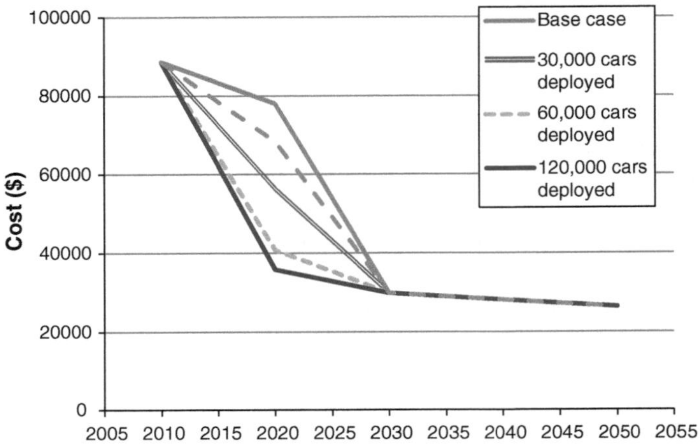

Fig. 5 Capital cost of a hybrid fuel cell vehicle under different early deployment scenarios

but are not deployed in sufficiently large quantities to reach their potential floor cost of $150/kWh. The cost of fuel cells in 2050 is reduced to less than a twentieth of the 2015 cost. To achieve these cost reductions, the transport sector requires a cumulative installed capacity of around 131,000 GW of fuel cells by 2050 worldwide; corresponding to a cumulative total of around 1.6 billion vehicles, with around 53 million new fuel cell vehicles added each year by 2050.

The investment (discounted to base year 2005) over the 35 years from 2015 to 2050 that achieves these cost reductions in fuel cells is a cumulative global total of $1200 bn (i.e. the cumulative total investment in fuel cell technologies globally). The figure for the 15 years from 2015 to 2030 is $64 billion (required to have a cumulative installed capacity of around 1860 GW of fuel cell by 2030). However, this cost is offset by the avoided investments in the conventional technology: petrol and diesel engines. As a result, the additional 'learning investments' required to bring down fuel cell cost are rather small, around $33 bn (discounted to base year 2005) for the 15 years.

As noted above, it is larger vehicles with higher annual mileage[2] that are deployed first, rather than cars. Nevertheless, the costs of fuel cell cars is reduced significantly in 2030 (Fig. 5), despite having had no deployment of fuel cells in cars by that date. Instead, roll-out of fuel cell buses and light-goods vehicles has driven down the costs of fuel cells and other EV components, reducing the capital costs of fuel cell vehicles. Even so, fuel cell vehicles remain too expensive in the near term

[2]Average annual mileages for buses and light goods vehicles are much higher than for cars. In the model, this is reflected in assumed average annual mileages specific to each vehicle mode.

to compete with conventional hybrids, which are deployed globally resulting in a significant reduction in global transport CO_2 emissions. Only from 2050 onwards, as emissions constraints bite further, does the transition to hydrogen passenger mobility begin.

The early deployment scenarios demonstrate a clear effect on near term costs, with early deployment of fuel cell technologies in cars or buses driving down costs of key components. This is shown in Fig. 5. However, despite these accelerated cost reductions in the near term, the early deployment scenarios do not have a sufficiently large impact on costs to accelerate adoption. Given the presence of other, cheaper abatement opportunities throughout the energy system, the model prefers to deploy hydrogen vehicles later, as carbon abatement costs rise.

6.4 Hydrogen Versus Electric Vehicles?

There is an on-going debate about the complementarity or competitiveness of hydrogen and electric vehicles (Bento 2010). In the results presented here, both hydrogen fuel cell vehicles and battery electric vehicles are deployed in all scenarios. At a global level then, the model does not support an absolute trade-off between hydrogen and electricity as transport fuels, since different markets in different regions may prefer one or the other,[3] and both are required to achieve global decarbonisation at least cost. There is also significant deployment of fuel cell plug-in hybrid electric vehicles (FCPHEVs) in all scenarios, representing a complementarity between fuel cell and battery electric technology at the level of the individual vehicle.

In the medium term, therefore, there appears to be synergy between vehicles using hydrogen and electricity as fuels, as scenarios with more hydrogen vehicles (FCVs and FCHVs) tend also to deploy more electric vehicles (BEVs, Petrol and diesel PHEVs), in part because of the shared cost reductions. By the end of the century, most passenger cars and light goods vehicles are fuelled with either hydrogen or electricity or both (FCPHEVs). In this heavily decarbonised transport sector, hydrogen and electricity become competitors in the sense that scenarios with more of one have less of the other (see Fig. 6). It should be noted from the axes of the diagram that in the long term (by 2095), more hydrogen than electricity is consumed by the transport sector in all scenarios.

[3]Technology costs are global, but fuel production costs and carbon intensities vary, reflecting different resource endowments, and this can result in different fuels being preferred in different regions.

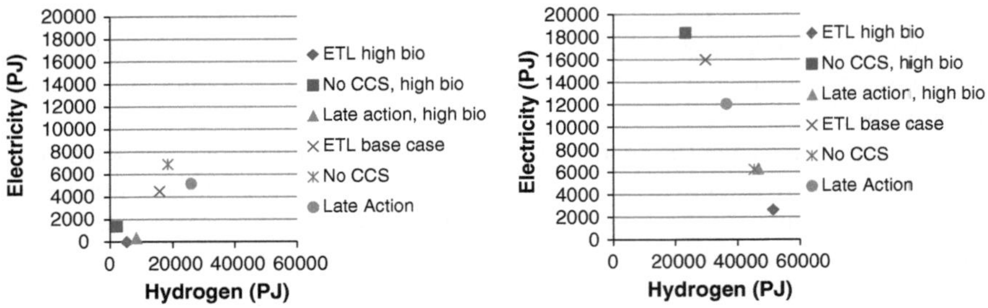

Fig. 6 Transport sector consumption of hydrogen and electricity under different scenarios, in 2050 (*left panel*) and 2095 (*right panel*)

7 Conclusions, Limitations and Policy Implications

The study concludes that electricity and hydrogen emerge as complementary fuels, rather than as strict competitors, with both deployed in all scenarios. This reflects the fact that hydrogen and battery electric vehicles share components: in the near term, deployment of hybrid cars reduces the costs of components that are used in fuel cell vehicles; and later deployments of fuel cell vehicles further reduce the costs of battery electric vehicle components, resulting in synergy rather than competition between hydrogen and electricity technologies. However, in the long term when the transport sector has been largely decarbonised, technology competition between hydrogen and electricity does arise, in the sense that scenarios using more electricity in the transport sector use less hydrogen and vice versa.

Methodologically, a key observation is that a multi-cluster approach appears to overcome a shortcoming found by many previous authors. Specifically, while many previous applications of ETL within MARKAL/TIMES models have observed either immediate and rapid or zero deployment of the learning technology, with a resulting need for transition rate constraints, the multi-cluster approach presented here results in a gradual and phased deployment of the learning technology. The multi-cluster approach thus appears to be a promising approach to improving the modelling of endogenous technological change.

However, there are limitations that should be borne in mind in considering the conclusions from a policy perspective. In particular, there is deep uncertainty relating to the learning curve specifications, including the value of the learning rate and potential changes to the learning rate over time. Moreover, real world multiple and divergent scale-dependent drivers of cost reduction have been modelled with a single factor. Similarly, a single global learning process has been modelled here, whereas in reality some components of learning tend to be location specific (e.g. related to local practices and institutions). These uncertainties and limitations are in addition to those inherent in all long-term energy system optimization, and the results are not intended to be predictive, but rather are intended to yield insights into possible dynamics and patterns in the energy system.

The messages for policymakers must therefore be drawn with caution. The current analysis suggests that, in the long-term, both hydrogen and electricity remain important options for long-term decarbonisation. The results also suggest that policymakers seeking to accelerate the deployment of hydrogen or electric vehicles through early deployments may be disappointed if the rest-of-the-world follows a least-cost abatement trajectory.

Acknowledgments TIAM-UCL was developed through the UK Energy Research Centre, while the analysis reported in this chapter was part of the UK Sustainable Hydrogen Energy Consortium. The RCUK Energy Programme funded both these initiatives.

References

Anandarajah G, McDowall W, Ekins P (2013) Decarbonising road transport with hydrogen and electricity: Long term global technology learning scenarios. Int J Hydrogen Energy 38 (8):3419–3432

Bento N (2010) Dynamic competition between plug-in hybrid and hydrogen fuel cell vehicles for personal transportation. Int J Hydrogen Energ 35(20):11271–11283

Bergek A, Jacobsson S, Carlsson B et al (2008) Analyzing the functional dynamics of technological innovation systems: a scheme of analysis. Res Policy 37:407–429

Criqui P, Mima S, Menanteau P et al (2014) Mitigation strategies and technology learning: an assessment with the POLES model, Technology Forecasting and social Science, article (in press)

de Feber MAPC, Schaeffer GL, Seebregts AJ et al (2003) Enhancements of endogenous technology learning in the western European MARKAL model. Report for the EU SAPIENT project, ECN, Petten

Eames (2000) The large combustion plant directive (88/609/EEC): an effective instrument for pollution abatement? University of Sussex

Erb KH, Haberi H, Krausmann F et al (2009) Eating the planet: feeding and fuelling the world sustainably, fairly and humanely—a scoping study (Commissioned by Compassion in World Farming and Friends of the Earth UK). Institute of Social Ecology and PIK Potsdam, Potsdam

Gritsevskyi A, Nakićenovic N (2000) Modeling uncertainty of induced technological change. Energy Policy 28:907–921

Grubb M, Köhler J, Anderson D (2002) Induced technical change in energy and environmental modelling: analytic approaches and policy implications. Annu Rev Energy Env 27:271–308

Grübler A, Nakicenovic N, Victor D (1999) Dynamics of energy technologies and global change. Energy Policy 27:247–280

Gül T, Kypreos S, Turton H et al (2009) An energy-economic scenario analysis of alternative fuels for personal transport using the global multi-regional markal model (GMM). Energy 34 (10):1423–1437

Kahouli-Brahmi S (2008) Technological learning in energy–environment–economy modelling: A survey. Energy Policy 36:138–162

Krzyzanowski D, Kypreos S, Barreto L (2008) Supporting hydrogen based transportation: case studies with global markal model. CMS 5(3):207–231

Krzyzanowski D, Kypreos S, Grutzwiller L, et al (2004) Implications of technology learning in energy-economy models of the transport sector. Report to the alliance for the global sustainability (AGS). Paul Scherrer Institute, Switzerland

Lipman T, Hwang R (2003) Hybrid electric and fuel cell vehicle technological innovation: hybrid and zero-emission vehicle technology links. In: 20th International Electric Vehicle Symposium and Exposition, 15–19 Nov, Long Beach, California

Loulou R, Remme U, Kanudia A et al (2005) Documentation of the TIMES model: Part II. Energy Technol Syst Anal Programme

Loulou R, Labriet M (2008) ETSAP-TIAM: the TIMES integrated assessment model part I: model structure. CMS 5:41–66

Mattsson N, Wene CO (1997) Assessing new energy technologies using an energy system model with endogenized experience curves. Int J Energ Res 21(4):385–393

McDonald A, Schrattenholzer L (2001) Learning rates for energy technologies. Energy Policy 29:255–261

McDowall (2012) Endogenous technology learning for hydrogen and fuel cell technology in UKSHEC II: Literature review, research questions and data. UKSHEC social science working paper 8. UCL Energy Institute

McDowall W, Dodds P (2012) A review of low-carbon vehicle and hydrogen end-use data for energy system models. UKSHEC working paper 5. UCL Energy Institute

Seebregts AJ, Kram T, Schaeffer GJ et al (1998) Endogenous technology learning: experiments with MARKAL, Contribution to Task 2.3 of the EU-TEEM Project. ECN, Petten

Seebregts A, Kram T, Schaeffer GJ et al (1999) Endogenous technological change in energy system models: synthesis of experience with ERIS, MARKAL and MESSAGE. ECN-C–99-025, PSI, IIASA, Laxenburg, Austria

Slade R, Saunders R, Gross R et al (2011) Energy from biomass: the size of the global resource. UKERC Report number: UKERC/RR/TPA/2011/001. UK Energy Research Centre, London

Totschnig G, and Keppo I (2007) CASCADE-MINTS Part 1: an analysis with MESSAGE. Final report to the energy–economics–environment modeling laboratory(E3MLAB) at the Institute of Communication and Computer Systems of the National Technical University of Athens, Athens, Greece

Watanabe C, Wakabayashi K, Miyazawa T (2000) Industrial dynamism and the creation of a "virtuous cycle" between R&D, market growth and price reduction: the case of photovoltaic power generation (PV) development in Japan. Technovation 20:299–312

Winskel M, Markusson N, Jeffrey H (2014) Learning pathways for energy supply technologies: Bridging between innovation studies and learning rates, Technological Forecasting and Social Change, vol 81, pp 96–114, ISSN:0040-1625

Winskel M, Markusson N, Jeffrey H et al (2013) between learning rates and innovation studies: learning pathways for emerging energy supply technologies'. Technol Forecast Soc Chang 81:96–114

Yeh S, Rubin E (2012) A review of uncertainties in technology experience curves. Energy Econ 34 (3):762–771

Zaetta R, Madden B (2011) Hydrogen fuel cell bus technology state of the art review. Element Energy report for the NextHyLights project, Cambridge

Modal Shift of Passenger Transport in a TIMES Model: Application to Ireland and California

Hannah E. Daly, Kalai Ramea, Alessandro Chiodi, Sonia Yeh, Maurizio Gargiulo and Brian Ó Gallachóir

Abstract Climate change mitigation clearly requires a focus on transport that should include improved representation of travel behaviour change in addition to increased vehicle efficiency and low-carbon fuels. Energy system models focus however on technology and fuel switching and tend to poorly incorporate travel behaviour. Conversely, transport demand modelling generally fails to address energy and climate policy trade-offs. This chapter seeks to make energy systems analysis more holistic by introducing modal choice within passenger transport in a TIMES model, to allow trade-offs between behaviour and technology choices explicit. Travel demand in TIMES models is typically exogenous—no competition exists between alternative modes. A simple illustrative TIMES model is described, where competition between modes is enabled by imposing a constraint on overall travel time in the system. This constraint represents the empirically observed travel time budget of individuals, constraining the model choosing between faster and more expensive modes (e.g. cars) and slower but cheaper mode (e.g. buses or rail).

H.E. Daly (✉)
UCL Energy Institute, 14 Upper Woburn Place, London WC1H 0NN, UK
e-mail: hannah.daly@ucl.ac.uk

K. Ramea · S. Yeh
Institute of Transport Studies, University of California, Davis, USA
e-mail: kramea@ucdavis.edu

S. Yeh
e-mail: slyeh@ucdavis.edu

A. Chiodi · B. Ó Gallachóir
Environmental Research Institute, University College Cork, Cork, Ireland
e-mail: chiodiale@gmail.com

B. Ó Gallachóir
e-mail: b.ogallachoir@ucc.ie

M. Gargiulo
e4sma s.r.l., Turin, Italy
e-mail: maurizio.gargiulo@e4sma.com

G. Giannakidis et al. (eds.), *Informing Energy and Climate Policies Using Energy Systems Models*, Lecture Notes in Energy 30,
DOI 10.1007/978-3-319-16540-0_16

Further, a new variable is introduced, called travel time investment, which acts as a proxy for infrastructure investments to reduce the time associated with travel, to enable investment in alternative modes of transport as a means of CO_2 mitigation.

1 Introduction

Transportation contributes to 23 % of energy-related CO_2 emissions globally. With increasing demands especially for light-duty vehicles, freight, and aviation, global transport CO_2 emissions are expected to double by 2050 (IEA 2010). Reducing greenhouse gas emissions from the transport sector will require complementary policies in improving the efficiency of vehicles, introducing low-carbon fuels and advanced vehicles technologies, and better travel demand management (Schafer and Heywood 2009). Most of the growth in demand for cars will come from developing countries, as car travel in developed countries essentially saturated, and is projected to remain flat in the next few decades. On the other hand, public transport and aviation already play an important role in many developed (especially Europe) and developing countries. The importance of their role is expected to continue to increase given the need to drastically reduce on-road transportation emissions in order to meet stringent climate targets (Fulton et al. 2009; IEA 2012).

However, while most of the integrated assessment models (IAMs) that governments rely on for developing climate mitigation policies have been able to project portfolios of advanced fuels and vehicle technologies given climate goals, bottom-up models are currently ill suited to examine potential travel demand changes and travel mode shifts given climate policies and changes in fuel prices, and most importantly the necessary investments needed to reduce vehicle travel, increase public transport shares, and non-vehicle infrastructure given climate goals (Schafer 2012). Most IA models use scenarios describing future travel modal shifts without explicitly linking demand changes to drivers (e.g. fuel price changes) or infrastructure and technology investment decisions. This is despite the many studies which show that technological change is not sufficient for the transportation sector to develop in a way that is consistent with long-term climate targets (Hickman and Banister 2007; Bristow et al. 2008; Johansson 2009; Åkerman and Höjer 2006).

The aim of this chapter is to describe a methodology of modelling transport mode shift behaviour in TIMES models, which allows the model to more realistically represent the dynamics of mode choice behaviour and allows investment into public transport infrastructure as a mitigation option. A paper by Schafer (2012) provides a critical review of the (lack of) modelling of behavioural changes in transportation in energy, economy, environment, engineering (E4) models, compares common methodologies employed in IA models, their shortcomings and gives recommendations for future improvement. This paper argues that introducing behaviour change in transportation in these models is indispensible for exploring holistic approaches to mitigation, while being feasible and intellectually rewarding.

This chapter explores some of the recommended methodologies and applies them for the first time in the bottom-up optimization modelling framework using the TIMES model and implements this in two case studies based on the Californian TIMES model and the Irish TIMES model.

This chapter reviews the role of transport in energy models and key underlying concepts of travel behaviours and travel time budgets in Sect. 2, introduces a new methodology for energy system models in Sect. 3, introduces and compares the case studies in Sect. 4, presents results in Sect. 5 and discusses results and concludes in Sect. 6.

2 Transport Modeling and Energy Systems Models

Transport modelling is a very well established discipline used widely by decision-makers for planning infrastructure such as airports, roads and railways, for cost-benefit analyses, and environmental impact assessments. Transport planning models typically simulate travel trips by origin and destination, trip purpose, mode of travel and household demographics. Multinomial logit (MNL) modelling is often used to compute mode choice for trips between each origin and destination (de Dios Ortúzar and Willumsen 2001). This methodology expresses the utility associated with alternative modes and includes the variables that describe the attributes of alternatives, which influence the utility of all members of the population, and variables that influence people's preferences, or choices, among alternatives. Infrastructure and land use play a critical role in the patterns of travel demand, and accessibility to transport infrastructure is a strong determinant of mode choice and travel demand (Kockelman 1997). Therefore behaviour is a strong element of transport models, as is detail of the transport network. There is generally very little or no treatment of energy demand in transport planning models: They can be suitable for projecting travel (and hence energy) demand, but not for analysing trade-offs in climate mitigation policymaking.

On the other hand, E4 models such as TIMES explicitly look at the energy system to examine issues ranging from macroeconomic interactions to looking at pathways to meeting climate mitigation scenarios, with very rich technological detail of the entire energy system, from fuel production and imports to energy conversion and demand technologies. A common use of TIMES/MARKAL models is developing least-cost pathways for meeting long-term climate targets, but the nature of the model restricts these pathways to showing only fuel and technology options. Travel demand for each mode is individually inputted into the model over the time horizon, and technologies within that model compete to meet the demand at least cost, subject to system-wide constraints. This deficiency in representing travel behaviour is common in technology-rich linear optimisation models.

Several energy models have included a mode choice module using different modal choice methodologies: For example, the Global Change Assessment Model (GCAM), developed at the Pacific Northwest National Laboratory, is a general equilibrium model that solves for prices, supply and demand for all markets (Kyle and Kim 2011). Mode choice in this model is endogenous, using a MNL approach, and responds to fuel price, wage rate and the cost of transport services. The Canadian Integrated Modelling System (CIMS) also includes a logit sub-model for mode and fuel choice (Horne et al. 2005). A third hybrid model with transport behaviour is IMpact Assessment of CLIMate policies-Recursive version (IMAC-LIM-R), developed at CIRED, which maximises a utility function subject to travel budget constraints. Infrastructure is endogenous: a decrease in supply leads to congestion and lower speeds, which feeds back into the model (Waisman et al. 2013). From the reviewed transport models, this is the only study that includes transport infrastructure endogenously as a determinant of travel demand.

Pietzcker et al. (2014) compares transport decarbonisation from five energy-economic models, and finds that for the linear optimisation models based on TIMES have less flexibility than other models for mitigation, because mode choice is not endogenous. One model from the study (GCAM) includes the value of time in determining travel patterns. This study also points out that targeting behaviour through infrastructure can have a major impact on travel demand patterns, and should be considered in developing mitigation policies.

2.1 Travel Time Budget (TTB)

An important attribute of the passenger transport sectors of the hybrid energy models such as GCAM, where modal choice is simulated, is that travel time is modelled. Representing travel time explicitly is at the core of our approach. We use the conception of a fixed travel time budget to constrain overall travel time in the model: Empirical research has shown that averaged over a country or region, people spend a fixed amount of time travelling per day. Studies suggest that region-wide average personal travel time is constant and is estimated as 1.1 h per person per day (Zahavi and Ryan 1980). This "travel time budget" as such is a stable characteristic and is considered a constant in our model.

Other studies have used the notion of a travel time budget to simulate travel demand and modal split: Schafer and Victor (2000) uses a fixed travel time and money budget to forecast future global mobility, assuming a constant shift towards faster travel modes. Metz (2010) comes to a different conclusion, observing that daily travel demand is saturating in Britain, while the daily travel time budget has been constant, because of the diminishing marginal utility of the value of the extra choice associated with more mobility. Girod et al. (2012) also uses fixed travel time and money budgets to simulate travel demand and modal share. The fixed travel time has implications for travel demand and speed: Studies have shown evidence that reducing travel time of journeys through increasing capacity and improving infrastructure induces increased travel demand (Noland and Lem 2002).

3 Methodology

This section describes the basic model structure of the methodology and its implementation in a simple illustrative TIMES model. In this model, different transport modes compete on the basis of fuel and capital costs to deliver overall travel demand, while a constraint on overall travel time in the system, representing the travel time budget (TTB) of individuals, ensures that faster and more expensive modes can also compete. We introduce a new variable, travel time investment (TTI), a proxy for investments to reduce the time associated with travel. This model is then tested under a reference scenario (to 2030), an investment scenario and a CO_2 emissions reduction scenario. To the authors' knowledge, while TTB has been used in other energy models, this is the first time this parameter has been used to represent modal choice in a linear optimisation model, which has the advantage of being technologically rich and comprehensively covering the whole energy system.

3.1 Model

Motorised travel demand is represented by passenger kilometres travelled (PKT), which is the sum of demands of car (CKT), bus (BKT) and train (TKT). PKT for a technology is given by the vehicle kilometres travelled (VKT) multiplied by the load factor (LF, or occupancy of the vehicle). PKT is divided into long and short distance demand (PKT_L and PKT_S) in order to capture the characteristics of the different technologies servicing the different demands: High-speed train and buses can service long distance travel, while city buses and electric trams can service short distance; cars serve both. Furthermore, the speed of technologies serving long and short distance differs significantly: For example, for longer distance a rail trips, the required waiting time is absorbed by the speed of the overall journey and is more significant in shorter trips.

The model is based on a least-cost linear programming approach. It determines $PKT_{t,d}$, the travel demand d for long and short distance of each of the technologies t such that the overall system cost is minimised. The cost of technology activity, $c_{t,d}$ is the cost in €/PKT of travel in each technology producing long or short distance travel demand d, given by the sum of the fuel, investment and operation and maintenance (OM) costs in €/PKT.

The concept of a travel time budget (TTB in million hours, mhs) is introduced to the model to represent the empirically observed fixed travel time per-capita in the real world, as described in Sect. 2.1. This enables competition between different transport modes based on travel time in addition to cost. Without this the model will be likely to switch modes immediately to the cheaper but slower and more time–costly public transit modes, which does not reflect travel behaviour.

Ideally, speed and infrastructure would be endogenous to the model, so that the model could invest into decreasing travel time. We introduce a variable travel time investment (TTI) which is a proxy to endogenise this relationship.

The model determines $PKT_{t,d}$ and $tti_{t,d}$ subject to Eq. 1:

Minimize total cost:

$$C = \sum_{t,d} PKT_{t,d} \cdot c_{t,d} \tag{1}$$

where $PKT_{t,d}$ is the travel demand of technology t for long or short distance travel demand d, and $c_{t,d}$ is the sum of fuel, investment, OM and TTI cost in €/PKT:

$$c_{t,d} = f_{t,d} + i_{t,d} + om_{t,d} + tc_{t,d}$$

Fuel cost $f_{t,d}$ is a product of the price per unit of energy of fuel and the energy intensity of the technology, divided by the load factor, and the cost of travel time investment $tc_{t,d}$ depends on vehicle speed (Eq. 2):

$$tc_{t,d} = \frac{tti_{t,d} \times \tau}{s_{t,d}} \tag{2}$$

τ is the TTI cost in €/h and $s_{t,d}$ is the speed in kilometres per hour of technology t.

The model is subject to two main constraints, firstly, that technologies meet the exogenously defined travel demand for long and short distance demand d, and secondly, that the total yearly travel time of the system minus the travel time investment (a proxy for a reduction in the travel time of modes) does not exceed the yearly travel time budget (TTB) (Eq. 3 and 4):

$$\sum_{t,d} PKT_{t,d} = D \tag{3}$$

$$\sum_{m} s_m \times PKT_m + TTI \leq TTB \tag{4}$$

3.2 Implementation in TIMES

Within the new Reference Energy System, as shown in Fig. 1, we introduce just two travel demand commodities: long distance demand (TLDD) and short distance demand (TSDD) expressed in PKT/year. In order to produce energy service demands all technologies such cars, trains and buses have two inputs: the fuel input and the time input. Here the TIME input describes the travel time from origin to destination, which is dependent on the modal speed, waiting and transfer time. This depends on technology, infrastructure, reliability, congestion, accessibility, etc.

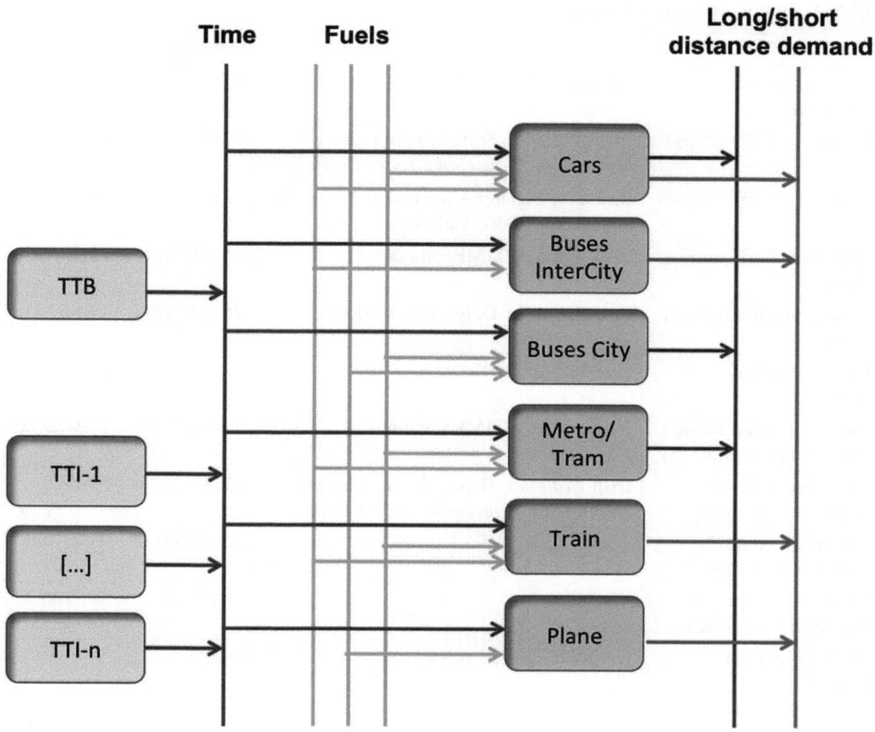

Fig. 1 New reference energy system

4 Case Studies: Ireland and California

The above methodology is applied to two case studies, Ireland and California, two regions for which TIMES models already exist.

Passenger cars are predominantly used as the preferred mode of transport in California. Public transit, that includes all the commuter trains and buses in the state, comprises about 4.4 % of the total trips (California Department of Transportation 2013). In this study we define short distance PKT demands as those trips within the metropolitan areas in the state, with population greater than 1 million.

For the Irish model, short distance travel demand is defined to be trips of 30 km or less. Total annual travel demand and the base-year modal split of demand by car, bus and train for short and long demand were derived from microdata from Ireland's Central Statistics Office Pilot National Travel Survey (Central Statistics Office 2011) conducted in 2009. This used a travel diary methodology to survey travel characteristics, including distance, mode, time and trip purpose, for a cross section of the population. Total annual travel demand in PKT for this modelling exercise was calculated using the average daily distance (by car, bus or train) per

Table 1 Important input parameters

	Source	California	Ireland
Travel time budget (h/person/day)	Zahavi and Ryan (1980)	1.1	1.1
Motorized TTB (2009)	Irish *National Travel Survey* and US *Nationwide Household Travel Survey*	1.02	0.91
Motorized TTB (2030)	Based on Schafer-Victor model (Schafer and Victor 2000; Daly et al. 2014)	1.07	1.03
Per-capita PKT (annual, 2009)	Irish and CA TIMES models	18,803 km	12,305 km
Per-capita PKT (annual, 2030)	Calculation in Daly et al. (2014)	26,209 km	19,829 km
Travel demand elasticity	Girod et al. (2012)	1	1
2009 motorized mode share (bus/car/train, %)	Irish and CA TIMES models	1.9/97.9/0.2	5.2/1.2/3.6
Car speed (miles/h) (long/short distance)	Irish *National Travel Survey* and US *Nationwide Household Travel Survey*	37/32	59/28.8
Bus speed (miles/h) (long/short distance)		15.3/14.6	47.1/13.9
Train speed (miles/h) (long/short distance)		NA/24.7	55.7/20.2
2030 population (million)	CA/Irish TIMES model	44.57	

person for this survey. The speed of each mode for long and short distance demand was calculated as the weighted average quotient of trip distance and trip time.

In order to calculate load factors for cars and buses, vehicle kilometres travelled (VKT) were used: Total private car VKT for 2008 was derived from national car test odometer readings (Daly and Gallachóir 2011); bus VKT were sourced from the Central Statistics Office, and VKT for Dublin's light rail system (Dart and Luas) was used for short distance demand (CSO 2008).

The physical characteristics of transport technologies—costs and efficiencies of different modes—for each region is derived from the TIMES models that exist for California, CA-TIMES (McCollum et al. 2012), and Ireland, Irish TIMES (Chiodi et al. 2013). A detailed description of the data inputs and derivation of baseline travel demand is described in Daly et al. (2014), and Table 1 summarises the main input parameters used.

5 Results

The modal-share model is run for four scenarios for each case study. The first scenario is a reference case which represents the previous state of modelling in TIMES, including no TTB. The following three scenarios describe the mode share (in total PKT) when introducing TTB, TTI and a constraint on CO_2 emissions. A detailed description of each scenario follows.

S0: *Reference*. This reference scenario represents the outcome of standard TIMES model structure. The model is first run without the limit on travel time budget, which implies the passenger has no bound on travel time. The model chooses freely between modes on the basis of technology and fuel costs. As shown in Fig. 2 once the existing car capacity retires, the model chooses bus technology for both regions, which is the slower and cheaper mode of transport according to our assumptions.

S1: *No TTI*. A constant travel time budget is introduced into the model based on projected annual passenger kilometres travelled (PKT) and assumed modal speeds. In both regions, PKT grows faster than TTB, therefore pushing the model to choose faster modes of travel within the given time budget. The models quickly become unfeasible as cars, the fastest mode, are already saturating travel demand and the model has no faster mode to switch to. Results for this scenario are shown in Fig. 3.

S2: *Including TTI*. Travel Time Investment (TTI) is introduced in this scenario, allowing the model to invest in increasing the overall travel time budget.

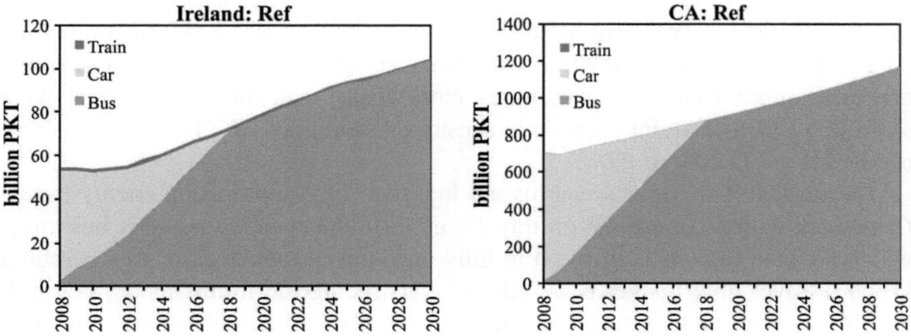

Fig. 2 Modal share results for S0 (bPKT), illustrative of approach without TTB

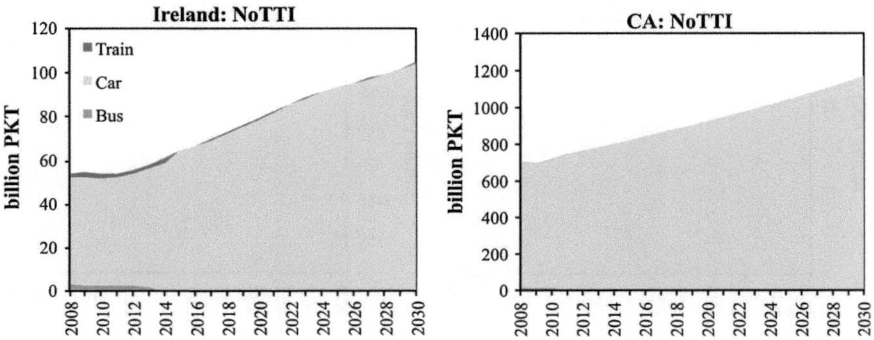

Fig. 3 Modal share results for S1 (bPKT), illustrating the impact of including TTB and not TTI

This variable acts as a proxy for the investment required to encourage modal shifting, for example through improving public transport speeds. The cost of TTI impacts significantly on results: For low TTI costs (e.g., €2/h), the model for both regions invests heavily in slower public transport, because the modes' investment, fuel and OM costs are sufficiently low that investment in TTI is cost effective. At low TTI cost, the model for both regions also chooses a level of rail transport, which has a higher cost but greater speed than bus transport. When TTI cost is sufficiently high (e.g., €7/h), shown in the results here, the model invests in new private cars exclusively in Ireland, while using the installed capacity of buses and trains, and invests in some new bus technology in California as well as mainly private cars. At very high TTI costs, the model chooses exclusively private cars in meeting travel demands, and the current capacity of bus and rail is not used. Figure 4 shows results for TTI cost at €7/h.

S3: *TTI + CO_2 constraint*. This scenario introduces a 20 % CO_2 emissions reduction constraint, relative to S2 emissions. The constraint is applied to 2030 emissions from S2 and linearly interpolated from 2010. In this scenario, there is a tradeoff between speed and emissions: the slower public transport modes are invested in both regions so that the emissions constraint is met, but a minimal amount of TTI is invested in. New rail is invested in this scenario for both regions for short distance travel, with new capacity for long distance buses also featuring. At a very high TTI cost, rail is chosen exclusively over busses, as the slower speeds consumes more TTI and makes buses more costly than trains. Thus, the modal share in a CO_2 constraint scenario is sensitive to the price of TTI. Figure 5 shows results for a TTI cost of €7/h.

The results of the four scenarios are intuitive: In an optimising energy system framework with no constraint on travel time (S0), the cheapest mode is bus travel, which for both regions is invested in fully once the current stock of cars is retired. When a travel time budget is introduced, cars, being the fastest mode, dominate (S1). Mode shift under emissions constraint without TTI is infeasible in the model because no mode exists which is sufficiently time- and carbon-efficient to meet both

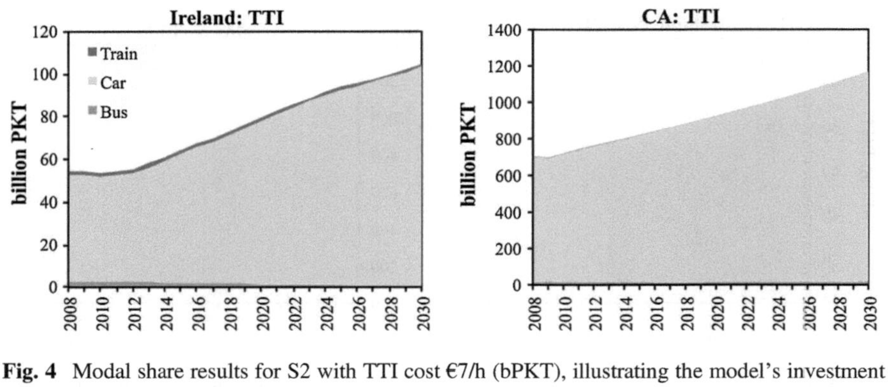

Fig. 4 Modal share results for S2 with TTI cost €7/h (bPKT), illustrating the model's investment in infrastructure to enable further travel demand growth

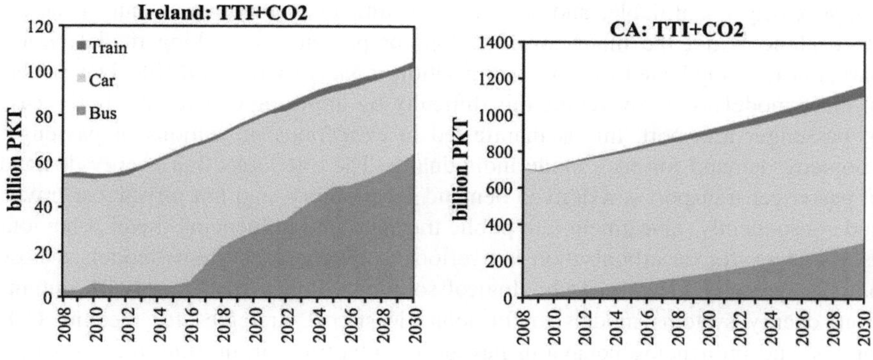

Fig. 5 Modal share results for S3 with TTI cost €7/h (bPKT), illustrating the case of modal shift, enabled by an investment into infrastructure

demands. S2 illustrates a realistic baseline scenario with no emission constraint: private cars dominate both cases, with no significant shift to public transport, because incomes increase, causing a greater per cavity travel demand with no per capita increase in travel time. S3 illustrates the potential for mode shifting when investments into public transport infrastructure is allowed to lower the time associated with these modes and increase the attractiveness to users. Both rail and bus travel are selected in this scenario, along with additional passenger cars.

6 Discussion and Conclusion

The results presented in the previous section show how this methodology portrays the competition between transport modes in a least-cost linear framework. In particular, results show a higher penetration of efficient, public transport modes when a CO_2 constraint is imposed. In this case, there is a trade-off in the model between the cost of investing in higher TTI, and so reducing the travel time associated with these modes to make them more attractive to passengers, and an emissions constraint. The reference scenario shows why a TTB constraint and a TTI cost is necessary to the model: Without imposing a restriction on travel time, the model would choose the most efficient and cheapest mode, which are buses in both Ireland and California. This reflects the real-world drawback of public transport, namely, the associated additional time and inconvenience, and the cost required of government to make efficient transport modes more acceptable to the public. These results are not intended to project realistic travel behaviour, but rather act as an illustration for how the mitigation potential of public transport infrastructure can feasibly be introduced to E4 models.

Many parameters influence modal choice. Some, such as the cost of fuel for a car or price of public transport or the travel time of different modes are objective and easily modelled. Other parameters—social status and comfort, for example—are not so easily quantifiable, and so are more difficult to incorporate into a model. Price alone is not the main consideration for passengers, making modal choice particularly complicated for cost-optimisation models such as TIMES. Developers of these models often overcome this difficulty by imposing constraints: In the case of passenger transport, this is manifested in exogenous projections of passenger kilometre demand for each mode individually. The overlooks that energy demand in passenger transport is a derived demand for mobility, and not private car travel, and consequently, investment into public transport and influencing travel behaviour as a strategy for decarbonisation is overlooked by energy systems models, whose outputs typically focus on technological solutions. Policy makers rely on outputs from energy systems models to formulate least-cost strategies for meeting CO_2 targets, and influencing behaviour has an important role in meeting these goals.

This model makes a first step towards incorporating competition between modes in linear optimisation energy models. Novelly, it uses a methodology based on the empirically observed, stable and global daily travel time budget to realistically represent the modal choice in a reference case, and introduces a new parameter, travel time investment, which is a proxy cost for investment into public transport, representing the cost to decision-makers of reducing the barrier to more public transport use. While TTB has been used in other energy models, this is the first time known to the authors this parameter has been used to represent modal choice in a linear optimisation model, which has the advantage of being technologically rich and comprehensively covering the whole energy system.

This prototype model requires further work to be fully useful, in particular, an extension of the TTI parameter to distinguish investment costs for each mode, and the inclusion of the methodology into a full energy systems model. However, the approach presented here is a significant step towards incorporating behaviour into energy systems models. In particular, it represents the feedback from transport infrastructure investment to travel time and quality, and therefore modal choice.

References

Åkerman J, Höjer M (2006) How much transport can the climate stand?—Sweden on a sustainable path in 2050. Energy Policy 34(14):1944–1957. doi:10.1016/j.enpol.2005.02.009

Bristow AL, Tight M, Pridmore A, May AD (2008) Developing pathways to low carbon land-based passenger transport in Great Britain by 2050. Energy Policy 36(9):3427–3435. doi:10.1016/j.enpol.2008.04.029

California Department of Transportation (2013) 2010–2012 California Household Travel Survey Final Report

Central Statistics Office (2011) National travel survey. Central Statistics Office, Information Section, Skehard Road, Cork, Ireland

Chiodi A, Gargiulo M, Deane JP, Lavigne D, Rout UK, Gallachóir BPÓ (2013) Modelling the impacts of challenging 2020 non-ETS GHG emissions reduction targets on Ireland's energy system. Energy Policy 62:1438–1452

CSO (2008) Transport omnibus. Central Statistics Office, Information Section, Skehard Road, Cork, Ireland

Daly HE, Gallachóir BPÓ (2011) Modelling private car energy demand using a technological car stock model. Transp Res Part D Transp Environ 16(2):93–101

Daly HE, Ramea K, Chiodi A, Yeh S, Gargiulo M, Gallachóir BÓ (2014) Incorporating travel behaviour and travel time into TIMES energy system models. Applied Energy 135(0):429–439. doi:10.1016/j.apenergy.2014.08.051

de Dios Ortúzar J, Willumsen LG (2001) Modelling transport, 3rd edn. Wiley, New York

Fulton L, Cazzola P, Cuenot Fß (2009) IEA Mobility Model (MoMo) and its use in the ETP 2008. Energy Policy 37(10):3758–3768

Girod B, van Vuuren DP, Deetman S (2012) Global travel within the 2C climate target. Energy Policy 45:152–166

Hickman R, Banister D (2007) Looking over the horizon: transport and reduced CO_2 emissions in the UK by 2030. Transp Policy 14(5):377–387

Horne M, Jaccard M, Tiedemann K (2005) Improving behavioral realism in hybrid energy-economy models using discrete choice studies of personal transportation decisions. Energy Econ 27(1):59–77

IEA (2010) World energy outlook 2010. International Energy Agency, Paris

IEA (2012) Energy technology perspectives. International Energy Agency, Paris

Johansson B (2009) Will restrictions on CO_2 emissions require reductions in transport demand? Energy Policy 37(8):3212–3220

Kockelman KM (1997) Travel behavior as function of accessibility, land use mixing, and land use balance: evidence from San Francisco Bay Area. Trans Res Rec J Trans Res Board 1607 (1):116–125

Kyle P, Kim SH (2011) Long-term implications of alternative light-duty vehicle technologies for global greenhouse gas emissions and primary energy demands. Energy Policy 39(5):3012–3024. doi:10.1016/j.enpol.2011.03.016

McCollum D, Yang C, Yeh S, Ogden J (2012) Deep greenhouse gas reduction scenarios for California—strategic implications from the CA-TIMES energy-economic systems model. Energy Strat Rev 1(1):19–32. doi:10.1016/j.esr.2011.12.003

Metz D (2010) Saturation of demand for daily travel. Trans Rev 30(5):659–674

Noland RB, Lem LL (2002) A review of the evidence for induced travel and changes in transportation and environmental policy in the US and the UK. Trans Res Part D Trans Environ 7(1):1–26

Pietzcker RC, Longden T, Chen W, Fu S, Kriegler E, Kyle P, Luderer G (2014) Long-term transport energy demand and climate policy: alternative visions on transport decarbonization in energy-economy models. Energy 64(0):95–108. doi:10.1016/j.energy.2013.08.059

Schafer A (2012) Introducing behavioral change in transportation into energy/economy/environment models. Draft Report for "Green Development" Knowledge Assessment of the World Bank

Schafer A, Heywood JB (2009) Transportation in a climate constrained world. The MIT Press, Massachusetts

Schafer A, Victor DG (2000) The future mobility of the world population. Trans Res Part A Policy Pract 34(3):171–205

Waisman H-D, Guivarch C, Lecocq F (2013) The transportation sector and low-carbon growth pathways: modelling urban, infrastructure, and spatial determinants of mobility. Clim Policy 13:106–129

Zahavi Y, Ryan JM (1980) Stability of travel components over time. Transportation Research Record (750). Trans Res Board. ISSN: 0361–1981

The Role of Energy Service Demand in Carbon Mitigation: Combining Sector Analysis and China TIMES-ED Modelling

Wenying Chen, Xiang Yin, Hongjun Zhang, Ding Ma, Jincheng Shi, Weilong Huang and Nan Li

Abstract China's primary energy consumption increased from 1.46 btce (billion tons of coal equivalent) in 2000 to 3.25 btce in 2010, greatly influenced by energy service demand growth. For example, crude steel production rose from 152 to 637 million tons, urban per capita floor space from 10 to 21.5 square meters, passenger transport turnover from 1226 to 2789 billion passenger km (pkm), and freight transport turnover from 443 to 14,184 billion tons km (tkm). This trend in energy service demand will be a critical factor in the level of energy consumption and carbon emissions in the future. In this chapter, multiple approaches, including the stock-based model, the saturation model, the discrete choices model, and so on, are used to project energy service demands from different demand sectors. The projections of energy service demand are used as inputs in the China TIMES-ED model to generate a reference scenario. Several carbon constraint scenarios have been designed to analyze the role of energy service demand reductions in industry, building and transport in the mitigation of carbon emissions in China.

1 Introduction

Over the past three decades China's economy has experienced rapid development, with annual growth rates of around 10 %. GDP per capita reached 4400 US$ in 2010, with an annual growth rate of around 7 % (NBS 2011a). The value-added contribution of the tertiary industry to total GDP increased by 21.6 % points between 1980 and 2010, but the value-added contribution of secondary industry still accounted for 46.67 % of total GDP in 2010. Finally, the urbanization rate reached 51.3 % in 2010, on the back of an average annual increase of around 1 percentage point since 1980.

W. Chen (✉) · X. Yin · H. Zhang · D. Ma · J. Shi · W. Huang · N. Li
Institute of Energy, Environment and Economy, Tsinghua University, Beijing, China
e-mail: chenwy@mail.tsinghua.edu.cn

G. Giannakidis et al. (eds.), *Informing Energy and Climate Policies Using Energy Systems Models*, Lecture Notes in Energy 30,
DOI 10.1007/978-3-319-16540-0_17

These changes, as expressed in industrialization and urbanization, led to the rapid expansion of industrial production, transportation and building throughout the country. For example, the production of crude steel and cement was 637 and 1882 million tons respectively in 2010, 17.2 and 23.4 times the level of 1980 (NBS 2011a). Freight and passenger transport turnover increased to 14,184 billion ton km and 2789 billion passenger km respectively, and car ownership rose to 57 vehicles per thousand people in 2010 (NBS 2011a). Urban residential, rural residential, and commercial floor space increased to 24.4, 14.4, and 7.9 billion square meters respectively by 2010. The result is that final energy consumption increased to 2.28 btce (billion tons of coal equivalent) in 2010, with the industrial sector consuming around 70 % of this. Primary energy consumption increased to 3.25 btce in 2010, having recorded an average annual growth rate of 5.78 % in the past 30 years (NBS 2011b). However, with coal dominating energy supply (70 % of the total), the downside of this growth is that carbon dioxide emissions reached 7.2 billion tons in 2010.

With economic growth and living standard improvements, China's energy consumption and carbon emissions are expected to continue to grow without strong climate mitigation efforts. Critical to China's efforts to achieve low carbon development are structural adjustments in the economy towards producing more higher value-added and less energy intensive products and services, energy saving and energy efficiency improvements, the development of new renewable energy, and improvements in consumer behavior. This chapter contributes to the debate on these changes by using multiple approaches including the stock-based model, the saturation model, the discrete choices model and so on, to project energy service demands from different demand sectors. The chapter also presents the China TIMES-ED model, which is used to generate a reference scenario and several carbon mitigation scenarios. Finally, the role of energy service demand reduction in industry, transport and building sectors in carbon emission mitigation is analyzed.

2 Methodology

2.1 China TIMES Modelling

TIMES (The Integrated MARKAL and EFOM Model) is a combination of the MARKAL (Market allocation) and Energy Flow Optimization Model (EFOM) models developed by the Energy Technology Systems Analysis Program (ETSAP) of the International Energy Agency (Loulou et al. 2005). China MARKAL, a dynamic linear programming energy system optimization model, was developed to study China's future energy development and carbon mitigation strategies beginning in 2000 (Chen 2005; Chen et al. 2007, 2010). On the basis of China MARKAL, the China TIMES model was developed for 5-year intervals extending from 2010 to 2050. This development is based on a reference energy system (RES), which incorporates the full range of energy processes, i.e. exploitation, conversion, transmission, distribution and end-use (Chen et al. 2013). The five demand sectors of agriculture, industry, commercial, residential (divided into urban and rural), and transportation are considered and further divided into over 40 sub-sectors (Fig. 1). More than 400 technologies, including existing and advanced technologies such as poly-generation with carbon capture and storage (CCS), which may be deployed in the future, are included in the model.

Modeling using China TIMES first determines the least-cost mix of technologies and fuels to meet projected energy service demands for sectors and sub-sectors generated by the Energy Service Demand Projection Model (ESDPM) for a given social economic development scenario. This leads to the detailed fuel and technology mixes for both the demand and supply sides, as well as for the carbon emissions pathway from 2010 to 2050 for the reference scenario. Carbon constraints are then introduced into the model with elastic demand, and the supply/demand equilibrium where both the supply side and the demand side adjust to change in prices to maximize net total surplus, is computed (Eq. 1):

$$\begin{aligned} &\text{Max} \quad \sum_i \sum_t \left(p_i^0(t) \cdot \left[DM_i^0(t)\right]^{-1/\mathrm{E}_i} \cdot DM_i(t)^{1+1/\mathrm{E}_i} / (1 + 1/\mathrm{E}_i)\right) - \mathrm{c} \cdot \mathrm{X} \\ &\text{s.t.} \quad \sum_k CAP_{k,i}(t) \geq DM_i(t) \qquad i = 1, 2, \ldots, I; \quad t = 1, \ldots, T \\ &B \cdot X \geq b \end{aligned} \tag{1}$$

where

DM is a vector of variable demands;
p_i is the marginal cost of procuring demand DM_i;
E_i is price elasticity of demand DM_i;

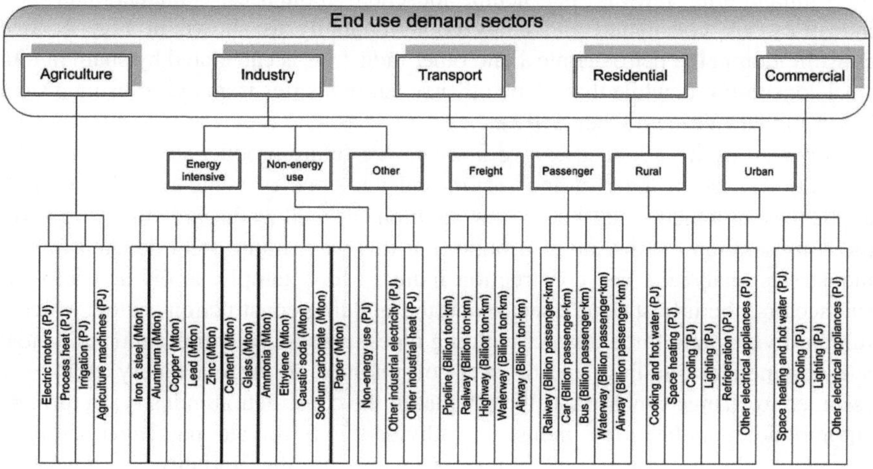

Fig. 1 End-use demand sectors and subsectors in the China TIMES model

$CAP_{k,i}$ is the capacity of end-use technology k to meet demand DM_i;
X is the vector of all TIMES variables with associated cost vector c;
DM_i^0 is the energy service demands from the ESDPM model as in the reference scenario; and
p_i^0 is the marginal cost of demand DM_i generated from the reference scenario.

In the carbon constraint scenarios, DM_i will be obtained based on the endogenous p_i, which is affected by the choices of technology, fuel, and so on. Therefore, in the China TIMES model with elastic demand, carbon mitigation can be achieved not only by technology and fuel substitution, but also by energy service demand reductions. Different price elasticities of energy service demand for each end-use sector are assumed (Kesicki and Anandarajah 2011). For example, −0.37 to −0.49 is assumed for different energy intensive industrial products, −0.32 to −0.41 for different energy service demands in building, and −0.18 to −0.4 for different transport modes.

2.2 Energy Service Demand Projection

2.2.1 Industry

The energy service demand projection for the industry sector is calculated to project production amounts of energy-intensive products such as steel, cement, ammonia, aluminum, paper, and so on, and a bottom-up stock-based approach is applied. This chapter takes steel as an example, to describe how to build the projection model for industry. Nine main steel consumers, including construction, machinery, automobile, shipbuilding, railway, petroleum, household appliances, containers and other industries, are considered and analyzed individually as shown in Fig. 2. Steel consumption in the petrochemical and other industries is calculated by share in total steel consumption, while that of the other seven industries is analyzed using a stock based model (Yin and Chen 2013).

For most of these industries, we first analyze future product stocks, such as the total floor space in the building sector, and the stock of vehicles and household appliances, and then study future new additions as well as discarded products with the consideration of lifetime distribution; in this way, future steel demand in each industry is analyzed. The construction industry for example, is divided into two sub-sectors: the infrastructure sector and the building construction sector, which is further divided into three distinct building types: urban residential, rural residential, and commercial buildings. Also, steel consumption in the machinery industry is assumed to change synchronously with that of the construction industry. In turn, the automobile manufacturing industry is divided into private passenger vehicles, business vehicles, buses and trucks. Considering the variance in household

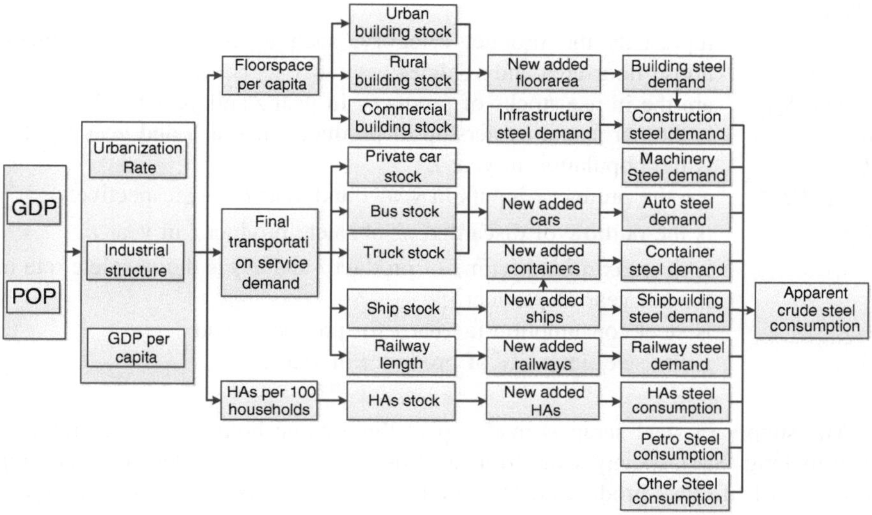

Fig. 2 A bottom-up analysis model of steel demand

appliance (HAs) possession, usage and discard between urban and rural areas, these are analyzed separately.

The stock based model was developed by employing the Material Flow Analysis (MFA) method. The stock based model can be described mathematically with four equations as follows. Equation 2 describes the driving forces of the model; here the stock of products is driven by population and lifestyle representing the engine of the system. Equation 3 describes the interaction between the inflows/outflows and stocks; stocks increase when the inflows exceed the outflows. Equation 4 indicates the obsolete outflow at time t and can be expressed as the function of the inflows and obsolete rates. Equation 5 is used to calculate steel consumption in each industry.

$$S_{i,t} = SP_{i,t} \times P_t \tag{2}$$

$$F_{i,t}^{in} = (S_{i,t} - S_{i,t-1}) + F_{i,t}^{out} \tag{3}$$

$$F_{i,t}^{out} = \sum_{k=1}^{L_i} F_{i,t-k}^{in} \times d_{i,k} \tag{4}$$

$$ST_{i,t} = F_{i,t}^{in} \times M_{i,t} \tag{5}$$

where

i	represents the product category, such as household appliances, house floor area and vehicles;
$S_{i,t}$ and $S_{i,t-1}$	are the in use stocks of product i in year t and year $t-1$;
$SP_{i,t}$	is the per capita ownership of product i in year t and year $t-1$;
P_t	is the population in year t;
$F_{i,t}^{in}$ and $F_{i,t-k}^{in}$	are the product i inputs in year t and year $t-k$, respectively;
$F_{i,t}^{out}$	is the outflow of discarded or obsolete product i in year t;
L_i	is the maximum lifetime of product i and $d_{i,k}$ is the obsolete rate in the kth year of product i;
$ST_{i,t}$	is steel consumption in year t for product i; and
$M_{i,t}$	is the steel intensity of product i in year t.

The supply of steel scrap is made up of three parts: home scrap generated in steel-making (SM), society scrap from steel-processing (SP) and depreciation scrap from end-of-life steel produces (SD), and imported steel scrap. SM, SD and SP can be calculated using Eqs. 6–9:

$$SC = SM + SP + SD \tag{6}$$

$$SM_t = ST_t \times \alpha_t \tag{7}$$

$$SP_t = RS_t \times \beta_t \tag{8}$$

$$SD_{i,t} = \gamma_t \times \sum_{k=1}^{L_i} ST_{i,t-k} \times d_{i,t-k,k} \tag{9}$$

where

ST_t	is crude steel production in year t;
RS_t	is the rolled steel production in year t;
α_t	is the scrap production rate in steel making;
β_t	is the scrap production rate in steel processing; and
γ_t	is the collection rate in year t.

The values of α_t, β_t, γ_t were about 5.5, 5.6 and 40 % in 2010 respectively, and α_t, β_t were assumed to be constant during 2010–2050; γ_t was assumed to increase to 50 % in 2050 (Yin and Chen 2013).

A normal distribution is applied with respect to the lifetime of floor space and household appliances, and the standard deviations are 20 % of the mean values. The real observed life of urban and rural buildings is only about 30 years and 25 years respectively, as a result of both the low quality of construction in the past and the rapid urbanization of recent years. They are both assumed to reach their design lifetime of 50 years by 2030. The average product lifetime of refrigerators, washing machines, air conditioners and microwave appliances is assumed to be 10, 12, 12 and 10 years respectively. In the analysis of the lifetime of vehicles, a Weibull distribution was applied. The average lifetimes of private LDVs, buses, heavy duty, medium duty and light duty trucks were assumed to be 14.46, 13.11, 12.8, 10.09 and 8.02 years respectively (Yin and Chen 2013).

The intensity of the use of steel in buildings depends upon a range of factors such as the structure and height of the buildings. The average steel intensity was assumed to be 95 kg/m^2 for both urban residential and commercial buildings in 2010. It will increase to 97.1 kg/m^2 in 2020. Thereafter it decreases by 10 % per decade from 2025 to 2050, while steel intensity in rural buildings will be 13.7 % of that in urban buildings during the modeling time horizon. Current steel intensity for private LDVs is assumed to be 842 kg/vehicle; 7566, 2552, 1033 and 727 kg/vehicle for large, medium, small and mini passenger vehicles respectively; and 9164, 3624, 1606, and 766 kg/vehicle for large, medium, small and mini trucks respectively. This is projected to decrease by 20 % from 2010 to 2020, and 10% per decade from 2020 to 2050. The steel intensity for refrigerators, washing machines, air conditioners, and microwave ovens was assumed to be 30, 18, 26 and 8 kg/unit respectively in 2010, and to decrease by 10 % per decade in the future.

2.2.2 Transportation

Passenger transport is divided into five services, and freight into four as displayed in Fig. 3. Passenger services based on business LDVs owned by government bodies and companies is treated separately from private passenger services, as these do not generally compete with each other. Private passenger transport was disaggregated into four distinct inland passenger transport service indicators, based on geographic coverage and travel purposes (intercity (pass_intercity), urban (pass_urban), rural (pass_rural), and business (pass_business—refers to government and company owned LDVs) and one international passenger service, i.e. international aviation (pass_intl_aviation). Freight transport encompasses two inland freight transportation services—domestic freight (freight_domestic) and rural freight (freight_rural)—and two international freight transportation services—international ship (freight_intl_ship) and international aviation (freight_intl_aviation). Within each type of transportation service multiple subsectors representing available modal choices are created. Passenger transport employs motorcycles, walking, cycles, LDV, buses, rail, high-speed rail, and air, whereas freight transport modes are truck, rail, ship, air and rural vehicles (3 and 4 W).

The discrete choices model is applied to project energy service demand for every transport mode (Mishra et al. 2013). The demand for transportation services is determined by income, population, and the weighted average service cost of various transportation modes and technologies. Passenger transportation services (passenger kilometers) in period t is given by:

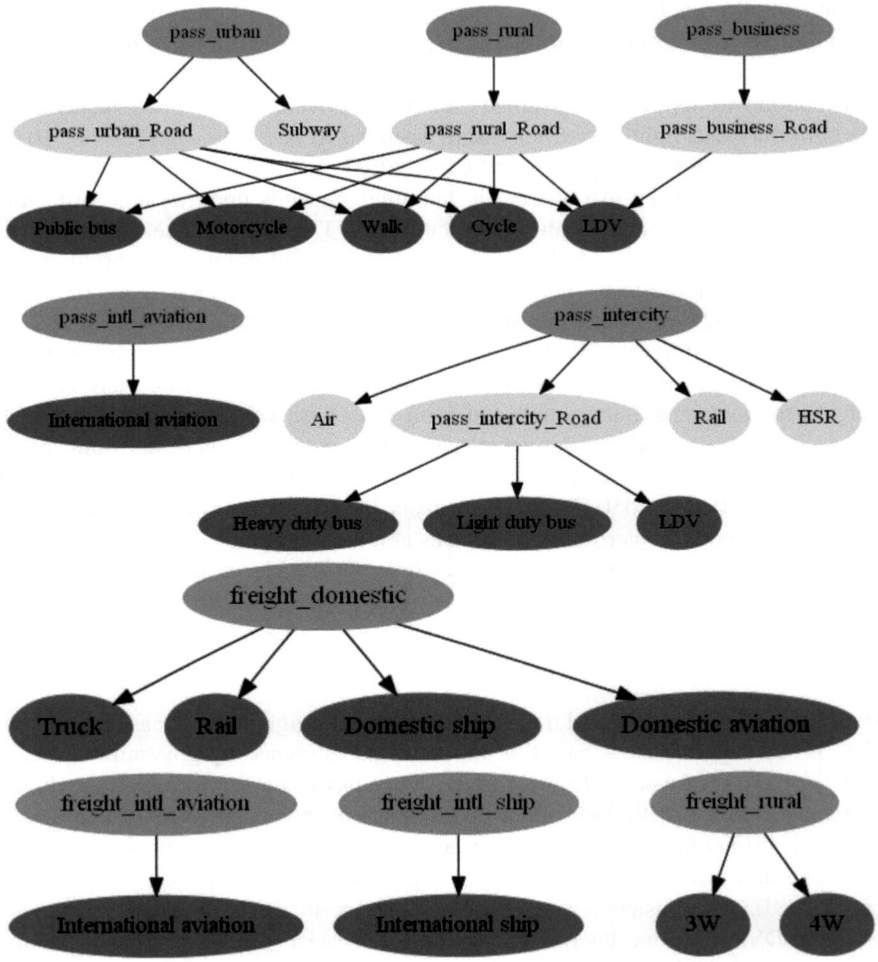

Fig. 3 Representation of transportation services and modes. *Top* passenger. *Bottom* freight

$$Passenger_{r,t} = A \times Income.p_{r,t}^{E\_income_{r,t}} \times C_{r,t}^{E\_TSC_{r,t}} \times Pop \tag{10}$$

where

A	represents a calibration coefficient;
$Income.p_{r,t}$	is per capita income or regional income (for urban and rural transportation);
$C_{r,t}$	is weighted-average service price;
Pop	is total population or regional populations (for urban and rural transportation); and
$E\_income_{r,t}$ and $E\_TSC_{r,t}$	are income and price elasticity, respectively.

Freight transportation service demands, which rely on the aggregate level of economic activity, are similarly formulated but are scaled by total income rather than per capita income and population. Freight transportation service in period t is given by Eq. 11:

$$Freight_{r,t} = A \times Income_t^{E\_GDP_{r,t}} \times C_t^{E\_TSC_{r,t}} \tag{11}$$

The transportation service price is expressed by the cost per unit of service demand. This is the weighted average of technology-specific service prices, which includes a technology's capital and fuel costs, and the time value of its use; it is given by Eq. 12:

$$C_t = \sum_m \sum_j share_{m,j,t} \times P_{m,j,t} \tag{12}$$

where

$P_{m,j,t}$ represents the general transport service price of technology j in mode m in period t; and

$Share_{m,j,t}$ is the share of technology j in mode m in period t.

The service price of using a transportation mode in period t is given by Eq. 13:

$$P_{m,j,t} = \frac{\sum_i (FuelPrice_{m,j,i,t} \times FuelEconomy_{m,j,i,t}) + Non\_FuelCost_{m,j,t}}{LF_{m,j,t}} + \frac{GDP_{r,t}}{Speed_{r,m,t}} \tag{13}$$

where

$FuelPrice_{m,j,i,t}$ is the fuel price (\$/MJ);

$FuelEconomy_{m,j,i,t}$ is the vehicle fuel intensity (MJ/VKM)

$Non\_FuelCost_{m,j,t}$ is the non-fuel price (\$/VKM);

$LF_{m,j,t}$ is the load factor (in persons or tons per vehicle);

$GDP_{r,t}$ is the wage rate (\$/(person-hour)), which is related to economic behavior; and

$Speed_{r,m,t}$ is the vehicle speed (km/h).

Fuel prices, including carbon prices are endogenous, and all the other variables are exogenous for different technologies. For freight transportation modes, where hauling time may not incur direct opportunity costs, time value is excluded.

In turn, $Share_{m,j,t}$ is given by Eq. 14:

$$Share_{m,j,t} = \frac{(SW_m)(P_{m,t})^{-\lambda_r}}{\sum_j (SW_m)(P_{m,t})^{-\lambda_r}} \tag{14}$$

where: λ_r is the price sensitivity constant in region r, which determines the degree to which future price changes will be reflected in modal shifts and varies from different service demand sensitivity; and SW_m is share weight, a calibration parameter.

In this discrete choices model, higher general transport service prices will lead to lower market share, but those modes with high prices will not totally disappear, and the share of modes with low prices will not increase sharply to dominate the market. While competition among modes does exist, all modes will have some market share.

2.2.3 Building

Buildings are divided into urban residential, rural residential, and commercial categories, and energy demand is further divided into space heating, cooling, water heating and cooking, lighting and electric appliances. With respect to different climate conditions and building design standards: four regions, Severe Cold (SC), Cold (C), Hot Summer Cold Winter (HSCW) and Hot Summer Warm Winter (HSWW), are considered separately, based on the Standard of Climatic Regionalization for Architecture (GB 50178-1993) (MOHURD 1993). Per capita floor space is the basis for the projection of space heating, cooling, lighting and similar types of energy demand sources. This is expected to increase with the improvement of living standards, but a saturation level is recognized with the application of the Gompertz model as follows (Eq. 15):

$$PFS = ae^{-be^{-cPGDP}} \tag{15}$$

where

PFS	represents per capita floor space;
$PGDP$	is per capita GDP;
a	represents the ultimate saturation level of per capita floor space; and
b and c	are two parameters that determine the shape of the curve.

The following approach from the literature Eom et al. (2012) is used to project energy service demand for space heating and cooling. The service demand per floor space is given by Eq. 16:

$$d_j = k_j \cdot \overline{q_j} \cdot \phi_j(P_j, i) \tag{16}$$

where

j	is a given service, such as space heating, cooling, lighting, etc.;
k_j	is a calibration parameter;
$\bar{q}_j$	is the saturation demand level;
$\varphi_j(P_j, i)$	represents the effect of income and price for the demand;
P_j	gives the price of service j; and
i	is per capita income.

The price and income effects are represented by Eq. 17:

$$\phi_{P,j} = 1 - \exp(-\frac{\ln 2}{\mu_j}\frac{i}{P_j}) \tag{17}$$

where

μ_j is referred to as the saturation impedance.

Demand saturation level for space heating and cooling is given by Eqs. 18 and 19:

$$\overline{q_H} = HDD \cdot \eta \cdot r - \lambda_H \cdot IG \tag{18}$$

$$\overline{q_C} = CDD \cdot \eta \cdot r + \lambda_C \cdot IG \tag{19}$$

where

HDD and CDD	are heating and cooling degree days, which represent the annual requirement of space heating and cooling to achieve comfortable indoor temperature which, in China is summer 26 °C for all four regions, and in winter 16 °C for the HSWW region, and 18 °C for other regions;
η	is the thermal conductance of buildings [GJ/(m^2 day °C)];
r	is the building's floor to surface ratio;
IG	represents the amount of building internal gains (GJ/m^2); and
λ_H and λ_C	are both calibration parameters.

2.3 The Decomposition Approach

To assess the contribution of energy service demand reduction to carbon mitigation, the following approach is applied (Eq. 20):

$$CO_2 = \sum_i Demand_i \times \frac{CO_{2i}}{Demand_i} \tag{20}$$

where

CO_2	is total carbon emission;
$Demand_i$	is energy service demand i; and
CO_{2i}	is carbon emissions for energy service i.

Using the Laspeyres decomposition approach (Ang 2004), change of carbon emission is given by Eq. 21:

$$\Delta CO_2 = \Delta Demand_{effect} + \Delta(\frac{CO_2}{Demand})_{effect} \tag{21}$$

where

ΔCO_2 is the change in carbon emissions;

$\Delta Demand_{effect}$ is the change of total carbon emissions from energy service demand; and

$\Delta(\frac{CO_2}{Demand})_{effect}$ is the change in total carbon emissions from carbon intensity.

$\Delta Demand_{effect}$ is given by Eq. 22:

$$\Delta Demand_{effect} = \sum_i \Delta Demand_i \times (\frac{CO_2}{Demand}) + \sum_i \Delta Demand_i \times \Delta(\frac{CO_2}{Demand})/2 \quad (22)$$

where

$\Delta Demand_i$ represents the change of $Demand_i$ compared to the reference scenario.

3 Scenario Design

3.1 Main Assumptions for Future Social Economic Growth

Economic and population growth, industrial structure adjustment and the urbanization rate are the four most important factors to impact on future energy consumption and carbon emissions. In this study, annual GDP growth rate is assumed to be 7.9, 7.0, 6.0, 4.5 and 3.0 during 2010–2015, 2015–2020, 2020–2030, 2030–2040 and 2040–2050 respectively. With the Chinese government's continued efforts at structural adjustment of the economy, the share of secondary industry value-added in GDP is projected to decrease from 45.75 % in 2010, to 36 % in 2050, while the share of the tertiary industry will increase from 43.14 to 62 %. Also, China's population is expected to peak at around 1.47 billion in 2035, and then decrease to 1.44 billion in 2050. There is strong empirical evidence that the urbanization rate is correlated to GDP, so the urbanization rate in China will increase as per capita GDP increases. Hence, we assume the urbanization rate to be a function of per capita GDP, and is therefore projected to increase from 49.9 % in 2010 to 74.0 % in 2050.

3.2 Scenario Design

Besides a reference scenario, four carbon constrained scenarios were considered; that is, M10, M20, M30 and M40. The cumulative carbon emissions from China during 2010–2050 are assumed to reduce 10, 20, 30 and 40 % relative to the reference scenario for M10, M20, M30 and M40, respectively.

4 Modeling Results

4.1 Emission Pathways in Different Scenarios

In the reference scenario, policies and measures related to carbon mitigation planned and implemented in China, such as energy savings and the development of new renewable energy technologies have been considered. Carbon emissions in 2050 are expected to increase to around 14.5 $GtCO_2$, and the accumulative carbon emissions between 2010 and 2050 would be around 480 $GtCO_2$ in the reference scenario. Carbon emissions from industry are expected to peak around 2025, mainly as a result of peak of energy-intensive products and greater energy efficiency improvements. Carbon emissions for the power sector are expected to almost stabilize after 2040 due to large-scale use of new and renewable energy. However, carbon emissions in buildings and transportation are expected to grow steadily, since emissions reduction from technology improvement and fuel substitution cannot offset emission growth from the expected increase in building floor space and transport turnover.

Each sector behaves differently in the mitigation scenarios as displayed in Fig. 4. Compared with the reference scenario, carbon emissions will reduce by 14–55 % or 0.5–1.8 billion tons for industry by the year 2050, and 2–54 % or no more than 0.7 billion tons for buildings, in carbon constrained scenarios. CO_2 emissions in

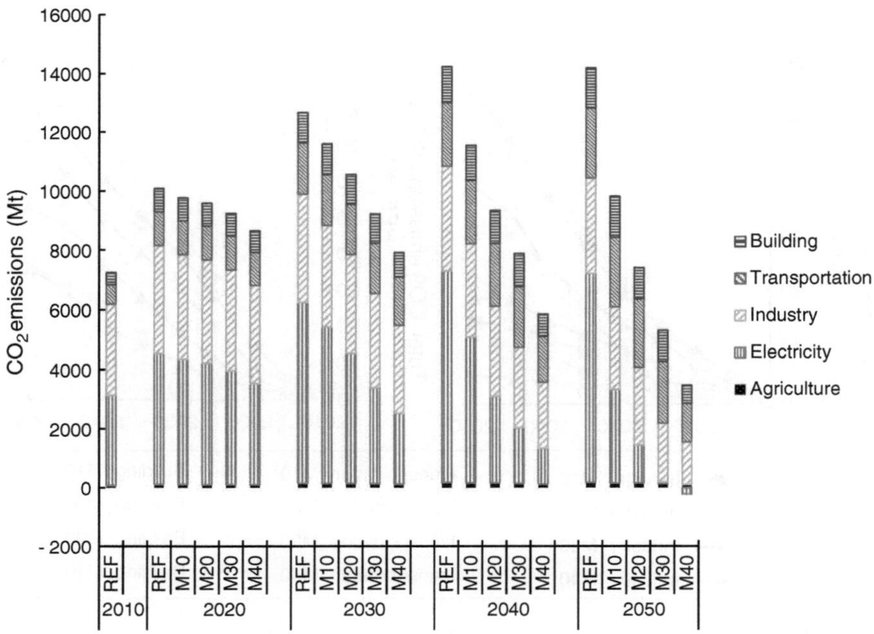

Fig. 4 Carbon emission mitigation for different sectors

transport will only reduce by 2–13 %, or about 0.1–0.3 billion tons in the M10, M20, and M30 scenarios due to heavy dependence on oil, while it will increase to 46 % in M4 (to nearly 1.1 billion tons). Reductions will be a result of large decreases in transport turnover, and rapid expansion in fuel cell, electric and biofuel vehicles, and so on. Overall, the end-use sectors can only reduce emissions by 0.6–3.7 billion tons of CO_2 in 2050, far below the 3.9–7.3 billion tons of reduction that will take place in the power sector.

Direct emissions account for the carbon emissions from coal, oil and gas for final energy consumption for each end-use sector. While for consumption of electricity and heat indirect carbon emissions are used to account for the carbon emissions from power and heat production. When indirect CO_2 emissions are considered, the total carbon reduction rate in the building sector will be 37, 63, 78, and 88% in M10, M20, M30, and M40 respectively, similar to those in the industry sector (36–81 %), as shown in Fig. 5. For the transport sector, this reduction will only be 6–19 % in M10, M20 and M30, and 50 % in M40, closer to direct emission reduction rates as a result of lower electricity consumption than in the two other sectors.

With improvements in the country's final energy mix, carbon intensity is expected to decrease from 2.01, 1.92 and 1.27 tCO_2/tce in 2010, to 1.96, 1.41 and 0.92 tCO_2/tce in 2050, for the transport, industry and buildings respectively (Fig. 6). The carbon intensity in the industry and buildings sectors will begin to decrease visibly after 2025. However, in the transport sector, significant decreases in carbon intensity will happen only after 2035, and its carbon intensity will still be

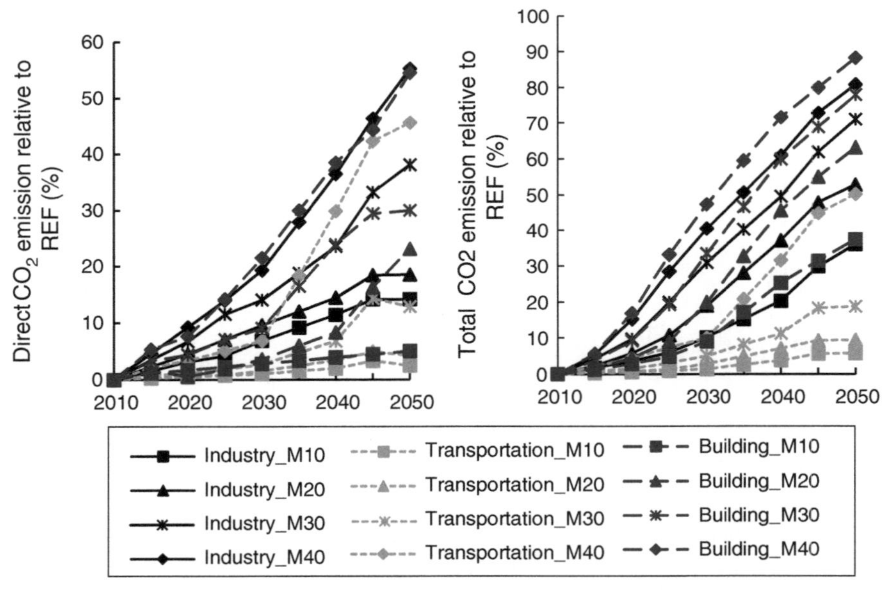

Fig. 5 Direct and indirect carbon emission reduction rates for different end-use sectors

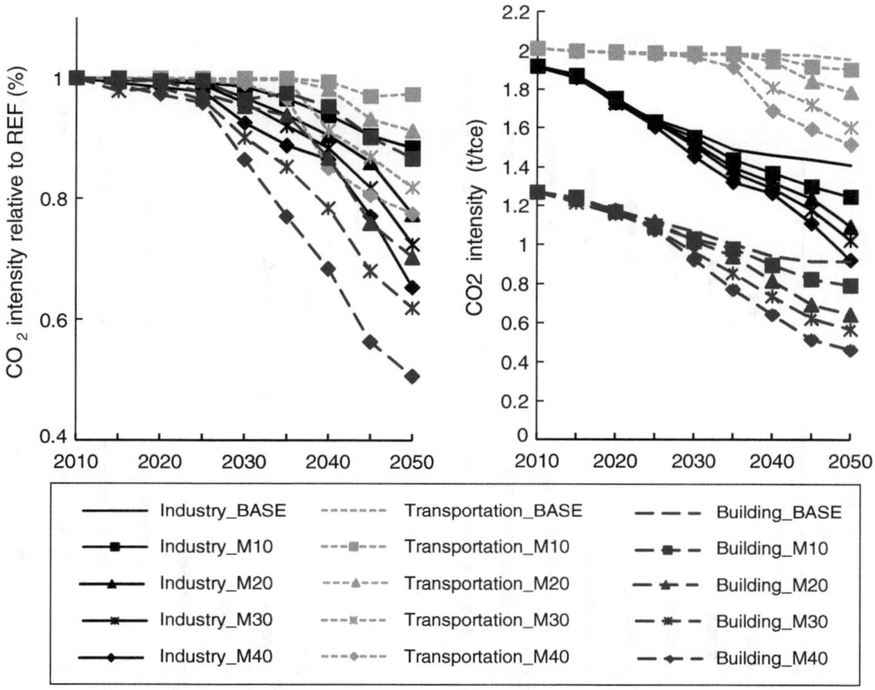

Fig. 6 Changes of carbon intensity in different end-use sectors

much higher than that of industry and building in 2050. Compared with the reference scenario, the carbon intensity of the industry, buildings and transport sectors will decline by 12–35 %, 13–49 % and 1–23 % in 2050, respectively.

4.2 Demand Reductions

In the ED version of the China TIMES model, carbon mitigation is achieved by both energy service demand reduction and the deployment of low and non-carbon technologies. Figure 7 compares the change of energy service demand in the industry, buildings, passenger transport and freight transport sectors under different carbon constrained scenarios, where the different symbols denote the deviation of energy service demand from the reference scenario for different energy services. The energy service demands of industry, especially the energy-intensive industries, record the greatest decrease. In 2050, the energy service demand in industry decreases by 12, 15, 23 and 30 % under M10, M20, M30 and M40 respectively, while the energy service demand in buildings, passenger transport, and freight transport decreases by only 7–25 %, 2–9 % and 3–17 % respectively. The finding of

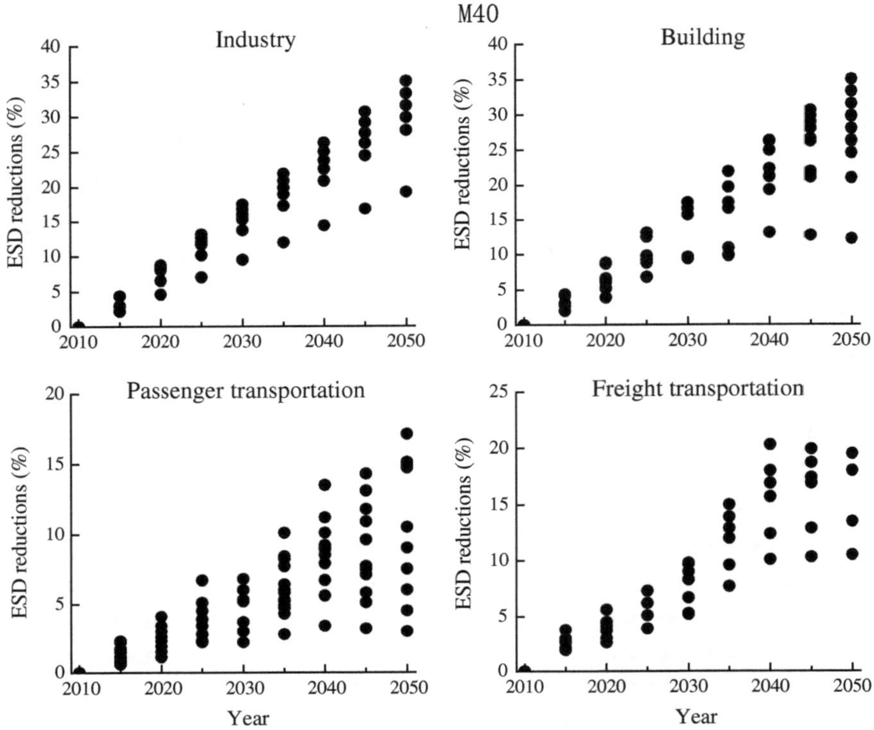

Fig. 7 Energy service demand reductions in M40

less energy service demand reduction in transport than the other two end-use sectors is consistent with the literature.

In the industry sector, taking the steel sector as an example, per capita steel consumption in 2050 decreases from 277 kg in the reference scenario, to 224 kg in M10, and 209 kg in M20, similar to the world average level in 2010 (207 kg), and lower than the current level of the developed countries (USA 277 kg, Japan 842 kg, Germany 541 kg and France 241 kg). In the M30 and M40 scenarios, per capita steel consumption decreases sharply after its peak in around 2015, to only 190 kg and 175 kg in 2050 respectively.

In the buildings sector in 2050, taking space heating as an example, demand for rural residential, urban residential and public buildings decreases by 12–25 %, 11–28 %, and 12–33 % respectively in the carbon constrained scenarios compared with the reference case. Considering that the current heating ratio of urban residential and public buildings is about 42 and 49 % of the total floor space respectively, the sharp decrease in the stringent carbon constraint scenarios will be difficult to achieve without significant breakthroughs in building thermal insulation technology. The total building floor space decreases from 90.3 billion square meters in the reference scenario, to 62.5–81.5 billion square meters in different mitigation scenarios, without considering the change of energy service demand per unit floor area. Per capita living space decreases from 42.6 m^2 in the reference scenario, to 35.1–36.5 square meters in M10 and M20 respectively, close to the current level in Japan (35.8 square meters in 2010). Under the M30 and M40 scenarios, however, per capita living space further decreases to 28.1–33.0 square meters. Assuming there are no actual reductions in floor space, the energy service demand per square meter needs to drop from 11.8 kgce/m^2 in the reference scenario to 8.0–11.2 kgce/m^2 in the constrained scenarios by 2050.

In the transportation sector, passenger and freight transport turnover in the mitigation scenarios decreases by 2–10 % and 2–12 % respectively in 2050. Within this pattern, turnover in those transport modes with higher energy intensities like airplanes and cars, decreases much faster than that of trains. Car turnover, for example, decreases by 3–16 % in 2050. If the load rate (persons per car) and the use intensity (kilometers per year) are consistent with the assumptions in the reference scenario, vehicle ownership per 1000 people in 2050 decreases from 415 to 350–400 (440 for Japan, 450–600 for the European Union, and 800 for the USA in 2010).

4.3 Contribution of Demand Reductions in CO_2 Mitigation

Figures 8 and 9 show the direct and total (including direct and indirect emissions) CO_2 emissions of end-use sectors in the four mitigation scenarios. With the increase in emission reductions, energy service demand reductions in end-use sectors will also contribute more to CO_2 emission reductions. In 2050, the decline of energy service demand contributes 420, 670, 1020 and 1460 million tons of direct CO_2 reductions in the M10, M20, M30 and M40 scenarios, respectively; accounting for

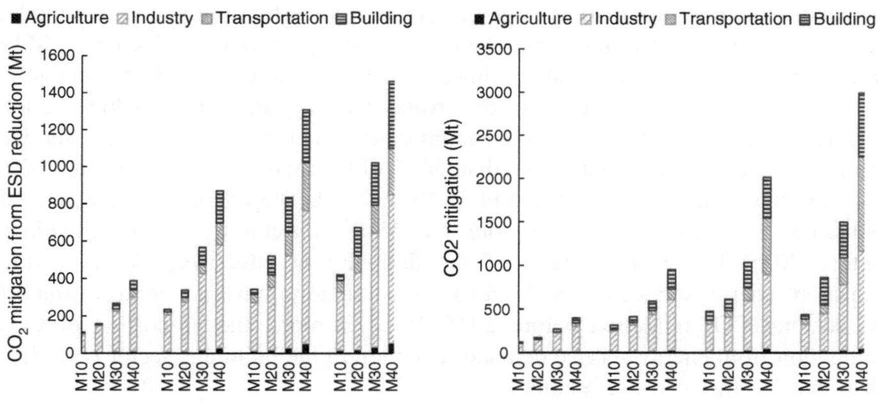

Fig. 8 Direct carbon mitigation from energy service demand reduction

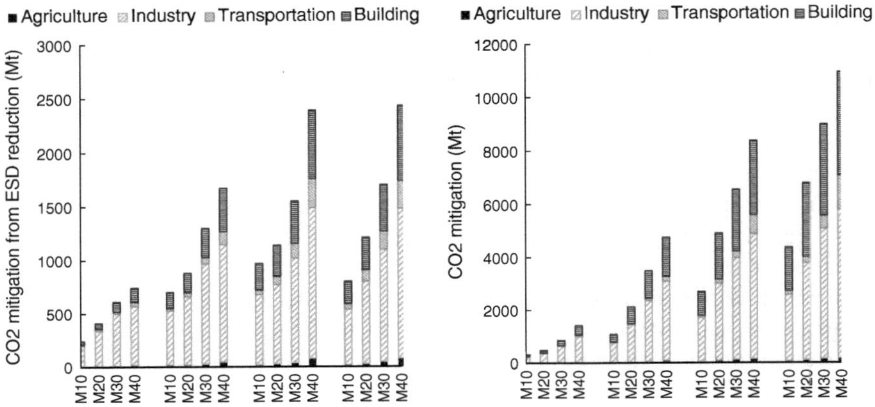

Fig. 9 Total carbon mitigation from energy service demand reduction

90, 75, 70 and 50 % of total direct CO_2 emission reductions. The total (direct and indirect) emissions reduction due to energy service demand reduction could be up to 800, 1200, 1700 and 2400 million tons in 2050. This contributes to 18, 18, 19 and 22 % of total CO_2 emission reductions in the four mitigation scenarios.

Among the end-use sectors, energy service demand reduction in industry makes up the largest proportion of total CO_2 mitigation, contributing 520, 770, 1050 and 1400 million tons of CO_2 reduction in the 4 different scenarios in 2050 (Fig. 9). However, with the increase in CO_2 mitigation, this proportion decreases from 64 to 58 % across these scenarios. Compared with the industry and buildings sectors, energy service demand reduction in transport have a relatively small effect on CO_2 emission reductions, with only 50, 170 and 260 million tons of emission reductions in M10, M20 and M30 in 2050, contributing between 6 and 11 % of total CO_2 mitigation. Energy service demand reductions in the buildings sector contribute 210–690 million tons of carbon reductions across all four scenarios in 2050, around 26 % of total reductions. However, although it is apparent that energy service demand reductions can make a large contribution to carbon mitigation, the model results also show that welfare loss from energy service demand reduction in M40 will be 6.5 times, 4.3 times, and 2.2 times that of M10, M20 and M30 respectively.

Due to the relatively high cost of advanced energy efficient and low carbon technologies, and lower mitigation requirements before 2020, energy service demand reductions contribute more than 50 % of the total CO_2 reductions in 2020. But this figure decreases to less than 25 % in 2050. The energy service demand reductions in industry contribute more than 55 % to sectoral emission reductions before 2025. However, because of the difficulty in effectively decarbonizing transport, energy service demand reductions continue to have a significant impact on sectoral CO_2 reduction before 2035. What is more, the proportion of CO_2 mitigation from energy service demand reduction in the buildings sector is far less than that in other end-use sectors.

5 Conclusion

China's energy service demand, total energy consumption and carbon emissions have experienced fast growth in the past three decades. However, due to its relatively low per capita income and per capita energy use, energy consumption as well as carbon emissions are projected to continue to increase in the future without strong carbon mitigation efforts. Carbon emissions in 2050 are expected to increase to around 14.5 $GtCO_2$, and cumulative carbon emissions between 2010 and 2050 will be around 480 $GtCO_2$. The 10–40 % reductions in cumulative emissions discussed in this chapter will require great efforts in both the low and non-technology deployment scenario, as well as transformation in both production and consumption modes to decrease energy service demand. Compared with the results derived from using the China TIMES without elastic demand (Chen et al. 2013), the marginal carbon abatement costs for similar levels of reduction will however be around 50 % lower.

Greater levels of carbon mitigation will require more reduction of energy service demand, but this would result in higher community welfare loss. It is therefore more important to control the current fast increases in energy service demand in the short term through transformation of both production and consumption modes to avoid lock-in. In the longer term, development of low and non-carbon energy will be more critical with respect to the achievement of significant carbon mitigation, as a result of the limited room for energy service demand reduction and the consequent higher community welfare loss. Apart from significant breakthroughs in both energy supply and end-use technologies, stronger policies and actions on the limitation of the export of energy intensive products, reasonable city layout planning, public transportation system improvement, building energy saving, housing property taxes, and so on, are necessary for the promotion of low carbon society development.

Acknowledgments We would like to thank Ministry of Science and Technology of China (2012BAC20B01), Ministry of Education of China (12JJD630002), and National Development and Reform Commission of China (2012011) for the support on model development and simulation.

References

Ang BW (2004) Decomposition analysis for policymaking in energy: which is the preferred method? Energy Policy 32(9):1131–1139

Chen W (2005) The costs of mitigating carbon emissions in China: findings from China MARKAL-MACRO modeling. Energy Policy 33(7):885–896

Chen W, Wu Z et al (2007) Carbon emission control strategies for China: a comparative study with partial and general equilibrium versions of the China MARKAL model. Energy 32(1):59–72

Chen W, Li H et al (2010) Western China energy development and west to east energy transfer: application of the Western China sustainable energy development model. Energy Policy 38:7106–7120

Chen W, Yin X, Zhang H (2013) Towards low carbon development in China: a comparison of national and global models. Clim Change. doi:10.1007/s10584-013-0937-7

Eom J, Clarke L, Kim SH et al (2012) China's building energy demand: long-term implications from a detailed assessment. Energy Policy 46:405–419

Kesicki F, Anandarajah G (2011) The role of energy-service demand reduction in global climate change mitigation: Combining energy modelling and decomposition analysis. Energy Policy 39:7224–7233

Loulou R, Remne U et al (2005) Documentation for the TIMES Model, PART I: Energy Technology Systems Analysis Programme. http://www.etsap.org/tools.htm

Mishra GS, Kyle P, Teter J et al (2013) Transportation module of global change assessment model (GCAM): model documentation. Institute of Transportation Studies, University of California, Davis

MOHURD—Ministry of Housing and Urban–Rural Development in China (1993) Standard of Climatic Regionalization for Architecture GB 50178–1993

NBS—National Bureau of Statistics (2011a) China statistical yearbook 2011. China Statistics Press, Beijing

NBS—National Bureau of Statistics (2011b) China energy statistical yearbook 2011. China Statistics Press, Beijing

Yin X, Chen W (2013) Trends and development of steel demand in China: a bottom up analysis. Resources Policy 38:407–415

Part III
Gaining Additional Insights Through Model Coupling

Soft-Linking Exercises Between TIMES, Power System Models and Housing Stock Models

J.P. Deane, Francesco Gracceva, Alessandro Chiodi, Maurizio Gargiulo and Brian Ó Gallachóir

Abstract Soft-linking TIMES models with carefully selected complementary models can provide useful additional insights into the results from the TIMES model and can usefully scrutinize specific TIMES results in greater detail with another model. This multi-model approach can take advantage of the individual strengths of different modelling approaches. This chapter collates methodologies and results from a number of soft-linking exercises with TIMES. Two specific examples are given; firstly the soft-linking of TIMES to a power system model to investigate the TIMES results and provide additional insights into power system flexibility, reliability and market issues. The second example comprises the soft-linking of a TIMES model to a power system and a housing stock model to explore the impacts of increased electrification of residential heating on the power system and associated emissions from the residential sector. These examples show how a

J.P. Deane (✉) · A. Chiodi · M. Gargiulo · B. Ó Gallachóir
Energy Policy and Modelling Group, Environmental Research Institute,
University College Cork, Cork, Ireland
e-mail: jp.deane@ucc.ie

A. Chiodi
e-mail: a.chiodi@ucc.ie

M. Gargiulo
e-mail: maurizio.gargiulo@e4sma.com

B. Ó Gallachóir
e-mail: b.ogallachoir@ucc.ie

J.P. Deane · A. Chiodi · B. Ó Gallachóir
School of Engineering, University College Cork, Cork, Ireland

F. Gracceva
European Commission Joint Research Centre, Institute for Energy and Transport,
The Netherlands and ENEA, Rome, Italy
e-mail: francesco.gracceva@enea.it

M. Gargiulo
Energy Engineering Economic Environment Systems Modelling and Analysis
(E4SMA s.r.l.), Turin, Italy

G. Giannakidis et al. (eds.), *Informing Energy and Climate Policies Using Energy Systems Models*, Lecture Notes in Energy 30,
DOI 10.1007/978-3-319-16540-0_18

multi-model approach and soft-linking can provide a strong complementary analysis to TIMES modelling exercises and generate insights into results that otherwise would be difficult to achieve with a single model approach.

1 Introduction

Soft-linking with TIMES is undertaken when the outputs from TIMES are scrutinized in greater detail with another model such as a dedicated power systems model, a macro-economic model, or a detailed sectoral models. The motivation for soft-linking is to provide a two-way transfer of information between the TIMES model and the linked model, in a manner that takes advantages of the strengths of each model. This exchange of information can provide additional insights and can improve and develop a deeper understanding of TIMES models' results. Part of this motivation is derived from a view that one specific energy modelling tool cannot address all aspects of the full energy system in great detail and greater insights and progress can be gained by drawing on the strengths of multiple modelling tools rather than trying to incorporate them all into one comprehensive model. A further motivation for soft-linking with sectoral models arises from the additional insights that may be gained regarding the timing for individual policy measures, thus facilitating a transition from technology roadmaps to policy roadmaps.

In the case of the electrical power system, both TIMES and power systems models address the modelling of complex systems, even though they are fundamentally different in their focus and application. Power systems models focus solely on the electrical power system and sometimes the gas network but do not consider the rest of the energy system. The primary inputs are generally exogenous in nature, including electricity load, fuel prices and power plant technical limits. Energy systems models examine the full energy system and in this case the electrical power system is by contrast completely endogenous and driven by the combined behaviour of supply sectors that provide primary fuels and end-use sectors driven by exogenous energy service demands. The focus is typically to provide a technology rich basis for estimating energy dynamics over a medium and long-term, multiple period time horizon. Because of the exclusive focus on electricity generation within power systems models, the problem description can be at a higher resolution, i.e. higher temporal resolution and with increased technical power plant operational detail (including ramp rates, minimum stable level, cold starts etc.) when compared to full energy systems model, which have to handle a much broader range of problems and sub-systems. Typically a power systems model can model from hourly to 5 min or higher resolution while energy systems models may have a limited number of temporally-independent "timeslices", which can be a limitation when looking at power systems with levels of fluctuating renewable energy.

The same applies in soft-linking with other model types. Regarding sectoral models, for example a dedicated housing stock model tends to have a focussed and detailed representation of housing stock in the residential sector while TIMES captures the housing stock in a more simplified manner. Soft-linking results from TIMES to a housing stock model can allow for results (in terms of energy) to be further scrutinised and translated into more meaningful units such as number of particular houses effected by a technology or policy.

This chapter collates methodologies and results from a number of soft-linking exercises including:

- The soft-linking of the Irish TIMES model to the power system model PLEXOS to scrutinise results in terms of power system flexibility and reliability.
- The soft-linking of TIMES Italy with a power system model to provide a complimentary dimension to TIMES analysis surrounding market issues.
- The soft-linking of the Irish TIMES model to a power system and housing stock model to examine the impact of increased electrification on the power system and associated emissions from the housing stock.

2 Why Soft-Linking to a Power System Model

The following sections highlights key areas of technical importance that benefit from soft-linking to a power system model.

2.1 Flexibility and Reliability

Power systems models can more readily take account of power system operation and be used to assess issues relating to flexibility and reliability. The benefit of higher resolution within power systems and energy systems modelling has been recognized where it was shown that optimal investment decisions derived from models can vary significantly depending on the timeslice selection used (Ludig et al. 2011). In Kannan (2011) the author has developed a temporal UK MARKAL model to investigate the role of electricity storage. The UK temporal MARKAL model has 20 annual timeslices compared to six in most standard MARKAL databases. In Pina et al. (2011) the authors have developed a high resolution temporal TIMES model by dividing each year into 4 seasons, with 3 days per season and 24 h per day. The results show that the increase in temporal resolution allows for more constraints to be taken into account, such as renewable resource availability, operational constraints, electricity demand dynamics and others.

Fluctuating renewable power such as wind, solar and ocean energy bring more variability and uncertainty to power system planning and operations and this can have an impact on power system reliability. Power system reliability is fundamentally composed of security and adequacy. A power system can be considered secure if it can withstand a loss (or potentially multiple losses) of key power supply components such as generators or transmission links. A power system is adequate if there is a sufficient installed capacity to meet demand. In general a number of key metrics are used to assess reliability. An overview of these can be found in Holttinen (2012). Briefly these are Loss of Load Probability (LOLP) which is a measure of the probability that demand will exceed the capacity of the system in a given period and the Loss of Load Expectation (LOLE) which is number of times in a given period that the load will be greater than the demand. LOLE can be used to set a security standard, generally given as a number of hours per year. If this is exceeded in, it indicates the system has a higher than acceptable level of risk. Expected Unserved Energy (EUE) is also a useful metric as it takes account of the extent of the shortages.

2.2 Unit Commitment and Dispatch

The security-constrained unit commitment and dispatch problem involves deciding the correct combination and power output of units for the economic and reliable operation of the power system, taking into account fuel and carbon costs, and reserve requirements required in case of forced outages of power plants or transmission lines and against demand uncertainty. Unit commitment being the decision of which units to turn on or off and dispatch being the decision of what level to run units at once they are on. The value of detailed unit commitment and dispatch modelling is that it captures many of the technical constraints and limitations of thermal power plant and quantifies the implications for variable renewable generation in terms of its impact on the probability of the system running short of generation and/or reserve requirements. This feeds back into the determination of the technical suitability and flexibility of the power system. While power systems models can model the unit commitment and dispatch problem at high resolutions (1 min–1 h), energy systems model generally assume a lower timely resolution for which the problem is solved. This is done so as to keep the problem computationally manageable. The unit commitment and dispatch problem can be relatively complicated to solve because the physical delivery of electricity is subject to the technical and economic constraints on generation. Some of these technical constraints may introduce integer variables into the linear programming formulation in order to track the on/off state of generation plant in time and to enforce important technical constraints minimum stable generation, minimum up and down times and start costs as a function of unit temperature.

2.3 Market Issues

Soft-linking can provide a complimentary dimension to TIMES analysis by allowing greater examination of the electricity market and impact of different portfolios on market prices and support mechanisms. A challenge for power systems is that the investments in flexibility required by a low carbon power system can be difficult to achieve if the market does not properly value the benefits of flexible resources. The problem here is if the market design benefits technologies that would help realize a system in line with political goals. A key characteristic of a market with large shares of renewables is its new market rationale, where the merit order is replaced by net demand (and the profile of the price curve is different from the demand curve) and the role of thermal plants changes substantially. There are many more periods of (temporarily) very low market prices, when there is a surplus of renewables and nuclear output, so that renewable electricity shifts the supply curve of conventional electricity virtually out of the market. Moreover, thermal plants have on average much lower load factors. Historically, in power market the ability to earn money on investments in new production facilities depends on whether the more expensive units can sell their electricity and recover more than their short run marginal cost. So, for conventional plants it was generally possible to recover the fixed costs when more expensive plants, usually gas-fired peaking units, set the price. But as the share of fix costs is considerably higher when full-load hours are low, in a high renewable market where renewables with virtually zero marginal costs set market clearing prices, this may no longer be the case. Power systems model generally can provide greater insight and analysis of these issues as they can simulate market configurations and allow for an understanding of market challenges to be developed.

3 Soft-Linking Methodology

The software used in these softlinking examples is PLEXOS Integrated Energy Model.[1] PLEXOS, developed by Energy Exemplar, is an electricity and gas systems modelling tool that uses mixed integer optimisation techniques to determine the least cost unit commitment and dispatch solution to meet demand while respecting generator technical-economic constraints. The software co-optimises hydro, thermal, renewable, and reserve classes; and no heuristic or sequential approach is taken. Modelling is carried out using mixed integer linear programming that aims to minimize an objective function subject to the expected cost of electricity dispatch and a number of constraints. The objective function of the model includes operational costs, consisting of fuel costs and carbon costs; start-up costs, consisting of a fuel off-take and a start cost; penalty costs for unserved energy and for failing to meet reserve requirements. System level constraints consist of an energy balance equation ensuring supply (net pumping demand) meets regional demand at each period. Water balance equations ensure water flow within the pumped storage units is conserved and tracked. Constraints on unit operation

---

[1] See http://energyexemplar.com/.

include minimum and maximum generation, maximum and minimum up and down time and ramp up and down rates. In chronological mode, the software solves for each period and maintains consistency across the full problem horizon.

The soft-linking methodology is described in detail in Deane et al. (2012). The initial step in the soft-linking methodology is to extract the power system from the energy system results. The power systems model is populated with an electrical portfolio, fuel prices and demand from the energy systems model while the energy systems model is enhanced with output from the power systems model. The goal of the methodology is ultimately to have an improved understanding of the energy systems model's results in relation to the electrical power sector and to understand what elements of the power system are important.

The steps in the soft-linking methodology are as follows:

1. Select the model, the scenario and the target year of the analysis for the energy systems model and execute the model.
2. Extract results from the energy systems model for the target year of interest for the electricity generation portfolio and populate the power systems model with this generation portfolio. Additional technical detail and data such as minimum stable generation, ramp rates and start costs, failure and maintenance rates are included in the power systems model. Fuel prices and carbon prices from the energy systems model are also provided to the power systems model.
3. Convert the annual electricity demand profile for the target year from the energy systems model into a half hourly chronological profile.
4. Initially run the power systems model for the target year using this data at half-hourly resolution without any additional technical constraints such as minimum stable generation, ramp rates and start costs. This is done to investigate the impact of increasing the chronological resolution of model.
5. Subsequently run the power system model with increasing level of technical constraints in order to determine the impact these technical parameters on model results.
6. Compare results between the two models, determine the differences and examine the reliability and flexibility of the power system.
7. Determine the implications of low wind production years on the reliability of the derived portfolio from the energy system model by running the power systems model with a number of different years of wind production profiles.
8. Use the insights gained from the results comparison to introduce constraints into the TIMES model to take account of the power system operation characteristics that are not readily captured within TIMES.

Figure 1 details a graphical representation of the methodology. Depending on differences that arise and insights that are gained, the energy systems model inputs or technical parameters can be adjusted to aim for improvement of results.

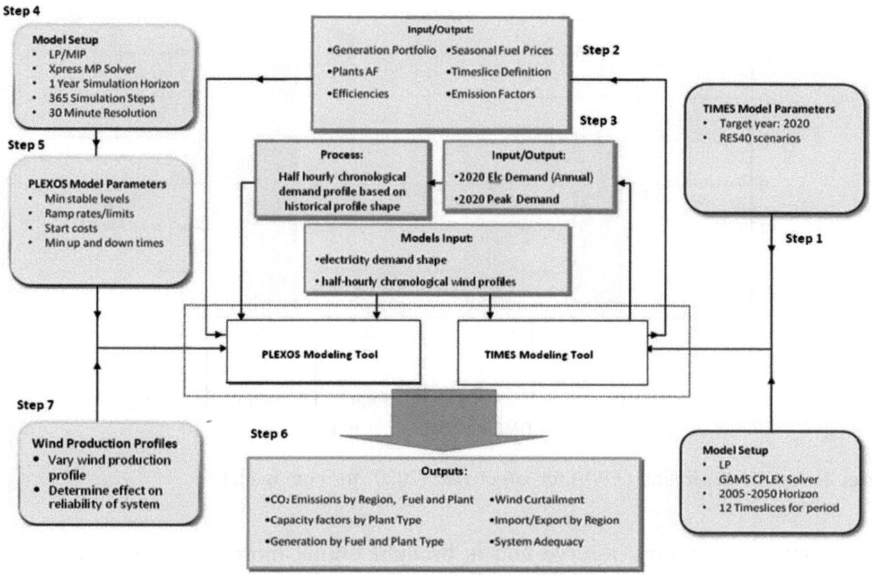

Fig. 1 Flow chart of soft-linking methodology

4 Power System Results

4.1 Flexibility

To demonstrate the soft-linking methodology as outlined above, we applied soft-linking to an energy systems model, Irish TIMES and a single year (2020) power systems model that was built using the results from a specific Irish TIMES scenario. This section describes summary results from the analysis.

Results of the detailed unit commitment and dispatch for a target year show that the power systems model commits more of the less efficient Combined Cycle gas Turbines (CCGT) units (*CC*-00) than the energy systems model across all technical scenarios examined. This is because these units come online when the newer CCGT units (*CC*-01) are out for maintenance or forced outages and are an important source of flexibility for the system. The energy model exploits the coal powered plant to its full capacity whereas in the power systems model these units are used less particularly with the inclusion of more technical parameters as the start cost gets incorporated into the objective function and coal generation is a 'pulled back' to allow gas and other generation to come online and run above their minimum stable level. As shown in Fig. 2, the distillate fuelled plants, while having a low capacity factor in the energy systems model run are shown to provide an import peaking ability and this value is only seen when higher levels of technical detail are modelled in the power systems model. Also pumped storage is an important

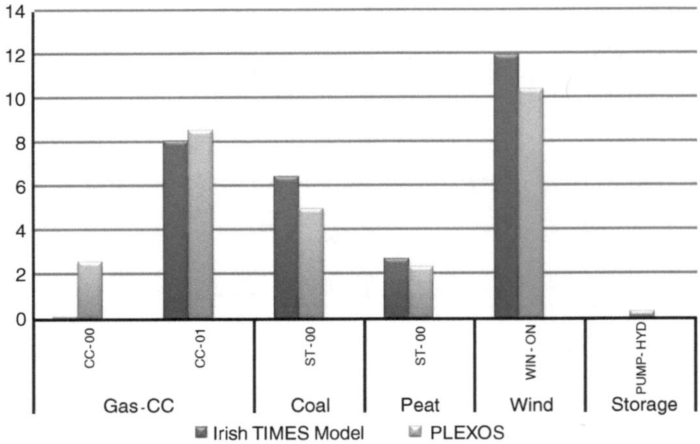

Fig. 2 Annual generation (TWh) for target year (2020) for both models

contributor to spinning reserve and is brought online more often to provide this service. Likewise the value of the pumped storage plant only becomes apparent in the power systems model. In relation to wind energy it can be seen that wind production is lower in the power systems model than the energy system model simulations indicating that wind curtailment is occurring. Results from the power systems model show annual wind curtailment of 8 % whereas The Irish TIMES model shows no wind curtailment. This stresses the importance of the correct modelling of flexible resources such as storage in the determination of system flexibility and suitability for renewable energy integration. These insights were fed back into the TIMES model by enforcing a constraint that limited the maximum annual production of wind generation on the power system and rerunning the system. Results for the low wind year simulations were broadly similar however as annual wind generation was lower an increase in thermal generation was seen. Equally results for the low wind year showed that system reliability was not compromised. This suggests that the power system portfolio in this analysis from TIMES is robust and resilient to changes in annual wind resource.

Table 1 shows the annual CO_2 emissions for both model runs. Looking at the power system scenario it is seen that the Irish-TIMES model has a greater

Table 1 Annual CO_2 emissions (Mt) for target year for both models

Fuel type	Irish TIMES model	Power systems model (PLEXOS)
Gas-CC-00	0.01	1.10
Gas-CC-01	2.95	3.12
Coal	5.77	4.35
Peat	2.48	2.20
Total	11.21	10.77

estimation of total annual emissions. This is because it has a higher level of coal and peat generation compared to the power systems model. The power systems model has higher emissions from gas plant but is offset by higher reduction in emissions from the coal and peat plant. In the absence of technical constraints the power systems model produces higher emissions as the baseload peat and coal plants are allowed to run longer.

In conclusion, the soft-linking of TIMES to a power systems model allows for greater technical scrutiny of the initial results from TIMES. Results in this analysis point to an overestimation of installed wind capacity in the original TIMES results. This insight was fed back into TIMES through a constraint on annual generation for this resource. This analysis also points to an underestimation of flexible resources such as pumped hydro storage.

4.2 Market Issues

This section applies the soft-linking methodology as described previously, to a case study in Italy. The objective of this particular exercise is to gain insights into the electricity market prices which can provide a complimentary dimension to analysis from TIMES. In this analysis we build a model of the Italian power system (PLEXOS-IT), using an energy system model (MONET). MONET is a six-region TIMES model of the Italian energy system developed by RSE (De Miglo et al. 2012) which is populated with detailed information on all main existing power plants and those under construction in Italy. In addition to detailed power plant technical characteristics, PLEXOS-IT also includes a representation of the 6 Italian market zones linked by transmission lines. The power system model contains data on transmission, in term of maximum/minimum flow, overloading ratings, resistance and reactance. PLEXOS-IT also includes linearised DC optimal power flow, which simply refers to the generator dispatch and resulting AC power flow that is minimum cost and feasible with respect to thermal limits on the AC transmission lines.

The MONET model is run with seasonal time slices and three diurnal time slices (day, night and peak), whereas PLEXOS_IT is run at half hourly time resolution and thus requires information in addition to that provided by MONET. The following characteristics apply to both models:

- The demand data for the 6 regions data has been scaled up to 2030, using the hourly demand profile data from 2010 (assumed the same one for all the regions).
- The half hourly renewable profiles are assumed the same in all the regions (in the absence of regional data).
- The model includes 6 nodes with transmission lines associated between relevant node and generators categorised by zone (and assuming current import and export transfer capacities).

The PLEXOS-IT model has also been populated with the data on the key technical characteristics of the functioning of power systems, i.e.:

- detailed characterization of power system operation, in terms of its key generation constraints;
- detailed characterization of the load, in terms of time granularity;
- detailed characterization of hydro resources (pumped storage as well as long- and short-term storages are optimized);
- a set of parameters/modules which are key for a proper representation of power system flexibility, in order to get insights into the flexibility requirement (e.g. impacts on the operation of the thermal system) of energy system scenarios characterized by a high share of variable renewables.

Key flexibility instruments have been added to the model, e.g. ancillary services (spinning, regulation and non-spinning reserves), demand response, pumped storage and hydro modelling. The models can also now be run at higher resolution time, up to 5 min, as previous research has shown the benefits provided by increasing the model temporal resolution (Deane et al. 2014).

Figures 3 and 4 show the hourly system marginal electricity price over the course of the year in the North region, in PLEXOS-IT–reference scenario and PLEXOS-IT–High renewables scenario. It is notable that (1) clearly the high VER

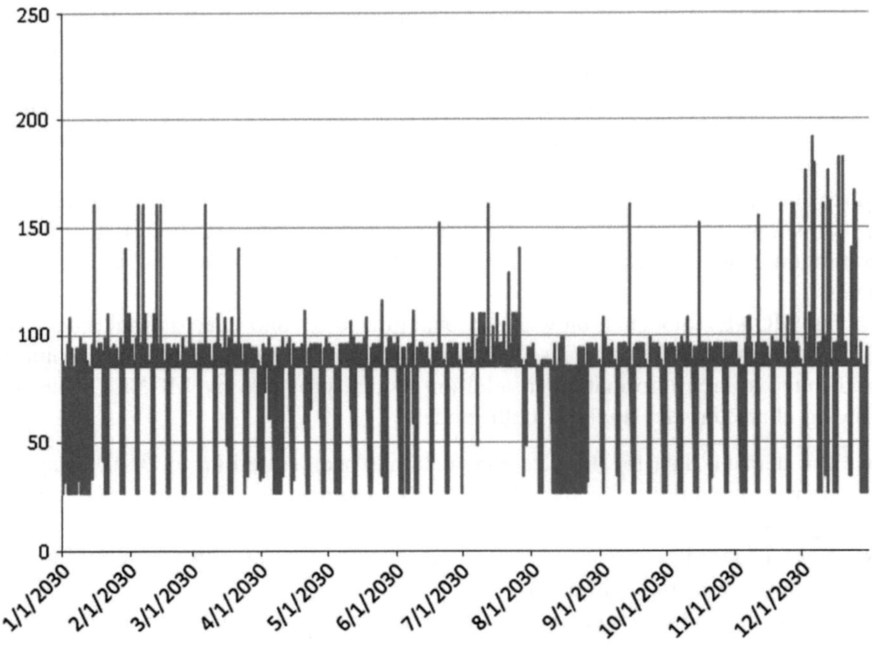

Fig. 3 Hourly electricity price over the course of the year, PLEXOS-IT—reference scenario, North region (€/MWh)

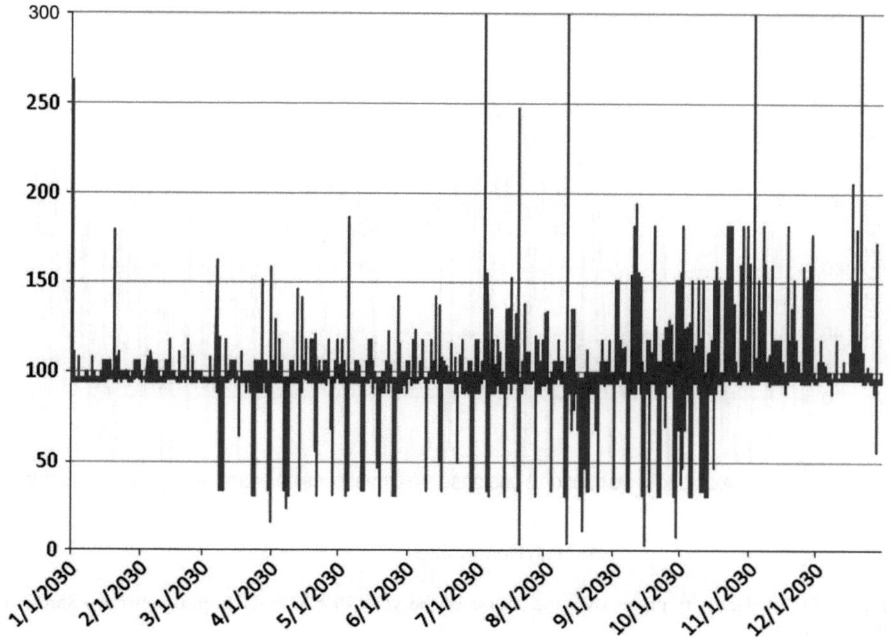

Fig. 4 Hourly electricity price over the course of the year, PLEXOS-IT—high renewables scenario, North region (€/MWh)

scenario presents a much higher volatility; (2) the volatility is higher during summer, when prices can even get close to zero.

This is further confirmed by Fig. 5, which shows the electricity prices in PLEXOS-IT High Renewables for Sardinia compared to the reference scenario, which is the region with the higher penetration of variable renewables. In this case the volatility becomes impressive, as well as the frequency of negative prices. This exposes an additional challenge for power systems with high levels of variable renewable generation. Results of simulations show that annual capacity factors from thermal fired gas plant drop from 58 to 28 % when moving from the reference scenario to the high renewables scenario. This poses great challenges in terms of financial remuneration for this type of plant and highlights the need for greater examination of this issue in terms of integrated energy system modelling.

The objective of this exercise is to demonstrate how soft-linking methodologies can be used to gain insight into market issues surrounding the integration of high levels of low marginal costs generation into current electricity market structures. It provides an extra dimension to a TIMES analysis by allowing an understanding of the market prices and market volatility to be developed. The above analysis does not answer the question on what market structure is best suited to power system with high level of variable renewables, however it provides a starting point in understanding this important issue.

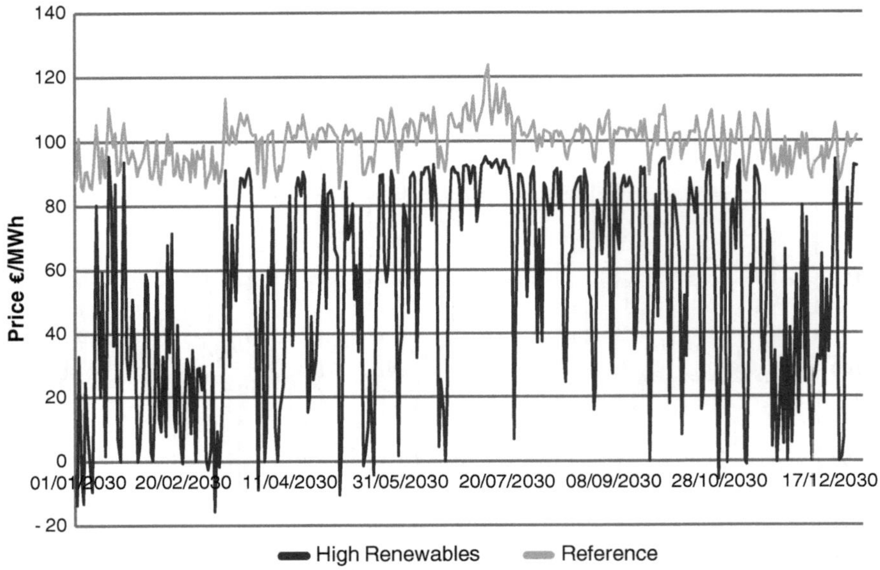

Fig. 5 Daily electricity prices over the course of the year, PLEXOS-IT high renewables Sardinia (€/MWh)

5 Soft-Linking TIMES to a Housing Stock Model

In this section we present a multi-model and soft-linking approach to assess the technical appropriateness of results for electrification of residential heating from TIMES.

5.1 Methodology

A number of models are used in this analysis to determine the impact of increased electric residential heating. In essence in this analysis each modelling tool, depending on its strength, asks and answers a different question. The questions can be summed up as follows:

1. What levels of electrification of residential heating form part of a least cost energy system in 2020 for Ireland to meet its national targets for emissions reductions in the Non-ETS sectors?
2. Can the power system operate with this extra level of electrification (provided by the answer to question 1) and what are the associated impacts, including the increase in power system CO_2 emissions? and

3. How many dwellings (and which type) should have heat pumps installed and how much oil based CO_2 emissions are offset as a result?

The methodology proceeds as follows (Fig. 6). The Irish-TIMES energy system model is used to assess the full energy system of Ireland under an emission mitigation scenario. The model assesses the cost optimal pathway for Ireland to achieve national emissions reduction targets in 2020. PLEXOS is then used to examine the impact and technical appropriateness of the half hourly heating requirement on the operation of the power system for the target year 2020 (Irish TIMES has a lower temporal resolution and more simplified representation of power system operation than the half hourly PLEXOS electricity dispatch model of the Irish power system). The ArDEM archetype dwelling model [previously used in Dineen and Gallachóir (2011)] is then used to determine the number of dwellings that could be served for a given amount of heat energy supplied.

Results for the Irish TIMES model suggest that electrification of residential heating will rise by the year 2020 in order for Ireland to meet its non-ETS emission reduction target in a cost optimal fashion. This is shown in Fig. 7, which presents the energy systems modelling results for the residential sector to the year 2020. The figure also compares results from a reference scenario (REF), which provides a least cost solution in the absence of a mitigation target, with those from a mitigation scenario, which seeks to deliver a 20 % emissions reduction relative to 2005 levels on non-ETS sectors and a 21 % on ETS CO_2 emissions by 2020 (in accordance

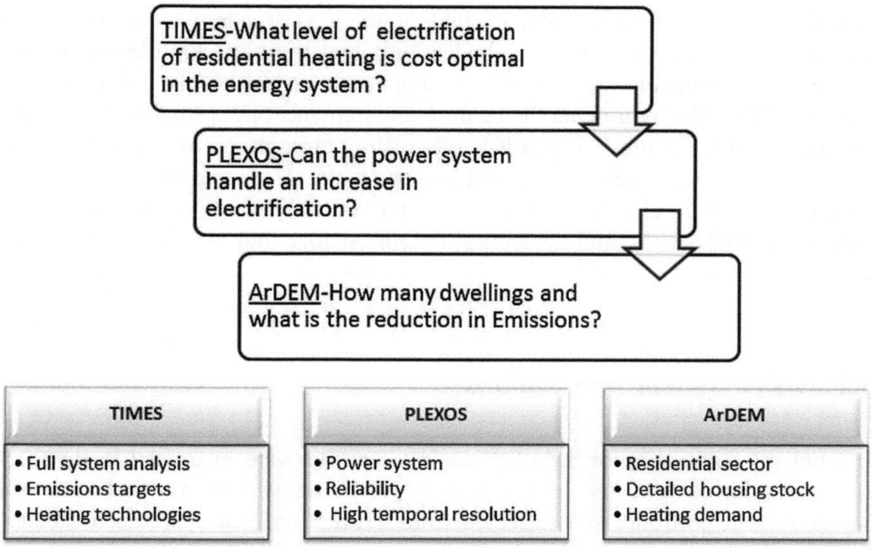

Fig. 6 How different models answer different questions

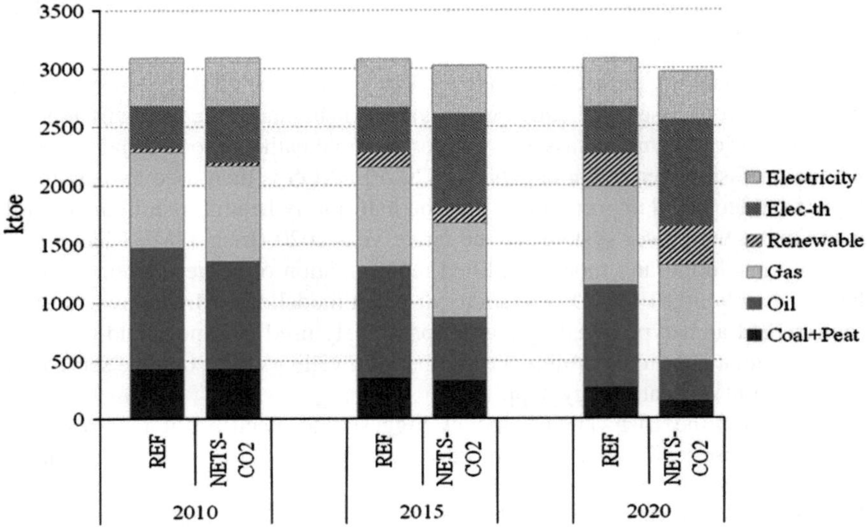

Fig. 7 Results from Irish TIMES for REF and emissions reduction scenario (NETS) to 2020

with current EU GHG policy frameworks through Directive 2009/29/EC[2] and Decision 2009/406/EC).

The REF scenario indicates that, in absence of emissions constraints, electrification of heating will almost remain stable in the next decade, while imposing the legally binding non-ETS emissions reduction target results in high levels of electrification. Electrification reaches a level of approximately 914 ktoe (10.6 TWh) by the year 2020. This represents the heating requirements of approximately 817,000 dwellings and the results suggest it is met mainly through the use of technologies such as direct electric heating and heat pumps mostly displacing oil and coal based systems. By 2020 electric heat accounts for 44 % of total residential heating demand in NETS-CO_2, and constitutes an almost four-fold increase on base year levels.

5.2 Power System Implications

A number of scenarios of installed heating capacity were examined in the 2020 power system using a half hourly heating profile derived from actual data. The power system portfolio was extracted from TIMES for that year. Each scenario

[2] The authors are cognisant that we have simplified how the ETS target is applied in this chapter, i.e. at Member State level rather than EU wide, while the Directive applies the target reduction across the entire EU.

represents installed electrical capacities ranged from 0 to 2000 MW and were examined in increments of 500 M. Results from the detailed power system analysis showed that the power system reliability (as derived by TIMES) was breached just above 1000 MW of installed Air Source Heat Pumps ASHP capacity. At levels above this, the reliability of the power system was compromised and extra capacity would be required. The use of a high resolution heating profile is important as it allows for the relationship between high heating demand (cold weather) and possible low renewable output (low wind speeds) to be captured.

5.3 How Many Homes?

To determine the CO_2 emissions, the ArDEM model was used to estimate the number of dwellings that could be heated with 1000 MW of installed ASHP electrical capacity. It is assumed for this analysis that the ASHP are replacing existing oil fired boilers that are at least 20 years old as it is unlikely that newer boilers would be replaced before the end of their useful life. Two retrofit scenarios are considered, the first where the ASHP would replace oil boilers and no other retrofit works would be carried out to the dwelling. As many of the dwellings considered are old and of poorer construction quality this would lead to situations where the ASHP would operate in poorly insulated inefficient dwellings. In the second scenario the ASHP is assumed to be installed and at the same time the roof and wall insulation of the dwelling are retrofitted to modern standard. Equally in this scenario it is assumed that appropriate heat emitters are installed for the dwelling. This would reduce the heating energy requirement for a 'typical' house from 18,709 to 14,904 kWh/year. This will allow greater efficiency and a greater number of dwellings to be converted from oil to electricity for the same load on the electricity generation system. The results of this analysis for 1000 MW of installed capacity are presented in Table 2. Note that the emissions associated with the '*Unaltered dwelling*' and '*Improved roof and wall insulation*' dwelling are different for the same energy delivered. This is due to the heterogeneous nature of dwellings in the ArDEM model and varying oil fired boiler efficiencies.

Table 2 Results from dwelling energy assessment model (ArDEM)

	Unaltered dwellings	Improved roof and wall insulation
Energy required for main space and water heating (GWh)	5087	5087
Energy requirement per dwelling (kWh/year)	18,706	14,904
Numbers of dwellings converted	271,951	341,315
Total CO_2 for oil existing oil boiler (kt/annum)	1841	1832
Total CO_2 with new ASHP (t/annum)	953	953
Net reduction in CO_2 (kt/annum)	888	879

The results in Table 2 shows that 1000 MW of ASHP's could provide the annual space and water heating requirements to meet the demand of 271,951 unaltered dwellings, but if these dwellings had shallow retrofits (such as wall and ceiling insulation) then this heat load can meet the requirements of approximately 341,315 dwellings. The associated reduction in emissions for the full system is approximately 879 kt of CO_2. This is in strong contrast to 817,000 dwellings converting to air source heat pumps using a single model approach with TIMES. In our analysis the TIMES model primarily underestimates the impact of ASHP on power system reliability particularly at times of high heating demand and low renewable energy output. To improve results from TIMES we fed the insights gained from this analysis back into the model by placing a constraint on the amount of electric heating that can be absorbed in the power system. When the analysis was rerun for this scenario, an increase in the use of bioenergy for heating and transport was observed. It was also noted that the power system portfolio did not significantly change.

In conclusion, this analysis provides a useful framework for providing complimentary analysis of results from TIMES by leveraging the strength of other models. The exercise shows that relying solely on an integrated energy systems model may lead to an overestimation of the extent of electrification of residential heating. Our multi-model approach suggests that between 270,000 and 340,000 existing oil fired residential dwellings could be with converted to air source heat pump technology (ASHP) without compromising the operation of the electrical power system. This is in contrast to 817,000 dwellings converting to air source heat pumps using a single model approach.

6 Conclusion

The examples presented here provide an indication of the benefits that a multi-model approach can bring in terms of both the additional insights it provides and how it can inform improvements in TIMES. There are many other examples of soft-linking TIMES with other models; chapters by Glynn et al. of this book provide some examples of soft-linking TIMES models with CGE models. This approach draws on the strengths of different models and develops innovative soft-linking methodologies in order to ensure robust data and communication flows between the models and is a useful alternative to trying to develop a model that tries to answer all questions.

References

Deane JP, Chiodi A, Gargiulo MÓ, Gallachóir BP (2012) Soft-linking of a power systems model to an energy systems model. Energy 42:303–312. doi:10.1016/j.energy.2012.03.052

Deane JP, Drayton GÓ, Gallachóir BP (2014) The impact of sub-hourly modelling in power systems with significant levels of renewable generation. Appl Energy 113:152–158. doi:10.1016/j.apenergy.2013.07.027

De Miglio R, Gargiulo M, Gelmini A, Lanati F (2012) The multiregional energy system model: MONET—a comprehensive tool for energy-environmental analysis at both regional and national level in Italy. Presented at the 12th IAEE European energy conference, Venice, Italy

Dineen DÓ, Gallachóir BP (2011) Modelling the impacts of building regulations and a property bubble on residential space and water heating. Energy Build 43:166–178. doi:10.1016/j.enbuild.2010.09.004

Holttinen H (2012) Wind integration: Experience, issues, and challenges. Wiley Interdiscip. Rev. Energy Environ 1:243–255. doi:10.1002/wene.18

Kannan R (2011) The development and application of a temporal MARKAL energy system model using flexible time slicing. Appl Energy 88:2261–2272. doi:10.1016/j.apenergy.2010.12.066

Ludig S, Haller M, Schmid E, Bauer N (2011) Fluctuating renewables in a long-term climate change mitigation strategy. Energy 36:6674–6685. doi:10.1016/j.energy.2011.08.021

Pina A, Silva C, Ferrão P (2011) Modeling hourly electricity dynamics for policy making in long-term scenarios. Energy Policy 39:4692–4702. doi:10.1016/j.enpol.2011.06.062

Economic Impacts of Future Changes in the Energy System—Global Perspectives

James Glynn, Patrícia Fortes, Anna Krook-Riekkola, Maryse Labriet, Marc Vielle, Socrates Kypreos, Antti Lehtilä, Peggy Mischke, Hancheng Dai, Maurizio Gargiulo, Per Ivar Helgesen, Tom Kober, Phil Summerton, Bruno Merven, Sandrine Selosse, Kenneth Karlsson, Neil Strachan and Brian Ó Gallachóir

Abstract In a climate constrained future, hybrid energy-economy model coupling gives additional insight into interregional competition, trade, industrial delocalisation and overall macroeconomic consequences of decarbonising the energy system. Decarbonising the energy system is critical in mitigating climate change. This chapter summarises modelling methodologies developed in the ETSAP community

J. Glynn (✉) · B. Ó Gallachóir
Environmental Research Institute, University College Cork, Cork, Ireland
e-mail: james.glynn@umail.ucc.ie

B. Ó Gallachóir
e-mail: b.ogallachoir@ucc.ie

P. Fortes
CENSE, Faculdade Ciências e Tecnologia, Universidade Nova de Lisboa, Lisbon, Portugal
e-mail: p.fs@fct.unl.pt

A. Krook-Riekkola
Department of Business Administration, Luleå University of Technology, Luleå, Sweden
e-mail: anna.krook-riekkola@ltu.se

M. Labriet
Eneris Environment Energy Consultants, Madrid, Spain
e-mail: maryse.labriet@enerisconsultants.com

M. Vielle
Ecole Polytechnique de Lausanne, Lausanne, Switzerland
e-mail: marc.vielle@epfl.ch

S. Kypreos
Paul Scherrer Institute, Villigen, Switzerland
e-mail: socrateskypreos@gmail.com

A. Lehtilä
VTT Technical Research Centre of Finland, Espoo, Finland
e-mail: antti.lehtila@vtt.fi

G. Giannakidis et al. (eds.), *Informing Energy and Climate Policies Using Energy Systems Models*, Lecture Notes in Energy 30,
DOI 10.1007/978-3-319-16540-0_19

to assess economic impacts of decarbonising energy systems at a global level. The next chapter of this book focuses on a national perspective. The range of economic impacts is regionally dependent upon the stage of economic development, the level of industrialisation, energy intensity of exports, and competition effects due to rates of relative decarbonisation. Developed nation's decarbonisation targets are estimated to result in a manageable GDP loss in the region of 2 % by 2050. Energy intensive export driven developing countries such as China and India, and fossil fuel exporting nations can expect significantly higher GDP loss of up to 5 % GDP per year by mid-century.

P. Mischke · K. Karlsson
Department of Management Engineering, Technical University of Denmark, Kongens Lyngby, Denmark
e-mail: peym@dtu.dk

K. Karlsson
e-mail: keka@dtu.dk

H. Dai
National Institute of Environmental Studies, Tsukuba, Japan
e-mail: dhc1434@gmail.com

M. Gargiulo
Energy Engineering Economic Environment Systems Modelling and Analysis (E4SMA s.r.l.), Turin, Italy
e-mail: maurizio.gargiulo@e4sma.com

P.I. Helgesen
Department of Industrial Economics and Technology Management, Norwegian University of Science and Technology, Trondheim, Norway
e-mail: per.i.helgesen@iot.ntnu.no

T. Kober
Energy Research Centre of the Netherlands (ECN), Policy Studies Department, Petten/Amsterdam, The Netherlands
e-mail: Kober@ecn.nl

P. Summerton
Cambridge Econometrics, Cambridge, UK
e-mail: ps@camecon.com

B. Merven
Energy Research Centre, University of Cape Town, Cape Town, South Africa
e-mail: brunomerven@gmail.com

S. Selosse
Centre De Mathématicues Appliquèes, MINES ParisTech, Paris, France
e-mail: sandrine.selosse@mines-paristech.fr

N. Strachan
Energy Institute, University College London, London, England
e-mail: n.strachan@ucl.ac.uk

1 Introduction

1.1 Why Link Energy-Economy Models?

In these two chapters the current state of the art of methods within the ETSAP community to couple energy systems models to macroeconomic models are presented. This chapter covers perspectives on the environmental rationale, model coupling development, outlines model coupling policy and research applications at the global and regional level. Next chapter of this book continues with national case studies, showing the UK's legislative use the coupled hybrid MARKAL[1]-MACRO (MM) model, and updates to the mathematical formulations of its successors TIMES[2]-MACRO (TM) and most recently TIMES MACRO-Stand-Alone (TMSA). The energy systems models discussed are bottom-up (BU) techno-economic linear optimisation engineering TIMES models, while coupled to top-down (TD) macroeconomic models. These range from single producer-consumer agent production function models, to multi-region structural computable general equilibrium (CGE) models. Both chapters collate the collective work that was presented at an IEA-ETSAP funded workshop in University College Cork in February 2014. They conclude synthesising common critical messages from the range of studies. The applied theory of what constitutes a consistent, pragmatic and heuristic model linkage is discussed. Soft-linking and hard-linking multi-model methods are introduced with attention paid to model structures, consequent data harmonisation and data transfer frameworks. Multi-regional models add insight into trade and competition effects upon delocalisation. Overall, maintaining a consistent paradigm throughout model coupling is critical in understanding the economic impacts of future changes to the energy system.

Affordable access to an acceptable energy supply is critical for a prosperous stable economy. Functional markets are theorised to price primary energy supply commodities, their refined products and final consumer energy products. Non market externalities such as green-house-gas (GHG) emissions or long term strategic policy decisions are difficult to fully include in near term commodity futures pricing, as a result of changing trends and resultant uncertainty. Half of all cumulative anthropogenic CO_2 emissions have occurred in the past 40 years. Increasing energy system carbon intensity between 2000–2010 has contributed to GHG growth increasing to 2.2 %/year when compared with 1.3 %/year over the previous three decades (IPCC 2014). Two thirds of global GHG emissions are produced by the energy system. The energy system analysis of International Energy Agency's (IEA) New Policy Scenario leaves the world on track for a long term average temperature increase of 3.6 °C, dangerously beyond the 2 °C limit (IPCC 2013; OECD/IEA 2013). A restructured low-carbon world economy is thus imperative (Capros et al. 2014; Krey et al. 2014).

---

[1] MARKAL—**MARK**et **AL**ocation model.

[2] TIMES—**T**he **I**ntegrated **M**ARKAL-**E**fom **S**ystem.

Internalising the energy system GHG environmental externality by appropriate pricing mechanisms via emissions permits trading markets and carbon taxation is seen as the primary means to drive decarbonisation in the energy system. In energy systems modelling, the marginal abatement cost of carbon is typically used as the scenario comparison yard-stick. Carbon pricing is critical to stabilise investor expectation to promote investment in marginal mitigation technologies. The European emissions trading scheme (EU-ETS) has made efforts to account for the environmental externality, but thus far has failed to be the causal force in reducing carbon emissions. It must be fixed, and other regions must similarly collaborate (Edenhofer 2014). Otherwise, climate change—essentially a commons problem—could become the modern era "tragedy of the commons" (Hardin 1968; Nordhaus 1994). Recently the UK has made efforts to correct this market failure with amending policy to introduce a carbon price floor (HM Revenue and Customs 2013). Revenue recycling schemes from carbon taxation can bring long term decarbonisation benefits to near term social good, tacking climate inequality, or achieve revenue neutrality. Policy-makers need tools to understand the effectiveness and the economic impact of policies whose purpose is to shift energy systems toward more environmentally desirable development pathways (Hourcade et al. 2006). Understanding energy-economy coupling is crucial in analysing regional effects of carbon tax, trade, competitiveness, and energy policy at large.

Accounting the cost of investment required to achieve least cost energy systems is achievable with technology rich BU energy systems models. The rationale behind linking engineering energy systems models with macroeconomic models is to include the feedback effect between energy cost and energy service demands. Coupling energy-economy models enables analysis of heterogeneous sectoral dynamics while providing a more suitable microeconomic framework (Bataille et al. 2006), that energy systems models on their own can only approximate with elastic demand. The objective is to estimate the changes in welfare and growth, where deviation from business-as-usual (BAU) in investment requirements induces productivity and consumption pattern changes through substitution effects. The potential magnitude of these effects vary considerably across differing economic schools of thought; from neoclassical to ecological economics; from growth opportunities to deep sustainability (Warr and Ayres 2006; Strachan and Kannan 2008; Jackson 2009; Ayres et al. 2013; Krey et al. 2014; The Global Commission on the Economy and Climate 2014). GHG emissions are typically the constraint driving redistribution of investment capital causing macroeconomic feedback, but of course this is not the only model scenario that could be considered. The macroeconomic cost of energy supply insecurity is an alternate use of model coupling, as is energy export and trade dynamics. The benefit of soft-linking energy system and macroeconomic models is in utilising the complementary strengths of both models to overcome the other's weaknesses. This allows additional insights of technological and economic detail to be gleaned that otherwise would not be quantified.

1.2 BU and TD Models

BU engineering models and TD macroeconomic models have evolved as the economically consistent means of assessing long term energy system dynamics and costs (Wene 1996; Hourcade et al. 2006). BU models include *optimisation, simulation, accounting and multi agent techniques* (Fleiter et al. 2011). Some TD methods include *input–output, econometric, computable general equilibrium* (CGE) and *system dynamic models*. This chapter is primarily focused on coupling TIMES optimisation and CGE models.

BU model methods are explicit in their data richness and outline detailed technology development pathways, interdependencies and costs. TIMES and it's forebear MARKAL form the primary constituent parts of a family of linear programming models supported by ETSAP under an implementing agreement of the IEA. TIMES is a techno-economic model generator for local, national or multi-regional energy systems, which provides a technology rich basis for estimating energy dynamics over a long-term (20–50 years), multi-period time horizon. TIMES computes a time varying inter-temporal partial equilibrium on inter-regional markets. The objective function maximises total surplus. This is equivalent to minimising the discounted total energy system cost while respecting environmental, technical and scenario constraints. This system cost includes investment, operation and maintenance and fuel import costs, less export income, terminal technology values and salvage values. This approach does not consider the same microeconomic theoretical underpinnings as a TD model and can be viewed as the optimisation by a clairvoyant energy planner with perfect information and perfect foresight over the total system, rather than maximising consumer choice preferences at a microeconomic level. Thus, TIMES models reference scenario pathways are driven by energy service demands exogenously defined by macroeconomic conditions and resource supply curves; while, subsequent dynamics are driven by environmental constraints under user consideration. The technical foundations of MARKAL is outlined by Fishbone and Abilock, while the full technical TIMES documentation is hosted online by ETSAP (Fishbone and Abilock 1981; Loulou et al. 2005).

TD CGE methods describe the whole economy, mapping and subdividing sectoral structures where substitution between factors of production is allowed. CGE models are built upon microeconomic theory to calculate prices and activities in all sectors of an economy to reach a general equilibrium. Consumers maximise their utility through demanding goods met by producers who maximise profits (Arrow and Debreu 1954; Johansen 1960). Historical national or global accounts data is required for calibration, where the Global Trade Analysis Project (GTAP) database is the most commonly used example. TD models in general, namely CGE models, do not include many technical aspects of the energy system. The energy system combined with the other factors of production, forms of capital and labour, are described in inter-related production functions to optimise consumer utility and economic growth. Capital value shares, elasticities of substitution, and autonomous energy efficiency improvement coefficients—estimating technological learning—and marginal technology cost curves (Kiuila and Rutherford 2013) enable estimation of technology choice and fuel switching dynamics.

The Lucas critique argues econometric models based on historic trends cannot model policy changes nor remain valid in future technology paradigm shifts (Lucas Jr 1976; Grubb et al. 2002). CGE models usually have smooth rates substitution, whereas poorly constructed optimisation models can display a "flip-flop" binary characteristic related to the capacity size of the marginal technology choices and level of model constraints (Grubler et al. 1999). The different approaches can provide differing solutions and result in differing policy conclusions. However, CGE models can give long term macroeconomic outlooks to drive TIMES energy systems models which can in-turn feedback energy costs adjustments to the CGE model, which upon iteration provides new energy demands (Hoffman and Jorgenson 1977). In a consistent framework the coupled hybrid model can build a more accurate representation of the system under scrutiny.

1.3 Hybrid Model Evolution

The linking of the Brookhaven Energy System Optimisation model (BESOM) with a CGE model is the first hybrid energy-economy model reported (Hoffman and Jorgenson 1977). The outputs of each of the individual models were transferred between each other manually by the user, in what has become known in the proceeding decades as *soft-linking*. Soft-linking is typically the simplest starting point by its transparency, flexibility, learning (Martinsen 2011), and practicality in establishing consistent common measuring points (CMP) in the overlap of model structures.

The alternative of programmatically linking of models to automate data transfer between models is known as *hard-linking*. MARKAL-MACRO is the first such reported hard-linked energy-economy model (Manne and Wene 1992), and is the basis for the subsequent TIMES-MACRO, TIMES-MSA and others (Manne et al. 1995; Wene 1996; Messner and Schrattenholzer 2000). Hard-linked models tend to establish optimum data transfer methods, enabling greater productivity, control, convergence and solution uniqueness. Historically hard-linking has come at a computational cost, requiring the model to be a reduced form single sector model (Manne and Wene 1992; Manne et al. 1995; Böhringer 1998; Messner and Schrattenholzer 2000; Bosetti et al. 2006; Strachan and Kannan 2008). This results in aggregated energy economy interactions, giving overall trends but limits its usefulness when applied to sector specific enquiries.

Combining BU and TD models in a mixed complementarity problem introduces a limited set of technological sectoral detail into a CGE framework (Frei et al. 2003; Sue Wing 2008; Proença and St. Aubyn 2013). The whole energy system cost optimisation problem could be integrated into a CGE model, with decomposition to improve solution algorithm performance and reduce computation time (Böhringer 1998; Böhringer and Rutherford 2008, 2009). However, the authors are not aware of such a model. Aside, the International Monetary Fund have made attempts to integrate oil supply dynamics into their global dynamic stochastic general equilibrium model GIMF (Benes et al. 2012; Kumhof and Muir 2014).

2 Linkage of the Global Energy Models TIAM-WORLD and GEMINI-E3

In order to assess climate mitigation agreements, an iterative procedure linking TIAM-WORLD and GEMINI-E3 is the first method proposed. TIAM-WORLD (TIMES Integrated Assessment Model) is a BU global multi-regional technology-rich optimisation model. GEMINI-E3 is a TD global multi-regional general equilibrium model (Loulou and Labriet 2008; Bernard and Vielle 2008). Recent work soft-linking the two models explores global and partial climate agreements (Labriet et al. 2015). An accurate representation of the energy and technology choices, and the macro-economic impacts, especially in terms of trade effects of climate polices, is critical in understanding future pathways to a climate constrained world.

TIAM-WORLD is part of the TIMES family of energy models and calculates a dynamic inter-temporal partial equilibrium on worldwide energy and emissions markets based on maximisation of total surplus (Loulou 2008). The version of the model uses in this application divides the world in 15 regions, driven by 42 energy service demands across all sectors. It covers the procurement, transformation, trade and end use of all energy forms, represented by over 1500 energy technologies and one hundred commodities in each region. Energy demands are calibrated by the user for the reference scenario, and each has its own price elasticity. Environmental emissions are endogenously modelled at the technology level. TIAM-WORLD integrates a climate module for the modelling of greenhouse gas concentrations, radiative forcing and temperature increase.

GEMINI-E3 is a multi-country, multi-sector, recursive computable general equilibrium model. It represents the world economy in 28 regions and 18 sectors. The standard model is based on the assumption of total flexibility on both macroeconomic markets, such as the capital and the exchange markets (the associated price are the real rate of interest and the real exchange rate, which are then endogenous), and microeconomic or sector markets (goods, factors of production). GEMINI-E3 is calibrated with the GTAP database which includes physical energy market data, social accounting matrices and bilateral trade flows.

2.1 Data Harmonisation

The initial harmonisation of the two very different model structures represents a critical challenge for hybrid model's theoretical consistency. Each of the model regions and commodities need to be paired. Furthermore, reference scenarios require harmonisation of the basic drivers of the energy system, being population growth, GDP trends, energy prices and energy policy constraints. Once harmonized, the reference cases of TIAM-WORLD and GEMINI-E3 propose similar CO_2 emission trajectory until 2030. Differing technological assumptions lead to longer term divergence of CO_2 trajectories. This effect has also been seen in similar modelling exercises (Labriet et al. 2012; Kanudia et al. 2014; Krey et al. 2014).

2.2 The Coupling Method

The purpose of the linkage of the models is to allow the strengths of each model (technological richness of TIAM-WORLD and macro-economic details of GEMINI-E3) to augment the overall analysis of energy and climate policies. The coupling approach optimises the data flow of common market points, from the model of relative more accuracy, to the other model. GEMINI-E3 receives data from TIAM-WORLD on energy and CO_2 prices, technical progress on energy use and capital consumption. TIAM-WORLD receives sector economic production data to recalculate energy service demands.

TIAM-WORLD only goes through one major modification: the removal of price elasticities of the energy service demands. This microeconomic behaviour is modelled by GEMINI-E3. GEMINI-E3 requires more numerous modifications to consistently utilise the data linkages: energy technologies that are not present in the standard version of GEMINI-E3, such as biomass, hydrogen, nuclear and other renewable energy sources are added to the model structure and the nested structure of the CES functions are rewritten; the CES functions relating to all energy consumption are replaced by Leontief function, whose coefficients representing the energy shares are computed on the basis of TIAM-WORLD results; technical progress is modified with energy efficiency improvements from TIAM-WORLD; finally, energy and carbon prices are computed by TIAM-WORLD.

The coupling procedure is carried out in a Gauss-Seidel method (Hageman and Young 2012) which seeks a fixed point for the useful demand vector through an iterative process. TIAM-WORLD is first run with useful demands from the harmonisation phase of the two models. TIAM-WORLD passes its results to GEMINI-E3, which is re-run. This is the first iteration. New macroeconomic output and industrial value added obtained from GEMINI-E3 are used to re-estimate the energy service demands. This process is repeated until model convergence is reached, defined as the Euclidean distance between the two last demand vectors over the norm of the last demand. Convergence is typically achieved in 6 iterations for climate constrained scenarios.

2.3 Results

Both global and partial climate agreements are studied with the proposed coupling methodology.

The comparison of the Iron and Steel production results obtained with TIAM-WORLD in a standalone manner with elastic demand and with the coupled models illustrates one of the added-value of the coupling: in a global climate agreement, while the iron-and-steel production decreases in all countries in TIAM-WORLD used in a standalone manner, several countries increase their production in the coupled models to compensate the production decrease in China and India. The combined analysis of trade, provided by GEMINI-E3, and energy dynamics, provided by TIAM-WORLD, helps understand these decisions: India and China prefer importing Iron and Steel from some other countries rather than producing it locally with clean energy and processes because of the lack of clean production opportunities in these countries compared with the others, more particularly biomass-fired power plants opportunities with carbon capture and sequestration.

However, the differences in sectoral emissions between TIAM-WORLD used in a standalone manner and the coupled models are smaller than 5 % over the model time horizon. This is an interesting result, showing that the inter-sectoral effects of climate policies have little effect on overall aggregated sectoral emissions.

In partial agreements, the coupled models help the assessment of the delocalisation of not only primary energy extraction (to Former Soviet Union and Africa), represented in TIAM-WORLD but also industrial production (to Asia), provided by GEMINI-E3. However, emission leakage remains small, mainly due to global lower oil demand.

The macroeconomic analysis from the coupled models also shows fossil fuel exporting countries, represented by the Middle East, Former Soviet Union and to a lesser degree Africa, are all extremely penalized by climate constraints. This simply occurs as a result of trade imbalances consequent to energy export revenue reductions while fossil fuel production declines.

2.4 Discussion

The two global models are coupled through an iterative exchange of data until convergence of energy demands. It builds upon the technology richness of TIAM-WORLD and the macro-economic details of GEMINI-E3. Technology changes, macroeconomic and inter-sectoral effects are assessed with the coupled models.

Although such an approach minimizes the number of structural changes of the original models compared to the full integration of models within a same optimization framework (Labriet et al. 2015), a meticulous examination and understanding of both models is crucial in order to define the correspondence between energy commodities, regions, economy sectors, to build the data exchanges between both models, and to avoid any methodological inconsistencies (Böhringer and Rutherford 2009).

An added value of the proposed coupling framework at a global scale is the understanding of the energy system transition interdependences upon trade and competition effects.

3 Global Energy Policies Analysed with TIAM-FR and IMACLIM-R

The hybrid linking of TIAM-FR and IMACLIM-R, while conceptually similar to linking TIAM-WORLD and GEMINI-E3 (summarised in Sect. 2), is fundamentally different in a specific assumption of perfect foresight. The CGE model IMACLIM-R allows the exploration of the differences in myopic technology pathways due to recursive time dynamics, i.e., the model is solved in sequential (yearly) time steps, linked through time by capital accumulation based on exogenous savings rates, while TIAM has perfect foresight of technology availability and development. This first section focuses on the reconciliation of these theoretical differences.

TIAM-FR, a version of the TIMES Integrate Assessment Model (TIAM) developed in France, is a typical BU TIMES model that has been widely used to assess sectoral and global energy and climate policy from both developed and developing countries perspective (Bouckaert et al. 2011; Assoumou and Maïzi 2011; Ricci and Selosse 2013). IMACLIM-R, is the recursive version of IMACLIM, a multi-regional multi-sector TD model that has been developed by CIRED to assess the long-term global economic impacts of climate policy (Guivarch et al. 2009; Sassi et al. 2010; Mathy and Guivarch 2010; Rozenberg et al. 2010; HAMDI-CHERIF et al. 2011).

The divergent viewpoints of models developed by energy engineers, or BU models, and those developed by economists, or TD models, can hinder effective dialogue and mutual understanding between researchers from different academic backgrounds. The purpose of this work is to promote a constructive dialogue between modellers from each side of the modelling paradigms, based on a comparative critique of the BU TIAM-FR model and the TD IMACLIM-R model.

3.1 Method

First and foremost, the conceptual frameworks (optimisation *vs.* recursive) of the two models must somehow be reconciled, and is done so with approaches to harmonise the theoretical structure, data and nomenclature of each model.

TIAM-FR is geographically aggregated in 15 world regions. It covers the time horizon from 2005 to 2100 to properly reflect the long-term nature of the climate constraint. Indeed, a climate module computes the change in CO_2 concentrations in atmospheric radiative forcing from anthropogenic activities and the temperature change relative to the pre-industrial period. The climate module does not induce retroactive energy services demands, which remain unchanged. More generally, TIAM-FR is driven by 42 exogenous end-use energy demands grouped into six sectors. Each energy demand is calibrated for the base year, and then follows a trend induced by some exogenous driver, *i.e.* regional economic and demographic projections and region-specific elasticities.

IMACLIM-R provides a more aggregated view of global economic activity, which it divides into 12 regions and 12 sectors. The base year of the model (2001) builds on the GTAP-6 database, a balanced Social Accounting Matrix (SAM) of the world economy although the original GTAP-6 dataset was modified to (i) aggregate regions and sectors according to the IMACLIM-R mapping, and (ii) accommodate the 2001 IEA energy balances (Sassi et al. 2010; Rozenberg et al. 2010).

IMACLIM-R's rationale stems from the necessity to understand better, amongst the drivers of energy-economy prospective trajectories, the relative role of (i) technical parameters, (ii) structural changes in the final demand for goods and services (dematerialisation of growth patterns) and, (iii) micro and macroeconomic behavioural parameters in open economies. This is indeed critical to capturing the mechanisms in the transformation of a given environmental alteration into an economic cost and in the widening or narrowing margins of freedom for climate mitigation or adaptation.

To fully exploit the potential of this dual representation requires abandoning the use of conventional aggregate production functions, which roughly represents the technological constraints impinging on an economy (Berndt and Wood 1975) and (Jorgenson 1982). It is indeed arguably impossible to find mathematical functions flexible enough to encompass all the contrasted scenarios resulting from the interplay between consumption styles, technologies and localisation patterns (Hourcade 1993), for small as well as for large departures from the reference equilibrium. This accounts for the already reported absence of formal production functions in IMACLIM-R.

IMACLIM-R and TIAM-FR use the same data and scenario with regards to the growth of population, from the United Nations. The global geographical division in TIAM-FR have been reprocessed from the simulation outcome of IMACLIM-R and re-aggregated in accordance with its 15 regions. The macroeconomic indicators were integrated into the TIAM-FR model to drive the energy service demand and, from it, determine the energy system in an optimisation framework. TIAM-FR model is then re-run with the macroeconomic output indices coming from IMACLIM-R to calculate the optimal outcome of the energy supply system and carbon emissions trajectories at the world level

Three Scenarios are considered, a business as usual scenario (BAU), and two climate scenarios (CLIM), one with BAU drivers, Clim_dBAU and the third scenario with drivers from a climate run of IMACLIM-R, Clim_dClim. More precisely,

BAU scenario from TIAM-FR is based on macroeconomic indicators extracted from the BAU scenario of IMACLIM-R. Concerning the climate scenario, CLIM_dBAU and CLIM_dCLIM refers to two different trajectories consistent with the 450 ppm target in 2100 for CO_2 emissions. CLIM_dBAU is derived from simulation based on the BAU growth indices in IMACLIM-R, whereas CLIM_dCLIM is driven by growth indices from the 450 ppm scenario in IMACLIM-R. The price elastic energy demand functions are not used in running TIAM-FR as the prices have not been harmonized between the two models.

3.2 Results

The results specifics are not in focus here but more so the relative impact between scenarios are of interest in investigating the demand reduction as a result of climate scenario in IMACLIM-R. CO_2 emissions paths induced by climate constraints are reported in Fig. 1.

The comparison of CLIM_dBAU and CLIM_dCLIM pathway shapes illustrates again the divergence between TIAM-FR and IMACLIM-R in terms of modelling philosophy. Under an inter-temporal optimized abatement trajectory (CLIM-dBAU), emissions may keep growing by 2040 then slightly drop until 2060 before declining sharply. By contrast, the agent cannot see this *optimal* abatement pathway in the IMACLIM-r. Therefore, the pricing signal must be very strong, to reflect the 450 ppm constraint to curtail the fossil-fuel dependent goods and services demand. The growth indices would be much lower than in the case of the *optimal* growth in the short and mid-term. However, in the long run, there would be more flexibility for emission growth in CLIM-dCLIM than CLIM_dBAU as the economy will be largely decarbonized and thus offers more room for an emissions increase. TIAM-FR and IMACLIM-R suggest different timing and arbitrage for sectoral emission abatement for a given climate target (Fig. 2).

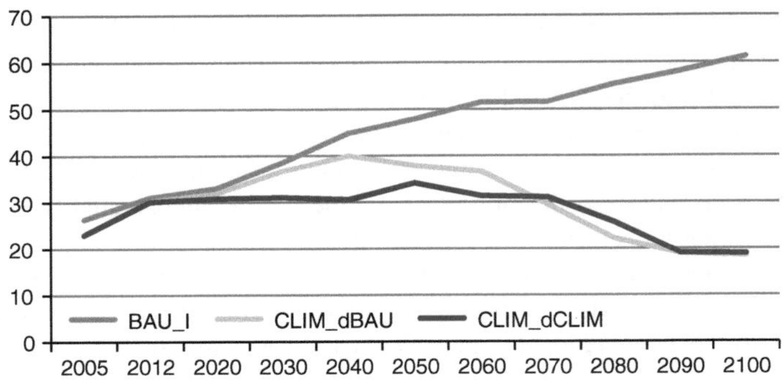

Fig. 1 World CO_2 emission trajectories under the three example scenarios (Gt)

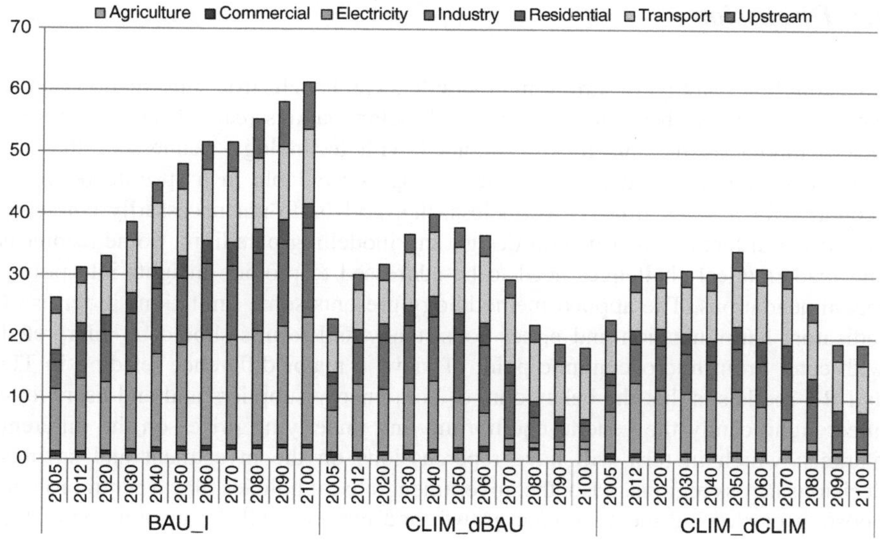

Fig. 2 World CO_2 emissions by sector (Gt)

In the CLIM_dBAU scenario, the CO_2 emitted by the electricity sector decreases from around 7 Gt in 2005 to 1.2 Gt in 2100. CO_2 emissions reach 0.6 Gt in 2100 in the CLIM_dCLIM scenario. CO_2 emissions represent nearly 21 Gt in 2100 in the BAU. The electricity sector share of total CO_2 emissions moves from 30 % in 2005 to 7 and 3 % respectively in CLIM_dBAU and CLIM_dCLIM. While CLIM_dCLIM appears more stringent in terms of decarbonisation for the electricity sector, it is interesting to note that the CO_2 emissions mitigation in the industry is more important in CLIM_dBAU than in CLIM_dCLIM with 2.6 Gt of CO_2 emitted in 2100 in the former against 3 Gt of CO_2 emitted in the latter scenario. CO_2 emissions in industry in 2100 represent 14 % in CLIM_dBAU and 16 % in CLIM_dCLIM of the total CO_2 emissions (24 % in BAU) against 19 % in 2005.

Other sectors impacted by the climate policies implemented in scenario are commercial and residential. In the BAU, these sectors account for 1 and 6 % respectively of the CO_2 emissions in 2100 (3 and 7 % in 2005). In CLIM_dBAU, they represent near to zero and 5 % respectively for commercial and residential sectors in 2100 and 1 and 16 % respectively in CLIM_dCLIM at the same period. The CO_2 emissions in commercial sector move from 0.8 Gt in 2005 to 0.007 Gt in 2100 (0.1 Gt in CLIM_dCLIM and 0.5 Gt in BAU) in 2100. Note that in the BAU, the CO_2 emissions from the commercial sector are less in 2100 than in 2005. As regard the CO_2 emissions in residential sector, they reduce from 1.9 Gt in 2005 to 0.9 Gt in 2100 (2.8 Gt in CLIM_dCLIM and 3.9 Gt in BAU in 2100).

3.3 Discussion

This coupling tentatively shows that modellers can benefit from information on the whole economy with the representation of factor markets (capital, labour) from a Macro model on the one hand, combined with technology richness of the BU models, which represent better the technologies available in a specific bounded economy for a given time. Nevertheless, the models do not necessarily converge due to the difference in structural design and modelling paradigm. Some technical and mathematical challenges need to be addressed to provide insights into policy recommendations. The applied methodology presents some limitations in terms of indicators harmonization and prices consistency and results should be interpreted with care. From microeconomic point of view, a major difference residing in TD and BU models is that the behaviours of both energy suppliers and end-users may affect significantly the general equilibrium and underlying prices on the different markets; which in turn will have repercussions on the investment and savings decisions across regions. Also, the government's fiscal policies play a central role in boosting or slowing the economic growth and influence all the institutions of the market.

4 From Global Modelling to Country Analysis: Focus on China with ETSAP-TIAM and AIM

China's economy and energy system developed rapidly since the 1980s, followed by an increase in CO_2 emissions. Analysing pathways for China's future development and associated global issues relies on complex global modelling tools that incorporate sufficient sub-regional details of China. Recent modelling exercises that account for such global and sub-regional economy and energy system features are however rarely described in the peer-reviewed academic literature (Mischke and Karlsson 2014).

This China soft-linking case study aims to bridge this knowledge gap between existing global and China-specific scenario studies, which are currently carried out by different academic institutions with multiple modelling tools (Mischke and Karlsson 2014). One example of such a modelling exercise for China was carried out by Chen (2005). Using a hybrid MARKAL MACRO model for China, (Chen 2005) concluded that the economic costs of a carbon emission reduction pathway in China towards 2050 are rather high, estimated at up to 2.54 % of GDP loss.

The soft-linking of a global TD economic model, the Asian-Pacific Integrated assessment Model (AIM/CGE) developed in the National Institute of Environmental Studies of Japan (NIES), with a global BU energy system model, the ETSAP-TIAM model with sub-regional China features developed in the Technical University of Denmark (DTU), is carried out here to establish a common global and China-specific reference scenario. On this basis, global, China national and China sub-regional economic, energy and emission pathways can be documented, analysed, and replicated simultaneously.

4.1 Methods

The two global optimization models are expanded with a sub-regional level of detail for China as per the country's regional geographic definitions of the 7th Five Year Plan (National People's Congress 1985). Both models represent the economy and energy system of 16 world regions plus China. China-specific base year data are calibrated against official Chinese government statistics, including provincial energy balances and input-output tables. The global AIM/CGE model represents moreover up to 30 provinces of China, with 22 economic sectors and three final demand sectors (Dai and Mischke 2014). A triangulation method to integrate provincial energy statistics for China into ETSAP-TIAM (Loulou and Labriet 2008) was established (Mischke 2013).

The soft-linking approach used in this study comprises the following three major steps, which are similar to other country case studies presented here:

Step 1: **TD to BU**
The AIM/CGE model provides initial inputs for the ETSAP-TIAM model for a direct or indirect linking of the sectors in both models. The outputs of the economic sectors from the AIM/CGE model are used as drivers for energy service demand in ETSAP-TIAM model. If required, alternative projections from other sources are used, such as population statistics.

Step 2: **BU to TD**
After ETSAP-TIAM calculates the optimal technology mix and final energy demand in different sectors, the energy efficiency parameters of the AIM/CGE model are adjusted so that the energy consumption matches the ETSAP-TIAM results.

Step 3: **Model iterations**
After these two steps, equivalent to the first iteration, the results of energy service demand in the AIM/CGE model might change. If the change in parameters is significant, new iterations are carried out until an acceptable convergence is found. The hybrid model developed in this study is named CGESL.

4.2 Common Reference Scenario

A common reference scenario is constructed and tested in various iterations. It follows the GDP and demographic trends of a newly developed, moderate Shared Socio-economic Pathways (SSP2) scenario (O'Neill et al. 2014). The SSP2

Table 1 Future economic growth increase for sub-regions of China under SSP2 (2005 = 1)

Region	2005	2010	2020	2030	2040	2050
East-China	1.0	1.5	3.5	6.5	9.8	12.3
Central-China	1.0	1.5	3.9	7.5	12.1	15.8
West-China	1.0	1.5	3.7	7.0	11.1	14.4

pathway is downscaled for China, following the principle that the existing socio-economic disparities within China will be narrowed towards 2050. Future GDP growth projections for China and other model regions are thus a main driver in both models. GDP pathways of East-, Central- and West-China are summarised in Table 1.

4.3 Reference Scenario Results

At a **global level**, the hybrid model (Fig. 1, marked in green) shows a 2–2.5 times increase in global power production, primary and final energy use and CO_2 emissions towards 2050. The pathway for final energy is thereby highly harmonised between the different modelling tools. The AIM/CGE model and the ETSAP-TIAM model (Fig. 3, marked in red and blue), if used stand-alone, diverge increasingly in their pathways for global power production, primary energy use and global CO_2 emissions.

At a **China national level**, the hybrid model (Fig. 4, marked in green) shows a 5 times increase in China's power production, primary and final energy use and CO_2 emissions towards 2050. A peak in these pathways is suggested around 2040 in the TD AIM/CGE and the hybrid CGESL model, however not in the BU ETSAP-TIAM model. As described above, the models stand-alone diverge increasingly towards 2050. While the TD AIM/CGE model calculates an almost 6 times increase

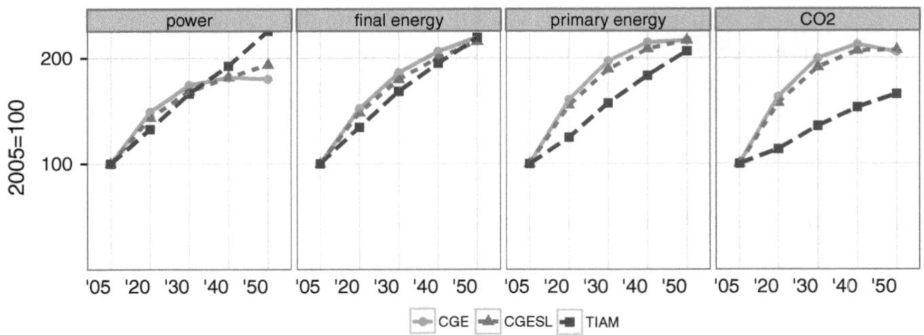

Fig. 3 World reference scenario in TD AIM/CGE, BU TIAM and hybrid CGESL models—pathways for power generation, primary and final energy use, and CO_2 emissions towards 2050

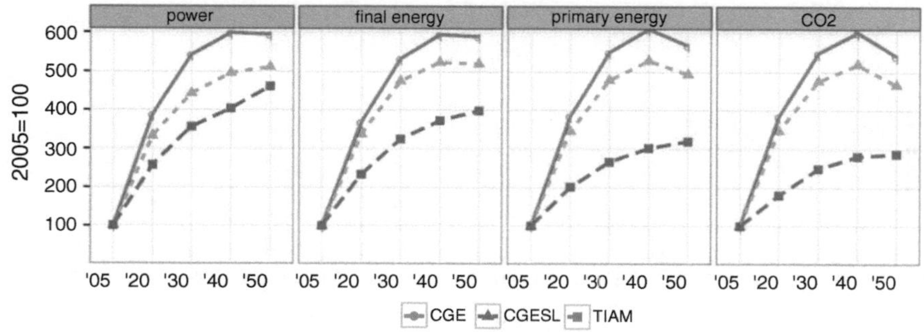

Fig. 4 China reference scenario in TD AIM/CGE, BU TIAM and hybrid CGESL models—pathways for power generation, primary and final energy use, and CO_2 emissions towards 2050

in all pathways towards 2050, the BU ETSAP-TIAM model calculates a much lower rate of increase of about 3–5 times.

Analyzing the modelling results for the **East-China sub-region**, which summarizes the highly developed coastal provinces of China, provides the further insights. The hybrid CGESL model (Fig. 5, marked in green) shows a 3.5–4 times increase in East-China's power production, primary and final energy use and CO_2 emissions towards 2050. A peak around 2040 is suggested in most pathways studied here, similar to the national-level results for China. As discussed before, the models stand-alone diverge increasingly.

The pathways for the **Central-China sub-region**, which comprises many resource-rich provinces of China, are provided in Fig. 6. The hybrid CGESL model (Fig. 6, marked in green) indicates a 6–6.5 times increase in Central-China's power production, primary and final energy use and CO_2 emissions towards 2050. The divergence in the pathways of the TD and BU models is highest for CO_2 emissions: the maximum increase in CO_2 emissions between 2005 and 2050 is about 7 times in the TD AIM/CGE model and only about 3 times in the BU ETSAP-TIAM model.

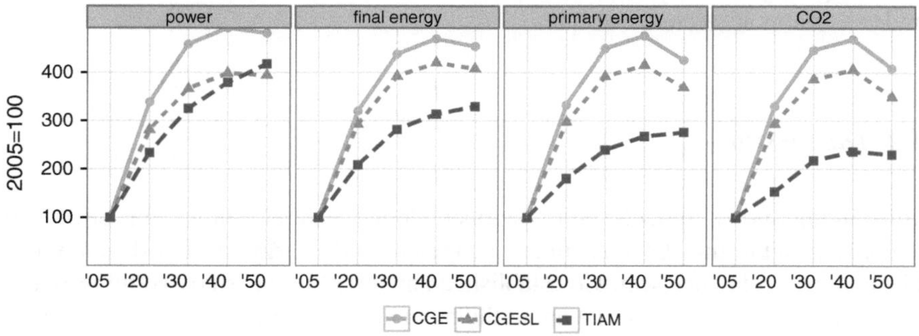

Fig. 5 East-China reference scenario in TD AIM/CGE, BU TIAM and hybrid CGESL models—pathways for power generation, primary and final energy use, and CO_2 emissions (2005–2050)

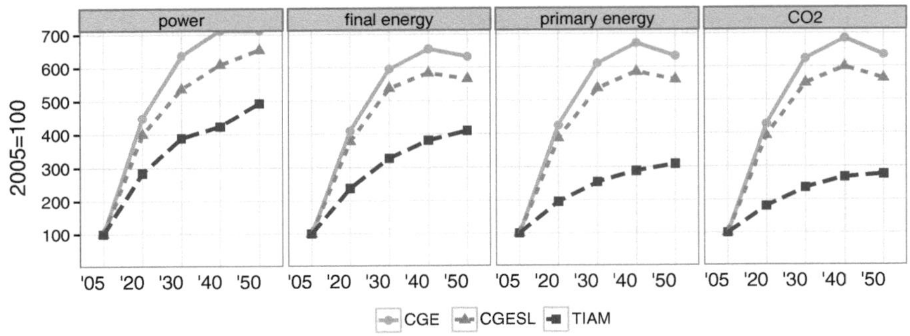

Fig. 6 Central-China reference scenario in TD AIM/CGE, BU TIAM and hybrid CGESL models—pathways for power generation, primary and final energy use, and CO_2 emissions towards 2050

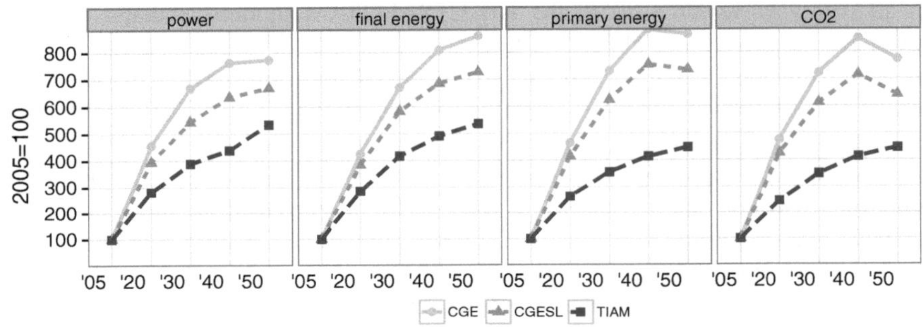

Fig. 7 West-China reference scenario in TD AIM/CGE, BU TIAM and hybrid CGESL models—pathways for power generation, primary and final energy use, and CO_2 emissions towards 2050

The **West-China sub-region** comprises many sparsely populated and economically less developed provinces of China. The corresponding future pathways are provided in Fig. 7. The results are similar to the other sub-regions of China, indicating major differences if models are not soft-linked and used stand-alone under a common reference scenario.

4.4 Discussion

Soft-linking global models with regional China features allows for new, sub-regional insights into China's future economic and energy system development. The common reference scenario established and tested in this study could provide a basis for future scenario studies about the potential global impacts of China-specific sub-regional and national energy and climate policies. These results, if replicable, reliable and transparent, could feed into an ongoing energy and climate policy debate in China, which is striving to balance global and China-specific regional development issues.

As previous scenario studies for China showed, the divergence in China-specific scenario results calculated by different modelling tools with different underlying assumptions is rather high (Mischke and Karlsson 2014). Our preliminary results confirm that China-specific modelling exercises should be sufficiently harmonised and documented first, before applying any modelling framework to study policy scenarios for China in a global context.

To cope with the range of uncertainty in China's future energy and emission projections, future work should focus on benchmarking such a global and China-specific modelling exercise with more leading global and China-specific scenario studies. More research is also needed to understand and explore uncertainty in underlying statistical differences that serve as inputs for this and other modelling frameworks.

5 From Global Modelling to Country Analysis: Focus on South America with TIAM-ECN and E3ME

Within the framework of the European research project CLIMACAP[3] the global energy system model TIAM-ECN and the global macro-economic model E3ME are linked in order to enhance the energy and economic analysis capabilities focusing on Latin American energy topics.

TIAM-ECN is the TIMES Integrated Assessment Model (TIAM) of the Energy research Centre of the Netherlands (ECN), used for long-term energy systems and climate policy analysis. It has a global scope with a world energy system disaggregated in 20 distinct regions. TIAM-ECN is a linear optimisation model, based on energy system cost minimisation with perfect foresight until 2100. It simulates the development of the global energy economy over time from resource extraction to final energy use.

E3ME is an econometric input-output model of the global economy, energy system and environment. It is maintained and developed by Cambridge Econometrics (CE), and is frequently applied to assess the macroeconomic impact of energy policies and technologies, as well as other energy-environment-economy (E3) interactions. In the CLIMACAP project is applied as a tool to assess the impact of whole energy system scenarios on the wider economy of selected Latin American countries. The model uses a combination of accounting identities and

[3] www.climacap.org.

empirically estimated econometric equations to assess the impact of these different energy system pathways on consumers, industries and the economy as a whole. Importantly, E3ME includes a technology defined approach to modelling the power sector, and therefore the scenarios can be made compatible with TIAM-ECN.

5.1 Methods

The two models are aligned in the sense that, firstly, they apply consistent assumptions for global parameters, including fossil fuel prices, carbon prices, technology efficiency and technology costs. Secondly, that the results from the TIAM-ECN model, including capacity and generation figures, energy demand and required investment costs, define model input data that is fed into E3ME. Energy sector results from TIAM-ECN are processed and input to E3ME including:

- Electricity capacity and generation development, by power sector technology;
- Hydrogen capacity and generation development, by hydrogen sector technology;
- Industrial energy consuming technology (production method) CCS capacity;
- Energy demand, by final user and fuel type;
- Energy system investment costs, by technology type;

These inputs are processed before being used in E3ME to convert to the required units of measurement and classifications. As the TIAM-ECN model is solved every 10 year interval to 2050 (focus in CLIMACAP project on horizon until 2050) and E3ME requires annual inputs, the figures for the intermediate years are interpolated from the TIAM-ECN results.

As explained above, a change in electricity prices is modelled in order to account for changes in the cost of power sector investment, transmission costs and CO_2 capture and storage. In all other cases it is also assumed that there is an increase in prices to finance the energy technology investment. There is an increase in prices in the industries that invest in carbon capture and storage (CCS) technology to fund investment in industry CCS. It is assumed that there is an increase in the price of vehicles that is sufficient to cover the investment cost to finance additional investment in vehicles.

Electricity prices, energy system investment, prices of energy-using capital, and fuel demand determine the overall economic impact. There are three channels through which the TIAM-ECN results impact on the economy:

- through the level of investment in energy technologies, and the upstream impact of that investment,
- through the electricity prices and industry costs, and the consequential impact on demand,
- through the mix of energy demand by fuel in the economy and the associated trade balance.

5.2 Results

The results in Fig. 8 show on the left side energy technology expenditures for Latin America and representative selected countries, and on the right side the corresponding macro-economic impact in term of GDP change decomposed by their main effects. The results refer to a scenario with a carbon tax on GHG starting at US$50 in 2020 and increasing by 4 % per year in real terms. The change of GDP is given versus the baseline development which does not impose any climate policy measures for the future.

For the macro-economic modelling with E3ME a dominating investment effect can be observed for Latin America. The investment is paid for, ultimately, by consumers who see an increase in real household consumption.[4] In net terms, GDP increases by 1.6 % in 2030, 2.0 % in 2040 and 1.3 % in 2050. The main driver for this dynamic is the shift in the structure of the economy, from fossil fuel supply chains to capital supply chains, which leads to stronger dynamic multiplier effects. A closer look at investments shows for Latin America as whole, and in particular for Brazil and Mexico, that additional investment in the power sector does not crowd out investment in the rest of the economy, since investment in productive assets is not constrained, because it can be withdrawn from investment in non-productive assets. As a result, the impact on GDP in E3ME is a net effect of the increase in investment. In principle, the positive investment impact could outweigh the negative price effects reducing real consumer spending since E3ME allows for spare capacity in the labour market and so demand-side (investment) stimulus can yield positive GDP results. Since many consumer goods are imported, the reduction in consumption leads to a reduction in imports which also impacts on GDP. For Mexico the net impact on GDP mostly reflects two competing factors in the longer term driven by the changing structure of the energy system. As more capital and less fuel intensive technologies come into the energy system a demand for these capital goods (investment) is offset by the extra price of these technologies. The technology outcome matters considerably in the determination of the results, in particular the overall cost and the relative weighting of the capital and operating cost components and the characteristics of those supply chains in the domestic economy. In the early period, the investment effects dominate substantially, but by 2050 the differences are much smaller and the net impact on GDP is only around 1 % at a CO_2 price of \$165/tCO_2 and emissions reductions of over 50 % compared to the baseline. Consumer spending in 2050 is 0.4 % higher than in the baseline due to the recycling of the carbon tax. Colombia's total production could be positive with an increase of up to 2.7 % by 2050, with negative GDP impacts from increasing imports (to meet increasing demand) and reducing exports (as a result of the price effects). The developments of employment under the carbon tax scenario show an increase of employment compared to the baseline by almost 5 million (net additional) jobs (+1.4 %) across Latin America by 2050. New jobs are created in particular in Brazil and in Argentina with a growth of more than 2 % each.

---

[4] In the modelling approach applied in this study the carbon tax revenues has been recycled to households.

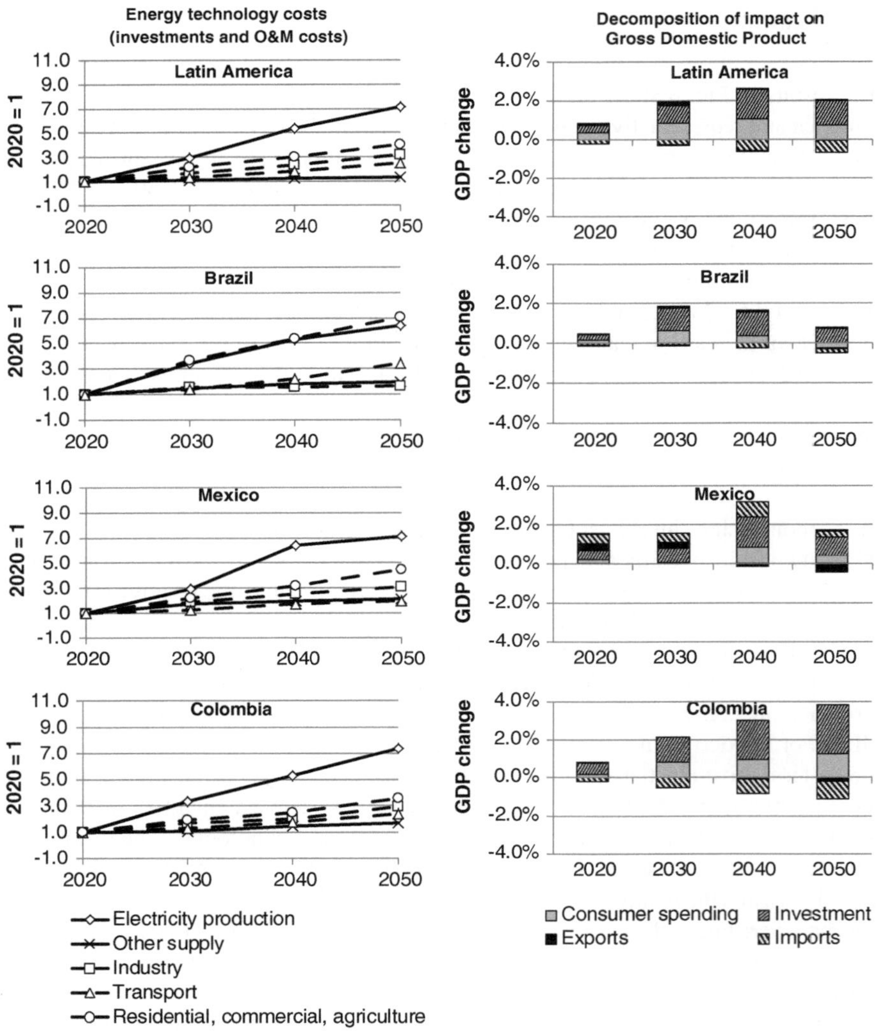

Fig. 8 Energy investments and GDP impact on Latin America under a high carbon tax scenario

5.3 Discussion

Comparing the results from the linkage of TIAM-ECN and E3ME with results from the CGE model, the consequences of increasingly higher carbon prices in terms of reduced consumer spending and GDP are linear in the CGE models and increase as the carbon price increases; but divergent and non-linear in the soft-linked modelling approach reflecting the explicit definition of physical characteristics of technology in TIAM-ECN and the economic impact of the technologies different economic characteristics as represented in E3ME

The model linkage approach captures detailed technology switching and this is reflected in the non-linearity of the economic results, but the model also yields different results because of fundamental differences in economic structure and approach that allows policy impacts that stimulate the demand side to lead to positive impacts on GDP even in the long term. The outcome of the combined model approach shows that both investments and consumer spending will increase under climate policy, which suggests that the price impacts of more expensive energy due to structural changes to the energy system can be compensated by the impact of the related changes to the structure of the energy system and economy.

References

Arrow KJ, Debreu G (1954) Existence of an equilibrium for a competitive economy. Econometrica 22:265–290. doi:10.2307/1907353

Assoumou E, Maïzi N (2011) Carbon value dynamics for France: a key driver to support mitigation pledges at country scale. Energy Policy 39:4325–4336. doi:10.1016/j.enpol.2011.04.050

Ayres RU, van den Bergh JCJM, Lindenberger D, Warr B (2013) The underestimated contribution of energy to economic growth. Struct Change Econ Dyn 27:79–88. doi:10.1016/j.strueco.2013.07.004

Bataille C, Jaccard M, Nyboer J, Rivers N (2006) Towards general equilibrium in a technology-rich model with empirically estimated behavioral parameters. Energy J Special Issue 2 (Hybrid Modeling):93–112

Benes J, Chauvet M, Kamenik O et al (2012) The future of oil: Geology versus technology. International Monetary Fund, Washington, USA

Bernard A, Vielle M (2008) GEMINI-E3, a general equilibrium model of international–national interactions between economy, energy and the environment. Comput Manag Sci 5:173–206. doi:10.1007/s10287-007-0047-y

Berndt ER, Wood DO (1975) Technology, prices, and the derived demand for energy. Rev Econ Stat 57:259–268. doi:10.2307/1923910

Böhringer C (1998) The synthesis of bottom-up and top-down in energy policy modeling. Energy Econ 20:233–248. doi:10.1016/S0140-9883(97)00015-7

Böhringer C, Rutherford TF (2008) Combining bottom-up and top-down. Energy Econ 30:574–596. doi:10.1016/j.eneco.2007.03.004

Böhringer C, Rutherford TF (2009) Integrated assessment of energy policies: decomposing top-down and bottom-up. J Econ Dyn Control 33:1648–1661. doi:10.1016/j.jedc.2008.12.007

Bosetti V, Carraro C, Galeotti M et al (2006) WITCH a world induced technical change hybrid model. Energy J 27:13–37

Bouckaert S, Selosse S, Dubreuil A, Assoumou E, Maïzi N (2011) Analyzing water supply in future energy systems using the TIMES integrated assessment model (TIAM-FR). Presented at the 3rd international symposium on energy engineering, Economics and policy: EEEP 2011, p 6

Capros P, Paroussos L, Fragkos P et al (2014) European decarbonisation pathways under alternative technological and policy choices: a multi-model analysis. Energy Strategy Rev 2:231–245. doi:10.1016/j.esr.2013.12.007

Chen W (2005) The costs of mitigating carbon emissions in China: findings from China MARKAL-MACRO modeling. Energy Policy 33:885–896. doi:10.1016/j.enpol.2003.10.012

Dai H, Mischke P (2014) Future energy consumption and emissions in East-, Central- and West-China: insights from soft-linking two global models. Energy Procedia 61:2584–2587. doi:10.1016/j.egypro.2014.12.253

Edenhofer O (2014) Climate change now—emissions, limits and possibilities. Presentation to the environmental protection agency, Dublin, Ireland

Fishbone LG, Abilock H (1981) MARKAL, a linear-programming model for energy systems analysis: Technical description of the bnl version. Int J Energy Res 5:353–375. doi:10.1002/er.4440050406

Fleiter T, Worrell E, Eichhammer W (2011) Barriers to energy efficiency in industrial bottom-up energy demand models—a review. Renew Sustain Energy Rev 15:3099–3111. doi:10.1016/j.rser.2011.03.025

Frei CW, Haldi P-A, Sarlos G (2003) Dynamic formulation of a top-down and bottom-up merging energy policy model. Energy Policy 31:1017–1031. doi:10.1016/S0301-4215(02)00170-2

Grubb M, Kohler J, Anderson D (2002) Induced technical change in energy and environmental modeling: Analytic approaches and policy implications. Annu Rev Energy Environ 27:271–308. doi:10.1146/annurev.energy.27.122001.083408

Grubler A, Nakićenović N, Victor DG (1999) Dynamics of energy technologies and global change. Energy Policy 27:247–280. doi:10.1016/S0301-4215(98)00067-6

Guivarch C, Hallegatte S, Crassous R (2009) The resilience of the Indian economy to rising oil prices as a validation test for a global energy–environment–economy CGE model. Energy Policy 37:4259–4266. doi:10.1016/j.enpol.2009.05.025

Hageman LA, Young DM (2012) Applied iterative methods. Courier Dover Publications, New York

Hamdi-Cherif M, Guivarch C, Quirion P (2011) Sectoral targets for developing countries: combining "common but differentiated re-sponsibilities" with "meaningful participation". Clim Policy 11:731–751. doi:10.3763/cpol.2009.0070

Hardin G (1968) The tragedy of the commons. Science 162:1243–1248. doi:10.1126/science.162.3859.1243

HM Revenue and Customs (2013) Carbon price floor reform and other technical ammendments. HM Revenue U Customs, London, UK

Hoffman KC, Jorgenson DW (1977) Economic and technological Models for evaluation of energy policy. Bell J Econ 8:444–466. doi:10.2307/3003296

Hourcade J-C (1993) Modelling long-run scenarios: Methodology lessons from a prospective study on a low CO_2 intensive country. Energy Policy 21:309–326. doi:10.1016/0301-4215(93)90252-B

Hourcade JC, Jaccard M, Bataille C, Ghersi F (2006) Hybrid modeling: new answers to old challenges. Energy J Special Issue 2 (Hybrid Modeling):1–12

IPCC (2013) Climate change 2013: the physical science basis. Cambridge University Press, New York, USA

IPCC (2014) Climate change 2014: mitigation of climate change. Cambridge University Press, Washington, USA

Jackson PT (2009) Prosperity without growth?—the transition to a sustainable economy. Sustainable Development Commission, London

Johansen L (1960) A multi-sector study of economic growth. North-Holland Pub. Co, Amsterdam

Jorgenson DW (1982) An econometric approach to general equilibrium analysis. In: Hazewinkel M, Kan AHGR (eds) Current developments in the interface: economics, econometrics, mathematics. Springer, Netherlands, pp 125–155

Kanudia A, Labriet M, Loulou R (2014) Effectiveness and efficiency of climate change mitigation in a technologically uncertain world. Clim Change 123:543–558. doi:10.1007/s10584-013-0854-9

Kiuila O, Rutherford TF (2013) Piecewise smooth approximation of bottom–up abatement cost curves. Energy Econ 40:734–742. doi:10.1016/j.eneco.2013.07.016

Krey V, Luderer G, Clarke L, Kriegler E (2014) Getting from here to there—energy technology transformation pathways in the EMF27 scenarios. Clim Change 123:369–382. doi:10.1007/s10584-013-0947-5

Kumhof M, Muir D (2014) Oil and the world economy: some possible futures. Philos Trans R Soc Math Phys Eng Sci 372:20120327. doi:10.1098/rsta.2012.0327

Labriet M, Drouet L, Vielle M, Haurie A, Kanudia A, Loulou R (2015) Assessment of the effectiveness of global climate policies using coupled bottom-up and top-down models. Les Cahiers du GERAD, G-2010-30 revised in January 2015, Montreal, Canada, p 22

Labriet M, Kanudia A, Loulou R (2012) Climate mitigation under an uncertain technology future: A TIAM-World analysis. Energy Econ 34(Supplement 3):S366–S377. doi:10.1016/j.eneco.2012.02.016

Loulou R (2008) ETSAP-TIAM: the TIMES integrated assessment model. part II: mathematical formulation. Comput Manag Sci 5:41–66. doi:10.1007/s10287-007-0045-0

Loulou R, Labriet M (2008) ETSAP-TIAM: the TIMES integrated assessment model part I: model structure. Comput Manag Sci 5:7–40. doi:10.1007/s10287-007-0046-z

Loulou R, Remme U, kanudia A, Lehtila A, Goldstein G (2005) Documentation for the TIMES Model. Energy technology system analysis programme (ETSAP), Paris

Lucas RE Jr (1976) Econometric policy evaluation: a critique. Carnegie-Rochester Conf Ser Public Policy 1:19–46. doi:10.1016/S0167-2231(76)80003-6

Manne A, Mendelsohn R, Richels R (1995) MERGE: a model for evaluating regional and global effects of GHG reduction policies. Energy Policy 23:17–34. doi:10.1016/0301-4215(95)90763-W

Manne AS, Wene CO (1992) MARKAL-MACRO: a linked model for energy-economy analysis. Brookhaven National Lab, NY

Martinsen T (2011) Introducing technology learning for energy technologies in a national CGE model through soft links to global and national energy models. Energy Policy 39:3327–3336. doi:10.1016/j.enpol.2011.03.025

Mathy S, Guivarch C (2010) Climate policies in a second-best world—a case study on India. Energy Policy 38:1519–1528. doi:10.1016/j.enpol.2009.11.035

Messner S, Schrattenholzer L (2000) MESSAGE–MACRO: linking an energy supply model with a macroeconomic module and solving it iteratively. Energy 25:267–282. doi:10.1016/S0360-5442(99)00063-8

Mischke P (2013) China's energy statistics in a global context: a methodology to develop regional energy balances for East, Central, and West China

Mischke P, Karlsson KB (2014) Modelling tools to evaluate China's future energy system—a review of the Chinese perspective. Energy 69:132–143. doi:10.1016/j.energy.2014.03.019

National People's Congress (1985) The seventh five year plan for national economic and social development. Peoples Education Press, Beijing, China

Nordhaus WD (1994) Managing the global commons: the economics of climate change, 1st edn. The MIT Press, Cambridge, MA

OECD, IEA (2013) World energy outlook 2013. International Energy Agency, Paris, France

O'Neill BC, Kriegler E, Riahi K et al (2014) A new scenario framework for climate change research: the concept of shared socioeconomic pathways. Clim Change 122:387–400. doi:10.1007/s10584-013-0905-2

Proença S, St. Aubyn M (2013) Hybrid modeling to support energy-climate policy: effects of feed-in tariffs to promote renewable energy in Portugal. Energy Econ 38:176–185. doi:10.1016/j.eneco.2013.02.013

Ricci O, Selosse S (2013) Global and regional potential for bioelectricity with carbon capture and storage. Energy Policy 52:689–698. doi:10.1016/j.enpol.2012.10.027

Rozenberg J, Hallegatte S, Vogt-Schilb A et al (2010) Climate policies as a hedge against the uncertainty on future oil supply. Clim Change 101:663–668. doi:10.1007/s10584-010-9868-8

Sassi O, Crassous R, Hourcade JC et al (2010) IMACLIM-R: a modelling framework to simulate sustainable development pathways. Int J Glob Environ Issues 10:5. doi:10.1504/IJGENVI.2010.030566

Strachan N, Kannan R (2008) Hybrid modelling of long-term carbon reduction scenarios for the UK. Energy Econ 30:2947–2963. doi:10.1016/j.eneco.2008.04.009

Sue Wing I (2008) The synthesis of bottom-up and top-down approaches to climate policy modeling: electric power technology detail in a social accounting framework. Energy Econ 30:547–573. doi:10.1016/j.eneco.2006.06.004

The Global Commission on the Economy and Climate (2014) Better growth, better climate—the new climate economy report. The Global Commission on the Economy and Climate, Washington, USA

Warr B, Ayres R (2006) REXS: a forecasting model for assessing the impact of natural resource consumption and technological change on economic growth. Struct Change Econ Dyn 17:329–378. doi:10.1016/j.strueco.2005.04.004

Wene C-O (1996) Energy-economy analysis: Linking the macroeconomic and systems engineering approaches. Energy 21:809–824. doi:10.1016/0360-5442(96)00017-5

Economic Impacts of Future Changes in the Energy System—National Perspectives

James Glynn, Patrícia Fortes, Anna Krook-Riekkola, Maryse Labriet, Marc Vielle, Socrates Kypreos, Antti Lehtilä, Peggy Mischke, Hancheng Dai, Maurizio Gargiulo, Per Ivar Helgesen, Tom Kober, Phil Summerton, Bruno Merven, Sandrine Selosse, Kenneth Karlsson, Neil Strachan and Brian Ó Gallachóir

Abstract In a climate constrained future, hybrid energy-economy model coupling gives additional insight into interregional competition, trade, industrial delocalisation and overall macroeconomic consequences of decarbonising the energy system. Decarbonising the energy system is critical in mitigating climate change. This chapter summarises modelling methodologies developed in the ETSAP community

J. Glynn (✉) · B. Ó Gallachóir
Environmental Research Institute, University College Cork, Cork, Ireland
e-mail: james.glynn@umail.ucc.ie

B. Ó Gallachóir
e-mail: b.ogallachoir@ucc.ie

P. Fortes
CENSE, Faculdade Ciências e Tecnologia, Universidade Nova de Lisboa, Lisbon, Portugal
e-mail: p.fs@fct.unl.pt

A. Krook-Riekkola
Department of Business Administration, Luleå University of Technology, Luleå, Sweden
e-mail: anna.krook-riekkola@ltu.se

M. Labriet
Eneris Environment Energy Consultants, Madrid, Spain
e-mail: maryse.labriet@enerisconsultants.com

M. Vielle
Ecole Polytechnique de Lausanne, Lausanne, Switzerland
e-mail: marc.vielle@epfl.ch

S. Kypreos
Paul Scherrer Institute, Villigen, Switzerland
e-mail: socrateskypreos@gmail.com

A. Lehtilä
VTT Technical Research Centre of Finland, Espoo, Finland
e-mail: antti.lehtila@vtt.fi

G. Giannakidis et al. (eds.), *Informing Energy and Climate Policies Using Energy Systems Models*, Lecture Notes in Energy 30,
DOI 10.1007/978-3-319-16540-0_20

to assess economic impacts of decarbonising energy systems at a national level. The preceding chapter focuses on a global perspective. The modelling studies outlined here show that burden sharing rules and national revenue recycling schemes for carbon tax are critical for the long-term viability of economic growth and equitable engagement on combating climate change. Traditional computable general equilibrium models and energy systems models solved in isolation can misrepresent the long run carbon cost and underestimate the demand response caused by technological paradigm shifts in a decarbonised energy system. The approaches outlined within have guided the first evidence based decarbonisation legislation and continue to provide additional insights as increased sectoral disaggregation in hybrid modelling approaches is achieved.

P. Mischke · K. Karlsson
Department of Management Engineering, Technical University of Denmark, Copenhagen, Denmark
e-mail: peym@dtu.dk

K. Karlsson
e-mail: keka@dtu.dk

H. Dai
National Institute of Environmental Studies, Tsukuba, Japan
e-mail: dhc1434@gmail.com

M. Gargiulo
Energy Engineering Economic Environment Systems Modelling and Analysis (E4SMA s.r.l.), Turin, Italy
e-mail: maurizio.gargiulo@e4sma.com

P.I. Helgesen
Department of Industrial Economics and Technology Management, Norwegian University of Science and Technology, Trondheim, Norway
e-mail: per.i.helgesen@iot.ntnu.no

T. Kober
Energy Research Centre of the Netherlands (ECN), Policy Studies Department, Petten/Amsterdam, The Netherlands
e-mail: Kober@ecn.nl

P. Summerton
Cambridge Econometrics, Cambridge, UK
e-mail: ps@camecon.com

B. Merven
Energy Research Centre, University of Cape Town, Cape Town, South Africa
e-mail: brunomerven@gmail.com

S. Selosse
Centre de Mathématicues Appliquèes, MINES ParisTech, Paris, France
e-mail: sandrine.selosse@mines-paristech.fr

N. Strachan
Energy Institute, University College London, London, UK
e-mail: n.strachan@ucl.ac.uk

1 Introduction—Regional Applied Hybrid Models

Global economic and environmental scenarios consistently show a trend of continuous decline in natural resource reserves, degradation of environmental quality, increasing vulnerability of economic growth as a result of environmental stresses, competition for natural resources, soaring energy prices and climate change. These scenarios partly rest on significant efforts by the scientific community over the past three decades to improve knowledge of the interactions between economic growth and the environment; particularly modelling methods have developed to become increasingly applied to the assessment of the environmental and economic consequences of various energy and greenhouse gas (GHG) policies. Policy makers need clear and consistent information concerning the real impact of energy and climate policies on the economy and the most cost-effective technology portfolio to achieve their goals. Separate use of top-down (TD) and bottom-up (BU) models do not adequately address all these aspects, which might lead to ineffective policies.

Hybrid models, that combine the technological detail of BU models with the economic framework of a TD, e.g. General Equilibrium (CGE) models, have been developed as an alternate method. Despite the extensive literature on hybrid models, there are few quantitative examples employing a 'full-link' (i.e. not focusing on only one sector) and 'full-form' BU and TD models. This chapter outlines several hybrid models considering both full-link, full form, and sectoral model developments as well as hard-linking MARKAL and TIMES MACRO models. All models presented are applied nationally within the Energy Technology Systems Analysis Programme (ETSAP) Community. The general rationale, motivation for regional and global model development are summarised in preceding chapter. This chapter focuses on the first national decarbonisation legislation, theoretical model updates, improvements and lastly learning outcomes from applied methods to national models.

2 Evidence Based UK Climate Legislation Using Hybrid Models

The energy modelling research community has long underpinned energy policy (Jebaraj and Iniyan 2006), in providing insight and numerate policy guidance (Huntington et al. 1982). The United Kingdom (UK) was the first government to legislate for mandatory GHG reduction targets, first aiming at a 60 % CO_2 reduction by 2050 relative to 1990 (BERR 2007). The ETSAP hybrid UK MARKAL-MACRO (UK MM) model was used extensively to provide the evidence base to guide discussion in the first iteration of analyses and represented a significant addition to UK energy-economy modelling capacity (FES 2003; DEFRA 2007; Strachan and Kannan 2008). UK-MM is a BU optimisation method that maintains sectoral technological detail, but endogenises aggregated price dependent energy service demand dynamics via the single sector neoclassical growth model. It is the first step in assessing the competing elements of hybrid energy modelling: technological explicitness, microeconomic-realism and macroeconomic completeness (Bataille et al. 2006). It gave insights while public debate was still ongoing as to the costs, benefits, opportunities and energy security concerns of climate change under long term uncertainty (Pearce 2003; Nordhaus 2007). UK climate policy had been primarily driven by scientific and political competition (RCEP 2000; Stern 2006), while macroeconomic impact was not a significant concern in the short term. The UKERC UK-MM studies showed that the short term impacts were manageable (Strachan and Kannan 2008). This enabled public and policy discussion to focus on sector specific impacts, social impacts and industrial effects. Further, it moved the policy discussion from whether the UK should decarbonise or not, to how to decarbonise. Four subsequent studies combined modelling effort of the AMOS, E3MG, MDME3 and MARKAL-MACRO models to continue to assess the technical feasibility of the 60 % CO_2 reduction target, finding critical technologies and reducing uncertainty (Allan et al. 2007, 2012; Strachan et al. 2009). These modelling activities highlighted the critical nature of developments in the power sector, marginal technologies, resource availability, the cost of carbon and behaviour in relation to the potential impact upon economic activity (GDP). As a result of the 2008 climate change act, the climate change committee was founded, providing legally binding carbon budgets for the UK, and is investigating stronger measures of 80 % CO_2 reductions, beyond the power sector, by 2050.

In the wake of the 2008 economic crisis, with the resultant austerity measures, risk aversion, and reduced investment capital, implementing the carbon budgets have been more difficult that initially expected. In previous studies, ex-post analysis has shown errors in model forecasting in the EU (Pilavachi et al. 2008), and US (Winebrake and Sakva 2006), and notes particular care should be taken to avoid model bias entering energy policy when energy models are directly applied by policy makers (Laitner et al. 2003).

2.1 Modelling Method Summary

Like TIMES, MARKAL is a dynamic, technology rich linear programming (LP) energy systems optimisation model. It's objective function minimises total discounted costs, including capital, fuel and operating costs for resource, process, infrastructure, conversion and end use technologies. It is a partial equilibrium model with perfect foresight. MARKAL was extended with a hard-link to MACRO. The objective function of the hybrid model is the maximisation of discounted log of utility summed over all periods (t) with an end of horizon terminal investment term. Utility is derived as the log of consumption. National production is from energy, capital and labour, substitutable in a nested constant elasticity of substitution (CES) production function. Capital and labour substitute directly for each other based on optimal capital value shares in their aggregate. Aggregated capital and labour is substitutable with a separate energy aggregate. Investment is recycled to build up a depreciating capital stock, while labour growth rates are defined exogenously.

The marginal change in production output is equivalent to the cost of changing its energy demand. This allows heterogeneous energy demand adjustment across sectors dependent upon marginal demand costs. However, shadow price responses need to be smooth to ensure marginal demand responses are realistic and allow model convergence. Autonomous energy service demand adjustment enables useful climate scenario analysis of demand responses that are decoupled from economic growth. A technical summary of the TIMES-MACRO model formulation follows in Sect. 3, while further technical detail of the UK-MM is available in Strachan and Kannan (2008).

2.2 *Evidence Base for Policy*

54 low-carbon "what if" scenarios were modelled with UK-MM to advise the UK energy white paper of potential costs of differing technology development pathways in a future with a 60 % reduction in CO_2 emissions (BERR 2007). The summary results are clustered into 4 representative scenarios, focusing on insights from the hybrid linkage, the timing of emissions constraints trajectories, fossil fuel costs and technology abilities (Strachan and Kannan 2008). The macroeconomic impact of the future changes to the UK energy system are summarised as percentage loss of projected GDP in Table 1. There is significant technical change across all sectors in all base case scenarios—before carbon constraints are applied—with car stock switch to hybrid vehicles and implementation of energy efficiency measures in building energy conservation. In the medium to long term (2030–2050) energy efficiency opportunities are exhausted and final energy demand grows, even with MACRO feedback. Higher or lower fossil fuel prices lead to lower (8 %) or higher (3 %) energy consumption respectively in 2050.

In carbon constrained scenarios, decarbonising the electricity sector is seen as the best technology pathway without behavioural change and demand adjustments, while allowing greater electricity consumption. The additional flexibility of demand endogeneity through MM is critical in accurately assessing the marginal cost of carbon. In MM 60 % CO_2 reduction scenarios, energy efficiency and conservation is maximised, with 10–15 % reductions in individual energy demand (compared to

Table 1 UK MARKAL-MACRO scenario analysis summary results

MARKAL-MACRO scenario run	% GDP loss			
	2020	2030	2040	2050
Central scenario	0.46	1.7	2.43	2.81
With accelerated technological change	0.45	1.6	2.35	2.58
With higher fossil fuel prices	0.45	1.54	2.27	2.64
With accelerated energy efficiency	−0.07	0.63	1.63	2.04

standard MARKAL runs) contributing considerably to lowering marginal CO_2 prices. In the short term it is noted that all carbon constrained scenarios have relatively benign impact upon GDP, while accelerated energy efficiency policies can have positive economic benefits via energy cost savings increasing alternative consumption. It is also noted that while there is a significant loss of GDP in the range of 2–2.8 % GDP in the long term to 2050, this impact is not seen as insurmountable. The marginal CO_2 price of the central scenario rises to €147/tCO_2 ($189/t$CO_2$), while this price is estimated at €189/tCO_2 ($243/t$CO_2$) without endogenous demand reductions from MM.

2.3 Discussion

UK energy policy makers have recognised the insights generated by hybrid energy-economy giving GDP and demand responses to energy system decarbonisation. Relevant policy makers were educated in formal energy-economic analysis and how to interpret decarbonisation scenario analysis results. Key staff members of the Committee for Climate Change were on the original UK-MARKAL project steering group. The additional flexibility of the MM demand endogeneity is seen as critical in estimating the marginal cost of carbon. There are notable trade-offs between optimum technological decarbonisation pathways and the impact that behaviour has on the marginal technology choices.

While seen as manageable, the cost impacts from the UK MM model are likely to underestimate the cost of CO_2 mitigation as a result of the lack of regional trade competitiveness or transitional effects. This is observed when comparing results from the studies in Sect. 3, and Sect. 2 in Chap. 19. Decarbonising faster than other nations creates a competitiveness disadvantage that UK MM does not account for. Resultantly inter-regional hybrid models are critical to account for global trade and competitiveness effects. Further experience from policy engagement sees the requirement for more detailed disaggregation of hybrid models to investigate spatial and socio-demographic effects. An extended treatment of natural capital stocks within nested CGE models is required to investigate realistic substitutability between natural and conventional capital as factors of production. A final lesson learned from the UK policy experience is the need for greater modelling transparency to enable replication of results. Next however, the theory behind the MACRO and MSA models—the work of Socrates Kypreos and Antti Lehtilla—are outlined in Sect. 3.

3 TIMES-Macro Stand Alone

Computer based models representing energy, economy and environmental interactions are specified, among others as non-linear (NL) optimization problems or as computable general equilibrium (CGE) simulation models (Arrow and

Debreu 1954). Optimization models when satisfying some maximization conditions give the same solution as CGE models (Capros et al. 1997). The multiregional bottom-up energy system model TIMES (Loulou et al. 2005), linked with the top-down macroeconomic module MACRO called TIMES-MACRO (TM) (Remme and Blesl 2006), is solved by maximizing an inter-temporal utility function for a single representative producer-consumer agent in each region. TM has been developed as part of the Implementing Agreement of the Energy Technology Systems Analysis Project (ETSAP) of the International Energy Agency to assess, among others, the whole energy system and climate change mitigation options and policies on the national, multiregional or global level. The multiregional TM models are large in size not solvable with direct NL optimization methods even when the most powerful commercial solvers and state of the art computers are used. On the other hand, a similar in size and structure model, the well-known MESSAGE-MACRO of IIASA (Messner and Schrattenholzer 2000), is successfully and efficiently solved by decomposition methods. The mathematics to decompose and solve TM with an iterative algorithm is outlined below. The decomposition method converts TM to an energy part (TIMES) and a small size NL macroeconomic model, called TIMES-MACRO Stand-Alone (TMSA), where the energy model TIMES is substituted by appropriate quadratic cost supply functions (QSF). This outline continues describing the demand projections for TIMES and explain the multiregional TMSA, the Negishi (1972) welfare function and the iterative procedure applied to solve the problem based on the sequential equilibrium algorithm of Rutherford (1992) (Negishi 1972; Rutherford 1992). Finally the performance of the algorithm is explained and some resultant conclusions discussed.

3.1 Energy Service Demand Projections

The ETSAP family of models defines demands that reflect past trends and exogenous assumptions on population, GDP, energy intensity and technology penetration based on demand drivers and their elasticities. As most of the efficiency improvement options are included in the engineering model explicitly, and are selected if they make economic sense, the specific selection of autonomous efficiency improvement factors (*aeeif*) applied below could be introduced to reflect mainly life style changes. A simple but useful relation for demand projections is Eq. 1:

$$\frac{D_{kt}}{D_{k0}} = \left[\frac{dr_{kt}}{dr_{ko}}\right]^{\alpha_i} \cdot \left[\frac{P_{kt}}{P_{k0}}\right]^{-\sigma_i} \cdot \prod_{\tau=1,t} (1 - aeeif_{k\tau})^{ypp_\tau} \tag{1}$$

where

D_{kt}	the demand projection for sector k and period t;
D_{k0}	the same demand for the starting year calibrated to energy statistics in line with the socio-economic assumptions and the efficiencies of the end-use devices valid in the starting year of analysis;
dr_{kt}	the demand driver;
α_k	the driver elasticity;
σ_k	the price elasticity;
$aeeif_{kt}$	the autonomous efficiency improvement factor per demand category;
ypp_τ	the years per period;
P_{kt}/P_{k0}	the index of relative price of demand in sector k.

TIAM (the global multiregional integrated assessment version of TIMES) assumes different growth rates and elasticities of demand drivers for each individual demand category. Usually some consistency checks of economic assumptions and the projections generated based on the equation above must be completed. IIASA for example adjusts projections to the results of MERGE (Manne et al. 1995), while ETSAP uses GEM-E3 (Capros et al. 1997).

3.2 The Multi-regional TIMES-SA Model

In the following section the global and multi-regional macroeconomic growth model is decomposed into a multi-regional partial equilibrium energy problem, e.g., TIMES and a multi-regional macroeconomic model maximizing the global welfare function.

3.2.1 The Macro Stand-Alone Formulation (MSA)

For the new stand-alone Macro formulation, the original Macro model had to be generalized to support multiple regions. In the multi-regional case the model is solved by maximizing the Negishi-weighted sum of regional utilities based on iterations between the stand-alone TM model (TMSA) and the standard TIMES model. The TMSA model explicitly considers only the trade of the numéraire good, as the trade in all energy products is defined in the TIMES model. The basic formulation of the original TM implementation can be rewritten by Eqs. 2–11:

$$\text{Max } U = \sum_{t=1}^{T} \sum_{r} nwt_r \cdot pwt_t \cdot dfact_{r,t} \cdot \ln(C_{r,t}) \tag{2}$$

$$Y_{r,t} = C_{r,t} + INV_{r,t} + EC_{r,t} + NTX(nmr)_{r,t} \tag{3}$$

$$Y_{r,t} = \left(akl_r \cdot K_{r,t}^{kpvs_r \cdot \rho_r} \cdot l_{r,t}^{(1-kpvs_r)\rho_r} + \sum_k b_{r,k} \cdot DEM_{r,t,k}^{\rho_r} \right)^{\frac{1}{\rho_r}} \tag{4}$$

$$K_{r,t+1} = tsrv_{r,t} \cdot K_{r,t} + \frac{1}{2}(d_t \cdot tsrv_{r,t} \cdot INV_{r,t} + d_{t+1} \cdot INV_{r,t+1}) \tag{5}$$

$$K_{r,T} \cdot (growv_{r,T} + depr_r) \leq INV_{r,T} \tag{6}$$

$$DET_{r,t,k} = aeeifac_{r,t,k} \cdot DEM_{r,t,k} \tag{7}$$

$$EC_{r,t} = qa_{r,t} + \sum_k qb_{r,t,k} \cdot (DET_{r,t,k})^2 + amp_{r,t} \tag{8}$$

$$\sum_r NTX(trd)_{r,t} = 0 \quad \forall \{ t, trd\} \tag{9}$$

$$aeeifac_{r,t,k} = \prod_{\tau=1}^{t} (1 - ddf_{r,\tau,k})^{\frac{d_t + d_{t+1}}{2}} \tag{10}$$

$$l_{r,1} = 1 \quad \text{and} \quad l_{r,t+1} = l_{r,t} \cdot (1 + growv_{r,t})^{\frac{d_t + d_{t+1}}{2}} \tag{11}$$

where

$C_{r,t}$	annual consumption in period t (variable)
$Y_{r,t}$	annual production in period t (variable)
$K_{r,t}$	total capital in period t (variable)
$INV_{r,t}$	annual investments in period t (variable)
$DEM_{r,t,k}$	annual demand in Macro for commodity k in period t (variable)
$DET_{r,t,k}$	annual demand in TIMES for commodity k in period t (variable)
$EC_{r,t}$	annual energy system costs in Macro in period t (variable)
akl_r	production function constant
amp_t	constant term to account for the full annualized investment cost of existing capacities in the starting period
$b_{r,k}$	demand coefficient for demand commodity k
$aeeifac_{r,t,k}$	autonomous energy efficiency improvement
dt	duration of period t in years
$ddf_{r,t,k}$	demand decoupling factor (calibration parameter)
$depr_r$	depreciation rate
$dfact_{r,t}$	utility discount factor for period t
$dfactcurr_{r,t}$	annual discount rate for period t
$growv_{r,t}$	growth rate in period t (calibration parameter)
$kpvs_r$	capital value share
$l_{r,t}$	annual labor growth index in period t
nwt_r	Negishi weight for region r

pwt_t	period-length-dependent weights in the utility function (to be introduced to in cases where the period lengths are not equal)
$qa_{r,t}$	constant term of the quadratic supply cost function
$qb_{r,t,k}$	coefficient for demand k in the quadratic supply cost function
$tsrv_{r,t}$	capital survival factor between periods t and t + 1
ρ_r	substitution constant
T	number of periods in the model horizon

The primary differences in relation to the standard Macro formulation are; (a) The use of Negishi weights in the objective function when the model is multi-regional; (b) The inclusion of the trade in the numéraire good NTX(nmr) in the production function; (c) The introduction of the trade balances on the global level (Eq. 9); (d) The Negishi iterations balance for inter-temporal discounted trade deficits of a region over the full time horizon of the analysis; (e) The replacement of the full TIAM LP cost accounting by quadratic supply-cost functions for each demand commodity (Eq. 8).

3.2.2 The Standard TIMES LP Formulation

The second part of the decomposed model, the TIMES LP model, uses the standard TIMES formulation, which can be written in short as:

$$\text{Min } NPV = \sum_{r=1}^{R} \sum_{y \in YEARS} (1 + d_{r,y})^{REFYR-y} \cdot ANNCOST(r,y) \tag{12}$$

$$A \cdot x = b \quad \text{and} \quad x \geq 0 \tag{13}$$

where

NPV	net present value of all energy system costs
YEARS	the set of years within the model horizon
REFYR	reference year for discounting
$d_{r,y}$	capital discount factor for region r in year y
ANNCOST(r,y)	annual energy system cost in region r and year y
A	coefficient matrix for all other model equations
x	vector of all model variables
b	RHS constant vector for all other model equations
R	number of internal regions in the model

For a comprehensive treatment of the standard TIMES LP formulation, see Loulou et al. (2005). In order to make the LP formulation more analogous with the Macro objective function, the objective function of the standard TIAM code can be rewritten in terms of period-wise average annual costs and period-specific discount factors, as follows:

$$\text{Min } NPV = \sum_{r=1}^{R} \sum_{t=1}^{T} pvf_{r,t} \cdot AESC(r,t) \tag{14}$$

where

$pvf_{r,t}$	present value factor for period t in region r
AESC(r,t)	annual energy system costs in region r and period t
T	number of periods t in the model horizon

The general specifications of the decomposition algorithm are described by Kypreos and Lehtila (2013).

3.2.3 The Algorithm and It's Performance

In both MACRO formulations, the use of the MACRO model for evaluating policy scenarios requires that the demand decoupling factors (*ddf*) and labour growth rates (*growv*) have first been calibrated with the baseline scenario and the corresponding GDP growth projections. The core part of the calibration procedure is the updating of the demand decoupling factors and labour growth rates between successive iterations of the calibration algorithm.

In the TMSA implementation, all the basic mathematical formulas for the initial specification and updating the demand decoupling factors and labour growth rates are fully equivalent to those in the standard TM formulation introduced first by Kypreos (1996). The TIMES-MACRO documentation (Remme and Blesl 2006) contains the details on the calibration algorithm and follow the description of Kypreos and Lehtila (2013) in the ETSAP documentation (Kypreos 1996; Kypreos and Lehtila 2013).

The initial Negishi weights are proportional to the regional output share while the updated ones balance for inter-temporal trade deficits following the sequential optimization algorithm of Rutherford (1992). The weights are adjusted using the normalized price of the traded products, the trade excess and the inverse of the marginal regional utility and in that case, according to Rutherford the solution obtained is Pareto optimal.

$$\begin{aligned} NW_r &= \sum_{t,trd} \pi_{trd,t} \cdot NTX_{r,t,trd} + \sum_{t} \pi_{nmr,t} \cdot C_{r,t} \text{ with} \\ nwt_r &= NW_r / \sum_{r} NW_r \end{aligned} \tag{15}$$

One significant test run for the algorithm was the solution of TM for a single region as the problem could be solved with a direct optimization and the decomposition method and results are directly comparable. The USA TMSA model validated well against the direct solution of the TM of USA as solutions are identical. However, the decomposed problem needs 2 min to be solved while the direct optimization takes more than 100 times longer. It is interesting to report the computer time needed to solve the calibration and the policy analysis case as function of the number of regions. The model starts in 2005 and covers up to 2060 in 7 time steps. A 6-region model takes about 32 min to be solved; a 10-region model needs 66 min and finally a 15-region model takes 100 min.

3.3 Conclusions

The large scale general equilibrium growth model TIMES-MACRO is solvable only when decomposed to the linear energy model TIAM and a non-linear macroeconomic stand-alone model (TMSA) where quadratic supply functions substitute for the energy system represented in TIMES.

The methodology is presented herein that allows projecting demands for energy services for a set of socio-economic assumptions, life style changes and energy intensities based on sectoral drivers, and its income and price elasticities. The regional demand decoupling factors (*ddf*) are introduced to calibrate the baseline case reproducing the same demands, although the MACRO model uses unitary income elasticity and the same elasticity of substitution across all sectors. The TMSA model then including these decoupling factors simulates the postulated GDP growth and the demands for energy. This is done with a minimum investment in respect of computation time. The execution times needed for low tolerance errors (less than 10^{-4}), is significantly reduced during both the calibration itself and when applying the model for a policy case. This can be done for either a single country model or for the multiregional and global TM model.

Although the quadratic supply cost function is a simple and approximate metamodel that substitutes for the full-scale energy model and the marginal prices are sensitive to small demand changes, the algorithm is able to give an exact calibration for the baseline case followed by good results for the carbon constrained case as the tolerance error in demand evaluation is below 10^{-4}. The prerequisite for a successful application of the QSF in representing energy and economy interactions is to have all the important system constraints determining the changes of the energy system linearized and included in TIMES. This is because the quadratic cost formulation allows for small changes around the demand variables when searching for optimal solutions and converges in small steps. For the first time the decomposition method proposed is able to solve the global TIAM-MACRO model with 15 regions in 1.5 h based on TMSA (in Windows 7, 64-bit workstation, solution in a single thread).

3.4 Ireland—Application of TIMES-Macro Stand Alone

The hybrid linking of the Irish Energy system model, Irish-TIMES is taking a two pronged approach. Firstly the linkage and calibration of the newly developed Macro Stand Alone model to form Irish-TIMES-MSA. Secondly a softlinking process is underway linking the National macroeconomic HERMES model to enable model comparison between the two approaches—aggregated production function and disaggregated sectoral production.

HERMES is a complete structural model of the Irish economy. The specification of the HERMES model is built on the assumption that firms are attempting to minimise their cost of production or maximise their profits and that households are attempting to maximise their utility. The energy system is no longer specifically modelled in the HERMES model. Energy is taken as an exogenously determined cost to firms and households through the international oil price taken from NIESR's NiGEM model. Carbon taxation is incorporated in the government's financial accounts as a revenue source paid by firms and households. It is through oil and carbon pricing, both of which are exogenously determined within HERMES, that energy system costs feedback into the economy.

The initial Irish-TIMES-MSA results outline energy system pathways for a reference scenario (REF), a carbon constrained scenario with CO_2 reductions of 80 % relative to 1990 levels (CO_2-80), and an equivalent scenario with the macroeconomic impacts integrated into the analysis. The MSA scenarios cause a 10 % reduction in final energy consumption by 2040 due to reduced demand as a result of increased energy system cost and a reduction of consumption in the economy. Interestingly this alters the fuel mix most notably in the transport and residential heating sectors as carbon constraints become less binding and so fuel switching is delayed. The loss of GDP in the CO_2-80 scenario rises to −1.5 %/year by 2050, with the CO_2-95 scenario at −2.5 %.

4 Portugal—HYBTEP

The lack of "full link", "full form" models integration in other modelling studies has been overcome by the development of an integrated methodology to soft-link the extensively applied BU TIMES model (Loulou and Labriet 2008), with the CGE GEM-E3 model (Capros et al. 1997, 2014), used by several Directorates General of the European Commission. The hybrid platform, named HYBTEP (Hybrid Technological Economic Platform), applied to the Portuguese case, is defined by the soft-link between single country versions of the two models: TIMES_PT and GEM-E3_PT (Fortes et al. 2013). HYBTEP overcomes the main limitation of CGE models—failure in represent technology choices—considering the energy profile and prices from TIMES, and minimizes the drawback of BU modelling—failure to represent adequately the link between energy and economy—as the changes in the sectors economic behaviour are set by GEM-E3 according to the BU technological choices.

4.1 Methods

HYBTEP was built by the following tasks, taking an approach close to Labriet et al. (2010).

(i) Defining coherence between the two models. Correspondence and harmonization between the models sets and variables were set up, namely the economic sectors and energy commodities. Additional energy carriers were also added to GEM-E3_PT, namely biomass. This process resulted in thirteen economic sectors in HYBTEP from the aggregation of eighteen sectors from GEM-E3_PT and more than sixty demand categories of TIMES_PT. Moreover, a crucial step to achieve consistency among the models is the definition of common scenario assumptions, namely fossil fuel import prices, interest rates, energy constraints and policy conditions.

(ii) A new energy module in GEM-E3_PT was programmed allowing the model to receive exogenously the energy consumption by energy carrier and sector. This was done by assuming fixed shares of total energy demand per sector with a Leontief technology (i.e. elasticities of substitution of the Constant Elasticities Substitution (CES) production function equal to zero) (Fig. 1). These changes further implied alterations to the definition of the price of the energy aggregate, which are also set exogenously according to the BU model energy system costs evolution per energy aggregate (ELFU).

(iii) The interaction algorithm (Fig. 1) and the conditions for convergence between the models require careful planning and definition. TIMES_PT physical energy consumption and system costs evolution per sector are 'translated' in GEM-E3_PT monetary units through an energy link module and inputted in the CGE model as energy demand and energy prices. In addition, GEM-E3_PT technological change, as measured as increased efficiency in the energy system was defined by the output of the BU model. When a market policy instrument is being considered in TIMES_PT, e.g. an energy tax or a feed-in tariff, the respective economic value is also included in GEM-E3_PT, associated with the respective payer and payee sectors. GEM-E3_PT than compute economic drivers, such as sector domestic production, which are converted in energy services demand through a demand generator. Energy services are inputted into TIMES_PT and the model sets the least cost technological profile of the energy system. This cycle establishes a single iteration of the linked models. It continues until convergence is achieved between the models results, which are reached by assuming a stopping threshold, reflecting minimal energy service demand differences from iteration n and the previous (n − 1) (Fig. 2).

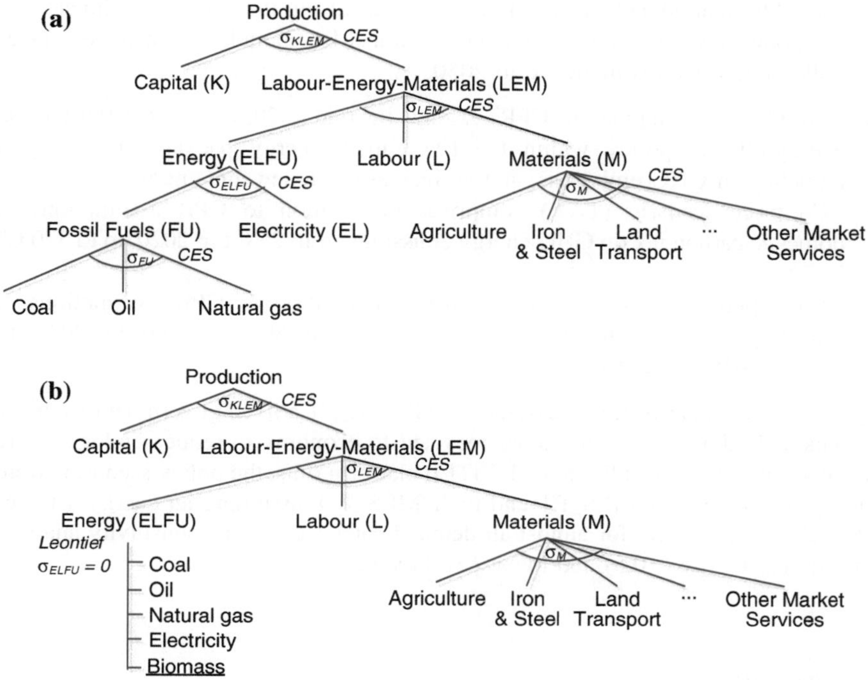

Fig. 1 GEM-E3_PT computable general equilibrium nested tree structure (*upper*—**a**) Original GEM-E3_PT structure (*lower*—**b**) adapted Leontief structure in HYBTEP

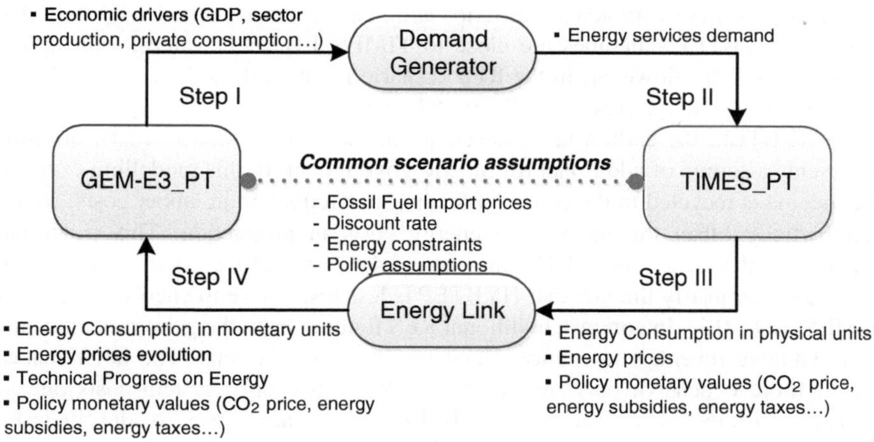

Fig. 2 HYBTEP soft-linking methodology (Fortes et al. 2014)

The additional advantages of HYBTEP in assessing the impact of climate and energy policies when compared with conventional BU model, were analysed under the following scenarios modelled to 2050:

- Current Policy Regulation (CPR) extends beyond 2020, the current Portuguese energy-climate policy within the EU climate-energy package, including a reduction in GHG emissions, and an increase in renewable energy.
- CO_2 price scenario (TAX) comprises in addition to CPR assumptions, a domestic carbon tax on GHG energy emissions from 25 €/t in 2020 up to 370 €/t in 2050.
- RES support scenario (RES) involves, in addition to CPR assumptions, a monetary incentive to renewable energy, from 50 $€_{08}$/MWh in 2020 to 191 $€_{08}$/MWh in 2050.

For all the scenarios it was assumed in GEM-E_PT a fixed government's deficit/surplus and additional revenues are recycled to economy to reduce endogenously social security tax. In addition to HYBTEP platform runs, the policy scenarios were run by the standard TIMES_PT and by TIMES_ED, assuming an energy service-price elasticity of −0.3 for almost all demand categories, and a sensitivity analysis considering higher (−0.5) and lower (−0.1) values.

4.2 Results

The HYBTEP results show, that under TAX and RES scenarios, the modelling tools present differences regarding energy consumption and GHG emissions. It is not possible to define a linear relationship between HYBTEP results and TIMES elasticities, as these vary across scenarios and in some cases years. Under the TAX scenario, HYBTEP outcomes are close to TIMES_ED(−0.1) values, with differences below 1 %. However, in the RES scenario the hybrid model reveals a lower endogenous elasticity, closer to TIMES_PT results.

In HYBTEP, the carbon tax induces an increase in production costs, but also represents a source of additional revenue to government. In this modelling exercise the income is recycled to the economy leading to a reduction in labour costs, which can partially offset the increase in energy costs in production. This economic framework that result in a GDP loss of −2.4 % in 2050 (versus a non-policy scenario), can justify the fact that HYBTEP is less responsive to energy prices than TIMES_ED(−0.3). In contrast, additional RES funding from the government means less available revenues to reduce social security contributions. The latter makes labour more expensive outweighing the decrease in energy system costs due to energy subsidies. The fact that HYBTEP results are close to the inelastic TIMES_PT, suggest that, the reduction of energy prices are offset by an increase in labour costs, leading to a small impact on demand for energy services. In 2050, RES scenario results in GDP gains of 2.8 %, mostly driven by exports increase. Besides ignoring this comprehensive economic context, and with exception of the energy sector (e.g. power or refinery), TIMES neglects the linkages between the sector, i.e., the intermediate consumption. Variations in the production price of one sector, also affect domestic demand in other sectors production, which are not considered by the BU model.

Moreover, the sensitivity analysis of TIMES energy services elasticities highlights the impact of this parameter on the energy system profile. The BU model final energy consumption presented differences [TIMES_PT vis-à-vis TIMES_ED (−0.5)] of up to 14 and −12 % in TAX and RES scenarios, respectively. The uncertainty of elasticity parameters, due to the lack of national studies, increases the uncertainty of the model results when comparing with a more transparent approach from HYBTEP.

4.3 Discussion

HYBTEP represents an evolution in the methodological complexity describing a method of soft-linking 'full-form', multi-sector BU and TD CGE models, resulting in an integrated modelling platform. Since the main structures of the models are maintained, HYBTEP can accommodate an extensive group of technologies and contains a sector detailed economic matrix, considering sectors own characteristics and specificities. The major conclusion concerns the increase of transparency and accuracy of modelling outcomes achieved with HYBTEP, since, by assuming the economic framework of each sector, it enables understanding of the mechanisms behind energy demand evolution while taking into account the cost-effective energy profile from a technological model.

5 Sweden—TIMES-Sweden and EMEC

The Swedish study describes development of full-form soft linkages between the models EMEC (Environmental Medium Term Economic Model—a TD CGE model) and TIMES-Sweden (a BU energy system model). A robust and transparent method to translate simulation results between the two models is developed, resulting in intermediate 'translation models' between EMEC and TIMES-Sweden. EMEC provides demand input to TIMES, while TIMES provides feedback on the energy efficiency parameters, the energy mix, and the prices of electricity and heat. These 'translations' can also be used stand-alone to feed into other energy system models. The presented soft-linking process demonstrates the importance of linking an energy system model with a macroeconomic model when studying energy and climate policy. With the same exogenous parameters, the soft-linking between the models results in a new picture of the economy and the energy system in 2035 compared with the corresponding model results in the absence of soft-linking.

EMEC is a static computable general equilibrium model of the Swedish economy developed and maintained by the National Institute of Economic Research (NIER) for analysis of the interaction between the economy and the environment (Östblom and Berg 2006). The EMEC model includes 26 industries and 33 composite commodities including seven energy commodities. There is also a public sector producing a single commodity. Produced goods and services are exported and used together with imports to create composite commodities for domestic use. Composite commodities are used as inputs by industries and for capital formation. In addition, households consume composite commodities and there are 26 consumer commodities. Production requires primary factors (i.e. two kinds of labour and capital) as well as inputs of materials, transports and energy. Households maximise utility subject to an income restriction, firms maximise profit subject to resource restrictions, the provision of public services is subject to a budget constraint and the foreign sector's import and export activities are governed by an exogenously given trade balance. The model differs from many other CGE models by having a detailed description of the energy use, environmental economic instruments as well as emissions.

The main structure of TIMES-Sweden was designed within the NEEDS and RES2020 projects, and has since been further developed (Krook Riekkola et al. 2011). TIMES-Sweden covers the Swedish energy system divided into six main sectors (Electricity and heat, industry, agriculture, commercial, residential and transport), based on the structure of EUROSTAT database. Each sector includes 60 different demand segments that drive the model. The structure and many of the assumptions are similar to the JRC-EU-TIMES model, documented in Simoes et al. (2013).

Even though the two models have different scientific bases, they both assume cost-minimising behaviour by producers and household demands based on optimising behaviour.

5.1 Methods

The recognition that difference sets of connection points are needed depending on which direction the information is being transferred during the iteration process resulted in two different approaches in mapping of the connection points—one when transferring information from EMEC to TIMES-Sweden and another when transferring information in the opposite direction.

Energy system models are not well suited to address changes in demand due to economic growth. Thus the EMEC model will be the provider of demand drivers from which the demand for goods and services to TIMES-Sweden is estimated. This approach will not differ from running TIMES-Sweden stand-alone, when the demand drivers always are based on results from CGE models like EMEC, the difference will be that they are re-estimated for each iteration-run. All demand segments cannot be treated in the same way and there are cases where no relationship exists between change in demand of a certain commodity and economic growth. Different approaches for translating the output from EMEC into usable input into TIMES-Sweden include; a direct approach based on economic development in a corresponding sector, an indirect approach based on an alternative activity economic development in one or several corresponding sectors, or an assumption of no connections.

Due to their broader focus, CGE models such as EMEC, are unable to explicitly address aspects of the energy system related to (i) changes in energy intensity due to introduction of new technologies, (ii) changes in the energy mix following changes in energy demand and, (iii) changes in electricity and heating prices due to competition of limited energy commodities between and within sectors. These aspects are the focus of the energy system output. To facilitate the transformation of results between TIMES and EMEC, the production function in the soft linked version of EMEC has been changed so that the elasticity between the different energy products in each sector is set to zero, i.e. the energy branch is assumed to be represented by a so-called Leontief structure with fixed input coefficients (Fig. 3).

5.2 Results

In EMEC, the reference scenario describes a possible outcome for the Swedish economy and energy demand in the long run. The reference scenario is based on the official macroeconomic forecast of NIER with the exception of energy efficiency

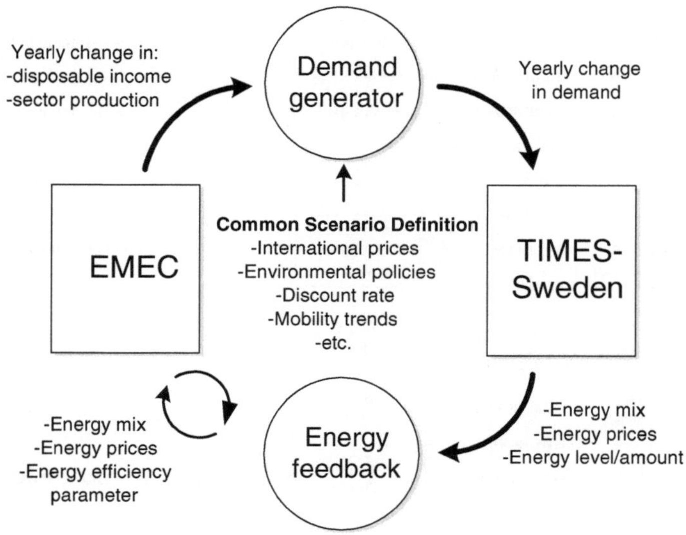

Fig. 3 Soft-linking between EMEC and TIMES-Sweden

parameters, which are determined by soft-linking the two models. In the climate scenario, the CO_2 tax is assumed to increase by 50 % and the CO_2 prices within the EU-ETS is increased from 16 to 30 €/tonne in 2020 and stays at this level to the end of the modelling period in 2035.

The iteration process (Fig. 4) starts with EMEC, whereby its macroeconomic outputs are fed into the translation model, providing a set of energy service demands for TIMES-Sweden. The models adapt to each other primarily in the first reference iteration R-2, and there-after only minor changes are made, while the models are considered converged within tolerance.

The lower demand in energy-intensive industries, after the reference iteration process, can be explained by a higher electricity price from TIMES-Sweden when compared to EMEC in isolation. TIMES-Sweden assumes fewer technology options in energy intensive industries to reduce their demand compared with EMEC, which assumes changes in energy demand based on substitution elasticities. Higher electricity prices and lower substitution possibilities imply increased production costs and a decreased demand for energy-intensive goods as their relative price increases. Soft-linking reinforces the trend towards higher increased demand for transport and services.

The climate scenario is analysed based on three different starting points: a non-linked reference scenario (Climate NL-ref), a non-linked climate scenario (Climate NL-Climate) and a soft-linked scenario (C-x Iteration). In the latter case, when the

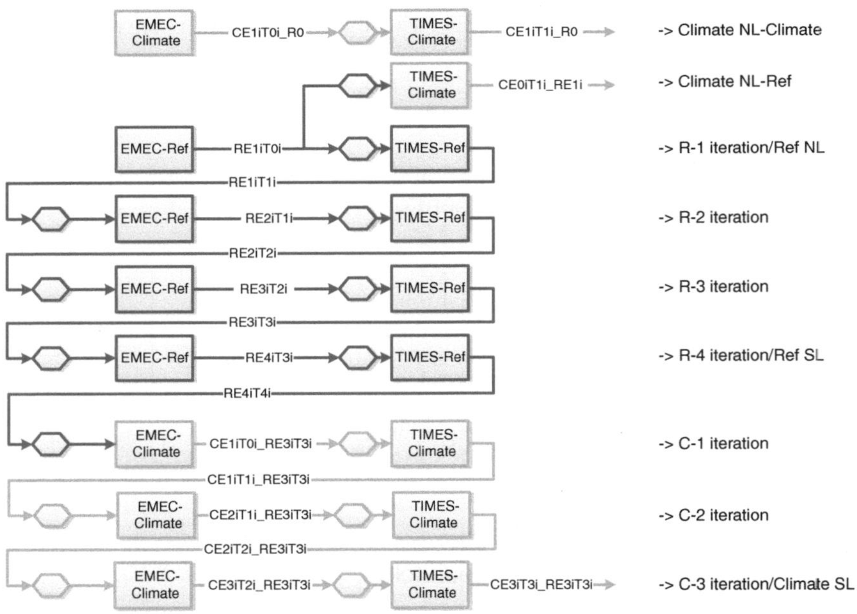

Fig. 4 The iteration scheme between EMEC and TIMES-Sweden

soft linked reference scenario is the starting point of the climate scenario iterations, the number of iterations does not affect the production level from EMEC to any greater extent. Hence, the differences between C-1 and C-3 are small compared with the differences between R-1 and R-2. The results of the EMEC model have already adjusted to mimic TIMES-Sweden's behaviour in the reference scenario. One reason is that the Swedish power system is almost carbon free, which in combination with the green electricity certificate scheme only gives marginal changes in the electricity price when the EU-ETS price is increased.

In order to test of the changes in the results from introducing the soft-linking process had a policy impact the resulting CO_2 trajectories from TIMES-Sweden were scrutinized. The results show the CO_2 emissions are significantly reduced with soft-linking. This is mainly a result of lower demand for energy services.

5.3 Discussion

Both EMEC and TIMES are based on national statistics which has permitted the build-up of detailed models. However the two models are based on two different statistical databases (national accounts versus energy statistics). The national account are structured to capture the main economic activities and thereby facilitate an robust analysis of the economy, while the energy statistics are structured in order capture the energy flows and thereby facilitate a robust energy analysis. When identifying connections points, several overlaps and mismatch were identified. Thus, instead of using common measuring points, we identify direction-specific 'connection points' to describe the interaction of model results from one model to the assumptions used in the other model.

The biggest challenge and uncertainty in soft-linking iteration is the price information from TIMES-Sweden to EMEC. The prices change between the base year in 2008 and the horizon end year 2035 were found to be exaggerated. The main explanation for this is that the calculated prices in the first modelling years do not include all costs. The optimization solves for the lowers total cost, but when the base years are fixed there is no need to include those cost figures when TIMES-Sweden is use stand-alone and comparing the results from different scenarios in a specific year. In contrast, the soft-linking process compares the price difference between two years with one scenario. This particular issue need to be solved in future studies.

Changes in investment flows, due to large structural changes in the energy system were aspects that could not be captured in a satisfactory way in this soft-linking methodology. The presence of a major restructuring of the economy, for example caused by the radical reduction of fossil fuel use, investment flows would most likely change substantially and affect the overall investment requirements and in turn give rise to significant general (dis)equilibrium effects.

6 South-African Electricity Sector—SATIM-el and SAGE

South Africa has a carbon-intensive economy. The energy sector is responsible for most of the country's emissions, with 78.9 % of total emissions from energy. These emissions have resulted from the extensive use of coal in the generation of electricity, the conversion of coal into liquid fuels, and coal for thermal uses in industry.

The Long Term Mitigation Scenarios (LTMS) study found carbon taxes to have the biggest emissions reduction potential compared to various other mitigation options (Winkler 2007). In a developing country like South Africa, it is important that policies and measures aimed at achieving the country's emissions reduction targets are not applied to the detriment of other national development objectives. The hybrid model linking the South African TIMES model (SATIM) to the extended South African General equilibrium model of the economy (e-SAGE) addresses this issue.

SATIM is an inter-temporal bottom-up optimisation energy model of South Africa built around the MARKAL-TIMES platform. SATIM uses linear or mixed integer programming to solve the least-cost planning problem of meeting projected future energy demand, given assumptions about the retirement schedule of existing infrastructure, future fuel costs, future technology costs, and constraints such as the availability of resources.

The e-SAGE model simulates the functioning of the economy and uses South Africa's 2007 Social Accounting Matrix (SAM) as data input, accounting for industries and commodities in South Africa, as well as factor markets, enterprises, households and the 'rest of the world'. The 2007 SAM has 61 industries and 49 commodities. It also has 9 factors of production, namely, land, 4 education based labour groups, and capital which is divided into 1 energy and 3 non-energy capital groups.

6.1 Methods

Alternate runs of SATIM and e-SAGE are performed from 2006 to 2040, each time exchanging information about fuel prices, demand, investment (capital growth), electricity production by technology group and electricity price. Given an initial demand, TIMES computes an investment plan, and a resulting electricity price projection, which is passed onto e-SAGE to see the impact, if any, that this new price projection has on the demand, which then go back to TIMES in the next iteration. The problem is that if both the price and capital growth are imposed onto e-SAGE for the entire model horizon, there is little room for demand to react. Demand tracks the investment (capital growth), which defeats one of the main points of using a CGE.

To circumvent this, only the price projection is imposed onto e-SAGE for the entire model horizon, and the production schedule and capital growth is only gradually imposed. The result of this is that by the end of the planning horizon, we have used a demand projection that is consistent with price, and can react to price changes. Based on this consistency, we can analyse the economic impacts of the investment decisions that were made in the power sector subject to constraints defined in that sector, such as a nuclear programme or a renewables programme, or how the energy and economy would respond to CO_2 mitigation policies.

The following scenarios are run as a demonstration of the linked models for the purpose of evaluating mitigation actions:

1. A set of TIMES runs without the CGE model, but assuming the same demand as the Reference linked model run for all scenarios:
   (a) A Reference case of the power sector without any mitigations actions (Reference).
   (b) A CO_2 tax runs starting at \$5 (R48)/ton CO_2 in 2016, increasing to \$12 (R120)/ton CO_2 in 2025, approximating Treasury's proposed carbon tax.
   (c) Two renewable energy scenarios:
      - 20 % share of centralised generation by 2030 and 30 % in 2040 (RE Prog 1); and
      - 30 % share of centralised generation by 2030 and 40 % in 2040[1] (RE Prog 2).
2. The same set of runs as above but this time with the linked CGE and TIMES models.

6.2 Results

Total capacity of the TIMES reference case reaches 103 GW in 2040, still dominated by coal with 55 GW (54 %). Coal also dominates production, maintaining the current share of around 81 % through to 2040. Gas (open cycle gas turbines and combined cycle gas turbines) capacity reaches 23 GW (23 %) for peaking and mid-merit loads. The remainder is made up of solar PV (13 %), hydro and pump storage (4 %) and nuclear and imports (6 %).

The currently proposed CO_2 tax level has a small impact on the system in this scenario. Total capacity is slightly higher at 106 GW in 2040, due to increased share of gas and solar PV that run at a lower capacity factor than coal. The coal share of capacity drops to 51 % and production to 79 %, whereas gas remains at around 23 % of total capacity. The coal production is mainly replaced by solar PV, increasing its share of production from 6 to 7 %.

[1] RE includes: centralised solar PV, solar thermal, wind, domestic and imported hydro, and biomass.

To reach a share of production of 30 % in 2040 in program 1 and 40 % in program 2, the RE share of capacity reaches 43 and 50 % by 2040. The high share of low-capacity technologies means that total capacity goes up to 120 and 126 GW, respectively. The RE program pushes the coal share of capacity further down to 30 and 19 % for the two programs, respectively. The gas share of capacity reaches 18 and 23 %.

The CO_2 emissions from the power sector of the reference scenario grow to almost double the 2010 levels reaching 430 Mton/annum in 2040. In the CO_2 tax scenario, the annual CO_2 drops by only 3 % relative to reference case. However, when using the more optimistic RE costs, a 20 % reduction is observed. When the penetration of low emission technologies is imposed directly with the RE programs, the CO_2 emissions drop more radically by 33 and 50 %, respectively by 2040.

Comparing the TIMES runs and the CGE-linked runs for the reference case and the CO_2 tax case, the reference cases are identical, given that they have the same demand, and fuel prices. In the CO_2 tax scenario though, there is a drop of the peak demand in the CGE-linked run, showing some demand response from the CGE to the higher electricity price.

All the policy scenarios result in slight GDP loss in 2040 relative to the reference case. In all the policy scenarios, the mining and metals sectors are the most negatively affected, mainly because of the electricity price increase, and the switch away from coal for some of the electricity production. The electricity sector grows quite significantly relative to the base with more investment taking place in this sector, however, not enough to avoid a net negative impact on GDP.

6.3 Discussion

The results so far indicate that the linked SATIM e-SAGE model is able to contribute to the goal of analysing the trade-off between mitigation and development objectives for South Africa. However, to gain further confidence in the results, more work is still needed in aligning both models, by ensuring consistency between other energy consuming sectors, not only in terms of their energy consumption, but also in terms of how the capital and labour costs computed in e-SAGE affect energy sector decisions in SATIM.

7 Danish—IntERACT

As a part of the Energy Agreement from 2012 all parties in the Danish Parliament except one agreed on an ambitious plan for phasing out fossil fuels for energy in Denmark. In 2035 the power and heating sector has to be without fossil fuels and all of the Danish energy system has to be independent of fossil fuels by 2050. As a part of the agreement and to support future planning, a new energy policy analysis model has to be developed.

The model outlined here is decided to be a combination of a CGE model for the Danish economy (CGE-IntERACT) linked with a TIMES model of the Danish energy system (IntERACT-TIMES-DK). The CGE and the TIMES model are being developed simultaneously to secure optimal structural fit and data harmonisation in the linking between the models. A soft-linking approach is chosen and energy demand in form of services are sent from the CGE to TIMES and fuel mix, energy use, energy cost and energy service prices are returned to the CGE.

The IntERACT project is developing a novel CGE approach modelling the energy service demand within its economic CGE model, rather than the typical approach of modelling specific energy goods such as oil, gas, coal or electricity. As has already been indicated in Sect. 5.3 the traditional approach is not well suited when analysing large scale technological changes such as in the case of a complete green transition and phase out of fossil fuels. The demands for comfortable room temperature, lighting, transport services and process energy are the basic needs of the economy, and it is the impact of the relative costs of these services that have significant influence on the economic behaviour.

The premise in the IntERACT model is that agents make economic decisions based on the relative prices of energy services, while the specific fuel use and the specific technology applied in order to obtain the energy service is secondary; i.e. economic utility or revenue is not derived from the amount of energy (PJ) of fuel consumed, but rather from the energy services the fuel actually delivers. This leads on from the concept of exergy and useful work as a productive element in the economy, as opposed to gross energy consumption. Agents maximise profit and utility using the costs of the energy service, using relative prices as usual. By using energy services in this method, the economic TD model creates an abstraction of energy and in a sense reduces the role of exact technologies. Indeed the TD model does not make any technological decisions to obtain a given amount of energy services. From the consumers perspective it does not matter how the room is heated (with an explicit technology choice), but rather how much the costs relative to inputs in the production or goods in the utility bundle vary.

8 Norway—Regional Effects of Energy Policy (RegPol)

The goal of the RegPol[2] project is to develop a hybrid energy-economy framework for Norway with special attention to the regional level, combining the technology rich bottom-up TIMES model with a top-down multi-sector economic computable general equilibrium (CGE) model. CGE-models focus on the interaction between different supply and demand sectors, and are developed to study effects of different policy proposals that apply different instruments within and across the sectors of an

[2] The RegPol project is financed by the Norwegian Research Council. Collaborative research partners are SINTEF Technology and society, NTNU and IFE.

economy. CGE-models usually do not include much technical detail, and have little information on the underlying infrastructure.

The majority of research has addressed the national and international level. The RegPol project focuses on the need to better understand how energy policies affect local decisions and how local advantages can be used actively in regional policy addressing implications for the energy sector. Both models will have a subnational geographical level with multiple regions. The TIMES model will have a geographical representation of the energy system, while the CGE model will describe the regional multi-sector economies plus trade and transport between regions. These models are called spatial CGE models (SCGE) and include modelling elements from new economic geography.

A regional model framework is needed to assess the effect of technology drivers on the deployment of technologies, localisation of new large scale production and changes in end use. Parameters, such as energy demand, population density, local electricity production, untapped resources, available energy infrastructure and geographical conditions influence the future regional development.

The model structures will be general, but a relevant geographical division for analysing energy policies consists of the Norwegian electricity price areas. Some areas have significant power surpluses while others have significant power deficits. Together with transmission constraints, this is relevant for location of both new production and new consumption. Some relevant analysis cases are:

- In Norway there is a political objective to build a substantial amount of renewable energy supported by green electricity certificates. Norway has excellent wind resources, and the RegPol project will analyse which project locations are advantageous, and how projects will affect regional development.
- The electrification of offshore oil and gas fields in order to avoid greenhouse gas emissions would constitute major electricity consumers. Such projects have created strained power situations, and should be analysed within a regional hybrid modelling framework such as RegPol.
- There has been increased focus on Norway's potential to store water in reservoirs. Norwegian hydropower could play a balancing role as a green battery within a European power system with a high share of power production from intermittent sources as wind and sun. This will require new production capacity and new interconnections to be built, both internally to access export links, and to the export markets.
- Development of the grid infrastructure is in itself an important question to analyse. Low transmission capacities may induce different price-levels between price areas, with corresponding consequences for regional industries and other demand.

The hybrid framework with TIMES and the SCGE model will be designed for efficient successive exchanges of adjusted solutions. Different designs for linking the models are investigated, both soft-linking, hard-linking and full integration. The higher data granularity, the more important it becomes to handle data exchange with automatic routines. RegPol starts with a soft-linking approach, but seeks to automate the linking and embed it in the hybrid framework.

Since production and consumption takes place in different locations, the spatial characteristics are important in order to find optimal solutions and effective policies. Various policies (like energy taxes and subsidies) also have regional rates and different regional impacts. The combination of technological and economical models with regional resolution is well suited to improve current analyses and provide the best guidance for future sustainable solutions.

9 Critical Messages from Applied Hybrid Methods

There are many useful points to note in this state of the art review of IEA-ETSAP hybrid energy-economy modelling. A final synthesis of the critical messages from all of the model applications and discussions are summarised below.

A restructured low carbon world economy is imperative to mitigate climate change. Modelling results repeatedly show global CO_2 emissions are significantly lower in hybrid model decarbonisation scenarios as a result of demand adjustments. The range of the differences between isolated energy system CO_2 emissions and their comparable hybrid model is between −5 and −13 % by 2050 depending on the carbon intensity of the region in question's economy.

Economic impacts vary regionally again dependent upon the energy intensity of a nation's economy, the trade partnerships, competitiveness and level of development. Loss of GDP can be as high as 5 %/year by 2050 in developing countries, while up to 3 %/year by 2050 in developed countries depending on the implemented mitigation mechanisms and revenue recycling schemes. Short term economic gains are to be made in energy efficiency measures.

Both energy system models and CGE models play an important role in the existing energy and climate policy analyses. Even when running the two kinds of models in isolation, the models use assumptions which are based on results from the other model (directly and indirectly). Thus, by soft-linking energy system models and CGE models the energy and climate policy analysis becomes more transparent.

Hybrid Models have already played a critical role in carbon mitigation policy and should continue to play a key role in policy advice in upcoming COP talks. Hybrid energy-economy modelling has an increasingly key role to play in accurately modelling the economic impact of climate mitigation, while addressing the most cost-effective technological solutions.

Furthermore, hybrid linking displays non-linear, sectoral non-uniform demand responses that cannot be captured with demand price elasticities, increasing the understanding and transparency of the model results. Model methodological and documentation transparency is a critical moving beyond publishing and presenting papers. Replicability is near impossible and makes difficult the traditional scientific process. A move to more open models is required for more rigorous validation of models and model results.

A challenge and source of uncertainty in soft-linking hybrid models is the price information from bottom up optimisation models to top down models. The price change between the base year and the end of horizon year are found to be exaggerated. The main explanation for this is that the calculated prices in the first modelling years do not include all costs. The optimization solves for the lowers total cost, but when the base years are fixed there is no need to include those cost figures. In contrast, the soft-linking process compares the price difference between two years with one scenario. This particular issue need to be solved in future studies.

Changes in investment flows, due to large structural changes in the energy system are difficult to satisfactorily capture in typical soft-linking methodologies. A major restructuring of the economy as a result of a radical reduction of fossil fuel use would most likely change investment flows substantially and affect the overall investment requirements. In turn this would give rise to significant general (dis) equilibrium effects resulting in model uncertainty.

References

Allan G, Lecca P, McGregor P et al (2012) The impact of the introduction of a carbon tax for Scotland. University of Strathclyde, Glasgow

Allan G, McGregor PG, Swales JK, Turner K (2007) Impact of alternative electricity generation technologies on the Scottish economy: An illustrative input-output analysis. Proc Inst Mech Eng Part J Power Energy 221:243–254. doi:10.1243/09576509JPE301

Arrow KJ, Debreu G (1954) Existence of an equilibrium for a competitive economy. Econometrica 22:265–290. doi:10.2307/1907353

Bataille C, Jaccard M, Nyboer J, Rivers N (2006) Towards general equilibrium in a technology-rich model with empirically estimated behavioral parameters. Energy J 93–112

BERR (2007) Energy white paper: meeting the energy challenge. Department of Business Enterprise and Regulatory Reform, London

Capros P, Georgakopoulos T, Van Regemorter D et al (1997) The GEM-E3 general equilibrium model for the European Union. J Econ Financ Model 4:51–160

Capros P, Paroussos L, Fragkos P et al (2014) European decarbonisation pathways under alternative technological and policy choices: a multi-model analysis. Energy Strategy Rev 2:231–245. doi:10.1016/j.esr.2013.12.007

DEFRA (2007) MARKAL MACRO analysis of long run costs of climate change mitigation targets. Department of Environment, Food and Rural Affairs, London

FES (2003) Options for a low carbon future—phase 2. Future Energy Solutions (part of AEA Technology plc), London

Fortes P, Pereira R, Pereira A, Seixas J (2014) Integrated technological-economic modeling platform for energy and climate policy analysis. Energy 73:716–730. doi:10.1016/j.energy.2014.06.075

Fortes P, Simões S, Seixas J et al (2013) Top-down and bottom-up modelling to support low-carbon scenarios: climate policy implications. Clim Policy 13:285–304. doi:10.1080/14693062.2013.768919

Huntington HG, Weyant JP, Sweeney JL (1982) Modeling for insights, not numbers: the experiences of the energy modeling forum. Omega 10:449–462. doi:10.1016/0305-0483(82)90002-0

Jebaraj S, Iniyan S (2006) A review of energy models. Renew Sustain Energy Rev 10:281–311. doi:10.1016/j.rser.2004.09.004

Krook Riekkola A, Ahlgren EO, Söderholm P (2011) Ancillary benefits of climate policy in a small open economy: the case of Sweden. Energy Policy 39:4985–4998. doi:10.1016/j.enpol.2011.06.015

Kypreos S (1996) The MARKAL-MACRO model and the climate change. Paul Scherrer Institut (PSI), Villigen

Kypreos S, Lehtila A (2013) TIMES-MACRO: decomposition into hard-linked LP and NLP problems. IEA-ETSAP

Labriet M, Drouet L, Vielle M et al (2015) Assessment of the effectiveness of global climate policies using coupled bottom-up and top-down models. Les Cahiers du GERAD, G-2010-30 revised in January 2015, Montreal, Canada, p 22

Laitner JA, DeCanio SJ, Koomey JG, Sanstad AH (2003) Room for improvement: increasing the value of energy modeling for policy analysis. Util Policy 11:87–94. doi:10.1016/S0957-1787(03)00020-1

Loulou R, Labriet M (2008) ETSAP-TIAM: the TIMES integrated assessment model part I: model structure. Comput Manag Sci 5:7–40. doi:10.1007/s10287-007-0046-z

Loulou R, Remme U, Kanudia A et al (2005) Documentation for the TIMES model

Manne A, Mendelsohn R, Richels R (1995) MERGE: a model for evaluating regional and global effects of GHG reduction policies. Energy Policy 23:17–34. doi:10.1016/0301-4215(95)90763-W

Messner S, Schrattenholzer L (2000) MESSAGE–MACRO: linking an energy supply model with a macroeconomic module and solving it iteratively. Energy 25:267–282. doi:10.1016/S0360-5442(99)00063-8

Negishi T (1972) General equilibrium theory and international trade. North-Holland Pub. Co, Amsterdam

Nordhaus WD (2007) A review of the Stern review on the economics of climate change. J Econ Lit 45:686–702. doi:10.1257/jel.45.3.686

Östblom G, Berg C (2006) The EMEC model: version 2.0

Pearce D (2003) The social cost of carbon and its policy implications. Oxf Rev Econ Policy 19:362–384

Pilavachi PA, Dalamaga T, Rossetti di Valdalbero D, Guilmot J-F (2008) Ex-post evaluation of European energy models. Energy Policy 36:1726–1735. doi:10.1016/j.enpol.2008.01.028

RCEP (2000) Energy—the changing climate. Royal Commission on Environmental Pollution, London

Remme U, Blesl M (2006) Documentation of the TIMES-MACRO model. ETSAP

Rutherford TF (1992) Sequential joint maximization. Boulder, Colorado

Simoes S, Nijs W, Ruiz P et al (2013) The JRC-EU-TIMES model assessing the long-term role of the SET plan energy technologies. Publications Office, Luxembourg

Stern N (2006) The economics of climate change: the Stern review. HM Treasury, London

Strachan N, Kannan R (2008) Hybrid modelling of long-term carbon reduction scenarios for the UK. Energy Econ 30:2947–2963. doi:10.1016/j.eneco.2008.04.009

Strachan N, Pye S, Kannan R (2009) The iterative contribution and relevance of modelling to UK energy policy. Energy Policy 37:850–860. doi:10.1016/j.enpol.2008.09.096

Winebrake JJ, Sakva D (2006) An evaluation of errors in US energy forecasts: 1982–2003. Energy Policy 34:3475–3483. doi:10.1016/j.enpol.2005.07.018

Winkler H (2007) Long term mitigation scenarios. Technical Report Energy Research Centre for Department of Environment Affairs and Tourism, Pretoria, South Africa

Assessing Climate Impacts on the Energy Sector with TIAM-WORLD: Focus on Heating and Cooling and Hydropower Potential

Maryse Labriet, Markus Biberacher, Philip B. Holden, Neil R. Edwards, Amit Kanudia and Richard Loulou

Abstract Much research is still needed to understand the climate vulnerability of the energy sector and to identify cost-effective adaptation options. This chapter explores the coupling of the World TIMES Integrated Assessment Model (TIAM-WORLD) with an emulated version of the climate model PLASIM-ENTS to assess the impacts of future temperature and precipitation changes on the heating and cooling subsector and available hydropower. An absence of climate feedback induced by the adaptation of the energy system to future heating and cooling needs was found for a 1.6–5.7 °C range of long-term global mean temperature increase: when aggregated at the global level, some changes compensate others, and heating and cooling represent a relatively small contributor to total energy consumption. However, significant changes are observed at the regional level in terms of additional power capacity, mostly coal power plants, to satisfy the additional cooling needs. Reduced needs for heating affect gas and coal heating systems more than

M. Labriet (✉)
Eneris Environment Energy Consultants, Madrid, Spain
e-mail: maryse.labriet@enerisconsultants.com

M. Biberacher
Research Studios Austria Forschungsgesellschaft mbH, Salzburg, Austria
e-mail: markus.biberacher@researchstudio.at

P.B. Holden · N.R. Edwards
Environment, Earth and Ecosystems, Open University, Milton Keynes, UK
e-mail: philip.holden@open.ac.uk

N.R. Edwards
e-mail: neil.edwards@open.ac.uk

A. Kanudia
KanORS-EMF, Noida, India
e-mail: amit@KanORS.com

R. Loulou
McGill University, Montréal, Canada
e-mail: richardloulou@gmail.com

G. Giannakidis et al. (eds.), *Informing Energy and Climate Policies Using Energy Systems Models*, Lecture Notes in Energy 30,
DOI 10.1007/978-3-319-16540-0_21

biomass and electric heaters, reflecting higher costs of these heating options in the longer term. Available hydropower is estimated to increase on a seasonal basis in most regions under future climate change. It could therefore contribute to supply the additional electricity needed for cooling in regions where both future cooling needs and hydropower potential are expected to increase. Hydropower results are however characterized by high uncertainty due to uncertainties in projected precipitation changes as well as the relatively coarse resolution of PLASIM-ENTS.

1 Introduction

Until recently, decision-makers within the energy sector have focused their interest on emission mitigation, given the contribution of energy to greenhouse gas emissions. However, the interest in climate risk management in the energy sector is growing, acknowledging that changes in weather patterns due to climate change can have severe implications for both the demand and supply sides of the energy sector (Mideksa and Kallbekken 2010; Ebinger and Vergara 2011; Schaeffer et al. 2012). The most recent Assessment Report of the Intergovernmental Panel on Climate Change concludes that "*the energy sector will be transformed by climate policy* (…) *but impacts of climate changes too will be important for secure and reliable energy supply*" (Arent et al. 2014).

Climate change may result in the following impacts on energy demand and production.

- Space heating and cooling requirements vary according to air temperature. Several studies assess these impacts often using engineering approaches, such as Wilbanks et al. (2007b) for the USA, Aebischer et al. (2007) for Switzerland and Europe, Akpinar-Ferrand and Singh (2010) for India, Isaac and van Vuuren (2009) and Mima and Criqui (2009) at global level. Impacts are expected to vary between different fuel sectors: on the one hand climate change may result in an increase in net annual electricity and electricity-peaking demand, driven, for instance, by additional cooling requirements and stressing the installed capacity and grids; on the other hand, demands for heating energy sources, possibly not electricity, may decline (Wilbanks et al. 2007a). The overall balance will depend on geographic, demographic, economic, building and technological conditions (Arent et al. 2014).
- Changes in water and air temperature modify the cooling efficiency of thermal and nuclear power generation, resulting in modified availability and efficiency of plants. Except in the case of extreme events, the average impact of future climate change is expected to remain small at the level of each plant (Durmayaz and Oguz Salim 2006; Linnerud et al. 2011; Rubbelke and Vogele 2011); however, the need for adaptation of the overall energy sector might be non-negligible

given the high share of fossil and nuclear power plants in some regions of the globe. Van Vliet et al. (2012) estimate a summer average decrease in the capacity of power plants of 6.3–19 % in Europe and 4.4–16 % in the United States, depending on cooling system type and climate scenario for 2031–2060.
- Changes in seasonal river flows and their variability, resulting from changes in precipitation patterns and surface water discharges, may affect hydropower potential and generation. Hydropower represents a large share of the electricity mix of several countries and of the renewable energy sources at the global level. Moreover, hydropower plants usually have a long lifetime. Given these different factors, the assessment of climate change impacts is likely to be crucial for this source of energy. Lehner et al. (2005) estimates that the hydropower potential for the whole of Europe could decline by 6 % by 2070 (20–50 % decrease around the Mediterranean, 15–30 % increase in Northern and Eastern Europe, stable hydropower pattern for western and central Europe). Hamududu and Killingtveit (2012) estimate that most of the high hydropower-producing countries in Northern regions (Canada, United States and parts of Europe and Russia) will have increased generation, while for most of the other regions, hydropower generation will decrease. Mima and Criqui (2009) estimate an average increase of the world hydro electricity generation of up to 7 % in 2100 resulting from climate change (+12 % in North America, +13 % in Commonwealth of Independent States, +7 and 6 % in Japan and Australasia, −2 % in Western Europe). Reduction in available capacity may reach 7 % in some regions of Brazil by the end of the century (Lucena et al. 2009).
- Changes in wind and solar conditions remain uncertain and will be highly dependent on regional characteristics (IPCC 2011). The relatively short lifespan of solar and wind technologies implies that the facilities would be replaced over time and therefore could spontaneously adapt to new local climate conditions or room would remain for relocation (Ebinger and Vergara 2011).
- The impact of altered soil conditions and precipitation on future available crops and bioenergy is expected to be relatively small on a global basis, but with large and uncertain regional differences (IPCC 2011). CO_2 fertilization as well as diet are considered as crucial factors of uncertainties on future bioenergy (Haberl et al. 2011).
- Finally, energy-related infrastructure is vulnerable to extreme events and sea level rise, which could affect localization of plants and security of supply (Craig 2011).

Much research is still needed to understand the climate vulnerability of the energy sector and to identify cost-effective adaptation options (Arent et al. 2014). Using MARKAL Norway, Seljom et al. (2011) assessed the impacts of climate change on the energy system of Norway. The objective of this chapter is to explore the coupling of the World TIMES Integrated Assessment Model (TIAM-WORLD) with an emulated version of the climate model Planet-Simulator coupled to the Efficient Numerical Terrestrial Scheme (PLASIM-ENTS) in order to assess the impacts of future temperature and precipitation changes on heating and cooling subsector and available hydropower.

The methodological framework is presented in Sect. 2, and results are described in Sect. 3.

2 Methodological Framework

2.1 TIAM-WORLD

The TIMES Integrated Assessment Model (TIAM-WORLD) is a technology-rich model of the entire energy/emission system of the World split into 16 regions,[1] providing a detailed representation of the procurement, transformation, trade, and consumption of a large number of energy forms (Loulou 2008; Loulou and Labriet 2008).

It is an incarnation of The Integrated MARKAL-EFOM System (TIMES) economic paradigm and computes an inter-temporal dynamic partial equilibrium on energy and emission markets based on the maximization of total surplus, defined as the sum of suppliers and consumers surpluses. In other words, the model finds the optimal (cost-efficient) energy and technology mix to satisfy demands for energy services like lighting, cooking, heating, cooling of houses, car usage, trucks, aluminum production, cement production, etc. Each demand may vary endogenously in alternate scenarios, in response to endogenous price changes.

The model contains explicit detailed descriptions of more than 1500 technologies and several hundred energy, emission and demand flows in each region. Such technological detail provides a precise description of technology and fuel competition in the entire energy system, where changes in one sector may have direct and indirect impacts on other sectors. The model is set up to explore the development of the World energy system until 2100. The model is calibrated to 2005 energy statistics of the International Energy Agency (IEA 2013a, b).

TIAM-WORLD integrates a climate module for the modeling of global changes related to greenhouse gas concentrations, radiative forcing and temperature increase. The module includes separate cycles for CO_2, CH_4, and N_2O, and also accounts for the additional forcing introduced by other causes, natural and anthropogenic. The total atmospheric forcing is then introduced into equations that simulate the changes in mean temperatures of two layers: surface, and deep ocean. The climate module provides a very useful means of simulating scenarios with specific climate targets, be they on concentration, forcing, or temperature.

---

[1] Africa (AFR), Australia-New Zealand (AUS), Canada (CAN), United States (USA), Mexico (MEX), Central and South America (CSA), China (CHI), India (IND), Japan (JAP), South Korea (SKO), Other Developing Asia (ODA), Middle East (MEA), Europe of 27 + Switzerland, Norway and Iceland (EUR), Other East Europe (OEE), Russia (RUS), Central Asia and Caucasia (CAC). OPEC and Non-OPEC disaggregation is considered within each region, when relevant.

2.2 PLASIM-ENTS

One of the principal obstacles to coupling complex climate models to the range of models needed to assess climate impacts in different sectors is the computational expense of the climate models. Replacing the climate model with an emulated version of its input/output response function circumvents this problem without compromising the possibility of including feedbacks and non-linear responses (Holden and Edwards 2010). The climate model emulator used here is PLASIM-ENTSem (Holden et al. 2014), an emulation of PLASIM (Fraedrich et al. 2005) coupled to the ENTS vegetation and land surface model (Williamson et al. 2006), here run at T21 resolution (approximately 5°).

PLASIM-ENTS has a 3D dynamic atmosphere, flux-corrected slab ocean and slab sea ice, and dynamic coupled vegetation (anthropogenic land use change is not represented in PLASIM-ENTS, but changes due to natural vegetation dynamics are represented). The seasonal and regional validations of both PLASIM-ENTS and PLASIM-ENTSem are described in detail in Holden et al. (2014). Figure 1 presents climate changes at 2100 under a radiative forcing corresponding to the representative concentration pathway RCP8.5 (Moss et al. 2010) where temperature increase reaches 4.7 °C in 2100. In summary, the emulator performs generally very well in capturing the spatial variability and magnitude of warming simulated by more complex models. The neglect of the sea-ice feedback in the configuration used in the current analysis results in understated warming in the Arctic in December-January-February. Although caution will be required, this error dominantly affects temperatures in sparsely populated high-northern latitudes and so may not be problematic for large-scale human impact studies. In terms of precipitation-evaporation, the increase is particularly strong in India in June-July-August as a result of a strengthening of the South-east Asian monsoon in PLASIM-ENTS, attributed as likely due to the neglect of aerosol forcing in the model. This increase should therefore not be regarded as robust.

The climate data required for the assessment of heating and cooling changes due to climate changes can be summarized in terms of Heating Degree Days (HDDs) and Cooling Degree Days (HDDs), which are the number of degrees respectively below and above the temperature levels from which heating or cooling are needed. Seasonal HDDs and CDDs are computed at each of the 2048 PLASIM-ENTS grid cells as described in Holden et al. (2014). The baseline temperature for both heating and cooling is fixed to 18 °C globally (discussion about this choice is included in Sect. 3.1). The mapping of the PLASIM-ENTSem degree-day data onto TIAM-WORLD regions relies on a population-weighted average over the grid cells that comprise a given region of TIAM-WORLD, considering 2005 population distribution data. In other words, while demographic changes *between* TIAM regions are considered in the assessment of energy needs, possible changes in distribution *within* TIAM regions are not considered. Such changes could have important impacts on the future needs for cooling and heating, and would deserve a better

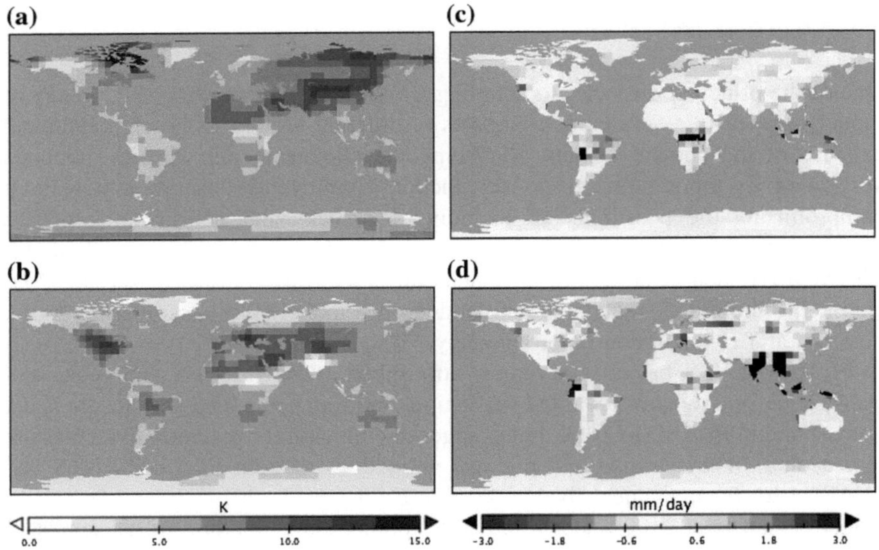

Fig. 1 Emulated climate change 2100–2000 under RCP8.5. **a** Dec-Jan-Feb warming, **b** Jun-Jul-Aug warming, **c** Dec-Jan-Feb precipitation minus evaporation increase, **d** Jun-Jul-Aug precipitation minus evaporation increase. Plotted data was calculated with the released version of PLASIM-ENTSem, which captures dynamic Arctic sea ice. *Note* Scales conceal 3K cooling and 14 mm/day increase in precipitation-evaporation in JJA India; these anomalous changes are driven by a simulated strengthening of the SE Asian monsoon which is not regarded as robust

consideration in future applications. Approximations due to different resolutions of data were addressed in the mapping (Holden et al. 2014).

2.3 Coupling of Models

Figure 2 summarizes the exchange of data between TIAM-WORLD and the emulator of PLASIM-ENTS, described in this section. Information exchange between models is handled by a fully automated script that launches models, reads output of one and creates input for the next.

2.3.1 Heating and Cooling

The drivers of future heating and cooling demands in TIAM-WORLD reflect changes in socio-economical characteristics of the countries, but do not consider changes in future temperature. Moreover, the climate module of TIAM-WORLD does not compute the regional or seasonal temperature changes required for a

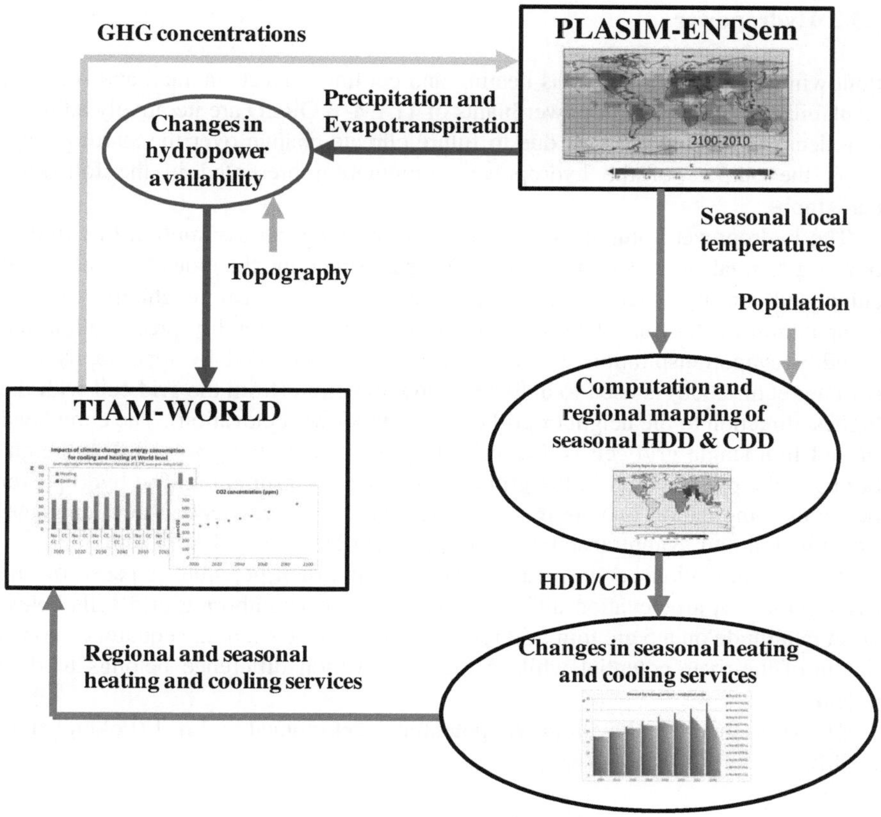

Fig. 2 Principles of the coupling between TIAM-WORLD and PLASIM-ENTSem for heating/cooling and hydropower

relevant representation of the possible heating and cooling adjustments due to climate change. The coupling of TIAM-WORLD with an emulator of the climate model PLASIM-ENTS provides this additional information.

In essence, there is an iterative exchange of data between the two models: TIAM-WORLD sends a time series of endogenously computed total greenhouse gas concentrations to the climate emulator. The climate emulator sends the seasonal and regional temperatures, converted into seasonal heating and cooling degree-days for each of the regions of the model, to TIAM-WORLD. These seasonal and regional degree-days are in turn used to compute new seasonal (3 seasons) and regional (16 regions) heating and cooling demands in TIAM-WORLD, by adjusting these demands proportionally to the changes of HDDs and CDDs of each region with respect to the values of the base year (Labriet et al. 2013). A new supply-demand equilibrium can then be computed by the model.

2.3.2 Hydropower

Following the same principle as heating and cooling impacts, annual and seasonal availability factors of hydropower plants of TIAM-WORLD are iteratively adjusted to reflect the relative changes due to future climate change over the starting year, using the outputs of the hydropower computation presented in the following paragraphs.

The hydropower computation is based on the physical assumption that hydropower potential at a certain location is determined by the potential energy of cumulated run-off water at this location relative to the near neighborhood. The computation of the run-off water relies on topography, monthly precipitation and monthly evapotranspiration. Elevation information provided by topography data (Fischer et al. 2008) is used to define the flow direction (from the grid cell with the highest direction to the neighbor grid cell with the lowest elevation). The cumulated run-off in a single grid cell is determined by inflow into the grid cell from neighboring cells, precipitation in the grid cell and evapotranspiration. The hydropower potential computation is done in a separate module which is coded in c language. Precipitation and evapotranspiration are provided by PLASIM-ENTSem.

The differentiation between run-of-the-river and dam potential is based on the assumption that an elevation difference between two neighboring grid cells below 50 m in altitude on a 5 arc min grid resolution (around 1 km at the equator) belongs to run-of-the-river potential while a higher elevation difference belongs to dam potential.

The gross theoretical hydropower potential is determined by Eq. 1 (Pokhrel et al. 2008):

$$E_i = m_i * g * \Delta h_i \quad \text{for all } i \tag{1}$$

where

E_i potential energy of run-off water in grid cell i
m_i mass of run-off water in grid cell i
g average gravity acceleration
Δh_i elevation difference between grid cell i and lowest neighboring grid cell

Land cover information was used to identify areas such as permanent snow and ice covered areas, protected areas or built-up areas in order to assume a realistic share of utilizable potential compared to the theoretically calculated potential.

This calculation provides a gross theoretically utilizable hydro power potential for each single grid cell, followed by dynamic aggregation of the resulting grid cell based hydropower potential over predefined regions of TIAM-WORLD.

Hydropower potentials computed with the above methodology are of the same order of magnitude as those obtained by Pokhrel et al. (2008) using the same approach except in Asia, where the potential reaches 37 TWh rather than 22 TWh. The high South-east Asian monsoon observed in summer (JJA) in PLASIM-ENTS certainly contributes to this higher potential, reinforced by the high elevation differences in the region. Indeed, small deviations in precipitation and evaporation could translate into much higher deviations in hydropower when multiplied by high elevation difference. In addition to this factor, geographic resolution of the computation of elevation and flow direction is expected to be a possibly high source of differences across studies: since flow direction has a direct impact on the assignment of hydropower potentials to certain locations, an averaging of the flow direction caused by weaker resolutions may result in wrong geographical assignments of the hydro power potential. Finally, not all factors that trigger hydropower potentials are considered, such as changes in sediment loads.

3 Results

3.1 Heating and Cooling

Scenarios. The assessment of climate change impacts on the energy system relies on a series of 12 different future states of the climate system. For the purpose of this exercise, focused on the understanding of the adaptation of the energy system to future climate changes, emission mitigation in the energy system is deliberately excluded and possible changes in the radiative forcing are artificially assumed to be due to non-energy factors.

In all Figures, CCx.x corresponds to scenarios with a long-term mean temperature increase of x.x °C at the global level. The range of long-term global mean temperature increase covered in the study is 1.6–5.7 °C. It is important to remember that regional temperature increases, as computed by PLASIM-ENTSem, will in general be different and these are used to assess the changes in heating and cooling. The case without considering the impact of climate change (NoCC) assumes the same global average temperature as today.

Based on Labriet et al. (2013), with kind permission of Springer Science +Business Media.

The long-term temperature increase obtained with the exogenous radiative forcing included in TIAM-WORLD is 3.3 °C. Regional HDD and CDD in this scenario, calculated with regional temperatures computed by PLASIM-ENTSem, are illustrated in Fig. 3, where different categories of regions can be identified: colder regions (high levels of HDD) where the main expected impact of climate change is a reduction of heating services, warmer regions (high levels of CDD) where the main expected impact of climate change is an increase of cooling services, regions with intermediate climate where both heating and cooling appear to be important and the net impact of climate change may depend on each region.

Global climate feedback. The first question concerns the magnitude of the feedback on the climate system of the changes observed in the energy system due to heating and cooling adaptation. Indeed, the increase of electricity generation for cooling, if not compensated by the decrease of energy use for heating, may be a

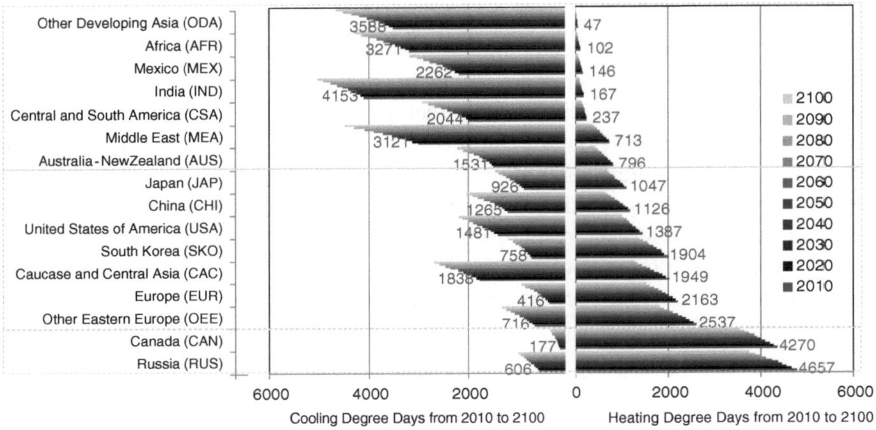

Fig. 3 Annual HDD and CDD corresponding to a long-term global average temperature increase of 3.3 °C. Numbers for 2010 are indicated in *red*. Based on Labriet et al. (2013), with kind permission of Springer Science+Business Media

source of additional greenhouse gases, which could accelerate climate change. Results demonstrate that changes in CO_2 emissions resulting from adjusted heating and cooling (Fig. 4) are not sufficient to have an impact on the climate system; in other words, no feedback between the energy and climate systems at the global level was discernible, on the time horizon considered (2100). This does not mean that the impacts of climate change on heating and cooling are negligible. It means that when aggregated at the global level, some changes compensate others, and that heating and cooling represent relatively small contributors to total energy consumption (Fig. 5).

Combined heating and cooling in the total energy balance. The share of combined heating and cooling energy consumption is small at the global level compared to the total energy consumption (less than 10 %), and varies from less than 3 % in regions like India and Africa, to more than 25 % in regions like Other Eastern Europe, Canada and Russia (Fig. 5). Changes of the share in the case without climate change reflect both socio-economic drivers in energy services (population growth, economic development) and technology dynamics (type and efficiency of technologies to provide the services). The difference between the shares obtained with and without climate change impacts illustrates a small net decrease of total energy consumed for combined heating and cooling needs in regions with a cold climate, and a small net increase of total energy consumed for combined heating and cooling needs in regions with a warm climate.

Fuel perspective. Impacts of heating and cooling adaptation to future climate change vary at the regional level (Fig. 6). In total, energy for heating and cooling decreases in China and Russia (domination of heating changes), increases in India, Central and South America and United States (domination of cooling change), and remains almost stable in Europe and at the World level (compensation).

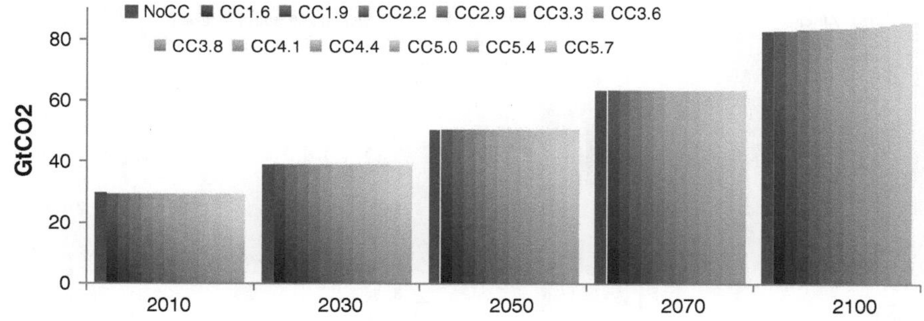

Fig. 4 Global CO_2 emissions from the energy system resulting from changes in heating and cooling in 12 different temperature scenarios

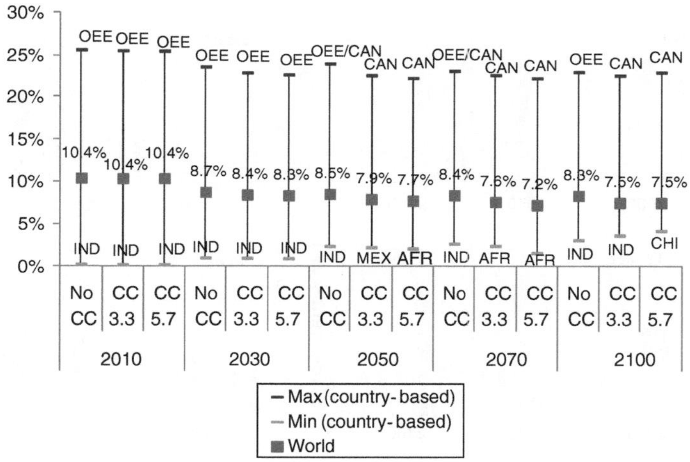

Fig. 5 Share of heating and cooling energy consumption in total final energy, in 3 cases: long-term global average temperature increase of 3.3 °C w/o climate changes (NoCC), with climate changes (CC3.3) and 5.7 °C with climate changes (CC5.7). Countries with the largest and smallest shares are indicated. Based on Labriet et al. (2013), with kind permission of Springer Science +Business Media

Reduced needs for heating affect gas and coal heating systems (reduced consumption of gas and coal for heating) more than biomass and electric heaters, reflecting higher costs of these heating options in the longer term. Solar energy does not appear in the results since it is used mostly for water heating and cooking in TIAM-WORLD.

In all regions, electricity consumption for heating and cooling increases, driven by cooling needs. The increase reaches up to 55 % over the case without climate change at the global level, and more than 60 % in Europe, Central and South America, and China. The seasonal impacts of climate change, especially on peak

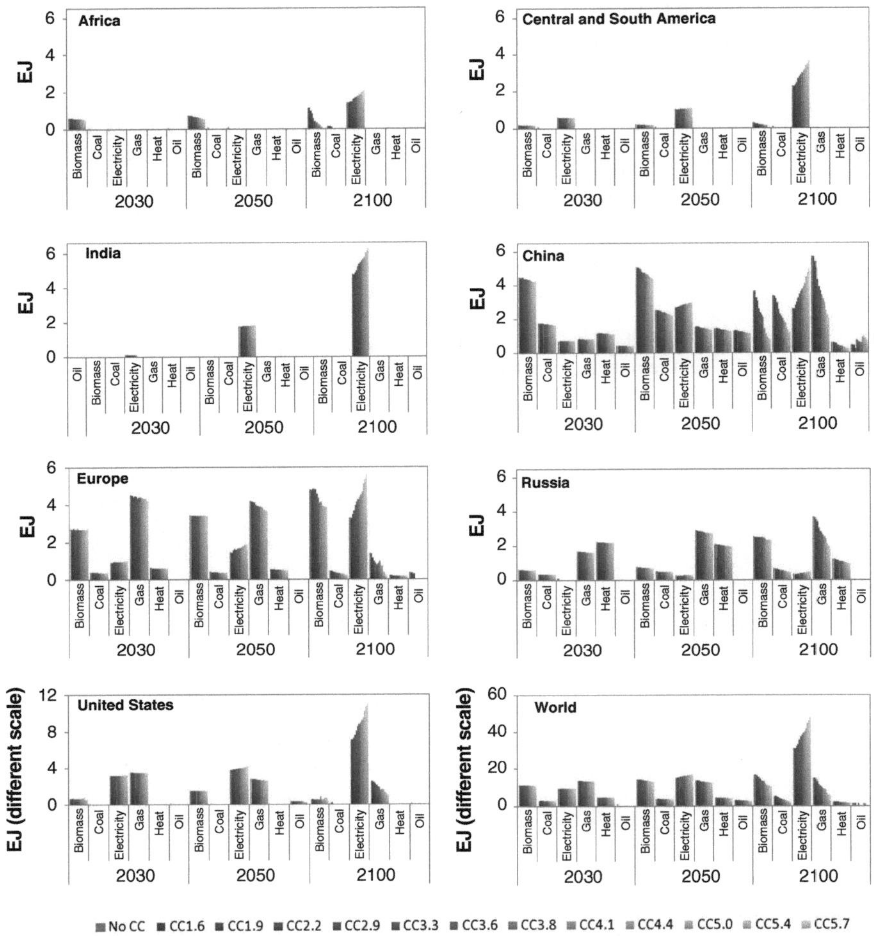

Fig. 6 Final energy consumption for heating and cooling in 12 different temperature scenarios (Results for other regions are available upon request)

electricity generation, are reflected in changes in electricity prices. Electricity prices in Europe increase by up to 45 % in summer days in the mid-term and 66 % at the end of the horizon in Europe (up to 30 and 50 % in the Reference case 3.3 °C scenario). The increase reaches 30 % during summer days in China, 10 % in USA, while electricity prices remain unchanged in Russia. In India, the season with the highest increase of electricity prices is the intermediate one (fall and spring), corresponding to the peak of temperature. The penetration of building shell improvement options, such as efficient windows and insulation, could contribute to the adaptation of the building sector to future increase of cooling needs. These options are however modeled via exogenous scenarios in this version of the model, and only device efficiency options are endogenous. Electric and geothermal heat pumps are the preferred technologies for cooling and represent the same shares of the cooling market in cases with and without climate change.

Not surprisingly, without any emission mitigation constraints, coal power plants appear to be the most cost-efficient power option. Resulting emissions are however compensated by the reduction in fossil fuel consumption for heating.

Threshold temperature. HDD and CDD computation requires the choice of a threshold temperature below/above which heating and cooling are needed. In order to understand the importance of the threshold temperature, CDD was computed for 4 threshold temperatures: 18, 22, 25 and 28 °C (Fig. 7). As expected, absolute values of CDD are smaller when threshold temperature is higher, over the entire time horizon. However, the increase of CDD relative to 2010 due to climate change is higher when threshold temperature is higher. In other words, climate change will result in bigger changes in cooling needs compared to the current situation when a higher reference temperature is used for cooling: if people start cooling after 22 °C, now and in the future, their absolute cooling needs will be smaller, but their cooling needs will increase more, due to climate change, than if they start cooling after 18 °C. In this context, the use of 18 °C to compute HDD and CDD is supported by two ideas. First, HDD and CDD are only an "indicator". Their computation based on 18 °C of course does not represent the real cooling needs, but this convention has the merit of being shared by all and makes comparison across studies possible. Second, in studies as the current one, HDD and CDD are not used to compute the absolute energy consumption but to compute relative changes over a situation without climate change. In conclusion, the use of a default threshold temperature of 18 °C follows the convention of similar studies.

3.2 Hydropower

Hydropower potential. The variation of potentials over time due to climate change was estimated in the reference case, corresponding to long-term temperature increase of 3.3 °C (Fig. 8). A global increase of 6 % in 2050 and 16 % in 2100 of hydropower power on an annual basis is estimated, with higher increases in spring (MAM). Hydropower potentials decrease at some seasons in China, United States and India, and increase in all other regions and seasons. The high increase of potential observed in India in summer (JJA) is associated with the strong SE Asian monsoon simulated by PLASIM-ENTS. These variations appear to be globally more optimistic than assessments proposed by other studies, usually closer to increases of less than 10 % by the end of the century at the global level (Hamududu and Killingtveit 2012; Mima and Criqui 2009). These studies also propose a decrease of hydropower in Europe, while an increase is obtained with our assessment, explained by an increase in Northern Europe higher than the decrease observed in Southern Europe. As mentioned in Sect. 2.3.2, several factors may contribute to these differences, such as the geographic resolution of the computation

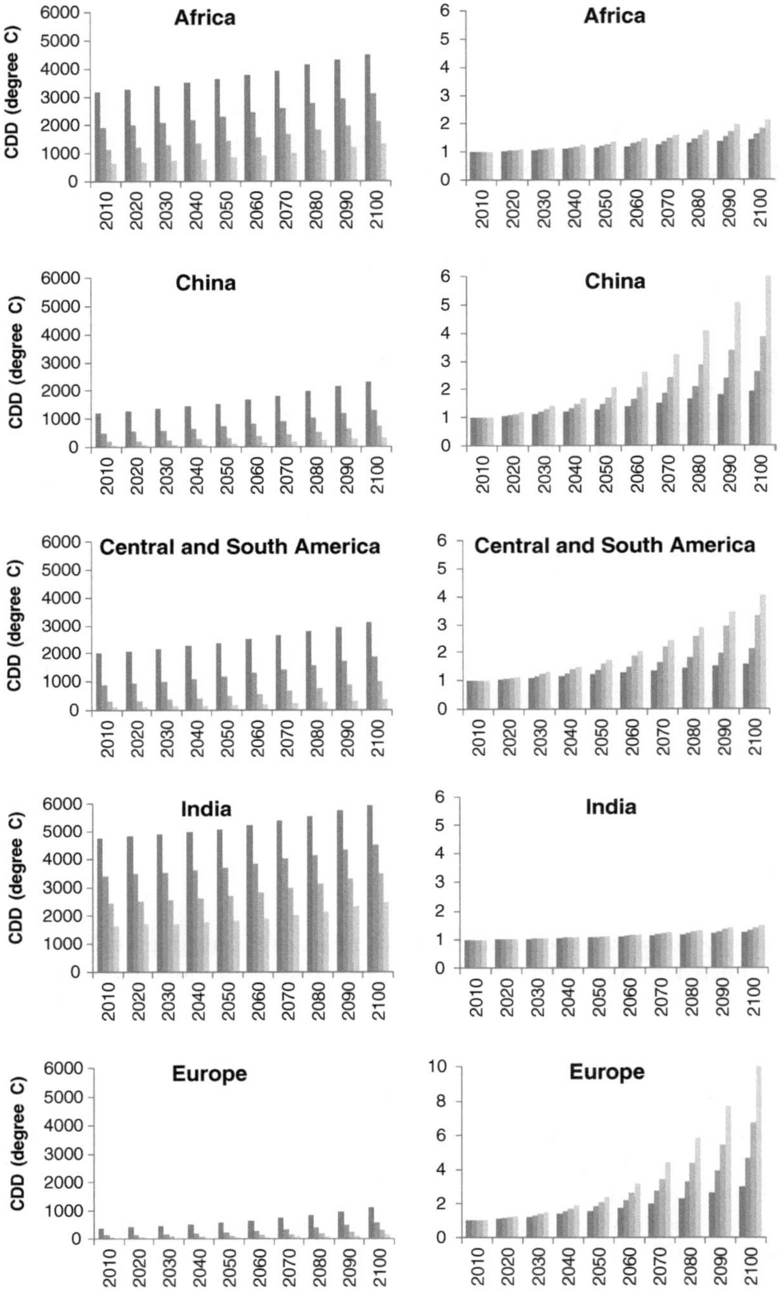

Fig. 7 Impact of temperature threshold on cooling degree days. *Left* Absolute values. *Right* Normalized to 1 in 2010 (Results for other regions are available upon request)

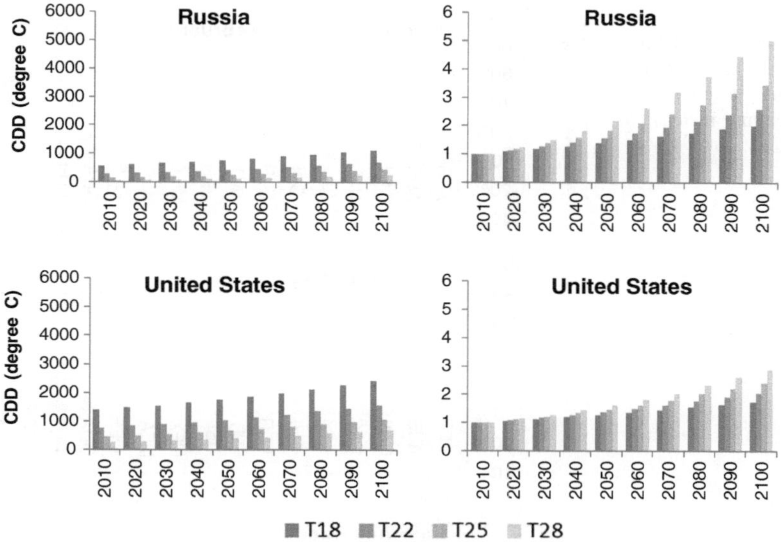

Fig. 7 (continued)

of the hydro potentials and the possibly high uncertainties in regions with high elevation difference in their geography. Numerical results presented below must therefore be considered as indicative of one of the possible futures only. Uncertainty resulting from the implementation at the global level of the analysis of the climate vulnerability of hydropower is also mentioned by Hamududu and Killingtveit (2012) in their study at the World level.

Changes in the energy system. Global increase in hydroelectricity generation reaches 135 TWh in the mid-century and 2000 TWh at the end of the century (Fig. 9), or respectively around 3 and 40 % more than when not considering the impacts of climate change on hydropower. Regions with highest absolute changes are Africa, Central and South America, as well as Other Developing Asia and Canada at the very end of the century. The increase in hydro potential observed in summer in India, acknowledged as not robust (see previous sections), does not produce a large increase of hydroelectricity generation.

Despite the increase of hydroelectricity generation, no change in total electricity generation is observed, neither at global nor regional levels. In other words, the higher availability of hydropower does not result in a higher electrification of the energy system, and additional hydroelectricity substitutes other forms of electricity: coal power plants as baseload power plants in Africa, and gas and wind power in other regions (Fig. 10b). The impact on CO_2 emissions is negligible given the limited degree of substitution (except in the national emission inventories of Africa and Japan in the longer term, where emissions are reduced by up to 15 %). However, the higher seasonal availability of hydropower contributes to the decrease of electricity prices in several regions, such as in Africa in summer.

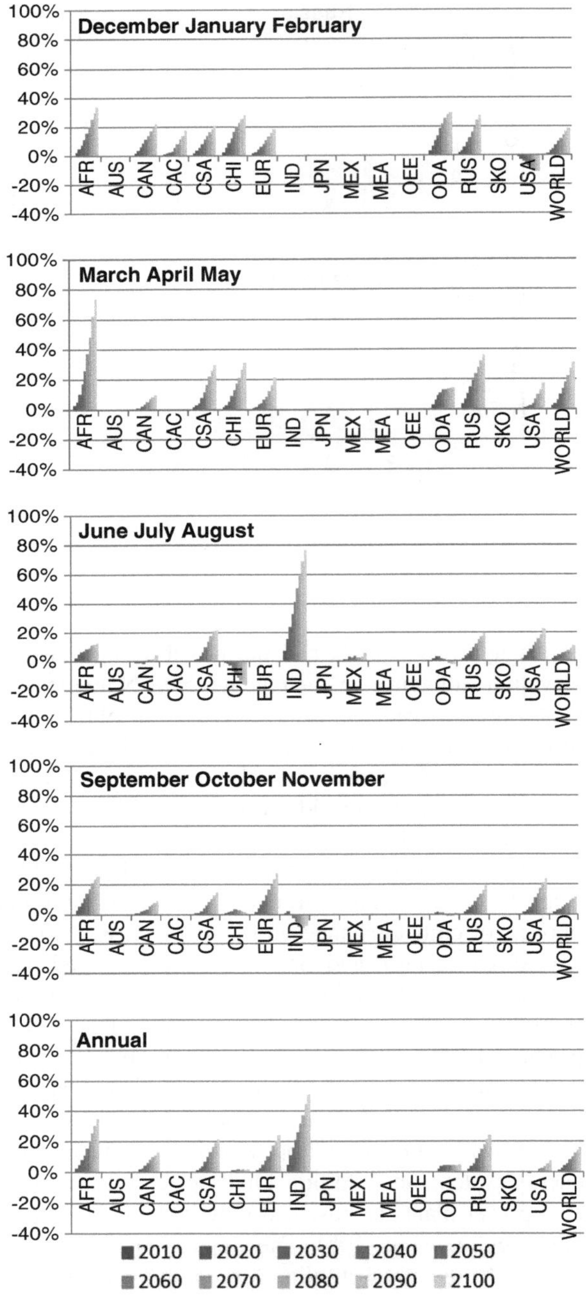

Fig. 8 Variations in hydropower availability in the reference case due to climate changes (long-term temperature increase of 3.3 °C)

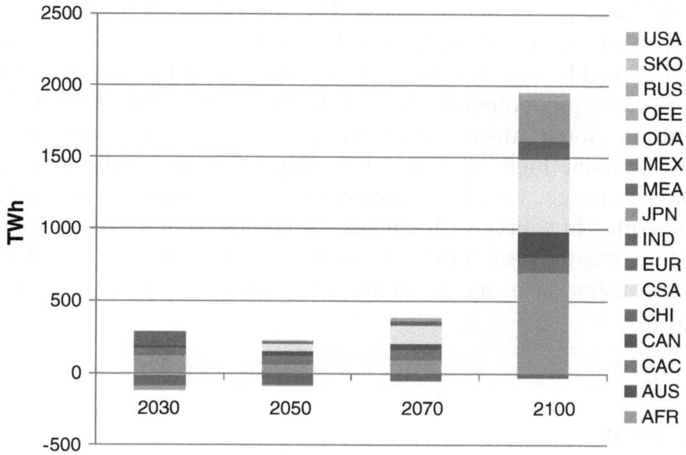

Fig. 9 Variations in hydroelectricity generation by region in the reference case due to climate changes (These variations correspond to the differences in hydroelectricity generation between the reference case without considering the impacts of climate changes, and the Reference case with impacts of climate changes) (long-term temperature increase of 3.3 °C)

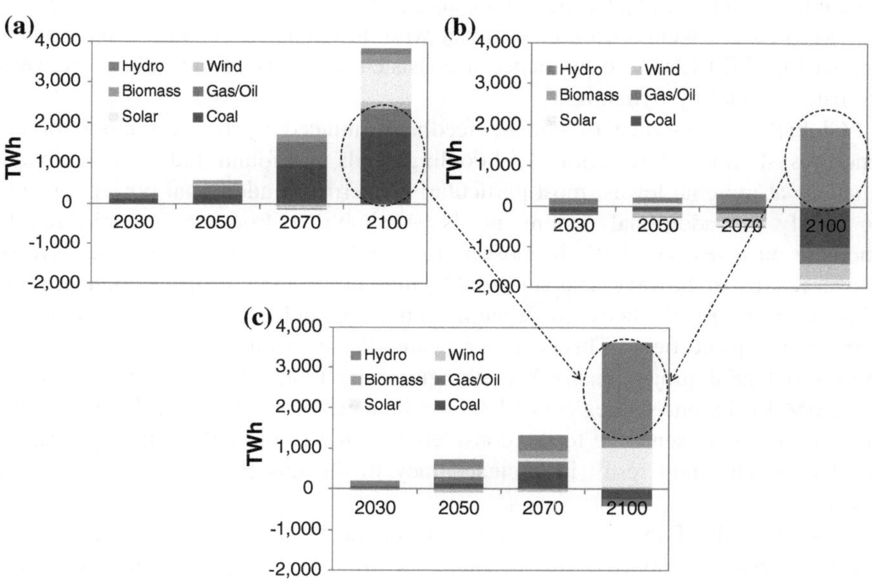

Fig. 10 Variations (These variations correspond to the differences in hydroelectricity generation between the reference case without considering the impacts of climate changes, and the Reference case with impacts of climate changes) in the electricity mix at global level in the reference case due to the impacts of climate change (long-term temperature increase of 3.3 °C)

Combined impacts of climate change. The analysis of the electricity mix at the global level shows that the increase in hydroelectricity availability could contribute to substitute the additional coal power generation needed to satisfy the additional needs in electricity for cooling due to climate change (Fig. 10). Regions like Africa and Central and South America particularly benefit from this substitution, being regions that combine high increases of cooling needs and hydropower potentials due to climate change. Given the important role that transmission and interconnections may play in coping with climate variations, more detailed analysis of the capacity of the energy system to adapt to future climate change would deserve an enhanced consideration of the geographical dispersion and capacity of the transmission grid.

4 Conclusion

The development and application of modeling tools are fundamental to support policy-makers and project implementers in understanding and planning not only the mitigation options but also the adaptation strategies of the energy sector.

The general objective of this chapter is to assess the changes in heating and cooling of buildings and in hydropower capacity and generation resulting from future temperature and precipitation changes. To achieve this, we have coupled the TIAM-WORLD techno-economic model with an emulated version of the climate model PLASIM-ENTS to guarantee a consistent analysis of the linkage between climate and energy dynamics.

Globally, an absence of climate feedback induced by the adaptation of the energy system to future heating and cooling needs was found, but with significant changes at regional levels, most particularly in terms of additional power capacity to satisfy the additional cooling needs. Available hydropower is estimated to increase on a seasonal basis in most regions under future climate change. Hydropower results are however characterized by high uncertainty: projected precipitation changes vary greatly between different climate models, much more so than for temperature projections. This is a significant source of uncertainty for the hydropower potential projections, especially given the relatively coarse resolution of PLASIM-ENTS and its neglect of land use change. Moreover, modeled watershed borders are quite sensitive to the considered spatial resolution of the topographic model, which could result in an inaccuracy in the modeled spatial hydropower potential.

The strength of the study is to assess climate impacts on the energy system taking a system perspective that accounts for impacts on the entire energy system (all sectors) and resulting fuel substitution effects. Future research may include the refinement of the computation of heating and cooling, for example with variable threshold temperatures, as well as the application of the hydropower methodology at a more detailed geographic resolution. Moreover, the PLASIM-ENTS emulator generates an ensemble of climate projections; the work described here has only considered the ensemble mean of these projections. In future work we will apply the ensemble to quantify the contribution of climate model uncertainties on impacts. Other impacts of climate change would of course deserve analysis, such as climate impacts on biomass and bioenergy, as well as on thermal power plants. In that sense, based on a more detailed representation of power plants, the climate vulnerability of thermal power plants could be considered, as well as the capacity of the transmission grid and interconnections to play an active role in the adaptation of the energy system to future climate change. The use of enhanced versions of the climate emulator, including sea-ice feedback and aerosol forcing, is expected in future applications. Finally, complementary to the assessment of techno-economic impacts of climate change on the energy system, macro-economic impacts may deserve more attention. Labriet et al. (2013) show that they are limited at global level but diverse across regions, mainly due to changes in terms of trade resulting from lower fossil fuel exports.

Acknowledgments The research leading to these results has received funding from the EU Seventh Framework Programme under Grant Agreement no. 265170 (Project ERMITAGE—Enhancing Robustness and Model Integration for The Assessment of Global Environmental Change).

References

Aebischer B, Henderson G, Jakob M, Catenazzi G (2007) Impact of climate change on thermal comfort, heating and cooling energy demand in Europe. ECEEE summer study, panel 5, energy efficient buildings, 859–870

Akpinar-Ferrand E, Singh A (2010) Modeling increased demand of energy for air conditioners and consequent CO_2 emissions to minimize health risks due to climate change in India. Environ Sci Pol 13(8):702–712

Arent D, Tol R, Faust E, Hella J, Kumar S, Strzepek K, Tóth F, Yan D (2014) Key economic sectors and services. In: Field, CB., Barros VR, Dokken DJ, Mach KJ, Mastrandrea MD, Bilir TE, Chatterjee M, Ebi KL, Estrada YO, Genova RC, Girma B, Kissel ES, Levy AN, MacCracken S, Mastrandrea PR, White LL (eds) Climate change 2014: impacts, adaptation, and vulnerability. part A: global and sectoral aspects. Contribution of Working Group II to the Fifth Assessment Report of the Intergovernmental Panel on Climate Change. Cambridge University Press, Cambridge

Craig R (2011) Energy system impact. Technical report, FSU College of Law, Public Law Research Paper No. 503

Durmayaz N, Oguz Salim S (2006) Influence of cooling water temperature on the efficiency of a pressurized-water reactor nuclear-power plant. Int J Energy Res 30(10):799–810

Ebinger J, Vergara W (2011) Climate impacts on energy systems—key issues for energy sector adaptation. The international bank for reconstruction and development the World Bank, Washington, D.C

Fischer G, Nachtergaele F, Prieler S, van Velthuizen HT, Verelst L, Wiberg D (2008) Global agro-ecological zones assessment for agriculture (GAEZ 2008). IIASA, FAO, Laxenburg, Rome

Fraedrich K, Jansen H, Kirk E, Luksch U, Lunkeit F (2005) The planet simulator: towards a user friendly model. Meteorol Z 14(3):299–304

Haberl H, Erb K, Krausmann F, Bondeau A, Lauk C, Mller C, Plutzar C, Steinberger J (2011) Global bioenergy potentials from agricultural land in 2050: sensitivity to climate change, diets and yields. Biomass Bioenergy 35(12):4753–4769
Hamududu B, Killingtveit A (2012) Assessing climate change impacts on global hydropower. Energies 5:305–322
Holden PB, Edwards NR (2010) Dimensionally reduced emulation of an AOGCM for application to integrated assessment modelling. Geophys Res Lett 37:L21707, doi:10.1029/2010GL045137
Holden PB, Edwards NR, Garthwaite PH, Fraedrich K, Lunkeit F, Kirk E, Labriet M, Kanudia A, Babonneau F (2014) PLASIM-ENTSem: a spatiotemporal emulator of future climate for impacts assessment. Geosci Model Dev Discuss 6:3349–3380
IEA (2013a) Energy Statistics of Non-OECD countries. International Energy Agency, Paris
IEA (2013b) Energy statistics of OECD countries. International Energy Agency, Paris
IPCC (2011) IPCC Special Report on Renewable Energy Sources and Climate Change Mitigation. In: Edenhofer O, Pichs-Madruga R, Sokona Y, Seyboth K, Matschoss P, Kadner S, Zwickel T, Eickemeier P, Hansen G, Schlömer S, von Stechow C (eds) Prepared by working group III of the Intergovernmental Panel on Climate Change. Cambridge University Press, Cambridge, 1075 p
Isaac M, van Vuuren D (2009) Modeling global residential sector energy demand for heating and air conditioning in the context of climate change. Energy Pol 37(2):507–521
Labriet M., Joshi SR, Babonneau F, Edwards NR, Holden PB, Kanudia A, Loulou R, Vielle M (2013) Worldwide impacts of climate change on energy for heating and cooling. Mitigation and adaptation strategies for global change, online
Lehner B, Czisch G, Vassolo S (2005) The impact of global change on the hydropower potential of Europe: a model-based analysis. Energy Pol 33(7):839–855
Linnerud K, Mideksa T, Eskeland G (2011) The impact of climate change on nuclear power supply. Energy J 32:149–168
Loulou R (2008) ETSAP-TIAM: the TIMES integrated assessment model part II: mathematical formulation. CMS 5:7–40
Loulou R, Labriet M (2008) ETSAP-TIAM: the TIMES integrated assessment model part I: model structure. CMS 5:41–66
Lucena A, Salem Szklo A, Schaeffer R, Rodrigues de Souza R, Soares Moreira Cesar Borba B, Vaz Leal da Costa I, Olimpio Pereira A Júnior, Henrique Ferreira da Cunha S (2009) The vulnerability of renewable energy to climate change in Brazil. Energy Pol 37(3): 879–889
Mideksa T, Kallbekken S (2010) The impact of climate change on the electricity market: a review. Energy Pol 38(7):3579–3585
Mima S, Criqui P (2009) Assessment of the impacts under future climate change on the energy systems with the POLES model. In: International energy workshop 17–19 June, 2009. Fondazione Giorgio Cini, Italy
Moss RH, Edmonds JA, Hibbard KA, Manning MR, Rose SK, van Vuuren DP, Carter TR, Emore S, Kainuma M, Kram T, Meehl GA, Mitchell JFB, Nakicenovic N, Riahi K, Smith SJ, Stouffer RJ, Thompson AM, Weyant JP, Wilbanks TJ (2010) The next generation of scenarios for climate change research and assessment. Nature 463:747–756
Pokhrel Y, Oki T, Kanae S (2008) A grid based assessment of the global theoretical hydropower potential. Journal of Hydraulic Engineering 52:7–12
Rubbelke D, Vogele S (2011) Impacts of climate change on european critical infrastructures: the case of the power sector. Environ Sci Pol 14(1):53–63
Schaeffer R, Szklo A, de Lucena A, Borba B, Nogueira L, Fleming F, Troccoli A, Harrison M, Boulahya M (2012) Energy sector vulnerability to climate change: a review. Energy 38(1):1–12
Seljom P, Rosenberg E, Fidje A, Haugen JA, Meir M, Rekstad J, Thore J (2011) Modelling the effects of climate change on the energy system—a case study of Norway. Energy Pol 39 (11):7310–7321
van Vliet MTH, Yearsley JR, Ludwig F, Vögele S, Lettenmaier DP, Kabat P (2012) Vulnerability of US and European electricity supply to climate change. Nature Climate Change 2:676–681
Wilbanks TJ, Romero Lankao P, Bao M, Berkhout F, Cairncross S, Ceron J-P, Kapshe M, Muir-Wood R, Zapata-Marti R (2007a) Industry, settlement and society. In: Parry ML, Canziani OF,

Palutikof JP, van der Linden PJ, Hanson CE (eds) Climate change 2007: impacts, adaptation and vulnerability. Contribution of working group II to the fourth assessment report of the intergovernmental panel on climate change, pp 357–390. Cambridge University Press, Cambridge

Wilbanks TJ, Bhatt V, Bilello DE, Bull SR, Ekmann J, Horak WC, Huang YJ, Levine MD, Sale MJ, Schmalzer DK, Scott MJ (2007b) Effects of climate change on energy production and use in the United States. Department of Energy, Office of Biological and Environmental Research, Washington, DC, p 160

Williamson M, Lenton T, Shepherd J, Edwards NR (2006) An efficient numerical terrestrial scheme (ENTS) for earth system modelling. Ecol Model 198(34):362–374

Coupling World and European Models: Energy Trade and Energy Security in Europe

Raffaella Gerboni, Daniele Grosso, Evasio Lavagno, Amit Kanudia and GianCarlo Tosato

Abstract Energy modelling can provide a knowledge basis for tackling the security of energy supply issue at different geographical levels. This chapter presents an application of the coupling of the global TIMES Integrated Assessment Model and of the Pan European TIMES model through a series of trade links described and characterised in the REACCESS corridor model. The coupling was developed during the EU FP7 REACCESS project and was further improved and updated during a follow-up phase. The application focuses on the analysis of security of supply to Europe via energy corridors. A new methodology for the assessment of energy security, addressing the risk associated to each supply, is presented together with a scenario analysis related to some of the most populated of the EU's Member States and to the European Union as a whole. The scenario analysis results show a sample of the possible assessments that stakeholders might be willing to rely on to address the effects of communitarian policies and targets: the preformed analysis, for example, unveils that a risk reduction at communitarian level may not univocally be translated into a benefit for individual Member States.

R. Gerboni (✉) · D. Grosso · E. Lavagno
DENERG - Politecnico di Torino, Torino, Italy
e-mail: raffaella.gerboni@polito.it

D. Grosso
e-mail: daniele.grosso@polito.it

E. Lavagno
e-mail: evasio.lavagno@polito.it

A. Kanudia
KanORS-EMR, Noida, India
e-mail: amit@kanors.com

G. Tosato
ASATREM, Rome, Italy
e-mail: giancarlo.tosato@gmail.com

G. Giannakidis et al. (eds.), *Informing Energy and Climate Policies Using Energy Systems Models*, Lecture Notes in Energy 30,
DOI 10.1007/978-3-319-16540-0_22

1 Background on the REACCESS Project

In the early 2000s, geopolitical instabilities, new threats and alliances, coupled with the increased availability of fossil fuels in key areas of the world, led the EU needing to strengthen a knowledge base via strategic studies in order to pave the way towards an efficient and pragmatic approach to guarantee (or improve or reinforce) the security of supply. The EU financed a set of research projects to provide strategic studies, overviews and analytical tools to policy makers, and it mostly used the Framework Programmes scheme to support these actions. ENCOURAGED, SECURE and REACCESS projects are examples of these efforts.

The Risk of Energy Availability: Common Corridors for Europe Supply Security (REACCESS) project was carried out under the 7th Framework Programme (FP7). Its main focus was the analysis of the security of energy supply in the European Union. This target was achieved by means of a modelling exercise performed adopting a detailed technical, economical, safety and environmental characterization of the energy corridors for the main commodities, i.e. hard coal, natural gas, crude oil, refined petroleum products, biomass, hydrogen, nuclear material, and electricity from concentrated solar power plants (CSP) (Pregger et al. 2011).

In particular, three TIMES models (Loulou et al. 2005)—two existing/adapted, that is the Pan European TIMES (PET36) and the KanORS TIAM-World, and one newly built (RECOR)—have been linked to define a global optimization model.

The Pan European TIMES (PET36) is a model that describes the whole energy system of 36 European countries (the 28 EU Member States plus Switzerland, Norway, Iceland, Bosnia Herzegovina, Former Yugoslav Republic Of Macedonia, Montenegro, Serbia and Albania), with five end-use sectors (Agriculture, Commerce, Industry, Residential and Transportation) and 70 exogenous demands for energy services. The release used within REACCESS is a revision of the previous version of the model (PET 27+), based on the EU27 countries plus Switzerland, Norway and Iceland (Biberacher et al. 2011).

The TIMES Integrated Assessment Model (TIAM) is a model that describes (in the original ETSAP-TIAM version) the whole energy system of the world divided in 15 macro-areas (Africa, Australia-New Zealand, Canada, Central and South America, China, Eastern Europe, Former Soviet Union, India, Japan, Mexico, Middle-East, Other Developing Asian Countries, South Korea, United States, and Western Europe), with five end-use sectors (Agriculture, Commerce, Industry, Residential and Transportation) and 42 exogenous demands for energy services. In order to satisfy the requirements of the REACCESS project, a new version of the model (KanORS TIAM-WORLD) was developed and some changes were made in the regional disaggregation. In particular, the Eastern Europe, Former Soviet Union and Western Europe regions were replaced by four new regions: Europe, Other Eastern Europe (including Ukraine, Belarus and Moldova), Central Asia and Caucasus and Russia (Biberacher et al. 2011). The region of Europe, for the purposes of the project, was then replaced with the finest description contained in PET36.

1.1 REACCESS CORridor (RECOR) Model

RECOR is the new model developed within REACCESS to fully describe (from the extraction fields to the supply entry point) all the present and planned/possible future energy infrastructures supplying the European countries, taking into account both captive (mainly pipelines, but also railways and electrical power lines) and open sea (ship routes from port to port) corridors. Besides all the European supply infrastructures, the main non-EU corridors have also been considered. For the extraction fields, data on extraction costs and on proven, probable and possible resources were provided. Each corridor has been divided into branches (Fig. 1) and each branch (implemented into the Model as a TIMES process) has been characterized by both technical (length, capacity, activity in the base year of the model, fuel-in, fuel consumption, life, etc.) and economical (investment cost, fixed and variable operating and maintenance costs, etc.) parameters. All along the corridors, supply branches stem as supply branches to the transit countries. The supply branch links the RECOR model to the Reference Energy System (RES) of a PET36 or a TIAM region. The number of the analysed connections by commodity is summarised in Table 1.

One of the main features of this kind of approach to the energy corridors description is the inclusion of their detailed spatial characterisation and the implementation of this topology into the model structure.

Furthermore, the code system adopted for each branch process and each commodity of a corridor allows the full traceability of an energy flow, from the extraction field to the supply point. If a single branch carries a commodity having two or more different origins, two kinds of processes are used:

- the infrastructure process describes the infrastructure itself and it is characterized by technical-economical parameters (capacity, investment cost, O&M cost,…); it has no input or output commodities and there is a single process for each branch;
- the commodity processes represent the topological link necessary for the traceability, without technical and economical features related to it; there is one process for each origin.

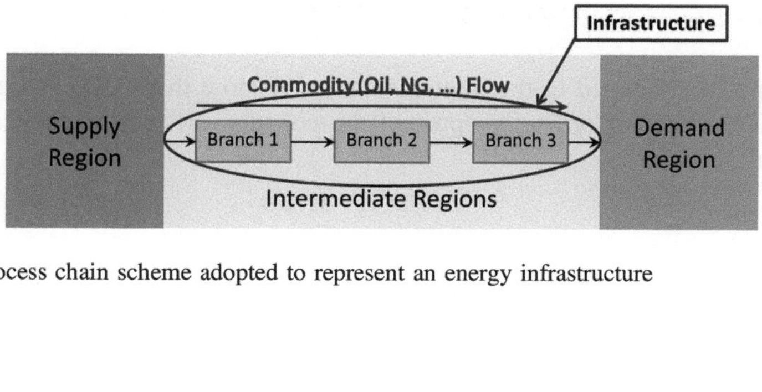

Fig. 1 Process chain scheme adopted to represent an energy infrastructure

Table 1 Number of connections characterised in the database of the RECOR model

Commodity	Number of connections		
Natural gas	No. of pipelines	EU	65
		Non-EU	13
LNG	No. of open sea connections	EU	91
		Non-EU	76
Crude oil	No. of pipelines	EU	34
		Non-EU	1
	No. of open sea connections	EU	321
		Non-EU	126
		Non-EU	1
Refined petroleum	No. of pipelines	EU	1
Products (RPP)	No. of open sea connections	EU	150
		Non-EU	70
Hard coal	No. of open sea connections	EU	210
		Non-EU	37
	No. of railways connections	EU	3
		Non-EU	6
Uranium	No. of open sea connections	EU	6
Biomass	No. of open sea connections	EU	21
Hydrogen	No. of pipelines	EU	5
	No. of open sea connections	EU	7
High voltage direct current (HVDC)	No. of electrical connections	EU	44

A constraint is used in order to link the total activity carried by the commodity processes to the capacity of the infrastructure process (Eq. 1).

$$\sum_{i=1}^{Num.CommodityProcesses} Activity_i \leq Capacity_{Infr.\,Process} \tag{1}$$

where:

i is the branch, and so it refers to a commodity process;
Activity is the activity carried by the branch i;
$Capacity_{Infr.\ Process}$ is the capacity of the infrastructure process.

This approach has led to the implementation of more than 3500 processes into the RECOR model in order to represent the corridors system synthetically enumerated in Table 1.

1.2 The Risk Evaluation

In the REACCESS project, a key achievement was the evaluation and use of risk indicators in order to identify weaknesses and threats for the security of energy supply to Europe. Two risk aspects were assessed: the technological risk (based on conventional risk analysis techniques, applied to each branch and part of the energy system) and the socioeconomic risk.

The socioeconomic risk was analysed at a country level by using a statistical technique known as Factor Analysis, assuming that the global country potential risk is the combination of 4 main risk vectors: Social, Political, Economic and Energetic.

For each of these vectors, a set of variables (38 for the Economic, 33 for the Political, 18 for the Social, 12 for the Energetic) has been firstly identified and then an iterative application of the Factor Analysis procedure has allowed the identification of the important variables and finally led to the evaluation of a factor score (ranging between 0 and 100) for each vector. The Overall Risk Index for each country was calculated as a mean of the four risk indexes: its value ranges between 5.4 for Norway and 79.4 for Afghanistan (García-Verdugo et al. 2011).

The worldwide representation of the overall Risk Indexes is shown in Fig. 2.

The RECOR model included both the socioeconomic Risk Indicators for the evaluation of the security of supply and the evaluation of the technological risk.

These indicators have been used in a so called "min/max" procedure that is a Multi Criterion Decision Method (MCDM). This procedure was adopted to encourage the diversification of the supply corridors (Biberacher et al. 2011).

After the end of the project in 2011, a fine-tuning follow-up phase started. During this period, a revision of the model involving both structural and numerical adjustments was performed.

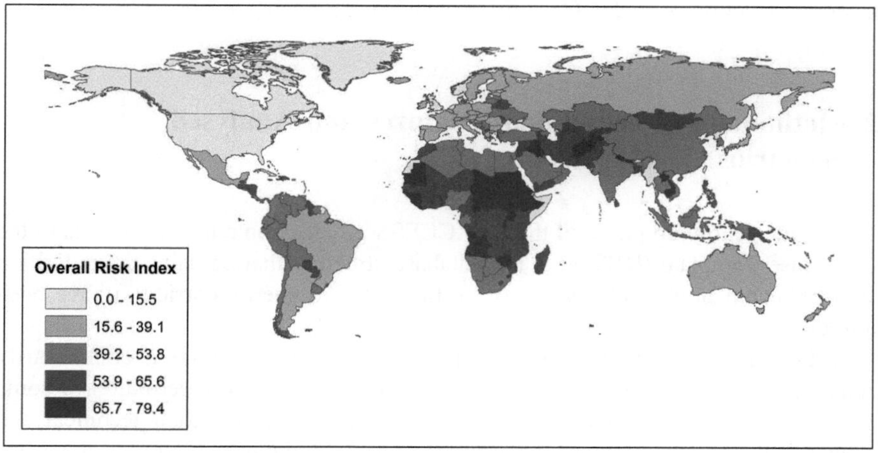

Fig. 2 Overall risk indexes by country, adapted from ESRI (2010)

1.3 Project Results

The REACCESS methodology was firstly used to perform a study on the EU's energy import by corridor from different supply countries, focusing in particular on the Gulf Cooperation Council (GCC) ones, i.e. Bahrain, Kuwait, Oman, Qatar, Saudi Arabia and United Arab Emirates (Kanudia et al. 2013). To achieve this aim four scenarios have been analysed: Reference, Risk avert (that minimises the EU27 risk indicator allowing a maximum increase of the total discounted system cost equal to 0.2 % with respect to the Reference one), Climate change mitigation (that assumes the Energy Modeling Forum target of a 50 % reduction of global emissions in 2050 over 1990) and Climate-Risk (that includes the 2050 targets of the Climate scenario but minimising the risk indicator for the EU27 with a maximum increase of the total system cost equal to 0.2 % in comparison with the Climate one).

The results show that a significant reduction of the risk related to the EU's energy supply can be obtained, with a corresponding little increase of the total system cost. Under the Risk scenario the contribution of GCC countries to the EU supply increases, as well as the diversification of the supply countries. In general, the EU27 shows a high import dependency from North Africa and Middle East (and in particular from GCC countries) in all the analysed scenarios, even if under Risk scenarios the total energy consumption and the fossil fuel imports decrease. Furthermore, cross-effects of risk and climate targets can be noticed.

The additional features introduced in the RECOR model allow a different approach to the risk evaluation—treated like a CO_2 emission, i.e. calculated by multiplying a sort of "emission factor" (corresponding to the risk index related to each supply) by the quantity of imported commodity—and, as a consequence, different kinds of analyses. Examples of scenario runs that might be performed are: the reduction of total CO_2 emissions in a single country or in a group of countries (like the European Union); the reduction of the risk value in the same areas; the simultaneous reduction of both CO_2 emissions and risk by using suitable constraints.

2 Methodology—Additional Features and Analysed Scenarios

During the follow-up phase of the REACCESS project, some major changes to the Data Base Template (DBT, it is the database structure that contains the definition and the technical characterization of all the analysed energy corridors) have been introduced.

In fact, as the international panorama on energy infrastructures is continuously changing, a full amendment of the existing corridors and the redefinition of some planned/possible future infrastructures (regarding their route, their technical and economical features, etc.) have proven necessary (e.g. the introduction of the Trans

Adriatic Pipeline carrying natural gas from Caspian region to Southern and Western European countries).

Another relevant point of the follow-up phase of the REACCESS project was the introduction of annual growth and decay coefficients for the main commodities (hard coal, natural gas, crude oil, refined petroleum products and biomass) delivered by energy corridors, for each supply branch and for each extraction field (only for the proven resources). According to their definition (Loulou et al. 2005), these coefficients allow the identification of a maximum range of variation for each supply by corridor and for each commodity production through the implementation of two typologies of constraints. The introduction of Growth/Decay coefficients on single supply branches provides some benefits that can be summarised as follows:

- to avoid unreasonable oscillation in the supply trends;
- to better simulate the supply composition of each demand region;
- to describe, in a customized way, the possible evolution of energy imports for all the analysed countries, taking into account potential stiffness deriving from long term supply contracts or specific import policies.

2.1 The New Risk Evaluation

The REACCESS project dealt with risk by adopting the min-max approach that is based on a three step procedure. The first step is a minimisation of the total system cost; the second step is a minimisation of the risk indicator (RI): this run is performed allowing a maximum variation of the total cost with respect to the value obtained in the first run; the third step is a new minimisation of the total system cost allowing a certain maximum percentage variation of the risk index in comparison with the value obtained in the second run. The risk indicator used in this procedure is estimated starting from the "Quantity of Risk weighted Energy" (QRE). This parameter is calculated—for each commodity, corridor branch, year and region—by multiplying the energy (expressed in PJ/y) flowing through a branch by the overall risk index associated with the departure country of the branch. The RI is then evaluated by firstly finding the maximum value of the QRE for each region, year and commodity and then by summing over all the regions, years and type of commodities.

The main effect of the min-max approach is to encourage the diversification of the supply, penalising the imports from a unique risky country (or from a limited set of risky countries). Furthermore, the minimisation of the risk indicator indirectly leads to a reduction in the import dependency, a modification of the fuel mix in both primary and end-use sectors and a reduction in the energy consumption.

In the follow-up phase of the project, the original Overall Risk Indexes have been maintained, but a new alternative approach was implemented. In particular, to quantify the total risk related to the activity delivered by energy corridors, two risk indicators and six commodities were introduced in the model. These parameters allow a risk estimation on the basis of two possible methodologies:

Probability of failure:
This approach is based on the introduction of the geopolitical risk indicator $R_{C,PoF}$, which is specific for each energy corridor and is defined by means of an application of elementary reliability theory for series networks. It can be interpreted as the likelihood that a corridor crossing a country will fail (whichever the reason: technological, as due to e.g. poor maintenance, or geopolitical as due to e.g. deliberated disruption). The risk indicator can be applied to all crossed countries or to the Non-EU only in accordance with the Lisbon Treaty. The $R_{C,PoF}$ risk indicator is expressed by Eq. 2.

$$R_{C,PoF} = 100 \cdot \left[1 - \prod_{i=1}^{n}\left(1 - \frac{R_i}{100}\right)\right] \tag{2}$$

where:

R_i (i = 1, 2,... n)	is the Overall Risk Index of the traversed country (n being the total number of crossed countries)

This means that the probability of success of the corridor is the product of the probabilities of success of the crossed countries, assumed independent.

By using the $R_{C,PoF}$ indicator, three additional commodities are defined.

RiskPoF	it is obtained—for each supply branch of the corridor *C*—by multiplying $R_{C,PoF}$ by the activity delivered to the demand country.
TotPoFRisk	it is defined for each demand region; it is the sum of all *RiskPoF* values for a region and it allows to estimate the global risk related to the supply by corridor for that country.
TotPoFRiskEU	it is defined for the 28 Member States of the European Union and, in the same way as *TotPoFRisk*, it is the sum of all *RiskPoF* values for each of the 28 EU countries.

Average:
This approach is based on the introduction of the risk indicator $R_{C,Average}$, which is specific for each energy corridor and it is defined as the average value of the Overall Risk Indexes of all the countries crossed by the corridor *C*.

By using the $R_{C,Average}$ indicator, three other additional commodities are defined.

RiskAverage	it is obtained—for each supply branch of the corridor *C*—by multiplying $R_{C,Average}$ by the activity delivered to the demand country.

TotAverageRisk it is defined for each demand region; it is the sum of all *RiskAverage* values for a region and it allows the estimation of the global risk related to the supply by corridor for that country.

TotAverageRiskEU it is defined for the 28 Member States of the European Union and, in the same way as *TotAverageRisk*, it is the sum of all *RiskAverage* values for each of the 28 EU countries.

Another indicator ($R_{C,Source}$) and two more commodities (*RiskSource* and *TotSourceRisk*) were introduced to quantify the risk related to the amount of activity exported through energy corridors for each supply country.

From the modelling point of view, all the risk commodities were implemented in the same way as a CO_2 emission commodity. For each technology, the CO_2 emissions are evaluated by multiplying the quantity of consumed fuel by a suitable emission factor; in the same way, the risk values are calculated by multiplying the quantity of imported commodity by a sort of "emission factor", corresponding to the risk index related to each supply. This means that risk reduction policy scenarios can be defined and introduced in the model by using the same method as for pollutant emissions reduction.

Referring to the risk reduction policy scenarios, the reduction of the total risk value (calculated by means of the *RiskPoF* approach) by a percentage α in a region r and in a milestone year t can be implemented through a fix type constraint.

Another parameter introduced in order to analyse the risk related to the supply of energy commodities is the Specific Risk (*SR*) for the total supply. This variable quantifies the risk associated to the single PJ/y delivered by corridors to the analysed region, thus allowing a comparison between different scenarios and/or countries, and it is defined as the ratio between the total Risk value (i.e. *TotPoFRisk* or *TotPoFRiskEU*) and the delivered activity, expressed in PJ/y (Eq. 3).

$$SR_{r,t} = \frac{TotPoFRisk_{r,t}}{\sum SupplyActivity_{r,t}} \quad (3)$$

where:

r is the region;

t is the milestone year.

2.2 Risk Scenarios

A scenario analysis using the new features on risk evaluation has been carried out, focusing on the effects on the Specific Risk of a policy on risk reduction performed at the Communitarian level or at the national level. For this purpose, the European Union as a whole and the six most populated EU's Member States (Germany,

Table 2 Scenario assumptions

Scenario (%)	Region	Commodity	Risk reduction (%)
Baseline	All regions	–	–
RiskDE15	DE	TotPoFRisk	−15
RiskES15	ES	TotPoFRisk	−15
RiskFR15	FR	TotPoFRisk	−15
RiskIT15	IT	TotPoFRisk	−15
RiskPL15	PL	TotPoFRisk	−15
RiskUK15	UK	TotPoFRisk	−15
RiskEU15	EU	TotPoFRiskEU	−15

France, Italy, Poland, Spain and United Kingdom) were considered, as they account for a large part of the European supply by corridors and represent more than 70 % of the total EU's population in 2013.

Eight runs (a baseline run and seven scenario runs) were performed. In each scenario run and for each milestone year, the risk commodity—*TotPoFRisk* or *TotPoFRiskEU*—value in the analysed region (the whole EU or one of the six EU's Member States taken into account) has been imposed to be less than or equal to the 85 % of the corresponding value obtained from the baseline run, thus simulating a 15 % risk reduction. The main assumptions for the above mentioned scenarios are reported in Table 2.

In each risk scenario run, the constraint on risk was implemented only from 2015 to 2040, while the results for the previous milestone years have been imposed equal to the ones obtained from the baseline run, in order to avoid unreasonable optimization effects on the supply in the past years.

3 Results

Figures 3, 4, 5, 6, 7 and 8 show for each country the comparison among the Specific Risk values related to the total supply by energy corridors in the three typologies of runs that have been performed (baseline, risk reduction for the country, risk reduction for the EU). Figure 9 shows instead the comparison between the baseline run and the scenario run results for the EU.

As expected, in the assumed time horizon, the specific risk value related to the global supply is almost always higher in the Baseline scenario than in the risk reduction scenarios. The only exception is the National risk reduction scenario for Italy: the long-term specific risk related to this scenario becomes slightly higher than the one related to the Baseline scenario (Fig. 6). This trend can be explained by the fact that, in the National risk scenario, the target of risk reduction is reached by a strong reduction in the amount of crude oil imported from Non-EU countries and re-exported towards EU Member States (in the form of crude oil itself or of refined petroleum products) rather than by a change in the supply composition. This is a

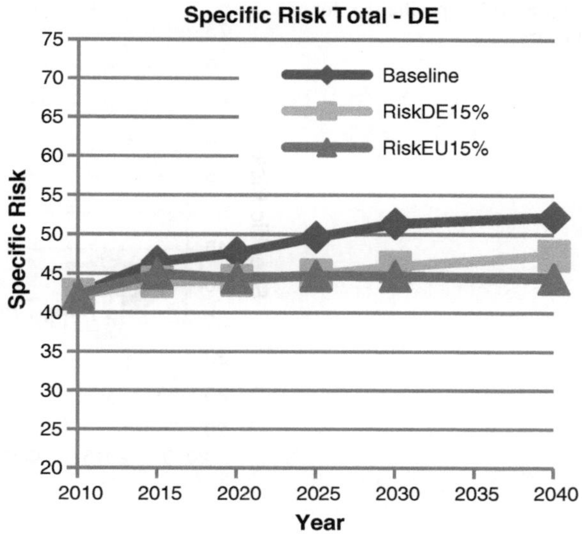

Fig. 3 Total specific risk for Germany

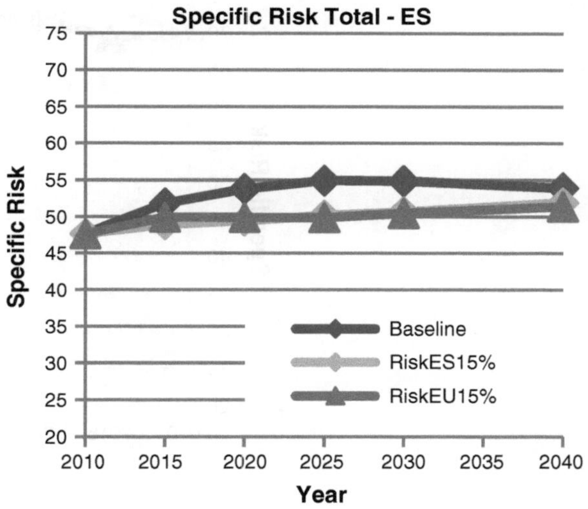

Fig. 4 Total specific risk for Spain

sort of "selfish" behaviour that brings to a national reduction of the total risk (due to the reduced import of commodities that use Italy as a "stop-over") although each PJ of energy imported is a bit more risky.

Comparing, for each region, the Communitarian risk reduction scenario and the National risk reduction scenario, it can be noticed that the first one leads to a significantly lower trend in Italy. Lower values are also observable in France and in Germany, while in Spain the two lines are almost overlapping. In Poland and in the

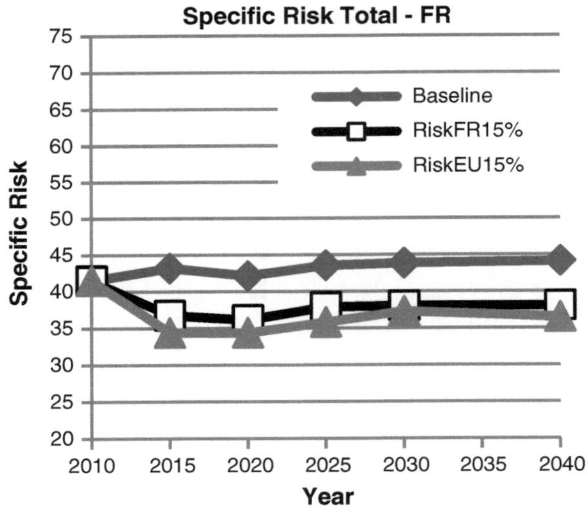

Fig. 5 Total specific risk for France

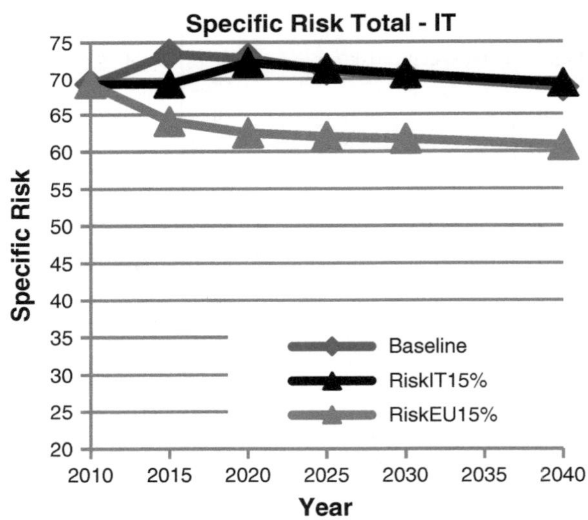

Fig. 6 Total specific risk for Italy

United Kingdom the reduction performed at the National level is more effective from the point of view of the specific risk reduction. Only in Poland the specific risk trend in the period 2015–2040 is monotonically decreasing in both the risk reduction scenarios.

These variations in the specific risk trends are due to the combination of two different effects: a change in the supply composition, that is a different use of the available energy corridors (Fig. 10) and/or fuel shift phenomena, and a change in the amount of the total import.

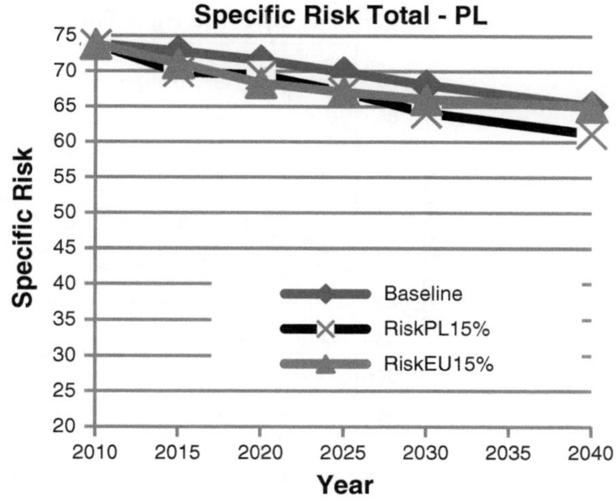

Fig. 7 Total specific risk for Poland

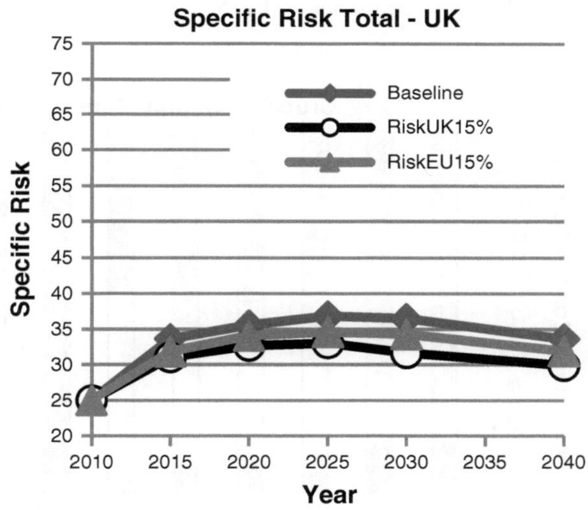

Fig. 8 Total specific risk for the UK

Referring to the last point, in particular, under the National risk scenarios, a significant reduction in the total supply by corridors can be noticed in all the analysed countries. This decrease also causes a slight reduction in the import dependency of each country in comparison with the one of the Baseline scenario over the time horizon 2015–2040, more relevant in Italy than in the other nations (Figs. 11 and 12). On the contrary, a risk reduction performed at a Communitarian level causes an increase in the total import by corridors in Germany, a non-unique behaviour in Italy and a decrease in the other countries lower than the one obtainable in the case of National reduction.

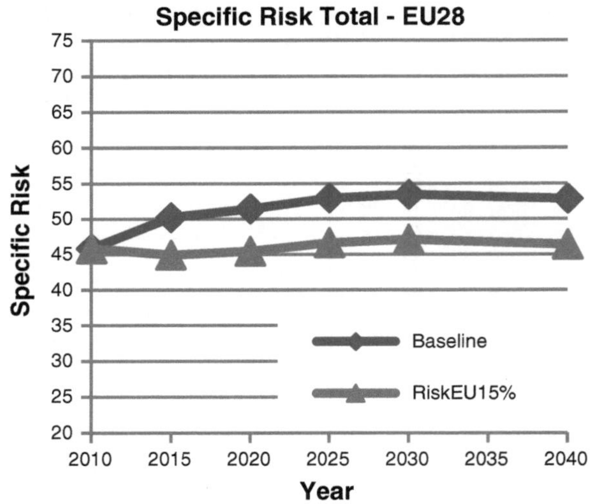

Fig. 9 Total specific risk for the EU-28

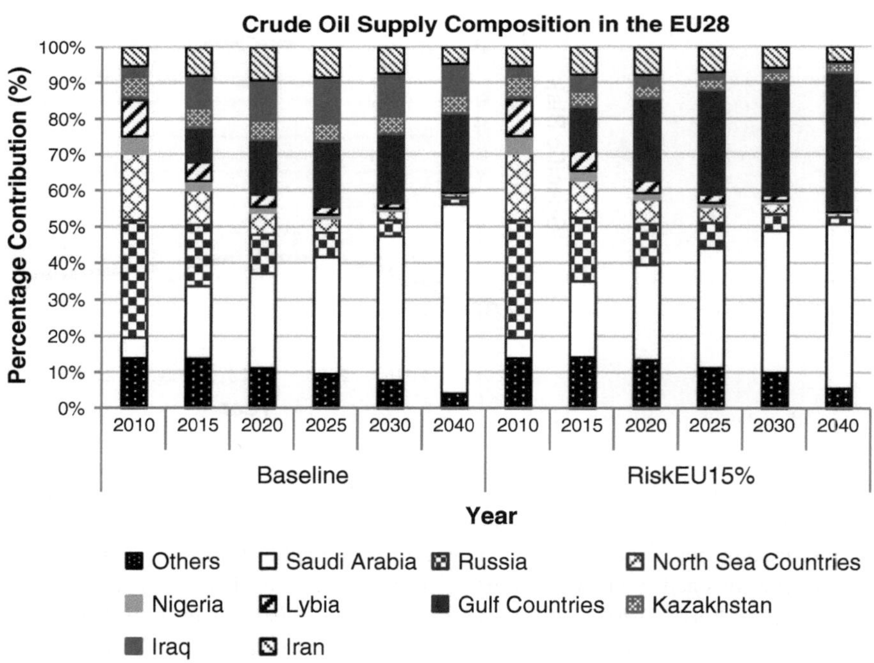

Fig. 10 Crude oil supply composition for the EU-28 (Gulf Countries = Kuwait + UAE; North Sea Countries = Norway + UK)

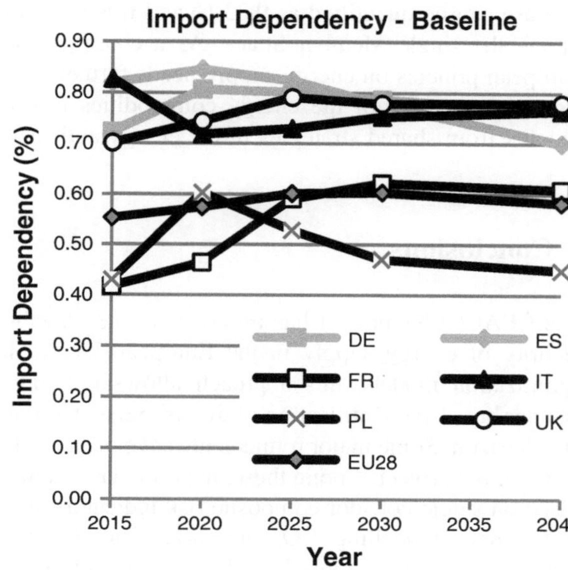

Fig. 11 Import dependency, baseline

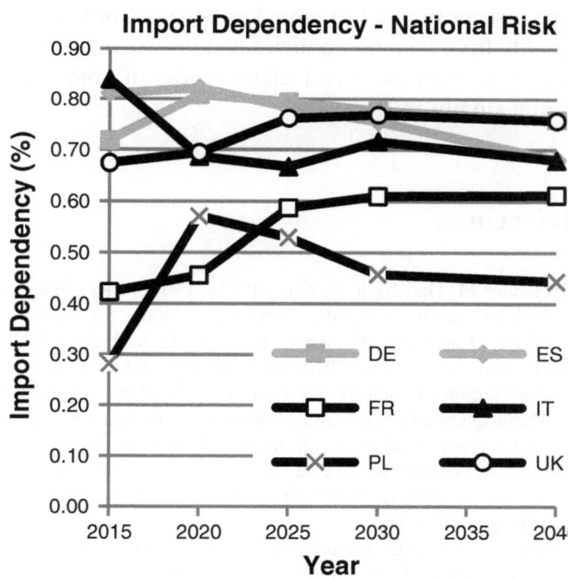

Fig. 12 Import dependency, national risk

The above results seem to suggest that a reduction in the risk of energy supply by corridors carried out at a Communitarian level may not univocally be translated into a benefit for the single Member States, while a predictable result is the increase of the cost for the entire European energy system. In the proposed analysis, this increase can be quantified as 0.23 % and it is shared (although inhomogeneously) among the single Member States. As a consequence, an effective application of European policies on energy supply needs further actions such as the promotion of a common market of the energy commodities in order to ensure also economic benefits from shared strategies in the energy and security field.

4 Conclusions

The REACCESS project has introduced a new methodology for investigating the security of energy supply in the European Union. In fact, by using forecasting optimization models, this approach allows not only evaluation in a qualitative manner but also quantification of the risk related to the supply over a mid/long-term time horizon. Some major refinements have been implemented during the follow-up phase of the project: among these, in particular, a new procedure for risk evaluation, based on single-corridor composite risk indicators and on new commodities similar to the ones modelling CO_2 emissions, and the introduction of Growth/Decay constraints on each supply branch can be mentioned. An application of the Model to compare the effects of risk reduction policies at Communitarian or national level from a security point of view has been performed. The results have shown unclear benefits from common policies and this fact seems to underline the need of further actions to promote a real effectiveness of common strategies on the security of energy supply in Europe.

References

Biberacher M, De Miglio R, Gargiulo M, Gerboni R, Lavagno E, Schranz L, Tosato GC (2011) Risk of energy availability common corridors for europe supply security—summary report, REACCESS Final Workshop, Brussels, 13 May 2011. http://reaccess.epu.ntua.gr/

ESRI Light grey canvas (2010) ESRI Inc., Redlands (CA). www.arcgis.com

García-Verdugo J, San-Martín E, Muñoz B (2011) Quantifying geopolitical energy risks. In: Marín-Quemada JM, García-Verdugo J, Escribano G (eds) Energy security for the eu in the 21st century: markets, geopolitics and corridors, Routledge, Oxon and New York

Kanudia A, Gerboni R, Loulou R, Gargiulo M, Labriet M, Lavagno E, De Miglio R, Schranz L, Tosato GC (2013) Modelling EU-GCC energy systems and trade corridors. Int J Energy Sect Manage 7:243–268

Loulou R, Remme U, Kanudia A, Lehtila A, Goldstein G (2005) Documentation for the TIMES model, Part I, II, III. http://www.iea-etsap.org/web/Documentation.asp

Pregger T, Lavagno E, Labriet M, Seljom P, Biberacher M, Blesl M, Trieb F, O'Sullivan M, Gerboni R, Schranz L, Cabal H, Lechon Y, Zocher D (2011) Resources, capacities and corridors for energy imports to Europe. Int J Energy Sect Manage 5:125–156